Principles and Practice of
RADIATION
THERAPY

Second Edition

Principles and Practice of

RADIATION THERAPY

Charles M. Washington, BS, RT(T), FASRT

Administrative Director
Radiation Therapy Services
The University of Texas MD Anderson Cancer Center
Houston, Texas

Dennis Leaver, MS, RT(R)(T)

Chairman and Assistant Professor
Department of Radiation Therapy
Southern Maine Community College
South Portland, Maine

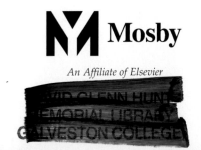

Mosby

An Affiliate of Elsevier

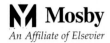

An Affiliate of Elsevier

11830 Westline Industrial Drive
St. Louis, Missouri 63146

NOTICE

Radiation Therapy is an ever-changing field. Standard safety precautions must be followed, but as new research and clinical experience broaden our knowledge, changes in treatment and drug therapy may become necessary or appropriate. Readers are advised to check the most current product information provided by the manufacturer of each drug to be administered to verify the recommended dose, the method and duration of administration, and contraindications. It is the responsibility of the licensed prescriber, relying on experience and knowledge of the patient, to determine dosages and the best treatment for each individual patient. Neither the publisher nor the authors assume any liability for any injury and/or damage to persons or property arising from this publication.

Previous edition copyrighted 1996

Library of Congress Cataloging-in-Publication Data

Principles and practice of radiation therapy/edited by Charles M. Washington, Dennis Leaver.—2nd ed.
   p. ; cm.
  Includes bibliographical references and index.
   ISBN-13: 978-0-323-01748-0   ISBN-10: 0-323-01748-7
    1. Cancer—Radiotherapy. I. Washington, Charles M. II. Leaver, Dennis T.
  [DNLM: 1. Neoplasms—radiotherapy. 2. Radiation Oncology—methods. WN 250 P957 2004]
  RC271.R3P734 2004
  616.99'40642—dc21

                     2003059915

ISBN-13: 978-0-323-01748-0
ISBN-10: 0-323-01748-7

Publishing Director: Andrew Allen
Executive Editor: Jeanne Wilke
Developmental Editor: Lisa Potts
Publishing Services Manager: Melissa Lastarria
Project Manager: Joy Moore
Senior Book Designer: Amy Buxton
Cover Design: Studio Montage

Last digit is the print number: 9 8 7 6 5

To those who have run and continue to run the race against cancer. We sincerely hope those who read this work will grow in the knowledge and understanding necessary to provide direction and compassion to their patients. Let us not grow tired in running our own race, but instead encourage those around us.

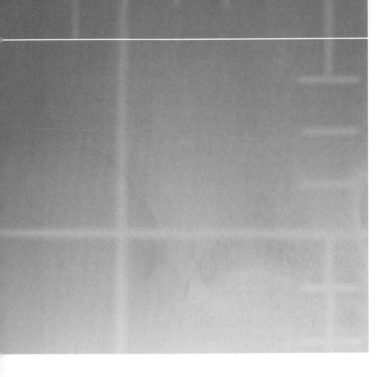

Contributors

Robert D. Adams, EdD, RT(R)(T), CMD
Program Director
School of Radiation Therapy
University of North Carolina
Chapel Hill, NC

Linda Alfred, BS, RT, MEd, MBA
Clinical Support Services Manager
Varian Oncology Systems
Palo Alto, CA

Julius Armstrong, MBA, RT(T)
Program Chairman
Radiation Therapy Program
Bellevue Community College
Bellevue, WA

Lisa Bartenhagen, BS, RT(R)(T)
Program Director
Radiation Therapy Education
University of Nebraska Medical Center
Omaha, NE

Lana Havron Bass, BS, RT(R)(T), CMD, FASRT
Dosimetrist
University of Texas Southwestern Moncrief Cancer Center
Ft. Worth, TX

E. Richard Bawiec, Jr., MS, DABR
Physicist/Department Coordinator
Saint Edward Mercy Medical Center
Fort Smith, AR

Susan B. Belinsky, EdD, RT(R)(T)
Associate Professor of Radiation Therapy
Director, Radiation Therapy Program
Massachusetts College of Pharmacy and Health Sciences
Boston, MA

Joseph S. Blinick, PhD
Chief Radiation Physicist
Maine Radiation Physics, Inc.
Portland, ME

Todd A. Blobe, BA, CMD, RT(T)
Certified Medical Dosimetrist
Mayo Clinic
Jacksonville, FL

Leila Bussman, BS, RT(R)(T)
Program Director
Radiation Therapy Program
Mayo School of Health Science
Rochester, MN

Annette M. Coleman, MA, RT(T)
Marketing Manager for Radiation Oncology
IMPAC Medical Systems, Inc.
Cambridge, MA

Stephanie Eatmon, EdD, RT(R)(T), FASRT
Program Director and Associate Professor
California State University, Long Beach
Long Beach, CA

Correen Fraser, BS, RT(T), CMD
Certified Medical Dosimetrist
Radiation Oncology Department
Henry Ford Hospital
Detroit, MI

Patricia J. Giordano, MS, RT(R)(T)
Assistant Professor/Program Director
Radiation Therapy Program
Gwynedd-Mercy College
Gwynedd Valley, PA

Sally V. Green, BS, RT(T)
Clinical Coordinator
Radiation Therapy Program
Bellevue Community College
Bellevue, WA

Patton Griggs, BS
Radiological Physicist
Department of Radiation Oncology
Central Maine Medical Center
Lewiston, ME

Christopher M. Hand, PhD
Medical Physicist
Department of Radiation Oncology
Abington Memorial Hospital
Abington, PA;
Adjunct Faculty
Radiation Biology
Radiation Therapy Program
Gwynedd Mercy College
Gwynedd, PA

Rosann Keller, MEd, RT(T)
Radiation Therapist II
Department of Radiation Oncology
Sinai-Grace Hospital
Detroit, MI;
Adjunct Assistant Professor
Wayne State University
Detroit, MI

Adam F. Kempa, MEd, RT(T)
Senior Lecturer
Department of Radiation Oncology
Wayne State University
Detroit, MI

Sean Ji-Won Kim, CMD, BS, RT(R)(T)
Senior Medical Dosimetrist
Radiation Oncology-Medical Physics
Flynn Cancer Center
Everett, WA

Deborah A. Kuban, MD
Professor of Radiation Therapy
The University of Texas
MD Anderson Cancer Center
Houston, TX

Linda Langlin, RT(R)(T)
Radiation Therapist and Clinical Supervisor
Central Maine Medical Center
Department of Radiation Oncology
Lewiston, ME

Dennis Leaver, MS, RT(R)(T)
Chairman and Associate Professor
Department of Radiation Therapy
Southern Maine Community College
South Portland, ME

Ronnie Lozano, MSRS, RT(T)
Chairman and Assistant Professor
Radiation Therapy Program
Southwest Texas State University
San Marcos, TX

Shirlee E. Maihoff, MEd, RT(T)
Independent Radiation Therapist
Brookwood Cancer Institute
Birmingham, AL

Valerie Marable, BS, RT(T), CMD
Dosimetrist III
Department of Radiation Oncology
Providence Hospital
Southfield, MI

Mary Ann McKenney, RT(R)(T)
Senior Radiation Therapist
Brigham and Women's Hospital
Boston, MA

†Alan C. Miller, MEd, RT(R)
Retired, Radiography Program
Program Director
Moultrie Area Technical College
Moultrie, GA

Tammy Newell, BS, RT(T)
Radiation Therapist
Department of Radiation Oncology
Elliot Regional Cancer Center
Manchester, NH

Timothy George Ochran, MS, DABR
Medical Physicist
Paris Regional Cancer Center
Paris, TX

Charlotte M. Prado, RT(R)(T), CMD
Medical Dosimetrist
Department of Radiation Therapy
The Methodist Hospital
Houston, TX

†Deceased.

Karl L. Prado, PhD
Associate Professor of Radiation Physics
Department of Radiation Physics
The University of Texas
MD Anderson Cancer Center
Houston, TX

Elizabeth G. Quate, MS
Director of Imaging Physics/RSO
Department of Radiology
Maine Medical Center
Portland, ME

Lynda Reynolds, MEd, RT(R)(N)(T), FASRT
Training and Development Specialist
IMPAC Medical Systems, Inc.
Edmond, OK

Pamela J. Ross, BS, RT(T)
Coordinator of Radiation Oncology
Radiation Oncology Department
New York Methodist Hospital
Brooklyn, NY

Janet Salzmann, RT(R)(T)
Radiation Therapist
Houston Northwest Radiotherapy Center
Houston, TX

Cheryl K. Sanders, MPA, RT(R)(T), FAERS, FASRT
Retired, Associate Professor
Formerly Director, Division of Radiation Sciences Technology
   Education
University of Nebraska Medical Center
Omaha, NE

Judith M. Schneider, MS, RT(R)(T)
Clinical Assistant Professor/Clinical Coordinator
Radiation Therapy Program
Indiana University School of Medicine
Indianapolis, IN

Donna Stinson, MBA, RT(R)(T)
Director of Client Services
WMSH Marketing Communications
Haddonfield, NJ

Nora Uricchio, MEd, RT(R)(T)
Director, Radiation Therapy Program
School of Allied Health
Hartford Hospital
Hartford, CT

George M. Uschold, EdD, RT(T), FASRT
Associate Professor of Radiation Oncology
University of Rochester
James P. Wilmot Cancer Center
Rochester, NY

Paul E. Wallner, DO, FACR
Chief, Clinical Radiation Oncology Branch
Radiation Research Program, DCTD, NCI
Rockville, MD

Charles M. Washington, BS, RT(T), FASRT
Administrative Director
Radiation Therapy Services
The University of Texas MD Anderson Cancer Center
Houston, TX

Jeffrey Young, MD
Medical Director
Radiation Oncology
Maine Medical Center
Portland, ME

Cara Zeidman, MSN, RN
Senior Client Services Coordinator
IMPAC Global Systems UK Limited
Staines, Middlesex, UK

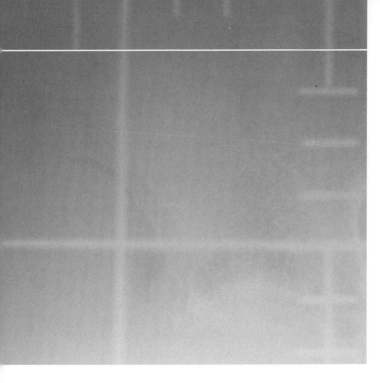

Preface

Since the first edition of this text was published in 1996, the field of radiation therapy has experienced tremendous growth. Improvements in three-dimensional treatment planning, intensity-modulated radiation therapy, brachytherapy, and patient immobilization have all allowed the radiation therapy team to enhance and improve clinical outcomes. More sophisticated electronic charting has allowed radiation therapists and medical dosimetrists to improve treatment-delivery documentation and quality-assurance practices. Although the face of radiation therapy has changed through these advances, the purpose and focus of this textbook has not. It is still designed to contribute to a comprehensive understanding of cancer management, improve clinical techniques involved in delivering a prescribed dose of radiation therapy, and apply knowledge and complex concepts associated with radiation therapy treatment planning and delivery.

The three separate volumes of the first edition, each designed to stand alone, have been combined into a single volume. Several chapters have been consolidated and additional information added, specifically in the areas of treatment planning, electronic charting, CT simulation, dose distribution, and education. As the methods of delivering a prescribed dose of radiation therapy have improved, so too has the effort to localize the patient, deliver an accurate dose, and reproduce the daily treatment fields.

Pedagogical features, designed to enhance comprehension and critical thinking, are incorporated into each chapter.

Elements include chapter outlines, key terms, and a glossary that includes significant terms from both editions. Of particular note are the Review Questions and Questions to Ponder at the end of each chapter. Review Questions reinforce the cognitive information presented in the chapter, helping the reader incorporate the information into the basic understanding of radiation therapy concepts. The Questions to Ponder are open-ended, divergent questions intended to stimulate critical thinking and analytic judgment. Answers to the Review Questions are found at the back of the book (Appendix B).

In addition, each chapter offers a reference list, giving the reader additional information sources. As in the first edition, the focus of each chapter is again to present the comprehensive needs of the radiation therapy management team. In fact, many experts in the field have contributed to this new edition, including radiation therapists, medical dosimetrists, physicists, radiation oncologists, nurses, and radiation therapy students.

We are grateful to the contributors of the chapters and for the reviewers who offered helpful feedback and suggestions. We also offer special thanks to the editorial staff at Elsevier for their patience and valuable contributions during the preparation and production of this work.

Finally, it is our hope the expanded knowledge and progress in treatment planning, delivery, and patient care outlined in this work will ultimately enrich the patient's quality of life and reduce suffering from the effects of cancer.

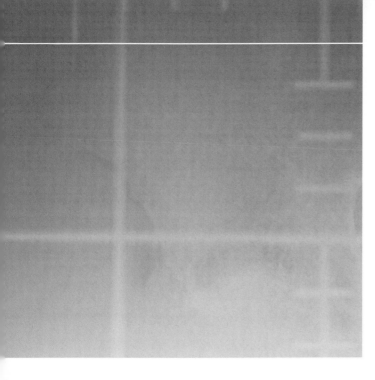

Reviewers

Lee Braswell, BAS, RT(R)(T)
Educational Director, Radiation Therapy Program
Pitt Community College
Greenville, NC

Teri L. DeLong, RT(T)
Radiation Therapist
Rutland, VT

Donna Kay Dunn, MS, RT(T)
Program Director
Indiana University School of Medicine
School of Allied Health Sciences
Radiation Therapy Program
Indianapolis, IN

Leia Levy, MAdED, RT(T)
Program Director
National-Louis University
Evanston, IL

Linda S. Lingar, MEd, RT, (R)(M)(ARRT)
Assistant Professor
University of Arkansas for Medical Sciences
Little Rock, AR

Brad Owen, BS, AS, RT(T)
Radiation Therapist
Central Maine Medical Center
Lewiston, ME

Sandy L. Piehl, MPA, RT(R)(T)
Program Director
Radiation Therapy
Indiana University Northwest
Gary, IN

Kristine Saeger, BS, RT(T)(R)
Program Director
Radiation Therapy—Clinical Science
University of Wisconsin–LaCrosse
LaCrosse, WI

Jess A. Smith, LVT, RT(T), AS, BS
Radiation Therapist
Maine General Medical Center
Augusta, ME

Mattie J. Tabron, EdD, RT(R)(T), FASRT
Associate Professor and Chairman
Department of Radiation Therapy
Howard University
Washington, DC

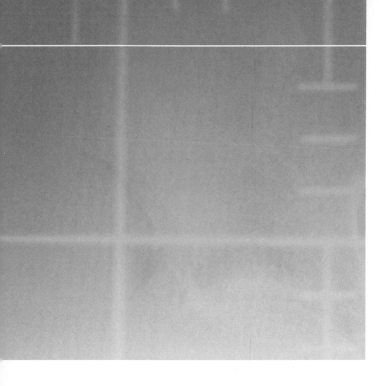

Contents

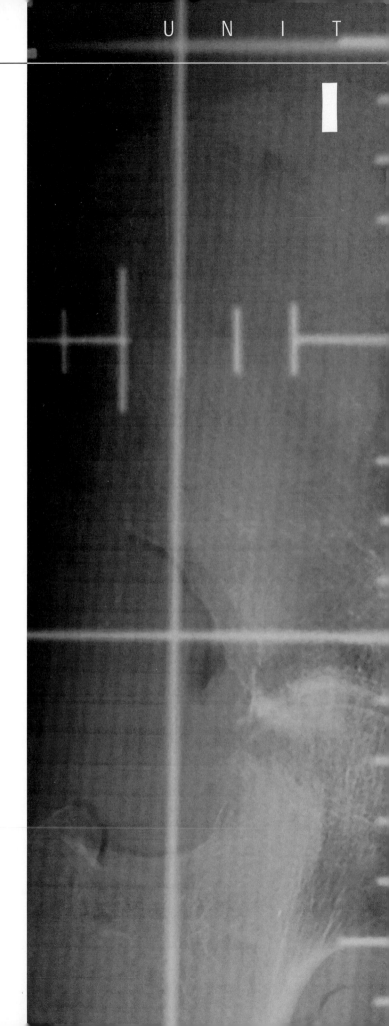

INTRODUCTION TO RADIATION THERAPY

Cancer: An Overview

Stephanie Eatmon

Outline

Key Terms

Adenocarcinoma
Anaplastic
Benign
Biopsy
Brachytherapy
Carcinoma
Cellular differentiation
Chemotherapeutic agents
Combination chemotherapy
Critical structures
Cytotoxic
Dosimetrist
Electrons
En bloc
Epidemiology
Etiology
Exophytic
False positive or negative
Gamma rays
Grade
Immunotherapy
Intraoperative
Intrathecal

Malignant
Metastasize
Multicentric
Natural history
Necrosis
NED (no evidence of disease)
Oncogenes
Palliation
Phase I, II, III studies
Photon
Prognosis
Prospective study
Radiation oncologist
Radiation therapist
Radioprotectors
Radiosensitizers
Retrospective studies
Sarcoma
Sentinel node
Simulation
Systemic treatment
Tumoricidal
Tumor staging

Throughout recorded history, cancer has been the subject of investigation. Lacking current surgical techniques and diagnostic and laboratory equipment, early investigators relied on their senses to determine characteristics of the disease. Investigators were unable to examine cells, so infections and other benign conditions were included in these early observations. Knowledge about early observations, including examinations, diagnosis, and treatment comes in part from Egyptian papyri dating back to 1600 BC.[6,8]

Initially investigators believed that an excess of black bile caused cancer. This belief defined cancer as a systemic disease for which local treatment (such as surgery) only made the patient worse.[6,8] In light of this, cancer was considered to be fatal with little possibility of a cure. When investigators could not prove the existence of black bile, the theory of cancer as an initially localized disease emerged. With this theory came the possibility of treatment and a cure.

The cause of this deadly disease remained a mystery, and, for some time, people thought that cancer was contagious. This theory brought isolation and shame to cancer victims, and, although this belief has long since vanished, patients not long ago expressed concern about spreading the disease to loved ones. Unfortunately today many cancer patients still suffer discrimination in the work place and when trying to obtain health insurance coverage.

In the fifth century BC, Hippocrates began the classification of tumors by observation and later the discovery of the microscope enabled early investigators to classify tumors on the basis of cellular characteristics.[8] Classification of tumors and their stages of growth will continue as technology advances.

BIOLOGIC PERSPECTIVE

Building on the work of early investigators and aided by technologic advances, researchers today are able to diagnose tumors in extremely early stages and examine tumor cell deoxyribonucleic acid (DNA) to determine mechanisms causing uncontrolled growth. Although knowledge about cancer has increased tremendously since early investigators began examining patients, much remains to be learned.

Theory of Cancer Initiation

Tumors are the result of abnormal cellular proliferation. This can occur because the process by which cellular differentiation takes place is abnormal or a normally nondividing, mature cell begins to proliferate. **Cellular differentiation** occurs when a stem cell undergoes mitosis and divides into daughter cells. These cells continue to divide and differentiate until a mature cell with a specific function results. When this process is disrupted, the daughter cells may continue to divide with no resulting mature cell, thus causing abnormal cellular proliferation.

The cause of this cellular dysfunction has been the subject of research for many years. Researchers now know that "cancer is a disease of the genes."[5] Normal somatic cells contain genes that promote growth and genes that suppress growth, both of which are important to control the growth of a cell. In a tumor cell, this counterbalanced regulation is missing. Mutations occurring in genes that promote or suppress growth are implicated in the deregulation of cellular growth. Mutations in genes that promote growth force the proliferation of cells, whereas mutations to the genes that suppress growth allow unrestrained cellular growth. For many tumors, both mutations may be required for progression to full malignancy.[4,5,10-12]

The terms for the genes involved in the cancer process are protooncogenes, oncogenes, and antioncogenes. Protooncogenes are the normal genes that play a part in controlling normal growth and differentiation. These genes are the precursors of **oncogenes**, or cancer genes. The conversion of protooncogenes to oncogenes can occur through point mutations, translocations, and gene amplification, all of which are DNA mutations. Oncogenes are implicated in the abnormal proliferation of cells. Antioncogenes are also called cancer-suppressor genes. Inactivation of antioncogenes allows the malignant process to flourish.

What causes these mutations to occur? For somatic cells, exposure to carcinogens such as sunlight, radiation, and cigarette smoke is implicated. In some situations, such as the familial form of retinoblastoma, gene mutations are passed down through generations. Random mutations that occur during normal cellular replication can also lead to unregulated cellular growth.

Researchers have identified several gene mutations, including the gene implicated in the familial form of breast cancer. With the use of gene mapping and advanced technology, study in this area will continue. To understand the principles of cancer treatment, a review of the cell cycle and an overview of tumor growth are necessary.

Review of the Cell Cycle

Mammalian cells proliferate through the process of mitosis or cellular division. The outcome of this process is two daughter cells that have identical chromosomes as the parent. The cell cycle is the period of time and activities that take place between cell divisions. The cell cycle is broken up into five phases called G0, G1, S, G2, and M (Fig. 1-1).

G0 is depicted outside of the cell cycle continuum because these cells are fully functioning but are not preparing for DNA replication. Most cells making up a tissue or organ are in the G0 phase. Given the proper stimulus, this reserve pool of cells can reenter the cell cycle and replicate.

G1, or the first growth phase, is characterized by rapid growth and active metabolism. The length of time that a cell remains in G1 is variable. Cells that are rapidly dividing spend little time in the first growth phase, whereas cells that are slow growing stay in G1 for a long period. The length of time spent in G1 varies from hours to years. During this time the cell synthesizes the necessary ribonucleic acid (RNA) and proteins to carry out the function of the cell. Later in the first growth phase, the cell will commit to replication of DNA.

S phase, or synthesis, is the period in which DNA is replicated to ensure that the resulting daughter cells will have identical genetic material. G2, or the second growth phase, is the period in which the cell prepares for actual division. Enzymes and proteins are synthesized and the cell continues to grow and moves relatively quickly into the M, or mitotic, phase.

Tumor Growth

When all cells are operating normally, there is a balance between cells that are dying and the replication of cells. Although tumor growth is a result of an imbalance between replication and cell death, the rate of growth is influenced by many factors. Malignant cells possess damaged genetic material, resulting in increased cell death. In addition, as the tumor grows larger the blood and nutrient supply is inadequate creating areas of **necrosis**, or dead tissue.

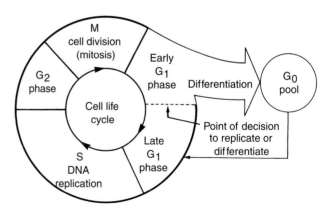

Figure 1-1. Cell generation cycle. *(From Otto SE: Oncology nursing, ed 2, St. Louis, 1994, Mosby.)*

Initially, tumor growth is exponential, but as the tumor enlarges and outgrows the blood and nutrient supply the rate of cell replication more closely equals the rate of cell death. This is demonstrated by the Gompertzian growth curve (Fig. 1-2). Tumors that are clinically detectable are generally in the higher portion of the curve. Treatment reduces the number of cells, thus moving the tumor back down the curve where the growth rate is higher. Tumor cells that were previously in the G0 phase are prompted to reenter the cell cycle. Cells that are rapidly dividing are more sensitive to the effects of radiation and chemotherapy.[3]

Tumor Classification

Tumors are classified by their anatomic site, cell of origin, and biologic behavior. Tumors can originate from any cell. This accounts for the large variety of tumors. Well-differentiated tumors (those that closely resemble the cell of origin) can be easily classified according to their histology. Undifferentiated cells, however, do not resemble normal cells, so classification is more difficult. These tumors are called undifferentiated or **anaplastic.**

Tumors are divided into two categories: benign or malignant (Table 1-1). **Benign** tumors are generally well differentiated and do not metastasize or invade surrounding normal tissue. Often, benign tumors are encapsulated and slow growing. Although most benign tumors do little harm to the host, some benign tumors of the brain (because of their location) are considered behaviorally malignant because of the adverse effect on the host. Benign tumors are noted by the suffix *oma,* which is connected to the term indicating the cell of origin. For example, a chondroma is a benign tumor of the cartilage.

Malignant tumors range from well differentiated to undifferentiated. They have the ability to **metastasize,** or

Table 1-1	General characteristics of benign and malignant disease	
Characteristics	**Benign**	**Malignant**
Local spread	Expanding, pushing	Infiltrative and invasive
Distant spread	Rare	Metastasize early or late by lymphatics, blood, or seeding
Differentiation	Well differentiated	Well differentiated to undifferentiated
Mitotic activity	Normal	Normal to increased mitotic rate
Morphology	Normal	Normal to pleomorphic
Effect on host	Little (depending on treatment and location of tumor)	Life threatening
Doubling time	Normal	Normal to accelerated

spread to a site in the body distant from the primary site. Malignant tumors often invade and destroy normal surrounding tissue and, if left untreated, can cause the death of the host.

Tumors arising from mesenchymal cells are termed **sarcomas.** These cells include connective tissue such as cartilage and bone. An example is a chondrosarcoma or a sarcoma of the cartilage. Although blood and lymphatics are mesenchymal tissues, they are classified separately as leukemias and lymphomas.

Carcinomas are tumors that originate from the epithelium. These include all the tissues that cover a surface or line a cavity. For example, the aerodigestive tract is lined with

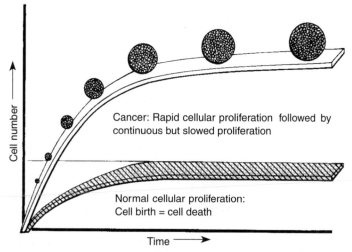

Figure 1-2. Gompertz' function as viewed by growth curve. *(From Otto SE: Oncology nursing, ed 2, St. Louis, 1994, Mosby.)*

squamous cell epithelium. Tumors originating from the lining are called squamous cell carcinoma of the primary site. An example is squamous cell carcinoma of the lung. Epithelial cells that are glandular are called **adenocarcinoma.** An example is the tissue lining the stomach. A tumor originating in the cells of this lining is called adenocarcinoma of the stomach. (Table 1-2 lists examples of nomenclature used in neoplastic classification.)

As in any classification system, some situations do not follow the rules. Examples include Hodgkin's disease, Wilms' tumor, and Ewing's sarcoma. This system of classification continues to change as more knowledge of the origin and behavior of tumors becomes available. (Table 1-3 lists histologies associated with common anatomic cancer sites.)

Cancer Outlook

The American Cancer Society[1] has estimated that 1,334,100 new cases of cancer were diagnosed in 2003 with more than 1500 individuals dying of the disease per day. Skin cancer and most in situ cancers are not included in these numbers. Today it is estimated that the 5-year relative survival rate for all cancers is 60%.[1]

Excluding carcinoma of the skin, the most common types of cancer include prostate; lung; and colorectal in men and breast, lung, and colorectal in women.[1] These statistics are not static and change with environmental, lifestyle, technologic, and other influences in society. Lung cancer in the 1930s was much less prevalent than it is today because of the increase in the number of cigarette smokers and improved diagnostic abilities. In addition, because of the more recent decline of smoking in the United States, the incidence of lung cancer has also dropped by approximately 17% in men.[1] Invasive carcinoma of the cervix decreased over the past 10 years as a result of the Papanicolaou (Pap) smear. Currently, more carcinoma in situ, or preinvasive, cancers of the cervix are found than invasive tumors.

Depending on the geographic location, the incidence of tumor sites also varies. For example, the incidence of stomach cancer is much greater in Japan than in the United States, and skin cancer is found more frequently in New Zealand than in Iceland.

Table 1-3	Histologies associated with common anatomic cancer sites
Site	**Most common histology**
Oral cavity	Squamous cell carcinoma
Pharynx	Squamous cell carcinoma
Lung	Squamous cell carcinoma
Breast	Infiltrating ductal carcinoma
Colon and rectum	Adenocarcinoma
Anus	Squamous cell carcinoma
Cervix	Squamous cell carcinoma
Endometrium	Adenocarcinoma
Prostate	Adenocarcinoma
Brain	Astrocytoma

PATIENT PERSPECTIVE

Although cancer is a curable disease, the diagnosis is a life-changing event. In studying the various aspects of neoplasia, care providers can easily lose sight of the person behind the disease. The patient must be the focal point of all of the radiation therapist's actions. The highest level of quality care results from an in-depth knowledge of the disease process, psychosocial issues, patient care, and principles and practices of cancer management, including knowledge of radiation therapy as a treatment option. This knowledge provides the radiation therapist with the tools necessary for optimal treatment, care, and education of the cancer patient. Providing care that does not consider the whole person is unacceptable.

The Person Behind the Diagnosis

When reviewing the large number of people who develop cancer, care providers can easily forget that the patient has a life outside of treatment with concerns and worries continuing and adding to the emotional, social, psychologic, physical, and financial burdens that come with the diagnosis. In addition, other medical concerns unrelated to cancer may complicate treatment and further burden the patient.

Factors such as age, culture, support systems, education, and family background play important roles in medical-treatment compliance, attitudes toward treatment, and responses to treatment. By knowing as much as possible about the patient and factors that influence the treatment outcome, the radiation therapist can provide quality patient care. For example, a female patient being treated to the pelvic region may insist that male physicians or therapist not be part of her treatment team. Although this would be an unusual situation and may present difficulties for the department, there may be some valid reasons for the patient's request such as a

Table 1-2	Classifications of neoplasms	
Tissue of Origin	**Benign**	**Malignant**
Glandular epithelium	Adenoma	Adenocarcinoma
Squamous epithelium	Papilloma	Squamous cell carcinoma
Connective tissue smooth muscle	Leiomyoma	Leiomyosarcoma
Hematopoietic	—	Leukemia
Lymphoreticular	—	Lymphoma
Neural	Neuroma	Blastoma

past history of sexual abuse. Once this information is obtained the specific needs of this patient can be met, with the patient receiving quality care. Another example would be the patient who requests a treatment time not convenient for the department schedule. For a therapist who has many patients to accommodate and a very tight schedule this request may seem unreasonable. It may turn out that a working relative is providing daily transportation to the clinic and does not have a flexible work schedule. An appointment time that interferes with the relative's work schedule may lead to the loss of employment. In this example there are three possible outcomes. One, the therapist gives the patient an appointment time that fits the treatment schedule and lets the patient work out the transportation issues. Two, the therapist gives the patient the requested appointment time and changes other patient appointments, or, three, the therapist refers the patient and relative to community transportation resources and works with all parties to develop a plan for treatment. For reasons such as these, an in-depth knowledge of available patient resources is essential to ensure that all patients receive the care and help they need to deal with the disease and resulting life issues. The actual radiation treatment is only part of the therapist's responsibility. A patient is not an organ with a cancer but a complete individual with a multitude of issues and needs that must be addressed. Because cancer affects the whole family, it is the responsibility of the therapist to provide information and available resources to assist the patient and family in dealing with all the issues and challenges that a diagnosis of cancer brings.

Cancer-Patient Resources

In each medical facility there is generally a myriad of cancer-support services. These services can include general education, cancer-site-specific education, financial aid, travel to and from treatment, and activity programs. Social work departments are available to assist with the financial, emotional, and logistic issues that arise, and community services through churches and other organizations are available to support individuals and their families. National organizations such as the American Cancer Society have established programs and information hot lines available to all patients. Caring for a cancer patient is often a 24-hour a day job and it is essential that resources are available at all hours. Radiation therapists must become familiar with the services offered in their communities and nationally to better serve the patients that they treat. This is especially true for therapists working at freestanding clinics not affiliated with a medical center. Educating patients and their families about available programs or referring patients to specific services to address specific needs is an important component of quality care.

ETIOLOGY AND EPIDEMIOLOGY

Today a tremendous amount of knowledge exists about factors that influence the development of cancer and the incidence at which it occurs. Etiology and epidemiology are the two areas of study that have contributed to the growing knowledge in these areas.

Etiology

Etiology is the study of the cause of disease. Although the cause of cancer is unknown, many carcinogenic agents have been identified. Experts use this information, as they have done with tobacco use, to establish prevention programs.

Etiologic and epidemiologic information is helpful in determining screening tests for early detection, producing patient-education programs, and identifying target populations. An example is the set of guidelines of the American Cancer Society for screening mammograms to detect breast cancer in its early stages.

Epidemiology

Epidemiology is the study of disease incidence. National databases provide statistical information about patterns of cancer occurrence and death rates. With this information, researchers can determine the incidence of cancer occurrence in a population for factors such as age, gender, race, and geographic location. Researchers can also determine which specific type of cancer affects which specific group of people. An example is the high incidence of stomach cancer in Japan compared with that in the United States. Epidemiologic studies also help determine trends in disease such as the recent decrease of lung cancer in men and the decline of stomach cancer in the United States.

DETECTION AND DIAGNOSIS

Early detection and diagnosis are keys to the successful treatment of cancer. The earlier a tumor is discovered, the lower the chance of metastasis or spread to other parts of the body. For some tumors such as carcinoma of the larynx, early symptoms cause the patient to seek medical care early in the course of the disease. As a result, the cure rate for early-stage glottic (or true vocal cord) tumors is extremely high. Cancer of the ovary, however, is associated with vague symptoms that could be the result of a number of medical problems. Therefore a diagnosis is often made late in the course of the disease. Cure rates for ovarian cancer reflect the results of late diagnosis.

Screening Examinations

To identify cancer in its earliest stages (before symptoms appear and while the chance of cure is greatest), screening tests are performed. Examples include the Pap smear for cervical cancer, fecal occult blood testing for colorectal cancer, and mammograms for breast cancer. For many cancer sites, screening examinations are not readily available because of the inaccessibility of the tumor and the high cost associated with the tests.

To be useful, screening examinations must be sensitive and specific for the tumors they identify. If an examination is sensitive, it can identify a tumor in its extremely early stages.

For example, a Pap smear is sensitive because it can help detect carcinoma of the cervix before the disease becomes invasive. If a test is specific, it can identify a particular type of cancer. Carcinoembryonic antigen (CEA) may be elevated because of a number of benign and malignant conditions. For this reason the test is not specific but is the most sensitive test available for determining recurrences of colorectal cancer.

Screening tests may also yield false-positive or false-negative readings. A **false-positive** reading indicates disease when in reality none is present. A **false-negative** reading is the reverse; the test indicates no disease when in fact the disease is present.

For a screening test to be highly useful, it should be sensitive, specific, cost effective, and accurate. The cost of the screening examination often limits its use to all but extremely high-risk populations.

Workup Components

After a tumor is suspected, a workup, or series of diagnostic examinations, begins. The purpose of the workup is to determine the general health status of the patient and collect as much information about the tumor as possible. To treat the patient effectively, the physician must know the type, location, and size of the tumor; the distance the tumor has invaded normal tissue; the presence of spread to distant sites; and lymph node involvement if any. These questions are answered in the workup.

The workup depends on the type of cancer suspected and the symptoms experienced by the patient. The workup for a suspected lung tumor is different than that for a suspected prostate tumor. The same questions are answered, but because the two tumors are extremely different, the tests are based on the specific tumor characteristics.

With advancing technology, more information is available to the physician than ever before. As new technologies emerge and prove useful in the information-gathering process, treatment becomes more effective. Before computed tomography (CT) became available, small tumor extension into normal lung tissues was not visible on chest radiographs. The physician had to make an educated guess about the extent of the tumor invasion and treat the patient based on the suspected condition. As a result, treatment fields had to be larger to encompass all the suspected disease. With CT, much of the guesswork is eliminated and treatment volumes can include areas of known disease while limiting even more the areas of normal tissue, therefore producing a more effective treatment.

Staging

Tumor staging is a means of defining the tumor size and extension at the time of diagnosis and is important for many reasons. Tumor staging provides a means of communication about tumors, helps in determining the best treatment, aids in predicting prognosis, and provides a means for continuing research. Staging systems have changed with advancing technologies and increased knowledge and will continue to progress as more information becomes known. For this reason, tumors that occur frequently have detailed staging classifications, whereas those that are rare have primitive or no working stages.

A common staging system adopted by the International Union Against Cancer (UICC) and the American Joint Committee on Cancer (AJCC) is the TNM system. The T category defines the size or extent of the primary tumor and is assigned numbers 1 through 4. A T1 tumor is small and/or confined to a small area, whereas a T4 tumor is extremely large and/or extends into other tissues. N designates the status of lymph nodes and the extent of lymph node involvement. A 0-through-4 designation exists depending on the extent of involvement, with N0 indicating that no positive nodes are present. N1 indicates positive nodes close to the site of the primary tumor, whereas N4 indicates positive nodes at more distant nodal sites. M is the category that defines the presence and extent of metastasis. Again, the M category is divided into a 0 or 1 designation depending on the extent of metastatic disease. The designation M0 indicates no evidence of metastatic disease found, whereas M1 indicates metastasis in multiple organs distant from the primary tumor (Fig. 1-3).

In the TNM staging are additional subcategories for commonly occurring tumors. Notations are often used to determine whether the staging was accomplished through clinical, surgical, or pathologic methods. Although the TNM system is widely used, numerous staging systems exist that more accurately detail important tumor characteristics for prognostic and treatment information. For example, the International Federation of Gynecology and Obstetrics (FIGO) system is used in the staging of gynecologic tumors.

Surgical Staging

Surgical staging offers the most accurate information about the tumor and the extent of disease spread. Although staging can be performed clinically, or without the use of invasive procedures, the status of the lymph nodes and micrometastatic spread would remain in question. During surgical staging the physician has the opportunity to perform a biopsy of suspicious-looking tissue, obtain a sample of lymph nodes for microscopic examination, and observe the tumor and surrounding tissues and organs. Although now very uncommon, performing a laparotomy for staging of Hodgkin's disease provides essential information in the determination of treatment below the diaphragm. At the time of surgery, lymph nodes are sampled, the spleen removed, and incisional wedge biopsies of the liver are performed. If no tumor is found in the abdomen, the patient is spared subdiaphragmatic radiation therapy.

Ovarian disease is also staged surgically through the use of a laparotomy because these tumors often spread by seeding into the abdomen. During the procedure the primary tumor site is identified, tumor is removed, suspicious areas

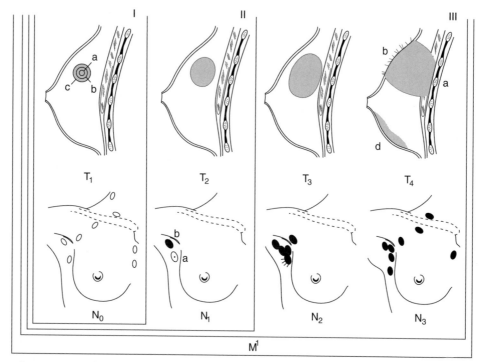

Figure 1-3. A diagrammatic depiction of the breast cancer staging system. *(From Rubin P: Clinical oncology, ed 7, Philadelphia, 1993, WB Saunders.)*

are biopsied, and fluid is introduced into the abdominal cavity to be removed and examined for cancer cells. The amount of tumor left behind following the surgery provides important treatment and prognostic information. The greater the amount of information obtained about the tumor the more accurate the staging is likely to be, resulting in more effective treatment. In addition, the more accurate the staging, the greater the ability to limit more aggressive treatment to only those patients who will benefit.

Grade

The **grade** of a tumor provides information about its aggressiveness and is based on the degree of differentiation. For some tumors, such as a high-grade astrocytoma, grade is the most important prognostic indicator.

The stage and grade offer an accurate picture of the tumor and its behavior. When physicians know the exact types of tumors with which they are dealing, treatment decisions can be made that effectively eradicate the tumors. (A detailed description of cancer detection and diagnosis is provided in Chapter 5.)

TREATMENT OPTIONS

Cancer treatment demands a multidisciplinary approach. Tumor boards were established to have cancer specialists work together to review information about newly diagnosed tumors and devise effective treatment plans. Participants of a tumor board can include surgeons, radiation oncologists,

medical oncologists, social workers, plastic surgeons, and other medical personnel. All these individuals play key roles in developing a treatment plan that effectively treats the tumor while helping the patient maintain a high quality of life (Fig. 1-4).

Surgery

As a local treatment modality, surgery plays a role in diagnosis, staging, primary treatment, **palliation,** and identification of treatment response. As a tool for diagnosis, surgery is used to perform a biopsy of a suspected mass to determine whether the mass is malignant and, if so, the cellular origin. Many biopsy methods exist, and the characteristics of the suspected mass determine the use of a particular method.

To provide the most effective treatment, the histology and cellular characteristics must be identified. A few questions that a biopsy will answer are as follows: Is the tumor growing at the primary site or has it spread from another area in the body? Is the tumor slow growing or very aggressive? Is the tumor malignant? Once this information is known an appropriate multidisciplinary treatment plan can be established.

Common **biopsy** methods include fine needle aspiration, core needle, endoscopic, incisional, and excisional. The information obtained through a biopsy is essential for appropriate treatment management. A fine-needle aspiration biopsy would be used to determine the histology of a suspicious breast mass. During the biopsy, sample cells are collected

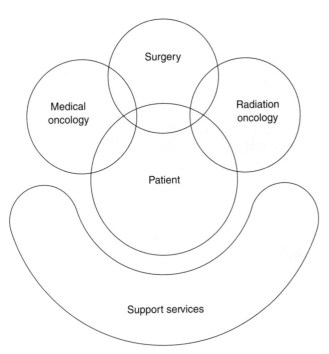

Figure 1-4. The cancer patient receives treatment and support from multiple sources during disease management.

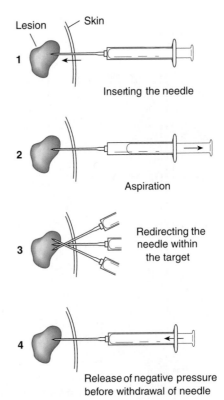

Figure 1-5. The steps in aspiration of a palpable lesion. Step 3 indicates the way that the needle should be redirected in the target, and step 4 emphasizes the importance of releasing the negative pressure before withdrawing the needle. *(From Koss LG: Needle aspiration cytology of tumors at various body sites. In Silver CE et al, editors: Current problems in surgery, vol 22, Chicago, 1985, Year Book Medical Publishers.)*

in the needle from several areas of the suspected tumor (Fig. 1-5). The cells are then transferred to a microscopic slide for further examination. This method of biopsy is relatively quick and easy with minimal patient discomfort and healing time. The disadvantage is that the collected cells are examined without the benefit of their neighboring cells to provide a glimpse of the tumor architecture. There is also the chance that malignant cells will be seeded along the needle track as the needle is withdrawn from the tumor.

A large-gauge needle (14 or 16) is used to perform a core-needle biopsy. As the needle is inserted into the suspected tumor, a core of tissue is collected. The tissue obtained can be sectioned and examined under a microscope. Using this method the tumor architecture is preserved allowing identification of the tumor tissue of origin (Fig. 1-6).

During endoscopic procedures, such as a bronchoscopy or colonoscopy, suspicious tissue can also be collected with the use of a flexible biopsy tool. The tool is passed through the scope, and tiny pincers are used to cut a small tissue sample. Tissue samples can then be frozen or imbedded in paraffin, sectioned, and examined under the microscope.

During an incisional biopsy, a sample of the tumor is removed with no attempt to remove the whole tumor. This method is often used with larger tumors or those that are locally advanced (Fig. 1-7). Excisional biopsies, on the other hand, attempt to remove the entire tumor and any possible local spread as in the case of malignant melanoma. When a nevi, or mole, becomes suspicious by changing colors or growing larger an excisional biopsy is performed. The nevi

and normal surrounding tissue to include a safe margin of underlying tissue are removed **en bloc,** or as one piece.

Surgery plays a major role in the treatment of cancer. With advances in knowledge, equipment, and techniques, procedures performed are now less radical and are apt to be part of a multidisciplinary treatment plan. The success of surgical intervention is dependent on the medical condition and wishes of the patient, the size and extent of the tumor, and the location of the tumor.

Not all patients are surgical candidates. Patients with preexisting medical conditions may have an unacceptable increase in surgical risk. For example, if the patient's pulmonary function is compromised, general anesthesia may be contraindicated and surgical procedures impossible. In addition, as with any treatment modality, the patient may decide not to have surgery in favor of another type of treatment or no treatment at all.

Because surgery is a localized treatment, it is most successful with small tumors that have not spread to neighboring tissues or organs. During surgery, the physician attempts

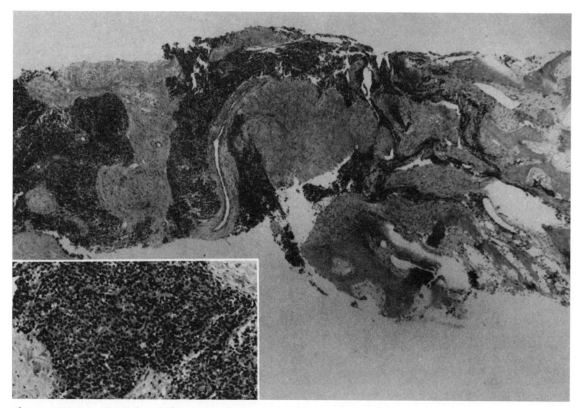

Figure 1-6. An example of the tissue core obtained by needle biopsy of a Ewing's sarcoma as seen microscopically. The insert demonstrates good preservation of cells. *(From del Regato JA, Spjut HJ, Cox JD: Ackerman and del Regato's cancer: diagnosis, treatment and prognosis, ed 6, St. Louis, 1985, Mosby.)*

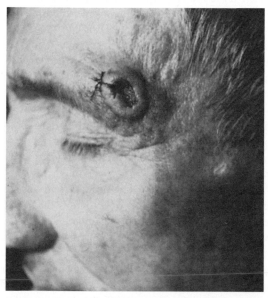

Figure 1-7. In an incisional biopsy, a specimen is removed from the edge of the tumor. *(From del Regato JA, Spjut HJ, Cox JD: Ackerman and del Regato's cancer: diagnosis, treatment and prognosis, ed 6, St. Louis, 1985, Mosby.)*

to remove the entire tumor and any microscopic spread, requiring the removal of normal tissue. As the size and/or extent of the tumor increases, more normal tissue must be removed, thus increasing the risk of the procedure. Surgical intervention may be the only treatment necessary if the tumor can be completely removed. If, however, the surgical margins are positive for cancer cells, the tumor has a high recurrence rate, or gross tumor was left, further treatment is necessary.

Before surgery, radiation therapy or chemotherapy may be given to increase the likelihood of a complete resection. The goals of radiation or chemotherapy in this case are to destroy microscopic and subclinical disease and shrink the tumor. Lower doses of radiation and/or chemotherapy are used to prevent complications during and following surgery.

The location of the tumor is an important factor in the success of surgical treatment. If a tumor is located in an area that is inaccessible or close to **critical structures** (vital organs or structures), surgery may not be possible. Damage to critical structures is incompatible with life or leaves the patient in worse condition than before treatment. A cancer of the nasopharynx is located in an area in which accessibility is difficult because the cancer is close to the base of the brain and the cranial nerves. For these reasons, patients with cancers of the nasopharynx are not good candidates for surgical intervention. With improved technology and procedures, however, location of the tumor continues to become less of a barrier to successful treatment.

Surgical palliation is used to relieve symptoms the patient may be experiencing as a result of the disease. An example is an obstruction of the bowel. The surgery does not have a curative effect on the disease but provides the patient with symptom relief for an improved quality of life. Cutting nerves to reduce or eliminate pain caused by the tumor is another example of palliative surgery.

Second-look surgeries are performed to determine treatment outcome. With an ovarian tumor, a second-look surgery provides information about tumor response to previous treatment. If the surgeon finds malignant cells during the second-look surgery, more treatment is indicated.

Radiation Therapy

Radiation therapy is a local treatment that can be used alone or with other treatment modalities. Benefits of radiation therapy include preservation of function and better cosmetic results. An early-stage laryngeal tumor can be effectively treated by surgery or radiation. Surgery may require removal of the vocal cords, thus leaving the patient without a voice. Radiation therapy, however, can obtain the same results while preserving the patient's voice. In the past, surgery for patients with prostate cancer commonly left the patient impotent with a high chance for incontinence. Radiation therapy can preserve function while providing an effective treatment.

Surgery and radiation therapy combined also obtain an optimal cosmetic result. In the past, breast cancer was usually treated with a radical mastectomy, leaving the patient disfigured. Currently, a common treatment consists of a lumpectomy with axillary node dissection followed by radiation therapy and leaves the patient with minimal disfigurement and an equal chance of cure. More recently, examination of the **sentinel node,** or the primary drainage lymph node, decreases the extent of an axillary node dissection. As a result, the patient experiences less range of motion deficits and lymphedema risks.

Radiation therapy plays a major role in palliation. An example is the treatment of bone metastasis. If the condition is left untreated, the patient experiences a great deal of pain and is at risk for pathologic bone fractures. Radiation therapy to these sites usually eliminates the pain and prevents fractures. If a tumor is pressing on nerves, radiation therapy is given to reduce the size of the tumor, thus eliminating pressure on the nerves and providing pain relief.

Radiation therapy is limited to a local area of treatment. Tumors that are diffuse throughout the body are not candidates for radiation therapy. Radiation therapy is further limited to areas in which a **tumoricidal** dose may be delivered without harming critical structures.

As with surgery, the patient's medical condition must be such that the patient can tolerate the treatment. If a patient is suffering from lung cancer and has little pulmonary function, radiation therapy may not be a suitable treatment option because it may further compromise the patient's ability to breathe. Numerous methods to deliver radiation exist. The two broad categories are external beam and brachytherapy.

External beam. Through the use of external beam x-rays, electrons or gamma rays can be delivered to the tumor. Linear accelerators are capable of producing x-rays of a specific energy. Some treatment machines can produce multiple x-ray, or **photon,** energies in addition to a range of electron energies. **Gamma rays** are produced by Cobalt 60 machines; although they were the primary treatment machine 30 years ago, their numbers are limited today.

High-energy x-rays are used to treat tumors that are deeper in the body, whereas **electrons** are effective at delivering energy to superficial tumors. For tumors, such as pancreatic cancer, electrons can be given at the time of surgery. **Intraoperative** radiotherapy is delivered directly to the tumor using a sterilized lucite cone that is positioned during surgery. The cone is then attached to the accelerator, treatment given, and the patient returned to surgery for incision closure. This method allows a high dose to be delivered to the tumor while sparing the normal surrounding tissues.

Treatment today is more precise and accurate than ever before. With the use of advanced treatment planning computers, sophisticated treatment equipment and much better imaging technology, a high dose of radiation can be safely delivered to the tumor with minimal damage to surrounding normal tissue. Conformal therapy and intensity modulated radiation therapy are two examples of recent advances. Very simply explained, these two techniques change the treatment field size and/or dose to vary with the shape of the tumor as the treatment machine is positioned or rotates around the body.

Brachytherapy. Brachytherapy, or "short-distance therapy," employs the use of radioactive materials such as cesium (^{137}Cs), iridium (^{192}Ir), or gold (^{198}Au). Through the use of brachytherapy, the radioactive sources can be placed next to or directly into the tumor. Because the energy of the radioactive sources is low, a high energy is delivered to the tumor, with the normal tissues close by receiving very little dose. Brachytherapy is accomplished using a multitude of techniques.

During an interstitial implant, radioactive sources are placed directly into the tumor. The sources may remain in place permanently or they may be removed once the prescribed dose has been delivered. Treatment of prostate cancer is a good example for both of these methods. For a permanent implant, tiny seeds of ^{198}Au are placed in the prostate. These seeds remain in the prostate, with their radioactivity decreasing over time. Because of the low energy of the radioactive material the patient poses no threat to his family and friends. Another patient with prostate cancer may be treated with a removable implant. At the time of surgery, needles are placed into the prostate through the perineum. Later, when the patient has left recovery and is in the appropriate hospital room, the radioactive sources are placed in the needles. The patient remains in the hospital with the sources in place until the prescribed dose has been delivered. Determination of the type of implant offered depends on the skill and preference of the radiation oncologist, the available resources, and the patient's wishes. Cancers of the head and neck and breast are amenable to interstitial implants.

Intracavitary implants are performed by placing the radioactive material in a body cavity, as in the case of treatment for cervical or endometrial cancers. Applicators are placed in the body cavity, often at the time of surgery, and later the radioactive sources are inserted and remain until the prescribed dose has been delivered. The prescribed dose can be delivered over several days as an inpatient (low-dose brachytherapy) or in one or more fractions as an outpatient procedure (high-dose brachytherapy).

Interluminal brachytherapy is used when the radioactive material is placed within a body tube such as the esophagus or bronchial tree. The radioactive material is positioned in the lumen at the tumor site and removed once the prescribed dose is delivered. Another brachytherapy technique, intervascular brachytherapy, is used to prevent restenosis of blood vessels following angioplasty or stent placement.

The tremendous arsenal of treatment delivery methods and the successful outcomes achieved makes radiation therapy a major weapon in the fight against cancer. As the ability to detect and image a tumor improves, the precision of the treatment delivery methods will continue to advance. Treatments that are commonly used today were only dreams 20 years ago.

Chemotherapy

Unlike surgery and radiation therapy, chemotherapy is a **systemic treatment.** Using **cytotoxic** drugs and hormones, chemotherapy is aimed at killing cells of the primary tumor and those that may be circulating through the body. Chemotherapy may be administered as a primary treatment or as part of a multidisciplinary treatment plan. As with the other major cancer treatments, chemotherapy is most successful when the tumor burden is small. Most chemotherapy agents affect the cell during a specific phase of the cell cycle. Tumors that are rapidly dividing provide more opportunities for the cytotoxic effects to take place because more cells are in the cell cycle.

Administration of chemotherapeutic agents is accomplished through a variety of methods depending on the drug prescribed. Oral administration is the easiest method but does require full patient compliance in taking the drug and in taking the drug at the correct times. Injections can be self-administered by the patient or the oncology nurse. Intraarterial administration requires an infusion pump connected to a catheter that has been placed in an artery near the tumor. Heparin, a blood thinner, is added to the cytotoxic agent to prevent clotting at the catheter site. Bladder cancer is often treated with an intracavity administration whereby

the chemotherapy drugs are instilled directly into the bladder. Cytotoxic drugs are introduced into the abdomen using an intraperitoneal administration through a catheter or implanted port. **Intrathecal** injection requires drugs to be instilled into the space containing cerebrospinal fluid. Although most chemotherapy drugs can be administered by the patient or a nurse, intrathecal administration is only done by a physician. One of the more common methods of drug installation is the intravenous (IV) route. Drugs may be administered using a syringe entering the vein directly or piggybacked with other fluids.

Chemotherapy agents are very toxic, and safety precautions must be taken during preparation and administration, such as the wearing of gloves, gowns, and face shields. Certain drugs have vesicant or blistering potential and if spilled on the skin or outside of the vein will cause ulceration, so extra precautions must be taken. For these reasons, patients coming to radiation therapy with IV lines for chemotherapy must be treated with extra care to preserve the patency of the IV line. Often these individuals have such small, weak veins so that finding a site for the IV is difficult at best. If a problem occurs with an IV line, the therapist should call the nurse charged with the care of that patient immediately to prevent total failure of the site.

Chemotherapeutic Agents

Chemotherapy agents are classified by their action on the cell or their source and include alkylating agents, antimetabolites, antibiotics, hormonal agents, nitrosoureas, vinca alkaloids, and miscellaneous agents[3,7,9] (Table 1-4).

Alkylating agents were the first drugs identified to have anticancer activity. This class of drugs is related structurally to mustard gas and are not cell cycle specific but rather work throughout the cycle. The mechanism of action is to bond with nucleic acids, thereby interfering with their action. Side effects include bone marrow depression, amenorrhea in women and azoospermia in men, and carcinogenesis. Administration of alkylating agents is associated with an increased risk of acute myelogenous leukemia and is related to the total drug dose. Examples of alkylating agents include nitrogen mustard, cyclophosphamide, and chlorambucil.

Antimetabolites act by interfering with the synthesis of new nucleic acids. They are cell cycle specific and are much more toxic to proliferating cells but are not associated with delayed bone marrow suppression or carcinogenesis. Side effects include gastrointestinal toxicity and acute bone marrow suppression. Examples of antimetabolites include methotrexate, often used with intrathecal administration, and 5-fluorouracil.

Anticancer antibiotics are derived from microbial fermentation. Antibiotics act on the DNA to disrupt DNA and RNA transcription. Although they are not cell cycle specific, the effects of the antibiotics are more pronounced in the S or G2 phase. Examples of anticancer antibiotics include dox-

Table 1-4	Chemotherapeutic drug classification with side effects
Drugs	**Major side effects**

ALKYLATING AGENTS

Busulfan	Nausea and vomiting, diarrhea, pulmonary fibrosis, bone marrow suppression, impotence, amenorrhea, and skin hyperpigmentation
Carboplatin	Nausea and vomiting, bone marrow suppression, ototoxicity, neurotoxicity, and hyperuricemia
Chlorambucil	Myelosuppression and interstitial pneumonia-pulmonary fibrosis
Cisplatin	Neurotoxicity, myelosuppression, nephrotoxicity, nausea and vomiting, hypokalemia, and hypomagnesemia
Cyclophosphamide	Myelosuppression, anorexia, stomatitis, alopecia, gonadal suppression, nail hyperpigmentation, nausea and vomiting, diarrhea, and hemorrhagic cystitis
Dacarbazine	Nausea and vomiting, anorexia, vein irritation, alopecia, myelosuppression, facial flushing, and radiation recall
Hexamethylmelamine	Nausea and vomiting, diarrhea, abdominal cramps, alopecia, myelosuppression, and neuropathy
Melphalan	Hypersensitivity, nausea, myelosuppression, amenorrhea, pulmonary infiltrates, and sterility
Nitrogen mustard	Nausea and vomiting, fever, chills, anorexia, vesication, gonadal suppression, myelosuppression, hyperpigmentation, and alopecia
Thiotepa	Nausea and vomiting, bone marrow suppression, mucositis, and gonadal dysfunction

ANTIMETABOLITES

Cytarabine	Myelosuppression, diarrhea, nausea and vomiting, alopecia, rash, fever, conjunctivitis, neurotoxicity, hepatotoxicity, pulmonary edema, and skin desquamation of the palms and soles of the feet
Floxuridine	Nausea and vomiting, diarrhea, oral and gastrointestinal ulcers, bone marrow suppression, alopecia, and hepatotoxicity
Fludarabine	Chills, fever, hyperuricemia, nausea and vomiting, bone marrow suppression, neurotoxicity, and pulmonary toxicity
Fluorouracil (5-FU)	Oral and gastrointestinal ulcers, nausea and vomiting, diarrhea, alopecia, vein hyperpigmentation, and radiation recall
6-Mercaptopurine	Nausea and vomiting, anorexia, myelosuppression, diarrhea, hepatotoxicity, and hyperpigmentation
6-Thioguanine	Anorexia, stomatitis, rash, vein irritation, hepatotoxicity, myelosuppression, and nausea and vomiting

ANTITUMOR ANTIBIOTICS

Bleomycin	Anaphylaxis, pneumonitis, pulmonary fibrosis, alopecia, stomatitis, anorexia, radiation recall, skin hyperpigmentation, fever, chills, and nausea and vomiting
Dactinomycin (actinomycin D)	Nausea and vomiting, stomatitis, vesication, alopecia, radiation recall, myelosuppression, and diarrhea
Daunorubicin	Myelosuppression, vesication, cardiotoxicity, stomatitis, radiation recall, nausea and vomiting, alopecia, and facial flushing
Doxorubicin	Myelosuppression, vesication, cardiotoxicity, stomatitis, alopecia, nausea and vomiting, radiation recall, and diarrhea
Idarubicin	Myelosuppression, alopecia, stomatitis, cardiotoxicity, nausea and vomiting, and vesication
Mithramycin	Myelosuppression, hepatotoxicity, hyperpigmentation, nausea and vomiting, facial flushing, and nephrotoxicity
Mitomycin	Myelosuppression, vesication, nausea and vomiting, alopecia, pulmonary fibrosis, hepatotoxicity, stomatitis, and hyperuricemia

HORMONAL AGENTS

Corticosteroids	
Dexamethasone	Nausea, suppression of immune function, weight gain, hyperglycemia, increased appetite, cataracts,
Hydrocortisone	impaired wound healing, menstrual irregularity, and interruption in sleep and rest patterns
Prednisone	
Solu-Cortef	
Antiandrogen	
Flutamide	Impotence and gynecomastia
Antiestrogen	
Tamoxifen	Nausea and vomiting, hot flashes, fluid retention, changes in menstrual pattern, increase in bone pain,
Zoladex	and hypercalcemia
Gonadotropin-releasing hormone	
Leuprolide	Impotence, decreased libido, increase in bone and tumor pain, genital atrophy, and gynecomastia

Studies that examine the effectiveness of treatment are classified by the study objectives. **Phase I studies** are used to determine the maximum tolerance dose for a specific treatment. The end point can be either acute or long-term toxicity. **Phase II studies** are used to determine if the Phase I treatment is significantly effective given the acute and/or long-term side effects to continue further study. **Phase III studies** are used to compare the experimental treatment with standard treatment using a randomized sample.

Randomized Studies

Clinical studies often include several methods of treatment to determine which method results in the best outcome. After meeting all eligibility requirements for the study, patients are randomly selected for one of the treatment arms. The purpose of randomization is to eliminate any unintentional "stacking of the deck" and increase the accuracy of results and conclusions. Although patients may have the same type, grade, stage, and extent of cancer, each person responds individually to the disease and treatment. Care providers cannot control these factors, but randomization helps minimize their effects on the end result. With randomization, each arm of the study has approximately equal numbers of individuals with varying reactions.

Survival Reporting

In the planning stages of a clinical trial an end point must be established. Otherwise the study can continue indefinitely with no data analysis. Rates of survival at a set end point are one type of information used to determine the benefit of one treatment over another. Survival reporting, however, can be accomplished with many methods. With absolute survival reporting, patients alive at the end point and those who have died are counted. Patients lost to follow-up are included, but the fact that patients may have died from other causes is not considered. Adjusted survival reporting includes patients who died from other causes and had **no evidence of disease (NED)** at the times of their deaths. Relative survival reporting involves the normal mortality rate of a similar group of people based on factors such as age, gender, and race.

In addition, survival reporting at the end point includes information about the status of the disease. At the end point the patient may be alive with NED, disease free, or alive with disease. Of equal importance is the information about treatment failures. Treatment failures are classified as local, locoregional, or distant and are based on tumor recurrences at the primary or nearby lymph node sites or metastatic disease. This information is valuable for ongoing clinical trials and for determining types of treatment techniques to prevent future failures.

THE RADIATION ONCOLOGY TEAM

The effectiveness of treatment is dependent on the teamwork of individuals in the entire radiation therapy department. From the receptionist to the physician, each individual has an important role in the goal of treating the person with cancer. Every day in every department each of the radiation therapy team members has the opportunity to improve the quality of life for the cancer patient and his or her family. It may be answering a question, referring the patient to a support group, or giving a family member a hug. Each of these small actions have the potential to have a huge positive impact on the patient and his or her family.

When a patient enters the radiation therapy department the first person he or she interacts with is the receptionist or secretary. Before the patient's arrival, this individual is involved in obtaining the patient's medical records and diagnostic images. The receptionist obtains insurance and the appropriate personal information and informs the other members of the radiation therapy team that the patient has arrived. The patient is taken to the consult/examination room to talk with the **radiation oncologist.** By the time the patient is in the examination room, the physician has become very familiar with the patient's medical history by talking with the patient's primary physician and reviewing all of the medical records. The physician reviews the medical findings with the patient and discusses treatment options that are available. The physician and patient will discuss the benefits of radiation therapy as well as the possible side effects. By the end of the consult and examination the physician will have a treatment plan in mind and the patient will be sent on for treatment planning and/or simulation. A **dosimetrist** is responsible for designing the patient's treatment to accomplish the physician's prescription using the most effective techniques possible. A dosimetrist is often a radiation therapist who has had additional education but may also be an individual with a physics or medical physics background. Before treatment, the patient will undergo a **simulation** or a procedure designed to delineate the treatment fields and construct any necessary immobilization or treatment devices. During a simulation, the **radiation therapist** is able to explain the simulation and treatment procedures and answer any questions the patient may have. Simulation provides an excellent time to assess the patient's medical condition and educational and support needs. Once the physician has approved of the treatment plan and simulation, the patient goes to the treatment machine. Depending on the purpose of treatment, the patient may be scheduled for 1 to 7 weeks of treatment. During treatment, the radiation oncologist generally sees the patient once a week to ensure that the treatment is progressing as expected. The radiation therapist sees the patient every day and is responsible for assessing the patient's reaction to treatment and the general medical condition. Radiation therapists and/or department nurses educate the patient about skin care, nutrition, and support services and provide appropriate referrals as necessary. Once the radiation therapy prescription has been completed the patient will be scheduled for a follow-up appointment. The radiation oncologist may see the patient in follow-up for many years, or the primary physician may follow the patient.

Depending on the size of the department, the team may be very small or very large. In a small outpatient facility the team may consist of a physician, therapist, receptionist, and part-time physicist (Fig. 1-8). The role of the team members in this scenario is vastly different in a large department with multiple doctors, treatment and simulation therapists, dosimetrists, physicists, nurses, and clerical and support staff. Generally, as the department grows larger the job description of the team members becomes more specific. In a large department a therapist's role may be limited to the actual treatment, and another therapist is responsible for simulations. The role of the radiation therapist in dosimetry might be limited to treatment planning, calculations, and quality assurance procedures. In a large department, the role of the physician may also be limited to one area of expertise. For example one physician might treat only those patients with head and neck tumors. In a small department, however, the therapist's role will include treatment, simulation, treatment planning, patient care, and quality assurance. For the therapist, there are opportunities of working in a number of different clinical sites from free-standing clinics to university medical centers. Each center offers different opportunities and challenges for the therapist who is willing to continue to learn and grow.

SUMMARY

Cancer has been a focus of scientific attention for decades. As technology improves and knowledge about the disease increases, detection, diagnosis, and treatment improve. The future of cancer management looks bright, with more sophisticated surgical techniques, more precise and advanced radiation therapy techniques, and improved chemotherapeutic agents. This is truly an exciting time to be joining the professional medical team in radiation therapy.

Review Questions

Fill in the Blank

1. _____ _____ occurs when a stem cell undergoes mitosis and divides with daughter cells.
2. _____ are also called cancer-suppressor genes.
3. Tumors arising from mesenchymal cells are termed _____.
4. _____ are tumors that originate from the epithelium.
5. _____ _____ is a means of defining tumor size, extent, and extension at the time of diagnosis.

Listing

6. List three classifications of tumors.
   a.
   b.
   c.
7. List five factors that play important roles in the medical compliance with, attitude toward, and response to the treatment of cancer.
   a.
   b.
   c.
   d.
   e.
8. Name four cancer-treatment options.
   a.
   b.
   c.
   d.

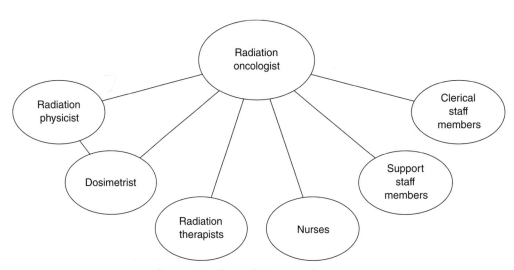

Figure 1-8. The radiation oncology team.

Questions to Ponder

1. What cancer patient resources are available in the hospital in which you work? What resources are available in your community?
2. Mr. Jones has a T2 tumor of the larynx, and Mrs. Smith has a T4 tumor of the larynx. What differences would you expect to see in the tumors and in the treatment plans for each of these patients?
3. What effects have etiology and epidemiology had on cigarette smoking?
4. How does a prognosis help or hinder a physician, care provider, or patient?
5. Analyze a clinical trial taking place in the hospital in which you work. What type of research is being done?
6. Discuss the process of carcinogenesis.
7. Discuss differences between benign and malignant neoplasms.

REFERENCES

1. American Cancer Society: *Cancer facts and figures 2003.* Available at http://www.cancer.org. Accessed March 2003.
2. Bunn PA: *New targeted therapies for lung cancer.* Available at http:www.medscape.com in *Medscape-Hematology-Oncology eJournal.* Accessed 8/20/02.
3. Cooper MR, Cooper MR: Systemic therapy. In Lenhard RE, Osteen RT, Gansler T, editors: *Clinical oncology,* Atlanta, 2001, The American Society.
4. Cotran RS, Kumar V, Robbins SL: *Robbins pathologic basis of disease,* Philadelphia, 1989, WB Saunders.
5. Henshaw EC: The biology of cancer. In Rubin P, editor: *Clinical oncology: a multidisciplinary approach for physicians and students,* ed 7, Philadelphia, 1993, WB Saunders.
6. Kardinal CG, Strnad BN: Confrontation with cancer: historical and existential aspects. In Gross SC, Garb S, editors: *Cancer treatment and research in humanistic perspective,* New York, 1985, Springer Publishing.
7. Otto SE: *Chemotherapy quick reference,* ed 2, St. Louis, 1997, Mosby.
8. Raven RW: The development and practice of oncology. In Gross SC, Garb S, editors: *Cancer treatment and research in humanistic perspective,* New York, 1985, Springer Publishing.
9. Shagam JY: Principles of chemotherapy, *Radiat Therapist* 10:37-53, Spring 2001.
10. Solomon E, Borrow J, Goddard AD: Chromosome aberrations and cancer, *Science* 254:1153-1159, 1991.
11. Weinberg RA: Tumor suppressor genes, *Science* 254:1138-1145, 1991.
12. Yunis JJ: The chromosomal basis of human neoplasia, *Science* 221:227-235, 1983.

BIBLIOGRAPHY

Aaronson SA: Growth factors and cancer, *Science* 254:1146-1152, 1991.

McCune CS, Chang AY: Basic concepts of tumor immunology and principles of immunotherapy. In Rubin P, editor: *Clinical oncology: a multidisciplinary approach for physicians and students,* ed 7, Philadelphia, 1993, WB Saunders.

Pajak T: Methodology of clinical trials. In Perez C, Brady L, editors: *Principles and practice of radiation oncology,* ed 2, Philadelphia, 1992, JB Lippincott.

Perez C, Brady L: Overview. In Perez C, Brady L, editors: *Principles and practice of radiation oncology,* ed 3, Philadelphia, 1998, JB Lippincott.

Ruben P, McDonald S, Keller J: Staging and classification of cancer: a unified approach. In Perez C, Brady L, editors: *Principles and practice of radiation oncology,* ed 2, Philadelphia, 1992, JB Lippincott.

Weiss DW: Immunological intervention in neoplasia. In Beers RF, Tilghman RC, Bassett EG, editors: *The role of immunological factors in viral and oncogenic processes. Seventh international symposium,* Baltimore, 1974, Johns Hopkins University Press.

2

The Ethics and Legal Consideration of Cancer Management

Janet M. Salzmann

Outline

Key Terms

Analytical model
Assault
Autonomy
Battery
Beneficence
Civil law
Collegial model
Consequentialism
Contractual model
Covenant model
Deontology
Doctrine of foreseeability
Doctrine of personal liability
Doctrine of res ipsa loquitur
Doctrine of respondeat superior
Engineering model
Ethics
False imprisonment

Incident
Informed consent
Invasion of privacy
Justice
Legal concepts
Legal ethics
Libel
Medical record
Moral ethics
Negligence
Nonmaleficence
Priestly model
Risk management
Scope of practice
Slander
Tort law
Virtue ethics

In radiation therapy, ethical issues arise daily in dealing with other health care professionals, patients, and families. In this fast-paced, changing world of health care, radiation therapists and students must be well versed in ethics and legal considerations of cancer management. The radiation therapist deals with patients who have specific needs related to their attempts to control catastrophic diseases that are taking over their lives and the lives of those close to them. Defining the roles and responsibilities of the radiation therapy student, the practicing radiation therapist, and other members of the radiation oncology team as they care for their patients is extremely important. In addition to developing technical skills necessary to practice in the profession, members of the radiation oncology team must develop an understanding of the basic theories regarding ethics, patients' rights, the scope of practice for radiation therapists, and the code of ethics for radiation therapy. The medical-legal aspects of informed consent, record keeping, and confidentiality are also important.

Radiation therapy has a code of ethics to guide students and therapists in professional conduct (see Box 2-1). However, the code does not list all principles and rules but only those that constitute the heart of ethically sound professional practice. A code of ethics serves two major functions: education and regulation. It educates persons in the profession who do not reflect on ethical implications of their actions unless something concrete is before them. It also educates other professional and lay groups concerning ethical standards expected of a given profession.[12] Understanding ethical concepts and legal issues and developing interpersonal skills through the study of the material in this chapter enables student therapists and practicing radiation therapists to care for their patients humanely and compassionately.

ETHICAL ASPECTS OF CANCER MANAGEMENT

Definitions and Terminology

Webster's New Collegiate Dictionary[13] defines **ethics** as (1) the discipline dealing with what is good and bad, moral duty, and obligation; (2) a set of moral principles or values; (3) a theory or system of moral values; and (4) the principles of conduct governing an individual or a group. Ethics for the individual derives from the person's experiences, teachings, and values. The individual gathers an understanding of right and wrong from the cumulative experiences of life and develops patterns of approaching situations in which the complexities of right and wrong must be addressed.[14]

In the study of ethics a person must distinguish between **moral** and **legal ethics.** Morality has to do with conscience. It is a person's concept of right or wrong as it relates to conscience, God, a higher being, or a person's logical rationalization. *Morality* can be defined as fidelity to conscience. **Legal concepts** are defined as the sum of rules and regulations by which society is governed in any formal and legally binding manner. The law mandates certain acts and forbids other acts under penalties of criminal sanction. The law is primarily concerned with the good of a society as a functioning unit.[7]

In dealing with ethical issues in cancer treatment, health care professionals should consider bioethics, which is based on four underlying principles: **beneficence, nonmaleficence, autonomy,** and **justice.** Beneficence calls on health care professionals to act in the best interest of patients, even at some inconvenience and sacrifice to themselves. Nonmaleficence directs professionals to avoid harmful actions to patients. Autonomy emphasizes that patients are independent actors whose freedom to control themselves is to be respected. Justice asks persons to ensure that fairness and equity are maintained among individuals.[10]

Ethical Theories and Models

Many persons believe that ethics simply means using common sense. Therefore a value system and appropriate behavior should be factors in any health care professional. However, ethical problem solving begins with an awareness of ethical issues in health care and is the sum of ethical knowledge, common sense, personal values, professional values, practical wisdom, and learned skills.[11] Although an individual's personal system of decision making may be developed from values and experiences, it generally involves some understanding and application of basic principles common to formal ethics.[14]

Ethical theories can be divided into the following three broad groups: (1) **consequentialism,** (2) **deontology,** and (3)

- The radiation therapist advances the principal objective of the profession to provide services to humanity with full respect for the dignity of mankind.
- The radiation therapist delivers patient care and service unrestricted by concerns of personal attributes or the nature of the disease or illness and nondiscriminatory with respect to race, color, creed, sex, age, disability, or national origin.
- The radiation therapist assesses situations; exercises care, discretion, and judgment; assumes responsibility for professional decisions; and acts in the best interest of the patient.
- The radiation therapist adheres to the tenets and domains of the scope of practice for radiation therapists.
- The radiation therapist actively engages in lifelong learning to maintain, improve, and enhance professional competence and knowledge.

Modified from the American Society of Radiologic Technologists: *The code of ethics for radiation therapists,* Albuquerque, NM, 1993, The American Society of Radiologic Technologists.

---

virtue ethics. Consequentialism, or the theory of utility, evaluates an activity by weighing the good against the bad or the way a person can provide the greatest good for the greatest number. Deontology uses formal rules of right and wrong for reasoning and problem solving. A few gray areas exist in this theory, which make it difficult to use in our society because varieties of life experiences make formal rules of right and wrong impossible to define. Virtue ethics is the use of practical wisdom for emotional and intellectual problem solving. Practical reasoning, consideration of consequences, rules established by society, and effects that actions have on others play important parts in applying the theory of virtue ethics. This approach to problem solving serves the health care professional by integrating intellect, practical reasoning, and individual good.[11]

Models for ethical decision making involve different methods of interactions with the patient. The **engineering** or **analytical model** identifies the caregiver as a scientist dealing only in facts and does not consider the human aspect of the patient. The engineering model is a dehumanizing approach and is usually ineffective.[11] For example, with the engineering model the radiation therapist considers the patient only a lung or brain rather than an individual who has thoughts and feelings. This type of approach in the care of cancer patients is cold, unfeeling, and extremely inappropriate.

The **priestly model** provides the caregiver with a godlike, paternalist attitude that makes decisions *for* and not *with* the patient. This approach enhances the patient's loss of control by giving the caregiver not only medical expertise but also authority about moral issues.[11] An example of this model is the therapist or student forcing a patient to comply with planning or treatment procedures regardless of the patient's pain or discomfort because the physician ordered it or because the disease is known to respond to treatment. Patients must be allowed to make decisions about their compliance to treatment.

The **collegial model** presents a more cooperative method of pursuing health care for the provider and patient. It involves sharing, trust, and consideration of common goals. The collegial model gives more control to the patient while producing confidence and preserving dignity and respect.[11] For example, the therapist takes the extra time required to get acquainted with patients and listen to their needs. This knowledge enables the therapist to help patients cooperate with demands of positioning for planning and treatment. The collegial model takes time and is crucial to the humane treatment of cancer patients.

The **contractual model** maintains a business relationship between the provider and patient. A contractual arrangement serves as the guideline for decision making and meeting obligations for services. With a contractual arrangement, information and responsibility are shared. This model requires compliance from the patient; however, the patient is in control of the decision making.[11] The contractual model is best represented by the process of informed consent. Complete information is given and explained thoroughly, and the patient makes decisions.

The **covenant model** recognizes areas of health care not always covered by a contract. A covenant relationship deals with an understanding between the patient and health care provider that is often based on traditional values and goals.[11] The covenant model is demonstrated by a patient trusting the caregiver to do what is right. This trust is often based on previous experience with health care, particularly cancer care procedures and treatment.

The role of the radiation therapist in regard to ethical decision making involves the application of professionalism, the selection of a personal theory of ethics, and the choice of a model for interaction with the patient. The difficulties encountered are the result of constant changes in health care, patient awareness, and evolving growth of radiation therapy in a highly technical and extremely impersonal world of health care.[11]

Patients should actively participate in their own care. Patients' awareness of their rights, their needs, and the availability of the many treatment options provide opportunities and complications. The American Hospital Association has published *The Patient Care Partnership: Understanding Expectations, Rights, and Responsibilities* (see Box 2-2), and

---

Box 2-2   **The Patient Care Partnership: Understanding Expectations, Rights, and Responsibilities**

When you need hospital care, your doctor and the nurses and other professionals at our hospital are committed to working with you and your family to meet your health care needs. Our dedicated doctors and staff serve the community in all its ethnic, religious, and economic diversity. Our goal is for you and your family to have the same care and attention we would want for our families and ourselves.

The sections below explain some of the basics about how you can expect to be treated during your hospital stay. They also cover what we will need from you to care for you better. If you have questions at any time, please ask them. Unasked or unanswered questions can add to the stress of being in the hospital. Your comfort and confidence in your care are very important to us.

WHAT TO EXPECT DURING YOUR HOSPITAL STAY

- **High quality hospital care.** Our first priority is to provide you the care you need, when you need it, with skill, compassion, and respect. Tell your caregivers if you have concerns about your care or if you have pain. You have the right to know the identity of doctors, nurses, and others involved in your care, as well as when they are students, residents, or other trainees.
- **A clean and safe environment**. Our hospital works hard to keep you safe. We use special policies and procedures to avoid mistakes in your care and keep you free from abuse or neglect. If anything unexpected and significant happens during your hospital stay, you will be told what happened and any resulting changes in your care will be discussed with you.
- **Involvement in your care.** You and your doctor often make decisions about your care before you go to the hospital. Other times, especially in emergencies, those decisions are made during your hospital stay. When they take place, making decisions should include:
  1. *Discussing your medical condition and information about medically appropriate treatment choices.* To make informed decisions with your doctor, you need to understand several things:
     - The benefits and risks of each treatment.
     - Whether it is experimental or part of a research study.
     - What you can reasonably expect from your treatment and any long-term effects it might have on your quality of life.
     - What you and your family will need to do after you leave the hospital.
     - The financial consequences of using uncovered services or out-of-network providers.

continued

| Box 2-2 | The Patient Care Partnership: Understanding Expectations, Rights, and Responsibilities—cont'd |

Please tell your caregivers if you need more information about treatment choices.

2. *Discussing your treatment plan.* When you enter the hospital, you sign a general consent to treatment. In some cases, such as surgery or experimental treatment, you may be asked to confirm in writing that you understand what is planned and agree to it. This process protects your right to consent to or refuse a treatment. Your doctor will explain the medical consequences of refusing recommended treatment. It also protects your right to decide if you want to participate in a research study.

3. *Getting information from you.* Your caregivers need complete and correct information about your health and coverage so that they can make good decisions about your care. That includes:
   – Past illnesses, surgeries, or hospital stays.
   – Past allergic reactions.
   – Any medicines or diet supplements (such as vitamins and herbs) that you are taking.
   – Any network or admission requirements under your health plan.

4. *Understanding your health care goals and values.* You may have health care goals and values or spiritual beliefs that are important to your well-being. They will be taken into account as much as possible throughout your hospital stay. Make sure your doctor, your family, and your care team know your wishes.

5. *Understanding who should make* decisions *when you cannot.* If you have signed a health care power of attorney stating who should speak for you if you become unable to make health care decisions for yourself, or a "living will" or "advance directive" that states your wishes about end-of-life care, give copies to your doctor, your family and your care team. If you or your family need help making difficult decisions, counselors, chaplains and others are available to help.

- **Protection of your privacy.** We respect the confidentiality of your relationship with your doctor and other caregivers, and the sensitive information about your health and health care that are part of that relationship. State and federal laws and hospital operating policies protect the privacy of your medical information. You will receive a Notice of Privacy Practices that describes the ways that we use, disclose and safeguard patient information and that explains how you can obtain a copy of information from our records about your care.

- **Help preparing you and your family for when you leave the hospital.** Your doctor works with hospital staff and professionals in your community. You and your family also play an important role. The success of your treatment often depends on your efforts to follow medication, diet and therapy plans. Your family may need to help care for you at home. You can expect us to help you identify sources of follow-up care and to let you know if our hospital has a financial interest in any referrals. As long as you agree we can share information about your care with them, we will coordinate our activities with your caregivers outside the hospital. You can also expect to receive information and, where possible, training about the self-care you will need when you go home.

- **Help with your bill and filing insurance claims.** Our staff will file claims for you with health care insurers or other programs such as Medicare and Medicaid. They will also help your doctor with needed documentation. Hospital bills and insurance coverage are often confusing. If you have questions about your bill, contact our business office. If you need help understanding your insurance coverage or health plan, start with your insurance company or health benefits manager. If you do not have health coverage, we will try to help you and your family find financial help or make other arrangements. We need your help with collecting needed information and other requirements to obtain coverage or assistance.

While you are here, you will receive more detailed notices about some of the rights you have as a hospital patient and how to exercise them. We are always interested in improving. If you have questions, comments, or concerns, please contact _____.

Courtesy American Hospital Association.

every medical institution has the responsibility to make this document available to its patients. Each patient's responsibility for the treatment process grows with patient education.[11]

PATIENT AUTONOMY AND INFORMED CONSENT

Cancer remains one of the most dreaded diseases and often evokes images of death, disfigurement, intolerable pain, and suffering. Approximately 35 years ago, the central ethical issue in caring for the cancer patient was whether to tell the patient the truth that the diagnosis was cancer. Today, advancements in treatment, surgery, chemotherapy, and radiation therapy have resulted in longer periods of remission, improved survival, and even cure. This has generated more complex ethical issues.[10] More than half of all cancer patients ultimately need radiation therapy. The physician and patient must weigh the benefits of therapy against possible complications.[2]

The health care professional's ability to listen to patients sensitively, grasp the patient's truth, and honor that truth is indispensable, even across social, cultural, and age barriers. To be effective and supportive, physicians and caregivers must in a sense be masters of each patient's personal language. This ability to listen and communicate is an extremely important clinical skill that must be learned, preferably from experts. Mastery of listening and communicating should be highly valued.[8]

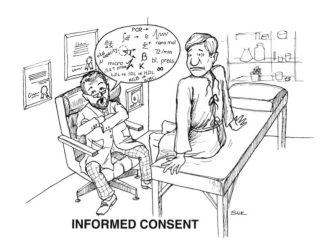

INFORMED CONSENT

Truth telling, which is required for informed consent, is an extremely curious principle. Persons have been taught from early childhood to tell the truth but doing so is often extremely difficult and sometimes even seems wrong. Not long ago, lying to a patient about the cancer diagnosis was the norm. Caregivers believed that telling the truth would be destructive and that patients preferred ignorance of their conditions. Studies over the years, however, have conclusively documented that cancer patients want to know their diagnoses and do not suffer psychologic injuries as a result of knowing.[10]

The claim that each person is free to make life-directing decisions is often known as the *autonomy principle.* The concept of autonomy, understood in this sense, is crucial to ethics. Without some sense of autonomy, no sense of responsibility exists, and, without responsibility, ethics is not possible.[15] In conventional cancer therapy, patient autonomy is protected further by the practice of **informed consent.** The American Medical Association's principles of medical ethics imply the following about informed consent: a physician shall be dedicated to providing competent medical service with compassion and respect for human dignity, shall deal honestly with patients and colleagues, and shall make relevant information available to patients. Patients should be informed and educated about their conditions, should understand and approve their treatments, and should participate responsibly in their own care.[2] The basic elements of informed consent are called patients' rights to know and participate in their own health care. Informed consent is a doctrine that has evolved sociologically with the changing times. Every patient is entitled to informed consent before any procedure is performed.[7] (See Box 2-3.)

Competency refers to the minimal mental, cognitive, or behavioral ability or trait required to assume responsibility. Generally the law recognizes only decisions or consents made by competent individuals. Persons older than the age of 18 are presumed to be competent; however, this may be dis-

puted with evidence of mental illness or deficiency. If the individual's condition prevents the satisfaction of criteria for competency, the person may be deemed incompetent for the purpose of informed consent. Mental illness does not automatically render a person incompetent in all areas of functioning. Respect for autonomy demands that individuals, even if they are seriously mentally impaired, be allowed to make decisions of which they are capable. Minors are not considered legally competent and therefore require the consent of parents or designated guardians.[2]

The rule directing that a patient may not sign a document or give informed consent for a procedure after being medicated was established to protect the person going to surgery. Persons who have been premedicated for procedures are considered incompetent. However, persons experiencing intractable pain may be incapable of exercising autonomy until after they are medicated and pain free or experiencing pain control.[14]

The responsibility for obtaining informed consent from a patient clearly remains with the physician and cannot be delegated. The courts believe that a physician is in the best position to decide which information should be disclosed for a patient to make an informed choice. The scope of disclosure in any situation is a physician's responsibility. Some states, however, also have legislative standards or state statutes that articulate the information the physician must tell a patient.[2]

Often a third person (a health care provider) is present during the informed consent session because patients are reluctant to question their physicians but will likely question the witness. The witness can then inform the physician about the patient's lack of understanding. The third-party signature is merely an attestation that the informed consent session took place and that the signature on the document is the patient's.[2] The patient must be able to understand the information as presented, and no attempt must be made to influence the decision. General agreement exists that informed consent is an active, shared decision-making process between the health care provider and patient.

Box 2-3   Informed Consent

To give informed consent, the patient must be informed of the following[7]:
1. The nature of the procedure, treatment, or disease
2. The expectations of the recommended treatment and the likelihood of success
3. Reasonable alternatives available and the probable outcome in the absence of treatment
4. The particular known risks that are material to the informed decision about whether to accept or reject medical recommendations

Confidentiality

A struggle exists in medical practice between confidentiality and truthfulness. According to Garrett et al.[3] truthfulness is summarized in two commands: "Do not lie and you must communicate with those who have right to the truth." Truthfulness must not be the only consideration in discussing patients' rights and caregivers' obligations to patients. One of the major restrictions a health care profession imposes is strict confidence of medical and personal information about a patient. This information cannot be revealed without the direct consent of the patient's physician.

Breach of confidence is one of the major problems encountered in providing patient care and can result in legal problems. Information should not be discussed with other department personnel, except in the direct line of duty if it is requested from one ancillary department to another or with nursing service to meet specific medical needs. In the radiation therapy setting, staff members must be especially careful not to discuss patients in hallways or around the treatment area unless the discussion is directly related to the treatment. Staff members should never discuss information with their own families or friends, even in the most general terms, because doing so is a violation of the patient's rights. The patient's treatment chart should be kept in a secure area, inaccessible to anyone not involved in the treatment. Confidentiality issues must be stressed in every educational program at every opportunity.[4]

State laws requires some exceptions to confidentiality. These exceptions may include particular types of wounds, certain communicable diseases, and abuse.[11] Subject to state law, confidentiality may be overridden when the life or safety of the patient is endangered such as when knowledgeable intervention can prevent threatened suicide or self-injury. In addition, the moral obligation to prevent substantial and foreseeable harm to an innocent third party usually is greater than the moral obligation to protect confidentiality.[11]

Roles of Other Health Care Team Members

Patients and families dealing with cancer may be suddenly thrust into a new and potentially threatening world of blood tests, scans, and specialists. A family physician or internist who is familiar with the patient's history and has established a trusting relationship with the patient can be a key member of the cancer-management team. This physician can help the patient and family make appropriate treatment decisions and can act as a liaison between the patient and other people involved in the evaluation and treatment. If a patient does not have a physician to act as an advocate at the time of the cancer diagnosis, a physician should quickly be chosen to serve in this capacity through the course of the illness.[1]

In most situations, other health care professionals are available to help patients cope with the emotional effects of cancer. Nurses who spend much time at a patient's bedside can provide important information to the patient and physician. Social workers are invaluable in assessing the level of a family's psychologic distress and its capacity to cope with the illness.[1] Community resources such as veteran patient programs (e.g., Reach to Recovery) that involve people who have coped with cancer in their own lives can provide valuable information and help reassure patients and their families. The local clergy may be able to provide spiritual guidance based on their knowledge of a particular patient's and family's needs.[1] The responsibilities and **scope of practice** of radiation therapists are shown in Box 2-4.

DYING PATIENTS AND THEIR FAMILIES

Care for the dying patient and family has changed dramatically over the years with improvements in technology. The evolution of terminal care changed curing to caring, beginning with the publication of Dr. Elizabeth Kübler-Ross's book *On Death and Dying*.[6] Because they deal daily with terminally ill patients, radiation therapists and their students must explore questions concerning patients' rights, refusal of treatment, and quality of life and must understand the emotional state of cancer patients. A basic fear of dying is present in all humans. Patients fear the diagnosis, the treatment, the disease, and the death associated with it.[9]

Although the final stage of a terminal illness is obvious, its beginning is less well defined. At some point during the treatment of patients who have metastatic cancer, the focus of management shifts from aggressive therapy to palliative care, from efforts to suppress tumor growth to attempts to control symptoms. Signals that the goals of treatment must be changed include the recognition of the tumor's progression, the failure of therapy to control the disease, the patient's deteriorating strength, and the patient's loss of interest in pursuing previously important objectives and pleasures. Rarely is this decision a difficult one; rather, it reflects the natural acceptance of the inevitability of patients' deaths on the part of families, caregivers, and patients themselves.[1]

Over the past decade, people in many countries have come to accept the notion that aggressive life support (i.e., prolonging life to the bitter end) is frequently not the right action to take. The ethic of allowing terminally ill patients to die with dignity has evolved. In recent years the concept of the individual's right of self-determination has been central in the resuscitation issue. The medical and legal communities have recognized that self-determination is no more than an extension of the patient's right of informed consent. Physicians in the past were placed in an extremely uncomfortable position of wanting to comply with the patient's wishes to die in peace and dignity but fearing a malpractice suit by family members for failing to do all that should, could, or might have been done to resuscitate the dying patient. The response to this dilemma was the living will. The purpose of the living will is to allow the competent adult to direct the course of a possible future medical condition when the individual might no longer be competent by reason of illness. The living will concept assumes that the individual who executes the directive does the following:

Box 2-4	The Scope of Practice for the Radiation Therapist

The American Society of Radiologic Technologists (ASRT) developed and published the scope of practice for the field of radiation therapy. It is imperative that every student therapist and every radiation therapist practicing their profession be knowledgeable regarding the scope of practice. It is the defining document to guide us through our day-to-day responsibilities as radiation therapists caring for our patients.

The structural elements of radiation therapy technology as a health profession in the contemporary health care delivery system in the United States include the following:
- A cognitive base
- A structured curriculum
- A professional credential
- A code of ethics
- Clinical practice autonomy
- Self-governance

The history of these elements combines in a complex structure that can be traced across historical time spans and contemporary functional boundaries. For example, in the history of radiography, radiation therapy was at one time an area of responsibility of the radiographer. This is no longer true today.

Curriculum of the discipline contains elements of physics, psychology, patient care, and pathology, among others, that cross horizontally through several medical specialties. The professional curriculum incorporates didactic and clinical elements and basic sciences that are reflective of contemporary practice in radiation therapy. The content and structural learning experiences facilitate attitudes and skills that prepare graduates to demonstrate a commitment to patient care and continued personal and professional development.

DESCRIPTION OF THE PROFESSION

Radiation therapy is the art and science of treatment delivery to individuals to restore, improve, and enhance performance; diminish or eradicate pathology; facilitate adaptation to the diagnosis of malignant disease; and promote and maintain health. Because the major focus of radiation therapy is the delivery of prescribed dosages of radiation to individuals from external beam and/or brachytherapy radiation sources or hyperthermia units, the radiation therapist's concern is with those factors that influence radiation dose delivery, individual well-being, and responsiveness to treatment, as well as those factors serving as barriers or impediments to treatment delivery.

The practice of radiation therapy is performed by competent radiation therapists who deliver care to the patient in the therapeutic setting and are responsible for the simulation, treatment planning, and administration of a prescribed course of radiation therapy and/or hyperthermia. Additional related settings where radiation therapists practice include education, management, industry, and research.

PROFESSIONAL CREDENTIAL

The initials RT(T) (ARRT) indicate a registered technologist in radiation therapy and certification as a radiation therapist by the American Registry of Radiologic Technologists.

SCOPE OF PRACTICE

The curriculum base for a radiation therapist is that outlined in the ASRT Professional Curriculum for Radiation Therapy. Education program standards are those defined in the Essentials and Guidelines of an Accredited Educational Program for the Radiation Therapist. Radiation therapy professional educational programs prepare the radiation therapist to do the following:
1. Provide radiation therapy services by contributing as an essential member of the radiation oncology treatment team through provision of total quality care of each patient undergoing a prescribed course of treatment
2. Evaluate and assess treatment delivery components
3. Provide radiation therapy treatment delivery services to cure or improve the quality of life of patients by accurately delivering a prescribed course of treatment
4. Evaluate and assess daily the physiologic and psychologic responsiveness of each patient to treatment delivery
5. Maintain values congruent with the profession's code of ethics and scope of practice as well as adhere to national, institutional, and/or departmental standards, policies, and procedures regarding treatment delivery and patient care

DOMAINS OF PRACTICE

Domain: Organizational and work role competencies
1. Coordinate and meet multiple patient needs and requests: set priorities
2. Participate effectively in a therapeutic team approach to provide optimal therapy
3. Adapt to contingency planning in response to variables that influence workload and/or schedule
4. Maintain a flexible stance toward patients, visitors, and staff, as well as technology and bureaucracy
5. Coordinate daily activities so as to devote complete attention to all necessary tasks involved in treatment delivery

continued

Domain: Administering and monitoring radiation therapy treatments

1. Implement and deliver a planned course of treatment
2. Administer treatment accurately and safely: monitor and report untoward effects, reactions, therapeutic responses, and incompatibilities
3. Withhold treatment when conditions warrant and consult with a radiation oncologist before proceeding
4. Participate in total quality management system to ensure safe and accurate patient care
5. Detect equipment malfunctions and take appropriate action
6. Accurately document details of treatment procedures and maintain daily treatment records
7. Apply principles of radiation protection at all times
8. Take appropriate action with regard to real or potential radiation hazards
9. Understand the function of equipment, accessories, treatment methods, and protocols and apply such knowledge appropriately
10. Simulate and plan a course of treatment by defining and identifying tumor volume, target volume, and treatment volume as directed and prescribed by the radiation oncologist
11. Construct and/or prepare immobilization devices, beam directional devices, and the like that facilitate treatment delivery
12. Perform daily and periodic quality assurance checks and related tasks as appropriate
13. Perform dosimetric calculations and treatment planning procedures
14. Monitor doses to normal tissues within the irradiated volume to ensure that tolerance levels are not exceeded
15. Prepare and/or assist in the preparation and use of brachytherapy sources

Domain: caregiving

1. Create a climate for and establish a commitment to healing and/or improving quality of life
2. Provide comfort measures and facilitate the preservation of patient self-image and dignity
3. Serve as a source of support and encouragement for each individual patient and family
4. Provide patient education to maximize patient compliance with the plan of care and provide family education as needed
5. Monitor and interpret patient side effects and/or complications to create a management strategy that fosters prevention, healing, and comfort
6. Monitor the patient's physical and psychologic response to treatment and refer the patient for appropriate management when indicated
7. Detect, document, and report significant changes in patient conditions
8. Understand the particular demands and experiences of a pathologic illness and anticipate related patient care needs
9. Participate in patient follow-up, statistical reporting programs, and clinical research
10. Practice techniques that prevent the spread of disease to provide a safe environment for patients, staff, and self
11. Provide basic patient care
12. Practice basic techniques of venipuncture and the administration of contrast media
13. Prepare patients for procedures to gain desired results and minimize anxiety
14. Work to make culturally avoided aspects of an illness approachable and understandable

Domain: effective management of rapidly changing situations

1. Perform skillfully in extreme, life-threatening emergencies; rapid grasp of a problem; contingency management; rapid matching of demands and resources in emergency situations involving patient or equipment applied in treatment delivery
2. Identify and manage a patient crisis until physician assistance is available
3. Take appropriate action in case of fire or other emergency situations to provide a safe environment for patients, visitors, and staff
4. Assist in the rehabilitation process or the loss of ability to provide self-care as a patient's lifestyle changes

Domain: professionalism

1. Demonstrate respect for confidentiality of medical records and privileged knowledge
2. Demonstrate respect for the Patient's Bill of Rights
3. Share expertise and knowledge with students and others while respecting their needs and rights
4. Pursue appropriate continuing education
5. Apply the profession's code of ethics in all aspects of practice
6. Adhere to any applicable standards, policies, and procedures
7. Refrain from practicing procedures for which appropriate training and/or education has not been obtained

Modified from the American Society of Radiologic Technologists: *The scope of practice for radiation therapists,* Albuquerque, NM, 1993, The American Society of Radiologic Technologists.

1. Demonstrates competency at the time
2. Directs that no artificial or heroic measures be undertaken to preserve the patient's life
3. Requests that medication be provided to relieve pain
4. Intends to relieve the hospital and physician of legal responsibility for complying with the directives in the living will
5. Has the signature witnessed by two disinterested individuals who are not related, are not mentioned in the will, and have no claim on the estate[2]

In practice, actions to carry out a living will may involve withholding or discontinuing interventions such as respirator support, chemotherapy, surgery, and even assisted nutrition and hydration.[8] The decision to withhold curative therapy is based on the conclusion that the course of the patient's disease is irreversible and extraordinary measures to sustain life are not in the patient's best interest. To nullify the routinely mandatory order for cardiopulmonary resuscitation in the event of a cardiac arrest, many hospitals require the physician in charge of a terminal care patient to issue a specific do not resuscitate (DNR) order. Plans for the patient's death, including issuance of the DNR order, should be made soon after the issue has been discussed with the patient and family. In most situations, patients and their families are relieved to know that every effort will be made to maintain the patient's comfort and that the death will be peaceful.[1] All hospitals must have written policies and procedures describing the way that patients' rights are protected at their institutions.

Hospice Care

In the Middle Ages a hospice was a way station for travelers. Today a hospice represents an intermediate station for patients with terminal illnesses. The hospice movement began with programs to provide palliative and supportive care for terminally ill patients and their families. Hospice services include home, respite, and inpatient hospital care and support during bereavement. In addition to providing 24-hour care of the patient, the goal of hospice care is to help the dying patient live a full life and to offer hope, comfort, and a suitable setting for a peaceful, dignified death. The hospice team assists family members in caring for the patient by providing physical, emotional, psychologic, and spiritual support. Several types of hospices are available, including freestanding facilities, institutionally based units, and community-based programs.[1]

Patients may enter the hospice on their own or may be referred by family members, physicians, hospital-affiliated continuing-care coordinators and social workers, visiting nurses, friends, or clergy. Although admission criteria vary, they usually include the following: a terminal illness with an estimated life expectancy of 6 months or less; residence in a defined geographic area; access to a caregiver from immediate family members, relatives, friends, or neighbors; and the desire for the patient to remain at home during the last stage of the illness. On the initial assessment visit a member of the hospice team obtains the patient's medical history and emotional and psychosocial histories of the patient and family and discusses nursing concerns. After the program begins, team members meet regularly to review the care plan for each patient and put into effect and supervise services for the patient and family.[1]

Most families prefer home care for dying relatives if they can rely on the supportive environment offered by a hospice. Institutionalization is perceived as impersonal and impractical, and acute care hospitals are not designed for the long-term care of terminal patients. A private home can be transformed to accommodate the level of care required, and nurses can instruct family members in physical care techniques, symptom management, nutrition, and medications. After the patient and family are made to feel confident and capable of managing the physical care, they can begin to address the emotional and spiritual issues surrounding death. During a patient's terminal illness, many problems arise, some of which test the hospice team's ingenuity and endurance. In general, however, simple remedies, common sense, good nursing care, preventive medicine, and generous use of analgesia should be used to help reduce the suffering of the patient.[1]

MEDICAL-LEGAL ASPECTS OF CANCER MANAGEMENT

Definitions and Terminology

Radiation therapists need to perform their duties with confidence even in today's litigious society. As consumers become more aware of the standards of care that they should receive and more cognizant about seeking legal compensation, health care professionals must become more knowledgeable about legal definitions concerning the standard of care.[7]

The type of law that governs relationships between individuals is known as **civil law.** The type of law that governs rights between individuals in noncriminal actions is called tort law. Torts are not easy to define, but a basic distinction is that they are violations of civil, as opposed to criminal, law. **Tort law** is personal injury law. The act may be malicious and intentional or the result of negligence and disregard for the rights of others. Torts include conditions for which the law allows compensation to be paid an individual damaged or injured by another. The two types of torts are those resulting from intentional actions and those resulting from unintentional acts.[7] Health care providers incur duties incidental to their professional roles. The law does not consider the professional and patient to be on equal terms; greater legal burdens or duties are imposed on the health care provider.[2]

Several situations exist in which a tort action can be taken against the health professional because of deliberate action. Intentional torts include civil assault, civil battery, false imprisonment, libel, slander, and invasion of privacy.

Assault is defined as the threat of touching in an injurious way. If patients feel threatened and believe they will be touched in a harmful manner, justification may exist for a charge of assault. To avoid this, professionals must always explain what is going to happen and reassure the patient in any situation involving the threat of harm.[7]

Battery consists of touching a person without permission. Again, a clear explanation of what is to be done is essential. If the patient refuses to be touched, that wish must be respected. Battery implies that the touch is a willful act to harm or provoke, but even the most well-intentioned touch may fall into this category if the patient has expressly forbid it. This should not prevent the therapist from placing a reassuring hand on the patient's shoulder as long as the patient has not forbidden it and the therapist does not intend to harm or invade the patient's privacy. However, a procedure performed against a patient's will may be construed as battery.[7]

False imprisonment is the intentional confinement without authorization by a person who physically constricts another with force, threat of force, or confining clothing or structures. This becomes an issue if a patient wishes to leave and is not allowed to do so. Inappropriate use of physical restraints may also constitute false imprisonment. The confinement must be intentional and without legal justification. Freedom from unlawful restraint is a right protected by law. If the patient is improperly restrained, the law allows redress in the form of damages for this tort. The proof of all elements of false imprisonment must be established to support the claim that an illegal act was done. If they are dangerous to themselves or others, patients may be restrained. An example of false imprisonment is a therapist using restraints on a patient without informing the family, particularly if a child is involved.[7]

Libel is written defamation of character. Oral defamation is termed **slander.** These torts affect the reputation and good name of a person. The basic element of the tort of defamation is that the oral or written communication is made to a person other than the one defamed. The law recognizes certain relationships that require an individual be allowed to speak without fear of being sued for defamation of character. For example, radiation oncology department supervisors who must evaluate employees or give references regarding an employee's work have a qualified privilege. Radiation therapists can protect themselves from this civil tort by using caution while conversing in the hearing of patients and their families.[7]

Invasion of privacy charges may result if confidentiality of information has not been maintained or the patient's body has been improperly and unnecessarily exposed or touched. Protection of the patient's modesty is vital during simulation, planning, and treatment procedures.[7] Maintaining that privacy is extremely important in regard to video monitors in treatment areas. No one should ever be in the viewing area except necessary staff members.

An unintentional injury to a patient may be negligent. **Negligence** refers to neglect or omission of reasonable care or caution. The standard of reasonable care is based on the doctrine of the reasonably prudent person. This standard requires that a person perform as any reasonable individual of ordinary prudence with comparable education and skill and under similar circumstances. In the relationship between a professional person and a patient an implied contract exists to provide reasonable care. An act of negligence in the context of such a relationship is called malpractice. Negligence, as used in malpractice law, is not necessarily the same as carelessness. A person's conduct can be considered negligent in the legal sense if the individual acts carefully. For example, if a therapist without prior education attempts a procedure and does it carefully, the conduct can be deemed negligent if harm results to the patient.[7]

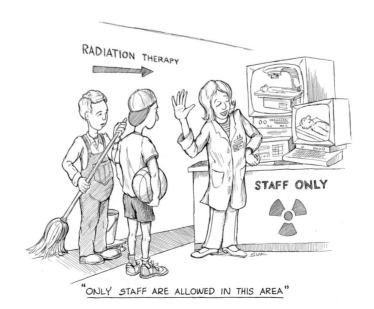

"ONLY STAFF ARE ALLOWED IN THIS AREA"

LEGAL DOCTRINES

Doctrine of Personal Liability

Radiation therapists should be concerned about the risk of being named as defendants in medical malpractice suits. Things can go wrong, and mistakes can be made. The legal responsibility of the radiation therapist is to give safe care to the patient.

The fundamental rule of law is that persons are liable for their own negligent conduct. This is known as the **doctrine of personal liability** and means that the law does not permit wrongdoers to avoid legal liability for their own actions even though someone else may also be sued and held legally liable for the wrongful conduct in question under another rule of law. Although they cannot be held liable for actions of hospitals or physicians, therapists can be held responsible and liable for their own negligent actions.[7]

Doctrine of Respondeat Superior

The **doctrine of respondeat superior** ("let the master answer") is a legal doctrine that holds an employer liable for negligent acts of employees that occur while they are carrying out orders or serving the interests of the employer. As early as 1698, courts declared that a master must respond to injuries and losses of persons caused by the master's servants. Nineteenth-century courts adopted the phrase *respondeat superior,* which is founded on the principle of social duty that all persons, whether by themselves or by their agents or servants, shall conduct their affairs in a manner not to injure others.[7] This principle is based on the concept that profit from others' work and the duty to select and supervise employees are joined in liability.[2]

Doctrine of Res Ipsa Loquitur

In a malpractice action for negligence the plaintiff has the burden of proving that a standard of care exists for the treatment of the medical problem, the health care provider failed to abide by the standard, this failure was the direct cause of the patient's injury, and damage was incurred. If the alleged negligence involves matters outside general knowledge, an acceptable medical expert must establish these criteria. A long-accepted substitute for the medical expert has been the **doctrine of res ipsa loquitur,**[4] which means "the thing speaks for itself." Courts have decided to resolve the problem of expert unavailability in certain circumstances by applying res ipsa loquitur, which requires the defendant to explain the events and convince the court that no negligence was involved.[2]

Doctrine of Foreseeability

The **doctrine of foreseeability** is a principle of law that holds an individual liable for all natural and proximate consequences of negligent acts to another individual to whom a duty is owed. The negligent acts could or should have been reasonably foreseen under the circumstances. A simple definition is persons reasonably foreseeing that certain actions or inactions on their part could result in injury to others. In addition, the injury suffered must be related to the foreseeable injury. Routine radiation therapy equipment checks are important in overcoming this doctrine.[7]

RISK MANAGEMENT

Conceived little more that a decade ago, the concept of risk control, or **risk management,** was believed to be the key element in loss prevention from adverse medical incidents. Risk management links every quality-improvement program with measurable outcomes necessary to determine overall effectiveness. Effectiveness here means success in reducing patient injury. An acute-care hospital or medical center has the duty to exercise such reasonable care in looking after and protecting the patient. The legal responsibility of any health care practitioner is safe care. Risk management, which is a matter of patient safety, is the process of avoiding or controlling the risk of financial loss to staff members and the hospital or medical center. Poor-quality care creates a risk of injury to patients and leads to increased financial liability. Risk management protects financial assets by managing insurance for potential liability by reducing liability through surveillance. It identifies actual and potential causes of patient accidents and implements programs to eliminate or reduce these occurrences.[7]

Hospital liability and malpractice insurance, also known as *patient liability insurance,* is intended to cover all claims against the hospital that arise from the alleged negligence of physician staff members and employees. Many have discussed whether radiation therapists should carry malpractice insurance. In making that decision, persons must determine the extent of provisions for malpractice coverage in their institutions. According to the doctrine of respondeat superior, the employer is liable for employees' negligent acts during work. The authority and responsibility of a physician supervising and controlling the activities of the employee supersede those of the employer according to the doctrine of the borrowed servant. Regardless of the way these legal doctrines may be applied, the fundamental rule of law that every therapist should clearly know and understand is the doctrine of personal liability; persons are liable for their own negligent conduct. A wrongdoer is not allowed to escape responsibility even though someone else may be sued and held legally responsible. In some situations, hospital insurers who paid malpractice claims have successfully recovered damages from negligent employees by filing separate lawsuits against them.[7]

Hospital employees are instructed to report any patient injury to administration through the department manager. An incident report is routinely used to document unusual events in the hospital. An **incident** is defined as any happening that is not consistent with the routine operation of the hospital or the routine care of a particular patient. It may be an accident or a situation that could result in an accident.[11] Hospitals use

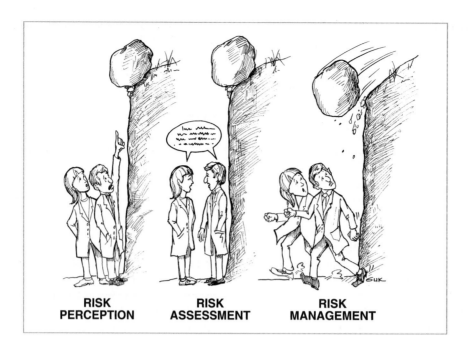

RISK PERCEPTION   **RISK ASSESSMENT**   **RISK MANAGEMENT**

incident reports in their accident-prevention programs to advise insurers of potential suits and prepare defenses against suits that might arise from documented incidents. Incident reports should be prepared according to the institution's published policies and procedures. An incident report is no place for opinion, accusation, or conjecture; it should contain only facts concerning the incident reported.[2]

MEDICAL RECORDS

The radiation oncology **medical record** is used to document chronologically the care and treatment rendered the patient. All components of the patient's evaluation and cancer must be documented in the radiation oncology record. The format usually includes the following: a general information sheet listing the names of pertinent relatives, follow-up contacts, family physicians, and persons to notify in an emergency; an initial history and findings from the physical examination; reports of the pathology examinations, laboratory tests, diagnostic imaging studies, and pertinent surgical procedures; photographs and anatomic drawings; medications currently used; correspondence with physicians and reimbursement organizations; treatment set-up instructions; daily treatment logs; physics, treatment planning, and dosimetry data; progress notes during treatments; summaries of treatment; and reports of follow-up examinations. These radiation oncology records must be maintained and secured in the department separate from hospital and clinic records to ensure ready access at any time.[5] Radiation oncology medical records are commonly maintained in both paper and electronic formats. Medical record entries should be made in clear and concise language that can be under-

stood by all professional staff members attending the patient. Handwritten entries must be legible. An illegible record is worse than no record because it documents a failure by staff members to maintain a proper record and may severely weaken a hospital's or physician's defense in a negligence action. Entries into the paper record should be typed or made in ink, and persons making entries should identify themselves clearly by placing their signatures after each entry. The hospital and physician should be able to determine who participates in each episode of patient care.[2] Entries should be made daily by the therapist operating the treatment machine. Any other therapist involved in that day's treatment of a patient should also check the entry for accuracy and initial the record.

Medical records are sometimes used by staff members to convey remarks inappropriate for a patient's chart. The following are examples of entries that should never be made:
- This is the third time therapist X has been negligent.
- Dr. A has mistreated this patient again.
- This patient is a chronic complainer and a nuisance.

Such editorial comments are inevitably used against the physician and hospital in any negligence action filed by the patient. In addition, as the trend moves toward access by patients to their own medical records, patients are more likely to read and react with hostility to such comments.[2]

The general rule is to avoid the need for making corrections, but because humans are not perfect, corrections must be made from time to time. In the paper record, a staff member should simply draw a line through an incorrect entry because doing so leaves no doubt about which item has been corrected. The staff member should initial the correction, enter the time and date, and insert the correct information.

Mistakes in the chart should not be erased because doing so may create suspicion concerning the original entry.[2]

Radiation therapists under the direct supervision of the radiation oncologist and medical physicist carry out daily treatments. All treatment applications must be described in detail (orders) and signed by the responsible physician. Likewise, any changes in the planned treatment by the physician may require adjustment in immobilization, new calculations, and even a new treatment plan. Therefore the therapist, physicist, and dosimetrist must be notified.[5]

SUMMARY

In addition to the development of technical knowledge and skills, the foundation of radiation oncology includes standards of conduct and ideals essential to meeting emotional and physical needs of patients. Radiation therapists must first view their profession as more than a job. Student therapists should not pursue a simple goal to just pass a series of examinations and eventually the registry or earn a degree. Student therapists should set goals establish them as professionals. An ideal professional has superior technical knowledge and works in harmony and cooperation with peers, physicians, and other health care personnel. With the appropriate educational background and determination to excel, a person can practice professionalism and achieve technical excellence. The patient, health care system, and therapist benefit, and the result is a large number of individuals working together to achieve the best possible treatment and care for their patients.[4]

CASE STUDIES

Case I

As a student therapist, Susan observes many clinical situations. She is assigned to a treatment area that has an extremely high volume of patients. Susan observes that a staff member has treated a patient without an important treatment device in place. When she approaches the staff member about the situation, he mumbles something about the patient being palliative. Obviously the treatment error must be corrected. How does Susan ethically and professionally handle this issue that her conscience dictates be addressed? Is this an ethical or legal issue?

Case II

Sam is a staff radiation therapist in a large center. He has a patient on his treatment schedule that is uncooperative and verbally abusive to the staff members. It is time for the patient's treatment, but once in the treatment room he is refusing to cooperate by getting into the position required and holding still. Sam knows the patient is uncomfortable and needs the treatment to relieve symptomatic disease. Should Sam restrain the patient and force him to have the treatment? What legal and ethical considerations are involved in Sam's final decision?

Case III

Mrs. Smith is a 50-year-old mother with three adult children. She has been admitted to the hospital for tests to rule out cancer. While the tests are being processed, her husband and children meet with the doctor and ask him not to tell Mrs. Smith if the results are malignant. They tell him that she is afraid of cancer and that if she is given the diagnosis, she will become severely depressed and give up all desire to live. The physician is not comfortable with this request, but the family insists. The physician reluctantly agrees. What ethical and legal concepts are implicated in the family's request and physician's decision to comply with it?

Case IV

Currently employed in a small radiation oncology center, Sandra has the task of orienting a new employee to the department and the treatment machine to which she is assigned. The new therapist, although older than Sandra, is newly graduated from an educational program and has recently taken the American Registry of Radiologic Technologists examination for Radiation Therapy. She has not yet received her credentials but is certainly qualified to begin her position in the department. In the course of working with Jane, Sandra begins to realize that there are some physical limitations for Jane. She has freely shared that she has a degenerative problem with her hands and has some loss of strength. When Sandra begins to make some suggestions for modifying the handling of the custom blocks and other heavy treatment devices over the patient lying on the table, Jane becomes extremely defensive. Sandra is aware that the safety of her patients is at risk and she must take some action. Discuss what that action might be and whether this might be an ethical or a legal situation.

Case V

A new patient is scheduled to start treatment on Jim's treatment machine on Monday. Everyone has warned him that the new patient is very angry and very difficult to schedule procedures with. He meets Mrs. Jones on Monday morning, greets her warmly, and does all that he can to put her at ease during the long process of starting her treatments. When the time comes for him to discuss her appointments, Mrs. Jones insists that she needs different appointment times daily. Jim carefully explains that they cannot accommodate quite that many changes in the schedule for the 7 weeks that she will be with them. Jim and Mrs. Jones reach an agreement that seems to satisfy them both. For the next several weeks Mrs. Jones arrives at a different time every day. Sometimes she calls to reschedule; sometimes she just comes in to the department. Jim and the other therapist he works with try very hard to accommodate their patient, but it is causing havoc with the rest of their schedule and inconveniencing most of their other patients. Jim approaches Mrs. Jones with the question of whether another appointment time would be better for her. Mrs. Jones quickly becomes verbally abusive, screaming that she wishes she had gone elsewhere for treatment. She shouts that she doesn't want to talk about this anymore and she is tired of being chastised every time she is 5 minutes late. Because this is the first time Jim or his partner has mentioned her tardiness, they are surprised at her reaction. Discuss how they should handle the situation. Consider whether or not they will be able to discuss this with Mrs. Jones or refer her to a supervisor, because she is so convinced that she has been harassed about her appointments since the beginning. What kind of legal or ethical issues does this case history contain?

Review Questions

Multiple Choice

1. Which of the following does not govern ethics?
   a. Professional codes
   b. Popular science
   c. Patient's Bill of Rights
   d. Technical practice
2. Which of the following rights does legal ethics include?
   a. Life
   b. Liberty
   c. Medical care
   d. All of the above
3. Moral ethics are based on which of the following?
   a. Right and wrong
   b. Institutions
   c. Legal rights
   d. Codes
4. Which of the following is an ethical characteristic?
   a. Justice
   b. Individual freedom
   c. Egoism
   d. Confidentiality
5. Professional ethics deals with personal character and which of the following factors that identifies professionals as caring and capable persons?
   a. Professional expertise
   b. Chosen profession
   c. Moral character
   d. All of the above
6. Confidentiality, truth telling, and benevolence are which of the following?
   a. Ethical principles
   b. Legal rights
   c. Ethical characteristics
   d. Legal doctrines
7. A tort falls under which of the following?
   a. Criminal law
   b. Statutory law
   c. Civil law
   d. Common law
8. *Res ipsa loquitur* means which of the following?
   a. Things speak for themselves
   b. The thing speaks for itself
   c. Do no harm
   d. The things speak for themselves
9. Which ethical theory group evaluates an activity by weighing the good against the bad?
   a. Deontology
   b. Consequentialism
   c. Virtue ethics
   d. Moral ethics
10. Which ethical model identifies the caregiver as a scientist dealing only with the facts and does not consider the human aspect of the patient?
    a. Engineering
    b. Priestly
    c. Covenant
    d. Collegial

Questions to Ponder

1. What does deontology emphasize?
2. Discuss the difference between legal and ethical, and describe a situation in which the two may be in conflict.
3. Discuss and compare the analytical and covenant models of ethical decision making. Discuss the way these models may be used in your profession and by whom.
4. What components are involved in ethical decision making for the radiation therapist?
5. Discuss the required elements that make up an informed consent.
6. Explain the purpose of the scope of practice as it pertains to your performance as a radiation therapist.
7. Compare and discuss the different settings available in hospice care.
8. Discuss the differences in assault and battery. What kind of action can be taken in response to either of these?
9. Analyze the difference between negligence and carelessness. Can careful behavior still result in a charge of negligence? Describe such an instance.
10. Explain the purpose of a medical record, and note the components of a complete radiation oncology record.

REFERENCES
1. American Cancer Society, Massachusetts Division: *Cancer manual,* ed 8, Boston, 1990, The American Cancer Society.
2. American College of Legal Medicine: *Legal medicine,* ed 5, St. Louis, 2001, Mosby.
3. Garrett T, Baillie HW, Garrett R: *Healthcare ethics: principles and problems,* ed 4, Englewood Cliffs, NJ, 2001, Prentice Hall.
4. Gurley LT, Callaway WJ: *Introduction to radiologic technology,* ed 4, St. Louis, 1996, Mosby.
5. Inter-Society Council for Radiation Oncology: *Radiation oncology in integrated cancer management, United States,* Philadelphia, 1991, The Inter-Society Council for Radiation Oncology.
6. Kübler-Ross E: *On death and dying,* New York, 1969, Macmillan.
7. Parelli RJ: *Medicolegal issues for radiographers,* ed 2, Dubuque, Iowa, 1994, Eastwind.
8. Roy DJ: Ethical issues in the treatment of cancer patients, *Bull World Health Organ* 67:341-346, 1989.
9. Slaby AE, Glicksman AS: *Adapting to life threatening illness,* New York, 1985, Praeger.
10. Smith DH, McCarty K: In the care of cancer patients, *Primary Care Cancer* 19:26-27, 822, 1992.
11. Towsley D, Cunningham E: *Biomedical ethics for radiographers,* Dubuque, Iowa, 1994, Eastwind.

12. Warner S: Code of ethics: professional and legal implications, *Radiol Technol* 52:485-494, 1981.
13. *Webster's new collegiate dictionary,* Springfield, Mass, 1976, G & C Merriam.
14. Winter G, Glass E, Sakurai C: Ethical issues in oncology nursing practice: an overview of topics and strategies, *Oncol Nurs Forum* 20:21-34, 1993.
15. Wright R: *Human values in health care: the practice of ethics,* New York, 1987, McGraw-Hill.

3

Principles of Pathology

Patricia J. Giordano

Outline

Key Terms

Cell cycle
Chromosomes
Cytoplasm
Endoplasmic reticulum
Genome
Golgi apparatus
Lysosomes
Mitochondria
Nuclear membrane
Nucleoli
Nucleotide

Nucleus
Oncogene
Organelle
Peroxisomes
Polypeptides
Proteins
Ribosome
Transcription
Translation
Tumor-suppressor gene
Vacuoles

Pathology is the branch of medicine devoted to the study and understanding of disease. More precisely, the discipline seeks to understand the effect of disease on the function of the human organism at all levels and relate functional alterations to changes perceived at the gross anatomic, cellular, and subcellular levels. This chapter considers briefly the history and evolution of the pathology of cancer,[1,3] discusses the cellular theory of disease, and examines the physiology of the neoplastic process. In addition, some of the practical aspects of establishing a pathologic diagnosis and using that information to classify and treat cancer are considered. Finally, this chapter provides an overview of subcellular molecular biology and its emerging effect on cancer.

Although the theory of disease and methods by which disease processes are studied have changed dramatically, humans have pursued these issues one way or another for well over 2000 years. As time passed, perceptions slowly changed. During the Middle Ages, semiscientific observations continued to be made and recorded, but evolution of the theory of disease was stagnant, and treatment was based mostly on superstition or witchcraft. Prevailing theory and recorded observations were not considered at odds until the sixteenth and seventeenth centuries. After these contradictions were recognized and old ideas challenged, the understanding of disease began to move rapidly forward assisted by new technology that opened unimaginable frontiers.

The introduction of the microscope in the early seventeenth century made possible the observation of unicellular human anatomy, thus propelling pathology from its infancy into its childhood. This also made possible correlations between clinical manifestations of disease and gross anatomic findings and between gross pathology and microscopic observations. These correlations were further developed and refined during the eighteenth and nineteenth centuries as physicians began to comprehend the roles individual organs played in the expression of illness and began to introduce new theories of disease and refine old ones. Practical application of these theories resulted in the development of the first scientifically sophisticated treatment of many diseases. A logarithmic growth has taken place in the twentieth century in medical technology and understanding of disease processes.

Since 1970, another great advancement has been made to understand more completely the physiology of disease. This movement into an unfamiliar and even smaller microcosm has revealed the world of molecular biology, in which disease may be studied at a subcellular level not previously appreciated. This advancement, which has permitted study and observation of function at the molecular level, is at least as great as the development in the seventeenth century that refocused observations from the gross anatomic to the cellular level. The rate at which knowledge is expanding in molecular biology is so fast that only a regular review of the current scientific literature on the subject can provide up-to-date information. This chapter offers an overview of molecular biology and related enterprises to help the student or practitioner of radiation therapy understand vistas that lie ahead.

CELLS AND THE NATURE OF DISEASE

Every clinical disease has its inception with some kind of cellular injury or malfunction that ultimately is expressed at the molecular level of cellular function. To understand this chapter, the reader should be familiar with basic principles of elementary mammalian biology. A general understanding of the structure and function of the mammalian cell, including the several organelles (nucleus, endoplasmic reticulum, ribosomes, Golgi apparatus, mitochondria, lysosomes, peroxisomes, and vacuoles) and plasma membrane, is particularly important. Details of cellular form and function may be obtained from any modern textbook of general biology.

Cells differ greatly concerning functions they perform; however, they have certain characteristics in common. All cells share the ability to produce energy and maintain themselves in a state of normal function by elaborating a vast array of proteins and macromolecules that facilitate adaptation to physiologic or pathologic stress. As long as cells can maintain themselves in the range of normal function, they exist in a state of homeostasis. The homeostatic state represents a set of circumstances in which cellular processes associated with life proceed normally and in accordance with the function genetically assigned to that cell. In a typical cell, these functions include processes that provide nutrition, protection, communication, and sometimes mobility and reproduction. All these processes are facilitated by the hundreds of macromolecules produced by each cell. Under prolonged or acute physiologic stress, this homeostasis may be maintained

only with great difficulty. When a cell's adaptive mechanisms fail, changes in cellular structure become identifiable and a pathologic or disease state ensues.

Changes in cellular structure can usually be seen under the microscope and may be broadly divided into two categories: irreversible and reversible. Irreversible changes represent cellular death or changes that eventually prove lethal to the cell. Changes representing reversible injury are consistent with cell survival if the precipitating cause is corrected. Dead cells are recognized under the microscope because enzymes begin to destroy them. These enzymes may be derived from the dead cell itself, or they may originate in other scavenging cells such as macrophages. Enzymatic action obliterates cellular detail. Irreversible changes signaling incipient cell death appear as a series of color alterations in typical cellular staining patterns and irregularities in the structure of the cell's nucleus. The nucleus under such circumstances may become fragmented, shriveled, or enzymatically destroyed. The changes of reversible cell damage may be subtler. They arise from internal loss of power caused by respiratory embarrassment. Cellular swelling is the hallmark of reversible damage and occurs as the damaged cellular membrane fails to regulate properly the concentration of sodium in the cell. As a consequence, water passes across the membrane to produce swelling. Swelling is followed by morphologic changes in the intracellular organelles and a decrease in the pH of the cell that can be identified by the application of special cellular stains. The radiation therapist must recognize that all these changes, whether reversible or irreversible, may occur in malignant and normal cells.

Inflammation

These changes in cellular form and function that represent a departure from homeostasis do not occur in a vacuum. They occur instead in the context of the aggregate physiology of the organism and therefore are subject to monitoring and response. In broad terms the monitoring of and response to tissue damage is called the inflammatory reaction.[9,11] Its clinical features have been known since antiquity and described as rubor, calor, tumor, and dolor (i.e., redness, warmth, swelling, and pain). Although the clinical syndrome has not changed since Celsius described these cardinal features in the first century AD, much more is known about its purpose and physiology.

The inflammatory response is a complex, immunochemical reaction initiated by normal cells that have been injured or damaged. It has implications for the defense of the organism and repair of the injury or damage that initially provoked the reaction. The reaction may be intense or subdued depending on the magnitude and nature of the precipitating stimulus. If the reaction evolves completely over a few hours or days, it is acute. If it persists for longer periods, it is chronic. In either situation, the features of the reaction account for the well-known cardinal signs.

Inflammation begins as local vascular dilatation that

permits an increase in blood flow to the affected tissue. The increase in blood flow accounts not only for the redness and warmth that accompany inflammation but also for increases in intravascular pressure and permeability of the vascular membrane. These changes in pressure and permeability expedite the escape of fluid into the interstitial space to produce swelling. This interstitial fluid, which escapes through gaps between the endothelial cells lining small veins, is mostly water-rich in proteins, polypeptides, and other low-molecular-weight substances called inflammatory mediators or cytokines. These latter substances, thought to be byproducts of tissue injury, seem to play a role in nerve stimulation and pain production.

Many white blood cells, mostly neutrophils, and other phagocytes, escape the vascular compartment with this fluid. These cells destroy bacteria and other microorganisms, neutralize toxins, and enzymatically destroy dead or dying tissue. When this phagocytic response accomplishes its physiologic objectives, it promotes the ingrowth of new capillaries and fibroblasts, which in turn facilitate tissue repair and a return to homeostasis. Tissue damage or injury initiates the cascade of events that constitute the inflammatory response. Without such an initiator, inflammation does not occur.

Many agents cause tissue damage leading to an inflammatory response. Among the most common agents are hypoxia, microbial infections, ionizing radiation, chemicals, allergic or immune reactions, and cancer.

The most common cause of tissue damage is hypoxia. Oxygen deprivation renders a living cell incapable of manufacturing energy. When insufficient energy is present to sustain the cell, intracellular organelles fail, the integrity of the cellular membrane is lost, and death results. Local hypoxia commonly results from vascular occlusive disease and trauma. Vascular occlusive disease is classically seen in acute myocardial infarction. Trauma is present, for example, in skin flap necrosis secondary to vascular damage at the time of a radical mastectomy. The radiation therapist sees generalized hypoxia as a result of cardiorespiratory compromise secondary to acute compression of the superior vena cava caused by lung cancer. If not promptly corrected, hypoxia of this magnitude results in death rather than localized tissue destruction and an ensuing inflammatory reaction. Similarly, other causes of generalized hypoxia such as carbon monoxide or cyanide poisoning, which prevent oxygen transport or use at the cellular level, do not involve inflammation.

Infections produced by bacteria and other microbes represent the most widely recognized cause of inflammation and commonly occur in patients undergoing radiation therapy. The many mechanisms of injury produced by microorganisms are complex and beyond the scope of this discussion; however, the bacterial cellulitis produced by minor injury to the edematous arm of a breast cancer patient who has undergone a radical mastectomy, an axillary lymph node dissection, and radiation therapy is often dramatic. Such an infection is frequently accompanied by all the cardinal signs of inflammation.

For the radiation therapist the most obvious and frequently seen cause of tissue damage is ionizing radiation. Radiation is an agent of tissue damage used medically in a sophisticated fashion to achieve carefully delineated objectives. The primary objective is to lethally damage all cancer cells in a predefined volume of tissue, thus rendering the surviving normal tissue free of neoplastic disease. In pursuit of this objective, some damage is inevitably inflicted on normal tissues incorporated in the radiation portal. Such damage, whether to normal or neoplastic tissue, elicits an inflammatory response. In patients undergoing radiation therapy, this response may be intense and easily identified. More often it is subtle or in deep tissues and not obvious.

Tissue Damage

Tissue damage produced by the use of chemicals or drugs is frequently encountered clinically. The list of agents responsible for such damage is long, and the mechanisms of injury are numerous. As with ionizing radiation, the judicious administration of certain chemotherapeutic agents may result in tissue destruction, thus having a tangible benefit for the patient. Chemical damage to superficial tissue may be observed after inadvertent extravascular extravasation of some chemotherapeutic agents. These extravasations provoke an intense local inflammatory response. Moreover, the application of some dermatologic agents to the skin of patients undergoing radiation therapy may contribute to an easily seen inflammatory reaction in and beyond the radiation portal.

Immune reactions protect the host organism from biologic agents. These agents or antigens may be encountered in the external environment of the host or generated less frequently internally. Under normal circumstances the intensity of the reaction confirms it to be a powerful mechanism of protection and tissue repair. Nevertheless, the reaction is often cytolytic and results in tissue damage. The normal immune reaction is subject to complex physiologic monitoring and control that promote the reaction's resolution when it is no longer a benefit to the host. Sometimes, however, when the reaction is caused by the presence of internally produced antigens, it can be a force that is destructive rather than beneficial to the organism.

A final and perhaps less obvious cause of tissue damage is neoplastic growth. One of the hallmarks of malignant tumors is local invasion and destruction of normal tissue. This destruction is accompanied by an inflammatory reaction that is usually of low intensity but microscopically identifiable. Occasionally the classical signs of inflammation may be encountered in clinical malignancies. Inflammatory breast cancer typically exhibits to a striking degree the four cardinal signs of inflammation but is unaccompanied at the microscopic level by typical inflammatory cells, thus emphasizing once more the role of tissue damage rather than macrophages in provoking the inflammatory response.

The six important causes of cell damage (radiation, hypoxia, chemicals, microorganisms, immunologic reactions, and neoplasms) often share a final common pathway in the production of their damage. This pathway leads to the formation of free radicals, which are highly reactive molecular species that are usually intermediary products of oxygen metabolism. Free radicals, which may be produced directly by agents such as ionizing radiation or indirectly by enzymatic reactions in tissue, are destructive to nucleic acids and other vital cellular components.

THE PATHOLOGY OF NEOPLASMS

Neoplastic Diseases

Of the diseases that afflict mankind, cancer is of major importance. In the United States, it claims more lives than any disorder except cardiovascular disease. Furthermore, it is the primary disease with which radiation therapists deal. Accordingly, an understanding of the pathology of neoplastic disease is vital to therapists in the performance of their jobs and in their quests for professional maturity.

The term *cancer* applies to many different disease processes that seem to share some common characteristics. In fact, over 100 types of cancer have been recognized and categorized.

The term *neoplasia* (meaning "new growth") applies to an abnormal process resulting in the formation of a neoplasm or tumor. In the neoplastic process, this new growth occurs beyond the limits of the normal growth pattern. The distinction between normal and neoplastic growth is usually though not always well defined and easily recognizable. Therefore the process of neoplasia can be appreciated as one of disordered growth.

For the patient the first and most important distinction between benign and malignant tumors involves the prognosis. Benign neoplasms seldom pose any threat to the host, even if left untreated. Several glaring inconsistencies notwithstanding, benign tumors usually carry descriptive names that end simply with -*oma*. These tumors tend to grow slowly and be composed of cells often appearing similar to the normal cells from which they arise. The size of benign tumors may persistently increase or inexplicably halt at a certain point. A benign tumor is usually surrounded by a distinct capsule of fibrous tissue that facilitates surgical removal if treatment is necessary. Although often large, these tumors do not invade surrounding tissue to produce direct destruction nor do they spread distantly to produce metastases.

However, characteristics of malignant tumors, which as a class are referred to as cancers, are much different. Cancers generally pose a serious if not fatal threat to the host. Therefore they are seldom left untreated after discovery. This class of tumors has two large subcategories (carcinoma and sarcoma) that designate the tissue of tumor origin. Cancers tend to grow rapidly, doubling in size over periods ranging from a few days to several months. They are composed of cells with microscopic characteristics decidedly different from normal cells that make up the tissue of origin. In fact, cancers may be so bizarre that they bear little if any resemblance to these cells. As cellular detail becomes more bizarre the cell is said to be poorly differentiated compared with tumor cells more closely resembling the cells of origin, which are said to be well differentiated. Growth is incessant and proceeds with invasion and destruction of nearby tissues. The speed of growth correlates roughly with the differentiation of the cells (i.e., well-differentiated cancers tend to grow more slowly than poorly differentiated ones). A true limiting fibrous capsule of the type in benign tumors is lacking. Distant spread, or metastasis, of the cancer results from malignant cells gaining access to blood and lymphatic channels. Not all such cells survive to colonize distant tissues. The metastatic process is only partially understood but clearly more complex than the passive transport of cancer cells through nearby lymphatics or veins. Most cells gaining access to vascular channels never produce viable deposits of tumor cells in regional lymph nodes or more distant tissues. Instead, they are immunologically destroyed by internal surveillance mechanisms. Cancer cells arising in certain organs have a predilection for metastases to specific sites (i.e., cancers of the prostate and breast have a tendency to metastasize to bone). This specific metastatic potential is influenced by the biochemical interaction between proteins and polypeptides produced by both the tumor cells and the cells' populating sites of potential colonization. (See Table 3-1 for a comparison of characteristics of benign and malignant tumors.)

Because benign tumors often require no treatment and have few radiotherapeutic implications, this chapter does not consider further their pathologic characteristics. Instead, subsequent attention is given to cancers, and their pathologic implications are considered from several points of view.

The term *cancer* in common usage applies to the entire spectrum of malignant neoplastic processes. Cancers are

Table 3-1	Characteristics of benign and malignant tumors	
Characteristic	**Benign**	**Malignant**
Growth rate	Slow	Rapid
Mitoses	Few	Many
Nuclear chromatin	Normal	Increased
Differentiation	Good	Poor
Local growth	Expansive	Invasive
Encapsulation	Present	Absent
Destruction of tissue	Little	Much
Vessel invasion	None	Frequent
Metastases	None	Frequent
Effect on host	Often insignificant	Significant

From Damjanov I, Linder J: *Anderson's pathology,* ed 10, St. Louis, 1995, Mosby.

broadly divided into carcinomas and sarcomas. The term *carcinoma* refers to a malignant tumor taking its origin from epithelial cells, which are widespread and generally considered to be cells that line surfaces. As such, epithelial cells cover most external surfaces, line most cavities, and form glands. From a functional standpoint therefore epithelial cells are protective, absorptive, or secretory. Because they are so widely distributed and metabolically active, epithelial cells give rise to a wide variety of tumor types that comprise most solid tumors encountered in clinical practice. Carcinomas tend to invade lymphatic channels more often than blood vessels; therefore metastases are frequently found in lymph nodes. The designation of carcinoma by the pathologist may be modified by a preceding phrase or prefix further identifying the tissue of origin. For example, a cancer arising from cells lining the upper air and food passages may be designated a squamous cell carcinoma to identify further the nature of the epithelial surface from which the cancer arose. Similarly, a cancer with its origin internally in an organ such as the pancreas (for which surfaces are difficult to imagine) is designated an adenocarcinoma to indicate origin from the secretory epithelium that lines the individual pancreatic glands.

In contrast, the term *sarcoma* describes a neoplasm arising from cells other than those forming epithelial surfaces. From a practical point of view, these cells reside in connective tissue or the nervous system. Although such cells constitute the majority of the body by weight, they spawn relatively few malignant neoplasms. Sarcomas tend to metastasize via blood vessel invasion. This accounts for the frequent appearance of metastatic sarcoma in the lungs. Sarcomas may also carry a pathologic prefix designating more precisely the tissue of tumor origin. For example, a malignant tumor arising in bone is termed an osteosarcoma, one arising in cartilage is termed a chondrosarcoma, and one originating from fat cells is termed a liposarcoma (see Table 3-2 for comprehensive nomenclature).

In describing carcinomas or sarcomas the pathologist provides additional commentary about the nature of the neoplasm. This commentary is designed to provide guidance in prognostication and treatment. In gross anatomic pathology, commentary is made about the size of the cancer and its apparent extent in tissues received from the surgeon. For example, a cancer of the kidney may be noted to have invaded the renal vein, a portion or all of which has been submitted to the pathologist along with the cancer. Comorbid changes in surrounding normal tissues such as abscess formations that might accompany perforated cancers of the colon are noted.

After examination under the microscope, cancer cells that exhibit no differentiation are called *anaplastic*. Similarly, the term *pleomorphic* describes the great variability in size and shape of these undifferentiated tumor cells. Nuclear abnormalities in cancer cells occur regularly. The nuclei of cancer cells may be assigned designations such as hyperchromatic, clumped, undergoing mitoses, and containing prominent nucleoli. These designations suggest circumstances that reflect malignant degeneration of cells.

Etiology

With so much descriptive terminology, it is perhaps surprising that so little is known about the causes of cancer. That unfortunate set of circumstances is, however, in rapid transition as a result of many advances in molecular biology. Nonetheless, the causes of cancer as presently understood are physiologically naive, incomplete, and more associative than precise. For example, some cancers are associated with exposure to certain chemicals such as those in tobacco smoke. Other cancers are associated with exposure to ionizing radiation in small-to-moderate doses. Still others are associated with viral infections. These associations are useful in describing possible risk factors in the environment, but they remain imprecise in elucidating molecular mechanics of carcinogenesis that allow useful therapeutic intervention.

Chemical carcinogenesis has been accepted as a clinical reality for many decades and was first suggested over 200 years ago.[4,10] In the mid-eighteenth century in England, Percivall Pott noted an association between scrotum cancer and the work done by chimney sweeps. In the early part of the twentieth century, this association between cancer and products of hydrocarbon combustion was confirmed in Japan by Yamagiwa and Ichikawa, who were able to induce cancers in the skin of laboratory animals by the chronic application of coal tar. Since that time, hundreds of chemicals that play roles in cancer induction have been identified and isolated.

Chemical carcinogenesis is not a simple process that proceeds in a linear fashion from point A to point B. Instead, it is a complex process in which interplay with other mechanisms of cancer induction is likely if not probable. The rate and intensity of these processes varies from one tumor system to the next. Chemical carcinogens are mutagens (i.e., they can cause unusual changes in the deoxyribonucleic acid [DNA] of cells they attack). Most chemical carcinogens are compounds containing atoms deficient in electrons and therefore chemically active in the relatively electron-rich milieu that characterizes ribonucleic acid (RNA), DNA, and their products. Many of these chemicals occur naturally, but some are synthetic. Most of them require metabolic activation to assume their carcinogenic statures. Their action is thus somewhat indirect compared with a few compounds such as chemotherapeutic alkylating agents that can directly induce neoplasia. The number of chemical carcinogens is great. Some of the more important ones include polycyclic hydrocarbons produced by the combustion of fossil fuels and tobacco, alcohol, asbestos, nickel compounds, vinyl chloride, and nitrosamines and aflatoxins (both of which may be found in food).

Any of these chemical compounds may react with the DNA of a normal cell to produce a mutation. Having undergone such a mutation, a cell is not necessarily committed to neoplasia. Many mutations are not carcinogenic and more

Table 3-2	Nomenclature of benign and malignant tumors		
Cell or Tissue of Origin	**Benign**	**Malignant**
TUMORS OF EPITHELIAL ORIGIN		
Squamous cells	Squamous cell papilloma	Squamous cell carcinoma
Basal cells	—	Basal cell carcinoma
Glandular or ductal epithelium	Adenoma	Adenocarcinoma
	Papillary adenoma	Papillary adenocarcinoma
	Cystadenoma	Cystadenocarcinoma
Transitional cells	Transitional cell papilloma	Transitional cell carcinoma
Bile duct	Bile duct adenoma	Bile duct carcinoma (cholangiocarcinoma)
Islets of Langerhans	Islet cell adenoma	Islet cell carcinoma
Liver cells	Liver cell adenoma	Hepatocellular carcinoma
Neuroectoderm	Nevus	Malignant melanoma
Placental epithelium	Hydatidiform mole	Choriocarcinoma
Renal epithelium	Renal tubular adenoma	Renal cell carcinoma (hypernephroma)
Respiratory tract	—	Bronchogenic carcinoma
SKIN ADNEXAL GLANDS		
Sweat glands	Syringoadenoma; sweat gland adenoma	Syringocarcinoma, sweat gland carcinoma
Sebaceous glands	Sebaceous gland adenoma	Sebaceous gland carcinoma
Germ cells (testis and ovary)	—	Seminoma (dysgerminoma)
		Embryonal carcinoma, yolk sac tumor
TUMORS OF MESENCHYMAL ORIGIN		
Hematopoietic/lymphoid tissues	—	Leukemias
		Lymphomas
		Hodgkin's disease
		Multiple myeloma
NEURAL AND RETINAL TISSUE		
Nerve sheath	Neurilemoma, neurofibroma	Malignant peripheral nerve sheath tumor
Nerve cells	Ganglioneuroma	Neuroblastoma
Retinal cells (cones)	—	Retinoblastoma
CONNECTIVE TISSUE		
Fibrous tissue	Fibroma	Fibrosarcoma
Fat	Lipoma	Liposarcoma
Bone	Osteoma	Osteogenic sarcoma
Cartilage	Chondroma	Chondrosarcoma
MUSCLE		
Smooth muscle	Leiomyoma	Leiomyosarcoma
Striated muscle	Rhabdomyoma	Rhabdomyosarcoma
ENDOTHELIAL AND RELATED TISSUES		
Blood vessels	Hemangioma	Angiosarcoma
		Kaposi's sarcoma
Lymph vessels	Lymphangioma	Lymphangiosarcoma
Synovia	—	Synoviosarcoma (synovioma)
Mesothelium	Benign mesothelioma	Malignant mesothelioma
Meninges	Meningioma	
Uncertain origin	—	Ewing's tumor
OTHER ORIGINS		
Renal anlage	—	Wilms' tumor
Trophoblast	Hydatidiform mole	Choriocarcinoma
Totipotential cells	Benign teratoma	Malignant teratoma

From Damjonov I, Linder J: *Anderson's pathology,* ed 10, St. Louis, 1995, Mosby.

important are likely to be detected by cellular surveillance mechanisms that lead to their detection and repair. Some mutations, however, produce strategic damage sufficient to have potential neoplastic consequences. The chemical compound provoking such a mutation is called an initiator; the cell has undergone initiation. Initiation only conveys new potential to the cell; it does not produce an immediate cancer. In fact, the time between the initiating event and clinical appearance of the tumor may be many years or decades. The time between the two events is termed the latent period. During the latent period, initiated cells may appear normal under the microscope. At the same time, they may display subtle changes in their capacity to respond to mechanisms that usually regulate cell growth. Programmed cell death, or apoptosis, may not occur as it normally does, cellular differentiation may become irregular, and the action of another group of chemicals (called promoters) may influence cellular growth. Promoters are seldom carcinogens but have the effect of hastening and intensifying abnormal growth characteristics set in motion by the initiator. As a result, cell division accelerates beyond that normally seen under the influence of the initiator alone to produce a clone of cells displaying increased metabolic activity and early abnormal growth characteristics. In this clone, genetic evolution continues to produce occasional cells that behave more like those of a clinical malignancy. These cells in turn become ascendant and produce daughter cells with even more aggressive features. Whether or not they are augmented by the action of promoters, all these phenomena, which are set in motion by the initiator, culminate in the development of a clinical malignancy if given sufficient time.

The physiologist Francis Peyton Rous first demonstrated viral carcinogenesis in 1911.[9] He induced the growth of soft tissue sarcomas in a strain of normal chickens simply by injecting the chickens with a cell-free filtrate made from a tumor in another bird of the same strain. Unfortunately, the importance of this experiment was not immediately recognized because the entire sequence could not be reproduced in mammals. Moreover, because the particulate nature of viruses was not comprehensively understood at that time, Rous' experiment was relegated to the realm of curiosity. In a few years, Twort and d'Herelle significantly advanced the scientific understanding of cell-free filtrates by presenting data documenting the true nature of viruses as small packets of genetic material having the capacity to infect and sometimes destroy living cells. Twenty years later, R.E. Shope and J.J. Bittner, working independently, reported viral tumor induction in rabbits and mice, thus inviting more understanding to viral carcinogenesis in mammals.

In scientific laboratories today, many mammalian cell systems exist in which viral tumor induction can be demonstrated.[6] In humans, no specific cancers have been shown to be caused by a viral agent acting alone. However, scientists have discovered strong associations between several cancers and specific types of viruses.

As suggested by Twort and d'Herelle, viruses are simply small packets of genetic material enclosed in capsules. This genetic material may be DNA or RNA, but with either the virus is an obligate parasite in need of a living cell to infect to reproduce itself. Some viruses can infect many kinds of cells in one or several species. For example, the rabies virus can infect rodents, dogs, and humans. Other viruses exhibit great specificity and can infect only certain cells in a single species. Regardless of the range of potential hosts, infection occurs after the genetic material in the virus gains access to the host cell. Inside the host cell, the viral **genome** assumes command of cellular function to replicate itself. In acute viral infections, this replication is rapid and not only produces hundreds of viral copies but also destroys the infected cell. Genes of viral derivation that have become incorporated into chromosomes of the host cell and are concerned with the regulation of cell growth are called viral oncogenes. A few human cancers are associated with certain viral infections. The four common viruses widely distributed in nature and implicated in human neoplasia are the Epstein-Barr virus (EBV), the human papillomavirus (HPV), the hepatitis B virus (HBV), and the human T-cell leukemia type I virus (HTLV-I).

EBV causes acute infectious mononucleosis. This virus has a predilection for lymphocytes. In some of the lymphocytes the genome of the virus may persist after the acute infection has resolved. Cell lines established from tumors in patients with Burkitt's lymphoma, immunoblastic lymphoma, and nasopharyngeal cancer frequently harbor this virus.

HPV is ubiquitous among higher vertebrates. Dozens of types have been recognized and recently classified. These viruses are associated with a variety of neoplasms ranging from simple warts to invasive cancer of the uterine cervix and probably play a role as initiator or promoter in a host of additional cancers arising from squamous cell epithelium.

HBV is endemic in Africa and Asia, continents in which chronic hepatitis is a major cause of mortality. In these same areas the incidence of hepatocellular carcinoma among those infected with HBV is many times that of uninfected persons. The transitional cascade from HBV infection to the development of hepatocellular carcinoma is complex and remains to be completely elucidated. However, the epidemiologic evidence for an association between the two is overwhelming.

HTLV-I is endemic in Japan, Africa, and the West Indies and is an example of a retrovirus that plays a causal role in the development of human malignancy. Retroviruses are RNA viruses that uniquely carry their own enzyme systems. After invasion of a host cell, this enzyme (reverse transcriptase) allows retroviruses to transcribe their own RNA into DNA, which is then inserted into chromosomes of the host cell. This transcription is necessary because DNA (not RNA) is the functional material of genes.

Although each of these four viruses is associated with human cancer in a significant way, they all require the operation of cofactors to permit neoplastic expression. Complex pathologic interactions are required to defeat the function of normal cells programmed to prevent carcinogenesis.

Most cancers seem to arise spontaneously for reasons poorly understood (i.e., they are not induced by pure chemical nor pure viral mechanisms). Such cancers are considered to be caused by environmental factors. Of course, chemicals and viruses are constituents of the environment, so the classification is somewhat contrived. Nonetheless, among environmental factors that can cause cancer, few are better documented than radiant energy. Ionizing radiation has been known for decades to be carcinogenic.[4,7] The increased incidence of cancer in radiation workers and survivors of atomic bombing is legendary. Most of the radiation workers, whose exposure was chronic, received many small doses of radiation over long periods and subsequently developed cancers of hematologic origin (i.e., leukemias and lymphomas). In contrast, atomic bomb survivors received single large doses of whole-body radiation, which in addition to hematologic malignancies, induced solid tumors of the thyroid, breast, colon, and lung. All these cancers became manifest after latent periods ranging from a few years to several decades. These long, latent periods suggest that many cofactors are operative in radiation carcinogenesis.

Similar latent periods occur in cancers induced by ultraviolet radiation. Sunlight (the principle environmental source of ultraviolet radiation) has been implicated in the induction of all common cancers of the skin (i.e., basal cell carcinoma, squamous cell carcinoma, and malignant melanoma). These cancers arise only in skin lacking protective melanin pigment and therefore rarely occur in African-Americans.

The mechanism by which radiant energy causes cancer is linked to its action as a mutagen. Energy absorbed by the cell's nucleus results in damage to the genetic material in the chromosomes, thus producing rearrangement or breakage in the strands of DNA. As in other situations that cause damage to DNA, intracellular mechanisms attempt to promote repair. When repair is incomplete in a cell surviving the radiation insult the derangement of the genetic material may be perpetuated in much the same way that the incorporated genetic material of the virus is replicated by cells surviving viral infections. During the ensuing latent period, these altered cells are subject to the action of the entire spectrum of carcinogens and may eventually, under proper circumstances, exhibit neoplastic growth.

ESTABLISHING A PATHOLOGIC DIAGNOSIS

Little if any reason exists to treat cancer without first establishing a pathologic diagnosis. This entails the recovery of cells that the pathologist can identify as malignant.[3] The probable nature of an anatomic abnormality detected in the clinic on physical examination or identified on any of the several imaging studies commonly used in modern medicine can be predicted with considerable accuracy. However, verification of the clinical suspicion usually has significant therapeutic implications for the patient and physician and satisfies minimally the standards required medicolegally before a full-scale assault on cancer can be recommended or planned. More important, the clinical suspicion is sometimes incorrect, thus resulting in major modification of the proposed treatment program. For example, carcinoma of the lung is a disease that can be diagnosed with great regularity before any cells are recovered for examination. By careful consideration of all other available information (including age, symptoms, signs, smoking history, blood test results, and results of imaging studies such as radiographs and computed tomographic scans), a malignancy of the lung can be diagnosed without much uncertainty. The conclusion might be made that little else is required. However, several types of lung cancer exist, and the ability of the previously mentioned determinants to discriminate among them is considerably more limited than their ability to simply suggest the presence of a pulmonary malignancy. Each of the types of lung cancer has its own clinical and biologic characteristics, and these characteristics determine the best treatment and influence the outcome. Accordingly, recovering tumor cells for study to make appropriate recommendations to the patient becomes extremely important. The likely outcome of tissue recovery is only the documentation of a specific type of lung cancer, but the implications could be enormous for all concerned if the typical lung cancer turns out to be something else (i.e., a metastatic cancer or even a benign tumor). Pathologists are not always correct, but their tools for establishing a diagnosis of malignancy are the most powerful available in the medical armamentarium.

The acquisition of living cells to establish a diagnosis of malignancy is obviously a maneuver that is invasive or requires internal encroachment on the site harboring the tumor. This intrusion may be major or minor. The three procedures most commonly used to make a diagnosis of cancer (listed in ascending order of invasiveness) are (1) recovery of exfoliating cells, (2) fine-needle aspiration of malignant cells, and (3) open biopsy of the tumor. Attention to detail is necessary to obtain consistently good results from any of these procedures. The diagnosis depends on submitting to the pathologist representative portions of the tissue suspected of being cancerous. If inadequate samples are submitted, unfortunate inaccuracies in diagnosis are inevitable.

Exfoliative cytology is the study of single cells obtained from various surfaces or secretions shed by the tumor. The foremost example of exfoliative cytology is the Papanicolaou smear, which is made for the early detection of cancer of the cervix and uterus. The usefulness of this technique has been proved over several decades.

Fine-needle aspiration is another recovery technique that results primarily in the acquisition of single cells. These cells are recovered through a fine needle inserted directly into the tumor. Because the needles are of small caliber, they can traverse most normal tissue without causing damage and therefore bring remote and relatively inaccessible tumors such as cancer of the pancreas in easy range.

Open biopsy (the most invasive of the three recovery procedures) is accomplished under direct vision. The tumor is surgically removed totally or partly.

Each of these procedures has its own set of variations, and some overlap of procedures is present from one to another. For example, a biopsy may be incisional with removal of only a piece of the tumor or excisional with removal of the entire tumor. Likewise, an incisional biopsy may be accomplished through a large-bore needle.

The tissue sample becomes the responsibility of pathologists who direct laboratory analysis of the specimen along several different pathways. Most important is the preparation of the sample for examination and study under the light microscope. This is usually accomplished by fixing the tissue or preserving its existing form and structure by immersing it in a solution such as formalin.

Specimens of solid tissue are fixed and then placed in hot, liquid paraffin. After the paraffin cools and hardens, the tissue can be cut in extremely thin slices by a machine called a microtome. These slices are placed on glass slides, which are then immersed in an organic solvent, thus dissolving the paraffin. The resulting tissue sections may be treated with any of a vast number of stains to demonstrate specific features of cellular detail. Using the microscope, pathologists search for evidence of malignancy previously mentioned in this chapter.

Specimens of exfoliating cells or those obtained by fine-needle aspiration are smeared thinly on microscopic slides before being appropriately fixed and stained. In these preparations of single cells, attention is given not only to the size and shape of individual cells but also to the specific features of the nucleus and cytoplasm. Cells lacking uniformity of size, shape, and nuclear configuration may be suggestive of malignancy.

In tissue sections, departures from cellular and nuclear uniformity are also abnormal. In addition, the presence of a malignant tumor usually disturbs normal tissue architecture.

This disturbance is the result of malignant cells invading and destroying surrounding tissue. Some of this invasion may be into blood or lymph vessels, therefore suggesting the metastatic potential of the tumor. However, no single microscopic abnormality is sufficient to establish the diagnosis of cancer in all instances. The job of pathologists often entails a highly complex and relatively subjective discrimination among a host of biologic variables, which together are predictive of the behavior of the process that is under study. Fortunately, pathologists have other tools to assist in this estimation. Among these tools is the flow cytometer, which is a piece of sophisticated electronic equipment that facilitates the extremely rapid passage of cells in suspension through a laser beam and past an array of detectors. These detectors analyze individual cells for predetermined characteristics such as size, DNA content, surface markers, cell-cycle position, and viability. In carefully selected test samples, abnormal DNA content, variation in cell size, and irregular

cell-surface markers can furnish additional evidence of malignancy, identify incomplete responses to therapy, or document early tumor recurrence after treatment. As the molecular biology of the cancer cell is dissected and understood, additional techniques to assist the pathologist in determining the parameters of cell growth have been and continue to be developed. A detailed discussion of this new pathology is beyond the scope of this chapter. However, some of these innovative approaches are referenced in this chapter in the section on the biology of the cancer cell.

CLASSIFYING CANCER

The classification of neoplastic diseases is far from an exact science. Published systems of classification are intended as communication guidelines for those involved in cancer management rather than absolute frames of reference for the pathologist. Virtually all these systems contain many inconsistencies that lack rational explanation but over decades have become entrenched in medical jargon. Only time and experience will convey to the inquisitive radiation therapist an understanding of the full spectrum and meaning of these inconsistencies.

In describing the histopathology of various cancers, the pathologist not only assigns the tumor to a subset but also assigns to that particular tumor a grade and sometimes a stage. Tumor grade and stage are intended to serve as indices of outcome and are therefore of clinical importance.

Tumor grade is a specification that describes the apparent aggressiveness of the cancer as determined by cytologic and morphologic criteria. High-grade tumors are apt to be more aggressive than low-grade tumors. Now in common usage is a system that assigns a numeric value from one to three. Tumors with low numeric designations are likely to be well-differentiated, of lower metastatic potential, and easier to control. Conversely, grade three, or high-grade, tumors appear poorly differentiated, may metastasize early, and may be extremely difficult to control.

Tumor stage is a description of the extent of the tumor at the time of diagnosis. Staging may be clinical, pathologic, or a combination of elements of both. Clinical stage is assigned on the basis of physical examination with or without the assistance of certain imaging studies depending on the tumor. It is based on recognition of tumor size, invasiveness, and local or distant metastases. The clinical staging of a cancer may be verified and therefore converted to a pathologic stage by recovering for study under the microscope appropriate tissue from one or more sites. A more advanced stage of disease generally implies a worse prognosis. High-grade tumors are likely to be more advanced in stage at the time of diagnosis than low-grade tumors. Most of the time, however, the principle determinate of prognosis is the stage of disease rather than the grade.

Presently, two staging systems predominate. The first of these (the AJCC system) was developed by the American Joint Committee for Cancer Staging and End Results

Reporting and represents the ongoing work of a consortium of specialty societies in American medicine. The other (the IUCC system) is the work of an international agency known as the International Union Against Cancer. The two systems bear similarities and employ the basic elements of TNM staging introduced over 50 years ago by Pierre Denoix. The TNM system specifies the extent or stage of a cancer by considering three categories: the primary tumor (T), the regional lymph nodes (N), and distant metastatic disease (M). In staging a particular tumor the initial of each category is given a numerical subscript designating the extent of disease found in that anatomic compartment. For example, an early breast cancer of less than 2 cm in diameter that has spread neither locally nor distantly is assigned a stage of T1N0M0. These staging systems have many permutations and variations with unique meanings regarding tumors of specific sites.

BIOLOGY OF THE CANCER CELL

Considering the cancer cell an absolute biologic renegade wreaking havoc on one system after another is tempting. This temptation is resisted, however, by recalling that to exist as an entity at all the cancer cell must participate in some of the same biologic processes sustaining the many normal cells around it.[5] Consequently, the biology of the cancer cell is best examined in the context of normal cellular function by noting deviations from normal function that cancer cells display.

Cells are diverse in size, shape, and function. Nevertheless, they have many common elements (Fig. 3-1). All mammalian cells are surrounded by a cell wall, or plasma membrane. All processes of life occur inside that membrane or on its surface and are accomplished by many specialized components called **organelles.** Within the plasma membrane is the **nucleus** of the cell containing the genetic material DNA that directs cellular metabolism. DNA is the material from which genes are made. Individual genes, which may number in the hundreds of thousands, are normally assigned specific positions or loci on protein structures called **chromosomes.** The cell nucleus also contains one or more **nucleoli,** which are organelles that facilitate **ribosome** assembly. A **nuclear membrane** encloses the nucleus. Between the nucleus and outer cell wall is a substance known as **cytoplasm,** which is a conglomerate of semiliquid material called cytosol and numerous extranuclear organelles. Woven throughout the cytoplasm is a filamentous membrane called the **endoplasmic reticulum,** which is continuous with the nuclear membrane and houses the ribosomes. Ribosomes are important organelles responsible for protein synthesis. Other important cytoplasmic organelles include the **Golgi apparatus, lysosomes, peroxisomes, vacuoles,** and **mitochondria.** The Golgi apparatus is important in the storage and management of intracellular chemical substances. Lysosomes play a role in intracellular digestion. Peroxisomes harbor specific enzyme systems, facilitating certain metabolic processes, and vacuoles function in cytoplasmic storage. Mitochondria

are the intracellular factories that produce adenosine triphosphate (ATP) from sugar and other organic fuels. ATP in turn is the source of energy that drives intracellular metabolism. Under ordinary circumstances, these components of the normal cell function together to maintain equilibrium, promote growth, and facilitate proliferation. All this occurs at one or more points during the cell cycle.

Classically, the **cell cycle** is the observable sequence of events pursued during the lifespan of a dividing cell.[2] The cycle is chronologically divided into four distinct phases: G1, S, G2, and M (Fig. 3-2). G1 is the period before the duplication or synthesis of DNA in the nucleus. This phase is extremely variable in length and may be indistinguishable from G0, in which living cells are fully functional but simply not programmed for mitosis. The S phase is the period during which nuclear DNA is synthesized and chromosomes are duplicated. The G2 phase of the cell cycle commences after DNA synthesis is complete and continues until the cell begins to divide during the M phase. During G2, G1, and S, the cell is growing, producing proteins and organelles, and discharging its metabolic responsibilities. The shortest phase of the cell cycle is M, during which mitosis occurs. Whereas other phases may be measured in days or weeks, mitosis usually occurs in about 2 hours. With completion of mitosis, two identical daughter cells have been made. They in turn enter G1 to repeat the same sequence of events that led to their production.

During G1 the young daughter cell grows (i.e., increases in mass) and undergoes differentiation, or the expression of structural and functional specialization. The cell may prepare to proliferate or divide once more, but G1 is usually a point of restraint in cellular proliferation. Ordinarily, proliferation and differentiation are closely controlled by interrelated physiologic processes. They also tend to be reciprocal (i.e., the greater the differentiation, the less the proliferation). When these complex, cell cycle–related, intracellular mechanisms break down, reciprocity may be expressed in the uncontrolled proliferation of poorly differentiated cells.

Ultimately, these processes are controlled by molecular events predetermined by gene expression. Through the study and understanding of gene expression, molecular biology has evolved and dramatically expanded over the last two decades, and molecular biology has contributed greatly to the understanding of normal and malignant cells. (For a detailed discussion of gene form and function, refer to a standard college textbook of biology.)

Genes that line chromosomes are composed of DNA, which is composed of a series of deoxyribonucleotides.[1,5] **Nucleotides** in general have three chemical components: a phosphate group, a molecule of sugar containing five carbon atoms, and a nitrogenous base. The five-carbon sugar may be deoxyribose or ribose, depending on whether the nucleic acid is DNA or RNA. Five nitrogenous bases—adenine, guanine, thymine, cytosine, and uracil—are in nucleotides. Adenine,

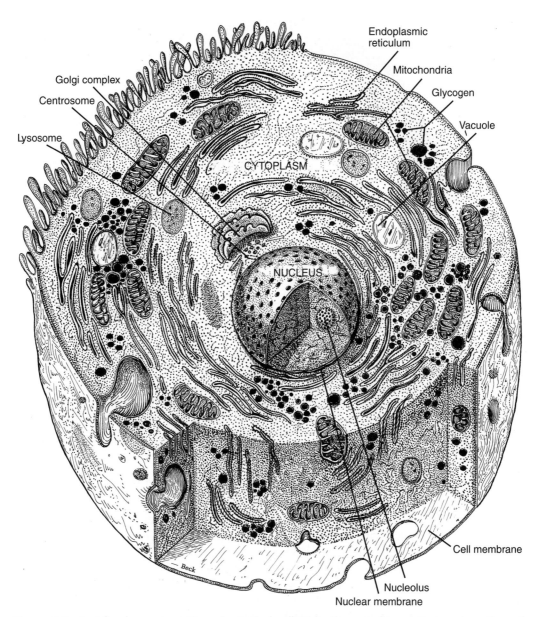

Golgi complex

Centrosome

Lysosome

Endoplasmic
reticulum

Mitochondria

Glycogen

Vacuole

CYTOPLASM

NUCLEUS

Beck

Cell membrane

Nucleolus

Nuclear membrane

Figure 3-1. A stylized representation of a typical cell. Note the membranes that enclose the cell proper and nucleus, respectively. A typical cell contains numerous organelles among which the endoplasmic reticulum, Golgi apparatus or complex mitochondria, and lysosomes are prominent. The ribosomes, themselves important organelles, are represented by the many dots bordering the endoplasmic reticulum. *(From Anthony CP, Kolthoff NJ: Textbook of anatomy and physiology, ed 9, St. Louis, 1974, Mosby.)*

guanine, thymine, and cytosine are in DNA. In RNA, uracil substitutes for thymine.

DNA is arranged in two complementary strands configured in the shape of a double helix (Fig. 3-3). Nucleotides are present in a specific and unique sequence as far as nitrogenous bases are concerned. These bases connect the two strands of DNA and are complementary because chemical bonds that can form between the nitrogenous bases are exclusive. Adenine on one strand can combine only with thymine on the other. Similarly, guanine can combine only with cyto-

sine. As a result, each strand bears in its structure the blueprint necessary to precisely reproduce the other strand. In the cell cycle during synthesis the strands are separated and each serves as a template to reproduce its complementary image; thus genetic replication is accomplished.

Proteins are the building blocks of life. They provide form and function for the organism and regulate growth and metabolism. Proteins are complex molecules composed of **polypeptides.** It is at the polypeptide level that the genetic expression has its impact, for it is the unique sequencing of

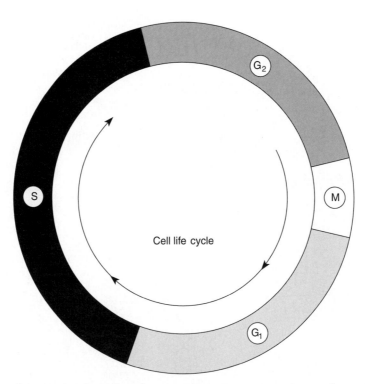

Cell life cycle

Figure 3-2. The cell cycle. Note that compartment G contains a subpopulation of cells in phase G0. These cells are indistinguishable from cells in G1 but are not programmed for mitosis and therefore will not enter S with other cells in G1. *(From Anthony CP, Kolthoff NJ: Textbook of anatomy and physiology, ed 9, St. Louis, 1974, Mosby.)*

the nucleotides along the length of a strand of DNA that determines the polypeptide configuration of all of the body proteins. Peptide information is encoded along the DNA strand in words called codons. Each codon is three nucleotides in length and represents a specific amino acid. Amino acids are the molecules from which peptides are made. RNA facilitates the transition from the code of DNA sequencing and codons to the structure of polypeptides and a protein molecule. In a process called **transcription,** enzymes in the cell nucleus facilitate the transfer of information from a strand of DNA to a strand of RNA. This particular type of RNA is called messenger RNA (mRNA). To become functional, this message-bearing strand of RNA undergoes splicing, during which the introns are excised. This excision results in a strand of RNA that contains only meaningful codons. After the splicing is complete, the mRNA leaves the nucleus for ribosomes in the cytoplasm.

Ribosomes are the site of **translation** at which the message borne by the mRNA is apprehended by another type of RNA termed transfer RNA (tRNA) and is restated in the language of peptides. Transfer RNA is the form of RNA that transfers amino acids from the cytoplasm to the ribosome. In the sequence prescribed by the incoming mRNA, the tRNA supplies the ribosome with the specific amino acids to con-

struct the required polypeptide. As the polypeptide grows in length, it begins to assume the three-dimensional configuration characteristic of the protein being constructed. After the required number of amino acids has been assembled and the three-dimensional folding and coiling has been completed, the resulting molecule may be a functional protein. In some situations the resulting protein undergoes enzymatic modification; in others, no such modification is required. In either situation, the result is a functional protein whose structure was determined by a unique sequence of nucleotides in the nucleus of the cell.

If the evident function of this newly made protein is to regulate cell growth by suppressing uncontrolled proliferation, such a protein is the product of a **tumor-suppressor gene.** Conversely, if the evident function is to accelerate cell growth, the responsible gene is termed an **oncogene** or perhaps its precursor, a protooncogene.[1,2] Tumor-suppressor genes and oncogenes are found in the normal genome. When both are properly located on the correct chromosome and accurately configured, cell growth and division proceed normally insofar as they are influenced by these proteins. If the genes become altered in location or configuration, the delicate balance between the proteins suppressing cell growth and those augmenting it may be destroyed.

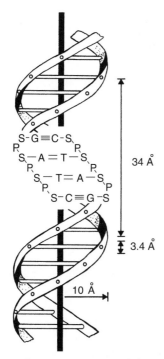

Figure 3-3. A schematic representation of the DNA double helix. *S,* The five-carbon sugar deoxyribose; *P,* phosphate group; *G,* guanine; *C,* cytosine; *A,* adenine; *T,* thymine. Note the sugar-phosphate backbone of each strand. The link between strands is uniquely accomplished by nitrogenous bases that form appendages of the backbone. *(From Boyd CM, Dalrymple GV: Basic science principles of nuclear medicine, St. Louis, 1974, Mosby.)*

DNA rearrangement occurs through mutations.[8] This rearrangement produces corresponding alterations in the resulting protein. In terms of neoplastic change the genes most sensitive to mutation are oncogenes and tumor-suppressor genes. Oncogenes may be of viral derivation or part of the normal genome. In either situation, they have the potential to trigger malignant growth. Protooncogenes have similar potential but require some modification, usually by mutation, to function as oncogenes. Mutations may result in several types of genetic aberration, including gene amplification, chromosome translocation, gene transposition, and point mutations.

After mutation, gene amplification occurs when DNA replication becomes selective, thus resulting in overproduction and therefore overexpression of any gene. Amplification of an oncogene results in augmentation of cell growth. The *erb*B-2 oncogene is often amplified in breast cancer, enhancing cell growth by elaboration of a protein that induces a favorable hormonal environment.

Chromosome translocation results from mutations that cause chromosome breakage. The broken fragments may be juxtaposed from one chromosome to another and function abnormally. They may also facilitate oncogene expression.

Translocations are frequently encountered in hematologic malignancies such as chronic myelogenous leukemia.

The pathology and pathophysiology of cancer are medical disciplines undergoing rapid expansion. Investigations of the molecular biologist have created a new understanding of the basic processes of life. With the discovery of each new gene and its protein product comes the potential to fit yet another piece into the biologic puzzle of cancer and its clinical management. To keep abreast of these developments the reader should monitor any of the several scientific publications devoted to providing understandable updates about cancer research.

Review Questions

Multiple Choice

1. An oncogene is a(an)
   a. Codon
   b. Exon
   c. Intron
   d. Protein
2. Which of the following terms is considered a genetic word?
   a. Codon
   b. Exon
   c. Intron
   d. Protein
3. Which of the following terms is best described by the word nonsense?
   a. Codon
   b. Exon
   c. Intron
   d. Protein
4. The nucleotide that is preserved during the splicing of the message-bearing RNA is the
   a. Codon
   b. Exon
   c. Intron
   d. Protein
5. Which of the following does not undergo transcription?
   a. Codon
   b. Exon
   c. Intron
   d. Protein
6. Etiologically, large cell lung cancer can be caused by
   a. Radiant energy
   b. Epstein-Barr virus
   c. Polycyclic hydrocarbons
   d. Asbestos
7. A common cause of malignant melanomas and basal cell carcinomas is
   a. Radiant energy
   b. Epstein-Barr virus

c. Polycyclic hydrocarbons

d. Asbestos

8. Transitional cell carcinoma of the bladder is closely related to exposure to
   a. Radiant energy
   b. Epstein-Barr virus
   c. Polycyclic hydrocarbons
   d. Asbestos

9. A common etiologic factor shared by infectious mononucleosis and Burkitt's lymphoma is
   a. Radiant energy
   b. Epstein-Barr virus
   c. Polycyclic hydrocarbons
   d. Asbestos

10. All of the following are characteristic of cancer except
    a. Metastases
    b. Blood vessel invasion
    c. Rapid growth rate
    d. Encapsulation

11. The study of cells by flow cytometry is not useful in defining which of the following?
    a. Physiologic function
    b. DNA content
    c. Cell-cycle position
    d. Surface markers

12. Cellular transformation from benign to malignant may result from all but which of the following?
    a. Mutation
    b. Initiation
    c. Promotion
    d. Apoptosis

13. All of the following are organelles except
    a. Nucleoli
    b. Ribosomes
    c. Golgi apparatus
    d. Endoplasmic reticulum

14. The shortest phase of the cell cycle is the _____ phase.
    a. G0
    b. G1
    c. S
    d. M

15. Malignant neoplasms arising from epithelial surfaces are best described as
    a. Carcinomas
    b. Adenocarcinomas
    c. Sarcomas
    d. Lymphomas

16. The bloodstream is a more likely route of spread for
    a. Carcinomas
    b. Sarcomas
    c. Adenocarcinomas
    d. Lymphomas

17. All of the following are nitrogenous bases in DNA except
    a. Adenine
    b. Guanine
    c. Uracil
    d. Cytosine

18. All of the following are nitrogenous bases in RNA except
    a. Adenine
    b. Guanine
    c. Uracil
    d. Thymine

19. A nucleoside differs from a nucleotide in that its composition does not include a
    a. Nitrogenous base
    b. Five-carbon sugar
    c. Phosphate group
    d. None of the above

20. The most invasive method of recovering cells to establish a diagnosis of cancer is
    a. Open biopsy
    b. Needle aspiration
    c. Exfoliative cytology
    d. None of the above

Questions to Ponder

1. What factors influenced historically the understanding of disease?
2. What is homeostasis?
3. Briefly discuss the metastatic process of malignant neoplasms.
4. Why is staging cancer important?
5. Describe the structure of DNA.

REFERENCES

1. Baserga R: Principles of molecular cell biology of cancer: the cell cycle. In De Vita VT Jr, Hellman S, Rosenberg SA, editors: *Cancer: principles and practice of oncology,* ed 6, Philadelphia, 2001, JB Lippincott.
2. Bonfiglio TA, Terry R: The pathology of cancer. In Rubin P, editor: *Clinical oncology,* ed 7, Philadelphia, 1993, WB Saunders.
3. Campbell NA: *Biology,* ed 3, Riverside, Calif, 1993, Benjamin/Cummings.
4. Hall EJ: Principles of carcinogenesis: physical. In De Vita VT Jr, Hellman S, Rosenberg SA, editors: *Cancer: principles and practice of oncology,* ed 6, Philadelphia, 2001, JB Lippincott.
5. Hill RP: The biology of cancer. In Rubin P, editor: *Clinical oncology,* ed 8, Philadelphia, 2001, WB Saunders.
6. Howley PM: Principles of carcinogenesis: viral. In De Vita VT Jr, Hellman S, Rosenberg SA, editors: *Cancer: principles and practice of oncology,* ed 6, Philadelphia, 2001, JB Lippincott.
7. Madri JA: Inflammation and healing. In Kissane JM, editor: *Anderson's pathology,* ed 10, St. Louis, 1995, Mosby.
8. Perkins AS, Vande Woude GF: Principles of molecular cell biology of cancer: oncogenes. In De Vita VT Jr, Hellman S, Rosenberg SA, editors: *Cancer: principles and practice of oncology,* ed 6, Philadelphia, 2001, JB Lippincott.
9. Sheldon H: *Boyd's introduction to the study of disease,* ed 11, Philadelphia, 1992, Lea & Febiger.

10. Shields PG, Harris CC: Principles of carcinogenesis: chemical. In De Vita VT Jr, Hellman S, Rosenberg SA, editors: *Cancer: principles and practice of oncology,* Philadelphia, 2001, JB Lippincott.

11. Vande Woude S, Vande Woude GF: Principles of molecular cell biology of cancer: introduction to methods in molecular biology. In De Vita VT Jr, Hellman S, Rosenberg SA, editors: *Cancer: principles and practice of oncology,* ed 6, Philadelphia, 2001, JB Lippincott.

BIBLIOGRAPHY

Anthony CP, Kolthoff NJ: *Textbook of anatomy and physiology,* ed 9, St. Louis, 1974, Mosby.

Boyd CM, Dalrymple GV: *Basic science principles of nuclear medicine,* St. Louis, 1974, Mosby.

del Regato JA, Spjut HJ, Cox JD: *Ackerman and del Regato's cancer: diagnosis, treatment, and prognosis,* ed 6, St. Louis, 1985, Mosby.

Kiemar V, Cotran RS, Robbins SL: *Basic pathology,* ed 5, Philadelphia, 1992, WB Saunders.

Overview of Radiobiology

Christopher M. Hand, Sean Ji-Won Kim,
Stephen M. Waldow

Outline

Key Terms

INTERACTION OF RADIATION AND MATTER

Since the discovery of x-rays by Roentgen in 1895, scientists and clinicians have investigated the interaction of **ionizing* radiations** and various target materials, including biologic tissue. *Radiation biology,* or *radiobiology,* has evolved since Roentgen's time and can be defined as the study of the sequence of events following the absorption of energy from ionizing radiations, the efforts of the organism to compensate, and the damage to the organism that may be produced.[61]

In evaluating the response of a living cell to ionizing radiation, the following must be considered[61]:

1. Radiation may or may not interact with a cell.
2. If an interaction occurs, damage may or may not be produced in the cell.
3. The initial energy deposition occurs extremely rapidly (much less than 1 second) and is nonselective or random in the cell.
4. Visible tissue changes after irradiation are not usually distinguishable from those caused by other traumas. (The only exception to this may be cataracts, which are discussed later.)
5. Biologic changes that occur after irradiation do so after some time has elapsed. The duration of this latent period is inversely related to the dose administered and can range from minutes to years.

---

*Ionization refers to the ejection of an electron from an atom, thus resulting in a charged particle or ion.

Types of Interactions

When radiation interacts with a cell, the ionizations are direct or indirect.[27] When a beam of charged particles (alpha particles, protons, or electrons) is incident on living tissue, direct ionization (the result of the incident particle itself) of a critical target (**deoxyribonucleic acid [DNA]**) is highly probable because of the relatively densely ionizing nature of most particulate radiations. Direct effects predominate when neutrons compose the primary beam because the secondary particles produced (protons, alpha particles, or heavy nuclear fragments) from the neutron's interaction with the nucleus of the atom may cause damage directly to the DNA or other important macromolecules (large molecules) in the cell.

The other form of ionization is indirect because of the effects of specific secondary particles on the target. This mechanism predominates when the incident beam is composed of x-rays, gamma rays, or neutrons. These indirectly ionizing radiations give rise to fast (high energy), charged secondary particles that can then directly or indirectly cause ionizations in the critical target. Indirect effect occurs predominantly when x-rays or gamma rays compose the primary beam, thus producing fast electrons as the secondary particles that interact with the cellular medium, water (H_2O). Indirect effects involve a series of reactions known as **radiolysis** (splitting) of water. The initial event in radiolysis involves the ionization or ejection of an electron from a water molecule, thus producing a water ion (charged molecule):

$$H_2O \rightarrow H_2O^+ + 1e$$

The ejected electron (e⁻), known as a *fast electron* because of its high energy, may now be absorbed by a second water molecule forming another water ion (H_2O^-):

$$e^- + H_2O \rightarrow H_2O^-$$

The pair of water ions produced are chemically unstable and tend to rapidly break down or dissociate into another ion and a **free radical** (a highly reactive species with an unpaired valence [outer shell] electron):

$$H_2O^+ \rightarrow H^+ + OH^\bullet \text{ and } H_2O^- \rightarrow H^\bullet + OH^-$$

The ion pair (H^+ and OH^-) may recombine, thus forming a normal water molecule with no net damage to the cell. The probability of recombination is high if the two ions are formed closely to each other. If these ions persist in the cell, they can react with and damage important macromolecules.

Free radicals may also recombine like the previous ion pair, thus forming a normal water molecule:

$$H^\bullet + OH^\bullet \rightarrow H_2O$$

Free radicals may also combine with other nearby free radicals, thus forming a new molecule like hydrogen peroxide that is toxic to the cell:

$$OH^\bullet + OH^\bullet \rightarrow H_2O_2 \text{ (hydrogen peroxide)}$$

Free radicals can participate in several other reactions involving normal cellular components, including DNA. Because the majority of the cell (80%) consists of water, the probability of damage by indirect effects is much greater than for direct effects with the use of indirectly ionizing radiations. Of the several reactions just presented for indirect effects, the predominant pathway that accounts for approximately two thirds of cellular damage involves the hydroxyl ($OH^\bullet$) radical. As discussed later, indirect effects predominate with sparsely ionizing or low **linear energy transfer (LET)** radiations and can be modified by physical, chemical, or biologic factors.

Linear Energy Transfer (LET) and Relative Biologic Effectiveness (RBE)

Depending on the composition of the incident beam of radiation, various secondary particles are produced in the cell. These secondary particles may directly or indirectly ionize the critical target. The physical properties of these secondary particles (mass and charge) give rise to a characteristic path of damage in the cell. Radiations can therefore be categorized by the rate at which energy is deposited by charged particles (incident or secondary) as they travel through matter. This is the LET of the radiation.[71] The LET is an average value calculated by dividing the energy deposited in kiloelectron volts (keV) by the distance traveled in micrometers (μm or 10^{-6} meters). Sparsely ionizing radiations such as x-rays and gamma rays are therefore classified as low LET because the secondary electrons produced are small particles that deposit their energy over great distances in tissue. Typical LET values for sparsely ionizing radiations may range from 0.3 to 3.0 keV/μm.[61] Densely ionizing radiations, which include charged particles such as protons and alpha particles, are classified as high LET because these particles are much bulkier in terms of mass than electrons and therefore deposit their energy over much smaller distances in the cell (Fig. 4-1). LET is therefore directly proportional to square of the charge (Q) and inversely proportional to the square of the velocity (v). The previously described relationship is expressed in the following equation:

$$LET = Q^2/v^2$$

Typical LET values may range from 30 to 100 keV/μm or greater, depending on the particle energy. Generally, a large, charged particle such as a proton or alpha particle does not penetrate nearly as far as a smaller, charged particle (electron) and not quite as far as an uncharged particle of equal mass (neutron). Neutrons usually have intermediate LET values (usually within 5 to 20 keV/μm). As the neutron's energy increases, its penetration in tissue also increases; therefore its LET decreases.

Knowing the LET of the radiation is important because

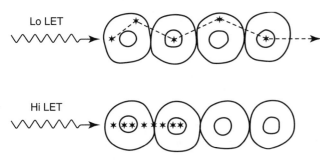

Figure 4-1. Comparative effects of low- and high-LET radiations on a population of cells. Low-LET radiation interacting with four cells emits an irregular path while the straight path of high-LET radiation only interacts with two cells. High-LET radiation has produced two hits in the nuclei of two different cells, whereas low-LET radiation has produced only one hit in the same number of cells. *(From Travis EL: Primer of medical radiobiology, ed 2, Philadelphia, 1989, Mosby, with permission.)*

the discovery was made early in the radiation therapy process that different LET radiations produce different degrees of the same biologic response. In other words, equal doses of different LET radiations do not produce the same biologic response. This is called the **relative biologic effectiveness (RBE)** of the radiation.[27] The RBE relates the ability of radiations with different LETs delivered under the same conditions to produce the same biologic effect. The equation for determining the RBE of a test radiation is as follows:

$$RBE \text{ of test radiation} = \frac{\text{Dose from 250-keV x-ray}}{\substack{\text{Dose from test radiation to produce} \\ \text{the same biologic effect}}}$$

The test radiation referred to includes any type of radiation beam being used. The effectiveness of the beam is determined by a historical comparison with a 250-keV x-ray beam that was the primary radiation beam available in the early days of radiation therapy. For example, if 400 cGy of 250-keV x-rays and 200 cGy of neutrons both result in 50% cell kill, the RBE of the neutrons equals 2. This means that the neutrons are twice as effective as the x-rays. In general, as the LET of the radiation increases, so does its RBE.

Radiation Effects on Deoxyribonucleic Acid (DNA)

The key molecule in the nucleus of the cell for radiation damage is thought to be DNA. Damage to a key molecule may be lethal to a cell and has led to the development of a target theory for radiation damage. This theory states that when ionizing radiation interacts with or near a key molecule (DNA), the sensitive area is termed a *target*. An ionization event that occurs in the target is termed a *hit*. These terms are applied only under conditions in which radiation interacts with the target by direct effects. This theory does not account for damage to DNA that is the result of free radical–mediated pathways.

Regardless of whether DNA is damaged by direct or indi-

rect effects caused by radiation, several types of damage can occur.[52] One form of damage involves the change in or loss of one or more of the four nitrogenous (nitrogen-containing) bases: adenine (A), thymine (T), cytosine (C), and guanine (G). A second form of damage may involve breakage of hydrogen bonds between the A-T and C-G base pairs, which function to keep the two DNA strands together. Bonds may also be broken between the components of the backbone of each DNA strand (i.e., between the deoxyribose sugar and phosphate groups connected to each base and known collectively as a *nucleotide*). This may lead to intrastrand or interstrand cross-linking of DNA.

The consequences of these types of DNA damage vary. Loss or change of a base results in a new base sequence, which can cause minor or major effects on protein synthesis. A change in base sequence not rectified by the cell is an example of a mutation (change in the genetic material). Agents such as ionizing radiation that cause mutations are mutagenic. Single-strand breaks in the DNA backbone (common after irradiation with low-LET radiations) may or may not be repaired. If they are not repaired, damage may occur. Single-strand breaks are more readily repaired than double-strand breaks, which are more apparent after exposure to high-LET radiations. The production of multiple-strand breaks compared with single-strand breaks correlates much more strongly with cell lethality. Radiation interaction with DNA does not always result in damage, and most of the damage can be and probably is repaired. Consequences of DNA damage in somatic (body) cells involve the irradiated organism or individual, whereas DNA damage in germ (reproductive) cells may also affect future generations.

Radiation Effects on Chromosomes

A review of the four phases of mitosis, which is a continuous process of organizing and arranging nuclear DNA during cell division, is helpful in understanding radiation effects on chromosomes. Fig. 4-2 shows the major events of mitosis. Because DNA molecules form genes and thousands of genes compose a chromosome, studying genetic damage from ionizing radiation in terms of gross structural damage to chromosomes is often easiest.[19]

Early studies in this area often involved plant chromosomes because their small diploid number (number of chromosomes in each somatic cell) and large relative size facilitated study under the light microscope. The fact that radiation is an efficient breaker of chromosomes by indirect or direct pathways is now well documented. Gross structural changes in chromosomes are referred to as *aberrations, lesions,* or *anomalies*. A distinction also exists between chromosome and chromatid aberrations. A chromosome aberration occurs when radiation is administered to cells in the G1 phase or before the cell replicates its DNA in the S phase. A chromosome aberration may involve both daughter cells after mitosis, because if the break is not repaired, the cell replicates it during the S phase. A chromatid aberration results when radiation is admin-

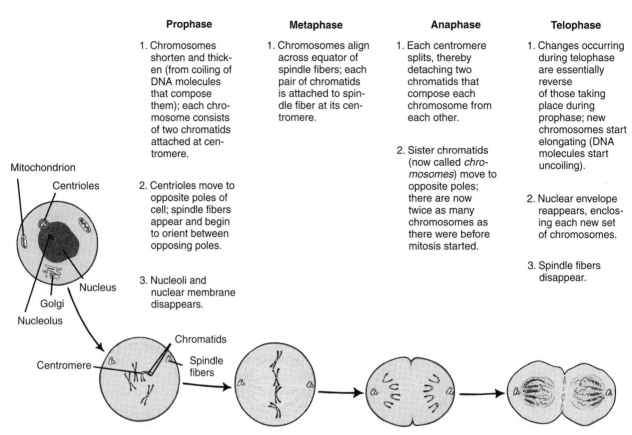

Prophase

1. Chromosomes shorten and thicken (from coiling of DNA molecules that compose them); each chromosome consists of two chromatids attached at centromere.

2. Centrioles move to opposite poles of cell; spindle fibers appear and begin to orient between opposing poles.

3. Nucleoli and nuclear membrane disappears.

Metaphase

1. Chromosomes align across equator of spindle fibers; each pair of chromatids is attached to spindle fiber at its centromere.

Anaphase

1. Each centromere splits, thereby detaching two chromatids that compose each chromosome from each other.

2. Sister chromatids (now called *chromosomes*) move to opposite poles; there are now twice as many chromosomes as there were before mitosis started.

Telophase

1. Changes occurring during telophase are essentially reverse of those taking place during prophase; new chromosomes start elongating (DNA molecules start uncoiling).

2. Nuclear envelope reappears, enclosing each new set of chromosomes.

3. Spindle fibers disappear.

Figure 4-2. The major events of mitosis. *(Modified from Thibodeau GA, Patton KT: Anatomy and physiology, ed 3, St. Louis, 1996, Mosby.)*

istered to cells in the G2 phase or after they have completed DNA synthesis. This term applies to the arms (chromatids) of a replicated (duplicated) chromosome. In this situation, only one of the two daughter cells formed after cell division is affected if the damage is not repaired.

Structural changes induced in chromosomes by radiation include single breaks, multiple breaks, and a phenomenon known as *chromosome stickiness,* or *clumping.* Consequences of these structural changes may include healing with no damage and loss or rearrangement of genetic material.

A single radiation-induced break in any part of a chromosome results in two chromosome fragments. One fragment contains the centromere (the place the mitotic spindle attaches during mitosis), and the other (known as the *acentric fragment*) does not.[61] The rejoining of these fragments, termed *restitution,* has a high probability of occurring because of their proximity.[19] Approximately 95% of all single breaks heal by restitution with the result being no damage to the cell.

If irradiation occurs in G1 cells and restitution does not occur, both fragments are replicated during the S phase, thus resulting in four fragments (each with a broken end).[61] Two of these chromatids contain a centromere, whereas the other two do not. The two centromere-containing chromatids may now join, thus forming a dicentric fragment. The other two

fragments may also join, thus forming an acentric fragment.

These structural aberrations become evident during the metaphase and anaphase stages of mitosis. Because the acentric fragment does not contain a centromere, the spindle fibers do not attach to it during the metaphase stage. Therefore the genetic material it contains probably will not be transmitted to either daughter cell. The dicentric fragment, however, has two centromeres and will therefore be attached to the mitotic spindle at two sites instead of one. Therefore this fragment is pulled simultaneously toward both poles of the cell. The fragment between the two centromeres therefore becomes stretched, thus giving rise to a characteristic anaphase bridge, which eventually tears by the end of the anaphase stage, thus resulting in an unequal transmission of genetic information to each daughter cell (Fig. 4-3).

A single break in one chromatid in two different chromosomes also produces four fragments. Two fragments contain a centromere and two do not.[61] Again, dicentric and acentric chromosomes may result by the joining of the broken fragments (Fig. 4-4, *A*). In addition, the acentric fragment from one broken chromosome may join to a centromere-containing fragment of the other broken chromosome, thus forming a new normal-appearing chromosome. This rearrangement is known as *translocation* (Fig. 4-4, *B*). Although translocation does not necessarily result in a loss of genetic information, the

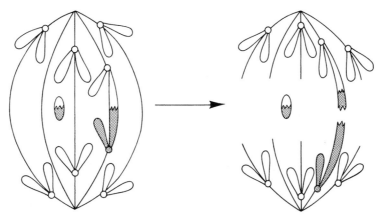

Figure 4-3. The fate of the dicentric and acentric fragments during anaphase, thus leading to anaphase bridge formation. The dicentric fragment attaches to the mitotic spindle at each centromere and is pulled toward both poles of the cell *(left)* and ultimately breaks again *(right)*. The acentric fragment does not attach to the spindle, thus resulting in loss of genetic material to the new daughter cells. *(From Travis EL: Primer of medical radiobiology, ed 2, St. Louis, 1989, Mosby.)*

sequence of genes in the new translocated chromosome is different from the original sequence before radiation damage. The consequences of radiation-induced translocations can vary from no effects in somatic cells to malformed or non-viable offspring if these translocations occur in germ cells.

A double break in one arm (chromatid) of a chromosome results in three fragments, each with a broken end.[61] Of these three, one fragment contains the centromere and the other two are acentric. The major consequences of a double break are known as *deletions* and *inversions* (see Fig. 4-3). A deletion of genetic material results when the fragment between the breaks is lost and the joining of the remaining two fragments join (Fig. 4-5, *A*). The effect of a deletion varies depending on the amount and significance of the genetic information that was in the lost fragment. An inversion of genetic material results when the middle fragment with two broken ends turns around or inverts before rejoining the other two fragments (Fig. 4-5, *B*). Although no loss of genetic material occurs after an inversion, the DNA base sequences and therefore the gene sequence are altered. This affects the types and amounts of critical proteins synthesized by the cell and can certainly affect the long-term viability of the cell.

Because of the random absorption of ionizing radiation in the cell, a single break can be induced in each chromatid of the same chromosome, thus again producing three fragments. The fragment with two broken ends contains the centromere and the other two fragments are acentric. This may result in the formation of a ring chromosome and an acentric chromosome (Fig. 4-6).[61] The ring chromosome is replicated and transmitted to the daughter cells, whereas the acentric fragment and its genetic information is not passed on. If a replicated ring chromosome becomes tangled before the

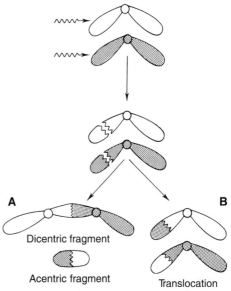

A — Dicentric fragment / Acentric fragment

B — Translocation

Figure 4-4. Two different chromosomes *(top)* may sustain a single break in one arm *(center)* and result in formation of dicentric and acentric fragments **(A),** or translocation of genetic material between the two **(B).** In the latter process, two complete chromosomes are formed. However, the exchange of chromosome parts and therefore genetic information should be noted. *(From Travis EL: Primer of medical radiobiology, ed 2, St. Louis, 1989, Mosby.)*

metaphase stage, unequal separation of each ring during the anaphase stage may result, so the daughter cells therefore do not inherit equal amounts of genetic information.

Several factors influence the type and extent of chromosome damage induced by ionizing radiations. The number of

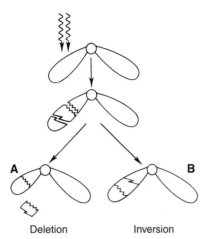

Deletion   Inversion

Figure 4-5. Two breaks occurring in the same arm of a chromosome *(top and middle)* may result in deletion of the fragment between the breaks **(A)** or inversion of the fragment, which is illustrated by the change in positions of the break lines **(B)**. *(From Travis EL: Primer of medical radiobiology, ed 2, St. Louis, 1989, Mosby.)*

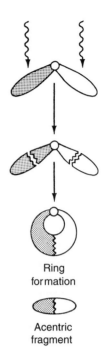

Ring
formation

Acentric
fragment

Figure 4-6. One possible consequence of breaks in both arms of a chromosome by radiation is that the broken arms join to form a ring. The remaining fragments join but are left without a centromere (acentric fragment). *(From Travis EL: Primer of medical radiobiology, ed 2, St. Louis, 1989, Mosby.)*

single breaks produced is directly proportional to the total dose of radiation administered. The frequency of single breaks, or simple aberrations, also increases as the LET of the radiation decreases. Therefore low-LET radiations such as x-rays and gamma rays produce simpler than complex (multiple break) aberrations.

Radiation Effects on Other Cell Components

Although nuclear DNA is the critical target for radiation-induced cell damage, other structures in the cell are also damaged by ionizing radiations and contribute to cell damage and death. Among these cellular components is the plasma or cell membrane. Absorption of energy by the structural components of the plasma membrane (i.e., the phospholipid bilayer and proteins) can result in membrane damage and therefore changes in the permeability of the membrane with regard to the transport of substances in and out of the cell. Damage to the mitochondrial and lysosomal membranes in the cytoplasm can also result in drastic consequences to the cell. All cellular components (including vital proteins, enzymes, carbohydrates, and lipids) can undergo structural and functional changes after irradiation that can be deadly to the cell. Because the deposition of energy from secondary particles (electrons, protons, or alpha particles) is random in matter, any site in the cell can be at risk for damage from radiation exposure.

CELLULAR RESPONSE TO RADIATION

Since the mid-1950s, when Puck and Marcus[44] first irradiated human cervical carcinoma cells in a Petri dish, the response of human, animal, and plant cells to radiation has been intensely studied. The response of cells after irradiation

can now be placed into one of three categories: division delay, interphase death, or reproductive failure.

Division Delay

Irradiated cells that involve a disruption in the mitotic index (MI), the ratio of the number of mitotic cells to the total number of cells in the irradiated population, is known as *division delay*. This results in cells in interphase at the time of irradiation to be delayed in the G2 phase. This is known as *mitotic delay*.

The consequence of mitotic delay is a decrease in the MI for the population, which means that fewer cells than normal will enter mitosis and divide. Therefore fewer new daughter cells will be produced. The magnitude of this response to radiation is dose dependent; the higher the radiation dose, the longer the mitotic delay and therefore the greater the decrease in MI. If the dose is less than 1000 cGy, most cell lines recover and eventually proceed through mitosis. This results in a higher than normal number of cells dividing and is termed *mitotic overshoot*.

Canti and Spear[12] first observed division delay in 1929 when they exposed chick fibroblasts in vitro to various doses of radiation. The mechanism behind division delay is thought to involve the inhibition or delay of DNA and/or protein synthesis after irradiation. Apparently, cells attempt to repair radiation damage before mitosis by stopping in the

G2 phase to confirm that the DNA and proteins are intact. Any damage found is repaired during this phase of the cell cycle so that it does not disrupt cell division or possibly lead to cell death.

Interphase Death

If irradiation of the cell during the G1, S, or G2 phase results in death, this mode of response is termed an *interphase death.*[61] Interphase death is defined as the death of irradiated cells before these cells reach mitosis. The form of cell death is also known as nonmitotic or nondivision death.[61] This form of cell response can occur in nondividing cells (such as adult nerve cells) and rapidly dividing cells. In general, radiosensitive cells (vegetative intermitotic [VIM] and differentiating intermitotic [DIM]) succumb to an interphase death at lower radiation doses than radioresistant cells (reverting postmitotic [RPM] and fixed postmitotic [FPM]). The exception to this is the lymphocyte, which is sensitive to interphase death at a dose as low as 50 cGy. The mechanism of interphase death is not clear but may involve damage to one or more biochemical pathways involved in cell metabolism. In most cell types, interphase death is not the primary mode of response to irradiation.

Reproductive Failure

The third and most common endpoint for response of cells to radiation is **reproductive failure** (also known as mitotic death), which is defined as a decrease in the reproductive integrity or cells' ability to undergo a limited number of divisions after irradiation.[44] This effect on the reproductive capacity of cells can be traced to the extent of chromosome damage induced by the radiation dose.

Apoptosis

Although unrelated to mitosis, because it is not an unsuccessful attempt by the cell to divide, another form of cell death that has been associated with the cellular response to radiation is apoptosis (programmed cell death). Cellular apoptosis appears to have gene (*p53* and *bcl-2*) involvement following exposure to radiation.[27] A characteristic apoptotic cell death involves nuclear fragmentation, cell lysis, and phagocytosis of the chromatin bodies by neighboring cells.[61]

Cell Survival Curves

The most common way of evaluating the cellular response to radiation was first introduced by Puck and Marcus[44] in 1956 when they irradiated human cervical cancer cells (known as *HeLa cells*) in vitro and plotted the results (number of colonies formed) on a semilogarithmic graph. Their results, termed a *survival curve,* was a plot of the radiation dose administered on the *x*-axis versus the surviving fraction (SF) of cells on the *y*-axis (Fig. 4-7).

This survival curve is characteristic of the survival of cells exposed to low-LET radiations such as x-rays or gamma rays. A shoulder region or flattening of the curve occurs at doses below 150 cGy and indicates that cells must accumulate damage in multiple targets to be killed. Because this survival curve is graphed on a semilog plot, the linear portion of the curve (above a dose of 150 cGy) indicates that equal increases in dose causes equal decreases in the SF of cells but the absolute number of cells killed varies[61] (Table 4-1).

This exponential response of cells to radiation is due to the random probability of radiation interacting with critical targets in the cell. On irradiation of a cell population with *n* targets/cell (with *n* > 1) several results are observed:

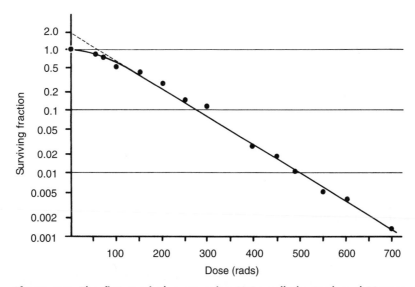

Figure 4-7. The first survival curve using HeLa cells by Puck and Marcus. Below 150 cGy the curve exhibits a shoulder region and becomes exponential (straight) at higher doses. *(From Puck TT, Marcus TI: Action of x-rays on mammalian cells, J Exp Med 103:653, 1956.)*

Table 4-1	The exponential relationship between a radiation dose and surviving fraction		
Original Cell Number	Dose Delivered (Gy)	Fraction of Cells Killed	Number of Cells Killed
1000,000	5	50	50,000
50,000	5	50	25,000
25,000	5	50	12,500
12,500	5	50	6,250
6,250	5	50	3,125

From Travis EL: *Primer of medical radiobiology*, ed 2, St Louis, 1989, Mosby.

1. Some cells are lethally damaged (all targets are hit)
2. Some cells are sublethally damaged (a few targets are hit)
3. Some cells are not damaged (no targets are hit)

As the radiation dose increases, the probability of cellular targets being hit also increases.

Three important parameters that allow interpretation of survival curves are the **extrapolation number (n), Do** dose, and quasithreshold dose **(Dq).** A characteristic survival curve for cells exposed to x-rays is shown in Fig. 4-8.[11]

The *n,* originally known as the *target number,* is determined by extrapolating the linear portion of the curve back until it intersects the *y*-axis. In Fig. 4-8, the *n* equals 2, which theoretically means two critical targets are in the cell and must be inactivated. For mammalian cells exposed to x-rays the *n* ranges from 2 to 10.

Another measure of cell response at low doses is the Dq. This parameter represents the dose at which survival becomes exponential. The Dq is a measure of the width of the shoulder region of the survival curve and is determined by drawing a horizontal line from an SF of 1 on the *y*-axis to the place it intersects the line extrapolated back from the linear portion of the curve for determination of *n*. The Dq is also a measure of the cell's ability to accumulate and repair sublethal damage.[7,21]

The third parameter, known as the *Do (or D37) dose,* reduces the SF of cells by 63%. In other words, 37% of the cells survive. The Do equals the reciprocal of the slope of the curve's linear portion and is a measure of the cells' radiosensitivity. Radiosensitive cells have a low Do, whereas radioresistant cells have a high Do. For mammalian cells the Do usually is between 100 to 220 cGy.[27]

Several equations describe the dose-response relationships expressed by survival curves.[11] The three survival-curve parameters are related by the equation $\log_e n = Dq/Do$. The SF can be calculated as $SF = 1 - (1 - e^{-D/Do})^n$. In this equation, *n* is the extrapolation number and *D* is the total dose.[11] This equation accurately predicts the response of complex cell types, including most mammalian cells in which the number of targets is presumed to be greater than one. (This is known as the *multitarget, single-hit model.*)

Factors Influencing Response

As proposed by Ancel and Vitemberger[3] in 1925, various external factors influence cellular response to radiation. This change in response is termed *conditional sensitivity.* Three groups of factors (physical, chemical, and biologic) can affect cellular radioresponse and therefore change the overall appearance of a cell line's survival curve and magnitude of the parameters n, Dq, and Do.

Physical factors. The response of cells to high-LET radiation differs from that seen after exposure to low-LET radiation.[9] The response of five mammalian cell lines to 300-kV x-rays and 15-MeV neutrons is shown in Fig. 4-9. The shoulder region (Dq) is usually decreased or even absent after irradiation with high-LET radiations such as alpha particles and neutrons. In addition, survival curves tend to be steeper (the Do is lower) after high-LET treatment. The effects of LET on biologic response are due to differences in the density of energy deposition in the cell. Because DNA is thought to be the critical target in cells, the most efficient radiation with the highest RBE induces two strand breaks in the DNA molecule, thus leading to a high probability of cell death. This optimal LET is thought to be approximately 160 keV/μm. Therefore all radiations with LETs above or below the optimal level are less efficient (having a lower RBE) in terms of cell killing (Fig. 4-10).

A second physical factor that influences cellular radioresponse is dose rate.[6] A dose-rate effect has been observed for reproductive failure, division delay, chromosome

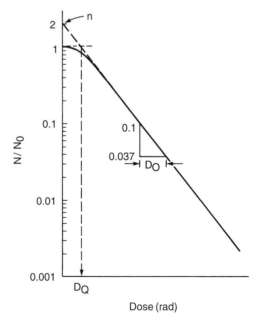

Figure 4-8. The multitarget, single-hit model of cell survival characteristic of low-LET radiations (x-rays and gamma rays). The parameters n, D_o, and D_q should be noted. *(From Bushong SC: Radiologic science for technologists: physics, biology, and protection, St. Louis, 1993, Mosby.)*

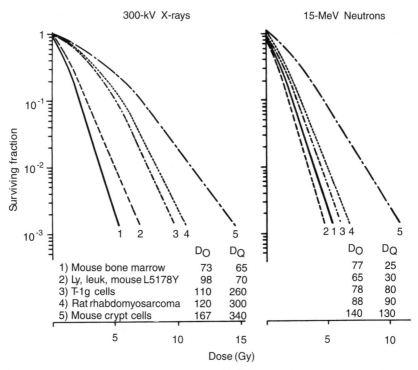

Figure 4-9. Survival curves for various types of mammalian cells irradiated with 33-kV x-rays or 15-MeV neutrons. The wide variability in the shoulder (D_q) and slope (D_o) seen in the x-ray survival curves is reduced after neutron irradiation. The D_o and D_q values shown are expressed in cGy. *(From Broerse JJ, Barendsen GW: Current topics, Radiat Res Q 8:305-350, 1973.)*

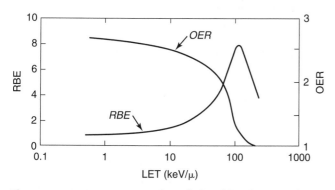

Figure 4-10. Demonstrates the relationship of OER and RBE as a function of LET. The data were obtained by using T1 kidney cells of human origin, irradiated with various naturally occurring alpha particles. *(Redrawn from Barendsen GW: In Proceedings of the Conference on Particle Accelerators in Radiation Therapy. LA-5180-C. Washington, D.C., 1972, U.S. Atomic Energy Commission, Technical Information Center.)*

aberrations, and survival time after whole-body irradiation. Low dose rates are less efficient in producing damage than high dose rates. Survival curves generally shift to the right, thus becoming shallower (Do increases), and the shoulder becomes indistinguishable at low dose rates (Fig. 4-11). This

change in the appearance of the survival curve is explained by the cells' ability to repair sublethal damage from radiation treatment during and after exposure when given at a low enough dose rates. This dose-rate effect is significant with low-LET radiations such as x-rays and gamma rays but is not observed with high-LET radiations.

Chemical factors. Two major chemical factors influence cellular response to radiation. Certain chemicals that enhance response to radiation are known as **radiosensitizers.** Other chemicals, termed **radioprotectors,** have the opposite effect (i.e., they decrease the cellular response to radiation).

The most potent radiosensitizer to date is molecular oxygen. The oxygen effect has been observed in all organisms exposed to ionizing radiation.[70] Although the exact mechanism of the oxygen effect is unknown, the presence of oxygen may enhance the formation of free radicals and "fix" or make radiation damage permanent that would otherwise be reversible. This is also known as the oxygen fixation hypothesis. Oxygen must be present during the radiation exposure for sensitization to occur. The sensitizing effects of oxygen are most significant with low-LET radiations in which indirect effects caused by free radical formation predominate over direct effects.

Cell survival curves differ for oxic (normal oxygen level) versus hypoxic (reduced oxygen level) cell populations.[10] As

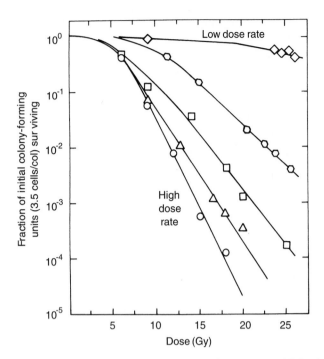

Figure 4-11. Dose-response curves for an established mammalian cell line irradiated with a wide range of dose rates from a high of 1.07 Gy/min to a low of 0.0036 Gy/min. Reducing the dose rate makes the survival curve more shallow and causes the shoulder to eventually disappear. *(From Bedford JS, Mitchell JB: Dose-rates effects in synchronous mammalian cells in culture, Radiat Res 54:316-327, 1973.)*

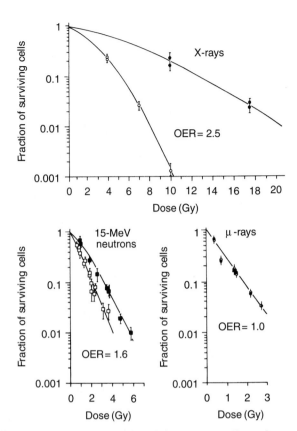

Figure 4-12. A comparison of the oxygen effect after x-ray, neutron, or alpha particle irradiation. The OER is highest after sparsely ionizing radiation (OER = 2.5), compared with densely ionizing radiations such as alpha particles (OER = 1.0). In the x-ray and neutron curves shown, the curve to the left represents the response of oxic cells and the curve to the right represents the hypoxic cell response. The oxic and hypoxic curves overlap when alpha particles are used. *(From Broerse JJ, Barendsen GW, van Kersen GR: Survival of cultured human cells after irradiation with fast neutrons at different energies in hypoxic and oxygenated conditions, Int J Radiat Biol 13:559-572, 1967.)*

the availability of oxygen decreases, cell response also decreases such that the survival curve shifts to the right because Dq and Do increase. This effect is most pronounced with x-rays and gamma rays. The effects are less as the LET of the radiation increases (Fig. 4-12). The magnitude of the oxygen effect is termed the **oxygen enhancement ratio (OER).**[27] The OER compares the response of cells with radiation in the presence and absence of oxygen. The equation for determining the OER for ionizing radiations is as follows:

$$OER = \frac{\text{Radiation dose under hypoxic/anoxic conditions}}{\begin{array}{c}\text{Radiation dose under oxic conditions to produce the}\\\text{same biologic effect}\end{array}}$$

One common endpoint used for determination of the OER is the Do. For example, if the Do = 300 cGy under hypoxic conditions but is reduced to 100 cGy under oxic conditions, the OER for the radiation in the experiment is 300/100 = 3.0. For mammalian cells the OER for x-rays and gamma rays is generally 2.5 to 3.0. This means that hypoxic cells are 2.5 to 3.0 times more resistant than oxic cells to a dose of low-LET radiation. The oxygen effect is less significant with neutrons[25] (OER = 1.6) and may not be observable with high-

LET radiations such as alpha particles (OER = 1.0). Fig. 4-10 illustrates a strong correlation between the OER and RBE as a function of LET. This figure illustrates that the maximum RBE and the rapid decrease in OER occurs at an LET of approximately 100 keV/μm.

Whereas oxygenation conditions are easily modifiable with cells in vitro, measurement of oxygen levels (known as *oxygen tension* or po_2) are more difficult to determine and modify in vivo. In vivo oxygen tensions of 20 to 30 μm Hg appear to render cells fully sensitive to low-LET radiations. The radiosensitivity of cells decreases as the po_2 decreases, thus limiting the response of hypoxic cells in tumors treated with radiation.

Other compounds have also been tested as radiosensitizers. Most notable among these are halogenated pyrimidines

and nitroimidazoles. Halogenated pyrimidines such as 5-bromo-deoxyuridine and 5-iododeoxyuridine are analogs of the DNA base thymidine.[28] These agents act as nonhypoxic cell sensitizers and are taken up by cycling cells during DNA synthesis (S phase). If enough of these compounds are substituted for thymidine, the DNA of the cell becomes more susceptible to radiation by a factor approaching 2. The rationale for the clinical use of these compounds is based on the shorter cycle times observed for tumor cells versus their normal cell counterparts. This should result in preferential uptake by tumors.

Nitroimidazoles such as misonidazole are oxygen-mimicking agents[1] (i.e., they behave chemically like oxygen in terms of indirect effects involving free radicals). In addition, nitroimidazoles may diffuse further than oxygen from blood vessels, thereby reaching radioresistant hypoxic cells in a tumor. These agents are classified as *hypoxic cell sensitizers.* The idea behind their use is to selectively increase the radiosensitivity of hypoxic tumor cells. This desired selective sensitization of tumors has not been achieved in the clinic. Two major reasons for this are that (1) neither of these sensitizing agents exclusively localizes in malignant tissue and (2) both of these agents cause side effects at therapeutic doses. New and improved sensitizing agents that localize in malignant tissues without toxic side effects are under development in the United States and England.

In some clinical situations, attempts have been made to protect normal tissues instead of sensitizing tumors to a dose of radiation. The agents used are known as *radiation protectors,* or *dose-modifying compounds.*[41] The most important group of protectors are sulfhydryls, agents that contain a free or potentially free sulfur (S) atom in their structure. Examples of sulfhydryls include cysteine, cysteamine, and WR-2721. Sulfhydryls act as free radical scavengers that compete with oxygen for free radicals formed after the radiolysis of water. If the sulfhydryl binds to the free radical before the oxygen does, the free radical can decay back to a harmless chemical species instead of causing damage to vital structures in the cell. The ability of a radioprotector to diminish the effects of a dose of radiation is called the *dose reduction factor (DRF).* The equation for determining the DRF is as follows[27]:

$$DRF = \frac{\text{Radiation dose with the radioprotector}}{\substack{\text{Radiation dose without the radioprotector} \\ \text{to produce an equal biologic effect}}}$$

As with the oxygen effect, radioprotectors must be present during the irradiation. In practice, radioprotectors are administered at short time intervals (within 30 minutes) before radiation therapy. In general, this allows uptake by normal tissues so that they are protected without allowing enough time for significant tumor uptake. This therefore precludes protection of the tumor. If the radioprotector is effective, a DRF of 2.0 to 2.7 may be achieved, depending on the normal tissue that is involved. Similar to the oxygen effect, protec-

tion by sulfhydryls is much more significant against low-LET radiations that depend on free radical mechanisms, whereas little or no protection against high-LET radiations can be achieved. As with radiosensitizers, therapeutic doses of radioprotectors often cause side effects in patients. This has limited the widespread clinical use of radioprotectors.

Biologic factors. Cellular response is also affected by two important biologic factors: position in the cell cycle and ability to repair sublethal damage. Cellular radiosensitivity is dependent on the specific phase of the cell cycle containing the cells at the time of irradiation. (This is also referred to as *age response.*) In general, cells are most sensitive in the G2 and M phases, of intermediate sensitivity in the G1 phase, and most resistant in the S phase, especially during late S[54] (Fig. 4-13). This variation in response of cells should not be discounted because the Do for late S-phase cells may be as much as 2.5 times higher than for the same cells in the G2 and M phases. During irradiation of asynchronous cells with low doses, the majority of survivors are expected to be S-phase cells.

In addition to the variation in sensitivity caused by position in the cell cycle, Elkind and Sutton-Gilbert[21] showed in 1960 that cell survival increases if a dose of radiation is administered in fractions as a split dose instead of as a single dose (with the total dose remaining the same). Elkind and Sutton-Gilbert showed that, depending on the time interval between each fraction, the survival curve parameters n, Dq, and Do can remain the same as expected after a single-dose treatment. With low-LET radiations, Elkind and Sutton-Gilbert showed that the shoulder on the survival curve repeated after each fraction. This indicated that cells were

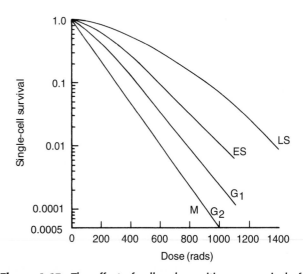

Figure 4-13. The effect of cell-cycle position on survival of a synchronous population of cells. The M and G$_2$ phases are the most radiosensitive, whereas the early S period *(ES)* and late S period *(LS)* are the most resistant. *(From Sinclair WK: Cyclic responses in mammalian cells in vitro, Radiat Res 33:620, 1968.)*

repairing sublethal damage from the first fraction before exposure to the second fraction. This repair of sublethal damage after low-LET irradiation appears to be completed in most cell lines tested within several hours of each exposure depending on the dose/fraction. This repair of sublethal damage in normal tissues during fractionated radiation therapy in the clinic may account for the sparing of normal tissues relative to tumors. In addition, hypoxia reduces a cell's capacity to repair sublethal damage. This may partially account for the favorable tumor responses after fractionation compared with single-dose radiation therapy.

RADIOSENSITIVITY

Law of Bergonié and Tribondeau

In 1906 two scientists named Bergonié and Tribondeau[8] performed experiments by using rodent testes to investigate reported clinical effects of radiation known at the time. Testes were chosen as the model for the experiments because they contain cells differing in function and mitotic activity. These cell types ranged from immature, mitotically active spermatogonia to mature, nondividing spermatozoa (sperm).

The results of the animal experiments indicated that immature, dividing cells were damaged at lower radiation doses than mature, nondividing cells. This result led to the formation of the **Law of Bergonié and Tribondeau,** which states that ionizing radiation is more effective against cells that (1) are actively mitotic, (2) are undifferentiated, and (3) have a long mitotic future. Bergonié and Tribondeau therefore defined radiosensitivity in terms of the mitotic activity and the level of differentiation. These two characteristics determined a normal cell's sensitivity to radiation. Therefore cells dividing more often are more radiosensitive than cells dividing less often or not all.

The level of maturity or differentiation of a cell refers to its level of functional and/or structural specialization. According to Bergonié and Tribondeau, cells that are undifferentiated (i.e., immature cells whose primary function is to divide and replace more mature cells lost from the population) are extremely radiosensitive. These cells are also known as *stem* or *precursor cells.* In the testes a spermatogonia is an example of a stem cell. A fully differentiated cell, known as an *end cell,* has a specialized structure or function, does not divide, and is radioresistant. Two examples of end cells are spermatozoa in the testes and erythrocytes in the circulating blood. In 1925 Ancel and Vitemberger[3] added to the findings of Bergonié and Tribondeau. Ancel and Vitemberger proposed that the environmental conditions of a cell before, during, or after radiation treatment could influence the extent and appearance of radiation damage. Current knowledge indicates that the expression of radiation damage generally occurs when the cell is stressed, usually during reproduction. The sensitivity of a cell to radiation can also be modified. This change in sensitivity is known as *conditional sensitivity.*

Cell Populations

In 1968 Rubin and Casarett[47] grouped mammalian cell populations into five basic categories based on radiation sensitivity (Table 4-2). The endpoint chosen was radiation-induced cell death. The most radiosensitive of these groups is known as *vegetative intermitotic (VIM) cells.* VIM cells are rapidly dividing, undifferentiated cells with short life spans. Examples include basal cells, crypt cells, erythroblasts, and type A spermatogonia.

The second most radiosensitive group is known as *differentiating intermitotic (DIM) cells.* These cells are also actively mitotic but a little more differentiated than VIM

Table 4-2	Classification of mammalian cells according to their characteristics and radiosensitivities		
Cell Type	**Characteristics**	**Examples**	**Radiosensitivity**
VIM	Divide regularly and rapidly, are undifferentiated, and do not differentiate between divisions	Type A spermatogonia, erythroblasts, crypt cells, and basal cells	Extremely high
DIM	Actively divide, are more differentiated than VIMs, and differentiate between divisions	Intermediate spermatogonia and myelocytes	High
Vessels/connective tissue	Irregularly divide and are more differentiated than VIMs or DIMs	Endothelial cells and fibroblasts	Intermediate
RPM	Do not normally divide but retain capability of division and are variably differentiated	Parenchymal cells of liver and lymphocytes*	Low
FPM	Do not divide and are highly differentiated	Nerve cells muscle cells, erythrocytes, and spermatozoa	Extremely low

From Travis EL: *Primer of medical radiobiology,* ed 2, St Louis, 1989, Mosby.
*Lymphocytes, although classified as relatively radioresistant by their characteristics, are extremely radiosensitive.
DIM, Differentiating intermitotic; *FPM,* fixed postmitotic; *RPM,* reverting postmitotic; *VIM,* vegetative intermitotic.

cells. In fact, VIM cells such as type A spermatogonia divide and mature into DIM cells such as type B spermatogonia.

The third group of cells, known as *multipotential connective tissue cells,* is intermediate in radiosensitivity. These cells (such as endothelial cells of blood vessels and fibroblasts of connective tissue) divide irregularly and are more differentiated than VIM and DIM cells.

The fourth group, *reverting postmitotic (RPM) cells,* normally do not divide but are capable of doing so. RPM cells typically live longer and are more differentiated than the three previously discussed groups. These cells, including liver cells, are relatively radioresistant. Another example of an RPM cell is the mature lymphocyte. This cell, however, is very radiosensitive despite its characteristics and is therefore an exception to the law of Bergonié and Tribondeau.

The most radioresistant group of cells in the body are known as *fixed postmitotic (FPM) cells.* FPM cells are highly differentiated, do not divide, and may or may not be replaced when they die. Examples include certain nerve cells, muscle cells, erythrocytes, and spermatozoa.

Tissue and Organ Sensitivity

Because radiosensitivities of specific cells in the body are now known, that information can be used to determine radiosensitivities of organized tissues and organs. Structurally, tissues and organs are composed of two compartments: the parenchyma and stroma. The parenchymal compartment contains characteristic cells of that tissue or organ. VIM, DIM, RPM, and FPM cells are examples of parenchymal cells. Regardless of the types of parenchymal cells in a tissue or organ, they also have a supporting stromal compartment.[61] The stroma consists of connective tissue and the vasculature and is generally considered intermediate in radiosensitivity, according to Rubin and Casarett.[47]

The radiosensitivity of a tissue or organ is a function of the most sensitive cell it contains.[47] For example, the testes and bone marrow are considered radiosensitive because of the presence of VIM stem cells in their parenchymal compartments. In these two organs, parenchymal cells are damaged at lower radiation doses than stromal cells (fibroblasts and endothelial cells). Radiation-induced sterility in males can occur after high doses because of destruction of immature spermatogonia cells that were destined to become mature spermatozoa.[69] A decrease in circulating erythrocytes in the blood after irradiation is due to destruction of the more sensitive stem cell (erythroblast) in the bone marrow.[59]

Tissues and organs that contain only RPM or FPM parenchymal cells are therefore more radioresistant. Examples include the liver, muscle, brain, and spinal cord. In this situation, stromal cells are damaged at lower doses than parenchymal cells. Blood vessels in these organs become damaged, thus decreasing blood flow and therefore the supply of oxygen and nutrients to the parenchymal cells. Therefore radiation-induced death of parenchymal cells in these organs is predominantly due to stromal damage. This form of indirect cell death is a significant mechanism of radiation damage in radioresistant tissues and organs.

SYSTEMIC RESPONSE TO RADIATION

Response and Healing

Response to ionizing radiation treatment refers to visible (detectable) structural and functional changes that a dose produces in a certain period. Response at all levels (whether in a cell, a tissue, an organ, a system, or the entire organism) is a function of the dose administered, the volume irradiated, and the time of observation after exposure. With the exception of cataracts of the ocular lens, radiation-induced changes are neither unique nor distinguishable from biologic effects caused by other forms of trauma.

Structural or morphologic response after irradiation is usually grouped into two phases: early or acute changes observed within 6 months of treatment and late or chronic changes occurring more than 6 months later.[61] The appearance of late changes is a consequence of early changes that were irreversible and progressive. The probability of late changes occurring depends on the dose administered, the volume irradiated, and the healing ability of the irradiated structure (organ).

Organ healing can occur after radiation exposure by the process of regeneration or repair.[61] *Regeneration* refers to the replacement of damaged cells by the same cell type. Regeneration results in partial or total reversal of early radiation changes and is likely to occur in organs containing actively dividing VIM and DIM parenchymal cells. Examples include the skin, small intestine, and bone marrow. Regeneration is the desired healing process and can restore an organ to its preirradiated state.

Irreversible early changes, however, heal by the process of repair. *Repair* refers to the replacement of damaged cells by a different cell type, thus resulting in scar formation or fibrosis. Healing by repair does not restore an organ to its preirradiated state. Repair can occur in any organ and is more likely after high doses (1000 cGy or above) that destroy parenchymal cells, thus making regeneration impossible. Repair is the predominant healing process in radioresistant organs containing RPM and FPM parenchymal cells that do not divide or have lost the ability to do so.

Under conditions that produce massive and extensive damage to the organ, neither healing process may occur and tissue death or necrosis results. Therefore the type of healing if any that occurs is a function of the dose received and volume of the organ receiving it.

The other important factor that must be considered is the time after the treatment. In general, radiosensitive organs (e.g., skin) respond faster and more severely than radioresistant organs.[61] The reverse situation may hold true at a later time. For example, irradiation of skin and lung tissue with a dose of 2000 cGy induces severe early skin changes but minimal early lung changes (within 6 months). However, if the same tissues are examined 6 to 12 months after irradiation, minimal late changes are found in the skin but severe late changes are observed in the lung. This rate of response depends mostly on the cell cycle or generation times of the parenchymal cells in each organ. Because most cells die when attempting to divide after irradiation, cells with short cycle times show radiation damage sooner than cells with long cycle times. In comparing skin and lung parenchymal cells, cycle times are considerably shorter for parenchymal cells of the skin.

General Organ Changes

The most common early or acute changes after irradiation include inflammation, edema, and possible hemorrhaging in the exposed area. If doses are high enough, these early changes may progress to characteristic late or chronic changes, including fibrosis, atrophy, and ulceration. These late changes are not reversible and therefore permanent. The most severe late response is tissue necrosis or death. The sensitivity of the most radiosensitive organ of a system determines the general response of that system in the body. The Radiation Therapy Oncology Group (RTOG) has summarized the acute and chronic effects of radiation into various categories or grades based on the severity of the clinical response (Tables 4-3 and 4-4).[62]

TOTAL-BODY RESPONSE TO RADIATION

This section involves specific signs and symptoms induced by exposure of the entire body at one time to ionizing radiation. The total-body response to radiation is presented in terms of three radiation syndromes.[27] Characteristics of each syndrome are dependent on the dose received and exposure

Table 4-3	RTOG acute radiation morbidity scoring criteria				
Organ/Tissue	Grade 0	Grade 1	Grade 2	Grade 3	Grade 4
Skin	No change over baseline	Follicular, faint or dull erythema; epilation; dry desquamation; decreased sweating	Tender or bright erythema; patchy, moist desquamation; moderate edema	Confluent, moist desquamation other than skin folds, pitting edema	Ulceration, hemorrhage, necrosis
Mucous membrane	No change over baseline	Injection/may experience mild pain not requiring analgesic	Patchy mucositis that may produce an inflammatory serosanguineous discharge; may experience moderate pain requiring analgesia	Confluent fibrinous mucositis; may include severe pain requiring narcotic	Ulceration, hemorrhage, or necrosis
Eye	No change	Mild conjunctivitis with or without scleral injection; increased tearing	Moderate conjunctivitis with or without keratitis requiring steroids and/or antibiotics; dry eye requiring artificial tears; iritis with photophobia	Severe keratitis with corneal ulceration; objective decrease in visual acuity or in visual fields; acute glaucoma; panophthalmitis	Loss of vision (unilateral or bilateral)
Ear	No change over baseline	Mild external otitis with erythema, pruritus, secondary to dry desquamation not requiring medication. Audiogram unchanged from baseline	Moderate external otitis requiring topical medication; serious otitis media; hypoacusis on testing only	Severe external otitis with discharge or moist desquamation; symptomatic hypoacusis; tinnitus, not drug related	Deafness
Salivary gland	No change over baseline	Mild mouth dryness; slightly thickened saliva; may have slightly altered taste such as metallic taste; these changes not reflected in alteration in baseline feeding behavior, such as increased use of liquids with meals	Moderate to complete dryness; thick, sticky saliva; markedly altered taste	—	Acute salivary gland necrosis

continued

			RTOG acute radiation morbidity scoring criteria—cont'd		

Table 4-3

Organ/Tissue	Grade 0	Grade 1	Grade 2	Grade 3	Grade 4
Pharynx and esophagus	No change over baseline	Mild dysphagia or odynophagia; may require topical anesthetic or nonnarcotic analgesics; may require soft diet	Moderate dysphagia or odynophagia; may require narcotic analgesics; may require puree or liquid diet	Severe dysphagia or odynophagia with dehydration or weight loss (>15% from pretreatment baseline) requiring NG feeding tube, IV fluids or hyperalimentation	Complete obstruction, ulceration, perforation, fistula
Larynx	No change over baseline	Mild or intermittent hoarseness; cough not requiring antitussive; erythema of mucosa	Persistent hoarseness but able to vocalize; referred ear pain, sore throat, patchy fibrinous exudate or mild arytenoid edema not requiring narcotic; cough requiring antitussive	Whispered speech, throat pain or referred ear pain requiring narcotic; confluent fibrinous exudate, marked arytenoid edema	Marked dyspnea, stridor, or hemoptysis with tracheostomy or intubation necessary
Upper GI	No change	Anorexia with ≤5% weight loss from pretreatment baseline; nausea not requiring antiemetics; abdominal discomfort not requiring para-sympatholytic drugs or analgesics	Anorexia with ≤15% weight loss from pretreatment baseline; nausea and/or vomiting requiring antiemetics; abdominal pain requiring analgesics	Anorexia with >15% weight loss from pretreatment baseline or requiring NG tube or parenteral support. Nausea and/or vomiting requiring tube or parenteral support; abdominal pain, severe despite medication; hematemesis or melena; abdominal distention (flat plate radiograph demonstrates distended bowel loops	Ileus, subacute or acute obstruction, perforation, GI bleeding requiring transfusion; abdominal pain requiring tube decompression or bowel diversion
Lower GI including pelvis	No change	Increased frequency or change in quality of bowel habits not requiring medication; rectal discomfort not requiring analgesics	Diarrhea requiring parasympatholytic drugs (e.g., Lomotil); mucus discharge not necessitating sanitary pads; rectal or abdominal pain requiring analgesics	Diarrhea requiring parenteral support; severe mucus or blood discharge necessitating sanitary bags; abdominal distention (flat plate radiograph demonstrates distended bowel loops)	Acute or subacute obstruction, fistula or perforation; GI bleeding requiring transfusion; abdominal pain or tenesmus requiring tube decompression or bowel diversion
Lung	No change	Mild symptoms of dry cough or dyspnea on exertion	Persistent cough requiring narcotic, antitussive agents; dyspnea with minimal effort but not at rest	Severe cough unresponsive to narcotic antitussive agent or dyspnea at rest; clinical or radiologic evidence of acute pneumonitis; intermittent oxygen or steroids may be required	Severe respiratory insufficiency; continuous oxygen or assisted ventilation

continued

Table 4-3	RTOG acute radiation morbidity scoring criteria—cont'd				
Organ/Tissue	Grade 0	Grade 1	Grade 2	Grade 3	Grade 4
Genitourinary	No change	Frequency of urination or nocturia twice pretreatment habit; dysuria, urgency not requiring medication	Frequency of urination or nocturia, which is less frequent than every hour. Dysuria, urgency, bladder spasm requiring local anesthetic (e.g., Pyridium)	Frequency with urgency and nocturia hourly or more frequently; dysuria, pelvis pain or bladder spasm requiring regular, frequent narcotic; gross hematuria with or without clot passage	Hematuria requiring transfusion; acute bladder obstruction not secondary to clot passage, ulceration or necrosis
Heart	No change over baseline	Asymptomatic but objective evidence of ECG changes or pericardial abnormalities without evidence of other heart disease	Symptomatic with ECG changes and radiologic findings of congestive heart failure or pericardial disease; no specific treatment required	Congestive heart failure, angina pectoris, pericardial disease responding to therapy	Congestive heart failure, angina pectoris, pericardial disease, arrhythmias not responsive to nonsurgical measures
CNS	No change	Fully functional status (i.e., able to work) with minor neurologic findings, no medication needed	Neurologic findings present sufficient to require home case; nursing assistance may be required; medications including steroids; antiseizure agents may be required	Neurologic findings requiring hospitalization for initial management	Serious neurologic impairment that includes paralysis, coma or seizures >3 per week despite medication; hospitalization required
Hematologic WBC (×1000)	≥4.0	3.0-4.0	2.0-3.0	1.0-2.0	<1.0
Platelets (×1000)	>100	75-100	50-75	25-50	<25 or spontaneous bleeding
Neutrophils	≥1.9	1.5-1.9	1.0-1.5	0.5-1.0	≤0.5 or sepsis
Hemoglobin (g %)	>11	11-9.5	9.5-7.5	7.5-5.0	—
Hematocrit (%)	≥32	28-32	≤28	Packed cell transfusion required	—

From Trotti A, Byhardt R, Stetz J, et al: Common toxicity criteria: version 2.0. An improved reference for grading the acute effects of cancer treatment: impact on radiotherapy, *Int J Radiat Oncol Biol Phys* 47:13-47, 2000.

CNS, Central nervous system; *ECG,* electrocardiogram; *GI,* gastrointestinal; *IV,* intravenous; *NG,* nasogastric.

Guidelines: The acute morbidity criteria are used to score and grade toxicity from radiation therapy. The criteria are relevant from day 1, the commencement of therapy, through day 90. Thereafter, the EORTC/RTOG Criteria of Late Effects are to be used.

The evaluator must attempt to discriminate between disease- and treatment-related signs and symptoms.

An accurate baseline evaluation before commencement of therapy is necessary.

All toxicities Grade 3, 4 or 5* must be verified by the principal investigator.

*Any toxicity that caused death is graded 5.

Table 4-4	**RTOG/EORTC late radiation morbidity scoring scheme**					
Organ/Tissue	**Grade 0**	**Grade 1**	**Grade 2**	**Grade 3**	**Grade 4**	**Grade 5**
Skin	None	Slight atrophy; pigmentation change; some hair loss	Patch atrophy; moderate telangiectasia; total hair loss	Marked atrophy; gross telangiectasia	Ulceration	Death directly related to radiation late effect for all tissue types
Subcutaneous tissue	None	Slight induration (fibrosis) and loss of subcutaneous fat	Moderate fibrosis but asymptomatic Slight field contracture <10% linear reduction	Severe induration and loss of subcutaneous tissue Field contracture >10% linear measurement	Necrosis	
Mucous membrane	None	Slight atrophy and dryness	Moderate atrophy and telangiectasia; little mucus	Marked atrophy with complete dryness; severe telangiectasia	Ulceration	
Salivary glands	None	Slight dryness of mouth; good response on stimulation	Moderate dryness of mouth; poor response on stimulation	Complete dryness of mouth; no response on stimulation	Fibrosis	
Spinal cord	None	Mild Lhermitte's syndrome	Severe Lhermitte's syndrome	Objective neurologic findings at or below cord level treated	Mono-, paraquadriplegia	
Brain	None	Mild headache; slight lethargy	Moderate headache; great lethargy	Severe headaches; severe CNS dysfunction (partial loss of power or dyskinesia)	Seizures or paralysis; coma	
Eye	None	Asymptomatic cataract; minor corneal ulceration or keratitis	Symptomatic cataract; moderate corneal ulceration; minor retinopathy or glaucoma	Severe keratitis; severe retinopathy or detachment; severe glaucoma	Panophthalmitis; blindness	
Larynx	None	Hoarseness; slight arytenoid edema	Moderate arytenoid edema; chondritis	Severe edema; severe chondritis	Necrosis	
Lung	None	Asymptomatic or mild symptoms (dry cough); slight radiographic appearances	Moderate symptomatic fibrosis or pneumonitis (severe cough); low grade fever; patchy radiographic appearances	Severe symptomatic fibrosis or pneumonitis; dense radiographic changes	Severe respiratory insufficiency; continuous O_2; assisted ventilation	
Heart	None	Asymptomatic or mild symptoms; transient T-wave inversion and ST changes; sinus tachycardia >110 beats/min (at rest)	Moderate angina on effort; mild pericarditis; normal heart size; persistent abnormal T wave and ST changes; low QRS	Severe angina; pericardial effusion; constrictive pericarditis; moderate heart failure; cardiac enlargement; ECG abnormalities	Tamponade; severe heart failure; severe constrictive pericarditis	
Esophagus	None	Mild fibrosis; slight difficulty in swallowing solids; no pain on swallowing	Unable to take solid food normally; swallowing semisolid food; dilation may be indicated	Severe fibrosis; able to swallow only liquids; may have pain on swallowing; dilation required	Necrosis; perforation; fistula	

continued

Table 4-4	RTOG/EORTC late radiation morbidity scoring scheme—cont'd					
Organ/Tissue	Grade 0	Grade 1	Grade 2	Grade 3	Grade 4	Grade 5
Small and large intestine	None	Mild diarrhea; mild cramping; bowel movement 5 times daily; slight rectal discharge or bleeding	Moderate diarrhea and colic; bowel movement >5 times daily; excessive rectal mucus or intermittent bleeding	Obstruction or bleeding requiring surgery	Necrosis; perforation; fistula	
Liver	None	Mild lassitude; nausea, dyspepsia; slightly abnormal liver function	Moderate symptoms; some abnormal liver function tests; serum albumin normal	Disabling hepatitic insufficiency; liver function tests grossly abnormal; low albumin; edema or ascites	Necrosis; hepatic coma or encephalopathy	
Kidney	None	Transient albuminuria; no hypertension; mild impairment of renal function; urea 25-35 mg%; creatinine 1.5-2.0 mg%; creatinine clearance >75%	Persistent moderate albuminuria (2+); mild hypertension; no related anemia; moderate impairment of renal function; urea >36-60 mg%; creatinine clearance (50%-74%)	Severe albuminuria; severe hypertension; persistent anemia (<10 g%); severe renal failure; urea >60 mg%; creatinine >4.0 mg%; creatinine clearance <50%	Malignant hypertension; uremic coma; urea >100%	
Bladder	None	Slight epithelial atrophy; minor telangiectasia (microscopic hematuria)	Moderate frequency; generalized telangiectasia; intermittent macroscopic hematuria	Severe frequency and dysuria; severe generalized telangiectasia (often with petechiae); frequent hematuria; reduction in bladder capacity (<150 ml)	Necrosis; contracted bladder (capacity <100 ml); severe hemorrhagic cystitis	
Bone	None	Asymptomatic; no growth retardation; reduced bone density	Moderate pain or tenderness; growth retardation; irregular bone sclerosis	Severe pain or tenderness; complete arrest of bone growth; dense bone sclerosis	Necrosis; spontaneous fracture	
Joint	None	Mild joint stiffness; slight limitation of movement	Moderate stiffness; intermittent or moderate joint pain; moderate limitation of movement	Severe joint stiffness; pain with severe limitation of movement	Necrosis; complete fixation	

From Trotti A, Byhardt R, Stetz J, et al: Common toxicity criteria: version 2.0. An improved reference for grading the acute effects of cancer treatment: impact on radiotherapy, *Int J Radiat Oncol Biol Phys* 47:13-47, 2000.

Cox, JD, Stetz J, Pajak TF: Toxicity criteria of the radiation therapy oncology group (RTOG) and the European organization for research and treatment of cancer (EORTC), *Int J Radiat Oncol Biol Phys* 31:1341-1346, 1995.

CNS, Central nervous system; *ECG,* electrocardiogram.

conditions. Three specific exposure conditions apply in dealing with radiation syndromes: (1) exposure must be acute (minutes); (2) total or nearly total-body exposure must occur; and (3) exposure must be from an external penetrating source rather than ingested, inhaled, or implanted radioactive sources.[61]

Radiation Syndromes in Humans

Although an abundance of animal data regarding the effects of total-body exposure to radiation exists, considerably less human data under the same conditions are available. However, human data are available from (1) industrial and laboratory accidents, (2) fallout from atomic bomb test sites,

(3) therapeutic medical exposures, (4) individuals exposed at Hiroshima and Nagasaki, and (5) the nuclear reactor accident at Chernobyl in the Soviet Union. As with lower animals, humans suffer the three radiation syndromes if the same exposure conditions are met.[27] Table 4-5 contains a summary of the acute radiation syndromes in humans after whole-body irradiation.

Hematopoietic syndrome. The hematopoietic syndrome in humans is induced by total-body doses of 100 to 1000 cGy.[27] The $LD_{50/60}$ for humans is estimated to be between 350 and 450 cGy but varies with age, health, and gender. Typically, females are more resistant than males, and the extremely young and old tend to be a little more sensitive than middle-aged persons. The prodromal stage or syndrome is observed within hours after exposure and is characterized by nausea and vomiting. The latent stage then occurs and lasts from a few days up to 3 weeks. Although the affected individual feels well at this time, bone marrow stem cells are dying. Peripheral blood cell counts decrease during the subsequent manifest illness stage at 3 to 5 weeks after exposure. Depression of all blood cell counts, termed *pancytopenia,* results in anemia (from a decreased number of erythrocytes), hemorrhaging (from a decreased number of platelets), and serious infection (from a decreased number of leukocytes).

The probability of survival decreases with an increasing dose. Most individuals receiving doses less than 300 cGy survives and eventually recovers over the next 3 to 6 months. As the dose increases, the survival time decreases. After 300 to 500 cGy, death may occur in 4 to 6 weeks. After 500 to 1000 cGy, death is likely within 2 weeks.[61] No record exists of human survival when the total body dose exceeds 1000 cGy.[27] The primary causes of death from the hematopoietic syndrome are infection and hemorrhaging after destruction of the bone marrow.

Gastrointestinal syndrome. If the total body dose is between 1000 and 10,000 cGy, the gastrointestinal syndrome is induced.[27] This syndrome may also be induced by a dose as low as 600 cGy and overlaps with the cerebrovascular syndrome above doses of 5000 cGy. The mean survival time for this syndrome is 3 to 10 days or up to 2 weeks with medical support and is largely independent of the actual dose received. The prodromal stage occurs within hours after exposure and is characterized by nausea, vomiting, diarrhea, and cramps. The latent stage then occurs 2 to 5 days after exposure. At 5 to 10 days after exposure, nausea, vomiting, diarrhea, and fever mark the manifest illness stage. Death occurs during the second week after exposure.

The gastrointestinal syndrome occurs as a result of damage to the gastrointestinal tract and bone marrow. As discussed previously, the small intestine is the most radiosensitive portion of the digestive system.[68] After exposure to doses in excess of 1000 cGy, severe depopulation of crypt cells leads to partial or complete denudation of the villi lining the lumen of the small intestine. Consequences of this damage include decreased absorption of materials across the intestinal wall, leakage of fluids into the lumen (thus resulting in dehydration), and overwhelming infection as bacteria gain access to the circulating blood. Significant changes in bone marrow also occur, highlighted by a severe decrease in circulating leukocytes. However, death occurs before the other peripheral blood cell counts significantly decrease. Despite attempts at regeneration of crypt cells in the small intestine, bone marrow damage likely leads to death as a result of the overwhelming infection, dehydration, and electrolyte imbalance.

Table 4-5	Summary of acute radiation syndromes in humans after whole-body irradiation				
Syndrome	**Dose Range**	**Time of Death**	**Organ and System Damaged**	**Signs and Symptoms**	**Recovery Time**
Hematopoietic	100-1000 cGy*	3 weeks to 2 months	Bone marrow	Decreased number of stem cells in bone marrow, increased amount of fat in bone marrow, pancytopenia, anemia, hemorrhage, and infection	Dose dependent— 3 weeks to 6 months; some individuals do not survive
Gastrointestinal	1000-5000 cGy†	3 to 10 days	Small intestine	Denudation of villi in small intestine, neutropenia, infection, bone marrow depression, electrolyte imbalance, and watery diarrhea	None
Cerebrovascular	> 5000 cGy	< 3 days	Brain	Vasculitis, edema, and meningitis	None

Modified from Travis EL: *Primer of medical radiobiology,* ed 2, St Louis, 1989, Mosby.
R, Roentgen.
*$LD_{50/60}$ for humans in this dose range (450 cGy).
†LD_{100} for humans in this dose range (1000 cGy).

Cerebrovascular syndrome.   The third and final radiation syndrome is the cerebrovascular syndrome. This syndrome, which was formerly known as the *central nervous system syndrome,* occurs exclusively above 10,000 cGy but can overlap with the gastrointestinal syndrome because it can be induced by a dose as low as 5000 cGy.[27] Death after such high total-body doses occurs in several days or less. The prodromal stage lasts only minutes to several hours (depending on the dose) and is characterized by nervousness, confusion, severe nausea and vomiting, loss of consciousness, and a burning sensation in the skin. The latent period (if distinguishable) lasts only several hours or less. Within 5 to 6 hours after exposure, the manifest illness stage begins and is characterized by watery diarrhea, convulsions, coma, and death.

The cause of death from the cerebrovascular syndrome is not completely known at this time. At autopsy, brain parenchymal cells appear almost completely normal despite the high dose. These parenchymal cells are extremely radioresistant FPM cells, according to Rubin and Casarett.[47] Autopsy findings show extensive blood vessel (stromal) damage in the brain, thus resulting in vasculitis, meningitis, and edema in the cranial vault. The resulting increase in intracranial pressure is probably the major cause of death. In addition, peripheral blood counts and the villi of the small intestine do not.exhibit significant changes in these individuals when examined at autopsy. This is due to the exposed person not living long enough for these effects to become evident.

Response of the Embryo and Fetus

Radiation exposure can also damage the developing embryo and fetus in utero. Generally, in utero radiation damage is manifested as lethal effects, congenital abnormalities present at birth, or late effects observed years later. These effects can be produced by (1) irradiation of the sperm or ovum before fertilization, thus resulting in inherited effects, or (2) exposure of the fetus to radiation, thus resulting in congenital defects. This section deals only with congenital abnormalities resulting from radiation exposure.

Stages of fetal development.   The husband-and-wife research team of Russell and Russell[49] divided fetal development into three stages: preimplantation, major organogenesis, and the fetal growth stage. Extensive mouse studies have established that the effect induced by radiation depends not only on the radiation dose, but also on the time of the exposure's occurrence during gestation.[48] In humans the preimplantation stage occurs from conception (day 0) to 10 days after conception. During this time the fertilized ovum is actively dividing, thus forming a ball of highly undifferentiated cells.

The newly formed ball of cells, known as the *embryo,* then implants in the uterine wall and begins the major organogenesis stage (from day 10 to week 6). During this time, on specific gestational days, embryonic cells differentiate into the stem cells that eventually form each organ in the body. At the end of the sixth week the embryo is known as a *fetus* and enters the fetal growth stage, in which it continues to grow until birth. The central nervous system in the fetus differs from that in the adult because the neuroblasts (stem cells) of the fetus are still mitotically active and not fully differentiated. Therefore unlike that in the adult, the fetal central nervous system is responsive to radiation and can be damaged at relatively low doses.

Radiation effects on humans in utero.   Radiation effects on human embryos have been investigated with data sources that were described previously (atomic bomb survivors in Japan after World War II, fallout exposures, occupational exposures, and diagnostic or therapeutic exposures of pregnant women).[26,32] A definitive cause-and-effect relationship between radiation and a specific abnormality is difficult to prove in human beings. Two major reasons account for this: (1) the background incidence of spontaneous congenital abnormalities is approximately 6% and (2) radiation does not induce unique congenital abnormalities (excluding cataracts). Therefore implicating a certain radiation exposure as the sole cause of a specific congenital abnormality is difficult. The results of animal studies have been extrapolated to humans to allow predictions with regard to effects that might occur in irradiated human embryos and fetuses (Fig. 4-14). However, the assumption should not be made that in utero effects in mice will be observed under the same conditions in human beings. Viable comparisons may indicate that the mouse embryo is slightly more radioresistant than the human embryo. In addition, the mouse gestational period ends in 20 days versus 270 days or more in human beings. Therefore although the same developmental stages occur for the most

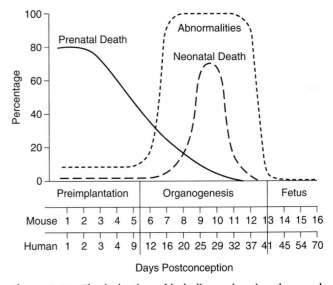

Figure 4-14. The induction of lethality and major abnormalities during in utero exposure on different gestational days in the mouse embryo using 2.0 Gy. Lower scale indicated Rugh's time estimates for the three stages in the human embryo. *(From Travis EL: Primer of medical radiobiology, ed 2, Philadelphia, 1989, Mosby, with permission.)*

part in mice and humans, they certainly occur much more rapidly in mice.[61] This should be taken into account during comparisons of animal and human radiation effects in utero.

Unfortunately, human data exist for radiation effects from in utero exposure. A report in 1930 by Murphy and Goldstein[38] described congenital defects (microcephaly) attributed to radiation exposure in utero. In one study of children born to 11 women who were pregnant and received high doses from the bomb dropped in Hiroshima, 7 of the 11 children (64%) had microcephaly and were mentally retarded.[43] In another study of 30 children were irradiated in utero at Nagasaki, 17 (57%) were affected (7 fetal deaths, 6 neonatal deaths, and 4 surviving children were mentally retarded).[39] Table 4-6 illustrates the correlation between gestational stage and the probability of developing congenital malformations.

Dekaban[18] in 1968 studied children born to women irradiated with a therapeutic dose of 250 cGy during various stages of gestation. The results of this study indicated that exposure to the dose during the first 2 to 3 weeks of gestation produced a high frequency of prenatal death but few severe abnormalities in surviving children who were brought to term (similar to the mouse studies). Irradiation between 4 and 11 weeks correlated with severe central nervous system and skeletal abnormalities. The same dose (250 cGy) administered between the eleventh and sixteenth week frequently resulted in mental retardation and microcephaly, whereas irradiation after the twentieth week resulted in functional defects such as sterility.

In summary, although difficult to prove conclusively, the embryo and fetus are considered to be the most radiosensitive forms of animals and humans. Radiation, if it must be administered during a known pregnancy, should be delayed as much as possible because the fetus is more radioresistant than the embryo. As mentioned previously, the most radiosensitive period for induction of abnormalities in humans is between days 23 and 37. These effects usually involve the central nervous system and most commonly include microcephaly, mental retardation, sensory organ damage, and stunted growth. Skeletal changes (bone) appear to be most prevalent when radiation is administered between weeks 3 and 20.

LATE EFFECTS OF RADIATION

The previous section dealt with the total-body response to high doses of radiation, which usually results in lethality. Of equal and possibly even more concern is the biologic response resulting from exposure to much lower doses of radiation. Because the latent period for an effect is inversely proportional to radiation dose, the biologic response to low doses is not observable for extended periods, ranging from years to generations.[27] These effects are therefore known as *late effects* and are termed *somatic effects* if body cells are involved or *genetic effects* if reproductive (germ) cells are involved.

Somatic Effects (Carcinogenesis)

Historical background. The most important late somatic effect induced by radiation is carcinogenesis.[14,63,65] Radiation is therefore classified as a *carcinogen,* or *cancer-causing agent.* In 1902 (only 7 years after Roentgen's discovery of the x-ray) the first reported case of radiation-induced carcinoma appeared in the literature. By 1910 at least 100 cases of skin cancer were reported in radiologists and radiation oncologists who were unaware of the potential hazards of this new modality.

Carcinogenesis is considered to be an all-or-nothing event. This means that any dose, no matter how low, has some potential of inducing cancer. Cancer induction is therefore a nonthreshold event with the probability of an effect increasing as the dose increases. Carcinogenesis is therefore an example of a stochastic effect, in which every dose carries some magnitude of risk.[27]

Sufficient human data exist to implicate radiation as a cancer-causing agent. Most of the early data involve occupational exposures by radiation scientists, clinicians, and therapists who were chronically exposed to various radiation sources before the risks of such exposures were known. Ionizing radiation has been implicated as a cause of skin cancer, leukemia, osteosarcoma, lung cancer, breast cancer, and thyroid cancer.

Leukemia. Radiation was first implicated as a cause of leukemia in 1911. That study involved 11 cases of leukemia in occupationally exposed individuals.[61] Atomic bomb survivors in Hiroshima and Nagasaki had higher incidences of leukemia than the nonexposed population.[27] Early radiologists in the United States who died between 1948 and 1961 had a much higher frequency of leukemia (300%) than the general population.[20,33] However, a similar study involving British radiologists showed no increased leukemia incidence

Table 4-6	Summary of radiation effects on the embryo and fetus*			
Stage of Gestation	**Growth Retardation**	**Death**	**Microcephaly and Mental Retardation**
Preimplantation	None	Embryonic death and resorption	None
Organogenesis	Temporary	Neonatal death	Very high risk
Fetal	Permanent	Approximately equal to the LD$_{50}$ in adult	High risk

*Summarized from Hall EJ: *Radiobiology for the radiobiologist,* Philadelphia, 2000, JB Lippincott.

in an early group (before 1921) compared with later groups who used some level of radiation safety.[13]

The latent period for leukemia induction by radiation is usually 4 to 7 years with peak incidence approximately 7 to 10 years after exposure. This period is much shorter than that observed for radiation-induced solid tumors, which have latent periods ranging from 20 to 30 years or longer.[27]

Radiation induction of leukemia is somewhat specific in that only certain types of leukemia show an increased incidence in irradiated individuals. For example, only acute and chronic myeloid leukemia types are more prevalent in irradiated adults, whereas acute lymphocytic leukemia is more common in irradiated children.[15] Radiation exposure does not seem to affect the incidence of chronic lymphocytic leukemia. The available evidence suggests that leukemia induction is a nonthreshold (stochastic), linear response to radiation[61] (Fig. 4-15). However, other cancers induced by radiation may follow linear-quadratic rather than a linear relationship to radiation dose.[27]

Skin carcinoma. The first reported case of radiation-induced skin cancer (which occurred on the hand of a radiologist) was in 1902.[40] Because early x-ray machines were crude, radiologists placed their hands in the beam path to check its efficiency. This led to early skin changes (erythema) that were used to gauge the output of the beam, but skin tumors were observed years later in many of these individuals. Patients treated with radiation for several benign conditions such as acne and ringworm of the scalp also showed an increased incidence of skin cancer year's later.[2] As a result of modern radiation safety procedures, skin cancers in radiation workers are no longer observed.

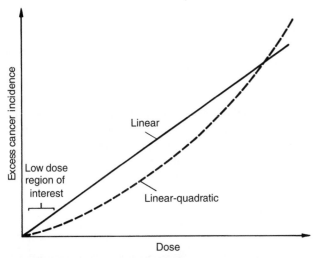

Figure 4-15. A schematic of the linear and linear-quadratic models used to extrapolate the incidence of cancer from high-dose data down to low doses. Both models fit high-dose data as well, but at low doses the estimated incidence depends on the model. *(From Travis EL: Primer of medical radiobiology, ed 2, St. Louis, 1989, Mosby.)*

Osteosarcoma. The most striking example of radiation-induced osteosarcoma, or bone cancer, is the group of young female watch-dial painters who used radium to paint clock faces for a company in northern New Jersey from 1915 to 1930.[34] These workers regularly licked their brushes (which contained radium paint) to make the brush tip come to a point before painting the watch dials. This resulted in chronic ingestion of radium, which is a bone-seeking radioactive element.[24] Of the several hundred workers exposed this way, approximately 40 cases of osteosarcoma were observed years later. The dose response for bone cancer in this group followed a linear-quadratic relationship that was dependent on the activities of the two radium isotopes (^{226}Ra and ^{228}Ra) contained in the paint.[46]

Lung carcinoma. German pitchblende miners in Germany more than 500 years ago suffered from a condition known as *mountain sickness,* which was later determined to be lung cancer.[27] Inhaling chronic amounts of radon gas in the air of the mines, these miners exposed their lungs to high-LET alpha particles that were emitted as the radon decayed. Uranium miners in the United States who were studied from 1950 to 1967 also had an increased incidence of lung cancer, most likely for the same reasons.[50] Radon gas and its decay products are now known to be significant contributors (200 mrem/yr) to annual background radiation levels and are the major risk factors for lung cancer in nonsmokers.

Thyroid carcinoma. Irradiation of enlarged thymuses in children before the 1930s over the dose range from 1200 to 6000 cGy was a popular treatment.[53,60] Unfortunately, a 100-fold increase in thyroid cancer was observed in these children. An increased incidence of thyroid cancer also occurred in individuals exposed as children from the bombs in Hiroshima and Nagasaki. Some of these individuals who developed thyroid cancer may have received doses as low as 100 cGy. Extensive follow-up is required to track the occurrence of these tumors because of their typical latent period of 10 to 20 years (which varies inversely with the dose that is received).

Breast carcinoma. Three major groups of irradiated women with increased incidences of breast cancer seem to implicate radiation as the causative agent[27]: (1) irradiated female survivors in Hiroshima and Nagasaki, Japan, (2) Canadian women in a Nova Scotia sanitorium who had tuberculosis and were subjected to numerous fluoroscopies, and (3) women treated for benign breast diseases such as postpartum mastitis. The best data that are available (with the Canadian study as the largest source) indicate that radiation induction of breast cancer most closely follows a linear dose-response relationship.[35]

Nonspecific Life-Shortening Effects

Research studies have shown that animals chronically exposed to low doses of radiation die younger than nonexposed animals.[45] Autopsy examinations (known as *necropsies* in animals) revealed a decreased number of parenchymal cells and blood vessels and an increased amount of connective tissue in organs. These changes resembled those seen in older animals and have been referred to as *radiation-induced aging.*[17] The effect on life span in these animals indicated a nonthreshold, linear relationship with radiation dose. However, more recent studies indicate that the life-shortening effect in these animals was probably due to cancer induction at moderate doses and organ atrophy, cell killing, and cell loss at high doses. Therefore the life-shortening result can be explained by the occurrence of specific rather than nonspecific effects. Most of the human data available support the statement that specific causes of radiation-induced life shortening are identifiable, although some exceptions to this probably exist.

Genetic Effects

Somatic late effects can occur in an irradiated individual, and exposure of reproductive (germ) cells in that individual may affect future generations. As mentioned previously, ionizing radiation is a known mutagen (i.e., it can induce mutations in the genetic material [DNA/genes] found in the cell nucleus). Mutations (which are permanent, heritable [transmittable to subsequent generations], and generally detrimental) occur spontaneously in genes and DNA. The number of spontaneous mutations that occur in each generation of an organism is described as the *mutation frequency,* which can be increased by any mutagenic agent, including radiation.[29] If the mutation frequency in a generation is doubled by exposure to radiation, the radiation dose is then known as the *doubling dose.*[51] In humans the doubling dose is estimated to range from 50 to 250 rem (0.5 to 2.5 Sv) with an average figure given as 100 rem (1.0 Sv).[27]

The classic study that demonstrated the mutagenic potential of radiation was performed by H.J. Müller[37] in 1927 and involved the use of the *Drosophila melanogaster,* or fruit fly. Müller irradiated male and female fruit flies under a number of conditions and observed the mutation frequencies in the next several generations. The fruit fly was used as the model for these experiments because it has a number of easily identifiable mutations such as those involving its wing shape and eye and body color. In addition, large populations of fruit flies can be maintained and bred relatively quickly and easily.

The results of Müller's fruit fly experiments (which have not been contradicted by subsequent studies with mice) include the following[37]:

1. Radiation does not produce new or unique mutations but increases the frequency of spontaneous mutations in each generation.
2. Mutation frequency is linearly related to radiation dose.
3. Radiation induction of mutations has no clear threshold; it is a stochastic effect like carcinogenesis.

In addition to Müller's experiments, subsequent animal studies have indicated that high dose rates can cause more genetic damage than low dose rates, males are more sensitive than females at low doses and low dose rates to genetic effects, and not all mutations show the same susceptibility to induction by radiation.[27] The estimated doubling dose for humans is based on extrapolations from the numerous animal experiments.

RADIATION THERAPY

Goal of Radiation Therapy

The goal of radiation therapy for cancer is to eradicate the tumor while not destroying normal tissues in the treatment field. This is easier said than done because radiation interaction in matter is a nonspecific, random process that does not distinguish between malignant and normal tissues. Biologic damage can be induced in tumor and normal tissues. Therefore the tolerance of the normal tissue in the treatment field limits the dose that can be administered to the tumor. Several methods have been attempted to deal with this limiting factor during treatment so that more effective tumor treatments can be given. Several of these methods are discussed in this section.

General Tumor Characteristics

Parenchymal and stromal compartments. Like normal tissues, malignant tumors are composed of parenchymal and stromal compartments. A tumor parenchyma may contain up to four subpopulations or groups of cells.[61]

Cells belonging to group 1 are viable, actively mitotic (cycling) cells that are responsible for tumor growth. The percentage of group 1 cells in a tumor type usually varies from 30% to 50% and is termed the *growth fraction (GF).*[36] The GF typically decreases as the size (volume) of the tumor increases.

Group 2 cells are typically viable but nondividing (not cycling). These cells, also known as *G0 cells,* have retained the ability to reenter the cell cycle and divide if properly stimulated.

Groups 3 or 4 are composed of nonviable cells. Group 3 cells appear structurally intact, whereas group 4 cells do not. Groups 3 and 4 cells therefore do not contribute to tumor growth.

The exact percentage of cells in each group varies with the size and type of tumor. In addition, each tumor contains a stromal compartment of blood vessels and connective tissue. In small, newly formed tumors the stroma may be entirely composed of normal host vessels, whereas large, older tumors contain a mix of normal and tumor vessels, or the supporting vasculature may be due to angiogenesis factors released by the tumor cells themselves. As discussed later, the tumor vasculature plays an important role in tumor growth and the oxygen effect.

Factors affecting tumor growth. The rate at which tumors grow depends on three major factors: (1) the division rate of proliferating parenchymal cells, (2) the percentage of these cells in the tumor (GF), and (3) the degree of cell loss from the tumor.[55] The division rate of factor 1 cells in a tumor tends to be faster than the division rate for normal parenchymal cells from the same tissue.[31] For example, malignant skin cells cycle faster than normal skin cells. This might seem to imply that tumors have short doubling times (the time it takes to double in volume), but tumor doubling times in vivo are actually much longer than expected. The two major reasons for this are GF and cell loss. Although factor 1 cells have short cycle times versus normal cells of the same origin, only an average of 30% to 50% of all cells in the tumor are included in this category.[36] In addition, of the new cells produced by mitosis at the end of each cycle, up to 90% may be lost from the primary tumor itself. This cell-loss factor *(f),* which is manifested by metastases, cell death, and exfoliation (shedding of cells as in gastrointestinal tumors), is thought to be the most significant in vivo factor with regard to tumor growth.[55] A high cell-loss factor slows the growth of the primary tumor, but if cells are lost by metastasis, new tumors form in other sites in the body and limit the curative potential of any treatment, including radiation therapy.

The oxygen effect. Tumor growth is characteristically unorganized compared with that of normal cells. During their early growth stages, tumors begin to outgrow their vascular supply. This results in differing levels of oxygen availability (known as *oxygen tension,* or po_2) for the tumor cells depending on their proximity to functioning blood vessels. This was first observed clinically in 1955 by Thomlinson and Gray,[58] who examined human bronchial carcinoma specimens. Thomlinson and Gray observed that the amount of necrotic (dead) tissue in the tumor was related to the size of the tumor itself. A tumor with a radius of less than 100 μm did not contain necrotic areas. A tumor with a radius of greater than 160 μm showed a necrotic area surrounded by a viable rim of cells approximately 100 to 180 μm thick.

Thomlinson and Gray concluded that tumor cells located more than 200 μm from the nearest blood vessels (capillaries) are anoxic (no oxygen available) and unable to proliferate. These cells then die, thus forming the necrotic area. Tumor cells closest to blood vessels, however, are well oxygenated (known as *oxic* cells), are actively dividing, and comprise the GF of the tumor. Between the oxic and anoxic cells are cells exposed to gradually decreasing oxygen tensions. These are known as *hypoxic cells.* Although hypoxic cells do not have normal levels of oxygen available to them, they are viable and capable of dividing. Data from animal tumors estimate that approximately 15% or more of the tumor-cell population may be hypoxic. This is known as the *hypoxic fraction* of the tumor.[64] Thomlinson and Gray's study estimated that the oxic, hypoxic, and anoxic populations in tumors were a result of the limited ability of oxygen to diffuse large distances in tissue. They estimated this diffusion distance of oxygen to be approximately 160 to 200 μm.[58] More recent studies indicate that a diffusion distance closer to 70 μm for oxygen may be more accurate.[27]

The vasculature network that forms in each growing tumor with factors such as division rate, GF, and cell loss ultimately gives rise to oxic, hypoxic, and anoxic cell populations in that tumor. The radioresponse of a tumor depends (among other factors) on these cell populations. Anoxic cells do not contribute to the GF and therefore do not affect clinical outcome. Cells that are fully oxygenated (oxic) are highly radiosensitive to low-LET radiations (see the previous discussion on OER). The third group (viable hypoxic cells) is resistant to low-LET radiations by a factor up to 2.5 to 3.0. The hypoxic fraction in each tumor is presumed to be responsible, at least in part, for tumor regrowth after radiation therapy. One of the reasons for the fractionation of a radiation dose is an attempt to increase the radioresponse of these hypoxic cells (see the discussion on reoxygenation).

Theory of Dose-Fractionation Techniques

Modern radiation therapy treatments are given in daily fractions over an extended period (up to 6 or 8 weeks) so that a high total dose is given to the tumor while ideally sparing normal tissues.[42] This technique, known as **fractionation,** originated in 1927 and replaced a single, high-dose radiation treatment. The type of tumor and tolerance of the normal tissue in the treatment field determine the total dose, size and number of fractions, and treatment duration.

A fractionated dose of radiation is less efficient biologically than a single dose. Therefore higher total doses are necessary during fractionation to produce the same damage compared with a single dose. For example, a single dose of 1000 cGy causes more damage than two fractions of 500 cGy separated by 24 hours, although the total delivered dose remains the same.

A typical fractionation scheme may involve a daily fraction size of 180 to 200 cGy given 5 times a week for 6 weeks for a total of 30 fractions. This results in a total treatment dose ranging from 5400 to 6000 cGy (54 to 60 Gy). Depending on the tumor to be treated, the actual total dose may be higher or lower than this.

The biologic effects on tissue from fractionated radiation therapy depend on the four Rs of radiation biology. These are repopulation, redistribution, repair, and reoxygenation.[67]

Repopulation. During protracted radiation therapy, surviving cells in the tumor and adjacent normal tissues may divide, thus repopulating these tissues partially or completely. Normal tissue repopulation is highly desirable and decreases the risk of late effects. Fractionated doses take advantage of normal tissue repopulation that occurs between fractions. This can result in the sparing of normal tissues in the treatment field.[67] In contrast, tumor repopulation is highly undesirable and contributes to tumor regrowth during or after treatment.

Redistribution. Irradiation of an asynchronous cell population (in which cells are distributed in all phases of the cell cycle) typically results in death to cells in the most sensitive phases (G2 and M), whereas more resistant cells (especially in late S) survive. This process, known as *partial synchronization,* results in a redistribution or reassortment of surviving cells after irradiation.[66] The ideal clinical situation for radiation treatment exists when tumor cells have moved into a sensitive phase and normal cells have moved into a resistant phase. Theoretically, the timing of each radiation fraction can be based on the progression of cells into a sensitive or resistant phase. However, because this cannot be determined clinically, the partial synchronization of cell populations by radiation and other modalities (e.g., hydroxyurea) that may occur has not yet been successfully exploited.

Repair of sublethal damage. Repair of sublethal damage has occurred within hours of radiation exposure in normal and tumor cells in vitro.[18] Fractionated radiation treatment takes advantage of repair processes in normal tissues active between radiation fractions. This partially accounts for the sparing effect on normal tissues that fractionation can achieve. Repair of sublethal damage is oxygen dependent (i.e., cells require a certain amount of oxygen to efficiently carry out repair mechanisms). Because a proportion of tumor cells are thought to be hypoxic, tumors in general are presumed to be incapable of repairing sublethal radiation damage as efficiently as normal tissues.[6] Although demonstrated in animal models, this differential repair between tumors and normal tissues may not be clinically significant in human tumors.

Reoxygenation. The fourth R of radiobiology, unlike the other three, is presumed to apply only to tumors. This phenomenon, termed *reoxygenation,* is the process by which hypoxic cells gain access to oxygen and become radiosensitive between radiation fractions.

As discussed previously, the OER for x-rays and gamma rays is 2.5 to 3.0 when delivered as a single dose. However, the OER decreases during fractionation of x-rays and gamma rays. This implies that a proportion of hypoxic cells reoxygenate and therefore become more sensitive to the next fraction. Although the exact mechanisms of reoxygenation are not clear, clinical trials of fractionated radiation therapy seem to indicate that tumor response is improved compared with that from single-dose treatment. During fractionation, the initial dose fraction should kill a significant proportion of well-oxygenated (oxic), radiosensitive cells near blood vessels in the tumor. The effects on hypoxic, radioresistant cells are considerably less from the same dose fraction. Therefore immediately after exposure the percentage of hypoxic tumor cells increases significantly and may even reach 100% for a short time. Within 24 hours, hypoxic cells somehow gain access to oxygen. Because cells nearest the blood vessels are likely killed by the radiation fraction, oxygen may diffuse beyond these dead cells and reach a percentage of the hypoxic cells. Studies on animal tumors have demonstrated that the hypoxic fraction reestablishes itself in the tumor, usually within 24 hours of treatment.[57] In other words, if a tumor had a hypoxic fraction of 15% before treatment, it eventually reestablishes this percentage after reoxygenation is complete. The standard time interval of 24 hours between radiation fractions in human tumors was extrapolated from animal experiments. This time interval coincides with the range of reoxygenation rates in animal tumors and presumably occurs in human tumors. Because healthy normal tissues do not usually have hypoxic cells, the process of reoxygenation does not apply to these tissues.

Methods of improving tumor radioresponse. Reoxygenation does not rid the tumor of all hypoxic cells. If it did, fractionated treatments using low-LET radiations would be highly curative. Unfortunately, some tumors remain resistant to fractionated radiation therapy. This has given rise to a number of methods to overcome this persistent oxygen effect.

One early method involved the use of a chamber of hyperbaric (high-pressure) oxygen.[61] Patients were placed in sealed chambers containing pure oxygen at a pressure of 3 atmospheres. The rationale behind this was that the diffusion distance of oxygen would increase as a result of the high pressure used in the chamber so that it might reach the hypoxic areas in the tumor. However, this technique did not produce improved clinical results.

A related method involved the administration of perfluorochemicals (drugs that can carry oxygen) with 100% oxygen or carbogen (95% O_2/5% CO_2) breathing before and during radiation treatment.[61] The clinical results seemed to indicate improved response for several tumor types (most notably head and neck tumors), but the overall results were disappointing.

Radiosensitizers, radioprotectors, high-LET radiations, chemotherapy agents, and hyperthermia (heat) have all been used with varying degrees of success in terms of improved tumor response. However, each method is limited by biologic or technical constraints.[27]

Concept of Tolerance

Strandquist isoeffect curves. Although the preference of fractionated radiation treatments over high single doses is now established, the exact protocol for administration of fractionated doses continues to evolve. In 1944 Strandquist[56] made the first attempt to establish a relationship between radiation dose and treatment time. He developed plots of total dose (on a logarithmic scale) versus treatment duration (time in days on a linear scale) and called them isoeffect curves (Fig. 4-16). These *isoeffect curves* related the treatment schedule in terms of total dose and time with the clinical outcome, including early effects, late effects, and tumor cure. The use of isoeffect curves led to treatment schedules for fractionated radiation therapy that gave a high probability of tumor control without exceeding the tolerance of normal tissue. Also during this time the discovery was made that the tolerance of normal tissue is more dependent on the number and size of fractions than on the overall duration between the first and last fractions.

Tolerance and tolerance dose. Because the radiation dose applied to the tumor mass is limited by the tolerance of

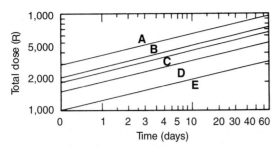

Figure 4-16. Isoeffect curves from Strandquist's data that relate various treatment schedules to the following clinical results: **A,** skin necrosis; **B,** cure of skin cancer; **C,** moist desquamation; **D,** dry desquamation; **E,** skin erythema. *(From Strandquist M: Studien über die cumulative Wirkung der Rπntgenstrahlen bei Fraktionierung, Acta Radiol 55[suppl]:1-300, 1944.)*

the normal tissue in the treatment field, identifying doses that can be used on normal tissues and factors affecting these doses is important. Tolerance doses have therefore been established for normal tissues in terms of the total dose delivered by a standard fractionation schedule that causes a minimal (5%) or maximal (50%) complication rate within 5 years ($TD_{5/5}$ or $TD_{50/5}$, respectively). These doses are commonly known as normal tissue tolerance doses (NTTDs). The $TD_{5/5}$ and $TD_{50/5}$ tolerance doses for various organs have been classified into mild to moderate and severe to fatal are presented in Tables 4-7 and 4-8, respectively.[30]

The NTTD is affected by two factors: the volume irradiated and fraction size. In terms of organ tolerance to radiation, the organ as a whole can tolerate higher radiation doses if the volume of the organ receiving that dose is small. As the volume of the organ affected by the treatment increases, the tolerance dose for the whole organ decreases. According to

Table 4-7	Organs in which radiation lesions result in mild to moderate morbidity			
Organ	**Injury**	**$TD_{5/5}$ (in cGy)**	**$TD_{50/5}$ (in cGy)**	**Whole or Partial Organ (Field Size/Length)**
Articular cartilage	None	>50,000	>500,000	Joint surface
Bladder	Contracture	6000	8000	Whole
Breast (adult)	Atrophy	>5000	>10,000	Whole
Ear				
Middle	Serous otitis	5000	7000	Whole
Vestibular	Ménière's syndrome	6000	7000	Whole
Endocrine glands				
Thyroid	Reduced hormone production	4500	15,000	Whole
Adrenal	Reduced hormone production	>6000	—	Whole
Pituitary	Reduced hormone production	4500	20,000-30,000	Whole
Esophagus	Ulceration, stricture	6000	7500	75 cm^2
Growing cartilage and bone (child)	Growth arrest	1000	3000	Whole
	Dwarfing	1000	3000	10 cm^2
Mature cartilage and bone (adult)	Necrosis	6000	10,000	Whole
	Fracture, sclerosis	6000	10,000	10 cm^2
Large arteries and veins	Sclerosis	>8000	>10,000	10 cm^2
Lymph nodes and lymphatics	Atrophy, sclerosis	5000	>7000	Whole node
Muscle (child)	Atrophy	2000-3000	4000-5000	Whole
Muscle (adult)	Fibrosis	6000	8000	Whole
Oral cavity and pharynx	Ulceration	6000	8000	50 cm^2
Ovary	Sterilization	200-300	635-1200	Whole
Peripheral nerves	Neuritis	6000	10000	10 cm
Rectum	Ulcer, stricture	6000	8000	100 cm^2
Salivary glands	Xerostomia	5000	7000	50 cm^2
Skin	Acute and chronic dermatitis	5500	7000	100 cm^2
Testis	Sterilization	100	200	Whole
Uterus	Stricture	7500	10000	5-10 cm

Modified from Rubin P, editor: *Clinical oncology: a multidisciplinary approach for physicians and students,* Philadelphia, 1993, WB Saunders.

$TD_{5/5}$: Tissue dose associated with a 5% injury rate within 5 years.

$TD_{50/5}$: Tissue dose associated with a 50% injury rate within 5 years.

Table 4-8	Organs in which radiation lesions are severe or fatal morbidity			
Organ	**Injury**	**$TD_{5/5}$ (in cGy)**	**$TD_{50/5}$ (in cGy)**	**Whole or Partial Organ (Field Size/Length)**
Bone marrow	Aplasia, pancytopenia	250	450	Whole
		3000	4000	Segmental
Brain	Infarction, necrosis	5000-6000	6000-7000	Whole
Eye	Blindness			
Retina		5500	7000	Whole
Cornea		5000	>6000	Whole
Lens		500	1200	Whole or part
Fetus	Death	200	400	Whole
Heart	Pericarditis and pancarditis	4500	5500	60%
		7000	8000	25%
Intestine	Ulcer, perforation, and hemorrhage	4500	5500	400 cm^2
		5000	6500	100 cm^2
Kidney	Acute and chronic nephrosclerosis	1500	2000	Whole (strip)
		2000	2500	
Liver	Acute and chronic hepatitis	2500	4000	Whole
		1500	2000	Whole (strip)
Lung	Acute and chronic pneumonitis	3000	3500	100 cm^2
		1500	2500	whole
Spinal cord	Infarction, necrosis	4500	5500	10 cm^2
Stomach	Perforation, ulcer, hemorrhage	4500	5500	100 cm^2
Uterus	Necrosis, perforation	>10,000	>20,000	Whole
Vagina	Ulcer, fistula	9000	>10,000	Whole

Modified from Rubin P, editor: *Clinical oncology: a multidisciplinary approach for physicians and students,* Philadelphia, 2001, WB Saunders.
$TD_{5/5}$, Tissue dose associated with a 5% injury rate within 5 years.
$TD_{50/5}$, Tissue dose associated with a 50% injury rate within 5 years.

Rubin and Casarett,[47] for example, the $TD_{50/5}$ for the heart is 55 Gy if 60% of the heart is irradiated. If only 25% of the heart is irradiated, the $TD_{50/5}$ increases to approximately 80 Gy.

The other factor that affects the NTTD is the size of the daily radiation fraction used. In general, as the size of the daily fraction increases, cell killing increases, and the cell's ability to repair sublethal damage decreases, thus resulting in a decrease in the radiation tolerance of normal tissues.

Nominal standard dose. In an attempt to design treatment schedules that result in optimal tumor response with acceptable normal tissue damage, Ellis[22] in 1968 proposed the concept of nominal standard dose (NSD). Ellis derived the following equation from the isoeffect curves of Strandquist that took into account several parameters of fractionated radiation therapy:

$$D = NSD \times T^{0.11} \times N^{0.24}$$

In the equation, D is the total dose, NSD is the nominal standard dose, T is the overall treatment time in days between the first and last fractions, and N is the number of fractions.[22] Ellis[23] proposed the unit of rets (rad equivalent therapy) for NSD, and in many situations NSD1800 rets was considered the standard for comparison. The NSD equation allowed radiation oncologists to enter their treatment data, calculate the NSD for their centers, and compare this with other centers. The limitations of this concept, however, include the following: (1) the equation is based on connective tissue response and therefore is not useful for late-responding normal tissues and (2) the equation does not take into account the volume irradiated, which is critical to determining the tolerance of normal tissues. Although the NSD concept was popular in the 1970s, it is now useful for only an extremely limited number of clinical situations in radiation therapy.

PRESENT STATUS OF RADIATION THERAPY

A number of treatment techniques combine the use of radiation therapy with other modalities. This is now the method of choice for many human malignancies. Because of the limited effect of low-LET radiations on hypoxic and S-phase tumor cells, the use of hyperthermia[4] and chemotherapeutic agents[27] in conjunction with radiation has increased with improved clinical results for a number of tumor types. In addition, the use of high-LET forms of radiation, such as protons, has certain benefits over conventional x-ray therapy.[5] The energy deposition of protons increases slowly with depth and reaches a sharp maximum near the end of the particles' range in a region called the Bragg Peak (see chapter on Radiation Therapy Equipment). Clinical applications have attempted to use this Bragg Peak region to maximize the delivery dose to the target organ while sparing the surrounding normal tissues. With the knowledge gained from clinical trials and preclinical experimentation, improvements in tumor responses and survival rates after radiation therapy continue to be realized.

Review Questions

Multiple Choice

1. What is the term describing certain chemicals or drugs that enhance the response of cells to radiation?
   a. Free radicals
   b. Radiosensitizers
   c. Radioprotectors
   d. Biologic rescue factors
2. What is applied to the tolerance of normal tissue in which a tissue dose of radiation is associated with a 5% complication rate in 5 years?
   a. Do
   b. Dq
   c. $TD_{5/5}$
   d. $TD_{50/5}$
3. Which of the following tissues is the least radiosensitive?
   a. Ovaries
   b. Ocular lens
   c. Small intestine
   d. Bone and cartilage
4. Which of the following is not one of the four Rs of radiation therapy?
   a. Reconfirmation
   b. Reoxygenation
   c. Redistribution
   d. Repopulation
5. Strandquist's isoeffect curves are related to which of the following?
   a. Oxygen enhancement
   b. Translocation of DNA
   c. Fractionation
   d. Radiation syndromes
6. According to the Law of Bergonié and Tribondeau, ionizing radiation is more effective against cells that are
   a. Actively mitotic, differentiated, and have a long mitotic future
   b. Actively mitotic, differentiated, and have a short mitotic future
   c. Not actively mitotic, undifferentiated, and have a long mitotic future
   d. Actively mitotic, undifferentiated, and have a long mitotic future
7. Which of the following particles do not contribute to the direct effect of radiation?
   a. Protons
   b. Positron
   c. Alpha particles
   d. Heavy nuclear fragments
8. Gross structural changes in chromosomes resulting from radiation damage are referred to as
   a. Chromosome stickiness or clumping
   b. Aberrations, lesions, or anomalies
   c. Deletions and inversions
   d. Interphase death or replication failure
9. What is another term for the cellular response that results in cell death after irradiation of the cell during G1, S, or G2 phase?
   a. Division delay
   b. Interphase death
   c. Reproductive failure
   d. Apoptosis
10. Which are the most important parameters that allow interpretation of survival curves?
    I. Extrapolation number (n)
    II. Surviving fraction (SF)
    III. Do (or D37)
    IV. Quasithreshold dose (Dq)
    V. Oxygen enhancement ration (OER)
    VI. Linear energy transfer (LET)
    a. II, V, and VI
    b. II, III, and V
    c. I, III, and IV
    d. III, V, and VI

Questions to Ponder

1. Discuss the interactions of radiation and matter (specifically, the indirect and direct effects on the cellular level).
2. Describe the relationship between LET, RBE, and OER. Be able to graphically support your answer.
3. How does radiation sensitivity relate to the goals of radiation oncology in terms of tumor control and the sparing of normal tissue structures?
4. Relate the three graphic components of the cell survival curve (n, Do, and Dq) to the administration of radiation treatments.
5. Briefly describe the three total-body responses to radiation. Remember to include the dose ranges that each of these responses occur.

REFERENCES
1. Adams GE, et al: Electron-affinic sensitization. VII. A correlation between structures, one-electron reduction potentials, and the efficiencies of nitroimidazoles as hypoxic cell radiosensitizer, *Radiat Res* 67: 9-20, 1976.

2. Albert RE, et al: Follow-up studies of patients treated by x-ray epilation for tinea capitis, *Arch Environ Health* 17:899-918, 1968.

3. Ancel P, Vitemberger P: Sur la radiosensibilitie cellulaire, *C R Soc Biol* 92:517, 1925.

4. Arcangeli G, et al: Tumor control and therapeutic gain with different schedules of combined radiotherapy and local external hyperthermia in human cancer, *Int J Radiat Oncol Biol Phys* 9:1125-1134, 1983.

5. Barendsen GW: Proceedings of the Conference on Particle Accelerators in Radiation Therapy pp 120-125. LA-5180-C. 1972, US Atomic Energy Commission, Technical Information Center.

6. Bedford JS, Mitchell JB: Dose-rate effects in synchronous mammalian cells in culture, *Radiat Res* 54:316-327, 1973.

7. Belli JA, et al: Radiation response of mammalian tumor cells. I. Repair of sublethal damage in vivo, *J Natl Cancer Inst* 38:673-682, 1967.

8. Bergonié J, Tribondeau L: De quelques resultats de la radiotherapie et essai de fixation d'une technique rationelle, *C R Acad Sci (Paris)* 143:983, 1906.

9. Broerse JJ, Barendsen GW: Current topics, *Radiat Res Q* 8:305-350, 1973.

10. Broerse JJ, Barendsen GW, van Kersen GR: Survival of cultured human cells after irradiation with fast neutrons at different energies in hypoxic and oxygenated conditions, *Int J Radiat Biol* 13:559-572, 1967.

11. Bushong SC: *Radiologic science for technologists: physics, biology and protection,* ed 4, St. Louis, 1988, Mosby.

12. Canti RG, Spear FG: The effect of gamma irradiation on cell division in tissue culture in vitro, part II, *Proc R Soc Lond B Biol Sci* 105:93, 1929.

13. Court-Brown WM, Doll R: Expectation of life and mortality from cancer among British radiologists, *Br Med J* 2:181, 1958.

14. Court-Brown WM, Doll R: Mortality from cancer and other causes after radiotherapy from ankylosing spondylitis, *Br Med J* 2:1327, 1965.

15. Court-Brown WM, et al: The incidence of leukemia after the exposure to diagnostic radiation in utero, *Br Med J* 2:1599, 1960.

16. Cox, JD, Stetz J, Pajak TF: Toxicity criteria of the radiation therapy oncology group (RTOG) and the European organization for research and treatment of cancer (EORTC), *Int J Radiat Oncol Biol Phys* 31:1341-1346, 1995.

17. Curtis HJ: *Radiation-induced aging in mice,* London, 1961, Butterworth.

18. Dekaban AS: Abnormalities in children exposed to x-irradiation during various stages of gestation: tentative timetable of radiation injury to the human fetus, *J Nucl Med* 9:471, 1968.

19. Dewey WC, Humphrey RM: Restitution of radiation-induced chromosomal damage in Chinese hamster cells related to the cell's life cycle, *Exp Cell Res* 35:262, 1964.

20. Dublin LI, Spiegelman M: Mortality of medical specialists, 1938-1942, *JAMA* 137:1519, 1948.

21. Elkind MM, Sutton-Gilbert H: Radiation response of mammalian cells grown in culture. I. Repair of x-ray damage in surviving Chinese hamster cells, *Radiat Res* 13:556, 1960.

22. Ellis F: Dose, time, and fractionation in radiotherapy. In Ebert M, Howard A, editors: *Current topics in radiation research,* Amsterdam, 1968, North Holland Publishing.

23. Ellis F: Nominal standard dose and the ret, *Br J Radiol* 44:101-108, 1971.

24. Evans RD, et al: Radiogenic tumors in the radium and mesothorium cases studied at MIT. In May CW et al, editors: *Delayed effects of bone-seeking radionuclides,* Salt Lake City, 1969, University of Utah Press.

25. Field SB: The relative biological effectiveness of fast neutrons for mammalian tissues, *Radiology* 93:915-920, 1969.

26. Griem ML, et al: Analysis of the morbidity and mortality of children irradiated in fetal life, *Radiology* 88:347-349, 1967.

27. Hall EJ: *Radiobiology for the radiologist,* ed 5, Philadelphia, 2000, JB Lippincott.

28. Kinsella T, et al: The use of halogenated thymidine analog as clinical radiosensitizers: rationale, current status, and future prospects—nonhypoxic cell sensitizers, *Int J Radiat Oncol Biol Phys* 10:1399-1406, 1984.

29. Krall JF: Estimation of spontaneous and radiation-induced mutation rates in man, *Eugenics Q* 3:201, 1956.

30. Kramer S: Principles of radiation oncology and cancer radiotherapy. In Rubin P, editor: *Clinical oncology: a multidisciplinary approach for physicians and students,* Philadelphia, 1993, WB Saunders.

31. Lyskin AB, Mendelsohn ML: Comparison of cell cycle in induced carcinomas and their normal counterparts, *Cancer Res* 24:1131, 1964.

32. MacMahon B: Pre-natal x-ray exposure and childhood cancer, *J Natl Cancer Inst* 28:231, 1962.

33. March HC: Leukemia in radiologists in a 20-year period, *Am J Med Sci* 220:282, 1950.

34. Martland HS: Occurrence of malignancy in radioactive persons: general review of data gathered in study of radium dial painters, with special reference to occurrence of osteogenic sarcoma and interrelationship of certain blood diseases, *Am J Cancer* 15:2435, 1931.

35. McKenzie I: Breast cancer following multiple fluoroscopes, *Br J Cancer* 19:1, 1965.

36. Mendelsohn ML: The growth fraction: a new concept applied to tumors, *Science* 132:1496, 1960.

37. Müller HJ: On the relation between chromosome changes and gene mutations, *Brookhaven Symp Biol* 8:126, 1956.

38. Murphy DP, Goldstein L: Micromelia in a child irradiated in utero, *Surg Gynecol Obstet* 50:79, 1930.

39. Otake M, Schull WJ: In utero exposure to A-bomb radiation and mental retardation: a reassessment, *Br J Radiol* 57:409-414, 1984.

40. Pack GT, Davis J: Radiation cancer of the skin, *Radiology* 84:436, 1965.

41. Patt HM, et al: Cysteine protection against x-irradiation, *Science* 110:213, 1949.

42. Peters LJ, Withers HR, Thames HD: Radiobiological considerations for multiple daily fractionation. In Kaercher KH, Kogelnik HD, Reinartz G, editors: *Progress in radio-oncology,* vol 2, New York, 1982, Raven Press.

43. Plummer C: Anomalies occurring in children exposed in utero to the atomic bomb at Hiroshima, *Pediatrics* 10:687, 1952.

44. Puck TT, Marcus TI: Action of x-rays on mammalian cells, *J Exp Med* 10:653, 1956.

45. Rotblat J, Lindop P: Long-term effects of a single whole body exposure of mice to ionizing radiation. II. Causes of death, *Proc R Soc Lond B Biol Sci* 154:350, 1961.

46. Rowland RE, Stehney AF, Lucas HF: Dose response relationships for radium-induced bone sarcomas, *Health Phys* 44:15-31, 1983.

47. Rubin P, Casarett GW: *Clinical radiation pathology,* vols 1 and 2, Philadelphia, 1968, WB Saunders.

48. Rugh R: X-ray-induced teratogenesis in the mouse and its possible significance to man, *Radiology* 99:433-443, 1971.

49. Russell LB, Russell WL: An analysis of the changing radiation response of the developing mouse embryo, *J Cell Physiol* 43(suppl 1):103-149, 1954.

50. Saccomanno G, et al: Lung cancer of uranium miners on the Colorado plateau, *Health Phys* 10:1195, 1964.

51. Schull WL, Otake M, Neal JV: Genetic effects of the atomic bomb: a reappraisal, *Science* 213:1220-1227, 1981.

52. Simic MG, Grossman L, Upton AC, editors: *Mechanisms of DNA damage and repair,* New York, 1986, Plenum Press.

53. Simpson CL, Hempelmann LH: The association of tumors and roentgen-ray treatment of the thorax in infancy, *Cancer* 10:42, 1957.

54. Sinclair WK: Cyclic x-ray responses in mammalian cells in vitro, *Radiat Res* 33:620-643, 1968.

55. Steel GG: Cell loss as a factor in the growth rate of human tumors, *Eur J Cancer* 3:381-387, 1967.

56. Strandquist M: Studien über die kumulative Wirkung der Roentgenstrahlen bei Fraktionierung, *Acta Radiol* 55(suppl):1-300, 1944.

57. Thomlinson RH: Effect of fractionated irradiation on the proportion of anoxic cells in an intact experimental tumor, *Br J Radiol* 39:158, 1966.

58. Thomlinson RH, Gray LH: The histological structure of some human lung cancers and the possible implications for radiotherapy, *Br J Cancer* 9:539, 1955.

59. Till JE, McCulloch EA: A direct measurement of the radiation sensitivity of normal mouse bone marrow cells, *Radiat Res* 14:213-222, 1961.

60. Toyooka ET, et al: Neoplasms in children treated with x-rays for thymic enlargement. II. Tumor incidence as a function of radiation factors, *J Natl Cancer Inst* 31:1357, 1963.

61. Travis EL: *Primer of medical radiobiology,* ed 2, St. Louis, 1989, Mosby.

62. Trotti A, Byhardt R, Stetz J, et al: Common toxicity criteria: version 2.0. An improved reference for grading the acute effects of cancer treatment: impact on radiotherapy. *Int J Radiat Oncol Biol Phys* 47:13-47, 2000.

63. Upton AC: Radiation carcinogenesis. In *Methods of cancer research,* vol 4, New York, 1968, Academic Press.

64. Van Putten LM, Kahlman LF: Oxygenation status of transplantable tumor during fractionated radiotherapy, *J Natl Cancer Inst* 40:441-451, 1968.

65. Warren S: Radiation carcinogenesis, *Bull N Y Acad Med* 46:131-147, 1970.

66. Withers HR: Cell cycle redistribution as a factor of multi-fraction irradiation, *Radiology* 114:199-202, 1975.

67. Withers HR: The 4 R's of radiotherapy. In *Advances in radiation biology,* vol 5, San Francisco, 1975, Academic Press.

68. Withers HR, Elkind MM: Microcolony survival assay for cells of mouse intestinal mucosa exposed to radiation, *Int J Radiat Biol* 17:261-267, 1970.

69. Withers HR, et al: Radiation survival and regeneration characteristics of spermatogenic stem cells of mouse testis, *Radiat Res* 57:88-103, 1974.

70. Wright EA, Howard-Flanders P: The influence of oxygen on the radiosensitivity of mammalian tissues, *Acta Radiol (Stockholm)* 48:26, 1957.

71. Zirkle RE: Partial cell irradiation, *Adv Biol Med Phys* 5:103, 1957.

5

Detection and Diagnosis

Dennis Leaver, Judith Bastin

Outline

Key Terms

Auscultation
Baseline
Excisional biopsy
Incisional biopsy
Inspection
Metastases
Palpation
Percussion
Premalignant

Prevention
Sensitivity
Sign
Screening
Specificity
Staging
Symptom
Syndrome

The practice of medicine is "not merely the application of scientific principles to a particular biologic aberration. Its focus is on the patient whose welfare is its continuing purpose."[31] Medicine today is an art based on the biologic, physical, and behavioral sciences. It is the accumulation of knowledge that has been developed through discovery, systematic scientific study, and research.

In the field of radiation oncology, physicians, radiation therapists, dosimetrists, physicists, and nurses use their medical skills to benefit the patient. Interpersonal skills are extremely important during interaction with the patient and professional staff members. The presence or absence of appropriate skills can affect the outcome in radiation oncology. This is especially important for the radiation therapist, who may evaluate, assess, and see the patient each day for up to 6 to 7 weeks if the goal of radiation therapy is curative.

A patient seeks the services of the radiation therapy team for consultation, physical examinations, delivery of a prescribed dose of radiation therapy for a specific symptom or set of symptoms, and follow-ups for previously treated conditions. The acquisition of data based on the patient's chief complaints and medical, personal, and family histories are an important part of the patient encounter. Additional patient information is obtained through results of current medical procedures and tests. Using the patient's database, the team puts the pieces of the medical puzzle together to obtain a diagnosis and treatment that fits the patient.

The routine physical examination is necessary to help maintain good health and detect conditions or diseases early so that intervention is possible before the patient demonstrates signs or experiences symptoms. Early detection has proved important in cancer management. According to the American Cancer Society (ACS),[1] **prevention** and early detection are two of the most important and effective strategies of saving lives lost from cancer, diminishing suffering resulting from cancer, and eliminating cancer as a major health problem. Prevention includes measures that stop cancer from developing. Early detection includes examinations and tests intended to find the disease as early as possible, before it has spread. The earlier a cancer can be found, the more effectively it can be treated and with fewer side effects. In fact, the relative survival rate for people with cancers for which the ACS has specific early detection recommendations (breast, colon, rectum, cervix, prostate, testes, and skin) is about 81%.[1] Early detection and effective **screening** (selecting appropriate tests, and studies to check for disease) programs translates into increased survival.

The actual physical examination (whether routine or a result of the patient experiencing signs or symptoms) is a methodical process of detection that covers all the systems. A **sign** is "an objective finding as perceived by an examiner." For example, the examining physician may notice signs such as a rash, feel a mass, or note the color of the patient's skin. A **symptom** is a "subjective indication of a disease or a change in condition as perceived by the patient."[11] For example, the patient may complain of pain, numbness, dysphagia, hematuria, dyspnea, difficulty in sleeping, or lack of appetite. These are symptoms.

If a patient is experiencing symptoms, it is usually an indication that the condition or disease process is more advanced. If a set of signs or symptoms arises from a common cause, it is referred to as a **syndrome.** Many diseases share the same signs and symptoms. Grouping signs and symptoms into a syndrome with results of tests and medical procedures helps the physician eliminate some diseases and narrow the choices for a correct diagnosis. A fever, night sweats, fatigue, general weakness, and weight loss can be indicative of many types of conditions and disease processes. However, with an additional finding of painless lymphadenopathy the choices for a diagnosis become fewer. The physician decides to perform a biopsy on a painless supraclavicular lymph node, and the pathology report indicates the presence of Reed-Sternberg (R-S) cells. Because R-S cells are found in a variety of infectious, inflammatory, and neoplastic disorders, the physician can concentrate on these areas for possible diagnosis and rule out other possibilities.

A diagnosis is defined as the identification of a disease or condition. A diagnosis can be subjective or objective. A subjective diagnosis is based on several factors. The patient's complaints and medical history are considered subjective. The physician's preliminary diagnosis with no hard evidence for support is also considered subjective. An objective diagnosis is based on results of current medical procedures and tests (such as a tissue biopsy or laboratory data) and observations of the physician and other medical personnel.

The process for obtaining an objective diagnosis begins with the interview and physical examination to help assess the patient's current status and determine necessary steps (if any) to take. During a physical examination the physician follows a methodical process that includes the acquisition of data through the interview process, a review of past medical records, a physical examination, a list of the patient's chief complaints, recommendations for further action, treatment recommendations, and follow-ups.[5]

THE INTERVIEW AS A DIAGNOSTIC TOOL

The most powerful diagnostic tool of the physician is the initial interview. By this means, one learns the chronologic events and symptoms of the patient's illness. Diagnostic hypotheses are generated and tested as the patient's history unfolds, resulting in the formulation of the most likely diagnoses at the completion of the interview.[31]

The physician must interview the patient to acquire accurate information. If the patient is too ill or handicapped to provide the information, the physician uses other sources such as family, friends, prior medical records, and other health care providers.

In the interview process the physician asks questions and the patient provides answers. The physician determines the patient's chief complaints and current status and obtains the patient's medical and psychosocial history. The interview is also used to establish the physician-patient relationship and demonstrate to the patient a caring, empathetic attitude.[6,25] In a study of 103 cancer patients by Sapir et al,[25] patients overwhelmingly expected their oncologists to be patient and skilled in diagnostic procedures (98%); tactful, considerate, and therapeutically skilled (90% to 95%); and skilled in the management of pain and the psychosocial consequences of cancer (75% to 85%). When there is bad news to be communicated, 92% of patients indicated that they would want disclosure, whereas 6% indicated that they would want the news withheld from them but passed onto a family member.[25] Evidence from studies like this reinforce the importance of the physician-patient relationship.

Allowing enough time for an interview is important. If the interview is rushed, the patient may feel that the physician is not empathetic. Not allowing enough time may limit the amount of information the physician is able to acquire. Interviewing requires active listening, which calls for no distractions. Distractions should be kept to a minimum if not eliminated. Phone calls, interruptions by staff members, and loud noises can interfere with good communication. Taking excessive notes during the interview can be a distraction for the patient and should be avoided.

The physician listens to the patient's own words and concentrates on the way the patient speaks (e.g., the choice of and emphasis on words and phrases). Equally important are the words the patient chooses not to say or cannot say. The patient may have a limited vocabulary and be unable to find the right word to describe the symptom or withhold information for a variety of reasons. The patient may lack the ability to communicate because of a stroke or mental deficit. A patient simply may not remember or may be afraid to describe all the symptoms because of the fear of a diagnosis. Patients may not give completely accurate statements. Fear of being judged or embarrassment may prevent young men and women from giving a complete history of their sexual activity. Patients may be reluctant to give much information to the physician for fear that it may affect their ability to get or retain a job. Some patients may feel that the physician's time is too important and may become hesitant in sharing their concerns.

The initial interview may be a long process in the radiation oncology setting, because the physician must not only assess the patient but also provide information regarding the goals, benefits, and risks involved in a course of radiation therapy. Radiation therapists and nurses may also interview the patient during the treatment process in an effort to obtain information about the patient's concerns and treatment-related side effects. The health care worker must select words that are clear and mean the same to the patient. The meaning of words is relative. A radiation therapist may ask, "What medications are you taking?" The response may be "None," although the patient is taking aspirin for pain and an antacid for indigestion. In the patient's mind, these are not medications because they were not prescribed.

Many factors can interfere with or facilitate the interview, such as the patient's physical senses and the ability to process and interpret information. The senses and ability to process and interpret information can be affected by age, inherited or acquired conditions, the disease process, treatment and medication, language, and environmental conditions such as loud noises or dim lighting in a room. Factors that help to facilitate the interview include the interviewer's ability to put the patient at ease, ask clear and concise questions, and use terminology having the same meaning to the patient and interviewer. Avoiding technical jargon can mean the difference between a successful interview and one that fails to help the patient.

The objective of the interview is to obtain as much accurate information as possible. During the interview the patient's ability to communicate, level of cognitive functioning, appearance, movement, and facial expressions should be assessed. One must also consider the reliability of the patient's responses. This requires skill in patient communication and observation, a technique that involves the use of verbal and nonverbal communication.

Verbal communication involves the manner, quality, and intonation of speech. Forms of nonverbal communication include personal appearance, facial expressions, posture, and manner of movement. The radiation therapist may be at a distinct advantage in assessing verbal and nonverbal communication from the patient because of daily interaction with the patient. Patients young and old will see their radiation therapist on average five to six times more often than their physician, assuming that the physician sees the patient during the

initial consultation and weekly thereafter. This increased exposure to the therapist allows a sense of mutual confidence and trust to develop. In many situations, the patient may divulge more information to the therapist, especially concerning treatment-related side effects, pain management, and other issues important to the patient.

Observing nonverbal communication while the patient is talking can help determine the real meaning of the patient's words. The patient may say one thing but really mean another. For example, the radiation therapist asks the patient, "Are you having any pain?" The patient says, "No." However, the patient's appearance, posture, and facial expressions contradict the verbal response. The patient sits slouched over, grimaces during movement, and moves slowly with great deliberation. These are all nonverbal signs of pain. These signs may be related to a medical problem other than pain or a psychologic problem, or they may simply have no significance. A slouched posture may indicate pain, low self-esteem, depression, or some other unexplained phenomenon. A grimace may be a psychologic response to the question or physician, a sign of indigestion, or a facial tic. Slow, deliberate movement may mean unfamiliarity with the surroundings, discomfort, or distraction. Observing this type of nonverbal communication requires probing further to rule out pain.

Some of the verbal responses that can facilitate the interview are minimal responses, reflecting feelings, and seeking clarification (Table 5-1). Responses that may hinder the interview are the use of social clichés, imposition of the interviewer's own values, and devaluing or minimizing the patient's feelings or responses (Table 5-2).

THE MEDICAL RECORD AND MEDICAL HISTORY

The medical record documents the patient's past medical experience. The format of the medical record may differ from institution to institution and according to whether the person was an inpatient or outpatient seen in the clinic or emergency room.

"The hospital medical record is a legal public document, in that it is available to the medical staff, medical departments of the hospital, clinic, insurance companies, or by subpoena to a court of law."[31] Patients do not own their medical

Table 5-1	Examples of facilitating verbal responses	
Type of Response	**Examples**
Minimal	"I see."
	"I understand."
Reflecting feelings	"I see you are very angry."
	"It is very scary"
Clarifications	"How bad did it hurt?"
	"This only bothers you at night?"

Table 5-2	Examples of hindering verbal responses	
Type of Response	**Examples**	
Social clichés	"You will feel better soon." "Don't worry: everything will be alright."	
Imposing values	"You should not be having sex out side of marriage." "Someone your age should be more responsible."	
Devaluing the patient's feelings or responses	"I wish I had a nickel for every time I heard this." "This is just part of the aging process."	

records, but they may review them on request and have copies released to other physicians. The medical record contains the medical history, results of laboratory tests and medical procedures, progress notes, copies of consent forms, correspondence and even films produced on the simulator and treatment machine.

The format for taking a medical history may vary from physician to physician but should always be done in a logical manner. Table 5-3 contains a summary of the type of information obtained that is important.

The Need for Demographic Data

Demographic data provide an overview of the patient, including information on the patient's age, gender, race, and possibly national origin. The reason for obtaining demographic data is that certain disease conditions are found to be more prevalent for groups according to age, gender, race, and national origin.

Table 5-3	Information gathered during the medical history interview	
Type of Data	**Information Obtained**	
Demographic data	Age, race, gender, marital status, and current occupation	
Chief complaints	Symptoms, current illness, and current condition	
Medical history	Childhood illnesses, allergies, immunizations, injuries, prior hospitalizations, psychologic problems, and medications	
Family history	Illnesses, causes of death, genetic disorders, and mental disorders	
Personal history	Occupation, lifestyle, and sexual activity and preferences	

For example, although cancer occurs at any age, the incidence is higher among older persons. However, certain types of cancer occur more frequently in other age-groups. The classic presentation of Wilms' tumor (a cancer of the kidney) is that of a healthy child in whom abdominal swelling is discovered by the child's mother, pediatrician, or family practitioner during a routine physical examination.[4,16]

Some types of cancer occur more frequently by gender. For example, men are affected twice as often as women by renal cancer, whereas the incidences of colon and rectal cancer are higher in women[29] (Table 5-4).

The incidence of cancer among races and nationalities varies. For example, the incidence of esophageal cancer is extremely high in the Bantu of Africa, China, Russia, Japan, Scotland, and the Caspian region of Iran.[16]

Determination of the Chief Complaints

When assessing the patient's chief complaints, the physician compiles a list of symptoms, known illnesses, and conditions. Listening to the patient's chief complaints helps determine necessary diagnostic decisions. This is important because certain symptoms, illnesses, or conditions may indicate the possibility of a predisposing factor, **premalignant** condition (physiologic characteristics or predisposing factors that may lead to malignancy), paraneoplastic syndrome, or other risk factors.

A predisposing factor given the correct stimuli has the potential of becoming malignant. Leukoplakia, an example of a predisposing factor, is identified as a white patch or patches in the mucosa of the oral cavity and on the tongue.

A premalignant condition eventually becomes malignant if left untreated. Premalignant conditions usually are manifested as dysplasia or atypical hyperplasia. Dysplasia is the abnormal development of cells in size and shape. Hyperplasia is an increase in the number of new cells. Dysplasia and hyperplasia can be determined only by microscopic examination. These types of changes are routinely assessed as a result of a Papanicolaou (Pap) smear test, in which cells from the uterine cervix are examined microscopically and may lead to detection of cervical cancer in women.

Some forms of cancer produce a paraneoplastic syndrome. Paraneoplastic syndrome is a term that describes certain metabolic disorders associated with cancer. These disorders indirectly result from the disease and are not caused by the spread of cancer to an organ or other tissues. The syndrome is a result of hormonal, hematologic, neurologic, and biochemical disturbances on the patient's physiology.

Hypercalcemia and hypoglycemia are part of the paraneoplastic syndromes associated with hepatic cell carcinoma.[14,16] Hypercalcemia is an excessive amount of calcium in the blood. Hypoglycemia is a reduced amount of sugar in the blood. Thrombophlebitis and antidiuretic hormone excess are part of the paraneoplastic syndromes associated with lung cancer. Thrombophlebitis is the inflammation of a vein caused by the development or presence of a blood clot in the

Table 5-4	Leading sites of new cancer cases and deaths—2003 estimates*			
	Estimated New Cases*		**Estimated Deaths**	
	Male	**Female**	**Male**	**Female**
	Prostate	Breast	Lung & Bronchus	Lung & Bronchus
	220,900 (33%)	211,300 (32%)	88,400 (31%)	68,800 (25%)
	Lung & Bronchus	Lung & Bronchus	Prostate	Breast
	91,800 (14%)	80,100 (12%)	28,900 (10%)	39,800 (15%)
	Colon & Rectum	Colon & Rectum	Colon & Rectum	Colon & Rectum
	72,800 (11%)	74,700 (11%)	28,300 (10%)	28,800 (11%)
	Urinary Bladder	Uterine corpus	Pancreas	Pancreas
	42,200 (6%)	40,100 (6%)	14,700 (5%)	15,300 (6%)
	Melanoma of the skin	Ovary	Non-Hodgkin lymphoma	Ovary
	29,900 (4%)	25,400 (4%)	12,200 (4%)	14,300 (5%)
	Non-Hodgkin lymphoma	Non-Hodgkin lymphoma	Leukemia	Non-Hodgkin lymphoma
	28,300 (4%)	25,100 (4%)	12,100 (4%)	11,200 (4%)
	Kidney	Melanoma of the skin	Esophagus	Leukemia
	19,500 (3%)	24,300 (3%)	9,900 (4%)	9,800
	Oral cavity	Thyroid	Liver	Uterine corpus
	18,200 (3%)	16,300 (3%)	9,200 (3%)	6,800 (3%)
	Leukemia	Pancreas	Urinary bladder	Brain
	17,900 (3%)	15,800 (2%)	8,600 (3%)	5,800 (2%)
	Pancreas	Urinary bladder	Kidney	Multiple myeloma
	14,900 (2%)	15,200 (2%)	7,400 (3%)	5,500 (2%)
	All sites	All sites	All sites	All sites
	675,300 (100%)	658,800 (100%)	285,900 (100%)	270,600 (100%)

From American Cancer Society, Inc., Surveillance Research, 2003.
*Excludes basal and squamous cell skin cancers and in situ carcinoma except urinary bladder.
Percentages may not total 100% due to rounding.

vein. Having any of these medical conditions does not necessarily mean that the individual has a malignant disease process. However, a patient who demonstrates several signs and symptoms of a particular syndrome must have a further workup to rule out those possibilities.

The Importance of the Medical History

The medical history provides a snapshot of the patient's prior medical problems and treatments. The determination of prior medical problems may establish risk factors for acquiring diseases in the future. For example, a patient who has a long history of indigestion and gastric reflux caused by a hiatal hernia may be at risk for ulcers or carcinoma of the esophagus.[14,16] A gastric reflux is the backward flow of contents of the stomach into the esophagus. A hiatal hernia is a congenital or acquired condition that is the result of movement of the stomach through the esophageal hiatus of the diaphragm into the thorax.

The medical history of immediate family members may determine additional risk factors. The immediate family consists of the parents, spouse, children, brothers, sisters, aunts, and uncles. The physician determines whether the parents are alive or deceased. If they are alive, the physician determines their ages and health status. If they are deceased, the physician must know the causes of death and the ages of the parents when they died. This is done to establish certain risk factors such as the acquisition of genetic disease and probability of developing medical conditions such as heart disease, arthritis, diabetes, and cancer.

Certain types of cancer appear to repeat in families. More than one sibling may develop leukemia. If the mother has breast cancer, the daughter is at a greater risk of developing the disease.[14,16]

The personal history encompasses the patient's lifestyle (past and present). The physician asks questions regarding dietary, exercise, alcohol, cigarette, and drug habits. The physician must also determine the patient's sexual activity frequency and preferences. Determining the patient's past occupations is also an important thing to do. For example, the patient may have been employed in an occupation that carried the risk of exposure to asbestos, disease, certain chemicals, or other carcinogens.

THE PHYSICAL EXAMINATION

The physical examination, medical history, and test results help the physician detect variations in the normal state of the patient. The physical examination is an extremely organized, detailed exploration of the patient's anatomic regions. Performing a physical examination requires all the physician's senses and skills.

The following paragraphs list some examples of aspects in the physical examination and information the physician may be seeking. The information in this section is extremely general and far from comprehensive regarding all aspects of the physical examination. Inspection, palpation, percussion, and auscultation are the four classic techniques of the physical examination.

Inspection

Inspection is the use of sight to observe. A distinction must be made between seeing and observing. Something may be seen but not observed. For example, a person may see a group of people, but on further observation of the group the person begins to make distinctions. The person may be able to say 10 people were in the group and may then observe differences in gender, race, age, appearance, and behavior.

The physician observes the color of the patient's skin, which may indicate signs of a disease condition. Many diseases and conditions affect skin coloration. The skin may be dark, pale, grey, flushed, jaundiced, or cyanotic. Dark skin may be natural or caused by irritation of another medical condition. Pale skin may be natural or caused by anemia. Flushed or reddened skin may be caused by hormones, a reaction to external beam radiation therapy, infection, or burns. Jaundice, a yellow coloration of the skin, may be caused by obstruction of the bile ducts. Cyanosis, a blue coloration of the skin, may be caused by an excessive accumulation of reduced hemoglobin in the blood.

The physician looks for scarring or lesions such as warts, moles, ulcerations, tumors, and asymmetry on the surface of the skin. Scarring is an indication of prior medical procedures or injury. The presence of lesions or changes in warts and moles may be benign, a sign of malignant transformation, or cancer. Asymmetry may be an indication of edema, thrombosis, hematoma, injury, or an underlying tumor. Edema is a swelling of the tissue caused by the accumulation of excessive amounts of fluid. Thrombosis is the abnormal accumulation of blood factors in a blood vessel that causes a clot. A hematoma is the abnormal accumulation of blood in tissue from a blood vessel that has ruptured. An inspection may use the sense of smell to help in making a diagnosis. For example, the smell of the patient's breath, wound, urine, or sputum may indicate infection, ketoacidosis, or some other condition.

Palpation

Palpation is the use of touch to acquire information about the patient. The physician palpates the patient by using the tips of the fingers. Light palpation is used for a superficial examination. Heavy pressure may be necessary for deep-seated structures. Through palpation the physician tries to distinguish between hard and soft, rough and smooth, and warm and dry. Vibrations in the chest or abdomen can be felt through palpation. Palpation of an artery can help determine the pulse. Palpation is also used to determine whether pain is present. For example, the patient may not experience pain from an inflammatory process until pressure is applied or applied and released quickly.

Percussion

Percussion is different from palpation in that percussion is the act of striking or tapping the patient gently. The purpose of percussion is to determine pain in underlying tissue or cause vibrations. Making a fist and pounding it gently over the kidney area does not normally produce pain. However, if the patient has an underlying kidney infection, percussion may produce pain.

Placing the examiner's third finger of one hand flat on the surface of the patient over the lung or abdomen produces another form of percussion. With the third finger of the other hand the examiner gently raps the dorsal surface of the third finger that is resting on the patient. Depending on the location of the percussion, different sounds are produced. For example, if percussion is done over the lung (which is an air-filled cavity), the vibrations have a different sound than that of the abdominal cavity. Percussion over a normal lung produces a resonant sound, whereas percussion over the abdomen produces a distinctively duller sound. For the radiation therapist, percussion is helpful in determining the place the abdomen ends and the lung begins. The radiation therapist may have to take a simulation film that requires centering over the diaphragm.

Auscultation

Auscultation is the act of listening to sounds within the body. With a stethoscope the physician performs auscultation by listening to the lungs, heart, arteries, stomach, and bowel sounds with a stethoscope. Sounds in the lungs vary depending on the presence or absence of air, fluid and disease, producing distinct sounds to the trained ear. A pumping heart produces sounds that can be altered by changes or abnormalities of its structure and function.

Vital Signs

Vital signs are almost always taken during the physical examination. Vital signs include the temperature, pulse, respirations, and blood pressure of the patient. Vital signs can vary from patient to patient depending on the time of day and physical activity, condition, and age of the patient. Taking **baseline,** or initial, values at various times to establish the patient's norm is important.

Temperatures are taken orally, rectally, in the ear, or in the axilla. Oral temperatures should not be taken on unreliable patients. This includes patients who are irrational, comatose, prone to convulsions, and young children. Patients in these categories should have rectal or ear temperatures taken. The rectal temperature is considered the most accurate. Devices most commonly used for taking temperatures are glass and electronic thermometers. Electronic thermometers give much quicker readings than glass thermometers. The electronic ear thermometer can be used on adults and children. Temperatures are measured in Fahrenheit (F) or Celsius (C), and some values are given in ranges. Textbooks may list slightly different values for normal and abnormal temperatures (Table 5-5).

Factors observed during the taking of a pulse are rate, rhythm, size, and tension. Rate indicates the number of beats per second. Rhythm is the pattern of beats. Size has to do with the size of the pulse wave and volume of blood felt during the ventricular contraction of the heart. Tension refers to the compressibility of the artery (e.g., soft or hard)[7] (Table 5-5).

Factors that are observed during the evaluation of respiration are rate, depth, rhythm, and character. Rate is the number of breaths that are taken in a minute. Depth refers to shallow or deep breathing. The deeper the breath, the greater the amount of air that is inhaled. Rhythm refers to the regularity of breathing (slow, normal, or rapid). Character refers to the type of breathing from normal to labored[7] (Table 5-5).

When taking a blood pressure, the systolic and diastolic pressures are noted. Systolic blood pressure represents the pressure in the blood vessels during the contraction of the heart and is the first sound heard through the stethoscope when taking a blood pressure. Diastolic pressure represents the pressure in the blood vessels during the relaxation phase of the heart after the contraction. The diastolic pressure is the last sound heard through the stethoscope when taking a blood pressure[7] (Table 5-5).

Recognizing pain as a major, yet largely avoidable, public health problem, the Joint Commission on Accreditation of Healthcare Organizations (JCAHO) has developed standards that create new expectations for the assessment and management of pain in accredited hospitals and other health care settings. According to (JCAHO) standards, pain is considered the "fifth" vital sign. Pain intensity ratings should be recorded along with temperature, pulse, respiration, and blood pressure. This should bring much needed attention to the undertreatment of pain. The JCAHO provides accreditation for more than three fourths of the hospitals and medical centers in the United States. New JCAHO standards have recently been developed for pain assessment and management. The new standards received final JCAHO approval in July of 1999 and were first scored for compliance in 2001. Details of the standards involving pain assessment and management can be reviewed on their web site (http://www.qmsonline.com/jcaho).

SCREENING

Cancer prevention that takes place in the United States is grouped in three levels. The first level of cancer prevention is devoted to helping people maintain good health through edu-

Table 5-5	Normal adult values for vital signs	
Vital Signs	**Values**	
Temperature		
Oral	96.8° to 98.6° F (36° to 37° C)	
Rectal	99.6° F	
Axillary	97.6° F	
Pulse	60 to 90 beats per minute	
Respirations	10 to 20 breaths per minute	
Blood pressure	110 to 140 mm Hg	
	60 to 80 mm Hg	
Pain	Subjective scales may be used indicating the intensity of pain	

cation that encourages changes in lifestyle. Immunizations to prevent cancer, if they existed, would be encouraged. The second level of cancer prevention is concerned with the early detection of conditions and disease. Early detection makes intervening and perhaps improving the outcome for the patient possible. The third level is devoted to rehabilitation.

Cancer screening is part of the second level of health promotion[29] Screening is the cornerstone of the diagnosis and management of the patient. It is done for large, asymptomatic populations at risk to detect deviations from the norm or signs of disease. Specific screening is performed for patients who are symptomatic, undergoing treatment, or being followed up. The determination to do mass screening is based on the results obtained, cost effectiveness, and risk to the patient. Areas of screening performed today are aimed at identifying cancer at its earliest stage, which translates into increased cure rates for most cancers.

Until the early 1960s the only routine screening that was available for asymptomatic patients included a chest x-ray film, an electrocardiogram, a complete blood count (CBC), a blood chemistry test, a urinalysis, and a stool examination for occult blood. With the development of multichannel automated analyzers, many laboratory tests could be obtained for the same cost as that of the few tests that had been performed before. Later studies questioned the value of doing such a large number of tests. Many of the tests that were performed did not improve the outcome in asymptomatic outpatients.[31]

Most screening studies can be grouped into two major categories: laboratory studies and medical imaging. Hundreds of laboratory tests and medical imaging procedures exist today. Discretion must be exercised in selecting appropriate tests to be done, and studies are not performed unless logical reasons exist for doing so.

The ACS believes that early detection examinations and tests can save lives and reduce suffering from cancers of the breast, colon, rectum, cervix, prostate, testes, oral cavity, and skin. Some of these cancers can be found by self-examination, physical examination, and laboratory tests (such as mammography, the Papanicolaou (Pap) smear, and the prostate-specific antigen [PSA] blood test).[1] Cancer screening can be effective if a disease has a high incidence or prevalence in a population and the test has the ability to produce results having the appropriate **sensitivity** (defined as the ability of a test to give a true positive result) and **specificity** (defined as the ability of the test to obtain a true negative result). Incidence is defined as the number of new cases of a disease over a period, and prevalence is defined as the total number of cases of a disease at a certain time. Screening may be set up to determine the incidence of new cancer cases over a period. Screening for the prevalence of cancer determines the number of cases at a certain time.[18]

In the United States, one of eight women develop breast cancer, and one in eight men develop prostate cancer.[3] Therefore a significant portion of the population benefits from mass medical screening. If the disease is caught early enough, morbidity and mortality rates may be reduced. Mass screening for breast cancer in China is not effective because the at-risk population is low. However, the reverse is true for cancer of the esophagus. The number of persons at risk for cancer of the esophagus is extremely high in certain regions of China. Because the population at risk for cancer of the esophagus is much lower in the United States, mass screening for esophageal cancer would not be beneficial in terms of outcome and cost effectiveness.

Areas where mass screening tools have received more attention in recent years include breast, lung, prostate, colon, cervix, gastric and others. Mass screening is based on the specific results obtained, cost effectiveness, and risk to the patient. Because areas of screening performed today are aimed at identifying cancer at its earliest stage, high-incidence cancers such as breast, lung, and prostate have received more attention.

For women 50 years and older the ACS recommends an annual mammogram, which can demonstrate lesions before they can be palpated. There are few controlled studies evaluating the effectiveness of screening by self-breast examination (SBE) alone.[23] However, research has clearly demonstrated that screening mammography can improve survival rates.[16,23,24] In addition, as a type of secondary screening tool, surgeons are judging the usefulness of sentinel lymph node biopsy (SNB) as a means of assessing axillary node status once the primary has been detected and evaluating current standards for the use of chemotherapy for micrometastases.[16,21,26]

Screening for lung cancer has been used for decades without demonstrating overall survival benefit. However, recent improvements in our biologic understanding of lung tumors, the advent of multislice spiral computed tomography (CT) scanning, and advances in the treatment of lung cancer have led many investigators to evaluate the use of CT in screening for lung cancer.* One Japanese study reviewed the results of a 3-year study (1996 to 1998) using low-dose spiral CT for annual lung cancer screening. The CT screening program detected suspicious nodules in 3.5% to 5.1% of those scanned (3878 to 5483 total patients). Eighty-eight percent (55/60) of the lung cancers identified on screening and later surgically confirmed were AJCC stage IA tumors.[28] Despite the small number of confirmed cancers overall, the use of low-dose spiral CT is able to detect cancers of the lung at a very early stage, when the cancer is more treatable.

Screening for prostate cancer, which is one of the leading causes of death in American men older than 50, remains controversial. The two most common methods used to screen for prostate cancer are digital rectal examination (DRE) and PSA blood test. Consensus is lacking on whom to screen, when to screen, and what to do if cancer is discovered.[10] Refinements to the sensitivity and specificity are needed to improve the effectiveness of the screening tool. PSA misses 18% to 25% of prostate cancers and provides false-positive results in a large percentage of the cases.[10,20]

In summary, the value of mass screening is determined by the number of the population at risk, cost of the studies, risks involved in the studies, and improvements in the morbidity and mortality rates.

Sensitivity, Specificity, and Predictive Values

Other measures for determining the value of a study are the sensitivity, specificity, and predictive values. Sensitivity is defined as the ability of a test to give a true positive result when the disease is present. In other words, a person who tests positive for cancer from a high-sensitivity test probably has cancer. Specificity is defined as the ability of the test to obtain a true-negative result. When the results of a high-specificity test are negative, that person probably does not have cancer.[12]

The ideal situation is for a test to yield a high sensitivity and high specificity. However, that is almost impossible. Because of the morbidity and mortality rates of cancer, the ability to detect cancer early in all individuals tested is important. High sensitivity is selected when the disease prevalence is low. A positive finding of cancer from a high-sensitivity test can be confirmed by subjecting the patient to a second test of high specificity. High specificity is selected when the disease prevalence is high. Determining the sensitivity and specificity of the test can affect its predictive value. The predictive value of a positive test increases with an increase in the sensitivity and specificity of the test. No single test should be relied on to establish a diagnosis of cancer.

Common Sources of Errors

The sources of errors in medical studies are many. Any medical examination always has a margin of error in the results.

---

*References 13, 16, 19, 22, 28, 30.

The possibility of errors exists in the ordering of a study Request forms must be filled out completely and correctly. The individual filling out the form must know places to obtain the necessary information that must be recorded on the requisition. This information includes the patient's demographic data, symptoms, or diagnosis if available and the purpose of the test.

Coordination of the patient's activities is important. Special consideration must be given to patients who are handicapped, disabled, diabetic, or infirm. Extra time may be necessary to accommodate these patients in scheduling a battery of activities before the study, preparing the patient, and performing the procedure. Care must be taken in the ordering of the study and test, coordination of activities, and preparation of the patient[9] (Table 5-6).

The tests require coordination so that they do not interfere with each other. For example, a glucose tolerance test takes place over 2 hours, at which time blood must be drawn. If the patient is not available when the blood is to be drawn, the results of the test are invalid. Some tests must be done before others because they may interfere with the next test. For example, an intravenous pyelogram (IVP) should be done before x-ray contrast studies of the upper and lower gastrointestinal (GI) systems. If the patient has an upper and lower GI study before the IVP, the contrast material left in the intestinal tract may obstruct the radiologist's view of the kidneys, ureters, and bladder. Improper coordination may result in the patient having to go through an uncomfortable preparation for the test again. (In the example just mentioned the preparation includes multiple enemas.) In addition, many of the tests are invasive, can be uncomfortable, and carry certain risks. Repeated radiographic procedures result in unnecessary exposure of the patient to ionizing radiation.[9]

THE AMERICAN CANCER SOCIETY'S RECOMMENDATIONS FOR DETECTING CANCER

The ACS strongly recommends mass screenings for colorectal, breast, cervical, prostate, and endometrial cancers. To date, results of mass screening for lung cancer have not proved beneficial in improving mortality rates. Getting people to stop smoking has the greatest effect on mortality statistics for lung cancer.[14]

Table 5-7 provides an excellent overview of recommendations for screening and detection by site and symptoms. New techniques for the diagnosis of prostate cancer (such as PSA blood testing and ultrasound) are listed in Table 5-7. The ACS recommends that the PSA blood test be performed yearly for men older than the age of 50. In addition, the ACS recommends prostatic ultrasounds for men who are at high risk.

LABORATORY STUDIES

Hundreds of laboratory studies are available today. Some studies are used to analyze the composition of the blood and bone marrow and rule out blood disorders. Blood studies are concerned with blood cells, whereas blood chemistry tests examine chemicals in the blood. Microbiologic studies are helpful in detecting specific organisms that may be causing an infection. Urine studies are done to analyze the composition and concentration of the urine. These are helpful in detecting diseases and disorders of the kidney and urinary system and endocrine or metabolic disorders. Fecal studies are done to examine the waste products of digestion and metabolic disorders. These studies are useful in detecting GI diseases and disorders such as bleeding, obstruction, obstructive jaundice, and parasitic disease. Studies are also done to investigate the immune system. Immunologic studies examine the antigen-antibody reactions. Serologic tests are done to diagnose problems such as neoplastic disease, infectious disease, and allergic reactions. Laboratory studies done to examine cells and tissue are discussed in the following section.

Baseline values should always be obtained to observe any deviation. Table 5-8 contains normal ranges for a CBC. The values may vary from institution to institution depending on the methods used.

MEDICAL IMAGING

The physiology and anatomy of the body can be imaged in many ways, and the procedures used can be extremely simple or complex. Every procedure provides some element of risk to the patient. Noninvasive procedures provide extremely little risk to the patient. Most invasive procedures provide some risk, but the exact amount of acceptable risk depends on many factors. The physician and patient must discuss the risks.

Electrical Impulses

Some medical imaging techniques use electrical impulses of the body to determine the ability of the heart, brain, and muscles to function. The electrocardiogram (ECG) demonstrates

Table 5-6	Actions that may alter test results	
Person Responsible	**Actions**	
Caregiver	Incomplete or inaccurately filled-out requisitions	
	Incomplete or inaccurate coordination of activities	
	Incomplete or inaccurate patient instruction	
	Incorrectly performed procedure	
	Incorrect labeling of specimens	
Patient	Incorrect interpretaion of instructions	
	Lack of cooperation	
	Inability to follow instructions or noncompliance	

Table 5-7	Summary of American Cancer Society Recommendations for the early detection of cancer in asymptomatic people
Cancer-related checkup	A cancer-related checkup is recommended every 3 years for people aged 20-40 and every year for people age 40 and older. This exam should include health counseling and depending on a person's age, might include examinations for cancers of the thyroid, oral cavity, skin, lymph nodes, testes, and ovaries, as well as for some nonmalignant diseases.
Breast	Women 40 and older should have an annual mammogram, an annual clinical breast examination (CBE) by a health care professional, and should perform monthly breast self-examination (BSE). The CBE should be conducted close to and preferably before the scheduled mammogram. Women 20-39 should have a CBE by a health care professional every three years and should perform monthly BSE.
Colon and rectum	Beginning at age 50, men and women at average risk should follow one of the examination schedules below: • Fecal occult blood test (FOBT) every year • Flexible sigmoidoscopy every 5 years • FOBT every year and flexible sigmoidoscopy every 5 years • Double contrast barium enema every 5 years • Colonoscopy every 10 years
Prostate	Beginning at age 50, the prostate-specific antigen (PSA) test and the digital rectal examination should be offered annually to men who have a life expectancy at at least 10 years. Men at high risk (African-American men and men who have a first-degree relative who was diagnosed with prostate cancer at a young age) should begin testing at age 45. Patients should be given information about the benefits and limitations of tests so they can make informed decisions.
Uterus	Cervix: All women who are or have been sexually active or who are 18 and older should have an annual Pap test and pelvic examination. After three or more consecutive satisfactory examinations with normal findings, the Pap test may be performed less frequently. Endometrium: Beginning at age 35, women with or at risk for hereditary nonpolyposis colon cancer should be offered endometrial biopsy annually to screen for endometrial cancer.

From *Cancer facts and figures*, Atlanta, 2001, The American Cancer Society.

Table 5-8	Normal ranges for complete blood count
Blood Component	**Range**
White blood cells	3.90 to 10.80 thousand/mm^3
Red blood cells	3.90 to 5.40 million/mm^3
Hemoglobin	12.0 to 16.0 g/dl
Hematocrit	37.0% to 47.0%
Differential white blood cells (WBC)	
Neutrophils	42.0% to 72.0%
Lymphocytes	17.0% to 45.0%
Monocytes	3.0% to 10.0%
Eosinophils	0.0% to 12.0%
Basophils	0.0% to 2.0%
Platelets	150 to 425 thousand/mm^3

the electrical conductivity of the heart muscle. This aids in the detection and diagnosis of heart disease. During the examination, wave patterns representing the electrical pulse are drawn on special paper. The physician studies the wave patterns to check for any deviations. The electroencephalogram (EEG) records brain-wave activity. The EEG helps detect and diagnose seizure disorders, brainstem disorders, brain lesions, and states of consciousness. An electromyogram (EMG) measures the electrical conductivity of the muscle, thus aiding in the detection and diagnosis of neuromuscular problems.

Nuclear Medicine Imaging

Nuclear imaging is achieved by the introduction of a radionuclide into the patient. A radionuclide, or radiopharmaceutical, is an isotope that undergoes radioactive decay. In doing so, it gives off radiation. It is an unstable element that attempts to reach stability by emitting several types of ionizing radiation. The radionuclide may be injected, swallowed, or inhaled. After the introduction of the radionuclide into the patient, it follows a specific metabolic pathway in the body. Several minutes to several hours later an imaging device is placed outside the patient's body, and the resultant radiation from the radionuclide is measured and imaged. Hot spot and cold spot imaging are the two major types of imaging done in nuclear medicine. Hot spot imaging involves an increase in the concentration of the radionuclide in the area compared with normal tissue. Cold spot imaging is the opposite.

The two most common imaging devices are the gamma camera and rectilinear scanner. The gamma camera does not move and views the whole area of interest at one time. The rectilinear scanner starts at the top or bottom of the area of interest and then scans from side to side until the entire area of interest has been imaged. Newer imaging modalities in nuclear medicine include single photon emission computed tomography (SPECT) and positron emission tomography (PET). These modalities make possible the viewing of the organ's function and blood flow in addition to the image of its anatomy.[4,16]

Scans of the kidney, liver, thyroid gland, lung, brain, and bone are commonly used to detect cancer. Scans demonstrate the function, anatomy, and size of a particular organ. Bone scans are especially helpful in evaluating metastatic disease.

Routine Radiographic Studies

Routine radiographic studies consist of contrast and noncontrast types. The use of contrast media such as barium, Telepaque, Oragrafin, Cholografin, Hypaque, and Conray helps to visualize anatomy that is radiolucent. If the anatomic structure is radiolucent, the x-rays are not completely absorbed by the structure and therefore cannot be demonstrated on a radiograph. For example, gas and fecal material in the colon may be visualized without contrast. However, to visualize the structure, position, filling, and movement of the colon, a barium-based contrast agent is necessary. For the esophagus to be visible, the patient must drink barium. Bone has a relatively high density and can be demonstrated on a radiograph without the aid of contrast media.

Routine noncontrast studies consist of chest x-rays; radiographs of the abdomen that include the kidneys, ureters, and bladder (KUB); and radiographs of the sinuses, skull, spine, and other bones. Contrast studies include but are not limited to the intravenous pyelogram (IVP), upper and lower GI tract, and arteriograms.

Mammography

The ACS recommends a baseline mammogram for women between the ages of 35 and 40 and an annual or biennial mammogram to be determined by the physician for women between the ages of 40 and 50. For women 50 years and older the ACS recommends an annual mammogram. The SBE is strongly recommended by the ACS. Women who regularly engage in SBE often detect lesions before their physicians. Mammography can demonstrate lesions before they can be palpated. SBE has not been proved to improve survival rates. However, research has demonstrated that screening mammography can improve survival rates.[16,23,24]

Computed Tomography

Seeing a complete 360-degree cross section of the body was not possible until 1972 with the development of the CT scanning unit. Initially, the first CT scanners were head scanners. Later generation scanners were able to demonstrate the whole body. CT scanners can demonstrate anatomic images in the transverse plane and the coronal plane.[8]

The CT scanner takes an x-ray image, digitizes it, and stores it in a computer. The computer can produce a high-resolution image.[27] Scanners that can produce a three-dimensional image are now available and being used for reconstructive surgery. Some of these units, found in radiation therapy departments, are used for simulation and three-dimensional treatment planning.

Routine radiographs can demonstrate differences between bone, air, and some degree of soft tissue. Because of the high-resolution capability of the CT scanner, radiologists can differentiate between bone, air, and soft tissue to a much higher degree than is possible with routine radiographs.[27] According to Levitt et al.,[17] "The CT has replaced upper GI series and pancreatic angiography in the detection of pancreatic cancer."

Magnetic Resonance Imaging

Until the mid-1980s, magnetic resonance imaging (MRI) was called nuclear magnetic resonance (NMR). The term *nuclear* was deleted because it was unpopular with the public. Unlike nuclear medicine and radiology, MRI does not use ionizing radiation. A major difference between the CT scanner and MRI is the ability of MRI scanners to obtain anatomical images in the sagittal plane. MRI units also have the ability to demonstrate soft tissue to a much greater degree than CT units. However, CT units can demonstrate bone better than MRI units.[8,16]

Ultrasonography

Ultrasonography is one of the least expensive imaging techniques. It is also quick and simple and usually causes only minimal patient discomfort. Ultrasound also differs from radiography in that its images are produced with high-frequency sound waves instead of ionizing radiation. Because of this, ultrasound has been used extensively in gynecologic and prenatal imaging. Fetal weight, growth, and anatomy can be studied without exposure to ionizing radiation. Ovarian tumors are often difficult to image and detect, but with ultrasonography the ovary can be seen. Ultrasound continues to play a major role in the management of prostate cancer.

The ability of ultrasound to demonstrate soft tissue structures is helpful in demonstrating gallstones, kidney stones, and tumors. Ultrasound is the imaging modality of choice for demonstrating tumors of the prostate. With the digital color Doppler, embolism can be diagnosed and occlusion of an artery can be identified by studying the blood flow.

CANCER DIAGNOSIS

Histologic evidence is vital in making a diagnosis of cancer. Tissue for diagnosis is obtained through scraping, needle aspiration, needle biopsy, incisional biopsy, and excisional biopsy.

Exfoliative cells can be found in all parts of the body. These are cells that have been scraped off deliberately or sloughed off naturally. They are found in the urine, sputum, feces, and mucus. Exfoliative cytologic studies are extremely helpful in identifying neoplastic disease, especially in the management of cervix and lung cancer. The only problem with cytologic studies is that individual cells are being viewed and the determination of cells as invasive or noninvasive is not possible.

Other methods of obtaining tissue are needle, incisional, and excisional biopsies. Needle biopsies and incisional biopsies can be done on an outpatient basis by using local anesthesia. Only small amounts of tissue can be obtained by needle and incisional biopsies. An **incisional biopsy** involves the removal of only a portion of the tumor for diagnosis. An **excisional biopsy** involves the removal of the entire tumor for diagnosis. This procedure provides for a more definitive diagnosis.[15]

When cancer is detected, determining the presence of metastatic disease is necessary. The use of a tumor marker may help detect widespread disease. A tumor marker is a substance manufactured and released by the tumor. Tumor markers "refer to a molecule that can be detected in serum, plasma, or other body fluid. No tumor marker has been shown to have a specificity or sensitivity that is adequate for the screening detection of malignancies in the general population."[14,16] Tumor markers are useful in detecting metastatic disease and determining the effect of the treatment.

STAGING SYSTEMS

After a histologic diagnosis of cancer has been made, the cancer must be staged. **Staging** helps determine the anatomic extent of the disease. Treatment decisions are based on the histologic diagnosis and extent of the disease. The natural growth for most cancers if untreated is that they extend beyond their original site by direct extension and then to the lymphatic and circulatory systems. They ultimately metastasize to distant sites. Staging systems are based on this concept.[2]

"Recommendations regarding staging of cancer by individual researchers, specialties, committees, and other groups have not been uniform."[2] The major groups who have been involved in staging and are working together to establish common terminology are the International Union Against Cancer (UICC), the International Federation of Gynecology and Obstetrics (FIGO), and the American Joint Committee for Cancer Staging and End Results Reporting (AJCC).[2]

The AJCC's general definitions of the TNM system are shown in Table 5-9 (subdivisions are not included). Another part of the staging system is the histologic type and histologic grade. Histologic type refers to cell type, and histologic grade refers to the differentiation of the cell. For example, the histologic type may be squamous cell carcinoma, and the histologic grade indicates the closeness of the cells' resemblance to a normal squamous cells. See Box 5-1 for the histopathologic grades.

Another aspect of the staging system is the use of stage 0

Table 5-9	TNM clinical classification
TNM Classification	**Description**

PRIMARY TUMOR (T)

TX	Primary tumor not assessable
T_0	No evidence of primary tumor
Tis	Carcinoma in situ
T_1, T_2, T_3, T_4	Increasing size and/or local extent of the primary tumor

REGIONAL LYMPH NODES (N)

NX	Regional lymph nodes not assessable
N_0	No regional lymph node metastasis
N_1, N_2, N_3	Increasing involvement of regional lymph nodes

DISTANT METASTASIS (M)

MX	Presence of distant metastasis not assessable
M_0	No distant metastasis
M_1	Distant metastasis

From *American Joint Committee on Cancer manual for staging of cancer,* ed 5, Philadelphia, 1997, Lippincott-Raven.

Box 5-1	Histopathologic grade (G)

GX	Grade not assessable
G1	Well differentiated
G2	Moderately differentiated
G3	Poorly differentiated
G4	Undifferentiated

through stage IV. Stage 0 usually indicates carcinoma in situ. Stages I and II indicate the smallness of the tumor and/or involvement of early local and regional nodes with no distant **metastases** (defined as the spread of cancer beyond the primary site). Stage III indicates that the tumor is more extensive locally and may have regional node involvement. Stage IV indicates locally advanced tumors with invasion beyond the regional nodes to other areas. The categorizations of stage 0 through IV are often grouped with the TNM system of staging. For example, stage 0, Tis, N0, M0 indicates an extremely localized early disease, whereas stage II, T2, N0, M0 indicates a more advanced disease. Stage IV, any T, any N, and M1 indicates an extremely late advanced disease.

There are several reasons for the precise clinical description and accurate classification of cancers, specifically:

■ To aid the physician and radiation therapy team in the planning of the treatment.

■ To provide some indication of prognosis. It may be one of many factors in determining prognosis.

- To assist in the evaluation of the results of treatment. It helps in comparing groups of cases, especially as it relates to various therapeutic procedures.
- To assist in the exchange of information from one treatment center to another.

SUMMARY

As stated earlier in this chapter, medicine is the accumulation of knowledge that has been developed through discovery, systematic scientific study, and research. These processes help detect, diagnose, treat, and manage disease. According to the ACS,[1] prevention and early detection are effective strategies of saving lives lost from cancer, diminishing suffering, and eliminating cancer as a major health problem. Prevention includes measures that stop cancer from developing. Early detection includes examinations and tests intended to find the disease as early as possible. After a diagnosis of cancer is made and the extent of the disease has been determined, appropriate treatment can be initiated.

Review Questions

Multiple Choice

1. Cancer screening can be effective if a disease has a high incidence or prevalence in a population and the test has the ability to produce results having the appropriate _____ and specificity.
   a. Incidence
   b. Sensitivity
   c. Range
   d. Cost factor
2. What are the factors that must be observed when taking the pulse?
   I. Rate
   II. Rhythm
   III. Size
   IV. Character
   V. Tension
   a. I and II
   b. I, II, III, and V
   c. III and IV
   d. I, II, IV, and V
3. What are the factors that must be observed for respirations?
   I. Rate
   II. Depth
   III. Character
   IV. Rhythm
   V. Tension
   a. I, II, III, and IV
   b. III, IV, and V
   c. I and II
   d. IV and V

4. Which of the following statements is not true?
   a. Ultrasonography uses high-frequency sound waves
   b. CT scans have a higher resolution than radiographs
   c. Electroencephalograms use ionizing radiation
   d. Most invasive procedures provide some risk to the patient
5. What is the normal adult range for blood pressure?
   a. 110 to 140 mm Hg over 60 to 80 mm Hg
   b. 130 to 160 mm Hg over 90 to 99 mm Hg
   c. 90 to 100 mm Hg over 60 to 80 mm Hg
   d. 115 to 150 mm Hg over 60 to 90 mm Hg
6. Exfoliative cytology is a means of collecting tissue through _____.
   a. Needle biopsy
   b. Scraping cells
   c. Incisional biopsy
   d. Excisional biopsy
7. Factors that help to facilitate the interview include all of the following except
   a. The interviewer's ability to put the patient at ease
   b. The asking of clear and concise questions
   c. The use technical jargon
   d. The use of terminology having the same meaning to the patient and interviewer
8. Some of the verbal responses that can facilitate the interview are
   I. Minimal responses
   II. Reflecting feelings
   III. Seeking clarification
   IV. Minimizing the patient's feelings or responses
   a. I, II, and III only
   b. I, III, and IV only
   c. II, III, and IV only
   d. III and IV only
9. Mass screening is based on the all of the following EXCEPT
   a. Specific results obtained
   b. Cost effectiveness
   c. Risk to the patient.
   d. Geographic location
10. All of the following are part of the medical record EXCEPT
    a. Results of laboratory tests
    b. Medical history
    c. Simulation and treatment-related films
    d. All of the above

Questions to Ponder

1. Describe the difference between an objective and subjective diagnosis.
2. Compare and contrast the elements of an interview in helping to make a diagnosis.
3. Describe nonverbal communication and give examples.

4. Predict the benefits of mass screening for at least three specific types of cancer.
5. Identify measures used to determine the value of a study.
6. Apply the general aspects of the TNM staging system in assisting with the treatment decision.
7. Compare the signs and symptoms for the following cancer sites: breast, prostate, lung, and colon.
8. Compare and contrast the screening, detection, and diagnostic tests for breast, prostate, lung, and colon cancer.

REFERENCES

1. American Cancer Society: http://www.cancer.org/ (Accessed 3/6/03).
2. American Joint Commission On Cancer: *AJCC cancer staging manual,* ed 5, Philadelphia, 1997, Lippincott-Raven.
3. *Cancer facts and figures,* Atlanta, 2003, The American Cancer Society.
4. Chao KSC, Perez CA, Brady LW: *Radiation oncology management decisions,* Philadelphia, 1999, Lippincott-Raven.
5. DeGowins RL: *Diagnostic examination,* ed 6, New York, 1994, McGraw-Hill.
6. Detmar SB, Aaronson NK, Wever LD, et al: How are you feeling? Patients' and oncologists' preferences for discussing health-related quality-of-life issues, *J Clin Oncol* 18:3295-301, 2000.
7. Du Gas BW: *Introduction to patient care: a comprehensive approach to nursing,* ed. 4, Philadelphia, 1983, WB Saunders.
8. Eisenberg RL: *Radiology: an illustrated history,* St. Louis, 1992, Mosby.
9. Fischbach F: *A manual of laboratory diagnostic tests,* ed 3, Philadelphia, 1988, JB Lippincott.
10. Gambert SR: Prostate cancer. When to offer screening in the primary care setting, *Geriatrics* 2001 56:22-26, 29-31, 2001.
11. Glanze WD, editor: *Mosby's medical and nursing dictionary,* ed 2, St. Louis, 1986, Mosby.
12. Henry JB: *Clinical diagnosis & management by laboratory methods,* ed 18, Philadelphia, 1991, WB Saunders.
13. Hirsch FR, Franklin WA, Gazdar AF, et al: Early detection of lung cancer: clinical perspectives of recent advances in biology and radiology, *Clin Cancer Res* 7:5-22, 2001.
14. Holleb AI, Fink DJ, Murphy GP, editors: *American cancer society textbook of clinical oncology,* Atlanta, 1991, American Cancer Society.
15. Hossfeld DK et al, editors: *Manual of clinical oncology,* ed 5, Berlin, 1990, UICC International Union Against Cancer, Springer-Verlag.
16. Lenhard RE, Osteen RT, Gansler T: *Clinical oncology,* Atlanta, 2001, The American Cancer Society.
17. Levitt SH, Khan FM, Potish RA, et al: *Levitt and Tapley's technological basis of radiation therapy: practical clinical applications,* ed 3, Philadelphia, 1992, Lea & Febiger.
18. Lewis SM, Collier IC: *Medical-surgical nursing,* New York, 1983, McGraw-Hill.
19. Locklear D: New CT scanner drives lung study, *Advance Rad Sci Prof* Mar 5, 2001.
20. Luboldt HJ, Bex A, Swoboda A, et al: Early detection of prostate cancer: a study using digital rectal examination and 4.0 ng/ml prostate-specific antigen cutoff, *Eur Urol* 39:131-137, 2001.
21. Noguchi M: Sentinel lymph node biopsy as an alternative to routine axillary lymph node dissection in breast cancer patients, *J Surg Oncol* 76:144-156, 2001.
22. Patz EF, Goodman PC, Bepler G: Screening for lung cancer, *N Engl J Med* 343(22):1627-1633, 2000.
23. Perez CA, Taylor M: Breast: stage Tis, T1, and T2 Tumors. In Perez CA, Brady LW, editors: *Principles and practice of radiation oncology,* ed 3, Philadelphia, 1998, Lippincott-Raven.
24. Rubin P: *Clinical oncology: a multidisciplinary approach for physicians and students,* ed 7, Philadelphia, 1993, WB Saunders.
25. Sapir R, Catane R, Kaufman B, et al: Cancer patient expectations of and communication with oncologist and oncology nurses: the experience of an integrated oncology and palliative care service, *Support Care Cancer* 8:458-463, 2000.
26. Singletary SE: Systemic treatment after sentinel lymph node biopsy in breast cancer: who, what, and why? *J Am Coll Surg* 192(2):220-230, 2001.
27. Sochurek H: *Medicine's new vision,* Easton, Pa, 1988, Mack Publishing.
28. Sone S, Li F, Yang ZG, et al: Results of three-year screening programme for lung cancer using mobile low-dose spiral computed tomography scanner, *Br J Cancer* 84:25-32, 2001.
29. Varricchio C, editor: *A cancer source book for nurses,* ed 7, New York, Boston, Atlanta, 1997, The American Cancer Society.
30. Wagner H, Ruckdeschel JC: Screening, early detection, and early intervention strategies for lung cancer, *Cancer Control* 2:493-502, 1995.
31. Wyngaarden JB, Smith LH, editors: *Cecil textbook of medicine,* Philadelphia, 1985, WB Saunders.

Radiographic Imaging

Dennis Leaver, Alan C. Miller[†]

Outline

Key Terms

[†]Deceased.

R adiographic imaging plays a critical role in helping the cancer patient. In radiation therapy it provides a way to view the interior of the human body. The x-rays used in this process can penetrate matter and create an image on film. This information helps members of the cancer-management team achieve an important goal in radiation oncology: to maximize the radiation dose to the diseased tissue (cancer cells) and minimize the dose to the surrounding normal tissue.

In this chapter, several concepts are introduced, including the history of x-rays, their production, the design of the tube from which they are produced, their interaction with matter, and the art of creating high-quality radiographic images.

HISTORICAL OVERVIEW

Approximately 100 years ago in November of 1895, a little-known German physicist tinkered in his laboratory at the University of Würzburg, Germany, with a fancy piece of glassware known as a Hittorf-Crookes tube. In communicating to his friend Theodor Boveri in early December 1895, Wilhelm Conrad Roentgen said, "I have discovered something interesting, but I do not know if my observations are correct."[10] After energizing his tube in the darkened laboratory, Roentgen noticed a strange green light emanating from a nearby piece of cardboard coated with phosphorescent material. This was hardly momentous because phosphorescence was a well-known event. However, when he passed a heavy piece of paper between the end of the tube and the cardboard coated with barium platinocyanide, the glow persisted. At that moment the scientist realized his newly found rays could pass through matter. He appropriately named them x-rays.

The essential elements of x-ray production have not changed in the intervening 100 years. However, x-rays have changed regarding their application in medicine. Modern x-ray tubes (Fig. 6-1) still require a source of electrons (the cathode), a current capable of liberating them from their tungsten filament home, a target toward which they can be directed (the anode), and the extremely high voltage necessary to persuade this reluctant electron cloud to flow at the velocity required to produce x-rays.

RADIOGRAPHIC IMAGING CONCEPTS

Radiographic imaging has rapidly expanded its role in diagnosing disease over the last half of the twentieth century. X-rays have a variety of diagnostic and therapeutic purposes, and, because of that, many modalities such as diagnostic radiology, nuclear medicine, mammography, cardiovascular imaging, and computed tomography (CT) scanning exist to aid the physician in the precise diagnosis of disease.

Several types of x-rays are used therapeutically in radiation oncology and its treatment of malignant disease. In the 40 to 300 kVp range, x-rays are used for two purposes. The first purpose is the treatment of skin cancers and other superficial tumors (most other tumors are treated with gamma rays and much higher energy x-rays above 1 million volts). The second purpose is the planning of a patient's treatment on the simulator. Two processes are used. With conventional simulation, x-ray fluoroscopy, radiographs and field defining system are used to obtain important patient anatomic information. During CT simulation, patient anatomic information and localization are obtained using CT images. That information gathered is then directly linked to a computerized treatment planning system.

Conventional simulation provides geometries similar to those found on treatment machines. This is done with x-ray equipment in the 50- to 120-kVp range. Diagnostic-quality images displayed on a radiograph or television monitor allow part of the cancer-management team to evaluate the geometry of the actual treatment. One of the radiation therapy department's essential functions is to ensure that all definitive (curative) and many palliative treatments are planned with meticulous detail to optimize the treatment's outcome (Box 6-1).[2] The radiographic imaging capabilities of the simulator allow the outlining of the tumor and a small volume of surrounding tissue to be documented and stored on a radiograph (Fig. 6-2).

The major components of an imaging system on a conventional radiation therapy simulator are an x-ray tube and a fluoroscope. Although these two components can be found hard at work in most diagnostic radiology departments, their purpose is somewhat different in radiation oncology. X-ray tubes in diagnostic radiology settings and those on radiation therapy simulators are essentially the same devices. Both can produce the same mysterious rays that Roentgen found interesting in 1895.

X-RAY TUBE

The electrical production of x-rays is possible only under special conditions, including a source of electrons, an appropriate target material, a high voltage, and a vacuum.[4] The production of x-rays occurs inside the tube because of high-speed electrons colliding with a metal object called the anode. The components of the tube, the cathode and anode, are enclosed in a glass envelope and protective housing.

Cathode

The **cathode** is one of the electrodes found in the x-ray tube and represents the negative side of the tube. It consists of two parts: the filament and focusing cup. As a first step in x-ray production, the primary function of the cathode is to produce electrons and focus the electron stream toward the metal anode.

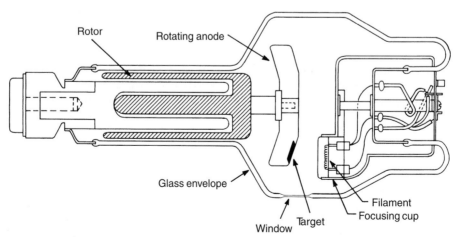

Figure 6-1. Diagram of a rotating-anode x-ray tube illustrating the fundamental parts. *(From Bushong S: Radiologic science for technologists: physics, biology, and protection, ed 7, St. Louis, 2001, Mosby.)*

Box 6-1	American College of Radiology (ACR) standards for radiation oncology equipment*

Radiation oncology assumes a significant role in the medical management and treatment of patients with cancer. Sixty percent of all cancer patients will be treated with radiation therapy as an integral component of their care. Optimal use of radiation therapy requires detailed attention to personnel, equipment, patient and personnel safety, and continuing staff. High-energy photon and electron beams, a computer-based treatment-planning system, simulation, dosimetry, brachytherapy, and the ability to fabricate treatment aids must be available to patients in all facilities, either onsite or through arrangements with another center. Regular maintenance and repair of equipment is also recommended as part of the *ACR Standards for Radiation Oncology.*

Treatment units, simulation equipment, and ancillary supporting equipment are an integral part of the *ACR Standards for Radiation Oncology.* This equipment should specifically include the following items:

1. Megavoltage radiation therapy equipment for external beam therapy: a linear accelerator or cobalt-60 teletherapy unit. If the cobalt 60 unit is the only megavoltage unit, it must have a treatment distance of 80 cm or more.
2. Electron beam therapy equipment or x-ray equipment for treatment of skin lesions or superficially placed lesions.
3. Appropriate brachytherapy equipment for intracavity and interstitial treatment (or arrangements in place for referral to appropriate facilities).
4. Computer dosimetry equipment capable of providing external beam isodose curves and brachytherapy isodose curves.
5. Simulator capable of duplicating the setups of any megavoltage unit and producing radiographs of the fields to be treated. Fluoroscopic capability is highly recommended.
6. Physics calibration devices for all equipment.
7. Beam shaping equipment.
8. Immobilization devices.

Modified from the American College of Radiology: *ACR standards for radiation oncology,* Reston, Va, 1999, ACR Publications Department.
*The standards of the ACR are not rules. Instead they attempt to define principles of practice that should generally produce high-quality patient care. The physician and medical physicist may modify an existing standard as determined by the individual patient and available resources. Adherence to ACR standards will not ensure a successful outcome in every situation.

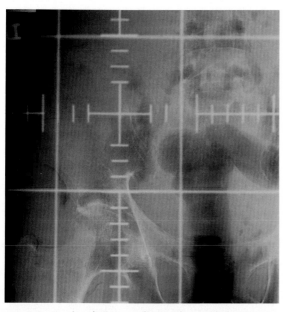

Figure 6-2. A simulation radiograph used for treatment-planning purposes. Note the field-defining wires outlining the tumor and a small volume of normal tissue.

Filament. The **filament** is a small coil of wire made of thoriated tungsten, which has an extremely high melting point (3380° C) (Fig. 6-3). The coil of wire is a smaller version of that inside a light bulb or toaster. A current, which heats the filament, is passed through the small coil of wire where electrons boil off and are emitted from the filament.

Most modern x-ray tubes have dual filaments, thus permitting the selection of a large or small source of electrons. The length and width of the filament control the ability of the x-ray tube to produce fine imaging detail. Most modern x-ray machines are equipped with a rotating anode tube having 0.6-mm (small) and 1.0-mm (large) focal spots. Other x-ray machines having focal spots as small as 0.1 mm and as large as 2.0 mm are also commercially available.[6] Using a small focal spot allows the radiation therapist to radiographically display fine detail. This is especially important in imaging the field-defining wires used to localize the treatment area during the simulation process.

Focusing cup. The selection of a small or large focal spot is associated with the small and large filaments, which are embedded in a small oval depression in the cathode assembly called a **focusing cup.** The negative charge of the focusing cup helps direct electrons toward the anode in a straighter, less divergent path.

Anode

The **anode** is the positive side of the x-ray tube. It receives electrons from the cathode as a target, dissipates the great amount of heat as a result of x-ray production, and serves as the path for the flow of high voltage. Aspects of the anode assembly include the composition of the anode, the target, and the line-focus principle.

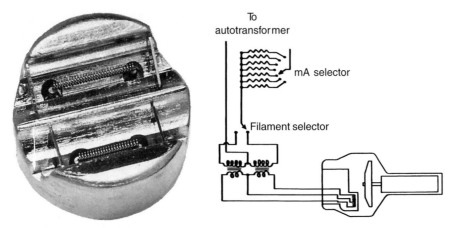

Figure 6-3. The dual-filament cathode in a focusing cup allows the selection of a small or large focal spot. *(From Bushong S: Radiologic science for technologists: physics, biology, and protection, ed 7, St. Louis, 2001, Mosby.)*

Composition. The anode is a circular disk composed of many different metals, each designed to contribute to the effectiveness of x-ray production (Fig. 6-4). The rotating tungsten disk serves as the target and can range up to 13 cm in diameter. Rhenium-alloyed tungsten serves as the target focal-track material because of its ability as a thermal conductor and the source of x-ray photons. The rotor, which allows most anodes to reach 3400 revolutions per minute, is an excellent device to help dispel the great amounts of heat created.

Target. Electrons from the cathode strike the portion of the anode called the target, or focal spot. This is the point at which x-ray photons are produced and begin to fan out in a divergent path. Divergence of the x-rays from their focal spot is similar to the sun's divergent rays seen on a partly sunny day. As the rays get closer to the earth, they fan out more from their source, which is 93 million miles away.

Line-focus principle. The **focal spot** is the section of the target at which radiation is produced. With the use of a small focal spot, more detail is seen on the simulation radiograph. Simultaneously, however, more heat is created by bombarding a smaller area of the target. To overcome the disadvantage of creating more heat and still maintain radiographic detail, the target is angled as shown in Fig. 6-5. In this way a larger geometrical area can be heated while a small focal spot is maintained. Fig. 6-5 displays the line-focus principle. The actual focal-spot size of the target is larger than the effective focal-spot size. Most x-ray tubes have a target angle from 7 to 20 degrees.[6,14]

Glass Envelope

The cathode and anode are in a vacuum in the x-ray tube. The removal of air from the glass envelope or x-ray tube permits the uninterrupted flow of electrons from the cathode to the

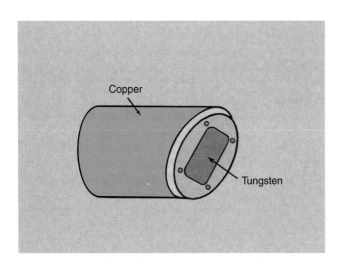

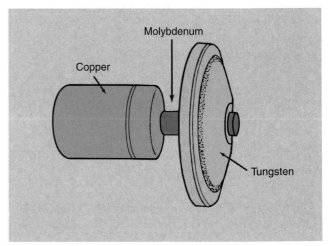

Figure 6-4. Composition of a rotating anode. *(From Bushong S: Radiologic science for technologists: physics, biology, and protection, ed 7, St. Louis, 2001, Mosby.)*

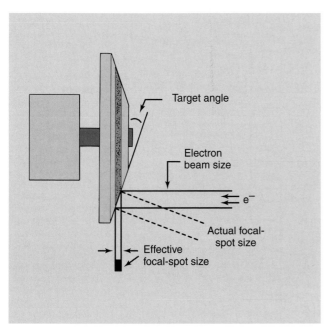

Figure 6-5. By angling the target of the rotating anode (thus taking advantage of the line-focus principle), a larger geometric area can be heated while a small focal spot is maintained. *(From Bushong S: Radiologic science for technologists: physics, biology, and protection, ed 7, St. Louis, 2001, Mosby)*

anode. The efficiency of the tube is increased because no air molecules are floating around inside the x-ray tube to collide with the accelerated electrons. The tube may measure from 20 to 30 cm in length and be as large as 15 cm in diameter at the central portion.

Protective Housing

To control unwanted radiation leakage and electrical shock, the x-ray tube is mounted inside the protective housing. Lead lining in the protective housing helps prevent radiation leakage during an exposure. A special oil fills the space between the protective housing and glass envelope to insulate the high-voltage potential and provide additional cooling capacity.

Recommendations for Extending Tube Life

Proper care and use by the radiation therapist can extend the life of the x-ray tube, the cost of which may range up to $120,000. Several practical steps may extend the life of the x-ray tube (Box 6-2). The manufacturer's warmup procedure should be followed to prevent excessive heat load on a cold anode; otherwise, serious damage can occur. Many systems have a digital display (measured in percent) of the heat capacity created on the tube after an exposure. This is a helpful tool in monitoring the heat units created. The rotor switch should not be held before an exposure. Most x-ray systems do not permit an exposure until the rotor has reached its full revolutions per minute. When the rotor switch is depressed,

thermionic emission of the electrons from the filament occurs and continues until an exposure is made. Any delay in exposure causes unnecessary wear on the filament and decreases the tube life. The use of a low mA (filament current) values during an x-ray exposure decreases filament evaporation, thus extending tube life. Finally, making multiple exposures near the tube limit should be avoided; otherwise, unnecessary heat stress on the anode may occur and cause serious damage.

X-RAY PRODUCTION

The essentials of x-ray generation are remarkably simple. They willingly follow the orderly progression of rules in the physical sciences. X-rays are just one of the many forms of electromagnetic energy organized according to wavelength on the electromagnetic spectrum (Fig. 6-6). Initially, x-rays may appear to have little in common with their spectral cousins: radio and microwaves, visible light, cosmic radiation, and a host of other energy forms. However, all these radiant energies share certain properties. They all travel at the speed of light (3×10^{10} cm per second); they all take the form of a wave, each with its own characteristic undulating pattern expressed as wavelength (the distance between the crests in the wave) and frequency (the number of complete wave cycles per second); and they all consist of photons, which are minute bundles of pure energy having no mass and no electrical charge. The concept of something made up of nothing may be difficult to appreciate because humans tend to think in terms of objects or things, even at the atomic level. However, photons (or quanta) exist and constantly roam around us at the speed of light.

Understanding the unique relationship that exists between photon wavelength and frequency is essential to understanding the dramatically different behaviors observed in various forms of electromagnetic radiation. For example, microwave television signals can transmit sound and image information across great distances, but they cannot readily pass through matter without being deflected. In contrast, x-rays are capable

Box 6-2	Extending x-ray tube life

1. Follow the manufacturer's warmup procedure to prevent heat damage to the anode.
2. Monitor the heat units created during repeated exposures.
3. Avoid holding the rotor switch before an exposure. Double-press switches should be completely depressed in one motion, and dual switches should have the exposure switch pressed first, and then the rotor switch.*
4. Use low mA (filament current) values whenever possible.
5. Avoid multiple exposures near the tube limit.

*From Carlton RR, McKenna-Adler A: *Principles of radiographic imaging,* ed 3, Albany, NY, 2001, Delmar Publishing.

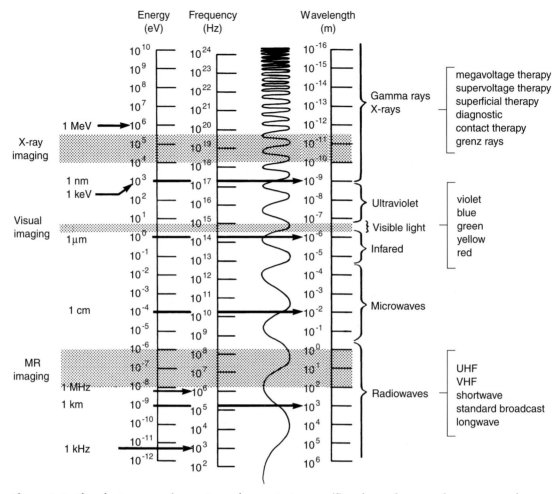

Figure 6-6. The electromagnetic spectrum demonstrates specific values of energy, frequency, and wavelength for some regions of the spectrum. *(From Bushong S: Radiologic science for technologists: physics, biology, and protection, ed 7, St. Louis, 2001, Mosby.)*

of penetrating matter and altering its atomic structure through a process called ionization (the ejection of orbital electrons). Because the velocity of all radiant energy forms is constant, the differing properties of radiant energy can be attributed only to variations in their wavelength and frequency.

X-ray radiations and gamma radiations are located at the high end of the spectrum and possess extremely short wavelengths. The relationship between wavelength and frequency is an inverse proportion (i.e., as wavelength decreases, frequency increases). In 1900 the German physicist Max Planck showed through his quantum theory that frequency and energy are directly proportional. Despite their constant velocities, different forms of electromagnetic radiation may have widely varying energies (from the low end of the spectrum [radio waves] to the high end [x-ray radiations, gamma radiations, and cosmic radiations]). As the wavelength decreases and frequency increases, so does the associated quantum energy.

X-rays are the classical form of artificially produced electromagnetic radiation. Unlike most spectral radiant energies,

no spontaneous equivalent for x-rays exists in nature. They are purely a human-produced phenomenon. As described earlier in this chapter, producing x-rays is simple and requires only a source of electrons, a target at which to direct the electron stream, a high-vacuum glass tube, and a source of electricity of sufficient voltage.

Thermionic Emission

In an oversimplification, x-rays are produced when a stream of electrons liberated from the cathode is directed across the tube vacuum at extremely high speeds to interact with the anode. These cathode electrons are freed from the tungsten filament atoms in a process called **thermionic emission.** This elaborate-sounding term makes perfect sense if broken down into its root forms (thermal refers to heat, ions are charged particles, and emission is release).

The process of liberating electrons through the application of heat is similar to that seen in an ordinary light bulb. An electrical current is applied to the filament, which because of its resistance, begins to glow. As the current increases, the filament reaches the white-hot state necessary for outer-shell electrons to leave their orbits. This is known as incandescence, and the resulting electrons are called thermions. Thermionic emission begins when the filament circuit (usually the first stage in a two-stage exposure switch) is energized.

Potential Difference

The electron cloud or space charge produced from the filament hovers in the vicinity of the cathode indefinitely unless something is done to encourage it to move. The motivating force comes the moment the exposure switch is depressed. High voltage, typically on the order of 70,000 to 120,000 V (70 to 120 kVp), is applied to create a high potential difference between the negative and positive anodes. According to the basic laws of electrodynamics, this causes the negatively charged electrons to be strongly repelled from the cathode and drawn at extreme speeds toward the attracting force of the positively charged anode. In modern three-phase radiographic equipment, the velocity of this electron stream can approach the speed of light.

Target Interaction

X-rays are produced when the kinetic energy of the moving electron stream is given up as it enters the nuclear field of the anode. As noted earlier in the discussion of x-ray tube design, the anode (or target) is composed of materials selected for their high atomic number and high melting point. The former factor largely determines the energy efficiency of x-ray production resulting from interactions that take place in the tube. The latter minimizes the potential for damage from the intense heat that those interactions produce. More than 99%

of the electrical energy applied to the tube is converted to heat, and only a tiny fraction (about 0.6% at diagnostic energy levels) becomes x-rays.

The principal interaction in x-ray production results in the output of **bremsstrahlung** (German for "breaking") radiation (Fig. 6-7). Bremsstrahlung accounts for approximately 75% to 80% of the tube's output and is produced by the sudden deceleration of the high-speed electron as it is deflected around the nucleus of the tungsten atom. The therapist should remember that electrons have mass and moving electrons possess kinetic energy. When any moving object is abruptly slowed, the surplus energy must be given off. The greater the angle of deflection around the nucleus, the more pronounced the degree of deceleration and the more energy released. A somewhat remote analogy may be found in an automobile rounding a bend in the road. As the automobile slows, some energy is converted to heat through friction with the brakes and tires. This same vehicle suddenly negotiating a sharp curve may have to slow almost to a stop, thereby giving off most or all its kinetic energy. In the target atoms of the anode the kinetic energy of the decelerating electron is given off as a bundle of pure energy, or an x-ray photon.

A second, lesser interaction also contributes to the production of x-rays. **Characteristic radiation** is created by the direct interaction of cathode electrons with inner-shell electrons of the target material. Some electrons may collide with tungsten orbital electrons that have sufficient energy to overcome their binding energy and eject them from orbit. This process is called ionization (Fig. 6-8). When an inner-shell electron is ejected from orbit, other electrons (generally from adjacent shells) move in to fill the hole left. The energy of

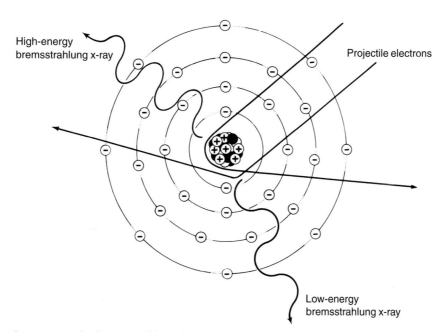

Figure 6-7. The bremsstrahlung interaction. *(From Bushong S: Radiologic science for technologists: physics, biology, and protection, ed 7, St. Louis, 2001, Mosby.)*

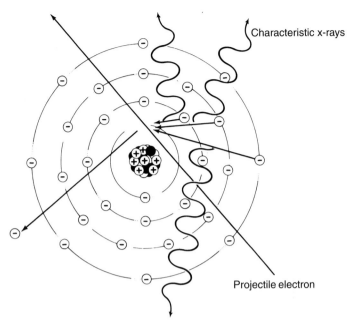

Figure 6-8. The characteristic interaction. *(From Bushong S: Radiologic science for technologists: physics, biology, and protection, ed 7, St. Louis, 2001, Mosby.)*

x-rays produced in this manner is dependent on the binding energy of the target atom's electrons. As the atomic number of an element increases, so does the energy level of each shell. This is the rationale for using materials of high atomic number (such as tungsten) in the targets of x-ray tubes. Binding energy drops with each successive electron orbit away from the nucleus. Outer-shell, or valence, electrons have an extremely low binding energy and are easily ejected from orbit. Therefore ionization events in the O or P shell of the tungsten atom do not produce characteristic x-ray photons of sufficient energy to be useful. Tungsten K-shell electrons, however, have a binding energy of 69.5 keV. When a K-shell electron is ejected from orbit and replaced with a tungsten L-shell electron, a surplus energy of 57.4 keV is released in the form of a characteristic x-ray photon.[3] Energies of this magnitude are well within the useful range for diagnostic x-rays.

Physical Relationships in X-ray Production

A basic premise of physics is that matter can be neither created nor destroyed; it can only change its state. Thanks to the efforts of Albert Einstein, matter's conversion to energy is now known. Einstein, the undeniable father of modern nuclear physics, proved mathematically the theoretical relationship between the kinetic energy of moving matter and the production of light quanta (photons). In his historic theory of relativity, Einstein demonstrated that matter accelerated to a sufficient velocity can become pure energy.

On a more practical level (applied to the production of x-rays) the velocity of the cathode stream is determined by the energy supplied in volts; as the voltage increases, so does the energy available for conversion into x-ray photons. As may

be expected, high-energy photons pass through matter more readily than low-energy photons. The ability of the photon stream to pass through matter such as human body tissues is critical to the production of a useful image on a radiograph. This ability is generally called penetration. A radiation beam of high energy penetrates structures with greater ease than a weak, low-voltage beam. Although this may appear obvious, the theory behind it is of great importance in diagnostic radiography and radiation therapy.

As the potential difference (voltage) is increased across the x-ray tube vacuum, the velocity of the cathode electron stream is increased. The greater the speed of the moving matter, the greater the resultant energy of the photon stream produced by target interactions. As noted earlier, when mass is slowed or stopped, its energy must be given up in some form. In this situation, mass is converted to heat and photons. Increasing voltage (kVp) increases photon energy.

This energy is commonly termed *beam quality*. A beam of radiation produced by using high kVp is a high-quality beam (i.e., it contains a large percentage of highly penetrating, extremely energetic photons). However, quality addresses only half of the x-ray beam equation. The number of photons in the beam must be considered, and the way quality and quantity may interrelate in radiographic image production must be examined.

From an extremely early age, children are taught a simple mathematical premise: if five oranges are given to a friend, the friend will have five oranges (quantity). Explaining that three of the oranges are nice and juicy (high quality) and the other two are dry and useless (low quality) is more difficult. Such is the relationship between x-ray tube current and x-ray production. The relationship is purely a question of the number of photons in the stream. Most students in radiation therapy find the concept of quantity easier to accept than issues involving the conversion of matter to energy.

Thankfully, the relationship between the number of cathode electrons released during thermionic emission and the production of x-ray photons is simple; they occur in direct proportion. As the operator of the radiation therapy simulation equipment increases tube current, a predictable increase in the number of electrons released occurs. The relationship between current (expressed in mAs) and the quantity of electrons liberated is a direct proportion. The relationship has no bearing on beam energy, penetrating ability, or any other variable necessarily useful. For example, it may be simply a question of producing 10-to-the-billionth-power photons for a certain mAs. If the mAs is doubled, 20-to-the-billionth power photons are produced. The fact that many of these photons will not have sufficient energy to contribute to any useful radiographic image (the dry oranges) is irrelevant, but an important correlation exists among energy, quantity, and image production.

X-RAY INTERACTIONS WITH MATTER

Overview

The ability of an x-ray beam to produce a latent radiographic image on film depends on certain key properties characteristic of extremely short-wavelength, high-frequency forms of radiant energy.[3,7,17] X-rays travel in straight lines and diverge from a point of origin. (This is critical in understanding the geometrical principals discussed in the previous section.) X-rays are capable of causing certain substances to fluoresce, ionizing materials through which they pass, and causing chemical and biologic changes in tissue. These properties are the basis of x-ray interactions with matter.

As it passes through matter, the x-ray beam undergoes a gradual reduction in the number of photons or exposure rate. This process is termed absorption or, more correctly, **attenuation.** Photons in the original or primary beam may also be scattered (i.e., they may change direction as they collide with atoms in their path). In the human body the rate of beam attenuation and degree of scattering is determined by tissue thickness, density, and effective atomic number. The net effect is a wide variation in the quantity of photons actually reaching the film. The nature of the tissues through which the beam must pass controls which photons strike and where they strike.

The human body is not a homogenous structure. It consists of varying quantities of air, fat, water, muscle, and bone, each with their own absorption properties. A radiograph of the abdomen (Fig. 6-9) provides an ideal demonstration of these differential absorption characteristics. Denser structures and those of higher-average atomic numbers appear as lighter areas on the radiograph because of their higher rates of attenuation. Air (as a result of its extremely low density) and fat (as a result of its relatively low atomic number) appear as dark areas, whereas bone (which is dense and has a high atomic

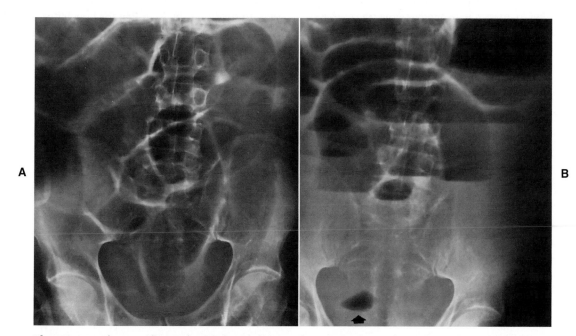

A

B

Figure 6-9. These radiographs of the abdomen demonstrate an obstruction of the small bowel. Large amounts of gas (shown as dark areas on the radiograph) are seen on supine **(A)** and upright **(B)** abdominal films. Note the small amount of gas in the colon. Bone (whiter areas) and other soft-tissue structures are also demonstrated in both radiographs. *(From Eisenberg RL, Dennis CA: Comprehensive radiologic pathology, St. Louis, 1995, Mosby.)*

number [z]) appears as a light shadow on the film. This range in differential absorption makes the viewing of anatomic detail possible. From a practical standpoint, the goal of the radiation therapist is to select technical factors (appropriate kVp and mAs) that maximize the rate of differential absorption and increase the visibility of detail in the image.

Interactions in the Diagnostic Range

For an appreciation of the importance of differential absorption, some understanding of x-ray photons at the subatomic level is important. In the diagnostic energy range, three interactions occur. Photons may be absorbed photoelectrically or undergo coherent (unmodified) or **Compton scattering** during an interaction. In general, a scattered photon is a bad photon. It rarely contributes to a useful image on the film, and therapists go to great lengths to minimize its detrimental effect. Technical factors are selected in an attempt to maximize differential absorption through photoelectric effect, minimize Compton scattering, and keep patient exposure within reasonable limits.

Unfortunately, the predominant interaction in the diagnostic energy range is the Compton effect (Fig. 6-10). Compton scattering is produced when an x-ray photon interacts with an outer-shell orbital electron with sufficient energy to eject it from orbit and alter its own path. The classic analogy is seen in the game of billiards, in which the cue ball collides with another ball and both fly off in different directions. In Compton scattering the freed electron likely travels only an extremely short distance before attaching to another atom. At high kVp settings the scattered photon may have enough energy remaining to interact with another atom (thus producing more scatter) or even exit the body part completely. If the

photon reaches the film, it strikes it at random, thus producing unwanted density because its path no longer corresponds accurately to the portion of anatomy through which it passed. In any situation, the scattered photon is a bad photon and detrimental to image quality.

Unmodified scattering (Fig. 6-11) is of relatively little importance to diagnostic imaging. This scattering occurs at low energy levels (generally below 10 keV), and the resultant scattered photons do not have sufficient energy remaining to be emitted from the part. Coherent scattering (also called Thomson or unmodified scattering) results in a change in the incident photon's direction but no change in energy. In this interaction, not enough energy exists to eject an electron from its orbit.

As noted earlier, the only interaction with the capacity to produce a useful image on the film is **photoelectric effect.** This interaction, sometimes described as *true absorption,* occurs when the incident photon penetrates deep into the atom and ejects an inner-shell electron from orbit (Fig. 6-12). Orbital electrons close to the nucleus have higher binding energies, and all the photon's energy is required to remove them from orbit. Because a photon is nothing more than a bundle of pure energy, it ceases to exist or is absorbed in the process if all its energy is given up. The energy is transferred to the electron, now termed a photoelectron, with a kinetic energy equal to the original energy of the incident photon. This photoelectron has sufficient energy to undergo a variety of other interactions that are beyond the scope of this chapter.

An atom is ionized when it loses or gains an electron. Ionization is an unstable atomic state, and the ionized atom seeks to stabilize itself by filling the hole left in its inner electron shell. This effort sets off a chain reaction that can lead to

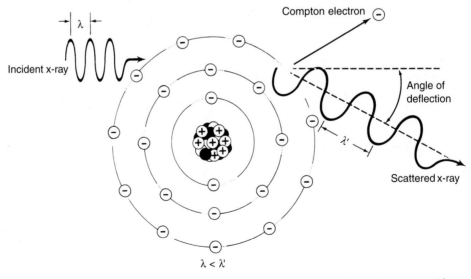

Figure 6-10. The Compton effect is produced when an x-ray photon interacts with an outer-shell orbital electron. The photon must posses sufficient energy to eject it from orbit and alter its own path. *(From Bushong S: Radiologic science for technologists: physics, biology, and protection, ed 7, St. Louis, 2001, Mosby.)*

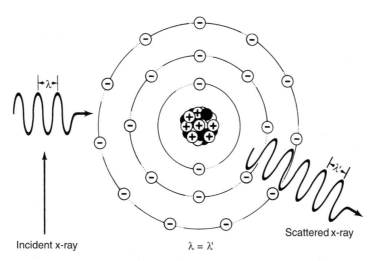

Incident x-ray

Scattered x-ray

$\lambda = \lambda'$

Figure 6-11. Unmodified scattering is an interaction between extremely low energy (generally below 10 keV) and is of little importance in radiation therapy. *(From Bushong S: Radiologic science for technologists: physics, biology, and protection, ed 7, St. Louis, 2001, Mosby.)*

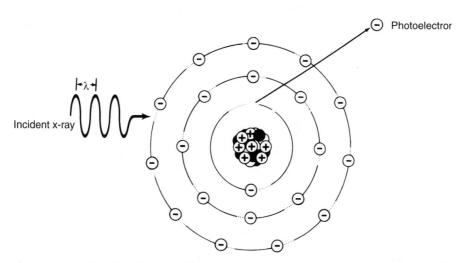

Photoelectron

Incident x-ray

Figure 6-12. The photoelectric effect, sometimes described as true absorption, occurs when the incident photon penetrates deep into the atom and ejects an inner-shell electron from orbit. *(From Bushong S: Radiologic science for technologists: physics, biology, and protection, ed 7, St. Louis, 2001, Mosby.)*

as many as six different ionizing events, each with its own subsequent release of pure energy (a new photon). In practice, most of these events possess insufficient energy to be of any radiographic significance. However, atoms of high atomic number with k-shell binding energies of 20 or 30 keV can easily produce secondary or characteristic photons energetic enough to reach the film or undergo additional ionizing events.

The human body is composed primarily of carbon, hydrogen, and oxygen atoms, and none of these materials has sufficiently high k-energies to produce secondary photons of any magnitude. For this reason, most photoelectric interactions in tissue result simply in absorption with no appreciable secondary effect. This is desirable because to clearly define anatomic structures of differing densities and atomic number on the radiograph, their relative variation in absorption rates, however slight, must be used to the fullest imaging advantage.

Normal human anatomy provides a predictable variation in tissue densities. For example, kidneys can be seen in a plain radiograph of the abdomen not because of their density difference compared with the greater surrounding tissue but because they are outlined by a thin band of fat called the adipose capsule. Contrast materials such as iodine, barium, and other agents of high atomic number may be used to enhance the visibility of structures with similar composition that would otherwise remain unseen. Advanced imaging modalities such as CT scanning and magnetic resonance imaging (MRI) have done much to overcome this limitation in conventional diagnostic radiography.

Imaging Pathology

Any diseased state in the body can dramatically alter the body's absorption characteristics. In many situations the changes that accompany pathology can actually improve radiographic demonstration. This phenomenon is of obvious value in diagnostic radiography and can also prove useful in

radiation therapy treatment planning. After all, localizing disease that is not visible radiographically is difficult.

Tissue changes that occur in pathology are often characterized as *additive* or *destructive* (Fig. 6-13). Additive pathologies are those with increased tissue density and therefore appear as light regions on the radiograph or CT image. (The opposite is true with the reverse image on the television monitor during fluoroscopy, in which densities such as bone and tumor appear darker.) Most nonmalignant disease entities are additive. They include edema, Paget's disease, atelectasis, abscesses, pleural effusions, and several other common illnesses. Hilar masses commonly associated with lung

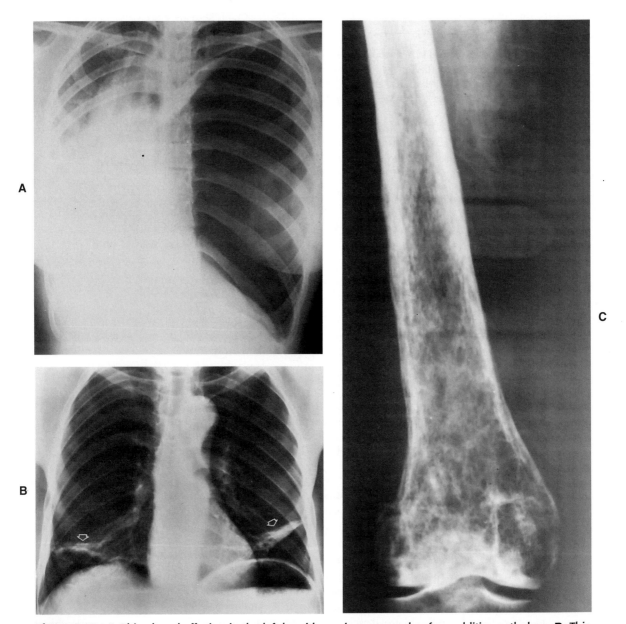

Figure 6-13. A, This pleural effusion in the left hemithorax is an example of an additive pathology. **B,** This illustration demonstrates atelectasis in the lower portion of both lungs (another example of an additive pathology [an opacity on the radiograph]). **C,** A Ewing's sarcoma has destroyed part of the distal femur. *(From Eisenberg RL, Dennis CA: Comprehensive radiologic pathology, St. Louis, 1995, Mosby.)*

tumors are universally additive, and any large, fluid-filled mass also appears as an additive pathology. Necrotic areas in a tumor are generally destructive in appearance (typical of astrocytoma), but the band of actively mitotic, highly vascularized malignant tissue that surrounds this dead mass is often seen as additive in density.

Unfortunately, definite rules for malignant disease imaging do not exist because several tumors can cause increased tissue density. Certain cancers follow predictable patterns that can reliably guide the radiation oncologist and radiation therapist in their efforts to localize the lesion. Most patients with multiple myeloma or any osteolytic metastatic disease have a destructive pathologic disease. Metastases from breast and prostate cancer can sometimes be seen as pathologically additive or destructive in the radiographic image when they are present in bone. Certain sarcomas and other soft tissue tumors frequently differentiate poorly from surrounding tissues and are best localized by palpation and visual observation, although they can be seen radiographically through the use of low-kVp techniques.

The individual nature of healthy and diseased body tissues makes generalizations on levels of absorption difficult and possibly unwise. Far more important is the radiation therapist's understanding that dense structures absorb more photons photoelectrically and produce more Compton scattering. Conversely, tissues that are thin, less dense, and aged result in dramatically decreased attenuation and thus produce a disproportionately darker image on the film.

FUNDAMENTALS OF IMAGING

Introduction to Concepts of Contrast and Density

The function of voltage (kVp) and current (mAs) in radiographic imaging involves the way more energetic photons (controlled by kVp) affect the film and the reason greater or lesser quantities of photons (controlled by mAs) make the film darker or lighter.[8,9] The explanation to these subjects focus on the two most important concepts in radiographic imaging: radiographic density and contrast.

Density.   **Radiographic density** is defined as the degree of darkening on the film. This is not to be confused with tissue density, which refers to the compactness of molecules in the atomic structure of different body parts. Radiographic density is a relatively simple concept to grasp because it is easy to visualize. A radiograph of high density is dark, and a radiograph of low density is light. The rules governing radiographic density are equally straightforward. When more photons reach the film, density increases; when fewer photons reach the film, density decreases.

Many authors suggest that the principal factor governing radiographic density is mAs (i.e., mAs equals the tube current in milliamperes multiplied by the time of exposure). Although mAs largely determines the quantity of photons in the primary beam, giving mAs an enormous amount of credit in the regulation of density is inaccurate because numerous other factors may have equal or greater effect. For example, source-film distance (SFD), kVp, and grid ratio are important factors. However, mAs has a clear and predictable role in radiographic density. When all other factors remain the same, the relationship between mAs and density is a direct proportion (i.e., as mAs is doubled, so is the resulting density on the film). This makes mAs an extremely useful tool in the control of density and one that therapists find easy to use. By virtue of its convenience, this tool is also subject to abuse because as mAs is doubled to increase density so is the dose of radiation exposure to the patient.

In addition, kVp may be used to change radiographic density. A far smaller increase in kVp is needed to significantly affect the film than is required by using mAs. When all other factors remain the same, a kVp increase of only 15% doubles the radiographic density. To put this in perspective, a scenario in which the therapist is involved in a prostate localization procedure may be considered. In the anteroposterior (AP) projection the therapist selects an mAs of 50 at 74 kVp. The resulting radiograph has insufficient density (too light) and must be repeated. The therapist may then use 100 mAs and 74 kVp or 50 mAs and 85 kVp to make the correction; either combination produces the same new radiographic density. One choice may be preferable to the other, and several variables yet to be discussed determine the more desirable combination.

When mAs is used to control density, the only direct effects are on density and patient dose. However, extremely high mAs exposures, particularly those made by using the small focal spot, can shorten tube life dramatically. In contrast, when kVp is used to adjust density, a change in radiographic contrast also occurs, and this may not always be desirable.

Another major extrinsic factor influencing density is distance, which refers to the gap between the focal spot of the x-ray tube and the recording medium or film. The terminology used to describe this gap varies with the equipment in use and its application. SFD, focal-film distance (FFD), and source-image receptor distance (SID) refer to the same idea.

Distance can have a profound effect on radiographic density (Fig. 6-14), and, although distance is a critical factor in diagnostic radiography when the radiographer may have to negotiate a variety of distance changes, it is less important to the radiation therapist who generally works with one or two fixed distances. Still, some discussion on the effect of distance is important, not only for its relationship to radiographic density but also because of its vital influence on occupational exposure. The relationship between distance and density follows the **inverse square law,** which states that the intensity of the beam of radiation is inversely proportional to the square of the distance. Put more simply, when distance is doubled, the quantity of radiation reaching the image receptor (or occupationally exposed personnel working with brachytherapy sources) is reduced to one fourth. From a practical standpoint, a film with a satisfactory radiographic density using 100 mAs at 80 cm SFD requires 400 mAs to produce the same density at 160 cm.

The inverse square law works because of the property of x-rays stating that they travel in straight lines and diverge from a point of origin. As distance is doubled, a quantity of radiation is spread over an area four times as great, therefore reducing the intensity of the beam in an area to one fourth its original value.

Contrast.   Perhaps no element of radiographic imaging is more important or more misunderstood than contrast. **Radiographic contrast** is the element of imaging that provides visual evidence of the all-important differential absorp-

tion rates of various body tissues. Radiographic contrast has been described as the tonal range of densities from black to white or the number of shades of grey in the radiograph. Neither of these definitions (nor any of the others that have appeared in print over the years) provides an adequate description of the significance of contrast in defining information on the film.

When most homes had black and white television sets, describing the effect of contrast on a visible image was easier. With these old sets, contrast could be arbitrarily increased or decreased by the twist of a knob. Today, a similar demonstration can be conducted through black and white photographs.

The dramatic variation in the three photographs in Fig. 6-15 is clear. Fig. 6-15 illustrates the difference between high and low contrast. The same ability to precisely define or destroy visible information exists in the medical imaging field and is the responsibility of the radiation therapist's correct application of technique.

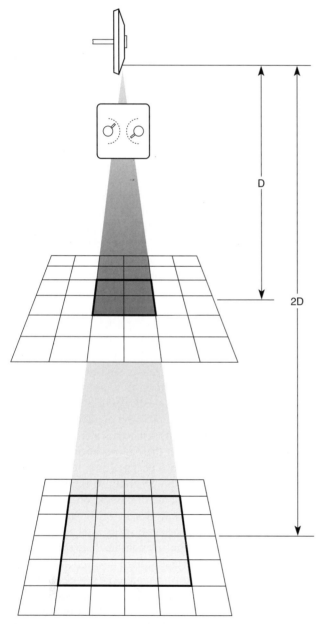

Figure 6-14. The inverse square law means as distance (D) is doubled. A quantity of radiation is spread over an area four times as great, therefore reducing the intensity of the beam in any area to one fourth its original value. *(Courtesy Eastman Kodak, Rochester, New York.)*

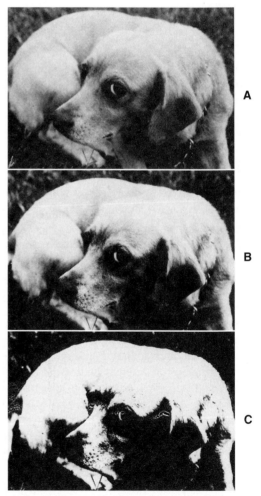

Figure 6-15. The dog pictured has been photographed to demonstrate differences in contrast. **A,** Low contrast. **B,** Moderate contrast. **C,** High contrast. *(From Bushong S: Radiologic science for technologists: physics, biology, and protection. ed 7, St. Louis, 2001, Mosby.)*

The skull radiographs shown in Fig. 6-16 also exhibit identical densities. However, even to the casual observer, the difference in visible information is readily apparent. Fig. 6-16, *A,* demonstrates clearly defined borders that may be pleasing to the eye, but it lacks detailed anatomic information. Fig. 6-16, *D,* is the opposite; the contrast is too low, and information is lost as a result of the overpenetration of the subject anatomy and increased production of scattered radiation. The other two images (Fig. 6-16, *B* and *C*) may represent optimal contrast. **Optimal contrast** results when technical factors (primarily kVp) are selected that maximize the rate of differential absorption between body parts of

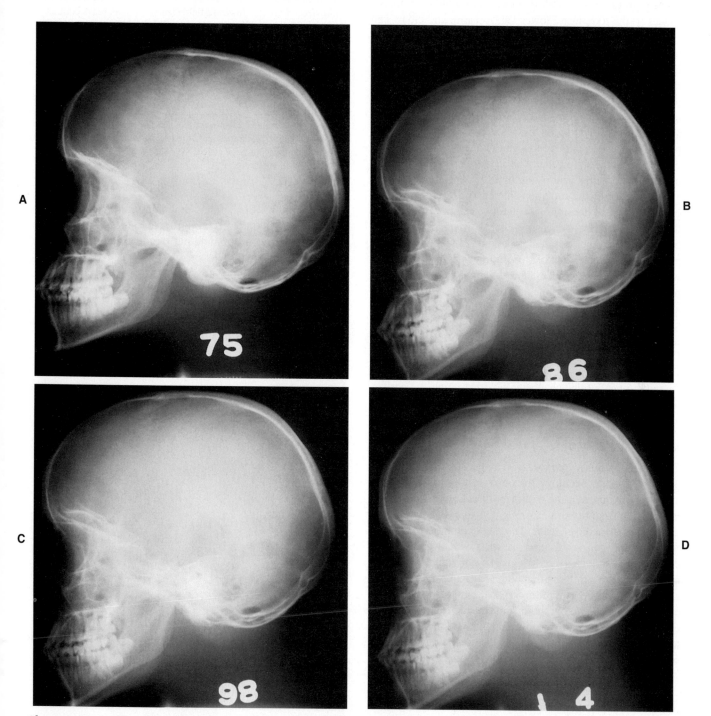

Figure 6-16. In this series of four radiographs, density remains constant. A 15% increase in kVp (**A,** 75 kVp; **B,** 86 kVp; **C,** 98 kVp; and **D,** 114 kVp) and reduction in mAs demonstrates visible changes in contrast. Note the loss of detail from image **A** to image **D,** especially near the sella turcica. In **D,** the contrast is low because of the overpenetration of the subject anatomy and increased production of scatter radiation.

varying tissue density and effective atomic number. Optimal kVp ranges exist for all body parts. The most important factor in determining optimal kVp is part thickness, but numerous other elements such as grid ratio and field size may also influence the selection (Table 6-1).

Generally, any time that the thickness of the body part exceeds 10 to 12 cm, a radiographic grid should be used. All tissues of the foot, hand, lower leg, forearm, and elbow can be adequately demonstrated without the use of a grid. In many situations the knee and upper arm may also be examined by using only screen-type radiographic techniques. Beyond this, a grid should be used to absorb the scattered radiation emitted from the thicker body parts and to allow the use of beam energies needed to maximize differential absorption between similar tissues. Chest and rib radiography may be an exception to this guideline but only under specific circumstances. In general, even these procedures should be performed with a grid using high kVp ranges.

The ability of the radiation therapist to exercise control over contrast and density in an effective manner is not something that is readily learned from books. Medical imaging is certainly a visual science, and no amount of text will take the place of experience. Persons operating imaging equipment who wish to fully exercise their skills must understand the physics of radiographic imaging and then use all the tools available to them to produce quality radiographs. The temptation is great for persons to consider only easy and predictable options, such as mAs in the control of density. Disregarding the enormous flexibility available through varying kVp, use of a grid, field size, and other factors discussed throughout this chapter is easy, but doing so deprives the true professional of the right to practice medical imaging as an art and a science.

RECORDING MEDIA

One of the primary purposes of diagnostic-quality x-rays used in radiation oncology (as opposed to extremely high-energy x-rays used in the treatment of cancer) is to transfer information from the simulator's x-ray beam to a member of the radiation oncology team. The most common method of receiving and storing this information is with x-ray film. The construction and characteristics of x-ray film and photographic film are similar in that both are sensitive to light and radiation. However, x-ray film has a spectral response different from that of photographic film. In addition to conventional recording media (processing film), modern imaging technology has developed many other radiographic image receptors such as fluoroscopic screens, image intensifiers, computer-linked detectors, scintillation and piezoelectric crystals, and selenium plates.[4,16] More recently, effort has been invested in developing and perfecting an imaging technology without the use of film.[14] With the use of CT simulation, fluoroscopy and film are replaced with digital reconstructed radiographs (DRRs), a type of computer image similar in appearance to a radiograph but displayed on a

Table 6-1	Factors influencing contrast and density		
Factor	**Change**	**Result**
Kilovoltage peak	Increase kVp	Decrease contrast
Part thickness	Increase thickness	Decrease contrast
Field size	Increase field size	Decrease contrast
Tissue density	Increase density	Decrease contrast
Grid ratio	Increase ratio	Increase contrast
Grid frequency	Increase frequency	Decrease contrast
Processing chemical	Increase temperature	Decrease contrast temperature
OFD	Increase OFD	Increase contrast

*Note that the change in contrast results when a single factor is modified alone and without compensation of other factors. Multiple concurrent changes can produce varying effects.
OFD, Object-film distance.

video monitor.[13] In digital radiography, radiation detectors whose electrical output is proportional to the radiation intensity are used to convert an output signal to a digital form the computer can display as an image (Fig. 6-17).[3]

Film

The conventional recording media (film, screens, and cassettes) used in capturing an x-ray image are discussed in this section. X-ray film has three major components: base,

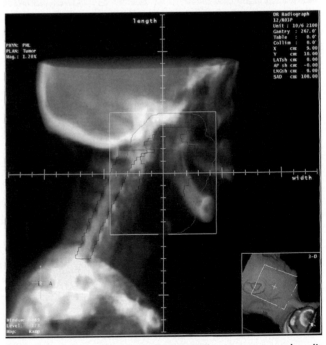

Figure 6-17. An example of a digitally reconstructed radiograph (DRR) demonstrating the treatment area on a lateral neck field of a radiation therapy patient with a tumor in the tonsillar fossa.

Supercoating
Emulsion
Adhesive

Base

Adhesive
Emulsion
Supercoating

150-250 μm

5-25 μm

Figure 6-18. A cross-sectional view of x-ray film. The base is a rigid, transparent plastic onto which the emulsion is coated. *(From Bushong S: Radiologic science for technologists: physics, biology, and protection, ed 7, St. Louis, 2001, Mosby.)*

emulsion, and protective coating. The base is a rigid, transparent plastic onto which the emulsion is coated (Fig. 6-18). An x-ray film base must be flexible enough to maintain its size and shape during processing (immersion in a chemical solution) and handling yet strong enough to withstand repeated viewing on a radiographic illuminator. To help reduce eyestrain during viewing of the radiographic image, a blue dye is added to the film during manufacturing. Before the film base is coated with the emulsion that contains the photosensitive crystals, a thin adhesive layer is applied to the base.

The emulsion is composed of gelatin and photosensitive silver halide crystals (Fig. 6-19). The photosensitive crystals are suspended in the gelatin in much the same way as fruit is suspended in Jell-O during the preparation of a gelatin mold. The emulsion is spread onto the x-ray film in an extremely thin, even coating. The silver halide crystals must be evenly distributed over the surface of the film so that one area of the film is not more photosensitive than another. The gelatin also allows the water and other chemicals to reach the silver halide crystals during the film processing.

About 95% of the photosensitive crystals are composed of silver bromide; the remainder consists of silver iodide. These crystals are the light-sensitive portion of the emulsion that allows it to interact with x-ray and light photons. These interactions are responsible primarily for the formation of the radiographic image on the film. To protect the image, a

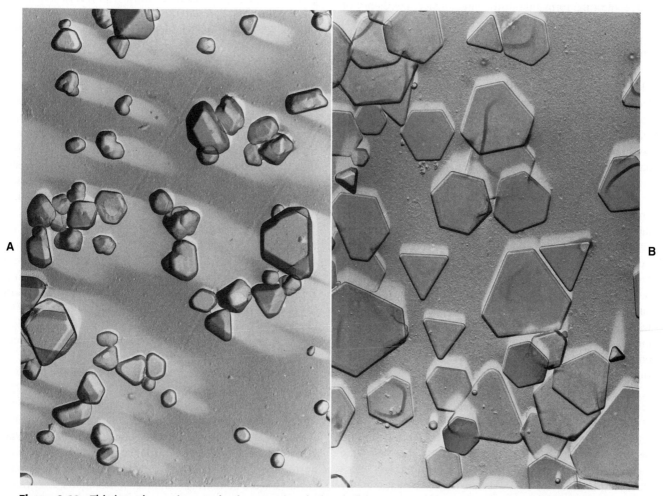

Figure 6-19. This is a photomicrograph of conventional silver halide crystals **(A)** and newer technology, tabular grain silver halide crystals **(B)**, which result in the coverage of a larger surface area. *(Courtesy Eastman Kodak Company.)*

durable coating is applied to the emulsion to reduce the chance of damage from scratches, abrasions, and skin oils from handling.

Latent image formation.   The remnant radiation (the amount of radiation leaving a patient after an x-ray exposure) that reaches the film's emulsion is responsible primarily for creating the latent image. The latent image is the image on the x-ray film that is not visible until the film is processed. The latent image exists on the film as an unseen change in the silver halide crystal's atomic structure. After processing, the invisible latent image becomes a manifest image, which contains a visible range of densities from black to white. The amount of radiation reaching the film after interaction with the patient greatly influences the degree of blackening on the film. This amount is proportional to the density and thickness of the anatomic part x-rayed. Denser and thicker parts of the body absorb more radiation and therefore allow less remnant radiation to reach the film. In many situations the x-ray photons and light photons are responsible for interacting with the atomic structure of the silver halide crystals. The affected silver halide crystals indirectly make up the image. Although much is still unknown about critical mechanisms that control the formation of the latent image, the theory of sensitivity specks and their essential involvement in the image-formation process (proposed by Gurney and Mott in 1938) remains almost unchallenged.[4]

Film characteristics.   Important characteristics of x-ray film are speed, contrast, and latitude. **Sensitometry,** which is the measurement of the film's response to exposure and processing, provides a mechanism to analyze these characteristics within the normal exposure range of the film. Sensitometric evaluation of the film may also be part of a quality-assurance program designed to monitor the simulator's exposure system and performance of the processing unit.

The **film speed** affects the degree of blackening (density) produced on the film for a certain amount of exposure. The thickness of the emulsion layer and size and shape of the silver halide crystals determine the speed of the film. For example, if two films with different speed are given similar exposures, one film would have less measured density. Several reasons may account for this. A film with large silver halide crystals produces a greater area of darkening than one with smaller crystals, given the same exposure. Similarly, a thicker emulsion layer provides more crystals in an area, thus producing more film density than a film with a thinner emulsion layer.

The speed of two films can be compared through a graphic relationship called a sensitometric, characteristic, or H & D curve (Fig. 6-20). Hurter and Driffield are two British photographers who in 1890 first described the relationship between exposure and density. This graph represents the measured density on a processed film compared with exposure. A special device called a **densitometer** measures the degree of blackening on the film. The readings from the densitometer, plotted on logarithmic graph paper, correlate to the

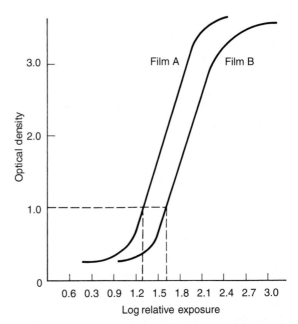

Figure 6-20. A characteristic curve shows the speed of a film. Film speed is the reciprocal of the exposure in roentgens, needed to produce a density of 1.0. Notice that film A is faster than film B. *(From Bushong S: Radiologic science for technologists: physics, biology, and protection, ed 7, St. Louis, 2001, Mosby.)*

characteristics of the film. Logarithmic paper keeps the graph to a reasonable size. Density increases with exposure sharply along the straight line portion of the graph for film A in Fig. 6-20 and less sharply for film B. Film A is faster than film B. Both curves are sigmoidal (i.e., they have a toe and shoulder portion and are not just straight lines). A characteristic, or H & D, curve also graphically expresses film contrast and latitude.

Another important characteristic of x-ray film is contrast, which is the ability of the film to record differences in density. Film emulsion manufactured to produce high contrast (mammography) or low contrast (a longer scale of greys) is designed to have its own unique response to exposure factors (kVp, mAs, distance). Low-contrast film provides more film latitude and is therefore more forgiving of errors in the selection of technical factors, whereas high-contrast film provides better image detail.[5]

Latitude is the range of radiographic exposures that produce densities in the diagnostically useful range (Fig. 6-21). Film A has a narrow latitude, whereas film B has a wider latitude and responds to an extended range of exposures. Film B is a more forgiving film because it allows a sizable variation in exposures while still displaying densities in the diagnostically useful range. An inversely proportional relationship exists between contrast and latitude. When contrast increases, latitude decreases. In other words, high-contrast film has narrow latitude and low-contrast film has wide latitude.

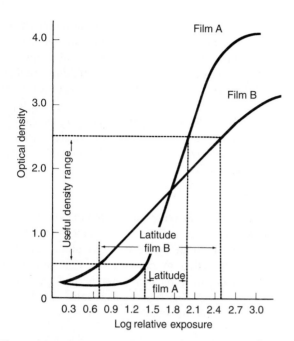

Figure 6-21. A comparison of two characteristic curves showing a difference in latitude. Relative exposure ranges are indicated for film A and film B. *(From Bushong S: Radiologic science for technologists: physics, biology, and protection, ed 7, St. Louis, 2001, Mosby.)*

Storage and handling of film. Several factors such as light, radiation, heat and humidity, shelf life, and proper handling influence the safe storage and handling of x-ray film. Most x-ray film must be stored and handled in the dark. A darkroom with an appropriate safelight (a special orange-red light that permits low-level illumination without fogging the film) is an essential component. A darkroom is needed not only for processing exposed simulation and port films but also for safely storing and handling the film. The unexposed film should be stored in a lightproof, lead-lined storage bin for added protection from light and radiation sources.

X-ray film is also sensitive to the effects of heat and humidity. Storage temperature should not exceed 68° F (20° C). Professional photographers know the benefits of refrigerating film, thus increasing its shelf life. Ideally, x-ray film should also be refrigerated. However, this is not always practical. Low humidity (below 30%) can cause unwanted static-discharge artifacts on the film, and high humidity (above 60%) may cause condensation or water spots on the radiograph.

The shelf life of x-ray film is determined by the expiration date stamped on each box of 100 sheets, much the same way a gallon of milk is stamped with an expiration date. Old film can cause a loss of speed and contrast as a result of an increase in fog (unwanted density on the film) from excessive heat, humidity, and background radiation. The fog on a film may reach a level at which it interferes with the quality of the radiographic image. Rotating film according to the expiration date reduces problems associated with old film.

Proper handling of x-ray film is also important in maintaining a high image quality. Storing boxes of film on end instead of stacked flat prevents the film from warping and sticking together. Care must be taken when cardboard inserts and paper interleaves are removed from around the film or when a new box of film is opened. Rough handling and quick movements, even with the proper humidity, can cause unwanted film abrasions from unnecessary pressure and static-discharge artifacts.

Film identification. All port films and simulation radiographs should be identified with the patient's name, date, institution at which the exposure was made, identification number, and additional treatment-related information. This can be accomplished in several ways. Most cassettes have a small rectangular space in one corner reserved for patient identification. A lead blocker prevents radiation from reaching this rectangular area during the exposure. Then patient information, usually included on a small index card (flash card), can be added to the film through a special daylight identification and cassette system. Information can also be added in the darkroom with a special flash-card device after the film is removed from the cassette but before the film is processed. China markers (wax pencils) frequently used in radiation oncology provide a method of adding critical treatment-related information on the film after processing. All the information on the film becomes part of the patient's medical record.

Intensifying Screens

Intensifying screens convert the invisible energy of an x-ray beam into visible light energy. About 99% of the latent image on the x-ray film is formed because of this visible light created by intensifying screens. The process of using intensifying screens with film is especially important in diagnostic radiology, where imaging detail and limiting the dose to the patient is more critical. Less exposure is required with film and screen systems than with direct-exposure film. These screens are commonly used in pairs to take full advantage of the double-coated emulsion on the film.

Screens used in radiation therapy. Three types of screens are used in radiation therapy: intensifying, lead, and copper screens. Intensifying screens, which are necessary in the production of diagnostic-quality radiographs, are used on the treatment-planning simulator. In contrast, lead and copper screens are primarily used in portal imaging.

Lead and copper screens are used primarily for port filming on high-energy radiation therapy equipment. They do not convert x-ray photons to light photons. The image quality of a port film is considerably poor compared with that of a chest x-ray or simulator film. However, the film must be good enough to determine field boundaries of the treatment area in relationship to anatomic or bony landmarks. Taking regular port films is good clinical practice and provides legal documentation of the patient's actual treatment area.

The thin metal screens can be used with screen-type or direct-exposure film. The lead and copper screens used in port filming can be mounted in a screen-type cassette with the intensifying screens removed or secured to a cardboard film holder. The screens can range in thickness from 0.1 to 0.5 mm for lead and up to 3 mm for copper.[15] The thin metal sheets act as an intensifying screen by ejecting electrons from the screen through photon interaction, thus providing an image on the film that represents the variation of beam intensity transmitted through the patient.[1] The ejected electrons from the screen do not have far to travel before reaching the film. High-energy photons used in port filming cause electrons produced further in the patient to travel greater distances to the film emulsion. This adds to geometrical blurring of the image. The copper screen absorbs some of these unwanted electrons and at the same time produces some of its own. Good screen-film contact is important to avoid poor image quality. Intensifying screens are used in the diagnostic photon range to produce simulation radiographs, whereas lead and copper screens are used in the megavoltage photon range to produce port films.

Cassettes and Film Holders

The **cassette** provides the light-tight conditions necessary for x-ray film and intensifying screens to work properly. The cassette, which opens like a book, is made of material with a low atomic number such as cardboard, plastic, and carbon fiber. Because of its low atomic number and strength, carbon fiber is also used as tabletop material for the radiation therapy simulator and CT couches. The x-ray film is loaded between the front and back intensifying screens, which are mounted inside the sturdy cassette. Pressure pads, usually made of felt or a spongelike material, are mounted between each intensifying screen and the cassette cover. This design helps maintain good film-screen contact when the cassette is closed and loaded with film. The location of the lead blocker in one corner of the cassette provides space on the film for patient-identification purposes.

The back of the cassette is designed differently than the front of the cassette. Lead or other metal backing prevents unwanted scatter radiation from returning to the simulator film after it has exited the cassette. This type of backscatter radiation can cause unnecessary fog and reduce image contrast.

Cleaning. The proper cleaning of cassettes and intensifying screens is important to total image quality. Dust, dirt, and other such materials inside the cassette can interfere with image quality by preventing light photons produced by the screens from reaching the film. Special antistatic cleaning agents, which reduce static electricity that can discharge and expose the film, are commercially available to clean intensifying screens. Mild soap and water can be used to clean the screens and cassette if the water does not contain high levels of minerals, which may leave unwanted stains and deposits.

The use of film, screens, and cassettes as conventional recording media in radiation therapy serves as a convenient, relatively inexpensive method of recording important patient information. Simulation and port films are legal documents considered part of the patient's medical record. Proper understanding of the tools used in creating these legal documents is essential to producing good-quality port films and high-quality simulation radiographs. Until an imaging technology without the use of film is perfected and widely available, close attention must be given to the principles of conventional recording media.

PROCESSING

Despite advances brought on by automation in the darkroom, some rudimentary understanding of film processing should remain a part of the future therapist's curriculum. The standard textbook definition of radiographic film processing describes the procedure as the conversion of the latent image to a visible image.[3,4,18] The visible image must also be reasonably well preserved for storage.

Developer

The latent image is created when the remnant radiation reaching the intensifying screens of the cassette is converted to light. The light exposes the film in a pattern that precisely corresponds to the intensity of the remaining radiation beam after it passes through anatomy. Without delving too deeply into the chemistry involved, when the exposed film is placed in a developer solution, a reducing agent converts the light-sensitive silver halide crystals in the emulsion to black metallic silver. Unexposed crystals are chemically restrained from involvement in this process. In manual film development the hazy, milky image taking shape on the film is visible even under the dim illumination of the safelight. However, if the film is exposed to white light at this time, the unfixed image is destroyed.

Fixer

The function of the fixer is to remove the unexposed silver halide from the film. (The silver washed off the film in this process is valuable, thus leading to the use of silver-recovery systems in most darkrooms.) The fixer also preserves the image by hardening the emulsion and neutralizing any developer remaining on the film. The film is then placed in a bath of running water to remove residual chemicals. In manual processing the entire cycle from development through washing and drying can take up to 2 hours.

Automatic Processing

Fortunately, modern diagnostic and simulation radiographic film development relies on a totally automated process requiring virtually no direct intervention from the therapist. The individual simply enters a darkened cubicle, removes the exposed film from the cassette, and places the film on a tray from which it is drawn into the complex inner reaches of the processor with its whirring rollers, various chemical baths, and heated blower system. About 90 seconds later, the completely processed and preserved image emerges, ready for viewing, analysis, and (ultimately) archival storage.

The diagram of a modern film processor (Fig. 6-22) is deceiving in its simplicity. Only a chain of rollers (the film-transport system) meandering through a row of three tanks is seen. However, this apparently simple processor took several major corporations nearly a generation to design and perfect.

The discussion on the construction of x-ray film in the previous section should be recalled. Film consists of a polyester plastic base coated with a gelatinous layer impregnated with light-sensitive compounds. For the chemicals involved in the development and fixing of the latent image to work effectively, the gelatin must absorb water, which serves as the chemical solvent. This is appropriately termed gel swell. In the days of manual processing, gel swell was of no significance because the increase in the thickness of the film was only a few microns. However, with the advent of primitive automatic processors, gel swell became the most important obstacle to a successful design. As it entered the water-based developer solution, the film promptly swelled sufficiently to become irretrievably lodged between the narrow gap of the rollers. Increasing roller separation proved ineffective because as the film passed to the fixer tank, it contracted so that it sat motionlessly between the now excessive roller play.

Automatic processing required the development of an entirely new set of chemicals, compounds that would limit gel swell and still provide adequate chemical penetration of the emulsion. The new chemicals also had to resist the increased oxidation that takes place at the higher processing temperatures necessary in rapid automatic equipment.

Troubleshooting

Modern film processors are usually remarkably reliable. However, having some limited troubleshooting skills for rare malfunctioning occasions is useful. In general, the condition of the film exiting the processor gives a good indication of the problem.

When the film feels sticky or greasy, probable causes include the following:
1. The fixer solution is exhausted.
2. The flow in the wash water is inadequate. (Check for plugged filters.)
3. The developer solution is contaminated.

In departments in which the demand placed on the processor is relatively low (including many therapy services, operating room darkrooms, and small medical office practices), developer exhaustion is a common problem. This is caused by insufficient replenishment of solutions. Each time a film is fed into the processor, a microswitch is tripped, thus activating the replenisher pumps for the fixer and developer. Low-volume periods prevent fresh solutions from being pumped regularly into the tanks. This may not be obvious because the deterioration of the chemicals is relatively gradual. The therapist simply finds necessity in making increases

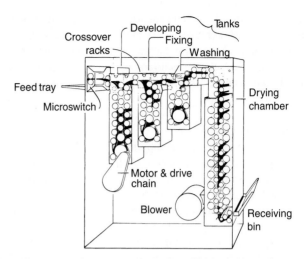

Figure 6-22. A diagram of a modern film processor demonstrating the major components. *(From Bushong S: Radiologic science for technologists: physics, biology, and protection, ed 7, St. Louis, 2001, Mosby.)*

in exposure factors to compensate for the loss of film density. This leads to excessive patient dose and general poor technique.

Film fogging can also be a problem. Fog results in an overall greying of the image and loss of contrast. Although fog can have many causes, the leading ones include the following:
1. The safelights are too bright. The bulbs may be of too high a wattage, or the safelights may be located too close to the work area.
2. The darkroom technique is poor. (Limit the time the film is exposed to the safelight.)
3. The film is stored too long or at excessive temperatures.
4. The film is exposed to ionizing radiation.
5. The chemical temperatures are too high.

One of the most common problems is related not to the automatic processor at all but to the humidity conditions in the darkroom. Excessively dry air (below about 50% relative humidity) may cause a buildup of static electricity. When this static electricity is discharged on the film, the result is dramatic black artifacts that resemble lightening bolts or Christmas trees.

A strict program of preventive maintenance and quality control can eliminate almost all processor problems. Although it is not a common practice in some departments, sensitometric evaluation of the processor should be conducted regularly. This relatively simple and economic testing regimen detects problems before they become serious and substantially improves the technical proficiency of simulation and port-film radiography.

APPLICATIONS IN RADIATION ONCOLOGY

Producing quality radiographs is not an easy task. Many components should be considered, such as geometrical factors, control of unwanted scatter radiation, and problems associated with contrast and density on the radiograph. An understanding of the many factors affecting the production of good-quality simulation radiographs and port films is essential. In this section, a practical-application approach to these issues is explored.

Geometrical Factors

Some principles in photography apply to radiography. Both areas require a certain intensity of light or x-ray energy and proper exposure time to create an image on the film. A recorded image is possible in both situations because x-ray and visible-light photons travel in straight, divergent lines. This principle of divergence, in which photons move in straight but different directions from a common point (focal spot), contributes greatly to the magnification and distortion seen on simulation radiographs and port films. Three geometrical factors are important in radiation oncology: magnification, distortion, and proper selection of focal-spot size.

Magnification. All images on a radiograph or port film appear larger than they are in reality. This condition is known as magnification. The images on the film represent objects in the path of the beam. These objects can be located closer to the common point source (e.g., objects on or near the block tray) or nearer to the film (anatomy in the patient). Fig. 6-23 illustrates the principle of divergence, in which more tissue is exposed at the level of the lumbar vertebrae *(B)* than at the skin surface *(A)*. The degree of magnification depends on several factors, all of which have to do with the geometrical arrangement of the x-ray target, the patient (object), and the radiographic film on which the image is displayed.[19]

Magnification can be measured and expressed as a factor. Magnification on a film is directly proportional to the distance of the object from the target or source and is dependent on the distance of the object from the film. The magnification factor is defined as follows:

Magnification factor = Image size/Object size

Example: If an object in the patient, such as the maximum width of a vertebral body, measures 5.3 cm and its image on the simulator film measures 7.5 cm, what is the magnification factor?

Answer:

Magnification factor = 7.5 cm/5.3 cm = 1.415

Another method of determining the magnification factor is using the geometrical relationship between similar triangles. Two triangles are similar if the corresponding angles are equal and corresponding sides are proportional. Fig. 6-23 illustrates a typical divergent x-ray beam used on the simulator. In many radiation therapy imaging procedures, determining the size of an object (especially in a patient) is not possible. In these situations the magnification factor can be calculated by using the ratio of SFD and source-object distance (SOD):

Magnification factor = SFD/SOD

Example: A radiograph taken at 140 cm SFD during a simulation procedure produces an image measuring 6.5 cm on

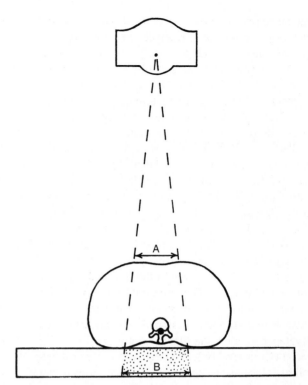

Figure 6-23. Divergence of an x-ray beam. More tissue is exposed as the beam exits the patient than at the anterior skin surface.

the radiograph. The distance from the target (source) to the object is 100 cm. What is the magnification factor?

Answer:

Magnification factor = 140 cm/100 cm = 1.4

Magnification, expressed as a factor or ratio, is inherent in the production of all simulation radiographs and port films. This is due in part to limitations of the simulation and treatment equipment used in radiation oncology. A greater degree of magnification is tolerated in radiation oncology than in diagnostic radiology, in which loss of radiographic detail from magnification is more critical to image quality. The radiation therapist should posses an understanding of the practical applications of magnification and demonstrate the ability to measure its effects in the clinical setting.

Distortion. Distortion is a change in the size, shape, or appearance of the structures being examined. Magnification is a good example of size distortion. More magnification occurs with large SODs. Conversely, the greater the SFD, the less the magnification of the object on the image. For minimal distortion, the distance and angulation of the x-ray beam in relationship to the anatomic part (object) and image receptor must be given special attention.

Shape distortion is the misrepresentation by unequal magnification of the actual shape of the structure being examined.[4] This occurs when the object plane or part examined is not parallel with the image plane. If these two planes are parallel, only size distortion occurs, and that distortion is directly proportional to the SOD and SFD. Because of unequal magnification, shape distortion can be the result of the following two factors:

1. The angulation of the x-ray beam is in relationship to the part examined.
2. The object and image planes are not parallel in common anatomic projections such as AP, posteroanterior (PA), and lateral.

In radiation therapy treatment planning, angling the beam to avoid treating sensitive normal tissue structures is frequently necessary. When this occurs, a certain amount of shape distortion is observed on the image. No formula exists (as it does in magnification) to assess the amount of shape distortion. Instead, the assessment is based on the radiation therapist's understanding of normal radiographic anatomy in various situations. Fig. 6-24, *A,* illustrates a common radiographic projection (AP), in which the object and image planes are closely parallel. Fig. 6-24, *B,* illustrates shape distortion of a vertebral body when the simulator beam is angled 25 degrees. Greater shape distortion of an image is illustrated in Fig. 6-24, *C,* in which the beam is angled 40 degrees from the vertical. The distortion that occurs in the thoracic

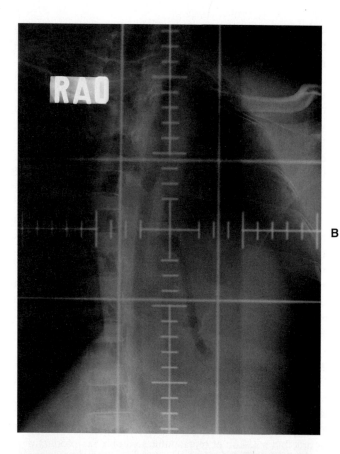

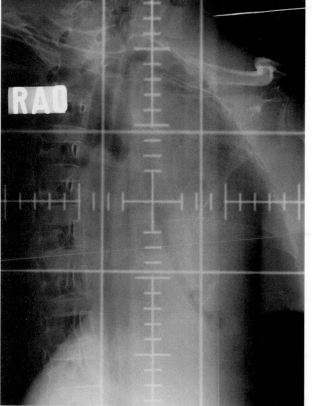

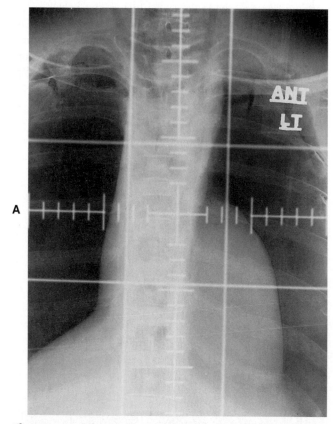

Figure 6-24. These three radiographs illustrate the normal anatomy of a thoracic vertebral body in the AP projection **(A)**, distorted anatomy with a 25-degree angulation of the beam **(B)**, and distorted anatomy with a 40-degree angulation of the beam **(C)**.

vertebrae should be noted. In this situation the objective in treatment planning may be to treat a lung mass while avoiding the spine (a sensitive critical structure).

Shape distortion can also occur when the object and image planes are not parallel. For example, in the pelvic region the obturator foramina are normally of equal size when radiographed in the anterior or posterior projection. If the pelvic bones are rotated slightly, shape distortion can be detected in the image, especially in the shape of the obturator foramina openings. Fig. 6-25 compares the amount of shape distortion as a result of unequal magnification when the object (the pelvis) and image planes are not parallel.

For reduction of the effects of distortion, the distances used for a specific procedure and angulation of the x-ray beam deserve particular attention. Otherwise, a misrepresentation of the size and shape of the anatomic part occurs. This misrepresentation, classified as size or shape distortion, can affect radiographic image quality. Other factors such as the selection of the focal-spot size can also contribute to distortion on the radiographic image.

Focal-spot selection. Focal-spot size and the line-focus principle (see Fig. 6-5) influence radiographic image quality.[12] X-rays are not emitted from a common point source but from a measurable area on the anode, which is commonly referred to as a spot or common point. Thus the focal spot (which can measure from 0.1 to 2.0 mm) is not a true point source but a square or rectangular area of x-ray production.

The **penumbra** is the area of unsharpness or fuzziness at the edge of the beam. This is a result of photons emanating from various locations on the target area and intersecting the object at different angles. Penumbra is undesirable, but a certain amount of it is unavoidable because of the geometry of image formation. Three situations can contribute to unwanted penumbra: large focal spot, large object-film distance (OFD), and short SFD.

The umbra (Fig. 6-26, A) is the central, sharper portion of the image influenced by the size of the focal spot. The penumbra surrounds the umbra, or area of greater detail. Fig. 6-26, B, illustrates the penumbra as a result of the selection of a large focal spot or mA station to produce a radiograph. Penumbra increases and image sharpness decreases as the focal spot becomes larger. Fig. 6-26, C and D, illustrate the effect of small and large OFDs on image size and resolution. A large OFD increases penumbra and reduces image detail. Fig. 6-26, E and F, illustrate the effect SFD has on penumbra. As SFD decreases, penumbra increases and resolution decreases.

Using a small focal spot in radiation therapy reduces the effects of penumbra, especially on the field-defining wires located in the collimator head of the simulator gantry. The large OFDs created by the field-defining wires located in the collimator head is unavoidable. Therefore to reduce the effects of penumbra, a small focal spot should be selected when possible. Any unsharpness or fuzziness of the field-defining wires on the radiographic image adds to the uncertainty of the treatment field outlined on the patient's skin. The difference in the width of the field-defining wires on the simulator radiographs should be noted in Fig. 6-27. The exposure factors for each radiograph used the same mAs and kVp. However, Fig. 6-27, B, shows the use made of a large focal

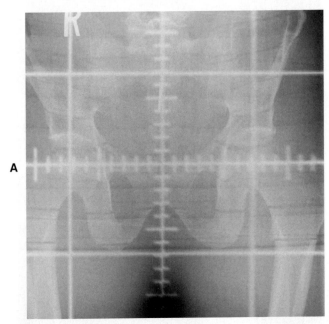
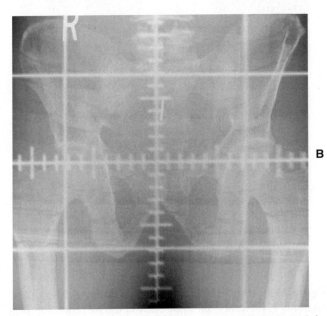

Figure 6-25. These two radiographs compare an anteroposterior (AP) projection of the pelvis **(A)** and shape distortion of the obturator foramina as a result of unequal magnification when the image and object plane are not parallel **(B).** One obturator foramen appears smaller than the other because of rotation of the pelvis.

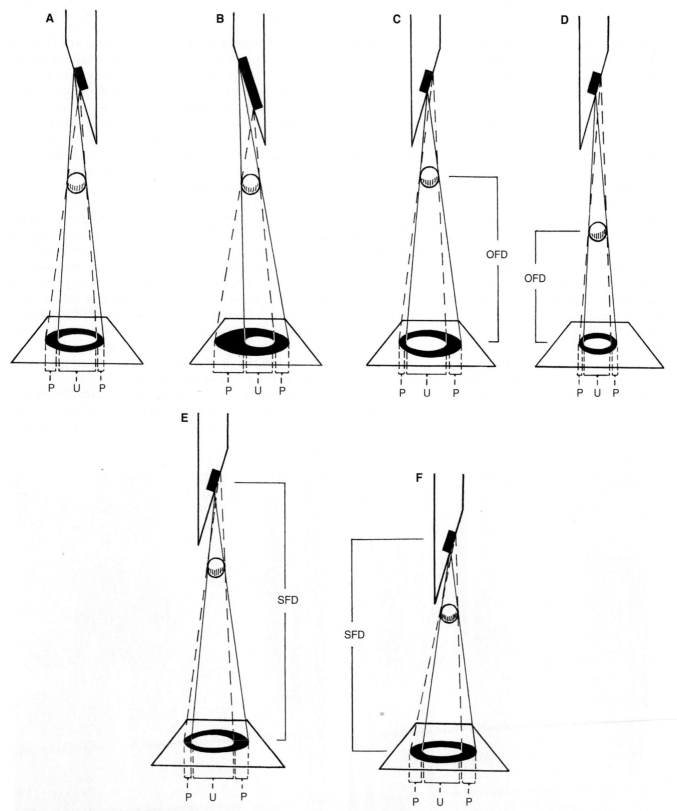

Figure 6-26. The umbra **(A)** is the sharper central portion of the image influenced by the size of the focal spot. The penumbra surrounds the umbra, or area of greater detail. **B,** The penumbra as a result of selecting a large focal spot or mA station to produce a radiograph. Penumbra increases and image sharpness decreases as the focal spot becomes larger. **C** and **D,** The effect of small and large object-film distances (OFDs) on image size and resolution. A large OFD increases penumbra and reduces image detail. **E** and **F,** The effect source-film distance (SFD) has on penumbra. As SFD decreases, penumbra increases and resolution decreases. *(From Carlton RR, McKenna-Adler AM: Principles of radiographic imaging, ed 3, Albany, NY, 1992, Delmar Publishing.)*

spot. An unnecessary amount of penumbra produced on the field-defining wires with the large focal spot can compromise the precision and accuracy demanded in radiation therapy.

Magnification, distortion, and the focal-spot size are controllable factors that affect radiographic image quality. A knowledge of these geometrical factors and an understanding of their application is necessary to produce quality radiographs. Other factors such as the control of scatter radiation can also improve radiographic image quality.

Control of Scatter Radiation

During an exposure, some x-rays are absorbed photoelectrically, and others pass through the patient to reach the film. This is partially a result of the kilovoltage. If more photons pass through the patient, the radiographic image has a greater density. The opposite is true if fewer photons reach the film and more photons are absorbed in the body, radiographic density decreases. A considerable amount of the radiographic density on the film is due to scatter radiation, in which photons arrive at the film after bouncing off matter haphazardly. However, the density on the film from scatter photons does not directly correlate to the anatomic structures of interest. Instead, the unwanted scatter radiation decreases contrast and reduces image quality.

Reducing scatter or secondary radiation, which is created

during a Compton interaction, is essential to improving image quality. Scatter photons are produced when an incoming primary photon interacts with an outer-shell electron and is forced to change direction. Sometimes that scattered photon never reaches the film or image receptor. Other times it does. When it reaches the film, scatter radiation reduces contrast by causing additional density on the film and fogging the image. The radiation therapist can create a better image by restricting the amount of scatter radiation reaching the film. Collimating the x-ray beam and using a grid reduces the effects of unwanted scatter radiation.

Less scatter radiation is produced by restricting the beam through careful collimation of the x-ray shutter blades. If fewer primary photons are emitted from the collimator head, fewer scatter photons are created. Collimating the primary x-ray beam is the first line of defense in controlling unwanted secondary radiation.[18] A grid absorbs scatter photons as a second line of defense. The grid, which acts like a filter by absorbing some photons, is placed between the film and patient. On some simulator models, the grid is built into the cassette holder. Other models require the manual positioning of a grid in the cassette holder before exposure.

Several other factors influence image quality. The following four primary factors influence the amount of scatter radiation reaching the film: kilovoltage, irradiated material, lead

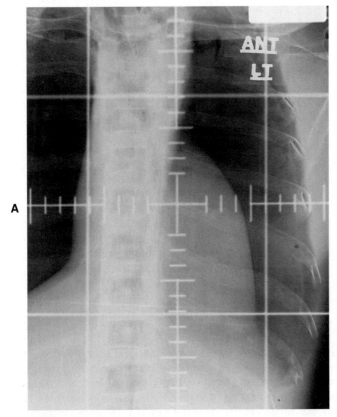 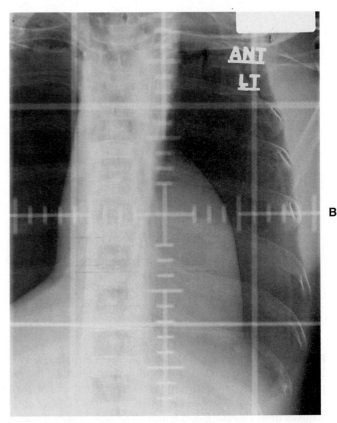

Figure 6-27. Penumbra, demonstrated on the field-defining wires of a simulation radiograph, as a result of focal-spot selection. **A,** Less penumbra as a result of a smaller focal-spot selection than shown in **B.**

REFERENCES

1. Bentel CG: *Radiation therapy planning,* New York, 1993, McGraw-Hill.
2. Bomford CK, Dawes PJ, Lillicrap SC et al: Treatment simulators, *Br J Rad Suppl* 23:4-32, 1989.
3. Bushong SC: *Radiologic science for technologists: physics, biology, and protection,* ed 7, St. Louis, 2001, Mosby.
4. Carlton RR, McKenna-Adler A: *Principles of radiographic imaging,* ed 3, Albany, NY, 2001, Delmar Publishing.
5. Chow MF: The effect of a film's sensitivity to its speed, contrast, and latitude, *Can J Med Radiat Technol* 19(4):147-148, 1988.
6. Cullinan AM, Cullinan JE: *Producing quality radiographs,* ed 2, Philadelphia, 1993, JB Lippincott.
7. DeVos DC: *Basic principles of radiographic exposure,* Philadelphia, 1990, Lea & Febiger.
8. Fuchs AW: Relationship of tissue thickness to kilovoltage, *Radiol Technol* 19(6):287, 1948.
9. Fuchs AW: The rationale of radiographic exposure, *Radiol Technol* 22(2):62, 1950.
10. Glasser O: *Dr W.C. Roentgen,* ed 2, Springfield, Ill, 1972, Charles C Thomas.
11. Hufton AP, et al: Low attenuation material for table tops, cassettes and grids: a review, *Radiography* 53(607):17, 1987.
12. Hunt M: Localization & field design using a CT simulator. In Coia L, editor: *A practical guide to CT simulation,* Madison, Wis, 1995, Advanced Medical Publishing.
13. Karzmark CJ, Nunan CS, Tanabe E: *Medical electron accelerators,* Princeton, NJ, 1993, McGraw-Hill.
14. Khan FM: *The physics of radiation therapy,* ed 2, Baltimore, 1997, Lippincott Williams & Wilkins.
15. Kodera Y, Kunio D, Hwang-Ping C: Absolute speeds of screen-film systems and their absorbed-energy constants, *Radiology* 161:229-239, 1984.
16. Malott JC, Fodor J III: *The art and science of medical radiography,* ed 7, St. Louis, 1993, Mosby.
17. Nation Council on Radiation Protection and Measurements: Medical x-ray, electron beam, and gamma-ray protection of energies up to 50 MeV (equipment design performance and use), NCRP Rep 102, Bethesda, Md, 1989, The Council.
18. Selman J: *The fundamentals of imaging physics and radiobiology physics,* ed 9, Springfield, Ill, 2000, Charles C Thomas.
19. Stears JG, et al: Radiologic exchange: resolution according to focal spot size, *Radiol Technol* 60:429-430, 1989.

Treatment Delivery Equipment

Dennis Leaver, Linda Alfred

Outline

Key Terms

HISTORICAL OVERVIEW

The discovery of x-rays by Wilhelm Roentgen in 1895 and the subsequent therapeutic use of radiation has generated a variety of equipment. The features of each system mirrored the technology of the day while addressing the radiobiologic needs of the patient as closely as deemed necessary with the knowledge then available. In the relatively short period since the discovery of these mysterious rays, a great deal of specialized equipment has emerged. The application of this equipment has had most of its success in the treatment of malignant diseases.

This chapter discusses several aspects of related radiation therapy equipment, low-energy machines such as grenz rays, contact therapy, superficial equipment, and orthovoltage machines. In addition, an overview of high-energy machines, including the Van de Graaff generator, betatron, cyclotron, linear accelerator, and cobalt unit are introduced. This chapter concludes with a discussion of positron emission tomography (PET) studies, remote afterloading, and future outlooks concerning radiation therapy equipment.

EQUIPMENT DEVELOPMENT

Conventional low-energy equipment, which typically uses x-rays generated at voltages up to 300 kVp, have been used in radiation therapy since the turn of the twentieth century. These kilovoltage units (low x-ray voltage radiation therapy treatment machines) include grenz, contact, superficial, and orthovoltage machines. The use of this equipment dramatically decreased after 1950. This was due in part to the increased popularity of cobalt 60 units and subsequent development of the **linear accelerator** (a radiation therapy treatment machine that uses high-frequency electromagnetic waves to accelerate charged particles such as electrons to high energies via a linear tube). However, kilovoltage equipment is still part of many departments today, partly because of the low cost and simplicity of design compared with megavoltage units. The primary application of kilovoltage equipment is in the treatment of superficial lesions.

The introduction of megavoltage therapy equipment, which generated x-ray beams of 1 MV or greater, was a natural progression from low-energy units. Although kilovoltage units were and are beneficial, they still have two principle limitations that are clinically essential: they could not reach deep-seated tumors with an adequate dosage of radiation, and they did not spare skin and normal tissue. As a result, manufacturers began concentrating their efforts on addressing these and other shortcomings of low-energy equipment.

The early to middle part of the twentieth century marked a period of tremendous development of equipment used to treat tumors (Fig. 7-1). The physics community began experimenting with the acceleration of electrons, protons, neutrons, and heavy ions. The attempt was being made in medicine to find a better way to deliver a lethal dose of radi-

ation therapy. In North America the Van de Graaff (1937), betatron (1941), cobalt 60 (1951), and linear accelerator (1952) were introduced.[19]

Until the early to mid-1950s, most cancer patients undergoing radiation therapy were treated with low-energy equipment. Physicians did their best with the equipment available to them. Surgery was still the treatment of choice for most cancers.

CHARACTERISTICS OF KILOVOLTAGE X-RAY EQUIPMENT

Central-axis-depth dose and physical penumbra are related to beam quality. In treatment planning, the central-axis-depth dose distribution for a specific beam depends on the energy (Fig. 7-2). The depth of an isodose curve increases with beam quality. For example, a 50% isodose curve (a line representing various points of similar value in a beam along the central axis and elsewhere) for a 200-kVp beam reaches a deeper tumor than a 50% isodose curve of a 100-kVp orthovoltage beam. The shape of the isodose curve also bulges sideways, as illustrated in the isodose distribution for the 200-kVp x-ray beam in Fig. 7-2. Orthovoltage beams show increased scatter dose to the tissue outside the treatment

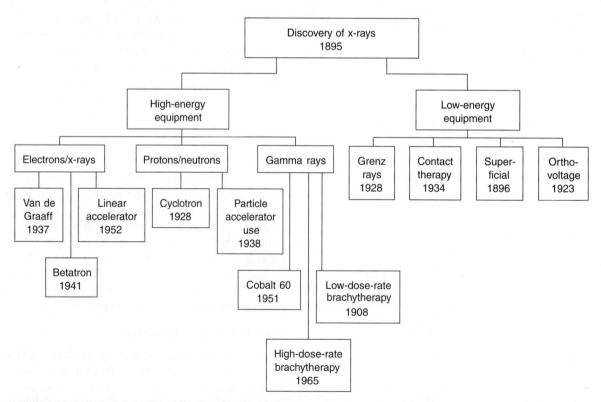

Figure 7-1. A timetable chart illustrates the development of high- and low-energy treatment equipment since the discovery of x-rays in 1895. Every effort has been made in researching the accuracy of the information in this table. However, several sources and experts in the field sometimes disagree about the exact dates that equipment was introduced clinically. *(For more information, refer to the following: Bentel C: Radiation therapy planning, New York, 1993, McGraw-Hill; and Grigg EM: The trail of the invisible light, Springfield, Ill, 1965, Charles C Thomas.)*

region, thus exhibiting a marked disadvantage compared with megavoltage beams.[33] In other words, the absorbed dose in the medium outside the primary beam is greater for low-energy beams than for those of a higher energy[25,30] (Fig. 7-2). In orthovoltage radiation, isodose curves become distended and tend to bulge sideways. Conversely, limited scatter outside the field for megavoltage beams occurs because of predominantly forward scattering of the beam. This is illustrated in the isodose distribution for the 25-MV beam in Fig. 7-2.

CLINICAL APPLICATIONS OF KILOVOLTAGE EQUIPMENT

Grenz-Ray Therapy

In 1923 Gustav Bucky constructed an x-ray tube with a lithium borate window (Lindemann glass). The window permitted the transmission of long wavelength x-rays, the physical properties of which Bucky later studied. Consequently, the rays became Bucky rays, or **grenz rays** (low-energy x-rays having an energy of 10 to 15 kVp). This term comes from *grenz,* a German word meaning "border." This was an accurate description because grenz rays were thought at the time to lie within a grey zone between x-rays and ultraviolet radiation.

The construction of a grenz-ray tube and superficial tube is similar. In a grenz-ray tube, the envelope is glass and the window is beryllium. Inherent filtration is approximately 0.1 μm aluminum (Al). Like the superficial and orthovoltage

units, the quality of grenz-ray measurements in terms of half-value layer (HVL) is expressed in millimeters of aluminum. Sometimes in dermatology, copper is the metal used to designate the HVL. The intensity of the radiation decreases when the kVp and mA decrease. This intensity also decreases when the distance is increased as a result of the inverse square law. Grenz rays are almost entirely absorbed in the first 2 μm of skin and have a useful depth-dose range of about 0.5 μm. The intensity falls off rapidly after this. Less than 2% is capable of reaching the sebaceous glands of the skin.

The application of grenz rays characteristically is safe and painless for the patient and often yields visible results in 48 to 72 hours. The recommended fractionation involving approximately 200 roentgens (R) per session at weekly intervals totals 800 to 1000 R, followed by a 6-month period before additional treatment may occur. Grenz rays are especially effective for the treatment of inflammatory disorders, namely those involving Langerhans' cells. Grenz rays have also yielded positive results for Bowen's disease, patchy-stage mycosis fungoides, and herpes simplex.[13]

Contact Therapy

Clinical data on contact therapy is scarce. Fig. 7-3 illustrates a handheld contact therapy unit. Historically, contact therapy was primarily used to treat superficial skin lesions. The treatment machine derived its name because the treatment unit actually came in contact with the patient. Another use of contact therapy relates to endocavitary treatments for curative

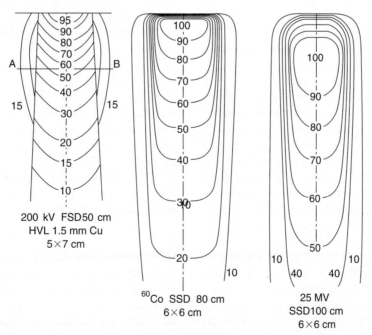

Figure 7-2. Isodose distributions for several beams: *left,* 200 kVp, HVL 1.5 μm Cu, SSD 50 cm, field size 5 cm × 7 cm; *middle,* cobalt 60, SSD 80 cm, field size 6 cm × 6 cm; *right,* 25 MV, SSD 100 cm, 6 cm × 6 cm. *(Redrawn from Johns HE, Cunningham JR: The physics of radiology, ed 4, Springfield, Ill, 1983, Charles C Thomas.)*

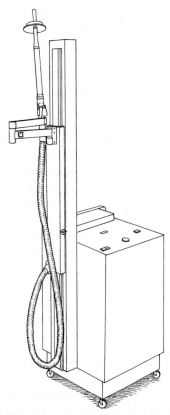

Figure 7-3. A handheld contact-therapy machine used to treat superficial skin lesions. The operators, one to monitor the patient and the other to hold the applicator, must wear protective shielding during the treatment application.

intent. This involves a limited group of patients with cancers of the low to middle third of the rectum.

The rectal cancers treated are confined to the bowel wall in most situations. Papillon has established several criteria for treating rectal lesions by using low-energy x-rays.[43] These criteria are as follows: a maximum tumor size of 3 × 5 cm, a mobile lesion with no significant extension into the anal canal, and a well differentiated to moderately well differentiated exophytic tumor that is accessible by the treatment proctoscope (≤10 cm from anal verge). This treatment is especially desirable for the patient because it preserves the anal sphincter. (This may not be true with other methods.) On an outpatient basis, patients received four treatments of 3000 cGy each, separated by a 2-week interval. Papillon used a 50-kVp Philip's contact unit. The source-skin distance (SSD) used was 4 cm with 0.50 to 1.0 mm aluminum filtration at a dose rate of 1000 cGy per minute. A 3-cm applicator cone can deliver treatments directly to the rectal mucosa via the rectum. Overlapping fields existed if the size of the lesion exceeded the diameter of the applicator.[41] Chapter 32 provides additional details about the use of contact therapy in the treatment of rectal lesions.

Historically, Chaoul contact therapy was the treatment of choice for hemangiomas, especially in the dermatology department of the University Hospital in Munich, Germany. Fractionated doses of 300 to 500 R and total doses ranging from 1200 to 1500 R were delivered to patients in intervals of several days. Most patients showed visible improvement as evidenced by diminished lesion size and less elevation within 8 weeks of treatment. The Chaoul radiation technique was less hazardous than previously used orthovoltage techniques.[14] The popularity of this technique has decreased dramatically since 1975 because large studies have proved conclusively that spontaneous involution of strawberry angiomas (hemangioma simplex) occurs in 95% of cases after several years.[14]

Superficial Treatments

Superficial therapy relates to treatments with x-rays produced at potentials ranging from 50 to 150 kV. Usually, 1- to 6-µm thick aluminum filters insert in a slot in the treatment head to harden the beam to the desired degree. The degree of hardening, as with other units, is measured in HVLs. Typical HVLs used in superficial treatments range from 1 to 8 mm of Al.[30] Superficial-treatment administration uses a cone or applicator. Cone sizes are generally 2 to 5 cm in diameter. Lead cutouts are tailored to fit the treatment area if needed. The cone lies directly on the skin or lead cutout and generally provides a source-skin distance (SSD) of 15 to 20 cm. Skin cancer and tumors no deeper than 0.5 cm are treated as a result of the rapid falloff of the radiation.

Three parameters are set at the console area for treatment delivery: kVp, mA (x-ray current measured in milliamperes), and treatment time. Superficial treatment and orthovoltage units are extremely reliable and free of electromechanical problems. This contributes to a lack of downtime, which is a problem more often with linear accelerators. The main difficulty encountered with the use of superficial units arises from having to lock down the unit after the cone is in position. Usually, the unit has a variety of handles or knobs (depending on the model) that require tightening while keeping the cone in place. This can be a challenge. Because no standard treatment table comes with the system, the patient can lie on a stretcher or sit in a chair for treatment, thus amplifying the difficulty of locking down all the knobs.[20]

Orthovoltage Therapy

Orthovoltage therapy describes treatment with x-rays produced at potentials ranging from 150 to 500 kV. Most orthovoltage equipment operates at 200 to 300 kV and 10 to 20 mA. Much like the superficial units, orthovoltage units use filters designed to achieve HVLs from 1 to 4 mm Cu.[9,30] Orthovoltage units can use external or del Regato cones to collimate the beam. In addition, a movable diaphragm consisting of lead plates can be used to adjust the field size. Conventionally, the SSD is 50 cm.

The types of tumors treated with orthovoltage units include skin, mouth, and cervical carcinoma (with the use of cones inserted into the patient). As with superficial treatments, the average treatment time can be seconds to several minutes depending on the filtered kV, prescribed dose, collimator, or cone size. The penetrating depth depends on the kV and filter. Usually, orthovoltage units experience limitation in the treatment of lesions deeper than 2 to 3 cm.

Orthovoltage units are still popular in many clinics and hospitals. They are reliable alternatives to the use of electrons in the treatment of many superficial skin lesions. Most skin lesions treated with orthovoltage units are squamous cell and basal cell cancers. Some clinicians prefer the orthovoltage unit for treating skin tumors because of beam characteristics, especially treatments requiring small fields.

In many departments in which kilovoltage equipment still exists, several treatment units may operate out of the same treatment room. Much of the equipment is older, compared with the design and appearance of modern megavoltage equipment. Historically, when orthovoltage was the highest energy available, treatments were limited by the skin's radiation tolerance. This limitation made the skin-sparing properties of cobalt teletherapy especially desirable and became the major reason for the modern trend to megavoltage beams.

MEGAVOLTAGE EQUIPMENT

X-ray beams of 1 MV or greater can be classified as **megavoltage equipment.** Examples of clinical megavoltage machines are accelerators such as the linear accelerator (Fig. 7-4), Van de Graaff generator, betatron, and cyclotron. Teletherapy units such as cobalt 60 are also classified as megavoltage treatment units.

Linear Accelerator

The term *linear accelerator* means that charged particles travel in straight lines as they gain energy from an alternating electromagnetic field. The linear accelerator (Fig. 7-5) is distinguished from other types of particle accelerators such as the **cyclotron,** in which the particles travel in a spiral pattern, and the betatron, in which the particles travel in a circular pattern.[29] According to a 1997 report by Owen and Hanks,[39,40] on the structure of radiation oncology facilities in the United States in cities with population over 25,000, there were a total of 2744 megavoltage treatment machines, 7167 full-time employee (FTE) radiation therapists, 2777 FTE radiation oncologists, 1349 FTE physicists, and 1314 FTE dosimetrists who treated 560,262 new patients and reported that 60% were treated with curative intent. Much of this work was accomplished with the administration of high-energy x-rays and/or electrons produced in a linear accelerator.

In the linear accelerator, x-rays and electrons are generated and used to treat a variety of tumors.[6,11,19] The **accelerator structure,** which resembles a length of pipe, is the basic element of the linear accelerator. The accelerator structure allows electrons produced from a hot cathode to gain energy until they exit the far end of the pipe.[29,55] Understanding the proper use of this equipment is significant to the radiation therapist because it is one of the essential tools enabling the radiation therapist to deliver a prescribed dose of radiation.

Aspects of the linear accelerator that are discussed in this section include a history of the electron accelerator, its design features, and a description of the major components. An explanation of the key components in a linear accelerator provides a basic overview of its operation and will aid in the student's understanding of this complex piece of equipment. These components include the klystron, waveguide, circulator, water-cooling system, electron gun, accelerator structure,

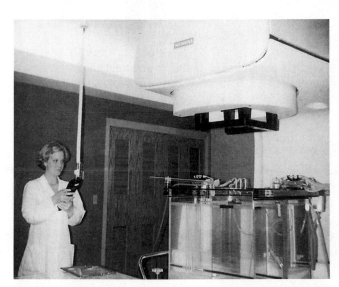

Figure 7-4. A, Linear accelerator, the Siemans Primus with rectangular water phantom used for measuring radiation beam characteristics.

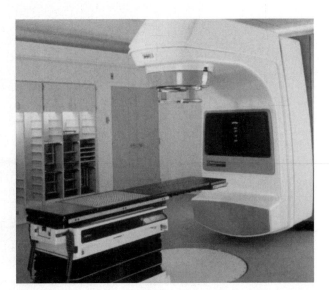

Figure 7-5. A linear accelerator, the 2300 CD. *(Courtesy Varian Medical Systems.)*

bending magnet (used in high-energy linear accelerators to bend the electron stream, sometimes at right angles so it is pointed at the patient), flattening filter, scattering foil, and other accessories.

History. The first 100-cm source-axis-distance (SAD), fully isocentric linear accelerator was manufactured in the United States and installed in 1961 (Fig. 7-6). With the linear accelerator, higher energy beams can be generated with greater skin sparing, field edges are more sharply defined with less penumbra, and computer technology shapes the treatment beam and personnel receive less exposure to radiation leakage.

Development. The development of the linear accelerator has its roots in the United States and England. In these countries, many men and women have contributed significantly to the research and development of the linear accelerator. Its development can be traced to the work of several key individuals.

The magnetron and klystron (Fig.7-7) proved invaluable in the development of and is an important component in the high-energy linear accelerator. The **klystron** is a form of radiowave amplifier and multiplies the amount of introduced radiowaves greatly. The magnetron and klystron are two special types of electron tubes that are used to provide microwave power to accelerate electrons. Microwaves are similar to ordinary radiowaves but have frequencies thousands of times higher. Microwave frequencies needed for linear accelerator operation are about three billion cycles per second (3000 MHz).[28] A major difference between the klystron and magnetron is that a klystron is a linear-beam microwave amplifier requiring an external oscillator or radiofrequency (RF) source (driver), whereas the magnetron is an oscillator and amplifier. The introduction of the magnetron and klystron assisted in the transfer of energy needed to accelerate electrons, which in turn were converted to high-energy x-rays used in the medical application of the linear accelerator in the treatment malignant disease.

Medical application. In the late 1940s the chief radiologist of Stanford's x-ray department, Dr. Henry Kaplan, became interested in the medical application of the linear accelerator. In addition, a working 1-MV linear accelerator was installed in 1948 at the Fermi Institute in Chicago. The mile-long waveguide, which ran under University Boulevard at the University of Chicago, provided photon and electron beams.[36] Work had also begun in England, but the Stanford University project proved most practical, partly because of the support of President Eisenhower in 1959 and subsequent funding by the U.S. Congress in 1961.

In 1948 the British Ministry of Health brought together the three main groups in England who were working on the linear accelerator project: the Medical Research Council (Dr. L.H. Gray et al), the Atomic Energy Research Establishment (D.W. Fry), and the Metropolitan Vickers Electric Company (later Associate Electrical Industries) (C.W. Miller et al). The resulting linear accelerator was installed at Hammersmith Hospital in London in June 1952. The first treatment was delivered on August 19, 1953, with an 8-MV photon beam. Another 4-MV linear accelerator was installed at Newcastle General Hospital (August 1953) and Christie Hospital in Manchester, England (October 1954). The first single gantry

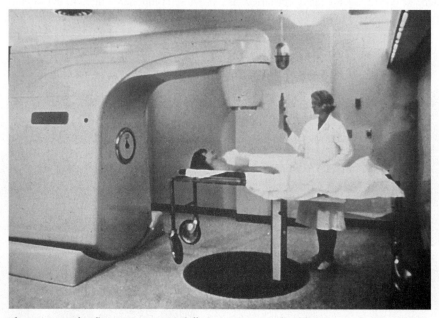

Figure 7-6. The first 100-cm SAD fully isocentric medical linear accelerator manufactured in the United States in 1961 by Varian Associates. *(Courtesy Varian Medical Systems.)*

Figure 7-7. Inspecting an early klystron that proved invaluable in high-energy linear accelerator development are (clockwise from lower left) Russel and Siguard Varian, Professor David Webster, William Hansen, and John Woodyard. *(Courtesy Varian Medical Systems.)*

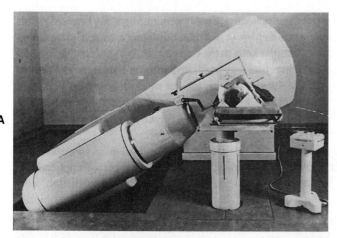

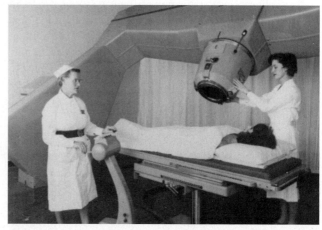

A

B

Figure 7-8. A, The first single gantry unit installed at Christie Hospital in Manchester, England, in October 1954. It could rotate over an arc of 120 degrees by lowering part of the treatment floor. **B,** The first clinical linear accelerator manufactured by Mullard (later purchased by Philips Medical Systems) in the United Kingdom, circa 1953. *(**A,** Courtesy Christie Hospital, Manchester; **B,** courtesy Philips Medical Systems, Shelton, Connecticut.)*

unit (Fig.7-8) could be rotated over an arc of 120 degrees by lowering part of the treatment room floor.[29]

The linear accelerator was introduced in England and the United States in the 1950s. In England a 2-megawatt magnetron and 3-m stationary accelerator were used to produce an output of 100 cGy/min with the 8-MV machine.[16,29] This was a major achievement, even by today's standards. In the United States a linear accelerator was first clinically used at Stanford University Hospital in January 1956 to treat a child suffering from retinoblastoma. The patient was still disease-free 32 years later.[18]

A joint venture between the British industrial work and

the Stanford University group under the direction of C.S. Nunan produced the first ergonomic linear accelerator (a 6-MV, isocentric linear accelerator with the ability to rotate 360 degrees around a patient lying supine on the treatment couch).

The evolution of the linear accelerator is discussed in this section with reference to three types of linear accelerators: the early linear accelerators (1953 to 1961); second-generation, 360-degree rotational units (1962 to 1982); and new computer-driven, third-generation treatment machines.

Early accelerators.   The early linear accelerators were extremely large and bulky compared with today's design features. In 1952 the first linear accelerator was installed at Hammersmith Hospital in London and had an 8-MeV x-ray beam and limited gantry motion. Several other linear accelerators with improved design features were also installed in England in the early to mid-1950s. As mentioned previously, the Stanford University linear accelerator in the United States treated its first patient in 1956. Since then, several manufacturers have designed and built linear accelerators for clinical purposes.

Second-generation accelerators.   Second-generation linear accelerators can be referred to as the older 360-degree rotational units, which are less sophisticated than their modern offspring. These isocentric units, some of which are still operational today, allow treatment to a patient from any gantry angle. They offered an improvement in accuracy and dose delivery over the extremely early models, primarily because of their 360-degree rotational ability around an isocenter.

If two linear-accelerator models built between 1962 and 1982 were compared, many more similarities than differences would be observed, regardless of the manufacturer. Fig. 7-9 illustrates two linear accelerators produced by different manufacturers. The similarities in design are related to their major features, such as gantry, treatment couch, and control console.

Second-generation linear accelerators are like some older cars on the road today. They may have more bumps, dents, and high mileage. They may work well at times but usually require a considerable amount of maintenance. An older car has the same basic components as a newer one, such as an engine, transmission, and operator's panel (with fewer knobs and buttons), to accomplish the task. A third-generation linear accelerator is like the newer car of today. The newer car is equipped with many of the basic components of the older, less-sophisticated automobile but has added features such as aerodynamic design, antilock brakes, and computer-integrated components.

Third-generation accelerators.   In general, third-generation accelerators have improved accelerator-guide, magnet systems, and beam-modifying systems to provide wide ranges of beam energy, dose rate, field size, and operating modes with improved beam characteristics. These accelerators are highly reliable and have compact design features.[29] Table 7-1 describes improvements in the technology of medical linear accelerators from the first- to third-generation treatment units.

Third-generation, computer-driven linear accelerators are available with a wide variety of options, which may include dual photon energies, multileaf collimation, a choice of several electron energies, and electronic portal verification systems. Because of the advances in three-dimensional treatment planning, some new linear accelerators provide additional features. Before some of these newer features are discussed, a basic understanding of components and design features of a linear accelerator are necessary.

Linear Accelerator Components

A typical linear accelerator (Fig. 7-10) consists of a drive stand, gantry (treatment couch), and console electronic cabinet. Some linear accelerators may also have a modulator cabinet, which contains components that distribute and monitor primary electrical power and high-voltage pulses to

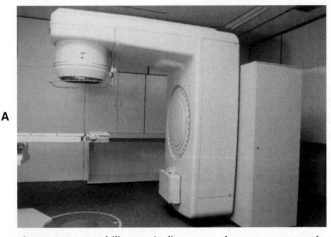
A

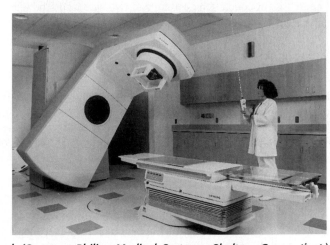
B

Figure 7-9. A, Philips 75/5 linear accelerator gantry and stand *(Courtesy Philips Medical Systems, Shelton, Connecticut.)* **B,** Siemens Mevatron gantry, stand, and treatment couch. *(Courtesy Siemens Medical Systems, Concord, California.)*

Table 7-1	Improvements in medical linear accelerator technology from the 1950s to present day			
Item (accelerator guide type)	**Early** (traveling wave)	**Modern** (standing guide)	**Result** (doubled guide efficiency)	
MV per meter of guide (shunt impedance, megohms/meter)	4 (13-47)	12-18 (86-112)	Shorter guide; simpler, more compact machine; and 360-degree gantry rotation	
Bending magnet	Nonachromatic	Achromatic	Stable treatment	
X-ray field size	Modest	Large	Full mantle at isocenter	
X-ray dose rate (centigray per minute)	100-200	250-500	Short exposure, even with wedge filters	
X-ray energies, MeV (number of modes)	4-6 (1)	4-24 (2)	Optimal for thin and thick sections of the patient	
Electron energies	None or low	Low to high	Full useful penetration	
Isodose distributions and their stability	Fair	Excellent	Protection of normal tissue and dose precision	
Microwave tube life	Months	Years	Machine up-time and lower cost	
Cleanliness	Oil pumps	Ion pumps and brazed guide	Freedom from arcing High-energy gradients	
Electronics	Tubes and relays	Solid state modulator	Reliability and ease of service	

From Karzmark CJ, Nunan CS, Tanabe E: *Medical electron accelerators*, New York, 1993, McGraw-Hill.

the magnetron or klystron. Each of the components is critical to the total function and operation of the linear accelerator.

Design Features

In the treatment room the major components of a linear accelerator can be divided into three specific areas: drive stand, gantry, and treatment couch (Fig. 7-10). A typical treatment room is designed with thick concrete or lead walls for shielding purposes. In this space the gantry is mounted to the stand, which is secured to the floor. Most radiation therapy machines have three rotating parts: gantry, collimator, and couch.[4] The treatment unit is positioned in a way that permits 360-degree rotation of the gantry. A treatment couch is mounted on a rotational axis around the isocenter. This permits the positioning of a patient lying supine or prone on the treatment couch. One ceiling and two side lasers project small dots or lines onto predetermined marks (established during the simulation process) on the patient. Sometimes a fourth midsagittal laser is mounted opposite the drive stand, high on the wall in a way that directs a continuous line along the sagittal axis of the patient. This laser may be used to position the patient's midsagittal plane along the long axis of the treatment couch. One or more closed-circuit television cameras may be mounted on the wall of the treatment room to enable the radiation therapist to monitor the patient during treatment.

Drive stand. The **gantry** rotates on a horizontal axis on bearings within the drive stand, which is firmly secured to the floor in the treatment room. The drive stand appears as a large, rectangular cabinet, at least as large as the gantry. As its name indicates, the drive stand is a stand containing the apparatus that drives the linear accelerator. The drive stand is

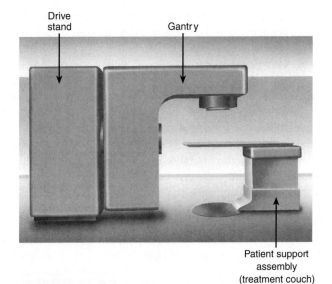

Drive stand   Gantry

Patient support assembly (treatment couch)

Figure 7-10. The major components of a linear accelerator include a drive stand, gantry, patient support assembly (treatment couch), control console (not shown), and modulator cabinet (also not shown). *(Courtesy Robert Morton and Medical Physics Publishing Corporation, Madison, Wisconsin.)*

usually open on both sides with swinging doors for easy access to gauges, valves, tanks, and buttons. Four major components are housed in the stand: the klystron, waveguide, circulator, and cooling system (Fig. 7-11).

The klystron, provides the source of microwave power used to accelerate electrons.[29] This microwave power is

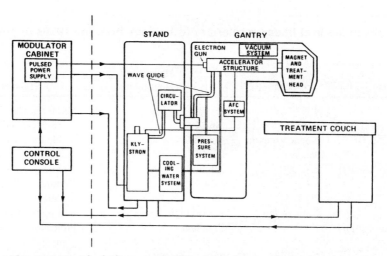

Figure 7-11. Block diagram of a linear accelerator illustrating the major components, including the stand, gantry, treatment couch, modulator cabinet, and control console. *(Courtesy Robert Morton and Medical Physics Publishing Corp, Madison, Wisconsin.)*

directed into the circulator and out to the **waveguide,** much like a copper wire delivers electricity to an outlet in a home. However, the waveguide is usually a hollow, tubelike structure. A circulator is placed between the klystron, directs the RF energy into the waveguide, and prevents any reflected microwaves from returning to the klystron. The **circulator** acts much like the valves found in human veins and the lymphatic system, which are designed to prevent the backflow of blood and lymphatic fluid. The water-cooling system, which is actually a thermal-stability system, allows many components in the gantry and drive stand to operate at a constant temperature. Components cooled by circulating water include the accelerator structure, klystron, circulator, target, and other important assemblies and components.

Gantry. The gantry is responsible primarily for directing the photon (x-ray) or electron beam at a patient's tumor. It can accomplish this through a single-rotational or multiple-fixed fields positioned the isocenter. For isocentric-type treatment, this point is usually positioned in the patient's tumor. The three translations of the **treatment couch** (left/right, up/down, and in/out) move the patient in relationship to the isocenter, thus allowing for precise patient positioning (Fig. 7-12).

The controls to the gantry motions are located on a control pendant(s) or the dedicated keyboard outside the room at the console area. Digital readings are also displayed. Gantry angle, collimator rotation, and field size (defined by the X and Y collimators) are commonly displayed for easy reference at the throat of the gantry (Fig. 7-13).

The major components in the gantry are the electron gun, accelerator structure (guide), treatment head (Fig. 7-14), and optional beam stopper.

Electron gun. The **electron gun** is responsible for pro-

ducing electrons and injecting them into the accelerator structure. Electron production in a diagnostic x-ray tube is similar to that in a linear accelerator.

Fig. 7-15 illustrates the design of a diode electron gun. The cathode is a spherically shaped structure made of a material with a high atomic number, such as tungsten. Tungsten is the element of choice because of the high temperatures required (between 800° and 1100° C). The anode, which carries a positive potential, is separated from the cathode to allow the focus electrode to direct the accelerated electrons through the beam hole in the anode.

Accelerator guide. The accelerator guide, sometimes called the accelerator structure, can be mounted in the gantry horizontally, as illustrated in Fig. 7-16 (high-energy machines), or vertically, as illustrated in Fig. 7-17 (low-energy machines). Microwave power (produced in the klystron) is transported to the accelerator structure, in which corrugations are used to slow up the waves (sometimes analogous to small jetties at a beach used to break up ocean waves). As a result, the crests of the microwave electric field are made approximately synchronous with the flowing bunches of electrons.[29,48] After the flowing electrons leave the accelerator structure, they are directed toward the target (for photon production) or scattering foil (for electron production) located in the treatment head. In the gantry, x-rays are produced or a treatment beam of electrons is shaped.

Accelerator structure. From basic radiologic physics, microwave means "extremely small wavelengths." Because the length of waves is inversely proportional to its energy, energy is high. The microwave frequency needed for the linear accelerator is in the range of 3 million cycles per second. Amplification that occurs in the accelerator

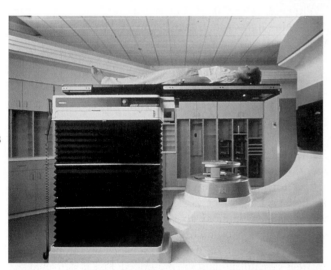

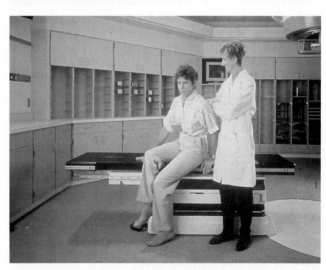

Figure 7-12. Three translations of the treatment couch are shown: **A,** In/out, up/down, and left/right. **B,** Newer treatment couches extend higher for greater posterior treatment distances. **C,** Travel lower to the floor for easy patient access. (**A,** Courtesy Siemans Medical Systems, Concord, Calif; **B** and **C,** Courtesy Varian Medical Systems.)

structure is in the closed-ended, precision-crafted copper cavities (Fig. 7-18). Here, the electrical power provides momentum to the low-level electron stream mixed with the microwaves. An alternating positive and negative electric charge accelerates the electrons toward the treatment head. Medical linear accelerators accelerate by traveling or standing electromagnetic waves of frequencies in the microwave

region. In the standing wave design, the microwave power is joined into the structure by side-coupling cavities, rather than through the beam aperture. This design tends to be more efficient than traveling wave design, but it can be more expensive.[44]

The length of the accelerator structure varies depending on the beam energy of the linear accelerator. The length may

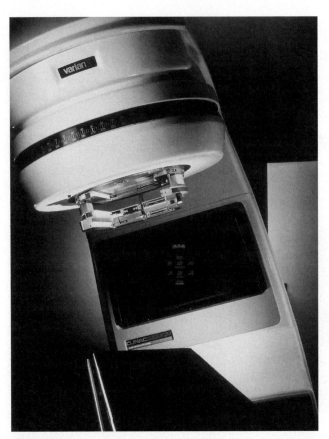

Figure 7-13. Readout displays for collimator angle, gantry angle, and upper and lower jaws (X and Y collimator) are digitally displayed at the throat of the gantry. *(Courtesy Varian Medical Systems.)*

vary from 30 cm for a 4-MV unit to 1 m or more for high-energy units.[28,29] For high-energy linear accelerators, up to five cavities are sometimes used to accelerate the electron bunch enough to generate the desired microwave energy. The therapist should remember that as more cavities are used, higher energy is derived. After electrons leave the accelerator structure, they are directed toward the treatment head. The treatment head may contain various beam-shaping devices, radiation monitors, and possibly a bending magnet if a horizontal accelerator structure is used.

Treatment head. Several components designed to shape and monitor the treatment beam are located in the treatment head (Fig. 7-19). For photon therapy, these components may consist of a bending magnet; x-ray target; primary collimator; beam-flattening filter; ion chamber; secondary collimators; and one or more slots for wedges, blocks, and compensators.

The horizontal accelerator structure required for an 18-MV photon beam needs a bending magnet to direct the electrons vertically toward a supine patient for an anterior treatment (otherwise, the electrons would continue straight out, horizontally through the treatment head of the gantry). A

magnet system may bend the electron group through a net angle of approximately 90 to 270 degrees and onto the x-ray target (or scattering foil for electron production).[29] After emerging from the x-ray target, the x-rays produced are shaped by a primary collimator, which is designed to limit the maximum field size. A beam-flattening filter located on the carousel with the scattering foil (Fig. 7-20) shapes the x-ray beam in its cross-sectional dimension. An ion chamber monitors the beam for its symmetry in the right-left and inferior-superior direction. Secondary collimation is achieved through the manual or remote control by using the setting knobs at the collimator head or pendant to adjust the upper and lower collimator jaws. On new units, secondary collimation may also be set from the treatment console outside the room. Additional beam-shaping and modifying devices such as a wedge, compensator, or custom shielding blocks can be placed in slots just below the secondary collimators.

In addition, a field light is located in the treatment head. Light from a quartz-iodine bulb outlines the dimensions of the radiation field as it appears on the patient (Fig. 7-21). This alignment of the radiation and light fields allows accurate positioning of the radiation field in relationship to skin marks or other reference points. When the secondary collimators are positioned to the desired width and length for the patient's setup, the reflected light field corresponds to the desired width and length of the radiation field. Multileaf collimators (MLCs) or Cerrobend blocking may further define the light field to correspond to the desired treatment field shape.

Control console. Monitoring and controlling of the linear accelerator occurs at the control console. Located outside the treatment room, the control console may take the form of a digital display, push-button panel or video display terminal (VDT) in which the machine status and patient-treatment information are incorporated into the computerized treatment unit. The ready state of the equipment allows the therapist to confirm the treatment parameters. All interlocks must be satisfied for the machine to allow the beam to be started. A lighted push-button or message on the VDT usually indicates the machine is in the ready state.

An indicator for the beam-on state (from a lighted push-button or message on the VDT) remains on throughout the patient's treatment until the prescribed dose is delivered.

Interlock displays can occur before or during a treatment. The interlock system is designed to protect the patient, staff members, and equipment from hazards. Patient-protection interlocks, including beam energy, beam symmetry, dose, and dose-rate monitoring, prevent radiation and mechanical hazards to the patient. For example, interlocks protect the patient against extremely high dose rates, especially if the treatment unit provides x-ray and electron beams. Because of the high electron-beam currents used for x-ray production, extremely high dose rates can result if the target or flattening filter do not intercept the beam. Machine interlocks protect the equipment from damage, which may include problems

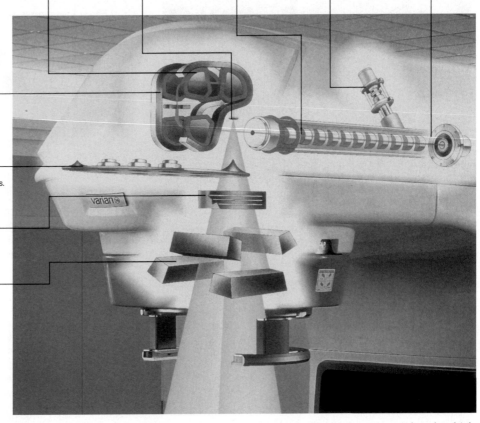

Steering System
Radial and transverse steering coils and a real-time feedback system ensure beam symmetry to within ±2% at all gantry angles.

Focal spot size
Even at maximum dose rate, the circular focal remains less than 3.0 mm, held constant by the achromatic bending magnet. Assures optimum image quality for portal imaging.

Standing Wave Accelerator Guide
Maintains optimal bunching for different acceleration conditions, providing high dose rates, stable dosimetry and low-stray radiation. Transport system minimizes power and electron source demands.

Energy Switch
Patented switch provides energies within the full therapeutic range, at consistently high, stable dose rates, even with low energy X-ray beams. Ensures optimum performance and spectral purity at both energies.

Gridded Electron Gun
Controls dose rate rapidly and accurately. Permits precise beam control for dynamic treatments since gun can be gated. Demountable, for cost-effective replacement.

Achromatic Dual-Plane Bending Magnet
Unique design with ±3% energy slits ensures exact replication of the input beam for every treatment. Clinac 2300C/D design enhancements allow wider range of beam energies.

10-Port Carousel with Scattering Foils/Flattening Filters
Extra ports allow future specialized beams to be developed. New electron scattering foils provide homogeneous electron beams at therapeutic depths.

Ion Chamber
Two independently sealed chambers, impervious to temperature and pressure changes, monitor beam dosimetry to within 2% for long-term consistency and stability.

Asymmetric Jaws
Four independent collimators provide flexible beam definition of symmetric or asymmetric fields.

Figure 7-14. The major components of the gantry include the electron gun, accelerator guide, and treatment head, which includes components such as the bending magnet, beam-flattening filter, ion chamber, and upper-lower collimator jaws. *(Courtesy Varian Medical Systems.)*

detected in the machine's high-voltage power supply, water-cooling system, or vacuum system.

Emergency off buttons, which can terminate irradiation and machine functions, are located on the control panel and at several other locations in the treatment room. These switches terminate all electrical power to the equipment and require a complete startup procedure before the treatment machine can produce an electron or photon beam.

Besides displaying the operational mode of the treatment unit, the control console serves several other functions. It may provide a digital display for prescribed dose (monitor units), mechanical beam parameters such as collimator setting or gantry angle, and possibly up to 50 other status messages.[29] Overall, the treatment-control console provides a central location for controlling and operating the linear accelerator.

Treatment couch. The treatment couch is the area on which patients are positioned to receive their radiation treatment. Several unique features of the treatment couch provide the tabletop with mobility. A standard feature allows the tabletop to move mechanically in a horizontal and lengthwise direction. This movement must be smooth and accurate with the patient in the treatment position, thus allowing for precise and exact positioning of the isocenter during treatment positioning. Many tabletops support up to 200 kg (450 lb) and range in width from 45 to 50 cm. If the couch width on the simulator is not similar to that of the treatment unit, reproducibility may become a problem, especially with large patients.

Unlike the tabletop on the simulator, patients may be positioned at either end of the treatment couch depending on the treatment plan (Fig. 7-22). At one end of the couch a

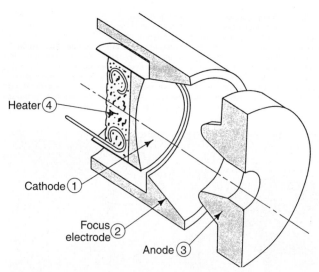

Figure 7-15. Cross-sectional view of a diode electron gun demonstrating the cathode and anode. *(From Karzmark CJ, Nunan CS, Tanabe E: Medical electron accelerators, New York, 1993, McGraw-Hill.)*

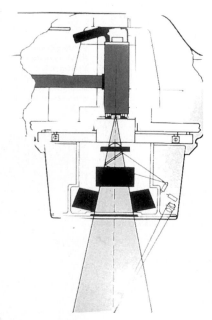

Figure 7-17. A low-energy linear accelerator demonstrates the vertically mounted, straight-through beam design, which eliminates the need for complex beam-bending magnet systems. *(Courtesy Varian Medical Systems.)*

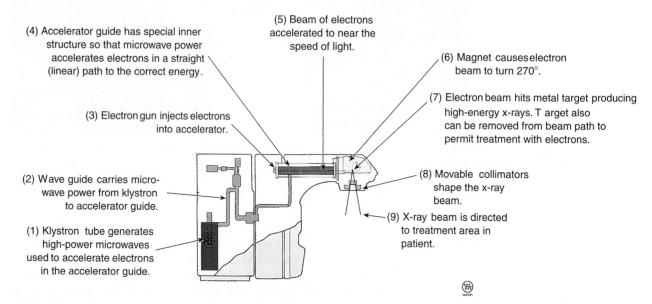

(4) Accelerator guide has special inner structure so that microwave power accelerates electrons in a straight (linear) path to the correct energy.

(5) Beam of electrons accelerated to near the speed of light.

(6) Magnet causes electron beam to turn 270°.

(7) Electron beam hits metal target producing high-energy x-rays. Target also can be removed from beam path to permit treatment with electrons.

(3) Electron gun injects electrons into accelerator.

(2) Wave guide carries microwave power from klystron to accelerator guide.

(1) Klystron tube generates high-power microwaves used to accelerate electrons in the accelerator guide.

(8) Movable collimators shape the x-ray beam.

(9) X-ray beam is directed to treatment area in patient.

Figure 7-16. This high-energy radiation therapy treatment machine illustrates the horizontally mounted accelerator structure and 270-degree bending magnet. *(Courtesy Varian Medical Systems.)*

rectangular or square segment of sturdy plastic or a frame with strings (similar to a tennis racket woven tightly together) can be located. After extended use, this racket-like section should be restrung to provide more patient support and reduce the amount of sag during treatment positioning. At the opposite end of the tabletop, some manufacturers have developed removable inserts (two, three, or more segments located to the left or right of a sturdy metal support). Patient-positioning and support devices such as an arm board, breast board, and treatment chair may be attached at the sides or end of the tabletop.

In addition, a set of local controls may be located on the

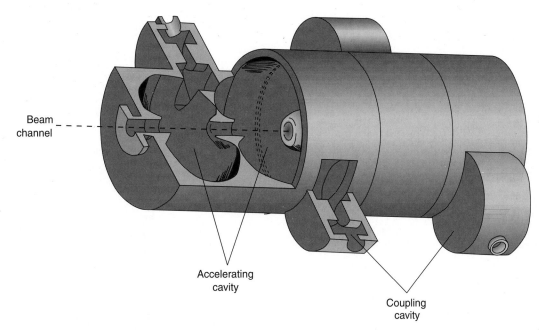

Figure 7-18. Cross section of a standing-wave accelerator structure used in high-energy treatment units. *(Courtesy Siemans Corporation, Concord, California.)*

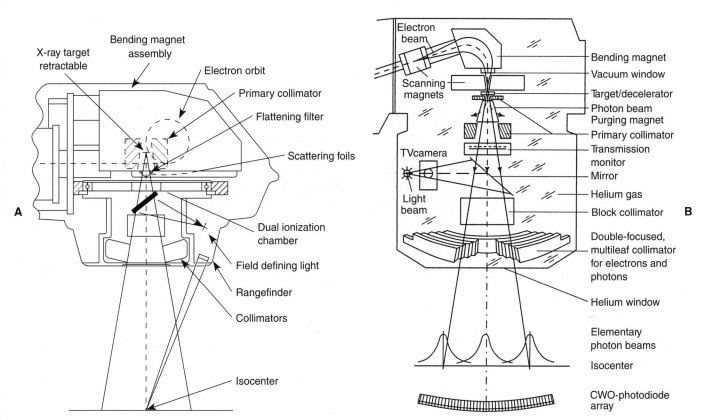

Figure 7-19. A, Cross section of the treatment head of a high-energy linear accelerator. **B,** Medical micotron. *(**A,** Courtesy CJ Karzmark and Varian Associates, Palo Alto, California; **B,** courtesy A. Brahme and Scandinavian University Press, Stockholm.)*

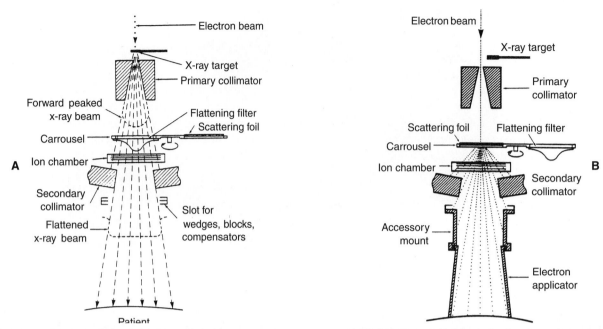

Figure 7-20. The subsystem components with the treatment head of a high-energy linear accelerator. **A,** Note the beam subsystem is in the x-ray mode, indicated by the position of the flattening filter. **B,** The subsystem in the electron mode is indicated by the position of the scattering foil. *(Courtesy Robert Morton and Medical Physics Publishing Corporation, Madison, Wisconsin.)*

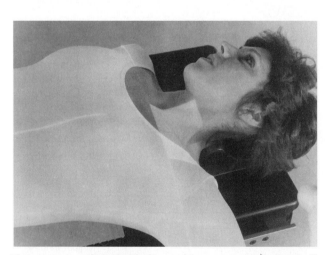

Figure 7-21. A light field, directed from a quartz-iodine bulb in the treatment head, corresponds to the radiation field in this anterior supraclavicular field. *(Courtesy Varian Medical Systems.)*

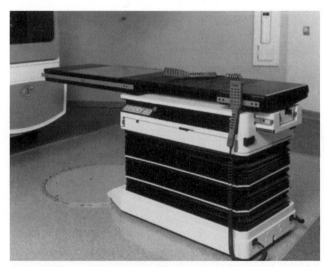

Figure 7-22. This couchtop contains removable side-rail and centerspine sections for treating posterior fields and posterior oblique fields. The side-rail posterior support panel provides a 47 × 61 cm treatment window, and removable couch panels may be shifted over 30 cm to adjust to variances in patient size and tumor location. *(Courtesy Varian Medical Systems.)*

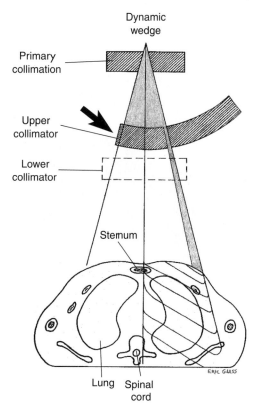

Figure 7-25. The upper collimator moves during treatment to create a dynamic wedge effect. *(Courtesy Varian Medical Systems.)*

the MLC information is transferred and duplicated in the treatment room without the therapist entering the room to change blocks between treatments. The MLC replaces the need for custom blocking in many but not all situations.

Several **multileaf collimator (MLC)** systems exist that

shield blocked area by using approximately 52 to 120 leaves. These heavy, metal collimator rods slide into place to form the desired field shape by projecting 0.5-cm to 2-cm beam widths per rod.[29] Fig. 7-27 compares the dose distribution for a prostate treatment field with multileaf collimation and custom Cerrobend blocks. Equivalent dose distributions are achieved with both methods.

Dynamic wedges are designed in such a way that wedge-dose distributions using varying fields sizes yield excellent wedged-isodose distributions compared with physical wedges.[32] This design relies strongly on computer software to vary the dose rate and mechanical motion of the collimator during treatment. When the beam is turned on, the dose rate and collimator setting are automatically set according to a pregenerated treatment plan. The field size changes to generate the desired wedge angle (see Fig. 7-25).

An electronic portal imaging device (EPID) is another method of improving treatment-field accuracy and verification. With conventional portal systems, cassettes are positioned in the slot under the treatment couch for antero-posterior (AP) films or placed in a cassette holder for posteroanterior (PA), lateral, and oblique field positions. With portal imaging technology, correct positioning of internal anatomic structures can be observed during the entire treatment process or checked by pretreatment imaging with the aid of computer software. Most electronic portal-imaging systems are lightweight and come with a retracted arm along the gantry's axis (Fig. 7-28). The arm is equipped with an image intensifier to improve the quality of the image. Despite the poor image quality common with regular port films (as a result of Compton and pair-production interactions), comparable quality images are possible (Fig. 7-29).

The position of the image detector in relationship to the patient can affect image quality through magnification and scatter radiation. Bissonnette et al[7] have shown that a magnification factor of 1.6 is optimal for TV based camera

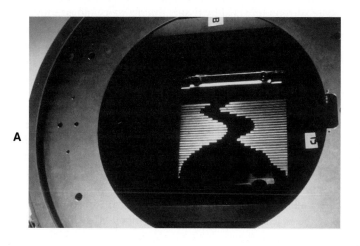

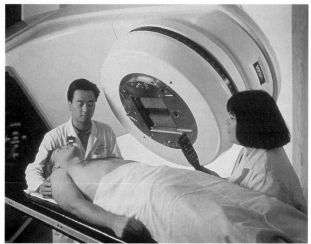

Figure 7-26. A, Multileaf collimator (MLC) mounted on the treatment head. **B,** Initial setup of the patient with MLC. **(A,** *Courtesy Siemans Medical Systems, Concord, California;* **B,** *Courtesy Varian Medical Systems.)*

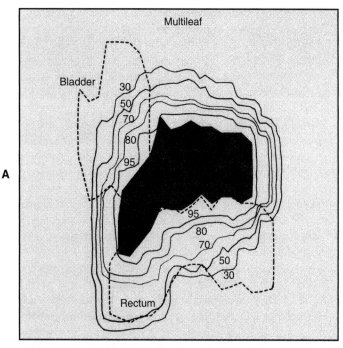

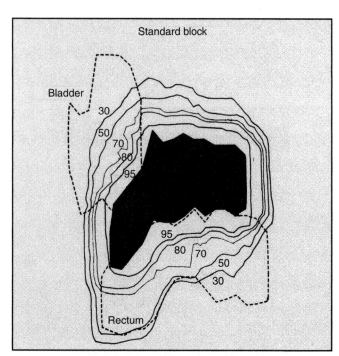

A

B

Figure 7-27. Comparison of dose distributions for lateral prostate treatment fields using multileaf collimator (MLC) and dose distribution for lateral prostate fields using custom cerrobend blocking (CCB). The isodose distributions are extremely similar. *(Courtesy Varian Medical Systems.)*

portal imaging systems. Swindell et al[57] found that an object-film distance (OFD) of 40 cm is sufficient to reduce the effects of scatter radiation on image quality. Attention to details such as scatter radiation and magnification are important factors in improving an already somewhat poor image quality.

Because it allows real time monitoring of patients during treatment, portal imaging is also used to detect movement during treatment and assess patient positional changes. In fact, in a study by Tinger et al,[58] who examined systematic and random setup errors in patients treated with pelvic irradiation, EPID images were used to document field displacements. In this study using 547 images, there was no documented intratreatment displacement in excess of 1 cm. However, intertreatment displacement exceeding 1 cm was documented in 23% of the patients in the AP, 16% in the superior/inferior, and 3% in the mediolateral direction. EPID are also used to detect patient movement, organ movement, and patient positioning in other areas such as the breast and abdomen. As technology improves so will its application in radiation therapy.

Verification and record devices. Computers have been introduced to assist the radiation therapist in the verification of treatment parameters. If the average number of patients treated on a linear accelerator is assumed to be between 30 to 35 patient per day and each patient may have an average of 20 separate parameters (gantry angle, treatment distance, field size, etc.), this equates to 600 to 700 parameters that must be matched each day. Verification systems not only allow incorrect setup parameters to be corrected before the

machine is turned on but may also provide data in other areas, such as computer assisted setup, recording of patient data, allowing for data transfer from the simulator or treatment planning computer, and assisting with quality control. See Chapter 24 on e-charting and image management for a more detailed discussion.

Stereotactic radiation therapy. Linear-based stereotactic radiation therapy (radiosurgery) involves the aiming and delivery of a well-defined narrow beam to extremely hard-to-reach places.[8,34] Because of the relatively high doses per fraction, stereotactic radiosurgery must at the same time spare surrounding healthy tissue. Brain tumors and arteriovenous malformations (AVMs) are conditions that benefit from this technology because of their anatomic location and the tendency for complications to arise with conventional treatment.[5] Most of the time necessary to complete a stereotactic treatment is spent in preparation, whereas the actual treatment time is comparatively small. The procedure is usually noninvasive, other than the impingement of the halo into the skull (small burr holes are drilled into the skull in several locations to secure the halo device). The halo device is used in immobilization and aids in treatment positioning. A finely collimated field is precisely aimed at the tumor volume. Here, a high dose of radiation is quickly delivered in a wide arc, thus ensuring an even dose distribution to the tumor volume (Fig. 7-30).

Computer-driven technology may provide more precise and accurate treatment in the future as more hospitals and clinics use these new technologies. As the technology

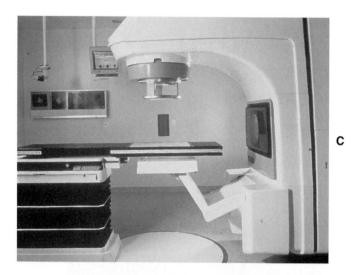

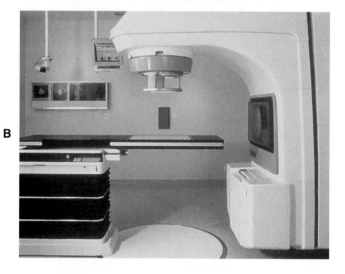

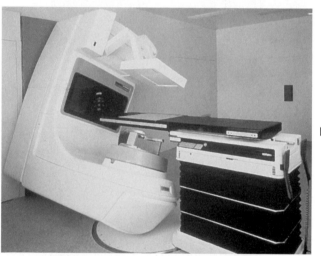

Figure 7-28. A, Fully retractable and collapsible gantry-mounted detector used in an electronic portal-imaging system. **B** to **D,** Retractable arm at various positions provides unrestricted room for patient positioning with an electronic portal-imaging system. (**A,** *Courtesy Siemans Medical Systems, Concord, California;* **B** to **D,** *Courtesy Varian Medical Systems.*)

becomes more available and costs are reduced, more patients will benefit from their use.

The sophisticated computer-driven linear accelerator can provide the patient with the benefits of these new technologies. Some of the equipment is expensive. Dual asymmetrical jaws act as beam splitters, thus eliminating the use of heavy custom-shaped blocking in some situations. Clinical evidence demonstrates that increased cure rates result from increased tumor doses greater than 7000 cGy in prostate cancer.[49] With the help of MLC and

electronic portal imaging, multiple fields and increased doses are achievable. In addition, sophisticated computer software allows the precise and accurate administration of IMRT.

IMRT has yet to reach its full potential in the field of radiation oncology. It represents a fundamental change in the way dose is delivered to the patient. IMRT combines the use of advanced computer programming with sophisticated treatment delivery equipment to plan a precise radiation dose in three dimensions. Using CT, magnetic resonance

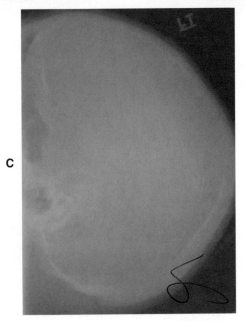

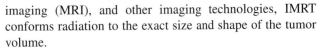

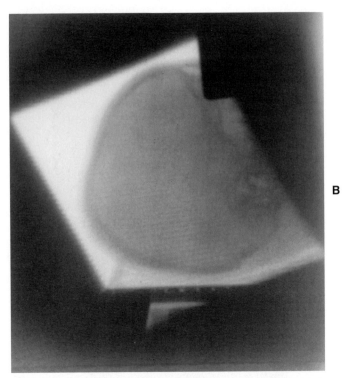

Figure 7-29. A, Monitor from Siemans Beamview Plus portal-imaging system demonstrates two processed images. **B,** Processed whole brain portal image from Siemans Beamview Plus portal-imaging system. **C,** Posttreatment whole brain port film taken with three to five monitor units on a 6-MV linear accelerator. (*A* and *B, Courtesy Siemans Medical System, Concord, California.*)

imaging (MRI), and other imaging technologies, IMRT conforms radiation to the exact size and shape of the tumor volume.

With the addition of computer-generated technology comes the added responsibility for quality assurance and safety. Equipment failure in linear-accelerator treatment units can result in serious radiation accidents, including overexposure.

Medical Accelerator Safety Considerations

With the increased use of multimodality treatment units, potential hazards exist that usually are not present in single-modality treatment units.[27,45] Monitoring and controlling safe operating conditions for a computer-driven linear accelerator is more difficult than for the more conventional, electro-mechanical type.

Emergency procedures. Emergency procedures, if implemented properly, can prevent a serious accident and possibly save a patient's life. Written emergency procedures

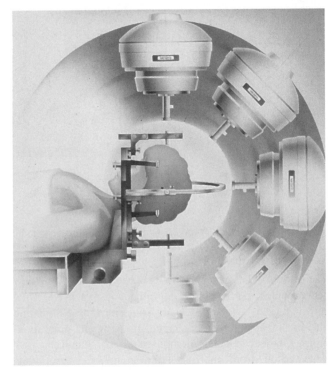

Figure 7-30. Stereotactic radiation treatment to an intracranial tumor from several angles. (*Courtesy Brain Lab Ag.*)

should be located at or near the treatment-control console. (Some state regulatory agencies require this.) Radiation therapists should be familiar with written procedures in the event of a patient emergency. Knowing the location of emergency stop buttons (inside and outside the treatment room) is critical in the event of a machine malfunction. Other emergencies involving the patient's medical condition may also require the therapist's attention.

Safety considerations. Electrical, mechanical, and radiation-safety considerations must be more elaborate with multimodality treatment units because of the accelerator's increased flexibility. An example may better portray the need for more elaborate safety considerations.

The failure of some software can allow the delivery of large doses. For example, if a large electron-beam current intended for x-ray production is used for an electron treatment, an extremely large dose rate can result. If the scattering foil is in place or the beam scanning operational, an estimated dose comparable to a typical 2-Gy dose fraction can be delivered to a patient in about 0.03 second at 4000 Gy/min. This dose rate can create hazards for the patient. To address this type of problem, digital logic and microprocessors have been incorporated into the linear accelerator control and monitor functions.[45]

Potentially dangerous problems can result from misadministration of a prescribed radiation dose. A **misadministration** (incorrect application or delivery of a prescribed dose of radiation therapy) can be minor or major and may cause death or serious injury to the patient depending on the extent of the dose. The Food and Drug Administration defines an accident that can cause death or serious injury as a class I hazard. If the risk of serious injury is low, because of human error or a linear accelerator malfunction, the accident is classified as a class II hazard.[45]

The American Association of Physicists in Medicine (AAPM) Radiation Therapy Committee Task Group Number 35 has developed a list containing most of the causes of potentially life-threatening problems associated with electrical, mechanical, human, and software errors involving medical linear accelerators[45] (Table 7-4).

Computer-operated linear accelerators provide more options for the radiation oncologist in treating benign and malignant disease. For example, electron arc therapy, x-ray arc therapy, and high-dose-rate (HDR) total-skin electron therapy are available on some units.[45] However, with the increased flexibility comes an added responsibility to ensure safe and proper operation of this equipment.

Linear accelerators continue to gain in popularity throughout the United States. Some authors estimate that in the industrialized world more than 75% of the treatment machines are linear accelerators.[29]

A comprehensive understanding of and familiarization with the design, characteristics, performance parameters, and control of the linear accelerator is essential for many of the members of the cancer-management team. In addition, the mechanical, electrical, software, and radiation-safety considerations are critical to applying the theory and operation of a linear accelerator to patients needing treatment.

Although the linear accelerator is the most widely accepted treatment machine in developed countries, it is worth discussing other methods of delivering a tumoricidal dose, especially the historic high-energy treatment machines, such as the betatron, Van de Graaff generator, and cyclotron. Also included in this discussion is the older cobalt unit and the more modern use of isotopes in HDR brachytherapy.

Betatron

The first betatron, developed by Kerst in 1941, produced x-rays of 2 MV.[35] **Betatrons** (megavoltage treatment units that can provide x-ray and electron therapy beams from less than 6 to more than 40 MeV) were initially used for radiation therapy in the early 1950s.[30,33] Besides medical uses, betatrons were applied to industrial radiography. Betatrons were used especially during World War II, when they provided the energy to x-ray thick castings and other metal sections of equipment used in wartime.

The operation of the betatron is based on the principle that an electron in a changing magnetic field experiences acceleration in a circular orbit (Fig. 7-31).

The accelerating tube is shaped like a hollow doughnut

Table 7-4	Medical accelerator hazards		
Type	**Cause**	**Consequences**	
Incorrect dose delivered	Electrical, software, and therapist	Serious injury, increased complicaions, genetic effects, second primary, and compromised tumor control	
Dose delivered to the wrong area	Mechanical, software, patient motion, and therapist	Serious injury, increased complications, genetic effects, second primary, and compromised tumor control	
Machine collision	Mechanical, software, patient motion, and therapist	Significant injury and death	
Incorrect beam	Electrical, software, and therapist	Serious injury, increased complications, genetic effects, second primary, and compromised tumor control	
General hazards	Electrical and mechanical	Significant injury and death	

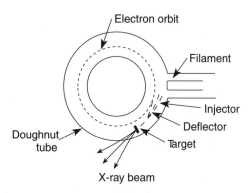

Figure 7-31. A schematic illustrating the operation of the betatron. *(From Khan F: The physics of radiation therapy, ed 2, Baltimore, 1994, Williams & Wilkins.)*

and is placed between the poles of an alternating current magnet. A pulse of electrons is introduced into this evacuated doughnut by an injector at the instant that the alternating current cycle begins. As the magnetic field rises, the electrons experience acceleration continuously and spin with increasing velocity around the tube. By the end of the first quarter cycle of the alternate magnetic field, the electrons have made several thousand revolutions and achieved maximum energy. At this instant or earlier, depending on the energy desired, the electrons are made to spiral out of the orbit by an additional force. The high-energy electrons then strike a target to produce x-rays or a scattering foil to produce a broad beam of electrons.[1]

One advantage of the betatron is the production of electrons for use with superficial tumors. In addition, x-rays can be used for hard-to-reach tumors at great depths. Betatrons capture and transport a smaller-than-average beam current compared with linear accelerators and are most often used for electron therapy. However, medical betatrons can produce x-ray beams with energies over 40 MV.[46]

The betatron generally used Lucite cones of various sizes, ranging from 15 cm × 15 cm to 8 cm × 8 cm at 100 SSD. Common tumors treated with the betatron included mostly gynecologic, bladder, and prostate carcinomas. The treatment times depended on the prescribed dose and diameter of the patient. They usually averaged 3 to 5 minutes and used a dose rate of 200 cGy/minute. To compensate for the characteristically noisy machine, therapists applied cotton balls and ear mufflers for patients wanting some noise reduced during treatments (Fig. 7-32).

Betatrons are suitable for electron production but cannot compare with the x-ray dose rates of a linear accelerator. Linear accelerators are also capable of much larger field sizes and electron therapy energies up to 20 MeV. The bulky and noisy betatrons will most likely continue to diminish in popularity as medicine demands more sophisticated and flexible equipment.

Van de Graaff Generator

Another historic medical accelerator, which has continued to diminish in popularity is the Van de Graaff generator. In 1937 R.J. Van de Graaff, while working at the Massachusetts Institute of Technology, developed the first electrostatic

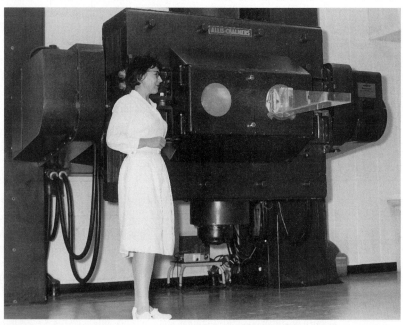

Figure 7-32. The Allis-Chalmers betatron. *(Courtesy M.D. Anderson Cancer Center, Houston, Texas.)*

linear accelerator. Accelerators may be circular or linear, and the linear type is electrostatic (such as the Van de Graaff) or electronic.[18]

The Van de Graaff is a constant potential electrostatic generator developed around the physical principle illustrated by the classical Faraday "ice bucket" experiment. The hemispherical high-voltage dome is analogous to the ice bucket (Fig. 7-33). In the ice bucket experiment, electrons deposited inside the electrically conducted metal bucket (presumably used for carrying ice in earlier days) quickly move to the outside. The process can continue until a specified potential is attained or until there is a coronal breakdown of the air outside the bucket.[33]

These 2-MV units have a steel dome of about 3 feet in diameter and 5.5 feet in height and are constructed nonisocentrically. Van de Graaff units use an external blocking tray to hold hand-placed blocks. Because no standard table is affixed to this unit, the patient lies on a stretcher underneath the machine or can even be placed in a chair if necessary. Blocking can be dangerous because blocks frequently require stacking to approximate the treatment area. Van de Graaff units can operate at 200 cGy/minute and provide a standard SSD of 100 cm, but they can also approximate much greater treatment distances. This was extremely useful in the treatment of extended fields needed to treat a variety of malignancies. The Van de Graaff unit (Fig. 7-34) was routinely used to treat seminoma (a lengthy field in the abdomen and pelvis is used to treat this type of testicular cancer), whole brain, and mantle field (used to treat lymph nodes in the neck and thorax for Hodgkin's disease).

Arcing was frequent for radiation therapists warming up these units, which could sometimes require as long as 1 hour. When setting up a patient for treatment, the therapist used a front-pointer device to measure the distance to the patient. No optical distance indicator was available.[22] However, the Van de Graaff unit could treat any tumor that other megavoltage equipment could treat. Its bulk made it cumbersome to use, and it was replaced by the isocentric linear accelerator, which are more popular today.

Proton Accelerator

On the other hand, an older treatment unit, such as the cyclotron has made a resurrection in the field of high-energy treatment machines. Current research in the use of protons, produced from a cyclotron, hold promise in the treatment of many types of malignant disease.

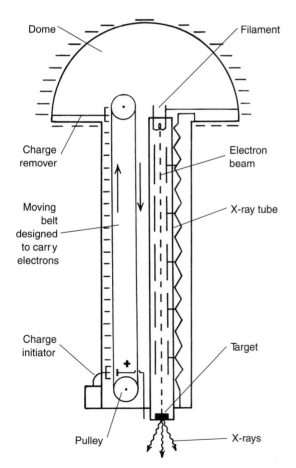

Figure 7-33. A schematic diagram of the Van de Graaff generator.

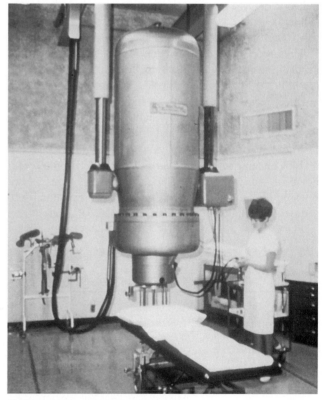

Figure 7-34. The Van de Graaff unit at the University Hospital in Oklahoma City, Oklahoma, was routinely used to treat seminoma, whole brain, and mantle fields. *(Courtesy University Hospital, Oklahoma City, Oklahoma.)*

In 1928, E.O. Lawrence developed the cyclotron.[18] A cyclotron is a charged particle accelerator used often for nuclear research. Early on, the use of the cyclotron for medical purposes was explored. Its use primarily relates to accelerating protons, neutron beams, light ions, and heavy charged particles used in radiation therapy.[56] In this section, three specific medical uses of the cyclotron are discussed briefly. This includes the production of radionuclides applied primarily in nuclear medicine and the use of neutrons and protons in radiation therapy.

Radionuclides. The cyclotron has been used recently as a particle accelerator for the production of radionuclides used in PET. This is a scanning technique that involves the systemic administration of a radiopharmaceutical agent labeled with a positron-emitting radionuclide. PET scanners are used in nuclear medicine studies to measure important physiologic and biomedical processes such as blood flow, oxygen, glucose and metabolism of free fatty acids, amino acid transport, pH, and neuroreceptor densities. A cyclotron is required to produce radionuclides such as carbon-11, nitrogen-13, and oxygen-15, which all have short half-lives. Today, nuclear medicine PET scanning occurs at more than 90 research centers around the world.[5]

Clinical application and characteristics of PET procedure. Unlike conventional radiographic or CT scanners that use x-rays passing through a person, PET scanners use radiation emitted from within the patient to produce images. While the patient is alert and conscious, distinct areas of the brain, for example, can be evaluated in microscopic detail. Patients receive a small amount of a radioactive pharmaceutical agent that closely resembles a substance naturally found in the body (such as sugar). The amount of radiation a patient receives varies with the radiopharmaceutical agent used. The most widely used radionuclides are listed in Fig. 7-35. Oxygen, carbon, and nitrogen are essential atoms to a majority of the body's physiologic processes.

PET imaging involves positrons emitted during the breakdown of the nuclei of certain radioisotopes. Pure energy, released as gamma rays, is a result of the collision and subsequent annihilation of matter and antimatter. Radiation from the positron-emitting isotope is detected by the PET scanner and displays in microscopic detail the chemical processes occurring. Two gamma rays of equal energy are produced when a positron meets an electron going in the opposite direction. The information is then delivered into a computer that performs complex algorithms, thus resulting in a detailed picture.[2] PET will probably expand to include the evaluation of patients with malignancy and those with psychiatric illnesses.[12,15]

Although the data strongly support the clinical applications of PET in certain brain and heart disorders, the future of PET will directly relate to reimbursement for these procedures. Other factors relate to the expense of a cyclotron, which can easily approach $1 million and is expensive to install and operate.[5]

The potential of PET imaging in the diagnosis of medical disorders is still being discovered. Cyclotrons are necessary components of a PET facility, mainly because many of the isotopes generated in the cyclotron have such short half-lives. This prohibits the transportation of the isotopes to any nonlocal distance. Most dedicated cyclotrons used in PET imaging are in place solely to produce PET radiopharmaceutical agents. Further advancements in superconducting technology may lead to smaller and more reasonably priced accelerators capable of heavy-particle radiation therapy using protons, neutrons, and heavy ions.

In addition to isotopes used for PET studies, cyclotrons produce the radiopharmaceutical agents used every day in hundreds of nuclear medicine departments for liver, bone, and other valuable diagnostic scans. These pharmaceutical agents include iodine-123, thallium-201, gallium-67, indium-111, and others.[63]

Components of the cyclotron. The cyclotron consists of a short metallic cylinder divided into two sections, which are usually referred to as dees, partly because of their shapes. These dees are highly evacuated and placed between the poles of a direct-current magnet producing a constant magnetic field. An alternating potential is applied between the two dees.[30]

An RF oscillator applies a high RF voltage to the dees. The voltage gradient in the gap between the dees reverses each time the dee polarities change. Inside each dee there is no electric field, but a particle is still subject to the magnet's field and therefore travels in a circular path. When the particle reaches the gap, it accelerates through the electric potential between the dees, and then coasts in a circular path through the other dee. By the time the particle has traveled 180 degrees, the oscillator has reversed the dee's polarity, so again, the particle accelerates through the gap. At each acceleration the radius of the orbit increases, so the particle spirals outward. The particles' final energy is the sum of the energy gained at each gap crossing.[46]

The machine does not have unlimited energy potential because of the theory of relativity. According to this theory, further acceleration causes the particle to gain mass. This

Radionuclide	Half-life
Carbon-11	20 min
Nitrogen-13	10 min
Fluorine-18	110 min
Oxygen-15	2 min
Gallium-68	68 min
Rubidium-82	1.3 min

Figure 7-35. Chart of radionuclides used in positron emission tomography (PET) studies. (From Bernier DR, Christian PE, Langan JK: Nuclear medicine technology and techniques, ed 4, St. Louis, 1997, Mosby.)

increase in weight causes the particle to slow down, thus ultimately causing the particle to be out of sync with the frequency of the alternate potential applied to the dee. This phenomenon is the reason electrons cannot accelerate in a cyclotron.[46]

Neutrons. As mentioned earlier, the cyclotron has been used not only for nuclear physics research but also to produce particles for clinical use. To produce neutron beams, deuterons ($^2_1H^+$) are accelerated to high energies and then forced to strike a suitable target (usually beryllium), thus producing neutrons (subatomic particles equal in mass to protons but without electrical charge) via nuclear reactions.[21] Because neutrons possess no electric charge, they are extremely effective in penetrating nuclei and producing reactions by a process termed stripping.[18] Fast neutrons were first used by Stone in 1938. Unacceptable late complications, mostly in fatty tissue in the patients treated, caused the study to be abandoned. These complications were due to the high concentration of hydrogen in the fatty tissue.[46]

Protons. A proton is a positively charged particle in the nucleus of all atoms that relates to the atomic number of the atoms. One of the earliest proton-producing, hospital-based cyclotrons was installed in 1949 at the Harvard Cyclotron Laboratory in collaboration with Massachusetts General Hospital and the Massachusetts Eye and Ear Infirmary (Fig. 7-36). A brief description of the production of protons at the Harvard cyclotron is presented to provide a basic understanding of the complex process of a proton accelerator (in this case a synchrocyclotron): to produce a usable beam of protons, we start with hydrogen gas. The basic unit, or atom, of hydrogen is composed of one proton and one electron. We strip off the electrons by subjecting the hydrogen gas to an electric current, which leaves us with an abundant supply of protons. These protons are then subjected to both an oscillating electric field, which accelerates them up to about $^1/_2$ the speed of light (approximately 300,000,000 miles/hr), and to a strong magnetic field, which keeps them contained in an ever-widening spiral configuration. At the end of each cycle (which takes 3/1000 of a second) the protons are channeled off into a beam pipe, which then leads into the treatment area. By using several magnets placed at various points along this beam pipe, the final proton beam attains a diameter about the size of a pencil and an intensity of some 109 protons/cm^2/sec (that is 1,000,000,000 protons hitting an area about $^1/_2$ inch square in 1 second's time).[10]

Proton radiation has proved effective in the treatment of benign and malignant lesions.[62] In 1961, under the direction of Dr. Raymond Kjellberg, the proton beam irradiated benign tumors of the pituitary gland. The program grew to include the treatment of AVMs. Almost 3000 patients have received a single high dose of radiation to a small, precise area with satisfactory results since the program ended in 1993.[59] Today, more than 6000 patients have received treatment to a variety of sites, including ocular melanoma; soft tissue and bone sarcomas; and prostate, head and neck, and other miscellaneous and metastatic tumors. A new proton facility with a rotational gantry was recently completed at Massachusetts General

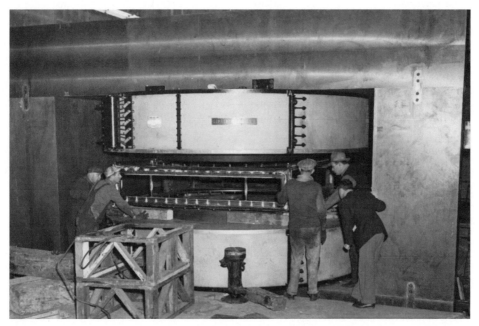

Figure 7-36. Construction of the 160-MeV synchrocyclotron at the Cyclotron Laboratory at Harvard University in 1947. Several workers are inspecting the coils, yoke, and dee. Although it was originally designed for physics research, the unit has treated thousands of patients with proton beams since 1961.

Hospital in 2003. Several new facilities for proton and ion therapy have been proposed worldwide. Table 7-5 describes current and proposed clinical programs using a variety of charged particles for the treatment of benign and malignant disease.

Protons are a valuable tool for clinical use for the following reasons: (1) they are precision-controlled; (2) scattering is minimal compared with that from x-rays, neutrons, and cobalt radiation; (3) they have a characteristic distribution of dose with depth; and (4) most of their energy is deposited near the end of their range, where the dose peaks to a high value and then drops rapidly to zero. This sudden change in dose distribution with depth is called the **Bragg peak.**

Fig. 7-37 illustrates the Bragg peak and compares two proton beams with a 10-MV x-ray beam. These reasons helped establish proton therapy as the treatment of choice for lesions close to sensitive areas of the body.[59]

Before treatment begins, a great deal of preparation is necessary. Patient positioning and immobilization are essential. Necessary pieces of equipment include various immobilization devices, an aperture (a 5-cm-thick brass cutout with a custom-shaped opening determined by the tumor volume [Fig. 7-38]), a modulator, and often a Lucite bolus compensator. The aperture has a purpose similar to custom-shielding blocks used with x-rays and gamma rays. With a compensator (a milled block of plastic carved out to various depths

Table 7-5	Current and proposed clinical programs using protons for the treatment of benign and malignant disease*					
Institution	**Where**	**Type**	**Date First Rx**	**Date Last Rx**	**Recent Patient Total**	**Date of Total**
Berkeley 184	CA, USA	p	1954	1957	30	
Berkeley	CA, USA	He	1957	1992	2054	June-91
Uppsala	Sweden	p	1957	1976	73	
Harvard	MA, USA	p	1961		9067	Jan-02
Dubna	Russia	p	1967	1974	84	
Moscow	Russia	p	1969		3445	Oct-01
Los Alamos	NM, USA		1974	1982	230	
St. Petersburg	Russia	p	1975		1029	June-98
Berkeley	CA, USA	heavy ion	1975	1992	433	June-91
Chiba	Japan	p	1979		133	Apr-00
TRIUMF	Canada		1979	1994	367	Dec-93
PSI (SIN)	Switzerland		1980	1993	503	
PMRC, Tsukuba	Japan	p	1983		700	July-00
PSI (72 MeV)	Switzerland	p	1984		3429	Dec-01
Dubna	Russia	p	1987		88	May-01
Uppsala	Sweden	p	1989		236	June-00
Clatterbridge	England	p	1989		1102	Dec-00
Loma Linda	CA. USA	p	1990		6672	Dec-01
Louvain-la-Neuve	Belgium	p	1991	1993	21	
Nice	France	p	1991		1590	June-00
Orsay	France	p	1991		1894	Jan-01
N.A.C.	South Africa	p	1993		408	Nov-01
MPRI	IN, USA	p	1993		34	Dec-99
UCSF-CNL	CA, USA	p	1994		284	June-00
HIMAC, Chiba	Japan	heavy ion	1994		917	Dec-99
TRIUMF	Canada	p	1995		57	June-01
PSI (200 MeV)	Switzerland	p	1996		99	Dec-01
G.S.I Darmstadt	Germany	heavy ion	1997		106	Jan-02
Berlin	Germany	p	1998		236	Dec-01
NCC, Kashiwa	Japan	p	1998		75	May-01
HARIMAC, Hyogo	Japan	P, (ion)	2001		30	Nov-01
PMRC, Tsukuba	Japan	p	2001		19	Jan-02
NPTC (Harvard)	MA, USA	p	2001		2	Jan-02

Courtesy Cyclotron Laboratory, Harvard University, Cambridge, Massachusetts.
Courtesy Janet Sisterson, Harvard Cyclotron Laboratory, Cambridge, Massachusetts.
*This information is taken in part from *Particles* (vol 29, 2002), a biannual newsletter published for those interested in proton, light-ion, and heavy-charged-particle radiation therapy.

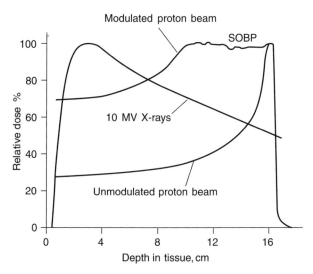

Figure 7-37. Depth-dose curves showing a Bragg peak (unmodulated) for a monoenergetic 160-MeV proton beam and an example of a modulated or spread-out Bragg peak (SOBP). Included for comparison is a depth dose curve for a 10-MeV x-ray beam. *(Courtesy LJ Verhey and J Munzenrider, Boston.)*

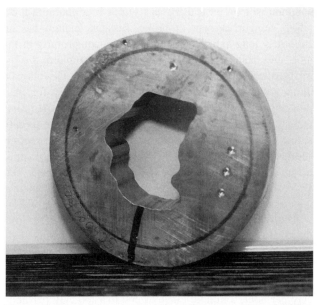

Figure 7-38. A brass aperture similar to custom-shielding blocks used with a linear accelerator is constructed individually for each patient treated with protons. This aperture measures about 8 cm in diameter and 5 cm in thickness and shapes the beam to conform to the tumor volume.

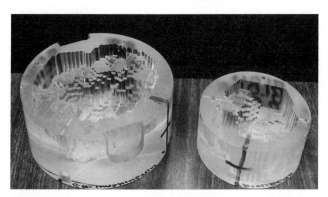

Figure 7-39. The Lucite bolus compensator, which is a milled circular piece of plastic, is used to even the dose distribution of the proton beam because of variations in tissue thickness and density.

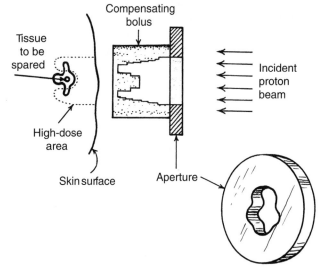

Figure 7-40. A cross section of a beam-defining aperture and compensating bolus, used with a high-energy proton beam, shape the proton beam. *(Courtesy Janet Sisterson, Harvard Cyclotron Laboratory, Cambridge, Massachusetts.)*

(Fig. 7-39) and modulator, the aperture controls the distance protons penetrate (Fig. 7-40). A spinning, circular Lucite modulator is positioned in the treatment beam to spread out the Bragg peak over a greater distance. This allows a larger volume of tissue to be irradiated because the treatment depth can be precisely controlled.

The treatments take approximately 2 minutes, but the setup time may vary from 30 minutes to 1 hour. Large fractions are usually given to extremely precise tumor volumes for which accuracy in millimeters is crucial. For example, a modulated proton beam can be directed to a tumor surrounding the brainstem and stopped within millimeters.

Remote Afterloading

Radiation exposure to staff members is still a concern in the application of brachytherapy isotopes used in radiation therapy. However, with low- or high-dose remote afterloading, radiation exposure is dramatically reduced. In the early days of brachytherapy an active radioisotope was preloaded in an applicator before being placed in a patient. Radium (the most common isotope used then) was sealed in a platinum tube, which sometimes bent or broke. Because radium has an extremely long half-life of 1620 years, a compromise of the tube presented a major radiation-safety problem. In the 1950s, afterloading applicators were developed. This allowed dummy sources to be evaluated radiographically for their proper position before the actual sources were loaded, thus reducing exposure to personnel. Cesium-137 began to substitute for radium during this time, mainly because of its shorter physical half-life of 30 years. Developments of applicators (including the Fletcher-Suite, Henschke, and Ter-Pogossian instruments) also occurred.[54] Many radionuclides commonly used in radiation therapy are listed in Fig. 7-41.

High dose rate and low dose rate. Parameters for **low-dose-rate (LDR) brachytherapy** versus **high-dose-rate (HDR) brachytherapy** are established in several ways. International Commission on Radiation Units and Measurement (ICRU) report 38 sets the range for LDR at 40 to 200 cGy per hour, a middle range at 200 to 1200 cGy per hour, and HDR at greater than 1200 cGy per hour or more than 20 cGy per minute. Brachytherapy sources such as iridium, cesium, cobalt, and radium are usually administered at dose rates of 50 to 500 cGy per minute. This rate commonly parallels that of a linear accelerator.[54]

Clinical considerations. Several important clinical considerations affect the decision to convert an established LDR brachytherapy program to one using HDR. Advantages for the HDR system are as follows: (1) treatment can be given on an outpatient basis; (2) treatment time is extremely short compared with that of an LDR system; (3) with this short treatment time the implant reproducibility is more precise than with manual systems; (4) complete radiation protection exists for staff members; (5) no general anesthesia or bed rest, which decreases complications, is needed; (6) the system has the ability to treat a large clinical patient volume; (7) individ-

ualized treatment can be done with source optimization; and (8) an increased level of comfort exists for the patient.[52]

LDR and HDR systems can improve dose distribution through multiple dwell positions. Optimal tumor dose distribution can be achieved while the normal tissue exposure is minimized. The danger of afterload applicators shifting in the pelvis, for example, during the several days usually involved in LDR treatment can negatively affect dose distribution. In HDR therapy the instruments are secured into place after the desirable position is attained. Packing or retracting protects the vaginal wall, bladder, and rectum over the several minutes of actual treatment time. A disadvantage of HDR therapy is that treatment plan changes are difficult to make before the treatment is completed because the time of treatment is several minutes instead of several days as with LDR. HDR is extremely labor intensive because it requires a complement of physicists, dosimetrists, therapists, nurses, and physicians for each insertion.[54]

Most HDR units use iridium-192 or cobalt-60 because of their high specific activity and ability to produce a gamma ray with sufficient penetration. Although iridium-192 offers smaller source size, a disadvantage is that the source needs replacing every 3 to 4 months because of the short 74-day half-life. The cost of exchanging an iridium-192 source is several thousand dollars. The justification for this ongoing expense is that the diameter of iridium-192 HDR sources is approximately 1 mm, whereas cobalt-60 and cesium-137 sources are more than twice the size.[38] The larger cobalt-60 and cesium-137 source diameter limits the application of HDR to intracavity (such as pelvic) and intraluminal (such as esophagus). The most common HDR remote afterloaders in North America use a single iridium-192 source on the end of a drive cable. The remote afterloader drives the source to specific locations in the applicator (dwell positions) and holds it in place there for a predetermined interval (dwell time).[38]

Radionuclide	Half-life	Photon energy (MeV)	Half-value layer (mm lead)	Exposure rate constant Rcm²/mCLh
^{225}Ra	1600 years (0.83 avg)	0.047-2.45	8.0	8.25*† Rcm²/Ci-h
^{222}Rn	3.83 days (0.83 avg)	0.047-2.45	8.0	10.15*‡
^{60}Co	5.26 years	1.17, 1.33	11.0	13.07‡
^{137}Cs	30.0 years	0.662	5.5	3.26‡
^{192}Ir	74.2 days (0.38 avg)	0.136-1.06	2.5	4.69‡
^{198}Au	2.7 days	0.412	2.5	2.38‡
^{125}I	60.2 days	0.028 avg	0.025	1.46‡

*In equilibrium with daughter products.
†Filtered by 0.5 mm Pt.
‡Unfiltered.

Figure 7-41. A chart of radionuclides used in brachytherapy. *(From Khan F: The physics of radiation therapy, ed 2, Baltimore, 1994, Williams & Wilkins.)*

Remote afterloading devices used for HDR contain many similar design elements, such as the following.[17,38]

1. A shielding safe to contain the source(s) when not in use and to reduce the radiation exposure around the unit to safe levels.
2. A source positioning system to move the source(s) from the safe to the treatment positions. This usually includes a drive mechanism, means of sensing the source position and timing its motion, transfer tubes connecting sections of the applicator to the treatment unit, and a method of directing a source to a selected transfer tube.
3. A safety system to ensure safe operation of the system, including dummy source(s) moved to and from the treatment positions before sending out the source to confirm the patency of the route; interlocks monitoring specific safety requirements such as treatment door closed, transfer tube connected to unit and route unobstructed; and backup batteries.
4. Emergency systems to withdraw the source(s) into the safe in an emergency, including a manual retraction method.
5. A control console to coordinate the operation of the unit's subsystems and provide start/stop functions, allow the programming of treatment positions and times, and produce hard copy documentation of the treatment as it progresses.

Radiobiology of high dose rate. Careful consideration of biologic effects must be included in the decision to move from LDR to HDR brachytherapy. HDR rates can be high enough that the exposure can be less than the repair half-time of sublethal damage (sometimes shorter than 2 hours). Ideally, the duration of an exposure does not exceed a small portion of the repair time for sublethal radiation injury (i.e., a few minutes).[37,54,60]

In the treatment of a head and neck tumor, for example, several preparatory procedures are necessary. Intravenous access is obtained after the patient's arrival to give the physician easy access for medications that may be required during the procedure. An endoscopic nurse helps the patient gargle and spray the nostrils with a special solution to numb that region in anticipation of scope insertion. The scope guides the catheter to the tumor site at which the radiation is directed. During the procedure the patient's heart and pulse are monitored, and oxygen is administered through the nostrils. An x-ray machine is positioned over the patient's head for localization purposes. After the scope is in place, a smaller tube (called a catheter) passes through the scope before scope removal. The scope is secured with tape, and then a radiograph is taken to verify position. The patient is moved from the examination room to the treatment room. The catheter, connected by tubing to the HDR unit, transports the appropriate radiation sources (Fig. 7-42). After the treatment is finished and the source secured, the patient is taken to the recovery room for usually less than 1 hour.[26] This is a typical HDR application for a tumor in the head and neck region.

HDR brachytherapy has been used successfully to treat tumors of the brain, esophagus, and rectum; tumors obstructing the biliary system; and gynecologic cancers (most notably, cervical carcinoma). Further work is needed to identify radiobiologic differences of this therapy compared with conventional LDR interstitial and intracavitary techniques.

Cobalt Unit

Today, less and less cobalt-60 (^{60}Co) units are used for the treatment of cancer in the United States. In the 1980s, ^{60}Co units were the mainstay of most radiation oncology departments.[39] The decrease began in 1960s with the introduction

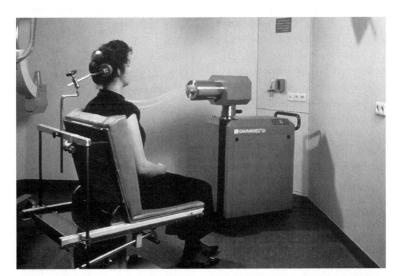

Figure 7-42. A remote afterloading system used to store and deliver high-dose-rate brachytherapy sources. Sources are delivered via a catheter located in the center of this portable device. Treatment time is generally in the range of minutes. *(Courtesy Gammamed and Frank Barker Associates, Pequannock, New Jersey.)*

of the linear accelerator because linear accelerators provided better isodose distribution (greater dose to the tumor and less dose to normal tissue), faster dose rate, and more manageable radiation protection concerns. Despite the decline in popularity of ^{60}Co units in the United States, they are the backbone of many radiation therapy departments in developing countries. This is probably due to the unit's cost, simpler design, and reliability.[53]

In the early 1950s, ^{60}Co units became popular because they could deliver a significant dose of radiation below the skin surface. Compared with earlier **teletherapy** (treatment at some distance) units such as radium and cesium treatment machines, ^{60}Co units were faster at delivering the dose and more cost effective at producing and using the isotope. At the time, mining the ore necessary to produce a small amount of radium was extremely expensive. The ^{60}Co units were the first practical radiation therapy treatment units to provide a significant dose below the skin surface and simultaneously spare the skin the harsh effects of earlier methods. This allowed the radiation oncologist and radiation therapist to deliver larger doses of radiation to greater depths in tissue. When a greater percentage of dose occurs below the skin surface, the term **dose maximum (D_{max})** is used to describe the process. D_{max} is the depth of maximum buildup, in which 100% of the dose is deposited. For ^{60}Co, D_{max} occurs at 0.5 cm below the skin surface. This was a tremendous advantage over the other types of equipment (especially orthovoltage) used to treat cancer at the time.

Unlike other types of equipment available in the early days of radiation therapy, ^{60}Co units were mechanically simple, compact, and reliable, usually requiring little maintenance.[53] Early radiation therapy equipment, such as the betatron or Van de Graaff generator, required a lot of space. In addition, most equipment (including some cobalt units) were stationary or wall mounted. For this reason, much of the early equipment was limited to a vertical beam direction. This meant the patient had to be positioned relative to the stationary equipment. Treatment with lateral beams (as in the case of head and neck cancer) was compromised somewhat because patients had to be placed on their sides and moved between the treatment fields.

To compensate for this shortcoming, some manufacturers designed stationary and rotational treatment models. With rotational units the source moved around the patient, thus improving positioning reproducibility and isodose distribution. These units rotated around an axis at a constant distance from the source, called the isocenter. Today, this type of unit is installed with wall and ceiling lasers that are designed to aid in accurately positioning a patient. The laser lights produce thin beams of light that intersect at the axis of rotation or isocenter and correspond to external patient marks. Linear accelerators operate on the same principle by using a rotational gantry to deliver multiple treatment fields from various angles (all aimed at the same target volume).

To protect personnel, the ^{60}Co source must be shielded when the source is in the off position. Compared with linear accelerators and other electrically operated therapy equipment, these machines constantly emit radiation. A great deal of high-density material, such as lead or depleted uranium, surrounds the source in the head of the machine (Fig. 7-43). To help the machine rotate smoothly and provide additional shielding, it must have a counterweight. In part, this is to balance the lead shielding in the head of the machine housing the radioactive ^{60}Co source. This counterweight, extending from the opposite end of the gantry in which the source is housed, is called a beam stopper. With the addition of a beam stopper, walls and ceilings in the treatment room do not require as much shielding. The beam stopper absorbs a significant amount of the radiation transmitted through the patient. Although it provides additional shielding and acts as a counterweight, the beam stopper has a number of drawbacks, including the difficulty associated with working around this cumbersome extension. The large beam stopper limits movement around the head of the gantry and can be a challenge at positioning a stretcher next to the treatment couch with the machine in the lateral position.

Application. Before the widespread distribution of linear accelerators, ^{60}Co units delivered radiation therapy treatments to all types of tumors. Because of its unique beam characteristics, the ^{60}Co unit is commonly used today to treat cancers of the head and neck area, breast, spine, and extremities. In addition, areas just below the skin surface (where a deep penetration of the beam is not necessary) can be effectively treated with ^{60}Co.

Anatomically, the head and neck area is not extremely thick. Therefore a ^{60}Co beam can provide an adequate distribution of dose by using **parallel opposed fields** (two fields treated 180 degrees from one another). The ^{60}Co beam is ideal in treating lymph nodes, which are superficially located in the cervical and subdigastric area. In addition, lymph nodes located in the axillary and supraclavicular areas, which may be involved with breast cancer, lie just below the skin surface and may require treatment only with a single portal field. Bone metastases from other primary sites commonly occur in the spine and extremities, thus making ^{60}Co a good choice for treatment in which a single portal field may be used. Some radiation therapy departments with several treatment units find the ^{60}Co unit provides a good balance to the treatment of a wide variety of diseases.

Production. ^{60}Co is an artificially produced isotope. Like many other isotopes used in the diagnosis and treatment of disease, ^{60}Co becomes radioactive when its atomic number is altered. This may happen in a particle accelerator called a cyclotron or nuclear reactor. The production of ^{60}Co begins with the stable form of cobalt, which has an atomic-mass number of 59. The atomic-mass number is the sum of protons and neutrons in the nucleus. After ^{59}Co is bombarded or irradiated in a nuclear reactor with slow neutrons, the nucleus of ^{59}Co absorbs one neutron and

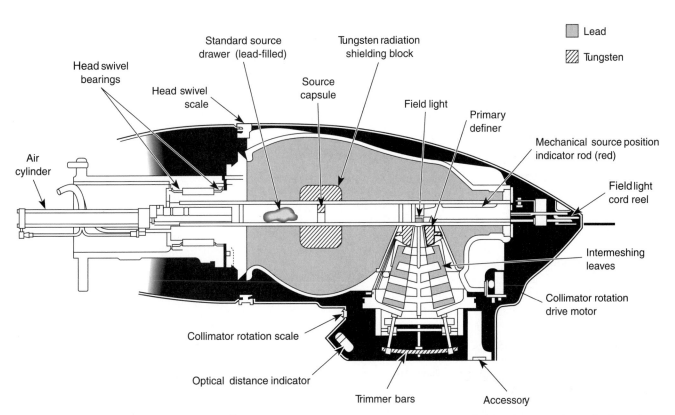

Figure 7-43. A cross section of typical ^{60}Co components. *(Courtesy Atomic Energy of Canada Limited, Medical Products, Kanata, Ontario, Canada.)*

becomes radioactive ^{60}Co. This can be expressed in the following formula:

$$^{59}Co + {}^{1}n^{60} \cong Co$$

As in any radioactive substance, ^{60}Co emits radiation in an effort to return to its more stable state.

^{60}Co activity may be expressed in curies (Ci), the historical unit of radioactivity, which equals 3.7×10^{10} becquerel (Bq).[10] Bq, the standard international (SI) unit of radioactivity equals 1 disintegration per second.[10] Most sources have an activity of 750 to 9000 Ci and may be referred to as kilocurie sources.[50] In addition, the activity may be defined in rhm units (1 rhm unit represents 1 roentgen per hour at 1 m). The quality of the radiation produced by the source does not depend on the number of curies or rhms. With a 3000-Ci source the equipment can be operated at an 80-cm distance and have a 10-cm depth dose of 56%.[24,30] Sources used in radiation therapy typically range from 3000 to 9000 Ci and have a specific activity of 75 to 200 Ci/g.

Specific activity is the number of transformations per second for each gram of radionuclide decaying at a fixed rate. Specific activity is the number of Ci per gram. The specific activity for a ^{60}Co source can be as high as 400 Ci/g, but, for radiation therapy treatment, it is usually 200 Ci/g. A smaller source at the standard 80 SSD produces a beam of lower intensity requiring longer treatment time.

The radioactive ^{60}Co source and its shielding (in the form

of a protective casing) is referred to as the cobalt capsule. The diameter of the capsule can range from 1 to 3 cm (Fig. 7-44). For radiation therapy purposes, 1.0 to 2.0 cm is preferred. The radioactive cobalt source contains disks, slugs, or pellets grouped in a cluster or solid cylinder, encased in a stainless steel capsule, and sealed by welding. The capsule is placed inside a second steel capsule that is also welded. The multiple layers of metal prevent leakage of the radioactive material and absorb the beta particles produced during the decay process.[30]

Characteristics. The radioactive ^{60}Co nucleus emits ionizing radiation in the form of high-energy gamma rays. ^{60}Co decays by first emitting a beta particle with an energy of 0.31 MeV that is absorbed in the source's steel capsule. After emitting the beta particle, the nucleus enters an excited state of nickel-60. The nickel-60 decays to a ground state by emitting two gamma rays per disintegration. Of the two gamma rays emitted, one has an energy of 1.17 MeV and the other 1.33 MeV.[50] The beam can be considered polyenergetic or heterogeneous because more than one energy is decaying from the isotope. For practical purposes the two energies are averaged to give an effective energy of 1.25 MeV.

Because ^{60}Co is a radioactive isotope, it has a half-life ($T^{1}/_{2}$), the time necessary for a radioactive material to decay to half or 50% of its original activity. ^{60}Co decays to 50% of its activity after a half-life of 5.26 years.[32] To compensate for the reduction in beam output each month, a correction factor

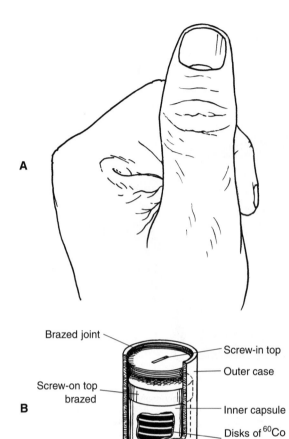

Figure 7-44. A, The radioactive ^{60}Co source or capsule can be compared in size to the end of a person's thumb. **B,** Double encapsulated teletherapy ^{60}Co source. *(From Meredith WJ, Massey JB: Fundamental physics of radiology, St. Louis, 1977, Mosby.)*

Table 7-6	Depth of maximum dose for various photon energies

Beam Energy	D_{max} (cm below skin surface)
Superficial	0.0
Orthovoltage	0.0
Cesium 137	0.1
Radium 226	0.1
Cobalt 60	0.5
4 MV	1.0
6 MV	1.5
10 MV	2.5
15 MV	3.0
20 MV	3.5
25 MV	5.0

From Stanton R, Stinson D, Shahabi S, editors: *An introduction to radiation oncology physics*, 1992, Madison, Wis, Medical Physics Publishing.

of approximately 1% per month must be applied to the output. The correction factor increases the treatment time necessary to deliver the appropriate dose. To maintain adequate output for patient treatment and thus eliminate longer treatment times, the ^{60}Co source should be replaced at least every 5.3 years.

Electron equilibrium is another term used to describe D_{max}. As energy increases, so does the depth of electron equilibrium. For ^{60}Co, this point occurs at 0.5 cm below the skin surface. Table 7-6 describes the depth of D_{max} for a variety of beams.

Penumbra is the area at the edge of the radiation beam at which the dose rate changes rapidly as a function of distance from the beam axis.[23,30] Penumbra describes the edge of the field having full radiation intensity for the beam compared with the area at which the intensity falls to 0.[55] Compared with the sharper field edge produced with linear accelerators, penumbra is a definite disadvantage in using ^{60}Co beams for radiation therapy treatments. Fig. 7-45 demonstrates the

difference between a ^{60}Co beam and a 6-MV linear accelerator beam. The sharp edge of the linear accelerator beam compared with the fuzzy edge of the cobalt beam should be noted.

The radioactive-source size contributes greatly to the degree of penumbra. The larger the source size, the larger the penumbra. The following formula is used to determine the penumbra (P equals the penumbra size, S equals the source size, SSD equals the source-to-skin distance, and SDD equals the source-to-diaphragm [collimator] distance):

$$P = S(SSD - SDD)/SDD$$

Penumbra can be applied in two ways. The first is geometric penumbra. This is the place where a lack of sharpness or fuzzy area occurs at the edge of the beam. The geometric blurring of the field edge occurs at the skin surface and greater depths in tissue. The geometric penumbra should be considered during the planning of the patient's treatment, especially where treatment fields will abut or match. An example can be made with the simulator. During the planning process on the simulator, the field-defining wires of the simulator outlines the treatment volume. The wires outline the treatment area anatomically on a radiograph and visibly on the patient's skin. Different field sizes (slightly larger with the cobalt unit) are necessary to cover the same amount of tissue adequately on the cobalt machine as compared with a linear accelerator.

The second type of penumbra, transmission penumbra, occurs as the radiation passes through the edge of the primary collimators. Transmission penumbra also occurs at the edge of the patient's shielding blocks mounted or placed below the collimator. The transmission penumbra correlates with the size of the collimator opening. Greater transmission penumbra occurs with larger collimator openings. As a result, larger field sizes have more transmission penumbra. If

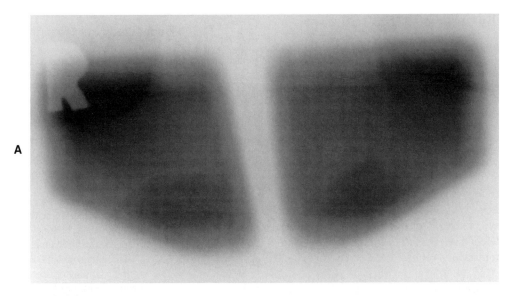

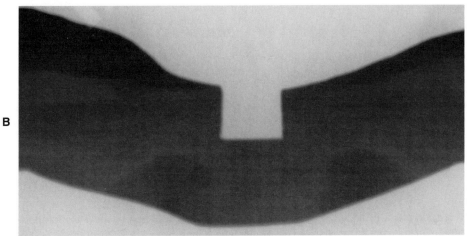

Figure 7-45. A, Port film taken with a ^{60}Co beam demonstrates the fuzzy field edges or penumbra. **B,** Port film taken with a 6-MV beam demonstrates the sharpness at the field edges or lack of penumbra.

the inner surface of the collimator or shielding blocks are parallel to the edge of the beam, the transmission penumbra can be reduced.[53]

To reduce this penumbra, a second set of smaller collimators (called satellite collimators, penumbra trimmers, or trimmer bars) can be added. Trimmers are metal bars that attenuate the edge of the beam, thus providing a sharper field edge. Trimmer bars should be located no closer than 15 cm from the patient's skin to reduce electron contamination by the metal devices.[47] The 15 cm of air between the trimmer bars and patient's skin provides enough distance for the secondary electrons produced by the trimmer bars to lose sufficient energy. If electron contamination occurs, it may add significantly to the patient's skin dose.

For radiation therapy beams, including ^{60}Co, shielding blocks are most commonly made of Lipowitz metal.

Cerrobend is a form of Lipowitz metal used for designing custom shielding blocks and consists of 50.0% bismuth, 26.7% lead, 13.3% tin, and 10.0% cadmium.[25,51] Cerrobend melts (70° C) at a much lower point than lead (327° C). Therefore Cerrobend is easier and safer to use. However, cadmium (a toxic metal) can get into the bloodstream of individuals working with Lipowitz metal. At a considerable greater expense, some manufactures have introduced a type of Lipowitz alloy without cadmium.

The Cerrobend used in custom block fabrication hardens quickly depending on the amount and degree of cooling applied to the alloy. Using the density ratio of Cerrobend to lead, a factor of 1.21 can be applied to the thickness of lead needed to attenuate 5% of the primary beam. For the most common megavoltage beams, a thickness of 7.5 cm of Cerrobend is used. This is equivalent to about 6 cm of lead.[30]

MACHINE DESIGN AND COMPONENTS

Source Positioning

Of the five methods to position the radioactive ^{60}Co source shown in Table 7-7, the two most commonly used are the rotating-wheel and air-pressure (piston) methods (Fig. 7-46). The rotating-wheel method moves the ^{60}Co source into the on position by rotating a metal disk 180 degrees while a motor holds the source in position over the collimator opening. If power is interrupted, the spring-attached wheel returns the source to the off position. The air-pressure method pushes a piston and thus the ^{60}Co source into the on position. A sliding draw allows the source to be positioned over the collimator opening. In the off position the source retracts back into the treatment head. In case of power failure the air-driven piston automatically returns the source to the off position.[20]

Travel time. The time necessary to deliver the source from the off, on, or treatment position is defined as the travel time. To compensate for the travel time, a correction (shutter error) must be added to the calculation to deliver the prescribed dose. The shutter error allows for the total advancement and retraction of the source from the off position to the on position and back to the off position again. Depending on the manufacturer and method of source delivery, this may take place in less than 1 second. If the travel time is neglected in the calculation used to deliver the prescribed dose, a small underdose may occur. Of course, the greater the number of fractions used to deliver the total dose, the greater the error in dose delivered.

Shielding. Because it constantly emits radiation, the ^{60}Co source must be shielded in a protective housing. The housing used for shielding and containing the device for positioning the source is referred to as the source head. The source head is a steel shell filled with lead or an alloy of lead, tungsten, and depleted uranium.[25] For adequate shielding the housing may be up to 2 feet in diameter.[50] Radiation leakage around the source head should conform to Nuclear Regulatory Commission (NCR) guidelines.[61]

Machine components. A multivaned or interleaf collimator is constructed as part of the source head to shape the size of the radiation beam. The collimator assists in reducing the penumbra associated with the source size. Trimmers or satellite collimators may be added to further sharpen the

Table 7-7	Five methods to expose the ^{60}Co source
Type	**Method**
Air pressure (piston)	The compressor generates air pressure by pushing the source horizontally into position over the collimator opening (often referred to as the *sliding drawer*).
Rotating wheel	The motor rotates a wheel 180 degrees by placing the source over the collimator opening.
Mercury reservoir	Mercury is withdrawn or returned to a reservoir located below the source at the collimator opening.
Chain driven	A sphere that is chain driven rotates a stationary source 90 degrees to place it at the collimator opening.
Moving jaws	Lead jaws located below the source open and close for exposure or shielding.

From Stanton R, Stinson D, Shahabi S, editors: *An introduction to radiation oncology physics*, 1992, Madison, Wis, Medical Physics Publishing.

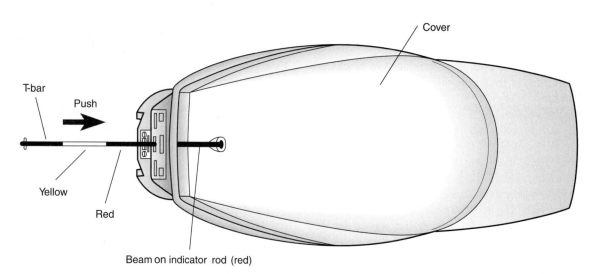

Figure 7-46. A ^{60}Co air-pressure (piston) drawer in the on position. *(Courtesy Atomic Energy of Canada Limited, Medical Products, Kanata, Ontario, Canada.)*

radiation-beam edge. Field size is defined by a light beam reflected from a light bulb to a small mirror. A tray holder is added below the collimators for field shaping by hand-placed lead or customized Cerrobend shielding blocks. Wedges made of lead, brass, or copper are placed in the path of the beam and shift or tilt the dose distribution from its normal shape. When needed, they are positioned in a separate slot in the block tray assembly.

Calibration and leakage. A qualified radiation physicist must perform full calibration testing for radioactive ^{60}Co units annually. Full calibration may be done more frequently if (1) the source is replaced, (2) a 5% deviation is noticed during a spot check, and (3) a major repair requiring the removal or restoration of major components is done. A monthly output calibration should be done for a set of standard daily operating conditions. Measurements taken during a full calibration include the following[3]:
1. Radiation and light field coincidence
2. Timer accuracy
3. Exposure rate or dose rate to an accuracy of ±3% for various field sizes
4. Accuracy of distance-measuring devices used for treatment
5. Uniformity of the radiation field and its dependence of the orientation of the useful beam position around the head of the unit cannot exceed 2 mrem/hr at 1 m, with a maximum of 10 mrem/hr at 1 m at any measurable location. The maximum permissible leakage in the on position cannot exceed 0.1% of the useful beam at 1 m from the source. The 0.1% of the useful beam is the percent of the actual output of the ^{60}Co source in cGy/min. For example, if the useful beam has an output of 197.3 cGy/min for the month of January, the maximum permissible leakage in the on position at 1 m from the source is 0.197 cGy/min.

A wipe test (or leak test) must be done twice a year on the sealed ^{60}Co source. If a source's seal is broken and leaking, it may have radiation contamination on the interleaf collimators. A wipe test is done, using long forceps, wiping the collimator edges with a filter paper, cloth pad, or cotton swab moistened with alcohol. A background radiation reading is done by using a survey meter calibrated with the same type material as the one being tested. A reading is then taken of the wipe to determine its activity, with the acceptable level of activity less than 0.005 mCi. If the activity is higher, radiation contamination or leakage may have occurred and the unit must be removed from service until decontamination and repair can be completed.

Radiation monitoring and light system. Because it is a radioactive source that emits ionizing radiation, ^{60}Co requires not only a light system to show when the machine is on and off but also a monitoring system to detect radiation. The machine on-and-off indicator lights must be on the console, at the head of the machine, and at the entrance to the treatment room. If the machine is on, a red light must be lit. When the machine is off, this light should show green. A radiation detector must be located in the treatment room. The detector is wired to a light outside the room near the console

and door. The light must be blinking red if radiation is present and must be in view of the radiation therapist. Before entering the room, the therapist must be sure the off light is green and the blinking red light has stopped. Because a moment is necessary for the ^{60}Co source to retract into its off position, the green light comes on first, before the blinking red light stops. If the red light continues to blink for longer than a few seconds, the therapist must be ready to carry out an established emergency procedure. The source may not have retracted fully or properly.

Emergency procedures. Emergency procedures must be established during the machine commissioning and before the unit is used for treatment. The emergency procedures must be posted at the machine console. These procedures must be developed by the radiation safety officer or radiation physicist and communicated to the radiation therapist and personnel responsible during a radiation emergency. No universal emergency procedure exists for a source that fails to return to the off position. Each department should develop and post emergency procedures. A sample procedure posted at the machine console is shown in the Box 7-1.

Another procedure may include retracting the ^{60}Co source into the head source area with a T-bar. A T-bar is a steel rod 18 to 24 inches in length shaped like a T. The first 7 inches opposite the end of the T is painted red with the next 7 inches painted yellow (see Fig.7-46). In case of an emergency in which the source does not retract, the T-bar is placed in the source drawer at the top of the machine or source head. With the T end of the bar held in hand, forward pressure is applied to push the drawer backward into the off position. The ^{60}Co source can be considered relatively safe if no red paint is showing on the T-bar outside the machine or source-head cover. Before the ^{60}Co source is in the fully safe position, the yellow portion of the bar must be entirely inside the machine or source-head cover. Because of the complexity of this procedure, any radiation therapy personnel performing it may be exposed to a higher dose of radiation than under normal working conditions.

SUMMARY

Ionizing radiation (in one form or another) has been used in the treatment of cancer almost from the time x-rays and radium were discovered. The equipment and competencies of the staff members involved in the quality delivery of patient treatments have undergone and will undergo continuous changes to keep pace with increasingly sophisticated treatment regimes. Historically, equipment evolved from low-energy, low-skin-sparing, unsophisticated systems (such as orthovoltage units) to today's computerized, megavoltage linear accelerators that can treat a variety of deep-seated tumors. New protocols are being formulated to reflect the enormous capabilities of radiation oncology equipment. The goal is to spare more normal tissue and deliver higher doses to the actual tumor volume. This will hopefully result in decreased morbidity and increased cure rates.

| Box 7-1 | Radiation Therapist Procedure for Cobalt 60 Emergency |

A. If the console timer fails to terminate exposure, do the following:
   1. PUSH EMERGENCY OFF BUTTON.
   2. TURN CIRCUIT BREAKER OFF.
B. If the source drawer fails to close by shutting off electrical circuits, do the following:
   1. OPEN TREATMENT ROOM DOOR.
      a. Use the hand crank if electrical power is off and if using a pneumatic door.
   2. REMOVE PATIENT FROM ROOM.
      a. Verbally request that the patient get off the table and come to the treatment door.
      b. If the patient is unable to respond to a verbal command, enter the treatment room and quickly remove the patient. Do not stand in the path of the primary beam.
   3. CLOSE TREATMENT ROOM DOOR.
      a. Use the hand crank if electrical power is off and if using a pneumatic door.
C. Notify the attending physician and radiation safety officer.
D. Secure the room against unauthorized entry by placing a DO NOT ENTER sign on the door, and secure or lock the door.
NOTE: This machine shall not be used unless the operating and emergency procedure manual is available in the control area. Operating personnel should familiarize themselves with this manual before operating this machine.

Many changes are yet to come concerning protons, IMRT, PET fusion studies, and remote afterloading that mirror the changing health care environment as much as the patient's needs. These changes will directly affect whether cyclotrons become realistic to operate and whether high-dose remote afterloading can rightly replace LDR facilities or become a practical boost alternative on a grander scale. Will IMRT replace conventional radiation therapy dose delivery?

Review Questions

Multiple Choice

1. Which of the following does not relate to beam quality?
   a. Penumbra
   b. kVp
   c. Central-axis depth dose
   d. mA
2. Protons are a valuable tool for clinical use for all except which of the following reasons?
   a. They have a characteristic distribution of dose with depth
   b. Scattering is minimal compared with x-rays, neutrons, or cobalt radiation
   c. Their energy range is similar to that of x-rays
   d. They are accelerated in a cyclotron
3. What is the half-life of ^{60}Co, a radioactive isotope?
   a. 1.25 years
   b. 5.25 years
   c. 10.5 years
   d. 30 years
4. What is the average energy with which ^{60}Co emits gamma rays used for radiation therapy treatments?
   a. 1.17
   b. 1.25
   c. 1.33
   d. 2.50
5. Because of the decay of the ^{60}Co source, a patient calculation correction of what percent must be made monthly?
   a. 0.1%
   b. 1.0%
   c. 5.0%
   d. 10.0%
6. Which of the following is a disadvantage in using a ^{60}Co beam for radiation therapy treatments?
   a. Penumbra
   b. Sharp field edge
   c. No skin sparing
   d. Computer driven components and accessories
7. When were linear accelerators first commercially available for clinical use?
   a. 1895
   b. 1930s
   c. 1950s
   d. 1970s
8. A scattering foil is placed in the path of the beam when which of the following are used for treatment purposes?
   a. Protons
   b. Electrons
   c. X-rays
   d. All of the above
9. What does a klystron or magnetron produce?
   a. Microwave power

b. Alternating current
c. Accelerated electrons and photons
d. Magnetic fields used to bend the beam

10. Trace the path of an electron in a linear accelerator by selecting the best route from the following.
    I. Electron gun
    II. Collimator
    III. Accelerator guide
    IV. Bending magnet
    a. I, II, III, IV
    b. I, III, IV, II
    c. II, I, IV, II
    d. III, I, II, IV

Questions to Ponder

1. List and discuss three specific medical uses of the cyclotron.
2. Discuss the application and use of the contact, superficial, and orthovoltage treatment units in radiation therapy.
3. Briefly explain the reason a clinical radiation facility may consider switching from an LDR to HDR brachytherapy program.
4. Why must a monthly calculation correction be made for the ^{60}Co unit?
5. Discuss an emergency procedure for a source that fails to retract.
6. Discuss the rationale for performing biannual leak or wipe tests on a ^{60}Co unit.
7. Discuss the integration of computerization and linear accelerator operation. What are the benefits and drawbacks?
8. Analyze the need, design, and operation of a linear accelerator cooling system.
9. What is ergonomy? Can you give some examples of other ergonomically designed tools in your department? What is the benefit of ergonomic designs?
10. Discuss the major components of the linear accelerator, including the klystron, waveguide, circulator, electron gun, accelerator guide, and bending magnet.
11. Describe the difference between a beam-flattening filter and a scattering foil.

REFERENCES

1. Ames JC: Personal communication, January 18, 1994.
2. Applied research, Triumf: Pet scanner. Canada, July 1992, Internal publication.
3. Arkansas State Board of Health: *Rules and regulations for control of sources of ionizing radiation,* Little Rock, 1994, The Arkansas State Board of Health.
4. Bentel GC: *Patient positioning and immobilization in radiation oncology,* New York, 1999, McGraw-Hill.
5. Bernier DR, Christian PE, Langan JK: *Nuclear medicine technology and techniques,* ed 4, St. Louis, 2000, Mosby.
6. Betti O: Treatment of arteriovenous malformations with the linear accelerator, *Appl Neurophysiol* 50:262, 1987.
7. Bissonnette JP, Jaffreay DA, Fenster A, et al: Optimal radiographic magnification for portal imaging, *Med Phys* 21:1435-1445, 1994.
8. Bomford CK, Walton L: The physics of stereotactic radiosurgery, *Fifth Varian European Clinac Users Meeting* 1(1):183-187, 1987.
9. Bushong SC: *Radiologic science for technologists: physics, biology, and protection,* ed 7, St. Louis, 2001, Mosby.
10. Coggeshall A, Johnson K, Sisterson J: *HCL: the Harvard cyclotron laboratory,* Cambridge, Mass, 1987, Harvard Cyclotron Laboratory.
11. Coia L, Moylan D: *Introduction to clinical radiation oncology,* Madison, Wis, 1991, Medical Physics Publishing.
12. Coleman E, et al: The future of positron emission tomography in clinical medicine and the impact of drug regulation, *Semin Nucl Med* 22(3):193-200, 1992.
13. Edwards IK Jr, Edwards EK, Edwards SR: Grenz ray therapy, commentary, *Int J Dermatol* 29:17-18, 1990.
14. Falco-Braun O, Schultze U: Contact radiotherapy of cutaneous hemangiomas *Arch Dermatol Res* 253-254:237-246, 1975.
15. Freeman L, Blaufaro DM: Letters from the editors, *Semin Nucl Med* 22(3):1-2, 1992.
16. Gington E: An informal history of the microwave electron accelerator for radiotherapy, *Proceedings Tenth Varian Users Meetings* 1(1):11-19, 1984.
17. Glasgow GP: Principles of remote afterloading devices. In Williamson J, Thomadsen B, Nath R, editors: *Brachytherapy physics,* Madison, Wis, 1995, Medical Physics Publishing.
18. Grigg FRN: *The trail of the invisible light: from x-olyahlen to radio (bio)logy,* Springfield, Ill, 1965, Charles C Thomas.
19. Hansen WF: The changing role of the accelerator in radiation therapy, *IEEE Trans Nucl Sci* 30:1781-1783, 1983.
20. Herbel L: Personal communication, June 14, 1994.
21. Horton JL, Otte VA, Schultheiss TE: Physical characteristics of the M.D. Anderson Hospital clinical neutron beam, *Radiother Oncol* 13: 17-22, 1988.
22. Ingram J: Personal communication, May 11, 1994.
23. Internal Commission on Radiation Units and Measurement: *Determination of absorbed dosed in a patient irradiated by beams of x and gamma rays in radiotherapy procedures,* ICRU report 24, Washington DC, 1976, The Internal Commission on Radiation Units and Measurement.
24. Jackson S: *Radiation oncology: a handbook for residents and the allied health professions,* St. Louis, 1985, Warren H Green.
25. Johns H, Cunningham J, Friedman M, editors: *Physics of radiology,* ed 2, Springfield, Ill, 1974, Charles C Thomas.
26. Jordan LN, Buck SS: A teaching booklet for patients receiving high dose rate brachytherapy, *Oncol Nurs Forum* 18:1235-1238, 1991.
27. Karzmark CJ: Procedural and operator error aspects of radiation accidents in radiotherapy, *Int J Radiat Oncol Biol Phys* 13:1594-1602, 1987.
28. Karzmark CJ, Morton RJ: *A primer on theory and operation of linear accelerators in radiation therapy,* revised, Madison, Wis, 1989, Medical Physics Publishing (originally published in 1981 by the Bureau of Radiologic Health).
29. Karzmark CJ, Nunan CS, Tanabe E: *Medical electron accelerators,* New York, 1993, McGraw-Hill.
30. Khan FM: *The physics of radiation therapy,* Baltimore, 1994, Williams & Wilkins.
31. Klein E: Higher doses, greater precision, *RT Image* 7(39):4-5, 1994.
32. Klemp PFB, et al: Commissioning of a linear accelerator with independent jaws: computerized data collection and transfer to a planning computer, *Phys Med Biol* 33:865-871, 1988.
33. Klevehagen SC, Thaites DI: *Radiotherapy physics in practice,* Oxford, England, 1993, Oxford University Press.
34. Lutz W, Winston KR, Maleki N: A system for stereotactic radiosurgery with a linear accelerator, *Int J Radiat Oncol Biol Phys* 14:373-381, 1988.
35. Mallory MI: Personal communication, January 18, 1994.

36. Miller RA: Personal communication, January, 1995.
37. Nais A: *An introduction to radiobiology,* New York, 1990, John Wiley & Sons.
38. Orton CG, Ezzell GA: Physics and dosimetry of high dose-rate brachytherapy. In Perez CA, Brady LW, editors: *Principles and practice of radiation oncology,* ed 3, Philadelphia, 1997, Lippincott-Raven.
39. Owen JB: Personal communication, July, 2001.
40. Owen JB, Coia LR, Hanks GE: Recent patterns of growth in radiation therapy facilities in the United States: a patterns of care study report, *Int J Radiat Oncol Biol Phys* 24:983-986, 1993.
41. Papillon J: Rectal and anal cancers: conservative treatment by irradiation: an alternative to surgery, Berlin, 1982, Springer-Verlag.
42. Palta JR, et al: Characteristics of photon beams from Philips SL 25 linear accelerators, *Med Phys* 17:106-116, 1990.
43. Palta JR, et al: Electron beam characteristics of a Philips SL 25, *Med Phys* 17:27-34, 1990.
44. Purdy JA: Principles of radiologic physics, dosimetry and treatment planning. In Perez CA, Brady LW, editors: *Principles and practice of radiation oncology,* ed 3, Philadelphia 1997, Lippincott-Raven.
45. Purdy JA, et al: Medical accelerator safety considerations: report of AAPM Radiation Therapy Committee Task Group no. 35, *Med Phys* 20:1261-1275, 1993.
46. Perez CA, Brady LW: *Principles and practice of radiation oncology,* ed 2, Philadelphia, 1997, Lippincott-Raven.
47. Rafla S, Rotman M: *Introduction to radiation therapy,* St. Louis, 1974, Mosby.
48. Rajan G: *Advanced medical radiation dosimetry,* New Delhi, India, 1992, Pentice-Hall of India Private Limited.
49. Sandler HM, McShan DL, Lichter AS: Potential improvement in the results of irradiation for prostate carcinoma using improved dose distribution, *Int J Radiat Oncol Biol Phys* 22:361-367, 1992.
50. Selman J: *Basis physics of radiation therapy,* ed 2, Springfield, Ill, 1976, Charles C Thomas.
51. Shahabi S: *Blackburn's introduction to clinical radiation therapy physics,* Madison, Wis, 1989, Medical Physics Publishing.
52. Speiser B: Advantages of high dose rate remote afterloading systems: physics or biology, *Int J Radiat Oncol Biol Phys* 20:1133-1135, 1991.
53. Stanton R, Stinson D, Shahabi S, editors: *An introduction to radiation oncology physics,* Madison, Wis, 1992, Medical Physics Publishing.
54. Stitt JA: High-dose-rate intracavitary brachytherapy for gynecologic malignancies, *Oncology* 49:59-70, 1992.
55. Stryker J: *Radiation oncology,* New Hyde Park, NY, 1985, Medical Examination.
56. Suit H, Vrie M: Review, proton beams in radiation therapy, *J Natl Cancer Inst* 84:159, 1992.
57. Swindell W, Morton EJ, Evans PM, et al: The design of megavoltage projection imaging systems: some theoretical aspects, *Med Phys* 18:651-658, 1991.
58. Tinger A, Michalski JM, Bosch WR, et al: An analysis of intratreatment and intertreatment displacements in pelvic radiotherapy using electronic portal imaging. *Int J Radiat Oncol Biol Phys* 34:683-690, 1996.
59. Travers M: Personal communication, May 5, 1994.
60. Travis E: *Primer of medical radiobiology,* ed 2, St. Louis, 1989, Mosby.
61. United States Nuclear Regulation Commission: Rules and regulations, part 170, Washington DC, 1994.
62. Verhey LJ, Munzenrider JE: Proton beam therapy, *Ann Rev Biophys Bioengin* 11:331-357, 1982.
63. Winn J: Personal communication, May 10, 1994.

Treatment Procedures

Annette M. Coleman

Outline

Key Terms

G rounded in the planning, simulation, and administration of a prescribed course of radiation therapy, the professional practice of radiation therapy is an essential component of quality oncologic care.[1] Conscientious attention to precision and reproducibility in simulation and treatment delivery and to the physiologic and psychologic needs of patients highlights the radiation therapist's contribution to the cancer-management team. Radiation therapists deliver radiation therapy treatments, monitor and operate sophisticated radiation producing and equipment, and maintain detailed treatment records.

Treatment delivery and patient care requires knowledge in a

variety of basic science and patient care principles and an understanding of and respect for the legal considerations of practice. Successful coordination of individual patient treatments in the context of a varied patient load requires the application of well-developed organizational and communication skills.

Accurate treatment delivery depends on the needs of the patient and the specialized knowledge and skills of the radiation therapist in the operation of equipment. The ability to reproduce daily treatment setups depends on abilities and limitations imposed by the equipment and geometry of the treatment beam and by the patient.

Daily patient treatment constitutes the foundation of the practice of radiation therapy. Proficiency in technical and patient care skills and a knowledge base in oncology, treatment planning, physics, and radiation biology are prerequisite to the formation of good clinical judgment. These are primary characteristics of the professional practice of the radiation therapist. The development of an action plan in the approach to treatment delivery assists the radiation therapist in ensuring thoroughness. A task analysis provides a simple method for organizing a plan of action (see Box 8-1).

TREATMENT CHART

Separate from the individual's medical chart, the treatment chart remains in the radiation oncology department as a record of the patient's radiation therapy history. It is the legal document of the patient's radiation treatment. Therefore its completeness, organization, and legibility are critical. Each page must clearly identify the patient by name and hospital identification number. The radiation therapist recognizes the ethical and legal responsibility to maintain the patient's privacy and right to confidentiality of medical records.

The treatment chart is a primary element of an institution's **quality-assurance (QA) program.** The QA program (see Chapter 17) consists of activities and documentation performed with the goal of optimizing patient care. The radiation therapist's primary role in the QA program is to ensure accuracy in the delivery of the radiation-treatment plan as prescribed by a radiation oncologist. This requires reviewing patient records, monitoring the functioning of radiation-producing equipment, maintaining accuracy in the reproduction of treatment parameters, monitoring changes in patient status, and maintaining complete and accurate treatment records. The radiation therapist communicates with the radiation oncology team through activities such as weekly chart reviews and through maintaining open verbal lines of communication. Because their participation in QA activities is integral to the accomplishment of program goals, radiation therapists are represented on the departmental QA committee.[6,11]

Traditionally dependent on the written records of each member of the treatment team, computerized patient-monitoring systems are rapidly becoming integrated into the fabric of radiation oncology. These systems monitor and document experiences of the patient with the department. They may be limited to the clinical record or increasingly they

Box 8-1	Task Analysis of Treatment Procedures

1. Review the chart.
2. Prepare the room.
3. Identify and prepare the patient.
4. Assist the patient onto a treatment table and locate surface landmarks.
5. Raise the couch, thus bringing the patient to correct source-skin distance (SSD).
6. Refine the patient position relative to the isocenter by using lasers.
7. Align the field light to surface landmarks.
8. Position beam-shaping accessories (blocks) and verify by using the light field.
9. Position beam modifiers (wedge, compensator, and bolus).
10. Inform the patient you are leaving and treatment will begin.
11. Monitor the patient.
12. Set appropriate machine controls and review the record and verification system.
13. Initiate the beam-on setting and monitor patient and equipment function.
   When multiple fields are to be treated, do the following:
14. Validate parameters downloaded to accelerator and enable accelerator motion, or enter the room and check the patient and field position.
15. Repeat steps 8 through 14 for all fields until the completion of treatment.
16. Assist the patient from the couch and room.
17. Complete a daily treatment record.
18. Prepare the room for the next patient.

are used to manage all aspects of the patient's experience with the treatment center including documentation of past and current treatment, response to treatment, schedules, communication with referring physicians, and billing information.

Quality-management programs require that the treatment chart include information regarding the patient's history, including a diagnostic evaluation, rationale for treatment, detailed description of the treatment plan, and documentation of informed consent and the treatment delivered.[4,6,11] Individual departments may identify specific documentation procedures demonstrating these requirements and quality-control procedures to verify their internal compliance. Normally, the radiation therapist does not begin treatment if any of this information is unavailable.

RATIONALE FOR AND DOCUMENTATION OF TREATMENT RESPONSE

The rationale for radiation treatment includes a written patient history documenting the results of diagnostic and staging procedures. Before receiving treatment, patients must receive an explanation of their status, treatment alternatives, and consequences associated with and without treatment and provide their consent to any procedures. This information must be presented in a manner that is understandable to the patient.[4] As patient advocate, the radiation therapist verifies patient understanding of education delivered and ensures that informed consent has been attained and documented.

Patient response to treatment is monitored and recorded throughout and following completion of treatment. The physician, nurses, and radiation therapists document observations. Assessment records from weekly on-treatment visits, records of the patient's weight and blood counts, and other indicators of treatment response are maintained. Radiation treatment responses often require medication or other intervention; all care activities are included in the chart. Other members of the treatment team such as nutritionists and social workers may also include their assessments and directions in the radiation therapy chart.

Treatment Record

The information necessary for the reproduction of the course of treatment by a qualified professional must include the patient's identification, a signed prescription, treatment-planning data, and the daily treatment record.[1,2,4,11] The **daily treatment record** documents the delivery of treatments, administration of daily and cumulative doses, use of portal films, and implementation of prescribed changes.

Before initiating daily treatment, the radiation therapist performs a review of the treatment section of the chart. A photograph of the patient should be included, thus providing a visual identification for caregivers. The treatment prescription, detailed patient- and equipment-positioning information, dosimetric plans, and calculations must be reviewed for completeness and accuracy. Any changes in the treatment plan must also be identified.

The written treatment chart is the traditional record of radiation delivery to the patient. Accessibility is limited and the accuracy of the treatment record dependent on conscientious attention to detail and the integrity of the radiation therapist. Even with great attention, the potential for charting errors is significant in written records. Addition errors, transposition of numbers, and other errors are possible at every entry and the variables tracked are necessarily minimized. As accelerators and treatment plans increase in complexity the paper record becomes increasingly limited in its capacity to track all treatment parameters. The current evolution in treatment delivery methods fuels an increasing use of verification and record (V&R, R&V, or RV) systems. V&R's integration with electronic medical records (EMR) changes the medium but not the requirements of charting. With industry's development of complete electronic charting tools, radiation therapists are witnessing the emergence of paperless and filmless radiation oncology departments and participating in the process and evaluation of these changes.

Prescription

Radiation may be delivered only under the direct order of a radiation oncologist. Similar to drug and other therapies, orders are written as prescriptions that must be signed by the radiation oncologist before the initiation of radiation treatment. No exceptions are allowed. The prescription must provide specific information to allow its interpretation by other qualified professionals, including the radiation therapist. The anatomic site and total radiation dose to be delivered with its **fractionation**[*] and **protraction**[†] schedule must be clearly stated. The prescription also identifies the **treatment technique**[‡] to be applied.[4] Information specifying beam energy, portal sizes and entry angles, and **beam modifiers** (devices that change the shape of the treatment field or distribution of radiation) may be included in the prescription and with patient-positioning information. The physician's signature and date must accompany any changes in the prescription or treatment plan. With the increasing acceptance of electronic charts, password or other protection for electronic physician signatures must be ensured.

The radiation therapist reviews the prescription immediately before the delivery of each treatment fraction. Changes in the treatment plan may be made any time during the course of treatment, and the radiation therapist is responsible for ensuring that changes are implemented as ordered. Common prescription changes include fractionation and total dose or the addition or deletion of a bolus or blocks. Changes affecting dose calculation require a review of the plan to ensure that corrections have been made before treatment delivery.

As the dispenser of the radiation prescription, the radiation therapist accepts a great responsibility. Radiation therapists must be knowledgeable of the effects of radiation on their patients, tumor-lethal doses, and limits of radiation tolerance for normal tissue. Prescriptions appearing to exceed these limits or deviate from standard practice should be reviewed with the physician before their implementation. Care must be taken to eliminate any errors and to ensure delivery of safe treatment.

Treatment Plan and Reference Imaging

Isodose distributions and monitor-unit calculations prepared by the dosimetrist are to be reviewed. All calculations should be reviewed and signed by at least two members of the treatment-planning team. Before treatment, the radiation therapist ensures consistency of calculation factors with treatment parameters. Field sizes, beam modifiers, and treatment depths must be consistent with those identified on the daily treatment setup instructions. Calculations may be further verified by dose measurements using diodes placed on

---

[*]Individual treatment doses.
[†]The time over which the total dose is to be delivered.
[‡]The number and orientation of treatment fields.

the patient in the **treatment field.** The treatment field, also called a *portal,* is the volume of tissue exposed to radiation from a single radiation beam.

Reference images displaying the beams eye view (BEV) of the treatment field shape and orientation are produced at simulation or as digitally reconstructed radiographs (DRRs) by treatment planning or virtual simulation systems. Beam-shaping devices such as blocks or multileaf collimator (MLC) plans are verified against these images before treatment.

Treatment Field Identifiers and Field Descriptions

The radiation therapist reviews the treatment description to ensure the availability of sufficient information for treatment-plan reproduction before the initiation of the treatment. If a verify and record system is in use in conjunction with a paper record, information must be consistent between the two records. Instructions include descriptive information with diagrams and/or photographs illustrating patient positioning and immobilization. Surface landmarks used to localize* the **target volume** (area of known and presumed tumors) must also be clearly identified. If adjustments have been made to the original information, they must be clearly identified, signed, and dated by the radiation therapist.

Each treatment field, or portal, is assigned an identifier and name indicating the prescription site and beam direction (Fig. 8-1). Identifier conventions vary; they may be numbered or lettered. Field identifiers are assigned only once to each patient, and new treatment fields are incremented sequentially as they are added to the patient record. Subletters, numbers, or prime marks (ˋ,ˋˋ) may be used to denote changes in the field size or shape from the original field when the prescription point has not changed. The field description follows describing field size,[†] angle of entry, and beam modifiers[‡] to be used. Changes involving beam direction or the placement of the isocenter generally are identified as new treatment fields.

Daily Treatment Record

The chart review continues with verification of previous entries. The most common charting errors are those of addition or transposition. Any corrections must leave the original entry legible. One line is drawn through the entry, followed by the correction, initials of the correcting individual, and the date. Because the chart is the primary document referenced in litigation processes, changes must be legible and accompanied by reasonable explanations. The use of correction

---

*To identify a hidden structure relative to observable or palpable surface landmarks.

[†]Portal dimensions are identified in centimeters, width by length.
[‡]Devices that change the shape of the treatment field or distribution of the radiation at depth.

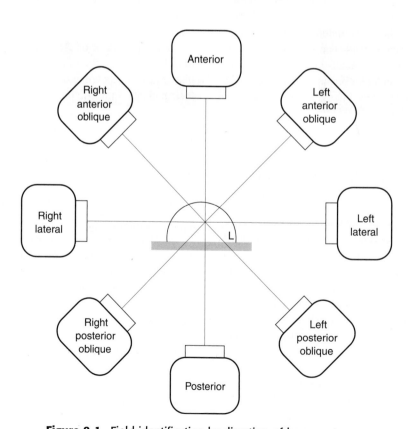

Figure 8-1. Field identification by direction of beam entrance.

fluid and other correction methods that hide original entries are viewed with suspicion and must therefore be avoided.

Although the treatment plan and prescription direct the treatment, and the daily treatment record documents the course of its implementation, an inspection of the daily treatment record directs each subsequent treatment. Records for individual treatments identify the date of treatment, **treatment number** (number of treatments delivered), and **elapsed days** (total time over which treatment is protracted). The daily and total dose delivered must also be included. The radiation therapist records the radiation dose and parameters under which it was delivered at the completion of each day's treatment. Notations are made regarding procedures completed on a particular treatment day, such as **portal verification** (the documentation of treatment portals through radiographic images or electronic portal imaging devices) films and the addition or deletion of a block. All treatment-record entries must be accompanied by the treating therapist's signature or initials and the date.

During this review the radiation therapist asks the following questions:
- "When was the last treatment?"
- "How far along is the patient in the course of treatment?"
- "Are verification films necessary?"
- "Have any changes in the treatment plan or prescription been ordered by the physician?"

By verifying the total dose delivered to the patient thus far, the radiation therapist appropriately monitors the administration of the radiation treatment. Radiation therapists maintain awareness of the dose being delivered to the target volume and **critical structures*** near or in the treatment volume and respond to or initiate necessary changes in the treatment plan through consultation with the radiation oncologist. The radiation therapist must document and sign treatment-plan changes in the daily treatment record.

Attention to the dose delivered also provides the therapist with expectations of the patient's physical reactions to the treatment. As the member of the treatment team who sees each patient daily, the therapist has a significant responsibility in monitoring these reactions. The radiation therapist possesses a firm understanding of radiation reactions and intervention methods for their management. The entire treatment team (including the oncologist and nursing staff members) monitors radiation reactions through review of blood counts, observation, and questioning of patients regarding their nutritional intake, skin reactions, and other associated symptoms. This understanding provides the foundation for the decision to proceed or withhold treatment pending consultation with the radiation oncologist.

Verification Images

The image file completes the treatment record. Portal images perform a critical role in QA by providing the means to eval-

uate and document reproduction of treatment **localization.** Verification images are taken on the treatment unit with the patient in the treatment position. These are compared to simulation or DRR reference images.

Portal image communication between the radiation therapist and radiation oncologist is critical to treatment accuracy. The radiation therapist creates images demonstrating the treatment localization, and the physician reviews them, approving or directing changes. Before daily treatment, the therapist reviews the status of images implementing and documenting any treatment modification orders.

TREATMENT PREPARATION

Treatment Room

The treatment room of the linear accelerator is engineered around isocenter. A well-planned treatment room facilitates accessibility to treatment accessories and movement by the therapists around this focal point. Shelves and storage cabinets form the perimeter; tables and counters do not obstruct access to and from the treatment unit. Treatment accessories are stored in consistent places and at heights that do not require therapists to use step stools or ladders. An organized system for custom block storage facilitates quick retrieval. The radiation therapist accepts responsibility for the maintenance of the treatment room as part of the department's QA program.

Laser systems use three to four sources to project points or lines of light to the isocenter. Projecting from the walls and from the ceiling (or opposite the gantry) the lasers coincide with the treatment unit's axes of rotation and intersect at the isocenter, providing visual guides to its location. The laser points or lines provide machine references to align with the external patient landmarks to align the accelerator's isocenter with the localized position within the patient. Helium neon (HeNe) lasers are used in either red or green. Green lasers project more sharply than red, their shorter wavelength scattering less at the skin surface. HeNe lasers are not harmful to skin but do have the ability to damage vision. The laser source must not be looked directly into.

Treatment rooms use standard and dim lighting. Standard lighting provides safety for patients entering and exiting the room and assists radiation therapists in locating accessory equipment. Reducing the light in the treatment room improves the visualization of lasers and field light, thus assisting the patient positioning and treatment setup process. While treatment is in progress, full lights are on for visualization of the patient on the monitors.

Treatment Unit

External-beam radiation therapy is accomplished through the use of sophisticated radiation producing equipment such as linear accelerators. These machines are engineered to facilitate the precise application of radiation beams to well-defined treatment volumes.

---

*Normal tissue with radiation dose tolerances that limit the deliverable dose.

Modern treatment units rotate around a fixed point. This point, or **isocenter,** is the point of intersection of the three axes of rotation (gantry, collimator, and base of couch) of the treatment unit (see Chapter 7 for descriptions of isocentric-treatment units). The isocentric mounting of treatment units facilitates the reproducibility of complex treatment plans. The accurate positioning of the treatment-unit isocenter relative to that of the treatment plan allows the rotation of the treatment unit (redirecting the treatment beam) to treat the target from multiple directions without moving the patient. These versatile units can treat extremely complex field arrangements.

The goal of radiation therapy treatment planning is to deliver an evenly distributed radiation dose to the target volume while minimizing the dose to surrounding normal tissue. Conventional and conformal treatment plans, including radiosurgery, accomplish this geometrically with the outline of each treatment field corresponding to the tumor volume. Relatively uniform dose is delivered to structures in the beam path. Normal tissue is protected by controlling beam direction and shape; areas in which treatment beams overlap receive an increased radiation dose relative to areas that receive radiation from only one field. (For a detailed discussion of radiation dose distribution, see Chapter 22.) **Intensity modulated radiation therapy (IMRT)** alters this model by delivering nonuniform exposure across the BEV using a variety of techniques and equipment. These nonuniform exposures create even dose distribution to target volumes with steep dose gradients to adjacent normal tissue. Full-field IMRT using accelerators with appropriate MLC capabilities differs little in the setup and delivery of treatment from conventional treatment methods. IMRT is an advanced form of 3-D conformal treatment planning that uses "inverse planning" techniques, where the clinical objectives are specified first and a computer program is used to automatically determine the optimal beam parameters needed for the desired dose distribution.

Many preparations are necessary before the arrival of the patient. The treatment setup dimensions, field size, gantry, collimator, and table positions are confirmed in the chart. The field size is typically set and the gantry positioned so lasers are visible and the field light crosshairs coincide with an axis of rotation (vertical or lateral). The table is raised or lowered to match the patient's transportation method. The proper treatment window is selected. Treatment couches are designed with two window options to allow various treatment fields to reach the patient without intercepting the couch. The primary window is supported by bars on either side of the table, thus providing stability while leaving an opening that allows treatment of posterior fields. The second window is supported down the center of the table, thus allowing treatment of oblique or rotational fields that intersect the side bars of the primary treatment window. A Mylar sheet covers windows to support the patient, and this support may be enhanced by a tennis racket beneath the Mylar.

Clean linens cover the treatment table, except over the treatment window. Treatment accessories, **positioning devices,** and **immobilization devices** matching those used at the simulation are prepared and placed in accessible places. These may include blocks, wedges, bolus, compensators, sponges, casts, masks, and/or bite blocks.

Standard collimation systems using adjustable, divergent, and opposing jaws, often with the ability to be positioned asymmetrically around the central axis, allow the customizing of fields into a square or rectangle. Field (or jaw) size indicates the size and dimensions of the radiation field at the isocenter. Many accelerators are also equipped with multileaf collimation systems that allow the customization of field shape without the use of shielding blocks. These systems contain an additional set of jaws that have been sliced into a series of opposing leaves. Leaf widths vary but are measured at isocenter. They are positioned independently, thus producing a variety of treatment field shapes. MLC leaf plans may be loaded at the time of room preparation or following patient positioning.

THE PATIENT

Identification

At least two methods of identification should be used to confirm patient identity because many factors contribute to the possibility of misidentification. Patients may have the same or similar names, and illness or anxiety may hinder their ability to respond to their own name. As a result, the radiation therapist must be extremely cautious when identifying patients. The consequences of misidentification can range from discontent in the waiting room to misadministration of treatment.

The treatment chart includes an identification photo for visual confirmation. Patients may be asked to state their own name. The most important piece of identification on inpatients is their wrist bracelet, which is checked before the patient is moved into the treatment room.

Patient Preparation and Communication

As a professional caregiver, the radiation therapist seeks to establish with the patient a relationship that encourages confidence and cooperation. Patients must entrust the radiation therapist with their care. The nature of their illness and anxiety surrounding the dangers of radiation make this no easy task. An individual may be treated over a period ranging from 2 to 8 weeks. Over this time the therapist has the responsibility to develop a constructive patient-professional relationship, which may provide the radiation therapist insight into the individual's experience and coping mechanisms. Observations of changes in patient behavior may also indicate changes in the disease state. In the event of such changes the physician must be notified. As a radiation oncology team member having daily contact with the patient, the radiation therapist becomes a liaison by directing the patient to resources designed to meet physical and psychosocial needs.

The radiation therapist demonstrates respect for the patient through the clear communication of directions at a level understandable to the patient. Age, mental status, and native language must be considered in the determination of the way messages can be presented most effectively. An understanding of what is expected during treatment empowers patients, thus fostering increased cooperation through feelings of mutual respect. Every effort must be extended to maximize patients' feelings of security. At the outset the patient is shown the audio and visual monitoring systems. Patients must be informed about safeguards to their privacy and reassured that although radiation therapists leave the room, contact will be maintained at all times.

If departmental practice requires the patient to undress before entering the treatment room, an explanation is given before the first treatment. The patient is informed of the necessity of removal of restrictive clothing that may alter the position of skin marks and inhibit reproduction of the patient's position. The location of gowns or robes and a secure place for their belongings is identified.

Radiation therapists greet patients and direct them into the treatment room. Here the radiation therapist initiates the rapport that characterizes the therapist-patient relationship. Throughout the course of treatment, the radiation therapist is a resource for the patient. The radiation therapist has a great deal of control over the extent of this relationship and hence the quality of care perceived by the patient. With this control comes the responsibility to create an environment sensitive to the patient's questions and concerns. At the same time, anticipation of these questions and concerns assists the radiation therapist to ease the anxiety associated with radiation treatments.

Patients must be counseled from the start of treatment in the proper maintenance of skin marks, general skin care, and nutritional guidelines. Radiation therapists provide these services while being mindful of the limitations of their scope of practice and make professional referrals when appropriate. Questioning skills may be used to discover the onset or severity of acute radiation reactions. Questions are chosen to encourage dialogue, and brief answers by the patient may be followed with gently probing questions to develop a fuller picture of the patient's reactions to treatment. The radiation therapist is responsible for assessing the patient's verbal and observable responses (e.g., skin reactions, weight change, and changes in demeanor) and evaluating whether treatment should continue or be withheld until the patient may be seen by the physician.

PATIENT TRANSFERS

Patients require varying assistance onto the treatment table. Many ambulatory patients may require only a stool to reach the top of the table. A treatment unit may be equipped with an extended-range treatment table, which may be lowered closer to the floor than a traditional treatment table, thus eliminating the need for step stools. Some patients may need a supportive arm to assist walking, whereas others may arrive in wheelchairs or on stretchers.

In evaluating the situation before transferring the patient onto the treatment table, the radiation therapist is mindful of the variety of auxiliary medical equipment the patient may be using. Although this equipment is most likely to be extensively used with inpatients, outpatients are not infrequently treated with oxygen or nutritional support and chemotherapy. Tubes and catheters must be recognized and carefully handled so as not to disrupt their placement or introduce infection.

Universal precautions are practiced with all patients. These precautions are methods of infection control in which any human blood or body fluid is treated as if it were known to be infectious. The radiation therapist is conscious that undiagnosed infections may be present in any individual, and the therapist handles all blood and body fluids as if they are infectious. Therapists also remember the immunodeficient state of their patients and take responsibility for the prevention of disease transmission. The most important practice toward this goal is thorough hand washing after patient contact. Linens must be replaced, and the treatment table and positioning accessories must be cleaned with disinfectant cleaners after each use.

For safe transfer of the patient to the treatment table, proper body mechanics of the patient and radiation therapist must be considered. In the initial planning of a patient transfer, the radiation therapist must assess the need for assistance. This is critical to the safety of the caregiver and patient. General rules for lifting require the maintenance of a wide base of support with the feet apart and one foot placed slightly in front of the other. The weight to be moved is kept close to the lifter, who bends at the knees and hips rather than at the waist while maintaining the normal curve at the lower back. Lifters should never twist nor bend sideways while supporting the weight.[8]

In the planning of any transfer the patient should be included when possible. Patients may be able to move themselves or have pain they wish the therapist to consider. They may also have other suggestions to facilitate their safe transfer.

Wheelchair Transfers

For patients unable to stand unassisted, the therapist prepares for the transfer by positioning the chair parallel to the table and locking the wheels. Foot rests are raised and the radiation therapist stands facing the patient. With the patient's feet together and therapist's feet on either side, the radiation therapist leans forward, bends at the knees and hips, and maintains the natural curve of the lower spine. The patient reaches around the radiation therapist's shoulders while the radiation therapist reaches under the patient's arms. The radiation therapist's arms are then locked around the patient's back. The patient is raised to his or her feet and pivoted 90 degrees so that the patient's back faces the table. Next, the patient is eased into a sitting position. With an arm behind the patient's shoulders and the other behind the knees, the therapist turns and eases the patient into the supine position in one smooth motion.

If for any reason (e.g., paralysis, pain) the patient requires more assistance onto the table, the patient should be transported to the department with a stretcher. This is a safety consideration for the patient and caregivers.

Stretcher Transfers

Stretcher transfers should be completed with a minimum of two caregivers. The stretcher is placed alongside the treatment table with the side rails lowered and wheels locked. The table is positioned at the same level as the stretcher. If the patient can slide over, one therapist may secure the stretcher while the other therapist stands opposite the treatment table, thus providing assistance and ensuring that the patient does not fall.

Immobile patients may be lifted from a stretcher to a table through the use of a draw sheet. The width of the treatment table next to the stretcher forces the lifters to breach rules of good body mechanics. At some point the weight is held away from the lifter's own center of gravity, and some must push rather than pull the weight. The reach may also make maintaining proper posture difficult. The use of a slide board for transferring stretcher patients reduces the risk of injury to the people performing the transfer. This option is preferred when insufficient staff members are available for a safe transfer. Slide boards are large enough to support the patient but are generally used to bridge the space between the stretcher and treatment table so that the patient may be pulled rather than lifted from one to the other. Patients are positioned with their hands on their chest. The slide board is positioned by rolling the patient from the treatment table and placing the board under the draw sheet. After the patient is eased back onto the slide board, the board is pulled to the treatment table or the patient is slid across the bridge created over the gap between the stretcher and treatment table. The slide board must be removed if it is in the path of a treatment beam.

Slide boards should not be used if rolling places the patient at risk for injury. In this situation, the assistance of several trained individuals is necessary. The appropriate number of lifters depends on factors such as the size of the patient or special considerations such as pain. Lifters position themselves to maintain support of the patient's head, shoulders, hips, and feet during the entire lift. Sheets are rolled and gripped firmly, and the team leader specifies a count so that everyone lifts at the same time. The patient is lifted just high enough to clear the treatment table and stretcher surfaces, moved over, and eased down. The radiation therapist ensures that the patient and any accessory equipment are secure before moving the stretcher away. Intravenous lines, catheters, oxygen, and other tubing are secured away from moving treatment machine parts.

PATIENT POSITION, ISOCENTER, AND FIELD PLACEMENT

Advances in imaging and treatment-planning computers encourage continued development in the precise planning of external-beam radiation treatments. With increasing confidence the physician, dosimetrist, and radiation therapist focus beams to the target volume while minimizing the radiation delivered to surrounding normal tissues. Verify and record systems communicate with the treatment unit to verify and document the reproduction of treatment-unit parameters for a specific plan. The clinical significance of these technical advances, however, will always be limited by the ability to translate them to the patient. Precision in the reproduction and immobilization of the treatment position, stability of surface landmarks, and exactitude in alignment of light fields with these references contribute greatly to variation in daily treatment delivery and thus represent the greatest obstacle to the application of advances in treatment planning. Management of these factors is a primary technical challenge for the radiation therapist.

The isocenter of the treatment unit is defined in a static position. The radiation therapist positions the patient daily relative to this point. Because neither the isocenter nor its planned position in the patient can be directly visualized during treatment setup, external tools must be used to guide the process. Lasers provide accelerator orientation references that must be aligned with surface references, localization landmarks, visible on or near the surface of the patient.

IDENTIFICATION OF LOCALIZATION LANDMARKS

While patient dignity is maintained with drapes, external landmarks are located by using the treatment description as the reference. References or **fiducial markers** may include natural anatomy or be artificial markers placed internally, at the skin surface, or fixed external to the patient. Landmarks may be maintained in a variety of permanent and nonpermanent forms.

The most common permanent references include visible and palpable anatomic landmarks (bones or other identifiable points that can be seen or felt and point to the location of hidden anatomy) or tiny permanent marks (tattoos) placed on the patient. Permanent marks are made using a small amount of dye introduced with a hypodermic needle under the surface of the skin, within the dermis. Permanent marks allow patients to bathe normally during treatment and provide references for follow-up assessment or subsequent treatment. Other permanent fiducial markers include implanted gold seeds that are visible radiographically. Implanted markers are useful for structures such as the prostate that are mobile relative to surface or radiographic landmarks.

Semipermanent references using ink or carfusion may be used during treatment to outline the field or mark the field center and corners. **Carfusion,** a dyelike liquid, varies in its formulation but generally contains silver nitrate and phenol in a fuchsin base, thus producing a magenta liquid that can be painted onto patients by using thin sticks or swabs. Marks created by this ink-like fluid are less easily removed than those of other markers. Concerns about toxicity and the accuracy of the marks have limited the use of carfusion. Semipermanent marks must be maintained throughout the course of treatment and have potential of removal or drift as they are reinforced.

External fiducial markers may also be applied to certain forms of immobilization devices. Stereotactic head frames that are screwed directly into the skull provide precise incremental references, which will not move relative to intracranial structures. Thermoplastic molds may also be designed with sufficient immobilization to ensure that marks will remain coincident with the treatment volume.

Patient Positioning

The positioning of patients with the isocenter of their treatment plan as close as possible to the center of the table provides the maximum clearance for techniques that require 360-degree gantry rotation around the patient.[6] Many oblique or tangential fields may be accommodated without rotation of the treatment table by making lateral shifts of the patient (consequently isocenter) relative to the table surface. For example, small angles off the vertical axis such as those used for lung boost fields may be accommodated by biasing the patient toward the side that the anterior field enters, or larger angles off the vertical axis (such as those used in breast tangents) may be accommodated by moving the patient closer to the treatment side.

The treatment description in the chart is used to reproduce a position consistent with that prescribed at the simulation (see Chapter 20). Configurations of positioning aids and immobilization devices must match those used at the simulation. External references rely on planar alignment; even slight variations of position can mean large discrepancies in the internal location that a surface landmark represents (Fig. 8-2). Tools assisting reproduction include descriptive statements such as supine versus prone, arm placement, and names and location of sponges or other positioning devices. Measurements indicating the relative position of anatomy (e.g., chin to suprasternal notch or slope of the sternum) may be used. Photographs taken at the simulation are often used to illustrate written descriptions. The precise reproduction of the treatment position is critical to the maintenance of the orientation of surface landmarks to internal targets.

Comfort significantly affects the patient's ability to maintain the treatment position. Care is taken at the time of simulation to define a treatment position that the patient can tolerate for daily treatment. Considerations at the simulation include the general condition of the patient (e.g., age, disability, pain), location of normal structures, skin folds in the treatment fields, ability to treat all fields in one position, and reproducibility. For treatment the goal is to reproduce the planned position to ensure the coincidence of surface landmarks relative to the internal target. Even with the best planning, however, discomfort is not avoided for every patient. In these situations the radiation therapist accommodates the patient's needs while maintaining the integrity of the planned position.

Immobilization devices reproduce treatment position while restricting movement. The complexity of this task varies depending on the mobility of the anatomic site. Long applied in the treatment of head and neck and extremities, improvements in treatment planning and portal image evaluation methods are demanding increased immobilization for all treatment sites. Improved devices are necessary to the accurate treatment of planning target volumes with increasingly narrow margins of normal tissue.

The common three-point positioning technique defines the plane of treatment on the patient and provides references with which the radiation therapist aligns the treatment plane

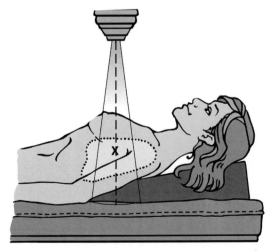 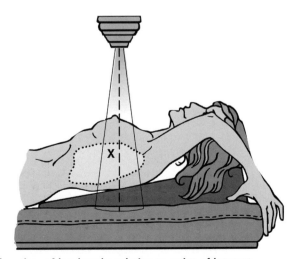

Figure 8-2. Change in patient position changes location of landmarks relative to point of interest.

with the axis of the gantry's rotation. With the patient in the approximate treatment position and the localization landmarks identified, the treatment table is positioned to bring the patient close to the location for treatment. The room lights are dimmed, and patient position is refined by using lasers and the treatment-field light. Through the alignment of three fiducial landmarks on the patient relative to three external references (lasers), the treatment position is reproduced.

A breast bridge (a two-legged device with a spirit level [Fig. 8-3]) or similar tool may be used to reproduce the position of two points relative to one another. For example, the rotation of the pelvis can be measured by placing each leg of the bridge on the anterior superior iliac spines of the pelvis. The incline of the thorax can be measured by placing one leg on the suprasternal notch and the other leg at the base of the sternum.

POSITIONING ISOCENTER

With the patient in the precise treatment position, the isocenter is positioned relative to the localization landmarks. In some situations the intersection of the planes identified by the three positioning points coincides with the localization points for the isocenter (Fig. 8-4). For many clinical situations, however, this is not practical. Anatomic references are seldom so conveniently located, and many sites do not lend themselves to the reproducible placement of localization marks. Examples include mobile skin surfaces such as those of the breast, of the axilla, and of older or obese persons; sloping surfaces such as those treated with tangential fields; irregular surfaces; and areas covered by dressings. For these situations a landmark and coordinate system may be used. The reproduction of isocenter placement is accomplished by aligning stable surface landmarks with lasers, defining a zero reference point. Table motions in the X, Y, and Z planes are

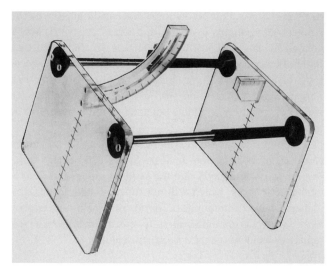

Figure 8-3. A breast bridge. *(Courtesy Arthur Swayhoover, Nuclear Associates, Carle Place, New York.)*

made from that point. Indexed couches with digital linear position readouts contribute valuable precision in making these adjustments. Z plane position may be determined from the table surface or the source-skin distance (SSD) from the gantry. Several methods may be used to determine SSD. An optical-distance indicator (ODI), or rangefinder, consists of a light that is projected onto the patient's skin and matched at the intersecting crosshairs.

Mechanical-distance indicators consist of incrementally marked rods or a measuring tape mounted to the collimator assembly extended to touch the patient's surface at the center of the treatment field. Couch movements direct the positioning of the isocenter, as demonstrated in Fig. 8-5.

Internal localization methods are increasingly applied in

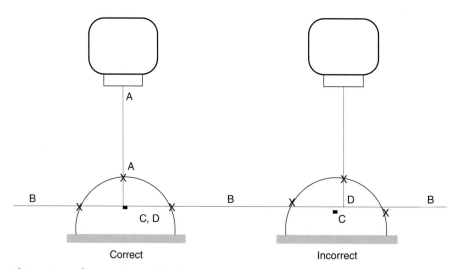

Figure 8-4. Three-point positioning: tattoos (x). **A,** Crosshairs. **B,** Lasers. **C,** Planned location of the isocenter. **D,** Actual location of isocenter.

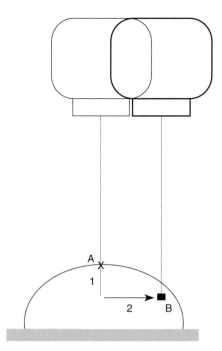

Figure 8-5. Landmark and coordinate method. **A,** Surface landmark (tattoo). **B,** Planned location of isocenter. *1,* Shift to depth; *2,* lateral shift.

the effort to further refine treatment volumes. Following traditional positioning and isocenter placement, normal anatomic or implanted radiopaque references may be visualized and positioning adjustments made. Ultrasound systems visualize internal structures such as the bladder/prostate margin. **Electronic portal imaging devices (EPIDs),** a system producing near real-time portal images on a computer screen for evaluation of treatment accuracy, can visualize implanted markers. Table position adjustments are applied as calculated from image findings and treatment proceeds.[5]

Beam Direction

The gantry and collimator are positioned to reproduce field requirements defined in the treatment plan. Before accepting the beam placement, the radiation therapist evaluates its accuracy. Using their knowledge of anatomy and information provided by the portal imaging, therapists assess the reproduction of the treatment setup daily. Considerations such as the sparing of a strip of tissue to preserve lymphatic drainage or sufficient flash for tangential fields must be included in this assessment. Portal films must be taken if any question exists about the accuracy of the treatment-field placement.

BEAM-SHAPING

Treatment units are designed to produce square and rectangular treatment fields delivering consistent doses of radiation across a field perpendicular to the central ray of the beam. Individuals and tumors, however, do not appear as squares and rectangles with flat surfaces. Further field shaping is required for most treatments and may be accomplished using static multileaf collimation and custom or standard blocking.

Blocks

Individualization of treatment volumes may also be accomplished through the use of shielding blocks. Whereas a supply of standard lead blocks may be maintained to accommodate emergency situations, modern radiation therapy requires the use of custom shielding or static multileaf collimation. To create custom blocks, molds are cut and filled with low-melting lead alloys. Cutting systems mimic the geometrical arrangement of the treatment beam, thus ensuring proper divergence and magnification at the treatment site. Drawbacks of these systems include space requirements for fabrication and storage and hazards associated with lifting heavy equipment and exposure to hazardous chemicals.

Shielding blocks, used to shape photon or electron fields, take several forms. Materials range from spent uranium to lead and lead alloys used in the production of customized shielding blocks. Blocks rest on or are screwed to plastic trays inserted into the accessory tray of the treatment-unit head. The shape and position of blocks are verified before the initiation of treatment by using portal imaging. The required thickness of actual blocks varies based on the energy of the treatment beam. Full-shielding blocks are constructed to transmit less than 5% of the original beam.

A supply of standardized lead blocks is among the necessary accessories in the treatment room. These occupy little space and accommodate emergency treatments until customized shielding can be created. Limitations include minimal variability in shape and size. Perpendicular block sides produce an increased **penumbra**[**] along the blocked field edges (see Fig. 8-6, *A*). Standardized lead blocks are often placed on trays without a means of being secured to the tray, and the radiation therapist is always careful to remove them before changing the gantry position.

Customized shielding blocks use lead alloys with low melting points. The most common material used is Cerrobend (Lipowitz metal). Cerrobend is comprised of bismuth, lead, tin, and cadmium. Lead and cadmium, potentially toxic and carcinogenic, must be handled with care. Safety precautions must be in place to prevent ingestion and inhalation of fumes; care with molten material must also be taken to prevent burns. These materials, Cerrobend and similar metals, allow molds to be cut from Styrofoam to match the size and shape defined by the physician at the simulation. These molds are filled with the molten alloy and allowed to cool. Cut block sides are parallel to the divergence of the treatment beam, thus reducing the penumbra caused by beam absorption through changing block thickness (Fig. 8-6, *B*). After completion of the individual's treatment, blocks are melted and the alloy is reused.

[**]Dose gradient caused by geometrical or physical factors.

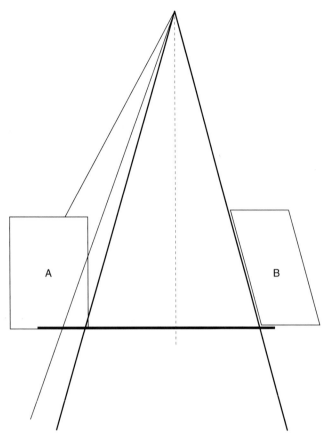

Figure 8-6. Blocks. **A,** Nondivergent (clinical). **B,** Divergent (custom).

Multileaf Collimators

Multileaf collimator (MLC) systems customize field shapes with the use of "jaws" that have been sliced into a series of opposing leaves. Each leaf is positioned independently, thus producing a variety of treatment field shapes. By reducing the need for the positioning of heavy blocks, MLC improves customization of treatment volumes while reducing treatment time and increasing safety for patients and radiation therapists. The radiation therapist will notice variations between MLC construction and control systems. Opposing banks of leaves form "leaf pairs." The number of pairs and the available widths vary with manufacturer with some manufacturers offering several models. Leaf width is measured at the isocenter and has an impact on the contour of the exposed field edge. Micro-MLC units provide greater refinement in field edge effects; these units are often removable. Space between leaves is a source of leakage radiation that may be minimized by manufacturer engineering of an interlocking leaf design or by positioning the primary jaws outside of the field as backup jaws during treatment delivery. Leaf end shape supports production of a divergent field edge and will be rounded on systems that move leaves on a single plane. Control systems may be integrated with the accelera-

tor console or may be separate; this has implications for selection of field parameters and MLC files as well as backup options should network access be interrupted. Because of the complexity of treatment procedures using MLCs, use of verification and record systems are usually in place.

MLCs have revolutionized the delivery of radiation treatment. In addition to conventional field shaping, MLCs may be configured for motion through beam delivery. As radiation intensity is varied, modulated across the exposed field, critical structures are protected. Areas of low dose in the target from one field are compensated by larger doses delivered through another gantry angle that does not intersect the protected structure. By producing several of these non-coplanar, intensity-modulated fields, the MLC can deliver high doses of radiation to targets that are irregularly shaped or close to critical structures.

Verification Imaging (Portal Imaging)

Portal images are taken at the start of treatment and at regular intervals during its course to verify placement of isocenter and beam position, including beam shape. Frequency of portal imaging is based on department policy and professional judgment and varies among institutions. Partially based on historical studies showing a reduction in treatment errors associated with increased portal imaging, weekly portal imaging for radical cases has become an accepted, although not universally implemented, standard.[6,7] Some clinical situations, such as unstable localization landmarks or the proximity of the treatment volume to critical structures, may require an increased frequency of portal imaging. Finally, weekly portal filming cannot document variations in daily positioning of treatment fields. A review of daily portal images taken with EPID has shown variations of greater than 1 cm in fields demonstrating excellent reproduction based on assessment of weekly films.[10] Awareness of these limitations spurs the desire for increased frequency and precision in portal imaging. The professional judgment of the therapist is central in determining an appropriate imaging schedule with the radiation oncologist.

Traditional film methods of portal imaging require attention to equipment and technique. Radiographic film is selected for its relative exposure sensitivity and must be properly supported when positioned for use. Portal film reacts more slowly to radiation exposure than diagnostic film, allowing images to be created using the energies and dose rates used in therapeutic radiation exposures. Cassettes provide film stability for the film, may be hard or soft, and are usually lined with lead and/or copper to reduce film fog caused by backscatter. Films are positioned perpendicular to the central ray of the treatment beam, and source-film distance (SFD) is minimized. Magnification markers, radiopaque indicators of known dimension, may be placed at the skin surface to determine magnification factors for an individual image. A graticule, however, is used more frequently. The graticule is a tray that fits into the collimator. Radiopaque markers within the tray project the position of the central ray and measured lengths along each axis.

Images may be created using single- or double-exposure techniques. Single-exposure images may be used when sufficient landmarks for verification are located within the treatment area. The single-exposure image may be created using the same film/cassette combination as the double image, or, alternatively, verification film (v-film) may be positioned throughout the treatment exposure. Verification film has a significantly slower exposure rate than that of standard portal film. The double-exposure technique yields a visualization of the treatment field and surrounding anatomy, thus increasing the number of landmarks available for interpretation. This technique is accomplished by producing a short exposure of the treatment area. A second exposure is taken after the removal of field-shaping blocks and opening of the collimators.

For multiple field treatment techniques using nonvertical or horizontal beam orientations, verification of isocenter is achieved through **orthogonal imaging.** Two images are taken at a 90-degree angle from one another, localizing isocenter in all planes. Orthogonal imaging is also applied in the verification process of IMRT.

Several options of obtaining portal images are now available, with traditional film remaining the most widespread. Digital image sources such as EPIDs or phosphor plates that are exposed in the same manner as film are gaining in popularity. Portal imaging systems that create static or real-time images of treatment volumes provide a means to improve daily treatment accuracy. A detector mounted opposite the head of the gantry converts the x-ray information into digital information that can be displayed as an image on a computer screen or through a laser printer to produce a hard-copy image. Computer manipulation of grey scales can enhance contrast. Some systems can superimpose simulation and on-treatment images to display measured variations from the simulation to the therapist. With this tool, therapists can implement precise adjustments before treatment delivery.

Image Communication

Portal and reference images (simulation or DRRs) are compared and clinical acceptance or changes are made. Portal image interpretation is mostly a subjective process with room for variation in assessment between individuals.[2] Therapists exercise clinical judgment when reviewing images within the context of department policies. Allowable decision making ranges from therapists reviewing and implementing positioning adjustments with image notations to the physician to therapists not reviewing images. Regardless, all images must be reviewed and signed by the physician; acceptance or change orders are noted on the image and returned to the radiation therapists for action.

Care must be taken in the evaluation of portal films to differentiate between systematic and random setup errors. **Systematic errors** are those resulting from variations in the translation of the treatment setup from the simulator to the treatment unit and remain constant through the course of treatment if not corrected. Portal images taken before the first treatment generally assess systematic errors. These include the localization of the isocenter relative to surface landmarks and the position and shape of blocks. Corrections may be made for these errors by adjusting setup parameters or blocks. **Random errors** are inherent variations in daily setup. The range of random errors varies with the anatomic site and must be accommodated in target-volume planning. A random error is minimized by careful patient positioning and treatment-plan reproduction. Increasing the rate of portal filming demonstrates the consistency of errors.

Time factors, poor image quality, and subjectivity in evaluation introduce limitations to precision with the use of traditional film portal imaging techniques. Images created by megavoltage beams have poor contrast, thus making landmarks difficult to delineate. Films often are evaluated after treatment, even on subsequent days, and offer no opportunity to correct for treatments already delivered. Even when portal films are taken immediately before treatment delivery, patient movement is possible while patients wait for the film evaluation. The time-consuming nature of the filming process also has an effect on schedule flow. Electronic portal imaging offers many advantages to the practice of radiation therapy by allowing the therapist and physician to verify portal field alignment and make adjustments much more quickly and accurately. Images are produced in seconds and displayed on a terminal at the **treatment console** (area located outside the treatment room), thus minimizing movement factors and the effect of frequent filming on the patient schedule.

BEAM-MODIFYING DEVICES

With assurance that the radiation is being directed to the prescribed volume, customization of dose delivery may require the addition of devices that modify the distribution of the radiation dose across the treatment field.

Bolus

In radiation therapy, **bolus** refers to materials whose interactions with the radiation beam mimic those of tissue. Bolus comes in many forms and has many applications. Common materials include paraffin wax, Vaseline gauze, wet gauze or towels, and water bags. Commercially available products developed specifically for use in radiation therapy are available in sheets of variable thicknesses (Fig. 8-7) and powder forms that can be mixed with water and formed to meet specific needs. Flexibility in shaping is an advantage because bolus must conform to the treatment surface without air gaps.

Bolus of a thickness equal to the depth of maximum dose eliminates the skin-sparing effect of megavoltage photon beams. Bolus may be applied with this goal over entire treatment areas or simply over scars, superficial nodes, or other areas of concern. When bolus is applied in this fashion, the

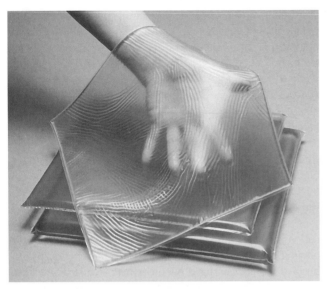

Figure 8-7. Bolus example: Superflab. *(Courtesy MED-TEC, Inc, Orange City, Iowa.)*

build-up of dose occurs within it, thus bringing the area of maximum dose deposition to the patient's surface.

Bolus may also be used to compensate for variations in surface contour or eliminate air gaps in cavities. For example, surgical procedures leaving anatomic defects such as those used for the removal of sinus or eye malignancies produce significant irregularities. Filling the cavity with bolus material such as Vaseline gauze or a water-filled balloon significantly improves the dose distribution in the target volume. This application is only useful in situations in which the loss of skin sparing is acceptable or desired. When skin sparing is to be maintained, the creation of individualized **compensators** (a beam-modifier that changes radiation output relative to loss of attenuation over a changing patient contour) should be evaluated.

Compensators

The design of megavoltage treatment units produces a radiation beam delivering a relatively even dose across the plane perpendicular to the radiation beam. Patients, however, rarely provide a flat surface parallel with this ideal. Skewing of dose distribution caused by irregular surfaces can be compensated by using bolus material to produce a level treatment area; however, a loss of skin sparing accompanies this technique. To retain this important effect, compensating filters may be positioned in the head of the treatment unit, thus modifying the radiation beam to accommodate the contour of the patient. Compensating filters can be made from a variety of materials as long as the materials' equivalence to tissue absorption is known. Common materials include copper, brass, lead, and Lucite.

Tissue deficits in need of compensation are usually most significant over one dimension (width or length), and a set of standardized two-dimensional compensators meets the needs of many treatment situations. Custom compensators can easily be built for special situations. Strips of attenuating materials of known thicknesses are layered and mounted onto a tray.

Three-dimensional compensators are created by using square blocks or special cutting units to complement the contour of the surface across the width and length dimensions. Care must be taken to position compensating materials on the tray so that their projection at the treatment distance corresponds to the area of tissue deficit. The complexity of their creation limits their use in most facilities. Alternative methods of creating three-dimensional compensators use equipment that can transfer the surface contour to a router system forming a Styrofoam mold designed to be filled with a specific compensating material such as bolus or Cerrobend. Three-dimensional Cerrobend compensators may also be generated for IMRT and modulate the intensity of the beam for IMRT. The plan for these compensators will be generated by a treatment planning system.

Wedges

The primary goal of treatment planning is treating a **target volume*** to an even (homogenous) dose while minimizing the dose delivered to normal tissue. The orientation of multiple fields to one another during treatment may produce inhomogeneous dose distributions over the target volume. The **isodose lines**† of a single treatment field on a flat surface are relatively parallel to the surface. When a second beam is positioned directly opposite this beam, the combined dose distribution is relatively even throughout the volume. However, as the **hinge angle**‡ (Fig. 8-8) decreases, doses delivered to overlapping areas vary significantly, thus creating areas of high- and low-dose regions in the desired target volume.

Wedges appear similar to compensator filters; however, their application differs significantly. The wedge is designed to change the angle of the isodose curve relative to the beam axis at a specified depth. Wedges reduce the dose in areas of overlap between fields that have hinge angles less than 180 degrees. The thick end of the wedge, referred to as the heel, attenuates the greatest amount of radiation, thus drawing the isodose lines closer to the surface. Attenuation decreases along the wedge to the thin end, or toe, where the dose delivered to the patient will be relatively greater than the dose at the opposite side of the treatment field. When wedges are used, heels should always be positioned together.

Standard wedge systems use externally mounted wedges that the radiation therapist must position when required by the treatment plan. The manufacturer usually provides these

---

*An area of known and presumed tumor.

†Lines connecting points of equivalent relative radiation dose.

‡The measure of the angle between central rays of two intersecting treatment beams.

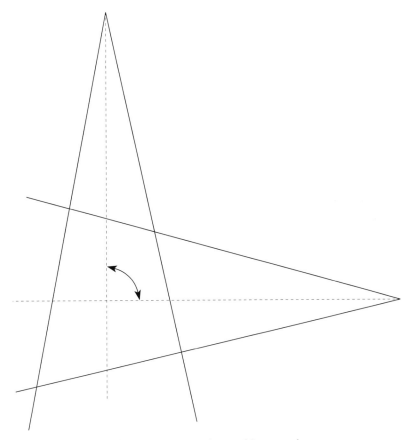

Figure 8-8. A 90-degree hinge angle.

wedges, which are customized for specific treatment units. Standard wedge sizes are 15, 30, 45, and 60 degrees.

Treatment units using internal wedging methods allow customizing of the wedge angle for each treatment plan. One system uses a 60-degree universal wedge placed in the beam path for a specified number of monitor units. The beam is interrupted to remove the wedge, and the remaining monitor units are delivered. Other systems use a dynamic jaw system in which a moving jaw starts at one side of the field and opens to a full field over the course of dose delivery. This effectively delivers a range of dose over the field. The side of the field at which the jaw starts its movement correlates with the wedge toe.

Field sizes are limited with the use of compensators and wedges. Care must be taken to ensure that treatment fields do not extend beyond the heel or sides of either beam-modification device (flash or extension beyond the toe is acceptable).

Transmission Filters

Transmission filters are designed to allow the transmission of a predetermined percentage of the treatment beam to a portion of a treatment field and may be used throughout the course of the treatment. This allows the physician to treat structures that have varying radiosensitivity in proximity to one another at different dose rates. For example, whole-abdomen radiation therapy induces significant gastrointestinal effects. By reducing the daily dose to the upper portion of the abdomen through the use of the transmission filter, patient tolerance is improved. The pelvis receives the dose at a higher rate, thus effectively completing the boost dose concurrently with the whole-abdomen treatment. When using a transmission filter, daily fraction and total doses for each area must be written in the prescription and documented separately in the daily treatment record.

Electron Contamination

The interaction of the photon beam with materials of beam modifiers produces scatter electrons that contaminate the photon beam and produce increased skin doses for patients. Low-energy electrons are absorbed in 15 cm of air; therefore all beam-shaping and modification devices for photon beams must be secured a minimum of 15 cm from the surface of the patient. In the treatment of head and neck cancer with lateral ports, patients who have metal fillings may benefit from the addition of internal shielding to reduce the dose on the buccal mucosa and tongue produced by increased electron scatter near the metal surface. A mouth guard made of wax and inlaid with a thin layer of tin can be prepared before the simulation and used throughout the treatment course to attenuate this scatter without significantly altering the dose distribution.

ELECTRON BEAM

Superficial treatment volumes may be treated using electron beams. The physical characteristics of these beams provide rapid dose build-up, an area of uniform dose deposition followed by rapid dose fall-off.

Collimation

The mass and charge of the electron give rise to increased interactions in air compared with those of the photon beam. This scattering of the electron beam necessitates the extension of **collimation** (field shaping) close to the treatment surface. Secondary collimation systems for electron therapy usually take the form of cones or trimmer bars attached to the treatment-accessory tray of the gantry. This equipment is usually secured before the patient is positioned (Fig. 8-9).

Field-Defining Apertures (FDAs)

Field-shaping requirements for electron-beam therapy differ significantly from photon requirements. Electron beams are attenuated much more efficiently than photon beams. Full shielding requires lead thicknesses of only several millimeters (general rule: $\frac{1}{2}$ energy in millimeters of lead). **Electron shields,** which are "cutouts" that collimate and shape the electron treatment field, may be cut and molded to the patient surface except in instances in which the field area makes the weight of the cutout uncomfortable.

As discussed earlier, collimation of electron beams is accomplished through the use of electron cones or trimmer bars. Electron cones or trimmer bars bring the collimation of these beams closer to the patient's surface, thus improving radiation-dose distribution by sharpening the dose gradient at the beam edges. Cones are limited to a few selected field sizes, generally squares. Trimmer bars attached to the collimator provide greater flexibility in field size, but the increased distance from the patient increases penumbra. To customize field areas, field-shaping cutouts can be designed to fit directly inside the electron cone or molded to fit the patient's contour, thus providing tertiary collimation at the treatment site. Planning of these field-shaping cutouts may be accomplished by using the simulator or a clinical procedure. For clinical customization the required field shape is drawn on a template positioned on the patient's surface with localization landmarks for later treatment reproduction. The template is then used to form a mold for creation of a Cerrobend cutout (Fig. 8-10), which fits inside the base of the cone.

Internal Shielding

Treatment sites such as the nares, auricle, eyelids, and lips are often treated with electron therapy. These structures are thin, and underlying normal tissue such as the medial nasal membranes, skin behind the ear, optic lens, and gingiva must be protected from unnecessary radiation exposure. Shields may be produced to achieve this goal. The interac-

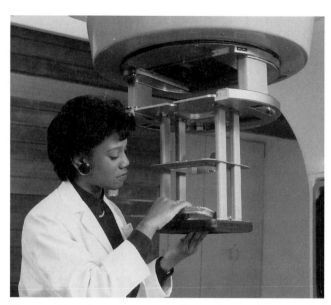

Figure 8-9. Electron cones. *(Courtesy Varian Medical Systems.)*

tion of the electrons with the metal of these shields, however, produces low-energy scatter radiation that increases the dose and reaction at the incident tissue surface. To absorb these low-energy photons, the shield must be covered with a low Z number material such as aluminum, tin, or paraffin wax.

Bolus

Although the materials used for bolus in electron therapy are the same as those used with photons, the applications differ. Three applications for bolus exist in electron therapy. First, because the dose deposition for electrons differs from

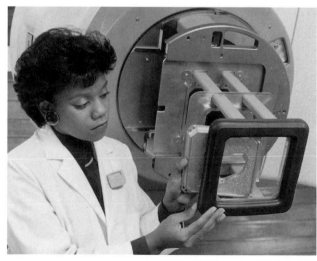

Figure 8-10. Electron cutouts. *(Courtesy Varian Medical Systems.)*

that of photons,* bolusing to eliminate skin sparing is only applied for low-energy electron beams. Second, the depth at which dose fall-off occurs can be customized by the choice of electron energy and by the use of bolus to decrease the depth of penetration. Third, irregular surfaces and air cavities play havoc with the dose distribution of electron beams, and bolus may be used to fill in these irregularities.

ASSESSMENT AND ACCEPTANCE OF TREATMENT PARAMETERS

The radiation therapist performs a final review of the treatment setup, verifying the patient positioning, beam direction, and use of beam modifiers. If arc therapy is being applied, the therapist ensures free clearance for gantry motion throughout the treatment rotation. Once satisfied that the set parameters meet those prescribed by the treatment plan, radiation therapists notify the patient that they will exit the treatment room to administer the radiation. The therapist reminds and reassures patients that they are being monitored at all times. An indication of the approximate time that the beam will be on is reassuring. On confirmation that the patient is the only person in the treatment room, the radiation therapists exit and securely close the door.

Console

Radiation delivery is controlled at the treatment console area located outside the treatment room. The configuration of the console varies widely among treatment units, from simple cobalt units with two timers and beam on-off lights to multiple computer-controlled screens displaying treatment unit and ancillary equipment parameters.

The console provides information to the radiation therapist regarding the status of the treatment unit. The use of beam modifiers may require verification of placement to release a safety interlock for treatment. **Interlocks** assist in meeting many safety parameters for treatment delivery, including (but not limited to) the closing of doors, placement of proper beam modifiers (wedges, compensators, electron cones), and machine-operation requirements (water, Freon, SF6). A lack of agreement with the requirements of any of these interlocks triggers a fault indicator on the console. Fault-light panels provide diagnostic information regarding proper functioning and the source of problems in the treatment unit.

The radiation therapist sets the parameters for treatment delivery, including the calculated primary and backup monitor unit (or timer) settings. Ion chambers within the beam measure radiation output, displaying relative dose delivered in monitor units (MU). Primary, secondary, and backup systems function to interrupt the treatment beam after the prescribed

dose has been delivered. Backup systems include secondary ion chambers calibrated a percentage lower than the primary ion chamber and timers that interrupt the beam after a set period of time. The accelerator is designed to deliver a dose at specified rates decreases in that rate may indicate problems. Backup systems may be manually or automatically set depending on the sophistication of the treatment unit and function as safety interlocks, terminating the beam if the primary counter malfunctions.

Gauges and light panels provide further information regarding machine operation, including the dose rate during beam operation. Although the maintenance of equipment is ultimately the responsibility of the radiation physicist, the monitoring of equipment functioning and reporting of problems to the physics or engineering department is a critical responsibility of the radiation therapist.[6] Any equipment malfunctions or setup errors affecting treatment delivery must be reported to the radiation oncologist, and corrective actions must be documented in writing. Malfunctions or errors resulting in misadministration must be reported following Nuclear Regulatory Commission (NRC) or state reporting requirements. Definitions of reportable events and misadministrations may change over time so determination of a reportable event must be made by the radiation safety officer. Equipment malfunctions causing serious injury or death are reported through the Food and Drug Administration's Medical Device Reporting Act.

VERIFICATION AND RECORD SYSTEMS

V&R systems provide machine setup parameters for treatment setup and delivery. They compare machine settings with those most recently prescribed for a particular field and prevent the initiation of the treatment beam if settings vary outside a certain tolerance range. Parameters typically monitored include monitor units, gantry position, collimator aperture and rotation settings, table position, arc versus fixed treatment, and use of beam modifiers.[9]

Care must be taken that parameters set on the first day of treatment are accurate because errors will continue on subsequent treatments.

V&R systems can provide significant functionality to aid in the accurate and efficient delivery of radiation therapy. The patient's entire course of external beam radiation therapy is defined and recorded on-line for access throughout the department. Treatment preferences are definable allowing selection of fields available for treatment and auto-setup of treatment parameters. Auto-sequencing of treatment fields presents the radiation therapist with the next set of treatment field parameters on completion of each field. For properly equipped accelerators, returning to the treatment room between fields is eliminated. Some accelerators are also capable of proceeding through an entire sequence of fields under the monitoring of the radiation therapist but without his or her intervention.

---

*The depth of maximum dose decreases with increase in energy followed by an area of homogenous dose and ending with an area of rapid fall-off.

TREATMENT DELIVERY

Beam On and Beam Off

The patient is informed that the radiation therapists are leaving the room for treatment delivery. With everyone except the patient out of the treatment room, the radiation therapist performs a final review of treatment parameters, the treatment beam is turned on, and the prescribed radiation dose delivered.

Initiation of the treatment beam requires turning a key, pressing a switch, or both. The console displays the dose rate and time or number of monitor units administered. Red "radiation on" lights in and outside the treatment room indicate the presence of radiation in the treatment room.

In the event of movement by the patient, improper machine motion, or failure of the unit to cease treatment at the prescribed dose, interruption of the treatment beam is necessary. Options for beam interruption include pressing the beam-off key, turning the operation key to the off position, or opening the door to the treatment unit. If these actions fail to stop the beam, an emergency off switch must be used, thereby completely turning off the treatment unit. The use of the emergency off switch usually requires a warmup period before reuse of the machine.

Geiger counters are required equipment in ^{60}Co treatment units. Visual (flashing light) and audible (clicks) indicators inform the radiation therapist of the radiation level in the treatment room. Source-position indicators located on the front of the treatment-unit head may include a dial for rotating sources or rod for sliding-drawer sources. In the ^{60}Co room, a note must be made of the return to normal exposure rate on entry into the treatment room after each treatment field is exposed. If the radiation source does not retract, radiation therapists must react quickly to ensure the safety of the patient and themselves. While staying out of the primary beam, the therapist moves the patient out of the beam's path and closes the collimator opening. An attempt may be made to manually retract the source by turning the dial on the head of the treatment unit or using a T-bar that fits over the rod and pushing the source into the retracted position. Any extra exposure time the patient receives must be noted in the chart.

Patient-Monitoring Systems

To protect the radiation therapist from radiation exposure, the patient must be left alone in the treatment room for the radiation delivery. However, to maintain patient safety and accuracy of treatment, audio and visual contact must be maintained at all times. A stop at the console area before the first treatment allows the radiation therapist to demonstrate monitoring systems, thus reassuring patients that they are being monitored during treatment delivery and that their privacy is being protected.

In some situations (orthovoltage or other low-energy treatments), the therapist may monitor treatment directly through leaded glass windows. This becomes impractical with megavoltage units, however, and indirect monitoring systems must be used. For standard radiation therapy treatment, at least two cameras are used to maintain visual contact with the patient. One camera provides a long view of the whole patient, thus allowing observation of general distress or movement. Another camera zooms in, thereby providing a closer view on the treatment field to observe subtle patient movement.

A two-way communication system between the treatment room and console remains continuously audible to the operator. A switch allows the communication into the treatment room when necessary.

Multiple Fields

Most treatment plans require radiation delivery through more than one port to achieve sufficient dose homogeneity through the target volume. Accuracy in multiple-field irradiation is greatly enhanced with the use of isocentric treatment techniques. With the isocenter of the treatment unit precisely positioned in the target volume, radiation beams can be aimed at the target volume from many directions without the patient being moved and accuracy compromised. The areas of overlap from these fields receive an increased dose relative to tissues receiving radiation from only one portal.

After radiation delivery to the first treatment port, the radiation therapist must assess the position of the patient and treatment unit for each subsequent field. Field size, table, gantry, and collimator angles are set, and treatment accessories are positioned. Capabilities of treatment units vary significantly. Some require therapist reentry to the treatment room between every field for positioning of the machine and placement of treatment accessories. As computer control of field shaping through MLCs and beam modification through dynamic wedges, MLCs, and so forth become more widely available, the operation of the accelerator from the console becomes more prevalent. Bidirectional communication with external V&R systems is increasingly exploited by accelerators that accept on-line parameters for treatment field setup. With prescribed position values downloaded to the accelerator, the therapist controls motion using motion-enabling functions at the accelerator console or on the pendant in the treatment room. Such auto-setup features reduce time for treatment and reduce potential for mispositioning of treatment variables.

Common Treatment Techniques

The choice of field arrangement depends on the location of the tumor and nearby critical structures. As a member of the treatment-planning team, the radiation therapist works with the radiation oncologist and dosimetrist to plan field arrangements within the capabilities of the treatment machine that cover target volumes while avoiding critical structures.

The most basic multiple-field technique is the parallel

opposed portal (POP). POP fields are defined as those with a hinge angle of 180 degrees. These fields may enter the patient from any two directions relative to the patient and are often identified by those directions. Examples include right-and-left lateral (laterals or "lats"), anteroposterior and posteroanterior (AP/PA), and anterior oblique and posterior oblique (obliques). These are used for a great variety of treatment sites and usually require few treatment accessories other than blocks and compensators. Superficial volumes on curved surfaces such as the breast or ribs may require opposing fields, which flash off the surface of the patient. These fields are called tangential fields, tangents or "tangs." The hinge angle between tangential fields may vary slightly from 180 degrees accommodating divergence of the beams and creating a coincident deep edge to the treated volume.

The four-field technique, sometimes referred to as a four-field box or brick, is commonly used in the treatment of deep-seated tumors of the pelvis or abdomen. These fields are arranged 90 degrees from one another and generally require no more than blocks for optimal dose distribution in the target volume.

The wedge-pair technique changes the volume receiving radiation by decreasing the hinge angle between two treatment fields. The relative dose in the area formed between the narrowing hinge angle increases. Overlapping isodose lines are not parallel to one another, and combining them produces extremely high dose deposition in the shallow portion of the target volume relative to the dose deposited more deeply. By reducing the amount of radiation delivered to this region, wedges distribute the dose more homogeneously throughout the target volume. Three-field techniques also often require the use of wedges to achieve the same dose-homogeneity goal.

Conformal therapy applies three-dimensional localization of the tumor volume. Using multiple fields possibly in a non-coplanar arrangement, the volume is defined through the BEV and the field shaped to include the target volume with minimal normal issue margins. Six or more fields are used to increase dose to the target while producing sharp fall-off of dose to surrounding tissue. Immobilization devices are carefully included in and treatment is delivered in the same manner as other multiple-field techniques. With high-energy beams, dose distributions are comparable to arc therapy.

Arc therapy demonstrates the ultimate multiple-field technique. In standard arc therapy, radiation is delivered as the gantry moves through its arc of rotation, thus effectively delivering radiation through a continuous sequence of individual overlapping treatment portals. Verification of clearance of the patient; accessory medical equipment; the treatment table; and all stretchers, chairs, and stools must be completed before initiating the treatment beam. Visual monitors must be positioned so that the patient and motion of the gantry can be observed. The changing gantry angle must not obstruct monitoring of the treatment at any time.

Stereotactic radiosurgery or radiation therapy uses sophisticated localization methods to reproduce the placement of the isocenter in the cranium with an accuracy of less than 1 mm. Non-coplanar arcs are directed at the tumor by changing the treatment-table rotation between treatment arcs. By distributing the dose delivered to normal tissue over an even greater area, the area of high relative dose is increasingly focused on the target volume. In radiosurgery a single large fraction of radiation dose can be delivered to the target without overdosing nearby normal brain tissue. With stereotactic radiosurgery the radiobiologic benefits of fractionation is combined with advances in localization and definition of dose distribution.

Total body irradiation (TBI) is accomplished through a variety of techniques. Patients must be positioned at an extended distance to produce a sufficiently large field size. On treatment units not specifically designed for this purpose, this usually means lying on the floor or standing or sitting against a treatment-room wall with the gantry rotated 90 degrees. To achieve dose homogeneity, patients must be treated with POP fields requiring repositioning halfway through the treatment. Several dedicated TBI treatment machines have been developed in centers with a high demand for this treatment. These machines simplify treatment by using fixed, extended distance, double-headed treatment units to deliver radiation through both surfaces with the patient in a comfortable, constant position.

IMRT requires a committed program for delivery. The program is highly physics intensive requiring specially equipped accelerators and/or MLC units, inverse treatment planning, and sophisticated dose measurement. For treatment delivery, immobilization is emphasized. Variations in positioning and isocenter alignment have increased significance in delivery of dose to volumes with highly defined margins. Orthogonal imaging is used to verify positioning of isocenter. An outline of the irradiated area may be imaged to display an outline of the "field" but does not offer the same information interpretable from traditional techniques.

Accelerators using MLCs to produce IMRT treatments may apply either of two methods. Segmental MLC (SMLC), or step and shoot accelerators, position leaves in the first position and the therapist initiates the beam. As the first **beamlet** (a small photon intensity element, also referred to as a *bixel,* used to subdivide an IMRT beam for calculation purposes) is delivered the beam turns off, the accelerator moves the leaves to the next position, turns the beam on and off, and so forth, proceeding through each leaf position until the treatment is delivered. The accelerator controls beam on/off throughout. An accelerator using dynamic MLC (DMLC) IMRT, sometimes called the *sliding window technique,* moves leaves through one beam on/off sequence. Operator intervention is similar in both accelerators with the radiation therapists positioning the patient and the accelerator and initiating the beam once.

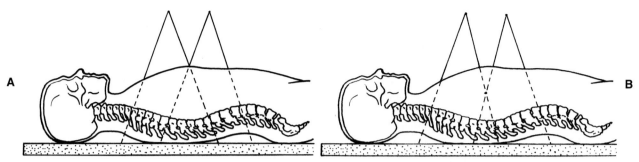

Figure 8-11. Matching adjacent treatment fields. **A,** Abutting a hot match. **B,** A calculated gap.

Adjacent Fields

The divergence of the radiation beam poses geometrical problems during the alignment of adjacent treatment fields. Matching methods vary with changing clinical objectives. Methods include abutting fields at the surface and the use of gaps between fields with or without coplanar alignment of treatment-beam edges. **Feathering** (migration of the gap through the treatment course) may be used to blur dose inhomogeneities in the gapped area. The choice of gap technique and positioning of the gap depends on the location of tumor and critical structures.

Abutting field edges produces a hot match in which the diverging beams overlap immediately below the surface (Fig. 8-11, *A*). This may be necessary in situations in which the tumor lies close to the skin surface near the position of the match. The primary example of this application is the treatment of head and neck cancer. The area of overlap must be carefully evaluated for the presence of critical structures and the dose delivered to them with this technique. Care must be taken to avoid the overdose of critical structures.

When an area of low dose is acceptable at and near the surface, adjacent fields may be separated by a gap (Fig. 8-11, *B*). Treatment fields overlap at a prescribed depth in the patient. The exact length of the gap must be calculated by knowing the length of each treatment field and depth at which the intersection of the fields is to be positioned (see Chapter 21 on dose calculations for more information).

Some clinical situations demand a precise alignment of the radiation beam. Areas of overdose and underdose arising from variations in the amount of overlap or space between fields may be unacceptable in these situations. Common examples include tangential breast techniques with matching supraclavicular fields and craniospinal irradiation (CSI). In each of these treatment techniques, positioning the planes of field edges coincident (coplanar) to one another is useful. This may be accomplished through the use of blocks, independent jaws or a gantry, a collimator, and couch rotations. A nondivergent beam edge is achieved through the placement of an independent jaw at the isocenter or through the use of a block to the same point (Fig. 8-12, *A*). These blocks may be called half-beam blocks,

central-axis blocks, or beam splitters. Two fields with non-divergent beam edges may be abutted or separated by a standard* gap. Limitations to the application of this method include techniques covering large target volumes because jaw openings must be double the length of the treatment area and concerns regarding beam transmission through blocks.

For large field sizes such as those used in CSI, the flexibility of motion designed in the treatment unit is used. The rotation of the gantry, collimator, and table can be used in the effort to align treatment-field edges. With CSI as an example the inferior field edges of the opposing cranial fields can be made coplanar through the rotation of the couch while a rotation of the collimator aligns the same edge with the divergence of the posterior spine field (Fig. 8-12, *B* and *C*). Although the abutting of these geometrically matched fields theoretically provides a perfect match without the inhomogeneity of other techniques, the risks of variations in daily setup must be recognized. Abutting may be desirable in clinical situations in which risks are low, but the presence of critical structures at the match may require the addition of a gap.

The use of a gap between geometrically aligned fields creates a low-dose area, or cold spot. This is reduced through the application of the feathering technique. The feathered gap moves through the course of treatment, thus varying the low-dose area and increasing the total dose that the area of the gap receives. Many methods are used with varied sequences, number of migrations, and gap sizes.[3]

Treatment-Room Maintenance

Maintenance of the treatment room and its contents is the domain of the radiation therapist. In addition to monitoring the performance of the treatment unit, the radiation therapist must inspect treatment accessories for signs of wear or damage. Supplies of nonreusable or disposal items such as tape, laundry, and some bolus materials must be monitored.

Cleanliness and orderliness are essential to providing a safe treatment and work environment. Treatment accessories

---

*Noncalculated because beam geometry no longer creates an overlap at depth.

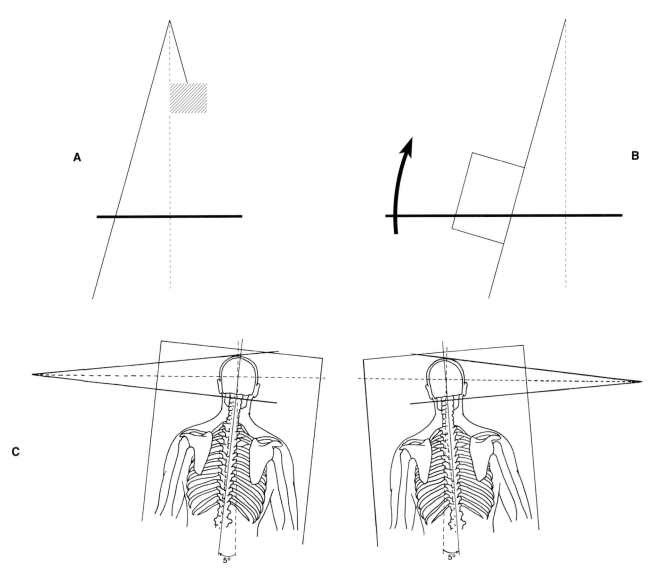

Figure 8-12. Geometrical field matching. **A,** Half-beam block. **B,** Collimator rotation. **C,** Couch rotation.

and positioning or immobilization devices coming in contact with patients must be cleaned and disinfected after each use. Sufficient shelf and cabinet space must be available to securely store equipment off the floor, and proper lighting levels must be maintained. Any unsafe conditions must be reported and corrected promptly.

SUMMARY

Through participation in the treatment-planning process and daily delivery of treatment the radiation therapist has a primary responsibility to the quality of care delivered to the patient. To meet the goals of treatment, whether palliative or curative, the radiation therapist remains vigilant in the accurate reproduction and administration of the treatment as prescribed by the physician. As the expert in treatment delivery, the radiation therapist is highly skilled in the use of megavoltage treatment units and accessories used to customize treatments for each patient. Through the documentation of treatment, monitoring of treatment-unit function, and inclusion on the departmental QA committee, radiation therapists actively participate in the ongoing goal of the radiation oncology team to continuously improve patient treatment and care.

As the treatment team member interacting with the patient on a daily basis, the radiation therapist applies knowledge of the physical and emotional reactions to radiation treatment by addressing the needs and concerns of patients within the guidelines of the scope of practice. Patients are directed to the physician or other professionals as specific needs are demonstrated.

Technical advances in diagnostic imaging, treatment-planning computers, and megavoltage treatment units have created great flexibility in the complexity of treatment plans that can be developed. Tumor volumes are identified and localized with greater confidence, and treatment beams are focused more narrowly. Normal tissue is increasingly spared from radiation exposure and damage. However, translation of the computer-generated plan to a living, breathing individual is still the primary challenge to reaping the benefits of these advances. Reduction in daily setup errors through the development and application of improvements in positioning, immobilization, and localization landmarks is attained through the diligence and precision of the radiation therapist.

Review Questions

Multiple Choice

1. Which of the following includes the area of a known and presumed tumor?
   a. Tumor volume
   b. Irradiated volume
   c. Critical volume
   d. Target volume
2. Beam modifiers that simulate tissue include which of the following?
   I.   Compensator
   II. Wedge
   III. Bolus
   a. I and II
   b. I and III
   c. II and III
   d. I, II, and III
3. What is the identification of the isocenter and field borders in relation to surface or bony landmarks?
   a. Definition
   b. Localization
   c. Dosimetry
   d. Simulation
4. Which of the following is included in the daily treatment record?
   I.   Treatment number
   II. Cumulative dose
   III. Patient position
   a. I and II
   b. I and III
   c. II and III
   d. I, II, and III
5. The period over which radiation is delivered is referred to as which of the following?
   a. Fractionation
   b. Exposure time
   c. Protraction
   d. Treatment time
6. Overlap of adjacent fields can be eliminated by using which of the following techniques?
   a. Half-beam blocks
   b. Gaps
   c. Feathering
   d. Abutting fields
7. The feathering technique is used to do which of the following?
   a. Eliminate overlap
   b. Increase dose to gapped region
   c. Decrease dose to gapped region
   d. Decrease dose in abutted fields
8. Patients are monitored during treatment delivery with megavoltage treatment units by using which of the following?
   I.   Closed-circuit television
   II. Direct visual
   III. Two-way audio
   a. I and II
   b. I and III
   c. II and III
   d. I, II, and III
9. What is the angle between the central axes of two treatment beams?
   a. Central angle
   b. Gantry angle
   c. Wedge angle
   d. Hinge angle
10. Which of the following may be used to shape electron fields?
    a. Cutouts
    b. Blocks
    c. Compensators
    d. Transmission filters

Questions to Ponder

1. Differentiate between an immobilization device and a positioning aid.
2. Analyze information to be included in the radiation therapy treatment chart.
3. Discuss factors contributing to decisions regarding portal imaging frequency.

REFERENCES

1. American Society of Radiologic Technologists: *The scope of practice for radiation therapists,* Albuquerque, NM, 1993, The American Society of Radiologic Technologists.
2. Denham JW, et al: Objective decision-making following a portal film: the results of a pilot study, *Int J Radiat Oncol Biol Phys* 26:869-876, 1993.
3. Digel C, et al: Dosimetric comparison of five craniospinal techniques, *Radiat Ther* 3:95-102, 1994.
4. Glatstein E: Radiation oncology in integrated care management. Report of the Intersociety Council for Radiation Oncology, December 1991.
5. Herman MG, et al: Clinical use of on-line portal imaging for daily patient treatment verification, *Int J Radiat Oncol Biol Phys* 28:1017-1023, 1994.
6. Kutcher GJ, et al: Report of the AAPM radiation therapy committee task group 40, *Med Phys* 21:581-618, 1994.

7. Marks JE, et al: The value of frequent treatment verification films in reducing localization error in the irradiation of complex fields, *Cancer* 37:2755, 1976.

8. Miller G, Hebert L: *Taking care of your back,* Bangor, Maine, 1984, IMPACC.

9. Podmaniczky KC, et al: Clinical experience with a computerized record and verify system, *Int J Radiat Oncol Biol Phys* 11:1529-1537, 1985.

10. Reinstein LE, Pai S, Meek AG: Assessment of geometric treatment accuracy using time-lapse display of electronic portal images, *Int J Radiat Oncol Biol Phys* 22:1139-1146, 1992.

11. Wizenberg MJ: *Quality assurance in radiation therapy: a manual for technologists,* Chicago, 1982, American College of Radiology.

Education

Pamela J. Ross

Outline

Key Terms

Accreditation
Advocate
Communication
Critical thinking
Life experiences

Protocol
Radiation therapy domain
Randomization
Transfer

E ducation is a vital part of radiation oncology because it seeks to dispel myths and overcome years of misunderstandings. Efforts to remove the stigmas attached to "CANCER" have been successful because there is a rapidly increasing public awareness and understanding of the disease. This, in great part, has been brought about through a commitment by the scientific community to disseminate essential facts that are required to produce a more knowledgeable populace. The misconceptions attached to radiation therapy, however, have been more difficult to dismiss and are still prevalent and frequently horrifying. Emphasis on education at all levels must be stressed so we can convert the skeptical and go forward into a new paradigm of radiation therapy.

Education is a multifaceted tool, essential for the professional growth of the radiation therapist. Education is comprised of two fundamental components: the conventional setting, which is composed of formal classroom learning at varying levels, and informal education, which consists of a large range of **life experiences.** Life experiences can be described as bits of information extracted from normal activities that collectively enhance an existing knowledge base. Using the basic concepts of traditional education as a foundation, life experiences play significant roles as a continuing education (CE) tool by expanding and refining rudimentary education. Life experiences are critical to the day-to-day activities of the radiation therapist because they are presently one of the best resources available to keep up with rapidly changing technology. The cumulative effect of life experiences can be correlated with performance improvement.

Interactive education over the past decade has been amplified through the existence of the Internet, which has opened up an infinite pathway to sharing of ideas and the circulation of information. Easy access to the World Wide Web (WWW), which contains an indeterminable amount of information, has illuminated the concept of unconventional education and is an important factor in increasing the scope of knowledge for educators and pupils. This is a dichotomy for the radiation therapist because the Internet is both an advantage and a challenge. The Internet gives the radiation therapist the advantage of having fingertip access to scientific information while at the same time gives the patient similar access to information. It is therefore more important than ever that the radiation therapist keep current with facts regarding cancer, all aspects of radiation therapy, and other available treatment options and alternative medicine. It is also necessary for the radiation therapist to have an understanding of social and financial aspects attached to patients undergoing cancer treatments. The radiation therapist is now, more than ever, looked on as a resource for the patient and must be knowledgeable enough to reinforce, debate, correct, and/or expand information that the patient has gained over the Internet or from other sources.

The educational evolution of radiation sciences can be traced as far back as 1646 with the invention of the first particle vacuum.[18] The study of radiation science was further advanced in the late nineteenth century when Antoine Henri Becquerel discovered radioactivity. These discoveries opened the door for Marie and Pierre Curie who, in 1898, performed scientific research on radioactive materials. It was during this time that Wilhelm Roentgen made the exciting discovery of x-rays in 1895. The first therapeutic use of x-rays was in 1896 when Dr. Emil Herman Grubbe first applied them to a breast cancer patient.[11] Despite the early history, education in radiation therapy lagged for many decades, mainly because of a lack of specialty identification. Professionals working in the field of radiation oncology continued the endeavor for recognition and the field has now advanced scientifically to a point where it functions as an important part of the study and treatment of cancer. As radiation therapy emerged as an independent area of practice, the need for educated personnel became apparent and the evolution of the radiation therapist commenced.

There were approximately 22.6 million radiation therapy visits in the United States during the year 2000. The radiation therapist is a key member of the medical team of experts in the care of cancer patients; thus a need exists for the therapist to have a strong, varied, and current education. Radiation therapists are highly respected professionals and an integral part of the scientific community because they serve as an authority for the education of others. The subsequent discussion describes the educational background of the radiation therapist, credentialing agencies in radiation therapy, patient education, and community education including necessary issues in radiation oncology that the radiation therapist must be capable of addressing.

THE EVOLUTION OF THE RADIATION THERAPIST

In the United States, radiation therapy education has been "recognized as a separate discipline within radiologic technology since 1964, when the first certifying examination was administered by the American Registry of Radiologic Technologists (ARRT)."[9] The first set of essentials for a formal school of radiation therapy were adopted by the American College of Radiology (ACR), the American Society of Radiologic Technology (ASRT), and the American Medical Association (AMA) in 1968. The essentials applied only to 1-year programs because almost all students entering radiation therapy at that time were recruited from radiography and nursing. In 1972, the ACR, ASRT, and the AMA provided guidelines for the first 2-year programs by adopting essentials for programs with a minimum entrance requirement of a high school diploma.[9] The 1968 didactic essentials for the first 1-year programs are compared with the 2002 didactic guidelines in Box 9-1.

The first radiation therapy education programs in the United States were strongly influenced by the earlier growth of radiation therapy that took place in England. The Royal Marsden School of Therapeutic Radiography currently hosts a 3-year program for radiation therapy that opened in 1963 in conjunction with the faculty of health and social sciences/school of radiography of Kingston University. They presently offer graduates of the program a Bachelor of Science degree in therapeutic radiography. The program includes a four-part clinical education (Introduction to Practice, Application of Skills, Localization and Dosimetry, and Competence and Practice). The didactic program has many courses that mirror course curriculum in the United States, but they also offer courses in research methods and ethics, research, and social psychology in health care.

On the heels of the English, the first 2-year certificate programs in the United States were credentialed in the mid-1960s. Courses at that time were offered at Mt. Sinai Hospital in New York City and Roswell Park Memorial Institute in Buffalo, New York. The first associate degree program in radiation therapy was offered in 1967 at the Upstate Medical Center in Syracuse, New York.[24]

GOVERNING AGENCIES

Three main agencies are directly involved in establishing educational standards, professional credentialing and the exchange of professional information for the discipline of radiation therapy. They are the Joint Review Committee on Education in Radiologic Technology (JRCERT), ARRT, and ASRT.

The JRCERT has been responsible for the development and review of educational standards in radiologic sciences since 1944. Not until 1964, 20 years after its inception, did the JRCERT recognize radiation therapy as a science distinguishable from other radiologic sciences. In 1975 the JRCERT established a set of essentials that incorporated both 1- and 2-year certificate programs as well as associate and baccalaureate programs in radiation therapy.

Currently the U.S. Department of Education recognizes the JRCERT as the organization for accreditation of education programs for radiographers and radiation therapists in

Box 9-1	Essentials

1968 SCHOOL OF RADIATION THERAPY CURRICULUM	2002 RADIATION THERAPY CURRICULUM
Introduction to course	Orientation to radiation therapy technology
Physics	Medical ethics and law
Mathematics	Methods of patient care
Elementary pathology	Medical terminology
Radiobiology	Human structure and function
Anatomy	Oncology pathology
Treatment planning	Radiobiology
Nursing procedures	Mathematics for health science
Radiation therapy	Basic physics
Protection and shielding	Radiation therapy physics I-II
Ethics	Radiation protection
	Principles and practice of radiation therapy I
	Principles and practice of radiation therapy II
	Radiographic imaging
	Dosimetry and treatment planning
	Quality management
	Introduction to hyperthermia
	Computer applications
	New modalities

The curriculum for radiation therapy programs has been revised over the years to reflect an increase in the professional status of the therapist. The radiation therapist has emerged as a critical player on the radiation therapy team, which makes it essential that the educational background reflect the scientific expanse of radiation therapy.

the United States.[19] **Accreditation** is the process of credentialing a learning institution to create a new program and giving formal approval to the merits for continuation of an existing program. The accreditation process includes a microscopic review of a program by a group peers and a comparison of the critiqued data to standards set down by that agency. The primary objective is to assure the public that all accredited programs have attained a satisfactory level of performance with the ability to educate a radiation therapist with the highest level of competence.

The accreditation process includes a self-study that is completed by the program staff requesting accreditation. The report is then submitted to the JRCERT before the second step, which is a site visit.

The self-study is an all inclusive document that has six main divisions: (1) *sponsorship* (describes the institution or institutions supporting the program), (2) *resources* (includes specifics regarding the program director, clinical coordinator, clinical supervisor, medical director of the school, didactic staff members, clinical instructors, financial resources, physical resources, equipment, supplies, and the library), (3) *curriculum* (includes the didactic courses offered and the specifics of the competency-based clinical program, including quality assurance, simulation procedures, dosimetry, treatment procedures, patient care and management, and periodic evaluation of the students), (4) *students* (describes the admissions criteria, program, health standards, and

guidance available for students), (5) *operational policies* (describes fair policies and student records), and (6) *continuing program evaluation* (includes an ongoing internal review process).

The site visit is the on-site review by the accreditation staff of a newly proposed program or a program requesting renewal of accreditation. This visit serves two purposes: to examine the didactic program and the competency-based clinical program and to compare the reality of the setting with the previously submitted self-study.

The number of JRCERT-accredited programs has grown since the 1960s and as of August 1, 2001, the JRCERT recognized 69 active and 2 inactive programs. Of the active programs, there are 44 college/university-based programs (20 baccalaureate, 18 associate, and 6 certificate) and 25 hospital/medical center based programs (1 baccalaureate, and 24 certificate).

A student considering radiation oncology as a career path can select one of four educational options: (1) a baccalaureate degree program in radiation therapy (2) a college-based associate degree in radiation therapy, (3) a 2-year, hospital-based certificate program, and (4) a 1-year certificate program in radiation therapy offered to graduates of an accredited 2-year radiology technology program. All options afford the graduate an opportunity to become nationally registered and/or state licensed.

The American Registry of Radiologic Technologists is

responsible for the credentialing examination that allows the radiation therapist to become nationally certified. The ARRT has the objective of "encouraging the study and elevating the standards of radiologic technology, as well as the examining and certifying of eligible candidates and periodic publication of a listing of registrants."[3] The ARRT was formed in 1922 after the Radiologic Society of North America (RSNA) agreed that x-ray technicians needed an organization to monitor education standards. The RSNA and the American Roentgen Ray Society (ARRS) worked together to form the ARRT.[9] Currently, the governing board of the ARRT consists of a nine member Board of Trustees; five Trustees are appointed by the ASRT and four Trustees are physicians appointed by the American College of Radiology (ACR).[5] The ACR is the organization primarily responsible for radiologists, radiation oncologists, and clinical medical physicists in the United States and has the following goals: (1) improve service to patients; (2) advance the science of radiology; (3) study the socioeconomic aspects of the practice of radiology; and (4) encourage CE for radiologists, radiation oncologists, medical physicists, and persons practicing in allied professional fields.[2] The ACR took over the responsibilities relating to the ARRT from the RSNA in 1944. In 1962 the ARRT recognized radiation therapy as a separate discipline from radiology and initiated the first examination. The first year that graduates from a radiation therapy program satisfied the essentials for the examination was in 1964 when 108 candidates took the examination with a passing

rate of 81%. Fig. 9-1 shows that the number of first-time test takers has suffered a decline over the past 8 years but Fig. 9-2 shows that over the past 3 years the number appears to be increasing.[5] The decline can be attributed to and correlated with the decrease in the number of available radiation therapy programs. There are presently approximately 12,457 registered radiation therapists in the United States. The eligibility requirement for a student to take the registry examination is the satisfactory completion of a formal radiation therapy course in a JRCERT-accredited program or equivalent institution. The equivalent institutions in radiation therapy are programs that fall under a category called "Regional or Institutional Accreditation." The candidate must complete both the didactic courses and clinical competencies at an acceptable level to be eligible for certification. Specific clinical competencies are stipulated by the ARRT and satisfactory completion is indicated by the program director's signature. A detailed list of the competencies can be found on the ARRT web site (www.arrt.org). All eligibility venues for ARRT certification for foreign educated therapists can also be found on the site.

The registry examination is now administered via computer. An eligible candidate must have completed the application process and, once approved, may take the examination on his or her time schedule. The first examination is set inside a 90-day window from the time of application approval; however, this window may be extended by the student as needed. Examinees can take the test at virtually any time after eligibility is established, not just at three set times. The examination is available in 400 test centers in 250 cities across the country and in five United States territories and

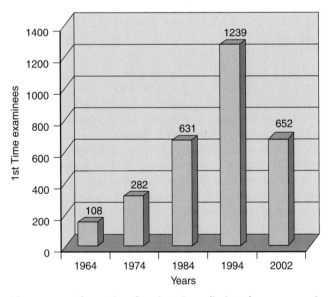

Figure 9-1. The national registry in radiation therapy experienced a 91.3% growth in the number of applicants accepted to take the registry examination over a 30-year period. The inaugural examination was given in 1964 with sequential examinations showing a steady and continuing increase up to the examination in 1994. The most alarming trend has been the enormous decrease in first time examinees from 1994 to 2002.

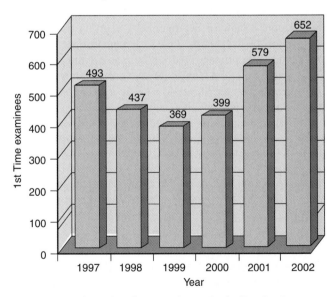

Figure 9-2. There has been a dramatic decline in the number of eligible students taking the radiation therapy certifying examination over the past 7 years, which can be correlated with the decreased number of radiation therapy programs. However, the number of first time examinees appears to be increasing over the past 3 years.

eight Canadian provinces. The ARRT examinations are also available internationally and can be taken in England, Germany, Italy, Japan, Korea, and Spain.[5] A policy was enacted in 1994 that limits the number of times that a candidate can fail the examination to three before he or she must show proof of remediation.

The core contents of the examination are continually updated and made available to program directors. The program directors can use this as a guide to update their curriculum. Changes made in the examination are instituted to reflect the evolving needs of the radiation therapist and the advancement in the field of radiation therapy.

Candidates who successfully complete the ARRT examination are awarded certification, which is renewable every 2 years. The renewal is based on the mandatory completion of CE credits. The 2-year cycle (biennium) starts on the birth date of the individual radiation therapist. The new graduate does not start the CE biennium cycle until the birth month of the second year postexamination. There is a minimum requirement of 24 CE credits, which must be completed for renewal. CE credits are defined as Category A and Category B. Of the 24 credits a minimum of 12 must be Category A and the remaining may be Category A or B. The distinction between A and B is based on the review process. A course must be reviewed and accepted by the recognized continuing education evaluation mechanism (RCEEM) (a quality control mechanism) or an organization approved by the RCEEM to be eligible for CE credit. The ARRT has defined an acceptable continuation activity as follows: "the learning activity must be planned, organized and administered to enhance the knowledge and skills underlying the professional performance that a technologist provide services to patients, the public, or the medical profession."[6] Credits are counted as 1 hour of activity equals 1 CE. Cardiopulmonary resuscitation (CPR) basic life support courses are awarded 3 Category A credits. It is the responsibility of the radiation therapist to satisfy their individual CE requirements. Any radiation therapist who does not meet the mandatory 24 CE credits is placed on "CE probation," which will be indicated on the credentialing card. Probationary status can be lifted by completing the missing number of credits to attain 24 credits as well as penalty credits.

The ASRT is a national organization that encompasses radiographers, radiation therapists, nuclear medicine technologists, and sonographers. The society originated in Chicago in October 1926 as the American Association of Radiologic Technicians (AART) and underwent a name change in 1930 to the American Society of Radiographers because of the possibility of confusion over the acronyms AART and ARRT. The society changed its name yet again in 1934 and was called the American Society of X-Ray Technicians (ASXT); and in July of 1963 the society changed its name once more to the present name, the ASRT. The final name change was meant to signify the professional status of the technologist and eliminate the connotation of on-the-job training.[4]

The ASRT is organized around a seven-member board of directors made up of the Chairman of the Board (past president), President, President-Elect, Vice President, Secretary, Speaker, and Vice Speaker of the House of Delegates. The House of Delegates consists of representatives from every chapter and affiliate society.

The first journal that was published for members of the Society was in 1929 under the name *The X-Ray Technician*. Later the publication title was changed to reflect the new name of the society, thus the title *Radiologic Technology*.[11] The advent of radiation therapy evoked a new journal, *The Radiation Therapist*, which is primarily concerned with the science of radiation oncology and the technical aspects of radiation therapy.

An important organizational step occurred in 1966 when the president of the society, Leslie Wilson, stated that the society would attempt to restrict professional status to technologists graduating from a formal 2-year program. A major development in the profession occurred in 1981 when President Reagan signed the Consumer-Patient Radiation Health and Safety Act, which "established standards for accreditation of educational programs and for certification of those who administer ionizing radiation procedures."[4] The Consumer-Patient Radiation Health and Safety Act has been amended and is now known as the Consumer Assurance of Radiologic Excellence (CARE) Act. The CARE act requires the government to establish educational and credentialing standards for personnel who plan and deliver radiation therapy and perform all types of diagnostic imaging procedures except medical ultrasound.[17] The CARE act was introduced by Representative Rick Lazio into the United States House of Representatives on September 25, 2000 and defeated, but on March 13, 2001 it was reintroduced into the United States House of Representatives by Congresswoman Heather Wilson.

In 1984 the society added an educational foundation, which uses contributions for projects focused on strengthening educational programs. The ASRT gained more momentum in 1992 when it was able to gain a majority of representation on the board of the ARRT and the board of the JRCERT.[23] This majority ensures a major voice in setting standards of practice. The chapter system, which was created in 1993, allows for the creation of specific focus groups such as radiation therapy, management, and education. Keeping up with the times and needs of its members, the ASRT offers directed readings in every journal that can be used to satisfy the mandatory education. The directed readings are available on-line and can be summarily graded and recorded. The ASRT tracks CE credits and automatically transfers them to the ARRT.

The continuing growth and education of the radiation therapist is due to the enduring and cooperative effort of the JRCERT, ARRT, and the ASRT working for the improvement of health care of the oncology patient through an increase in the educational status and the clinical ability of the radiation therapist.

FUNDAMENTAL HEALTH EDUCATION

The continuum of education is so consequential to the growth of the radiation therapist that a review of present scientific findings as it relates to the fundamentals of learning is a requisite. Recently research has established a scientific link between brain function and educational methods through a clearer understanding of the brain. The brain is a complex network of axons, neurons (nerve cells), and synapses. Information travels into the neurons from axons and then passes between neurons through synapses. Synapses are added through learning or mental exercises, and blood vessels are added through physical exercises. Two types of memory that have been described: declarative memory, which includes the memory of facts, and nondeclarative (procedural), which influences the memory of skills. It is believed that the physical composition of the brain changes during learning exercises.[16]

The goal of education has shifted from a focus on the basic reading, writing, and arithmetic to teaching people to be problem solvers and thinkers so that they are able to extricate knowledge from one set of circumstances and use it to deal with a different set of circumstances. The new model of education does not replace or eliminate the necessity for a person to have a strong factual base. A strong and deep knowledge of a subject will actually improve problem solving by first understanding the problem and then using fundamentals to resolve issues. One important goal of education is the transfer of knowledge, which is only possible through the understanding as opposed to the memorization of information. Understanding that leads to transfer actually expands our knowledge and increases our chances of solving a greater number of problems. This process makes us independent thinkers and gives us the ability to use formal education in other areas of life.

Another factor that influences learning is the amount and type of preexisting knowledge that a person has. Preconceptions influence a person's ability to learn and understand so it is recommended that, before embarking on an educational project, educators have a clear understanding of the student's background. The educator must also know the basic demographics of their audience including culture, gender, age, language, and ability to learn.

The National Research Council has defined four learning environments: (1) learner centered, which builds on preexisting knowledge; (2) knowledge centered, which focuses on creating knowledgeable students with an ability to understand; (3) assessment centered, which relies on feedback including summative assessment relying on outcome-based measurements and formative assessment that critiques the teaching format; (4) community centered, which involves the community as part of the learning process.[16] This is important because students spend the least amount of time during a 24-hour period in a classroom and a greater amount of time interacting in and with the community.

Regardless of age, not all people have the same initiative to learn. Motivation and factors that affect motivation for people to want to learn is an important issue that must be addressed to improve education. Motivation to learn can be influenced by defining the usefulness of the information being learned and by how challenged the student is by the information. Motivation becomes a factor because many tasks related to education are time consuming and people must be committed enough to dedicate the necessary time to be educated.

EDUCATIONAL BACKGROUND OF THE RADIATION THERAPIST

The role of the radiation therapist was created as a result of a specific need in the medical community. The education of the radiation therapist evolved from on-the-job training to condensed 12-month courses to a comprehensive 24-month program to more advanced associate and baccalaureate degrees. A student in an accredited radiation therapy program will be educated in two separate areas that merge and complement each other. The schooling consists of a didactic section as outlined in the 2002 Standards and a competency-based clinical section. The didactic program is easy to construct and to evaluate. Students attend classes that are organized according to the Standards, examinations are administered, and grades are awarded. These are familiar tasks for students who at this point have a minimum education level of high school. The clinical program is more difficult to prepare because the student is entering an unfamiliar area in which everything is different and at first a complex puzzle. The clinical component must teach a student to coordinate cognitive (knowledge), affective (behavioral), and psychomotor (physical) domains and then apply problem solving and critical thinking to function effectively in the clinical setting.[7]

The clinical program is based on technical competencies that are divided, according to the complexity of a setup, between junior- and senior-level students. Objectives of the program must be clearly stated and competencies clearly defined. Students are evaluated with regard to specific tasks and graded according to their ability to accurately, precisely, and safely complete a particular task. The principle of an evaluation system for all programs is based on the adeptness and efficiency with which the student performs a task using suitable patient care techniques, age-specific competencies, and the required safety methods. The evaluation process also includes social, communicative, and ethical considerations between the student and patient and the student and therapist. The ARRT created a task-inventory list that outlines responsibilities of the radiation therapist. Individually, each item seems insignificant, but collectively the items create a masterful therapist. The clinical aspect of radiation therapy should always be strengthened by didactic portions of the program. The combination of cognitive powers and technical abilities helps to reinforce accuracy and reproducibility incumbent daily on the radiation therapist.

Presently the ASRT is considering a restructuring of the

present educational options by creating the "Education Master Plan" (EMP) that would create a multitiered educational system producing radiation therapists with a variety of skills. The entry level or staff radiation therapist would be at the lower rung of the ladder, whereas the advanced practice radiation therapist would be at the higher end of the ladder and hold a baccalaureate or possibly a master degree. The EMP would help create better career opportunities as well as improve educational preparation for the radiation therapist.

It has been suggested that the addition of liberal arts courses produce a significantly higher level of critical thinkers. This suggests that graduates of baccalaureate and master's degree programs are more likely to be better problem solvers and better able to handle skills needed to be good educators and communicators.[14] These are obviously important skills for a radiation therapist to possess. It may, however, be that those interested in educational programs that involve a significantly longer investment of time are those that are more motivated. As mentioned earlier, a deep understanding of a subject leads to better understanding of the subject and greater problem-solving abilities. By virtue of the willingness to invest in the additional time in higher educational programs it follows that their knowledge base is stronger and students have a better opportunity to gain desired skills.

RADIATION THERAPIST EDUCATION

The radiation therapist acts as an educational resource for a diverse group of people including radiation therapy students, other radiation therapists, radiation oncology residents, radiation therapy patients, and the community. As such they are considered "health educators," and, according to the health educators' code of ethics, their "ultimate responsibility is to educate people for the purpose of promoting, maintaining and improving individual, family, and community health."[10]

Education in radiation therapy must empower the practitioner and afford experiences that foster analytical and critical-thinking skills. Rote memorization and recounting of facts and figures provide a basis for task-oriented scopes of practice. However, in today's health care environment, the radiation therapist must be able to solve problems and function effectively as a health care team member. Outcome-based education is a desirable form of instruction giving a radiation therapist an awareness that resolution involves organized analytical decisions and judgments.

The prescriptive methods of early educational philosophies are currently being replaced by outcome-based methodologies. This approach offers educators and educational institutions flexibility in developing educational curricula that suit their individual resources and philosophies in achieving the final product, a well-rounded therapist who is able to think critically.[22] Long learning curves after the completion of the educational process are not acceptable with the rapidity in health care delivery changes. Instead, a radiation therapist must have an ability to relate diverse experiences encountered in practical clinical education settings to a broad knowledge base obtained during didactic and clinical courses. A variety of experiences provide the therapist with opportunities to develop practical problem-solving skills, which are essential in practice today. This is an example of how the principle of **transfer** is important and used in daily activities. It is the responsibility of the radiation therapy program director to ensure that the curriculum and educators take the time to give students a strong knowledge base that is increased through understanding of the subject and will lead to transfer of didactic information to the clinical setting. Radiation therapists who are able to think critically are open-minded and therefore capable of analyzing and evaluating situations. **Critical thinking** can be defined as the freedom to use the cognitive process to allow mastery of theory and practical experiences. Critical thinking incorporates the use of cognitive, affective, and psychomotor domains. The art of critical thinking helps the therapist question and critique each step of a patient's treatment, thereby ensuring an understanding and accurate administration of the treatment. The therapist must be able to understand the function of the treatment plan and relate it to the function of the available equipment to ensure feasibility. As a part of the radiation therapy team, the radiation therapist must have the ability to make clinical judgments, offer alternative treatment arrangements, and relate all of this to other members of the team.

The three domains of learning—cognitive, affective, and psychomotor (Fig. 9-3)—illustrate the importance of integration of facts, attitudes, and physical skills to create an expert radiation therapist. The student advances through various steps of each domain as he or she progresses through the radiation therapy program and begins to see the necessity for information fusion. On a basic level the students are asked to memorize information that will be a necessary foundation,

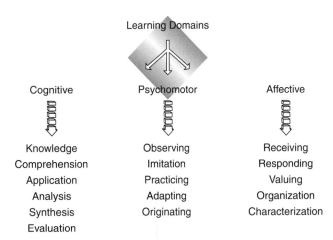

Figure 9-3. Representation of cognitive, affective, and psychomotor domains representing the three areas that must be combined to create a gifted radiation therapist. *(Data from ASRT Task Force on Educational Standards in Radiation Therapy. The Radiation Therapy Professional Curriculum. Copyright 1997 American Society of Radiological Technologists.)*

but on a higher level they must be able to use that basis to formulate relevant questions and make independent judgments.

Critical-thinking skills, such as reasoning and intuitiveness, give the therapist a knowledge base that allows a proactive approach to patient care. Higher thinking skills and diverse experiences allow the practitioner to anticipate problems. The evolution of education and educational standards that promote higher learning has greatly enhanced the effectiveness of today's practitioner.[21]

Educational Advancement

A student who has achieved the professional status of radiation therapist through completion of an accredited program and national certification by the ARRT will have several paths in his or her future to choose from. The student may first use the knowledge base and continue formal education to achieve an associate or baccalaureate degree if he or she graduated from a certificate program. This can be done in colleges during evening and weekend hours or can be done through distance learning. Distance learning has the advantage of offering a great variety of courses available with no time constraints, allowing daily work schedules to be uninterrupted. Distance learning has been facilitated with the addition and growth of the Internet. It allows easy transfer of information between the educator and student, and it provides interactive platforms for direct communication and participation of the student. Radiation therapists also have several career paths that they can follow. They may choose to further their education in the area of treatment planning and radiation physics toward a career as a medical dosimetrist or radiation physicist. Another career opportunity is in management and administration, which would necessitate the radiation therapist to continue education toward a baccalaureate or master's degree in hospital administration. Radiation therapists may elect to become educators in their own specialty. Teaching may include didactic courses, clinical competencies, or both and could eventually lead to a qualified individual becoming a program director or clinical coordinator. Some radiation therapists have chosen to pursue a medical degree and specialize in radiation oncology. One career path is for the radiation therapists to focus on the technology-based patient care area. This is an excellent choice in and of itself because clinical settings offer a variety of sophisticated technologies to work with and quality patient care is so important. The career choice is an individual one and need not be immediate because options are continually available. A new radiation therapist may take the opportunity to gain as much knowledge as possible during the clinical practice of radiation therapy over a period of several years before deciding to pursue a different career. A new graduate has a great deal of growth to achieve before becoming an accomplished radiation therapist and should benefit from all resources available. The therapist acts much the way an orbiting electron does, by interacting with various people including patients, colleagues, and physicians. As the electron does, so

the therapist goes through an endless process of absorbing useful information and participating in an infinite number of critical chain reactions.

PATIENT EDUCATION

The radiation therapist is expected to be an educator and a resource for the patient.

There is a distinction between patient teaching and patient education, which must be considered before embarking on an educational program. According to Einhorn that difference is that teaching is imparting information to have someone learn, whereas education is a plan that includes teaching, counseling, and behavior modification.[8] The education of the patient is an involved process, and, to make it effective, an educational model should be formulated including teaching, counseling, and behavior modification. All patients not being equal, several factors must be accounted for when creating an educational plan. This includes evaluation of the patient's physical and emotional condition; age; (refer to age-specific guidelines); and educational, cultural, religious, and social history. Once the program is constructed and implemented it must be assessed for effectiveness.[8] Program evaluation can be done verbally and/or through written questionnaires. Educational programs should be designed to address all aspects of cancer, including radiation therapy. Educational programs must be a multidisciplinary collaborative effort to meet the psychosocial, spiritual, dietary, and family needs of the patient. There are national programs arranged by the American Cancer Society (ACS), Cancer Care, and the National Cancer Institute that can be incorporated into a patient education program. They are large organizations that offer supportive care and educational resource for cancer patients. One example of this is a program called "Look Good Feel Good" that sets up meetings with women, supplies them with makeup, and uses this venue to bring patients together with similar concerns, allowing them to improve their emotional state by changing their physical condition. This is organized by the ACS. Hospitals have resources to fabricate and implement multidepartmental programs and make the information available to the public through printed brochures and/or on the Internet. Hospitals coordinate support groups and informational and educational programs that are focused on coping with cancer and grief. Churches and senior centers are examples of local groups that the patient can use as a resource for emotional and social support.

Patients in radiation therapy have special needs that must be defined and addressed. A diagnosis of cancer stirs many emotions including fear of the unknown, loss of control over life, and loss of dignity. In addition the patient is bombarded with information about medical treatment options that he or she is unfamiliar with and is expected in a short amount of time to select the destination. Once the patient has chosen radiation therapy as a treatment modality the goal of educational programs should be to ease the anxiety of the patient, to reinforce the need for continuation of treatments, and to guarantee continuous support both physical and emotional.

The advantage of living in a time of informational overflow is the job of gathering information to design an educational program is easy. Educational material includes printed pamphlets, videotapes, audiotapes, humor, music, newsletters, lectures, computer presentations, props, and web sites. One of the first steps when embarking on an educational project is to define the objective and the audience that will be helped in selection of the most productive methods and materials. The Internet is relatively a newcomer as an educational resource, but for patients that have access to computers there is invaluable information to be gained from it. One must caution that it is important to be selective when searching for information on the Internet and try to ensure that the information is accurate. Box 9-2 consists of some recommended web sites that may be useful to the radiation therapist and the patient.

The radiation therapist may not always be the direct source of education, but he or she must know enough basics to diagnose the patient's needs and direct the patient appropriately. Before the specifics about radiation therapy there are some basics that must be discussed with the patient. These include the Patient's Bill of Rights, which is at the core of patient care. The Patient's Bill of Rights is a tool that is available to the patient and the patient's family to help them retain control over life and define the decision-making process as a patient and help maintain the patient's dignity. The Patient's Bill of Rights is made available to the patient and the family in printed documents distributed to every patient, as well as displayed in prominent areas of the hospital. The Patient's Bill of Rights is listed in Box 9-3.

The Patient's Bill of Rights must be available in multiple languages that are appropriate for the patient population of the hospital. The language selections are made by using a mathematical analysis that is based on the acquisition of information from the U.S. Bureau of the Census regarding the demographics of the hospital's service area. Any non-English-speaking group that constitutes more than 1% of the patient population should have translator services and the Patient's Bill of Rights available in that group's language. An expert in communicating with the visually and hearing impaired should be available to relay the Patient's Bill of Rights to that population of patients.

PATIENT ADVOCATES

The patient **advocate** acts as a support mechanism for the patient and patient's family who believe that their rights have been violated and that the care is substandard. The patient representative is on the forefront of ensuring the patient's rights during a hospital visit. The role of the patient representative at The New York Methodist Hospital is defined as follows: "to assure that patients are provided with quality care given in a considerate, courteous and individualized manner without discrimination as to race, color, religion, sex,

---

Box 9-2	Recommended Internet Sites

The Internet is an excellent resource for comprehensive and fast access to cancer facts and figures. The Internet sites listed can be used as a reference for informational sources by both professional and lay persons.

http://www.radiotherapy.com
http://www.jrcert.org
http://www.asrt.org
http://www.arrt.org
http://www.oncolink.org
http://www.cancer.org
http://cancernet.nci.nih.gov
http://www.icare.org
http://www.cancercare.org
http://www.uihealthcare.com/depts/cancercenter/patients/publications
http://www.patientcenters.com
http://www.cancernet.co.uk
http://www.fda.gov/cder/cancer
http://www.mskcc.org
http://info.med.yale/edu
http://www.huntsmamcancer.org
http://www.bmi.net/mcaron/cancer.html
http://www.cancereducation.com/cancersyspagesnb/splash.cfm
http://www.cancerguide.org/online.html
http://www.icr.ac.uk/CAREINFO.htm
http://nlm.nih.gov
http://www4.ncbi.nlm.gov/Pubmed

These are some examples of web sites that are useful for both the radiation therapist and the oncology patient. There are many more sites that address specific cancers, and many hospitals have sites that can be explored for information regarding services and physician referrals. Doctors' backgrounds can be thoroughly checked. Finding sites is easily done through several search engines.

---

national origin, sexual orientation, or source of payment."[20] The patient representative assists the patient, family, and friends in understanding hospital policies and acts as an arbiter in cases of allegations of mismanaged health care and medical negligence. The patient representative may intervene in discussions regarding the signing of legal documents and activation of such documents as do not resuscitate (DNR) orders, health care proxy documents, and living wills.

A second group of hospital personnel, called social workers, has goals specifically focused on fulfilling the needs of patients. These needs change as the health status changes. The social worker intervenes when the needs of a patient lean toward psychosocial assessment, counseling, crisis intervention, financial problems, housing or home placement, home care, hospice arrangements, and support groups.[20] The social worker assists patients who are in some

Box 9-3	Patient's Bill of Rights

1. Understand and use these rights. If for any reason you do not understand or you need help, the hospital must provide assistance, including an interpreter.
2. Receive treatment without discrimination as to race, color, religion, sex, national origin, disability, sexual orientation, or source of payment.
3. Receive considerate and respectful care in a clean and safe environment free of unnecessary restraints.
4. Receive emergency care if you need it.
5. Be informed of the name and position of the doctor who will be in charge of your care in the hospital.
6. Know the names, positions, and functions of any hospital staff involved in your care and refuse their treatment, examination, or observation.
7. A no smoking room.
8. Receive complete information about your diagnosis, treatment, and prognosis.
9. Receive all the information that you need to give informed consent for any proposed procedure or treatment. This information shall include the possible risks and benefits of the procedure or treatment.
10. Receive all the information you need to give informed consent for an order not to resuscitate. You also have the right to designate an individual to give this consent for you if you are too ill to do so. If you would like additional information, please ask for a copy of the pamphlet "Do-Not-Resuscitate order—A Guide for Patients and Families."
11. Refuse treatment and be told what effect this may have on your health.
12. Refuse to take part in research. In deciding whether or not to participate, you have the right to a full explanation.
13. Privacy while in the hospital and confidentiality of all information and records regarding your care.
14. Participate in all decisions about your treatment and discharge from the hospital. The hospital must provide you with a written discharge plan and written description of how you can appeal your discharge.
15. Review your medical record without charge and obtain a copy of your medical record for which the hospital can charge a reasonable fee. You cannot be denied a copy solely because you cannot afford to pay.
16. Receive an itemized bill and explanation of all charges.
17. Complain without fear of reprisal about the care and services you are receiving and to have the hospital respond to you and, if you request it, a written response. If you are not satisfied with the hospital's response, you can complain to the New York State Health Department. The hospital must provide you with the Health Department telephone number.

The of Patient's Bill of Rights, as listed, is made available in accordance with the New York State Public Health Law and is distributed and posted in all public areas of the hospital in observance of this law.[4]

stage of recuperation from an illness or receiving treatment or at the end stage of life. Serving both inpatients and outpatients, the social worker assists the patient in applying for the most suitable financial resources. Patients who need continued outpatient services can be steered toward grants that can help pay for services such as home care assistance and transportation between the home and hospital. The social worker can assist the patient if family support is lacking and the patient's medical condition warrants admission to an adult care facility. They are also instrumental in arranging hospice care. In addition, the social worker can assist the family with necessary counseling about fears of unknown treatment and problems created by the interruption of daily life caused by an illness. The social worker is particularly important to oncology patients because this group of patients tends to have a great number and variety of needs. The National Association of Oncology Social Workers was formed to better fulfill the large scope of these needs.

The radiation therapist plays an important advocacy role for the oncology patient. The chances of a patient successfully completing a course of radiation therapy can be enhanced by the establishment of a strong patient-therapist relationship. The therapist can help create a comfortable environment for the patient by creating an atmosphere of mutual respect and understanding. The first step toward this is for therapists and patients to understand and use each component of the Patient's Bill of Rights as a framework for patient education in radiation therapy.

Communication

The first right with specific significance to the therapist-patient relationship relates to communication skills [12]:

> The patient has the right to understand and use these rights. If for any reason the patient does not understand or needs help, the hospital must provide assistance, including an interpreter.

Communication is a critical, basic skill that the therapist must possess. **Communication** is the art of transferring concrete and abstract information from one person to another. Humans communicate in two main ways: through verbal and nonverbal communication. Verbal communication uses utterances in such a way that a concept passes from one person to another with the same basic meaning. Nonverbal communication is a way to exchange mental images through body language using facial expressions, physical animation, or using written dialogue. The therapist must understand and use various forms of communication to enable appropriate interactions with the patient and enhance the patient-therapist bond.

The health care worker deals with such an array of people of different nationalities that verbal communication often yields to nonverbal communication as a matter of need. The health care worker can communicate in a variety of ways with a patient who does not speak English. The hospital may have a language roster enumerating different staff members who can translate different languages or each department may have direct access to translators through its own personnel. The AT&T language phone is a tool that can assist in communication by accessing translators for multiple languages and dialects over a phone line.

Patients who are hearing or speech impaired may need the support of staff members who are trained in the use of sign language and can also communicate through a relay teletype phone service. A means of written communication should be made easily accessible to the patient. A radiation therapist can also use nonverbal communication to express ideas to the hearing impaired.

Communication offers a way for patients to become involved in their own health care. Solid and honest communication can initiate and solidify a trusting interconnection between the radiation therapist and patient, thereby allowing treatment steps to proceed smoothly and effectively. Relationship formation is paramount, as is evident by the following tenet of the Patient's Bill of Rights[12]:

> The patient has the right to know the names, positions, and functions of any hospital staff members involved in the care and to refuse their treatment, examination, or observation.

The radiation therapist is only one in a line of personnel that the patient meets during the course of radiation therapy treatments. Members of the radiation therapy team include the radiation oncologist, radiation therapist, nurse oncologist, physicist, dosimetrist, dietitian, and others depending on the particular disease and needs of the patient.

Good communication skills must prevail, and all appropriate introductions between staff members and patients should be made at the earliest possible time. Patients have the right to question and understand the credentials of the professional team and they find comfort in knowing the educational background of radiation therapists and their credentials. The patient interacts with various people in the radiation department at different times. The nurse obtains basic information from the patient and explains the consultation process to the patient. The physician, attending or resident, obtains a history from the patient and examines reports and a variety of x-ray films or CT scans, magnetic resonance images (MRIs), and positron emission tomography (PET). The physician goes through a decision-making process and then discusses findings with the patient. The decision by a physician to treat with radiation alone or in combination with other modalities such as surgery, chemotherapy, hormones, or immunotherapy is given to the patient and family. The patient must make a determination and if the patient agrees to accept radiation as a treatment modality, the physician arranges a schedule for the patient to start the radiation therapy portion of the regimen. Now the patient becomes part of the radiation therapy family and from this point on the patient must be given clear instructions related to specific areas of treatment. This can come in the form of verbal and/or written instructions. The nurse may need to assist the patient with transportation arrangements to and from treatments. An initial assessment of the patient must be made by the physician, nurse, and therapist so that they may form a profile for outcome comparison during the treatment course. The Karnofsky scale is a standard assessment tool that is used throughout the medical community and will be helpful in determining the primary needs of the patient. The therapist, physicians, and nurse should have continuous interactions regarding the patient's care. A smaller department may be void of a nurse, dietitian, or social worker so those responsibilities will be transferred to the radiation therapist. The therapist is the single individual that the patient will interact with every day over several weeks of treatment. This makes the therapist the key player in observing and caring for the patient. The patient will rely on the radiation therapy team for complete disclosure of necessary information to deal with their cancer. This need is ensured in the following component of the Patient's Bill of Rights[12]:

> The patient has the right to receive complete information about the diagnosis, treatment, and prognosis.

This furnishes patients with the right to a clear understanding of the radiation treatment course that they are facing and the effects of the treatment. This prerogative is particularly important because radiation oncology patients need a clear depiction of the various steps that they will pass through during the treatment regimen, including a time line and a full explanation of diet and skin care and expected and unexpected reactions. The radiation oncologist carries the ultimate responsibility for the patient's care but they rely on the therapist as an independent, judgment-making professional to implement the radiation treatment and make continual evaluations of the patient. The patient usually starts the course of radiation treatments with a simulation. The therapist working in the simulator should know the patient's type of cancer, area to be treated, and general condition. This prepares the therapist for the amount and type of care the patient needs. This therapist is particularly important because they set the stage for the way the patient will view the department and forthcoming visits. The therapist should be compassionate, straightforward, and sincere with the explanation. The intervention of the family or friend may be required if the patient is unable to understand. Instructions should be simple and clear so that the patient does not need to use a complex thought process, which may cause confusion and distress. The patient should be told pertinent information about the simulation and treatment procedure. The therapist should allow the patient to ask questions and assess the patient's comprehension level. The therapist working in the simulator is the patient's first contact in the technical area and they must pave the way for the patient to be at ease and understand the treatment process. This initial therapist can help the patient begin to accept the reality of radiation therapy treatments. The simulation therapist will convey information to the patient that will be repeated and combined with additional facts by the treating therapist and supervisors during the course of treatment. The following are some examples of instructions and knowledge that is imperative for the patient:

1. Names of all personnel who will interact with the patient
2. The purpose of simulation
3. Specifics for the simulation and treatment (positioning, contours, contrast, rectal and vaginal markers)
4. The types of skin marks, including tattoos and skin care
5. Steps following simulation (treatment planning, verification simulations, treatment course)
6. Dietary recommendations
7. Explanation of the simulator and treatment machine (intercoms, monitors, gantry, lasers, blocks, wedges)
8. Expected and unexpected reactions
9. Setting of treatment schedules
10. Resources (transportation, translators, dietitians, social workers, support groups)
11. Define follow-up visits at treatment completion

The repetition of information from various members of the radiation therapy team is purposeful. It ensures the patient's full understanding regarding all aspects of the radiation therapy treatments needed for the patient to successfully complete the treatment course. This repetition is generally enhanced by the issuance of similar instructions by radiation oncologist, treating radiation therapist, and nurses. Repetition also eliminates the possibility for omissions of important information. The therapist should interact with the patient in a friendly and family-like manner while maintaining the professionalism necessary to gain the patient's respect and cooperation with instructions.

The daily interaction should foster a bond between the patient and therapist that helps gain the confidence and openness of the patient. This interaction allows the therapist to monitor firsthand the physical reactions and mental stability of the patient. The therapist has the duty of informing the relevant department personnel of any physical, psychologic, or mental changes in the patient. The therapist can assist the patient by describing various forms of available help, such as literature, videos, Internet, self-help support groups, social services, community education groups, financial support, and national groups that lend assistance through patient education such as the ACS and the National Cancer Institute. The therapist involvement in all aspects of the patient's care will create an important interdependence between the patient and therapist.

SOCIAL PERSPECTIVES RELATED TO THE RADIATION THERAPIST

The radiation therapy department is usually physically secluded from other departments and other hospital personnel because of the use of high-energy x-rays and the danger of unnecessary exposure to other personnel, patients, and visitors. By its nature, this seclusion affects the behavior of staff members and patients. For long periods of time the radiation therapy department becomes the home of the patient and staff members. The socialization and confinement process of a radiation therapy department can be described as a radiation therapy domain. The **radiation therapy domain** is defined by a limited physical environment in which a wide sample of strangers gather daily and create a miniature society. Social perspectives become an issue for the therapist because persons of a variety of ages, races, and nationalities all suffering from cancer coexist daily and must maintain harmonious interdependence. Many social interactions occur among clusters of patients and between patients and staff members illuminating the need for the following patient right[12]:

> The patient has the right to receive treatment without discrimination as to race, color, religion, sex, national origin, disability, sexual orientation, or source of payment. The patient has the right to receive considerate and respectful care in a clean and safe environment free of unnecessary restraints.

The professional commitment made by radiation therapists obligates them to fulfill this right, which is difficult as a result of the complexity of the patient population that has changed dramatically over the years. They tend to be smarter, better informed, and critical thinkers but less compliant to recommendations and requests. They demand suitable answers for their questions and they question everything. The problem that the therapist encounters is that even the most intelligent person is often unable to assimilate explanations and instructions while in a stressful situation. So answering questions does not always work to placate the patient.

Additional difficulties arise because the oncology population has decreased in age because of an emphasis on cancer education and detection. This young patient category has a set of special problems: family responsibilities, financial burdens, job obligations, and all other activities associated with being part of a household. These patients' needs (scheduling, child care, counseling, and others) must be accommodated to ensure patient compliance with treatment requirements and allow them an adequate quality of life. The protracted length of the treatment schedule makes it imperative that the radiation therapist gain the confidence of the patient technically and professionally.

The radiation oncology patient is scheduled for a series of treatments over a period of 2 to 8 weeks. The different interactions that are observable during this time are patient to patient, patient to therapist, patient's family to therapist, and patient's family to other patients and their family members. These interactions give patients a way to develop relationships (some lasting, some short term) with people who share similar circumstances. The patient may take this opportunity to extract information from others to acquire a knowledge base for the purpose of comparing personal treatment experiences and reactions to the disease. A variety of personalities emerge and people in the radiation therapy domain take on different roles. Family members and more capable patients become caregivers by helping less able patients. The freedom given to patients to fit into the radiation therapy domain as members of the extended family leaves them relaxed and amiable. This feeling allows for acceptance of the circumstances and often helps encourage patient compliance with treatment schedules and with adherence to necessary recommendations regarding care during various procedures. After patients experience this feeling of familiarity, they are able to set aside fears about daily treatments.

Radiation oncology departments are responsible for the patient's basic needs during treatment and should ensure some activities for the patient during the day. A television-viewing area with a videocassette recorder (VCR) may be set up for education or entertainment purposes, and reading material should be available. The patient should have access to a variety of refreshments (snacks, lunch, dinner). The department should provide available resources to accommodate patients by providing comfortable areas for relaxation. This becomes particularly important for a patient receiving multiple daily fractions of radiation. The fraction schedules vary, but in all situations the time the patient is in the department is substantially increased. These patients spend many hours interacting with radiation staff members and should be given special consideration for their circumstances.

The compliance of the patient to instructions and to treatment schedules is affected by the demeanor of the patient. Unfortunately, patients are not predictable. A competent therapist will individualize each situation by incorporating the peculiarities of each patient into the patient assessment looking at age, Karnofsky, and treatment objective (curative or palliative). Patients make their wishes for recovery known by complying with the treatment schedule. The attitude of patients and the social support they receive from family members and friends can affect the outcome of treatments. A patient who has a good physical and psychologic support system is better able to withstand the dehumanizing effects of the illness.

Patients begin a new learning experience when they are diagnosed with cancer. This diagnosis invariably creates an altered behavior pattern in the patient. The radiation therapist must be able to understand and help the patient through this transitional stage. Behavioral scientists have formulated many theories to explain human behavior. Abraham Maslow's theory, called the hierarchy of needs, bases all human behavior on needs.[13] This theory can be closely associated with stages that the patient passes through after a cancer diagnosis, and it can be a useful guide for the radiation therapist. The needs are divided into five categories: (1) physiologic, (2) safety, (3) socialization, (4) esteem, and (5) self-actualization. Theoretically, persons move consecutively from one category to the other and may at times revert back to a previous category, depending on their needs. Patients undergoing cancer therapy basically start from scratch on the hierarchy-of-needs chart. They must first fulfill physiologic

and safety needs by ensuring that the family receives care, financial problems are addressed, and housing needs are solidified. Then the patient can move to the category of socialization. During this stage, a patient may look for support and camaraderie from family and friends. Patients may seek people in similar situations to whom they can relate and on whom they can depend for social interaction. The next level on the hierarchy of needs is esteem. The patient looks for approval of the effect of the treatment from the physician and therapist to gain a feeling of empowerment over the disease. The last step in the needs theory is called self-actualization, the highest level of behavior. It is the most individualized of all the categories because its outcome depends on the personal aspirations and standards of the individual. Just as a musician must make music and an artist must paint, the radiation therapist must care for and accurately treat patients. This refers to their desire for fulfillment, namely, to become everything they are capable of becoming. Maslow indicated the belief that many people never reach this level because each time they approach it, they psychologically change their ideals. Therefore this level is unattainable for many. It may be unrealistic because it does not exist in a concrete form.

Legal Prerogatives of Patients

The factors in the Patient's Bill of Rights, which are important for the therapist to understand, clarify the patient's freedom to affect the outcome of treatment. This freedom applies to all aspects of patient care, including radiation therapy. The radiation therapist must learn to deal with the patient on various levels. The therapist can be properly prepared by becoming familiar with aspects of the health care system not directly related to radiation therapy but affecting the patient.

Patients have the legal right to affect the outcome of their treatment through the use of DNR orders, living wills, and health care proxies. It is the responsibility of the radiation therapy department (usually the nurse) to ensure that the patient is aware of the existence of these documents and that he or she has completed them. Although the radiation therapist may not be directly involved in the administration of these documents, awareness of them enhances the therapist's ability to respect the patient's wishes and offer some insight into the patient's circumstances.

The patient has the right to receive Do Not Resuscitate information.[12] A DNR order is a complex document, which, depending on the mental and physical capacities of the patient, can be signed by the patient, health care agent, or physician. A DNR order is a part of the Public Health Law and allows a legal avenue to withhold cardiopulmonary resuscitation in circumstances that warrant it if proper consent has been obtained. DNR policies may vary from hospital to hospital, and all personnel should familiarize themselves with the administrative directives regarding DNR as they relate to specific hospitals. The therapist should be aware of patients who have DNR orders signed to clearly understand the way to respond if the patient needs immediate and extreme medical care to sustain life.

The patient has the right to refuse treatment and be told what health effects this may have.[12] As long as they are of sound mind, patients have the complete and full authority on rights regarding decisions that affect their future. Family members' wishes, although they are important and should be respected, cannot override a patient's legitimate decisions. Patients may elect various means to express their wishes. A living will is one of the means by which people may take control over their future. A legal document may be completed at any time during the course of a lifetime. This document clearly states the wishes of the person initiating the will. A hospital must follow these wishes as long as the document is valid. The living will usually begins, "Being of sound mind, if I become incapacitated and there is no hope for my future recovery, I do not wish to be kept alive by extraordinary means."[20] This can be stated generally or more specifically by listing a variety of artificial means: cardiac resuscitation, respirator, tube feedings, and antibiotics. The living will may also include the refusal of life-sustaining treatment such as radiation therapy and chemotherapy. Many states have a standardized living will form that can be easily used; if this is not available, a legal document between the initiator and a lawyer may be created.

Persons may take affirmative action to ensure that their medical wishes are carried out by using a document called a health care proxy. A health care proxy is a legal document that appoints a person referred to as the health care agent, who may be a family member or friend. The health care agent is a legal appointee who has the authority to make critical decisions in the event that the initiator of the health care proxy becomes unable to make such decisions. The health care agent can make all medical decisions as they relate to treatment. The agent follows written instructions such as a living will and is obliged to follow the instructions in this document. In the absence of a living will the health care agent is bound to follow the moral and religious beliefs of the initiator of the proxy. This document may be written by a lawyer, or a standardized form can be used. Consideration should be given for early preparation of this document before its use may become necessary. A health care proxy is activated in the event that the initiator lacks the ability (mentally or physically) to make decisions regarding medical care. A health care agent is authorized to sign a consent form for radiation therapy on behalf of the patient.

These three documents allow patients to retain dignity during an illness by giving them responsibility for health care decisions.

Informed Consent

All documents, including those previously discussed, must be channeled through the proper personnel for signatures. The document called the consent form gives the patient the right to understand fully all tests or procedures that are part of the health care regimen and to accept or refuse them individually. The consent form protects the rights of the patient and integrity of the physician[12]:

> The patient has the right to receive all the information necessary to give informed consent for any proposed procedure or treatment. This information shall include the possible risks and benefits of the procedure or treatment.

The radiation oncologist has the full responsibility to explain to the patient all aspects of the radiation treatments, which include possible problematic conditions that can occur during the course of the treatment and late effects that can cause long-term complications. The explanation should include possible treatment options in combination with or separate from radiation therapy. The consent form can be written to be site-specific to ensure that pertinent information is given to the patient, or it may be presented in a more general form. The consent form may also request permission to take photographs during the course of the treatment. The consent form must be signed by the patient or appointed health care agent before the initiation of radiation therapy. The signature should be requested after the physician gives the patient or health care agent a complete disclosure of facts surrounding the radiation therapy treatments. The therapist at times may be asked to sign the consent form as a witness. In this situation the therapist should be a party to the discussion that takes place between the physician and patient or health care agent. If not witnessing the consent, the radiation therapist is responsible for ensuring that an appropriate consent form is completed before starting the course of radiation.

Clinical Research

Clinical research is an important activity, especially in academic departments that have residency-training programs. Clinical research usually entails treating patients according to a predetermined plan. Clinical studies offer the opportunity for eligible patients to be assigned to a particular study regimen according to random selection. Clinical trials may be conducted through national study groups or intramurally. The most prominent national study group for cancer-related trials is the Radiation Therapy Oncology Group (RTOG).

A clinical trial may compare existing treatments in different combinations or may compare new treatments or techniques with existing treatments. The goal of a clinical trial is to improve the patient's possibility of survival and quality of life through the discovery of more effective cancer treatments. Patients who meet the established requirements and agree to participate in clinical research are introduced to a component of the study called a protocol. A **protocol** is a specific regimen that dictates the type of treatment and manner in which it is administered to a patient. A protocol is divided into arms, which are specific formats of treatment. Patients are assigned randomly to participate in specific arms. This process is called **randomization.** There are no set number of arms per protocol; rather, the number depends on the objectives of the study. The process of randomized selection ensures that the patient's treatment-arm selection is chosen in a fair and equitable way. Patients may be informed about clinical trials from the primary physician, medical oncologist, or radiation oncologist. Information regarding trials can be acquired from physicians, community organizations, or professional organizations such as the National Cancer Institute. The patient has a right to a full disclosure of anticipated side effects and pros and cons of the treatment being offered through the protocol.

The Patient's Bill of Rights addresses the issue of clinical research and the prerogative the patient has in governing the selection of experimental treatments:

> The patient has the right to refuse to take part in research. In deciding whether or not to participate, the patient has the right to a full explanation.[12]

Patients who agree to participate in clinical research must sign an additional consent form specific to the protocol; however, this does not negate the patient's right to withdraw from the project anytime during the course of the treatment. The physician may also stop the treatment anytime during the course if the patient is not responding well to treatments.

The recruitment of many patients for clinical trials is important to ensure the participation of a substantial population of acceptable patients, make the trials meaningful, and increase the efficacy of future treatments. The therapist plays an important role in clinical research through the proper administration of radiation therapy. The treatment protocol is extremely specific regarding the patient's treatments, including describing the simulation, specifying exact areas that should and should not be treated, setting the daily and total treatment dose and number of fractions per day, and detailing any adjuvant therapy. The simulation and port films are sent for review to the coordinators of the trial and must comply with stipulations of the protocol. The therapist must ensure that all technical components of the protocol are followed precisely because any deviation can cause the department to be penalized and can jeopardize the validity of the study.

COMMUNITY EDUCATION

Addressing the education of the professional without also discussing the larger expanse of community education is impossible. Therapists can play an integral part in community education with their strong background in a variety of areas. The bill of rights written for the patient can be further expanded to be the bill of rights for the public. The public's right to be informed regarding cancer-risk reduction, the availability of cancer screenings, and various modalities of cancer therapy should be the objective of community education. Nearly 1.3 million new cancer cases are expected to be diagnosed in 2003, and almost 60% will be treated with radiation therapy for cure or palliation.[1]

Health education was defined by the Joint Committee on Health Education Terminology as the "continuum of learning which enables people, as individuals and as members of social structures, to voluntarily make decisions, modify behaviors and change social conditions in ways which are health enhancing"[15] Cancer is a disease that can often be linked to an active agent. Epidemiologic data have led to the belief that a number of many forms of cancers can be reduced through behavioral and environmental modification. The belief that the best offense is a good defense holds true in the world of medicine. The use of strong scientific data showing cause and effect to reduce the incidence of cancer is a good source for defensive ammunition. A decreased cancer incidence will reduce suffering and eventually benefit the society financially. Cancers that develop regardless of behavioral and environmental modification have a greater probability of eradication and better potential for control of the disease when the illness is diagnosed at an early stage. Human beings have the intellectual capability to make choices and therefore have the potential to reduce the risk of cancer or allow an early diagnosis. Humans can also exercise the privilege of an informed choice of therapy. The goal of an educated public is to allow selection of an aggressive and definitive course of treatment as early as possible after the diagnosis of a malignancy. The participation of the therapist in community education can be achieved through hospital-based programs, from programs in various freestanding institutions, and through professional organizations such as the ACS and National Cancer Institute.

The following are steps that should be followed to create an effective health education system:
1. Assess community needs
2. Identify and plan health education programs
3. Implement effective health education programs
4. Offer health education programs
5. Evaluate health education programs
6. Define health education needs and concerns

There are a number of models the radiation therapist can use as a template for creating health education programs. One very respected and most widely used model developed in 1980 is the PRECEDE model. PRECEDE is an acronym for predisposing, reinforcing, and enabling causes in educational diagnosis and evaluation. This model was update in 1991 to the PRECEDE/PROCEED model. PRECEDE is an acronym for predisposing, reinforcing, and enabling constructs in educational/environmental diagnosis and evaluation and PROCEED for policy, regulatory, and organizational constructs in educational and environmental development.[15] Other models include comprehensive health education model (CHEM), model for health education planning (MHEP), model for health education planning and resource development (MHEPRD), and generic health/fitness delivery system (GHFDS). Any of these models can serve as a tool for the radiation therapist to create a substantial foundation to create a health education program for cancer prevention and reduction.

Risk Reduction

Educating the public in cancer prevention is an untenable concept because cancer prevention is an idealistic and misleading term that is better defined as risk reduction. The term *cancer prevention* is misleading because it insinuates that measures capable of preventing cancer are available. *Risk reduction* is a more realistic term because it implies a greater chance of cancer prevention if people are willing to follow scientifically based advice. Risk reduction is one element of community education, the goal of which is to enlighten a large population.

Educating people in risk reduction is a twofold process: (1) to raise public awareness of a specific cause and effect and (2) to increase the awareness of primary care physicians and the public of recommendations for screening examinations made by nationally recognized cancer authorities such as the National Cancer Institute and ACS (Box 9-4). To be effective, the concept of risk reduction must reach a wide and varied population. This can be done by promoting cancer-risk reduction in existing groups, such as church meetings, Rotary clubs, Kiwanis clubs, parent-teacher organizations, groups helping homeless persons, and schools, or by setting up meetings to target a specified group of people.

Risk reduction can be targeted at different age-groups, starting with early childhood. Children may be trained to develop healthy eating habits, and teenagers may be taught specifically about the links between lifestyle (such as smoking and early sexual activity) and certain cancers (such as lung cancer and cancer of the uterine cervix). If children are educated during their most impressionable years to lead low-risk lifestyles, behavior modification may not be necessary when these children become adults. Pertinent areas of adult education include these risks and relevant aspects of early cancer detection and awareness. Community education includes the presentation of recommendations made by established professional organizations such as the ACS and National Cancer Institute. These organizations give fact-based information regarding screenings, follow-up examinations, and early warning signs of cancer and the way that they affect an early diagnosis of cancer.

Educational information can be disseminated through various forms: the routine verbal and written methods and

| Table 9-1 | American Cancer Society screening guidelines for early detection in asymptomatic people |

Test or Procedure*	Sex	Age	Frequency
Mammography	F	≥40	Annually
Clinical breast examination	F	20-39	Every 3 years
Clinical breast examination	F	≥40	Annually
Breast self-examination	F	≥20	Once a month
Prostate-specific antigen blood test (PSA)	M	≥50 for men expected to live at least 10 years	Annually
Prostate-specific antigen blood test (PSA)	M	≥45 for high-risk population	Annually
Digital rectal examination	M	≥50	Annually
Digital rectal examination	M	≥45 for high-risk population	Annually
Pap smear	F	≥18 or at inception of sexual activity, which ever comes first	Annually After 3 or more consecutive normal findings, the Pap smear may be done less frequently
Cervical examination	F	≥21 or at 3 yrs after inception of sexual activity, which ever comes first	Annually
Endometrial biopsy	F	35 with or at risk for hereditary nonpolyposis colon cancer (HNPCC)	Annually
Fecal occult blood test or flexible sigmoidoscopy	M, F	≥50	Annually or every 5 years
Fecal occult blood test and flexible sigmoidoscopy	M, F	≥50	Annually and every 5years
Colonoscopy	M, F	≥50	Every 10 years
Double-contrast barium enema	M, F	≥50	Every 5-10 years
Cancer-related check-up	M, F	20-39	Every 3 years
	M, F	≥40	Annually

Modified from American Cancer Society: *Cancer facts and figures—2003,* Atlanta, Ga, 2003, American Cancer Society.
*Screening examinations that are recommended by the American Cancer Society have been proved to have a direct relation to specific cancers. The aim of regular screening examinations is to increase the early detection of cancer.
F, Female; *M,* male.

newer methods such as videotapes and computer programs through the Internet, set up as patient information systems. These mediums can be combined to best meet the needs of a particular audience.

Community Screenings

Community screenings are another subdivision of the community education program. Cancer screenings are offered in the community through various hospital-based programs or community organizations. Organizations offer screenings based on the population they are serving, the means available to do the screenings, and the value of the examinations available. Screening programs are set up to offer the patient the appropriate physical examinations. They also offer an excellent forum for educating participants. The ACS approves of screening programs that are believed to have direct links to specific cancers and have an effective clinical or pathologic examination. The ACS's recommended screenings listed in Table 9-1 can be timed to draw maximal attention by having screenings tied in with national awareness months. The primary awareness months are April (cancer), September (prostate cancer), and October (breast cancer). Community or hospital screening programs can take advantage of this national exposure as free advertisement to emphasize the critical nature of timely medical care and the importance of an informed population.

Screenings benefit individuals in the community and those persons involved in the examinations. Screenings are offered free of charge and are usually run by volunteers. These volunteers include physicians, nurses, technologists, radiation therapists, and lay persons. The hospital or community organization that runs screenings and educational programs can raise money through grants established by professional organizations or from the government, or it can receive from the public through various types of fundraisers. Fund raising is sometimes an unpleasant and difficult task; however, it is necessary if medical awareness is to continue in an organized and constructive fashion in the community.

The radiation therapist can become involved in screening programs as part of the educational segment or can serve various other functions such as registering patients or assisting other professionals in preparation for the examination of the patient. The involvement of the radiation therapist in community screenings is yet another learning experience and gives the therapist a different perspective regarding care of the patient with cancer.

THE FUTURE OF THE RADIATION THERAPIST

The advancement of education and technology in radiation oncology is the responsibility of each successive generation of radiation therapists. Conceptually, the idea is to avoid complacency and pursue refinement and scientific advancement in the field of radiation therapy. This pursuit can be an individual or collaborative effort. The objective is to have radiation therapists with a strong scientific interest and thorough knowledge of job requirements. The therapist should be familiar with multiple facets of radiation therapy that directly or indirectly affect the role of the radiation therapist and how it relates to patient care. The ability of the therapist to excel in numerous areas and have an effect on their own future increases motivation and self-confidence. Radiation therapists who have a high opinion of their professional status are particularly inclined to play a direct, important role in the future direction and enrichment of the science of radiation therapy.

Review Questions

Multiple Choice

1. The _____ serves as a quality control mechanism to review and accept courses suitable for continuing education credits.
   a. ARRT
   b. RCEEM
   c. JRCERT
   d. ASRT

2. The brain is a complex network of _____, _____, and _____.
   a. Axons, neurons, synapses
   b. Grey matter, white matter, ventricles
   c. Cerebellum, cerebrum, pons
   d. Frontal lobe, parietal lobe, brainstem

3. The Consumer Assurance of Radiologic Excellence (CARE) Act establishes _____ and _____ standards for personnel who deliver radiation therapy and perform all types of diagnostic imaging procedures with the exception of ultrasound.
   a. Allowable radiation exposure, machine
   b. Environmental, air quality
   c. Educational, credentialing standards
   d. Patient care, age-specific criteria

4. The ARRT card will indicate "_____" for any radiation therapist who does not complete the required CE credits in a timely fashion.
   a. Not eligible
   b. No license renewal
   c. Delinquent CE
   d. Probationary status

5. One very respected model for creating health education programs developed in 1980 is the _____ and in 1991 it was updated to the _____ model.
   a. MHEP; MHEPRD
   b. PRECEDE; PRECEDE/PROCEED
   c. PRECEDE; PROCEED
   d. CHEM; GHFDS

6. Radiation therapy education was recognized as a separate discipline from radiography in _____.
   a. 1974
   b. 1964
   c. 1954
   d. 1970

7. The three main agencies responsible for governing the discipline of radiation therapy are _____, _____, and _____.
   a. AMA, JRCERT, ARRT
   b. ASRT, ARRT, AMA
   c. ARRT, JRCERT, ASRT
   d. ACR, AMA, ARRT

8. The radiation therapist plays the role of a/an _____ for the patient.
   a. Friend
   b. Therapist
   c. Social worker
   d. Advocate

9. The American Cancer Society gives credence to particular screening programs that are based on _____.
   I.   An effective clinical pathologic examination
   II.   The availability of doctors
   III. A direct link to specific cancers
   IV.   Cancer awareness months
   a. I and II
   b. I and III
   c. I and IV
   d. II and III

10. What steps are necessary to create an effective health education system?
    a. Assess community needs
    b. Evaluate health education programs
    c. Define health education needs and concerns
    d. All of the above

Questions to Ponder

1. Describe different ways that you can participate in professional organizations and how your participation can have a positive effect on your career and professionalism.
2. Discuss the importance of continuing education for the radiation therapist.

REFERENCES

1. American Cancer Society: *Cancer facts and figures—2003,* Atlanta, Ga, 2003, American Cancer Society.
2. American College of Radiology. *About the ACR: ACR governing structure,* Available at http://www.acr.org (Accessed September 10, 2001).
3. The American Registry of Radiologic Technologists: *ARRT educators handbook,* Mendota Heights, 1990, The American Registry of Radiologic Technologists, St. Paul, MN
4. The American Society of Radiologic Technologists: *The American Society of Radiologic Technologists historical background sketch,* Albuquerque, NM, 1995, The American Society of Radiologic Technologists.
5. The American Registry of Radiologic Technologists: Annual report to registered Technologists, April 2002. The American Registry of Radiologic Technologists, St. Paul, MN.
6. The American Registry of Radiologic Technologists: *Continuing education,* Available at http://www.arrt.org (Accessed September 3, 2001).
7. Clarke J, Biddle A: *Teaching critical thinking,* Englewood Cliffs, NJ, 1993, Prentice-Hall.
8. Einhorn C: *Steps of patient education,* Oncolink, University of Pennsylvania Cancer Center, Available at http://www.oncolink.upenn.edu/psychosocial/caregiver/pat (Accessed August 18, 2001.)
9. Fay M, Herda ML, Huffer BL et al: *JRCERT handbook for educational programs,* Chicago, 1991, The Joint Review Commission on Education in Radiologic Technology.
10. Gilbert GG, Sawyer RG: *Health education: creating strategies for school community health,* ed 2, Boston, 2000, Jones and Bartlett.
11. Grigg ERN: *The trail of the invisible light,* Springfield, Ill, 1995, Charles C Thomas.
12. Health Care Association of New York State: *Your rights as a hospital patient,* 1994.
13. Hersey P, Blanchard KH: *Management of organizational behavior,* ed 5, Englewood Cliffs, NJ, 1988, Prentice-Hall.
14. Leaver D: Advancing radiation therapy education and practice, *Radiat Ther* 9:80-96, 2000.
15. McKenzie JF, Jurs JL: *Planning, implementing, and evaluating health promotion programs,* New York, 1993, Macmillan.
16. National Research Council: *How people learn: brain, mind, experience, and school,* expanded ed, Washington, DC, 2000, National Academy Press.
17. Press Room: Care Act introduced in Congress, Available at http://www.asrt.org/other categories/press_room/care_act_pressrelease (Accessed September 15, 2001).
18. Rafla S, Rotman M: *Introduction to radiotherapy,* St. Louis, 1974, Mosby.
19. Standards for an Accredited Educational Program in Radiologic Sciences—Revised 2001, Available at http://www.jrcert.org (Accessed August 2, 2001).
20. The New York Methodist Hospital: Policies and procedures, revised July 1994, policy #762-056, revised October 1992, policy #762-027, revised July 1994, policy #762-091, revised June 1992, policy #762-064, revised March 1994, policy #762-111, revised May 1994.
21. Washington CM: Multiskilling, critical thinking and the radiation therapist: changing paradigms in education, Prepared for Varian's fifteenth user's meeting, The new journey begins, Session IV: the importance of investing in education in the new health care environment, document of proceedings published by Varian Associates, Inc, Palo Alto, California, May 1995.
22. Washington CM: Profession undergoing change, prepared for Education Consensus Conference, *Radiography: the second century,* document of proceedings published by the American Society of Radiologic Technologists, Albuquerque, NM, July 1995.
23. Wavelength: ARRT majority representation, *Wavelength* 3:1, 9, 1992.
24. X-ray Technology Bulletin: Update medical center offering degree course in therapy technology, *X-Ray Tech Bull* p. 3, 1967.

Infection Control In Radiation Oncology Facilities

Lana Havron Bass

Outline

Key Terms

Antibodies
Antigen
Autoclaves
Carrier
Colonization
Convalescence
Droplet nuclei
Epidemiology
Fomite
Immune serum globulin

Incubation
Mantoux tuberculin skin test
Nosocomial
Pathogenicity
Recombinant deoxyribonucleic
  acid
Skin squames
Titers
Vector
Virulence

The concept of trying to control infectious disease in medical settings has a relatively long history and is associated with famous names such as Florence Nightingale and Joseph Lister. The focus remains the same today; that is, health care workers (HCWs) promote the surveillance, control, and prevention of infectious disease. This chapter emphasizes measures taken to protect the HCW, patient, and public. Also, regulatory agencies and legal aspects of infection control are briefly discussed.

DEFINITIONS

In the hospital setting the epidemiology department is responsible for infection control. The term *epidemiology* is historically related to the study of epidemics, such as the bubonic plague of the Middle Ages.[101] Today, **epidemiology** may be defined as the study of the distribution and determinants of diseases and injuries in human populations. To familiarize oneself with terminology pertinent to epidemiology, the following definitions need to be reviewed.

Infection involves the reproduction of microorganisms in the human body. *Disease* is the collective term used to describe related clinical signs and symptoms associated with an infectious agent or unknown etiology. A person who becomes infected typically develops specific clinical signs and symptoms that can be detected externally, and the body initiates an immune response internally. If a person develops an infection but has no clinically observable signs or symptoms, the infection is referred to as a *subclinical infection.* It is important to note that a subclinical infection does initiate an immune response within the body. Another type of infection, which does not provoke an immune response, is known as colonization. **Colonization** involves the reproduction of an infectious microorganism, but there is no interaction between the body and the microorganism that would result in a detectable immune response. The microorganism is simply present in or on the body and it is multiplying. A person who is colonized but not ill is known as a **carrier.** Carriers may be a source of infection on a short-term or even permanent basis.

The relevance of these sources of infection is that disease is disseminated not just by people who are obviously ill but also by those with subclinical infections and by those who are carriers. *Contamination* is defined as the presence of microorganisms on the body (commonly on hands) or on inanimate objects. It is the movement of people from one environment to another that spreads disease, either directly from the infected person or indirectly through the things that he or she comes in contact with. By understanding the factors associated with the development of disease and its dissemination, control and prevention measures can be initiated.

Workers in the health care environment are especially interested in nosocomial infections. The term **nosocomial** was traditionally used to describe infections that developed in the hospital or to describe infections that were acquired in the hospital but did not develop until after discharge. Today, "hospital" is too restrictive and has been expanded to include ambulatory care settings and other health care settings. Nosocomial infections may be acquired not only by patients, but also by HCWs and visitors. Infections caught before a hospital admission, but in which symptoms do not become apparent until after admission, are not nosocomial; they are community related rather than hospital related. The primary goal of the epidemiology department is to decrease all preventable nosocomial infections. The hospital epidemiology team continuously monitors the number of infections that occur and investigates any abnormal occurrence or frequency to determine if some action could have been taken to prevent the infection.

The Centers for Disease Control and Prevention (CDC), a federal governmental agency located in Atlanta, has been actively involved in helping hospital infection control personnel in investigating epidemics since the mid-1950s. Over time this nationwide cooperative approach of hospitals and the CDC has to the formulation of very useful standards and guidelines, changes in federal law, and many studies to monitor effectiveness of infection control measures. The CDC has estimated that the nationwide nosocomial infection rate is 5.7%.[61] Investigators of the CDC Study of the Efficacy of Nosocomial Infection Control (SENIC) project, conducted from 1974 to 1983, estimated that nearly 2.1 million nosocomial infections occurred annually, that the infections cost more than one billion dollars, and that they lead to 25,000 deaths each year.[58] Since the SENIC project, which focused on overall hospital infection rate, a move toward specific outcome objectives has been adopted as recommended by Joint Commission on Accreditation of Healthcare Organizations (JCAHO) standards issued since the 1990s.[73] This newer concept focuses on lowering the infection rate of something specific, for example, the number of infections in central venous catheters in patients receiving chemotherapy infusions. Regardless of the focus, what is important to remember is that 30% to 50% of nosocomial infections are preventable and are primarily caused by problems in patient care practices such as handwashing.[60] Also emerging in the early 1990s from the voluntary public hospital experience of developing guidelines for infection control and surveillance associated with the SCENIC project is a new, formal federal advisory CDC committee, the Hospital Infection Control Practices Advisory Committee.

When compared with hospital inpatients, most ambulatory care setting patients are not exposed to the shear number of invasive procedures or to the variety of medical devices that are known to pose significant infection risks. Time spent at an ambulatory care setting is usually limited and also serves as a factor in reducing risk of acquiring a nosocomial infection. Nosocomial risk is low in ambulatory care settings overall, but special settings such as radiation oncology merit special attention because it may be important to identify those patients whose compromised immune status place them in a high-risk group. Droplet spread of viral respiratory infections is especially dangerous to this high-risk group. These patients may benefit from reduced contact with other patients and visitors in the waiting room. It may even be prudent to consider permitting selected patients to bypass the office waiting room entirely.

INFECTION CYCLE

Infectious disease cannot occur without the presence of an infectious agent, or *pathogen,* which is any of a wide range of small, primitive life forms. Pathogens may exist as bacteria; viruses; fungi; protozoans; algae; or lesser known agents such as chlamydiae, rickettsiae, and prions[49] (Fig. 10-1). Of these, bacteria and viruses are most often the sources of nosocomial infections, with fungi next and rarely protozoa or the other forms.[13] Several terms are associated with a disease and the infectious agent. **Pathogenicity** describes the ability of an infectious agent to cause clinical disease. In other words, some agents readily cause clinical disease, whereas others may be present but not cause clinical disease. The term **virulence** describes the severity of a clinical disease and is typically expressed in terms of morbidity and mortality. *Dose* refers to the number of microorganisms; thus an *infective dose* is one in which enough microorganisms are present to elicit an infection. Microorganisms are also selective as to their host or the location at which they cause disease. The infectious agent may cause disease in animals but not humans, vice versa, or in both. This selectivity is known as *host specificity.*

To remain viable, all microorganisms require a source and a reservoir; these may be the same or different. The *reservoir* is where the microorganism lives and reproduces. For example, the polio viral reservoir is human, never animal, whereas the rabies viral reservoir can be human or animal. The place from which the microorganism comes is known as the *source.* From the source it moves to the host; this transfer from the source to the host may be direct or indirect. In the case of the common cold transmitted through a sneeze, the reservoir and source are the same. An example in which the reservoir and source are not the same is histoplasmosis, which is a fungal infection. In this situation a chicken can serve as the reservoir. The chicken's fecal droppings are deposited on soil and serve as the source. Then the wind carries the remains of the droppings, and a human inhales them. Another example might be a case of hepatitis A (HAV), in which the reservoir is a cafeteria cook who handles food. The food serves as the source of the infection.

A *host* is the person to whom the infectious agent is passed. Whether the host develops clinical disease depends on the body location at which the infectious agent is deposited and on the host's immune status and related defense mechanisms. If disease develops in the susceptible host, the host goes through three disease phases: incubation, clinical disease, and convalescence. **Incubation** is the time interval between exposure and the appearance of the first symptom. The clinical disease stage is the time interval in which a person exhibits clinical signs and symptoms. **Convalescence** is the stage of recovery from the illness. Depending on the specific disease, a person may be infectious to others during any or a combination of the three disease phases. In some diseases, such as hepatitis from hepatitis B virus (HBV), in which a chronic carrier state exists, a person who is apparently well can actually be disseminating disease. For disease to be passed to others, a *portal of exit* is necessary. Examples include the respiratory tract, gastrointestinal tract, blood, and skin.

After an exit portal is reached, transmission can take place. *Transmission* is defined as the movement of the infectious agent from the source to the host. *Transmission routes* vary from one disease to another. Five transmission routes are identified: *contact, droplet, common vehicle, airborne,* and *vectorborne.* Box 10-1 displays an outline of transmission routes. A specific disease may use one or more transmission modes.

Contact spread can be *direct or indirect.* Contact transmission is the most frequent and most important transmission route for the spread of nosocomial infections. In direct contact transmission, the susceptible host makes physical contact with the source of infection, either an infected or a colonized person. Person-to-person spread can occur through simple touching, for example, by helping a patient out of a

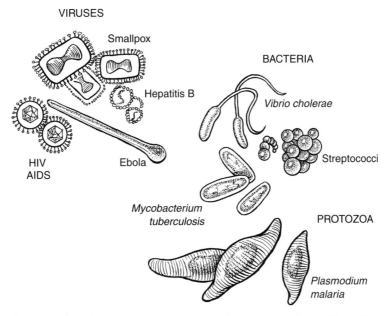

Figure 10-1. Microorganisms that cause disease come in a wide variety of shapes and sizes.

Box 10-1	Transmission Routes

	1. Contact
	    Direct
	    Indirect
	2. Droplet (large)
	3. Common vehicle (fomite)
	4. Airborne
	    Droplet nuclei
	    Dust particles
	    Skin squames
	5. Vectorborne

wheelchair and onto the treatment couch. Mononucleosis transmitted through kissing or acquired immunodeficiency syndrome (AIDS) spread through sexual intercourse also are examples of direct contact transmission. *Indirect contact* transmission involves an intervening object that is contaminated from contact with an infectious agent, which then comes into contact with another individual and results in a single infective episode. An example is a needlestick to a HCW after it has been used in a patient infected with human immunodeficiency virus (HIV).

Transmission by *droplet contact* involves the rapid transfer of the infectious agent through the air over short distances, such as in talking, coughing, or sneezing close to someone's face. The droplets consist of large, relatively heavy particles (larger than 5 mm in size) and thus are spread over short distances, typically 3 feet or less, and are deposited on the host's nasal mucosa, oral mucosa, and conjunctivae of the eye.[14] Rubella (also known as German measles or 3-day measles), colds, and influenza are commonly transmitted in this fashion. Suctioning of a patient with a head and neck cancer is another example of how large droplets can be created. Droplet contact involves large moist droplets and because of their weight they do not linger in the air for long periods of time; thus special air handling systems and ventilation are not required to prevent droplet transmission. Droplet contact transmission should not be confused with airborne transmission that is an entirely different transmission route.

Another route of transmission is common vehicle spread. This type of transmission involves a contaminated inanimate vehicle, known as a **fomite,** for transmission of the infectious agent to multiple persons. The number of people infected distinguishes this type of transmission from indirect contact, which involves the spread of infection to only one person. In common vehicle spread, all the people are infected from a common fomite. Fomites include food, water, medications, and medical equipment and supplies. An example of historical significance is blood that was contaminated with HIV or

HBV that went to several people before technology was developed to screen for the presence of these viruses.

Airborne transmission is spread that involves an infectious agent using the air as its means of dissemination and typically involves a long distance, which is described as typically 6 feet or greater or even up to miles away. These airborne pathogens are either the remains of droplets (5 mm or smaller in size) that have evaporated (**droplet nuclei**) or the infectious agent is contained in dust particles, or **skin squames** (the superficial skin cells). These infectious microorganisms may also remain in the air for hours or even days and may become inhaled by or deposited on a susceptible host within the same room or even miles away.[13]

Special air handling and ventilation are required to prevent airborne transmission when droplet nuclei are involved. Rubeola (measles) and varicella viruses (chicken pox and shingles) can be caught by a susceptible host just by being in the same room with an infected person. For these two infectious viral diseases, immune HCWs can safely care for infected patients; however, if susceptible HCWs must enter the room they should wear respiratory protection. Tuberculosis (TB) is also transmitted by droplet nuclei. TB has spread in hospitals because of air recirculation and low air-flow rate.[57] All HCWs need to wear respiratory protection in the presence of a known or suspected infectious pulmonary TB patient.[87]

A lesser known example is Legionnaire's disease, which can cause death. This acute bacterial disease is associated with air-conditioning cooling towers and evaporative condensers where the organism reproduces. Legionnaire's disease made the headlines again in 1994 when 1200 passengers were evacuated from a Royal Caribbean cruise ship. The pathogen was being carried throughout the ship through the air-conditioning system.[80]

Another airborne transmission route is that of skin squames. Our skin cells are always growing to replace aging cells that are located more superficially on our bodies and eventually sloughed off. If these sloughed skin cells are contaminated with a pathogen, they are capable of transmitting disease. In one study skin squames were found to be the cause of several outbreaks of streptococcal wound infections and were eventually traced to hospital staff personnel.[13]

Dust particles containing the infectious agent are another means of airborne transmission. One example is *Histoplasma capsulatum,* the infectious fungal agent of the disease histoplasmosis. This fungal agent grows as a mold in soil containing bird droppings, such as in a chicken coop or pigeon roost. On a windy day the dust containing the spores of this infectious fungal agent can be carried for miles to a susceptible host.[11]

In 2001, another airborne disease, anthrax, tragically made world headlines and took the life of a New York HCW and others. *Bacillus anthracis,* the infectious agent, is very resistant to adverse environmental conditions and disinfection and can remain viable in contaminated soil or on contaminated articles for many years.[11] Inhalation anthrax results from spore inhalation and there is no evidence of transmission by person to person contact. A cell-free vaccine containing the protective antigen is available from the CDC.[11] At present the number of vaccines is very limited, although measures are being taken to mass produce it for future widespread distribution if needed.

Vectorborne transmission involves a **vector** that transports an infectious agent to a host. An example of a vector is a fly that transports an infectious agent on its body or legs or an *Anopheles* mosquito that carries the malaria sporozoite, a protozoan parasite.[16] The malaria sporozoite enters the bloodstream of the human victim bitten by the mosquito. Other disease examples include Lyme disease and Rocky Mountain spotted fever, which are carried by ticks containing the infectious agent. Because mosquitoes, flies, rats, and other vermin are not commonly found in U.S. health care facilities, vectorborne transmission is not nearly as common as it is in other parts of the world.

To cause disease, the infectious agent must gain entrance to the body. The *entrance portal* can be through normal skin such as with leptospires or through broken skin such as with a needlestick in the transmission of HIV.[13] Agents also gain access through the respiratory system, gastrointestinal tract, urinary tract, or transplantation. Transmission of an infectious agent through these entry portals is also often associated with medications or equipment such as scopes or catheters. The complete cycle of infection is shown in Fig. 10-2.

DEFENSE MECHANISMS

Nonspecific Defense Mechanisms

To establish an infection, the pathogen must successfully get by the host's defense mechanisms. The human body comes equipped with a wide variety of nonspecific defense mechanisms. For example, skin serves as a mechanical barrier and contains secretions that have antibacterial qualities. The upper respiratory system is full of cilia that facilitate the removal of pathogens. If the cilia are not successful, mucus aids in catching and removing pathogens. The respiratory system also protects against invasion through its secretions and defensive white cells that engulf and destroy pathogens. The gastrointestinal and urinary tracts are acidic and thus serve as a hostile environment to possible invaders. Even tears exhibit antibacterial activity and aid in the removal of pathogens.

Other nonspecific defense mechanisms include local inflammatory action and genetic, hormonal, and nutritional factors. Personal hygiene and behavioral habits also influence the likelihood of developing disease. The age of a person also plays a role, with the extremely young and extremely old being most at risk. Alterations of any nonspecific defense mechanism through a skin break, surgery, chronic disease such as diabetes or immune deficiency disorders, or even medication to treat some diseases influence

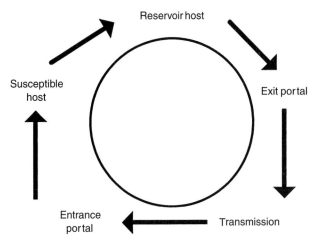

Figure 10-2. Diagram of the infection cycle. To stop disease, the cycle can be broken at any point.

the host's susceptibility by lowering resistance to infectious disease processes.

Specific Defense Mechanisms

Immunity plays a critical role in reducing host susceptibility. Immunity exists in two forms: natural and artificial. Box 10-2 displays an outline of the different types of immunity. *Natural immunity* develops as a result of having acquired a certain disease. For example, children who have had rubella will never have it again. This is a fairly general rule for most acute viral infections, and such immunity usually persists for the lifetime of the host. Natural immunity can also develop after subclinical disease, in which no readily apparent disease is observed. Unfortunately, all pathogens do not initiate lifelong immunity. Herpes simplex virus (cold sore) is a good example. After a herpes attack, the virus lies dormant until some event triggers another painful attack.

Artificial immunity can be further subdivided into active and passive immunity. Active immunization via vaccines against diphtheria, tetanus, and pertussis has been a mainstay of U.S. public health for many decades. Later, vaccines against poliomyelitis, measles, mumps, and rubella came

Box 10-2	Forms of Immunity

1. Natural immunity: active disease
2. Artificial immunity
   Active immunity: vaccine
   Passive immunity
      Maternal antibodies
      Antibody transferal to susceptible host

along. More recently, a vaccine against HBV was developed and must be offered to at-risk health care providers. Currently, immunologists have worked for two decades trying to develop an effective vaccine against HIV to curtail the worldwide AIDS epidemic. To date, several experimental vaccines have been developed, although their effectiveness has yet to be determined.

Vaccines come in several forms: killed, toxoid, and attenuated live vaccines. *Active immunization* consists of inoculation with the altered pathogen or its products. The vaccine serves as the **antigen** (foreign substance) and thereby triggers the human body's immune system to create **antibodies.** Antibodies are specific; they work only against a specific antigen. The physiologic basis of this specificity resides in the unique sequences of amino acids that makes a single antibody distinct from all other antibodies. T and B lymphocytes are the key white cells in the body's immune system. The immune response requires careful study and its complexity is beyond the scope of this chapter; however, it is well established that the B lymphocyte transforms itself into a plasma cell. Simply put, this cell is a highly active factory that synthesizes its own genetically unique type of antibody and sets it free into the body's fluids. The antibody then seeks the specific invading antigen. With some vaccines such as smallpox that were commonly administered in the past and hepatitis B used today, a booster is necessary after a period of time because the number of antibodies (**titers**) drops to a level insufficient to provide adequate protection.

Passive immunity, another form of artificial immunity, is defined as the transferal of protective antibodies from one host to a susceptible host. Examples include the administration of **immune serum globulin** (ISG) (e.g., a serum-containing antibody) for the prophylaxis of measles, tetanus, and HAV (infectious hepatitis). The transfer of maternal antibodies to the fetus through the placenta is another form of passive immunity. Other substances available for passive immunization include antiserum against rabies administered after animal bites and antibiotics in known contacts of cases of TB, gonorrhea, and syphilis. Although it protects the individual from the disease in most cases, passive immunization does not protect against infection nor does it prevent spread to others. Passive immunization typically has a short duration, usually several months at most, and thus active immunization is preferable whenever possible, such as in tetanus active vaccination.[13]

Environmental Factors Contributing to Nosocomial Disease

Environmental factors such as airflow, temperature, and humidity also influence links in the cycle of infection because they directly affect the pathogen and host. For example, measures directed at minimizing the risk of TB transmission within a hospital include the appropriate adjustment of airflow in designated rooms so that, in any high-risk area, negative pressure airflow occurs within the room. With the

recent increase of classic TB, AIDS-related TB, and antibiotic resistant strains of TB, the CDC has modified its guidelines. Hospitals are taking far greater protective measures to reduce the transmission of TB in the hospital environment.[28] Host susceptibility is also affected by environmental factors. For example, in winter, HCWs tend to stay indoors more often, with doors and windows tightly closed. The central heat tends to dry protective mucous membranes. This combination of reduced air circulation and dry membranes increases the risk of airborne diseases.

Many other environmental factors can contribute to nosocomial disease. A person may enjoy the comfort and beauty of carpets in a radiation oncology department, but carpeting greatly increases the microbial level when compared with linoleum-like surfaces.[3,96] The presence of carpet has little, if any, affect on the amount of bacteria in the air of the carpeted area, so if no contact is made with the carpet the risk of infection is negligible. However, carpets do present a greater infection risk to patients who use wheelchairs and pediatric patients who play or crawl on carpeted areas. Fresh flowers in water or in soil may enhance the beauty of surroundings but harbor a multitude of microorganisms such as spores and bacteria. For this reason, flowers and fruit are often banned as a theoretical risk from areas such as bone marrow transplant wards and intensive care units.[75] Following this philosophy, flowers and fruit should be banned from any area in which immunosuppression is a concern.

Laundry is a nosocomial concern after it has been used. HCWs should use caution in handling used laundry by making sure it is not vigorously shaken and never handling it without gloves if it is contaminated with blood or other body fluids. Fresh linen or paper should always be used for each patient.

Other items routinely used in radiation therapy should also be considered as possible infection control hazards. For instance, custom-made bite blocks should be disinfected between each use on a single patient and then dried and stored in a clean, closed container.[94] If a custom-made device is deemed unnecessary, disposable one-use-only bite blocks are commercially available. Also treatment tables and slide boards for transferring patients should be cleaned between each patient. Tattooing or placing permanent ink dots to identify treatment portals is a routine patient care procedure that presents risk to the radiation therapist as well as the patient. The ink bottle must be treated as if it was a sterile container. Each patient must be tattooed with a fresh syringe and needle. After being used, the needle should never be reintroduced to the ink container. Likewise, drawing ink into a syringe and then changing needles between the tattooing of patients is a dangerous and unacceptable technique. The major infection hazard associated with traditional tattooing supplies is the nonsterile ink reservoir. A welcome advance over traditional methods is a new tattooing device designed by a radiation therapist and being marketed as Steritatt. This device incorporates sterile, nontoxic ink that is contained in a sterile ink-dispensing pouch that looks somewhat like a mixture of an eyedropper and a syringe. This device is designed for single-patient use and thus is an ideal tool for tattooing from an infection control point of view.[84]

Ideally, bolus sheets should not be used on multiple patients. However, if bolus is to be reused, it must be wrapped in flexible plastic wrap to prevent the bolus material from being contaminated during use and then thoroughly disinfected before rewrapping for use on a subsequent patient. Another item often used on more than one patient is a pen or marker for drawing in a treatment port. If an item is contaminated by use on one patient, any harmful microorganisms can easily be spread to subsequent patients who need their treatment port markings reinforced. Some departments have solved this problem by issuing each patient a marker and placing it in a plastic, sealable bag that is kept with the patient's radiation treatment chart. The repeated use of marking pens and bolus would provide interesting data for epidemiologic studies.

To summarize, the best defense is a good offense. HCWs should take good care of their bodies to keep nonspecific defense mechanisms healthy, practice good personal hygiene and behavioral patterns, take advantage of active immunizations, and pay close attention to the work environment. Any strategy that workers can take to break a link in the cycle of infection helps protect not only themselves but also those for whom they care.

DRUG USE AND DRUG-RESISTANT MICROORGANISMS

Antibiotics have been in use for more than 50 years and have served as the main weapon in the medical world's arsenal against disease. Many of the once terrifying killer diseases have become mere health inconveniences that, if diagnosed early enough, can be cured with pills or injections. Not too long ago, some people envisioned a future free of infectious disease. Then things began to change. Mutated germs and emerging diseases such as AIDS and a mysterious respiratory illness caused by the Hanta virus, once unheard of, began making the media headlines.[69] This led to many questions about the origins of these new and resurgent diseases, and the reasons why antibiotics were not working as they once had. The answers to these questions require a review of the evolution of the use of antibiotics and other medications and a new understanding of the way that microorganisms function.

By changing their genetic makeup, microorganisms have found ways to resist the effects of medications. Many microorganisms have mutated and developed the ability to manufacture cell products that destroy the drugs that used to kill them[67,80] (Fig. 10-3). Mutations arise much faster in microorganisms than in humans because the time for a new generation to be created may be a matter of minutes compared with decades in humans. If in their relatively short evolutionary process mutations develop that are beneficial in the struggle to survive against medications, the mutants are

better suited to live and reproduce. Others have picked up protective genes from other microorganisms[70,80] (Fig. 10-3). People have also unwittingly helped in the development of drug-resistant microorganisms by not finishing prescribed medications and by demanding and receiving inappropriate antibiotics for illnesses. The tougher, remaining pathogens endure as the most fit to survive. Vaccines, like antibiotics, are challenged by mutating pathogens. This has been part of the problem in developing a successful vaccine for the continuously evolving HIV.

Because massive quantities of antibiotics and other drugs are used in medical settings, logic dictates that a large proportion of these new mutating pathogens are responsible for nosocomial infections. This causes great concern because the patients who are the sickest are also the poorest equipped to fight these "super infections." This is also alarming for HCWs and should serve as notice regarding the importance of the epidemiology department in helping to protect workers and their patients. The CDC's Hospital Infection Control Practices Advisory Committee has also been discussing approaches to control resistant microorganisms in hospitals.[26,27] Through stringent adherence to infection control protocols, nosocomial infections can be reduced, thus lowering the overall cost of health care.

HEALTH CARE FACILITY EPIDEMIOLOGY

The Hospital Infections Branch of the CDC was established to help hospitals deal with nosocomial infections. Today's hospitals are required to establish an epidemiology division if they wish to be accredited by and meet JCAHO standards.[74] Even in non-JCAHO-accredited facilities, state health departments or public health codes must be met for licensure, and requirements typically include some form of epidemiologic oversight.

State laws also govern the reporting of specific infectious diseases and the disposal of medical waste. In the past decade the Occupational Safety and Health Administration (OSHA) has focused its attention on health care facilities and the HCW more than ever before. In fact, OSHA mandated that employers of HCWs must offer the workers the HBV vaccine.[42] Although current mandates do not specifically address students, common sense suggests that students are also at risk and should be vaccinated. Today's HCW can expect to undergo an employment physical, an epidemiologically related health and safety orientation, ongoing in-services on a regular basis, and routinely offered health services such as TB testing and checking of disease-related titers.

Even hospital reimbursement by third-party payers such as Medicare or Blue Cross/Blue Shield is affected by a health care facility's attention to the quality of care and quality assessment (QA). This reimbursement association is influenced by external reviewers such as the Health Care Financing Administration. A staff radiation therapist, chief radiation therapist, or manager in a radiation oncology department can expect to participate at some level in the

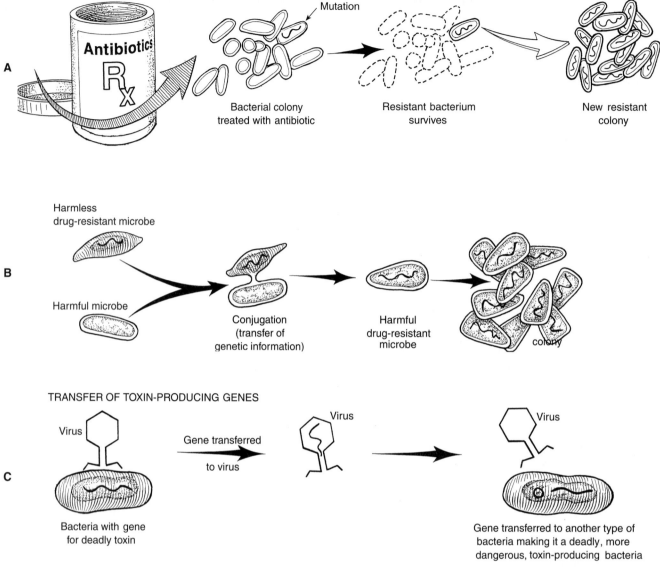

Figure 10-3. A, When antibiotics are used to treat a bacterial infection, most will die. However, mutated bacteria may survive and go on to produce more drug-resistant clones. **B,** The transfer of a drug-resistant gene from a harmless microbe to a harmful microbe through the conjugation process. **C,** A virus can carry a harmful trait to other types of bacteria, making them dangerous.

development or implementation of a QA or quality continuing improvement (QCI) program, with infection control being just one portion of the overall program.

PERSONNEL AND STUDENT HEALTH SERVICES AND PERTINENT INFECTIOUS DISEASES

The employee health clinic and the epidemiology division of a health care facility have a vested interest in their HCWs because the workers are at risk of exposure to infectious disease in the work place and the community. If workers develop an infection, they pose a risk to patients, coworkers, friends, and family members. Because of the nature of their chosen profession, HCWs have frequent and prolonged direct contact with patients who harbor a multitude of infectious agents; thus HCWs are at great risk of exposure.

A health placement evaluation should be completed for hiring or for a new student before contact is made with patients. Such an examination should determine that the potential HCW is able to perform the essential physical and mental functions of the position to ensure the safe and efficient performance of duties. The examination should also determine the worker's immunization status and medical history. A listing of recommended vaccines for HCWs is shown in Box 10-3. The following text highlights specific diseases that HCWs and their patients must be protected against.

HBV infection is the major infectious occupational hazard

Box 10-3	Recommended* Vaccines for Health Care Workers
Hepatitis B Influenza Measles Mumps Rubella Tetanus Pertussis Diphtheria Chickenpox	

*Should not be viewed as all-inclusive.

of HCWs. Its transmission occurs through contact with blood and body fluids. HBV is a highly transmissible virus, and evidence has shown that this potentially deadly virus can live on surfaces at room temperature for 7 days.[12] In response to HCWs' concerns, the Department of Labor, OSHA, and the Department of Health and Human Services issued a Joint Advisory Notice in 1987 and began the rule-making process to regulate HBV exposure.[44] In 1987 the CDC recommended that HCWs be vaccinated. The final rule proposed by OSHA was printed in the *Federal Register* on December 6, 1991, and mandated that the HBV vaccine be made available to all at-risk HCWs.[42] Workers should understand that the HBV vaccine protects only against hepatitis B, not hepatitis C, hepatitis D, hepatitis E, and so on, for which no vaccine is available at this time.[83] As with any rule, an implementation deadline is set; thus mandatory implementation did not occur until July 6, 1992.[42]

In the recent past, the CDC estimated that the total number of people infected annually in the United States with HBV was 280,000, with 8700 of these being HCWs. The annual CDC mortality rate for HCWs has been approximately 200.[42] Morbidity associated with HBV includes chronic hepatitis, which is highly associated with hepatocellular (liver) cancer and other types of progressive liver damage or associated complications such as liver failure and liver cirrhosis, both of which can lead to death.[17] In 1992, 5020 HCWs were infected. Of this number, 6 people died with acute cases and 300 developed chronic hepatitis.[83]

A safe HBV vaccine derived from human plasma became available in the United States in 1982 and is effective in producing an HBV antibody in most healthy, susceptible people. In 1987 a **recombinant deoxyribonucleic acid** (DNA) vaccine became available.[42] Both vaccines are remarkably free of side effects, the most common being soreness at the injection site.[92] The HBV vaccine is of no use in HBV carriers or individuals who are immune to HBV.[100] Postvaccinal testing should be performed 1 to 6 months after the three-part vaccination series to ascertain that immunity was conferred. Approximately 90% of healthy vaccinees develop protective

antibodies after the series of three injections.[91] With the HBV vaccine available by law to all at-risk HCWs, the morbidity and mortality rates in these workers will undoubtedly drop significantly.

Of increasing concern is the hepatitis C virus (HCV), which was identified in 1989.[2] As previously mentioned, no vaccine exists yet for HCV. Although the risks of transmission remain undefined, HCV appears to be transmitted not only through contact with blood and body fluids but also through household contact. Obviously, nosocomial and occupational exposure are of concern. Of particular importance is that HCV is associated with an extraordinarily high frequency of chronic infection leading to cirrhosis and primary hepatocellular carcinoma. The Food and Drug Administration (FDA) has recommended plasma screening for HCV since 1992.[2] Ongoing research should soon lead to the development of a vaccine.

Other diseases for which immunizations are recommended for HCWs are influenza, measles, mumps, rubella, pertussis, tetanus, and diphtheria. In diseases for which no vaccine is available or for which the HCW has not received a vaccine or does not respond to a vaccine, prompt prophylaxis is advised. Diseases included in this group are HAV, HBV, HCV, meningococcal disease, and rabies.

At the turn of the century, TB was one of the leading causes of death. As a result of improved housing and nutrition, TB decreased in frequency until 1985, at which time the decline leveled off. The primary transmission route is airborne droplet nuclei. The droplet nuclei are dispersed when people sneeze, cough, or talk. The risk of infection of a HCW depends on the number of droplet nuclei circulating in the air and the duration of time spent breathing the contaminated air. If exposed to TB, only about 10% of normal healthy individuals will actually develop the disease, half in the first 1 to 2 years after infection.[72] Around 1985, TB made a dramatic reappearance.[56] To a large degree, its emergence was related to the AIDS epidemic, increased immigration, and inadequate precautions being taken at health care facilities. In a study conducted at Parkland Memorial Hospital in Dallas, Texas, and published in 1989, one patient admitted to the hospital's emergency department in April 1983 contributed to the development of active TB in six employees and one other patient as well as positive conversion in at least 47 other employees.[57] Recirculation of air was deemed a major contributing factor in this specific transmission case. Based on the Parkland experience and CDC recommendations, many hospitals have redesigned air-flow systems, and the employee health clinics of such hospitals now make TB surveillance among HCWs a high-level priority.

Because of patient noncompliance with prescribed medications and lost follow-ups, multiple drug resistance (MDR) strains of TB developed. Even more frightening is the fact that the CDC has documented numerous cases of MDR TB in HCWs.[43] Some of these cases have resulted in death.[56] No effective vaccine exists for TB. The bacille Calmette-Guérin (BCG) vaccine, widely used outside the United States for several decades, confers varied and questionable degrees of protection, ranging from some degree of protection to no protection at all.[11] The CDC has issued several publications in recent years in response to the increase of TB. Titles include *Guideline for Infection Control in Hospital Personnel* (1983)[103]; *Guidelines for Preventing the Transmission of Tuberculosis in Health-care Settings, With Special Focus on HIV-Related Issues* (1990)[24]; *Guidelines for Preventing the Transmission of* Mycobacterium tuberculosis *in Health-care Facilities* (1994) and *TB Respiratory Protection Program in Health Care Facilities— Administrator's Guide* (1999).[34] Because these guidelines recommended special particulate respirators (face masks) to protect the HCW, it fell under federal laws implemented to protect workers and under the jurisdiction of OSHA. Jokes in the past about Darth Vader masks now had the ring of reality in the health care setting.

OSHA mandates that the minimum level of respiratory protection for TB will be a NIOSH certified N-95 half-mask respirator.[24,34,103] The National Institute for Occupational Safety and Health (NIOSH) is the governmental agency that actually assesses, recommends, and tests respirators for OSHA. The N-95 rating indicates that 95% of test particles will be stopped. OSHA also requires that HCWs who need to wear such masks be medically evaluated to wear them because of possible pulmonary- or cardiac-associated stresses on the user, receive training, and go through face fitting procedures.[24,34,103] It is important to note that simple surgical masks are not respirators and are not certified as such. Also of importance is that men with beards are precluded from using some of the NIOSH-approved masks because an adequate seal cannot be maintained.[24,34,103] Masks labeled N, R, or P meet CDC guidelines as do those that use hepatitis A (HEPA) filters and may be obtained with or without exhalation valves. Four main mask designs are available as described in Table 10-1.

TB screening should be part of the HCW's (or student's) initial evaluation and results should be read before the HCW has any direct contact with patients. For now, all new HCWs, including those with a history of BCG vaccination, should receive an intradermal **Mantoux tuberculin skin test** (purified protein derivative [PPD] of tuberculin) unless a previous positive reaction or completion of adequate therapy can be documented. The four-prong tine test is not recommended and has been deemed almost useless.[56] HCWs who document

Table 10-1	Types of OSHA and NIOSH approved respirators for protection against tuberculosis

DISPOSABLE PARTICULATE RESPIRATORS

Disposable, light weight
Negative-pressure design
Half mask or half mask with face splatter shield
Can be used in sterile field area if there is no exhalation valve

REPLACEABLE PARTICULATE FILTER RESPIRATORS

Half mask or half mask with face splatter shield
Reusable, with single or dual filters that are replaced
Negative-pressure design
Has to be disinfected and inspected
Cannot be used in sterile field area
Communication may be difficult
Also comes in full facepiece design which provides better seal and protection

POWERED AIR-PURIFYING RESPIRATORS (PAPRs)

Battery operated
Half or full facepiece designs
Has breathing tube and uses only HEPA filters
Usually more comfortable to wear and cooler
Easier to breathe
Cannot be used in sterile field area
Is not a true positive-pressure device, can be overbreathed when inhaling
Has to be disinfected and inspected
May be bulky and noisy
Communication may be difficult
Two types: tight fit and a loose fit, which does accommodate facial hair (beard)

POSITIVE-PRESSURE SUPPLIED-AIR RESPIRATORS

Uses compressed air from a stationary source delivered through a hose
Much more protective
Should be used when the other types do not provide adequate protection
Minimal breathing effort
Should not be worn during sterile procedures
Must be disinfected and inspected

Modified from Centers for Disease Control and Prevention: NIOSH TB respiratory protection program in health care facilities—administrator's guide, (DHHS Publication No. 99-143), Cincinnati, Ohio, 1999, National Institute for Occupational Safety and Health, HHS, CDC, pp vi-x, 1-37, 82-112.
HEPA, Hepatitis A; *NIOSH,* National Institute for Occupational Safety and Health; *OSHA,* Occupational Safety and Health Administration.

a positive history should be exempt from further screening unless they develop symptoms suggestive of TB. Periodic retesting of PPD-negative HCWs should be conducted to identify those who convert to positive. Current guidelines recommend at minimum an annual test for all HCWs and more frequent tests (as often as every 3 months) for those workers who are at high risk.[34] A positive screening Mantoux test is identified by a significant reaction, usually defined as 10 mm or more induration at the injection site, read 48 hours after injection.[17] Positive conversion is typically treated prophylactically with isoniazid (INH) for 6 months to 1 year with a monthly follow-up, whereas active TB is treated with at least two drugs such as INH, pyrazinamide (PZA), ethambutol (EMB), streptomycin (SM), or rifampin (RIF).[7]

All persons with a history of TB or positive TB test should be alerted that they are at risk of developing the disease in the future, even years later, and thus should promptly report any pulmonary symptoms. HCWs with active TB pose a risk to others and should be removed from work until adequate treatment is administered, cough has resolved, and sputum is free of bacilli in three consecutive smears.[88,92] In most infected workers or patients, respiratory secretions are no longer infectious 10 days after effective treatment.[92] Because of surveillance measures and changes in hospital practice the number of TB cases has been on the decrease since 1992 and the number of MDR TB has been declining since 1998.[31,34,,35]

With other diseases, infected HCWs should be removed from direct patient contact for variable time frames. These diseases include conjunctivitis, epidemic diarrhea, streptococcosis, HAV, herpes simplex of exposed skin areas such as the hands, measles, mumps, pertussis, rubella, rabies, *Staphylococcus aureus* skin lesions, and varicella zoster.

Of these diseases, varicella zoster virus (VZV) deserves special attention in a radiation oncology department. VZV is the pathogen that causes varicella zoster (chickenpox) and herpes zoster (shingles). VZV has an extremely high degree of communicability and is transmitted by the inhalation of small droplet nuclei or by direct contact with respiratory droplets or vesicle fluid.[59]

For children, chickenpox usually consists of a mild illness characterized by fever and a vesicular rash mainly on the body trunk. The rash may range from one or two vesicles to hundreds; thus extremely light or subclinical infections may go undiagnosed. The skin lesions appear in groups at different times, so late and early lesions can be seen at the same time. In adults, chickenpox is typically more severe and the risk of complications is higher. Infection early in pregnancy is associated with neonatal complications and congenital malformations. In cancer patients, chickenpox can be life threatening in children and adults as a result of an impaired immune system. If a cancer patient is exposed, varicella zoster immune globulin (VZIG) can be given to modify the disease.[19]

Shingles is a local manifestation of a recurrent, reactivated infection by the same virus. After a person has chickenpox, the VZV is thought to remain dormant in the cells of nerve root ganglia. Shingles usually is seen in middle age; however, children and even infants occasionally develop shingles. Lesions appear on the skin area supplied by the affected nerve. Clinically, especially in adults, pain and severe itching occurs and often lasts for long periods after the lesions have crusted over and healed. A significant number of transplant or cancer patients, especially those with leukemia, lymphoma, or AIDS-related cancers, develop shingles as a result of immunosuppression.[17]

Because VZV can be life threatening to cancer patients, HCWs, especially those in oncology or transplant departments, should have had documented varicella or should be able to show serologic evidence of immunity. Certainly only those workers who have a positive history should care for patients with VZV. If susceptible HCWs are exposed to persons with chickenpox or shingles, these workers should be considered potentially infective during the incubation period. They should be excluded from work beginning on the tenth day after exposure and remain away from patient contact for the maximum incubation period of varicella, which is 21 days.[19] Also, infected workers should not return to work until all lesions have dried and crusted, which is usually 6 days from the onset of the rash.[19] VZIG can be used after exposure in susceptible HCWs to lessen the severity of the disease if they develop it. If a worker receives VZIG after exposure, the incubation period is prolonged; thus the worker must be reassigned or furloughed for a longer time, typically 28 days after exposure.[19] A VZV vaccine has been available for many years outside the United States. In March of 1995 the FDA approved a vaccine by the trade name of Varivax for use in the United States.[10]

Viral respiratory infections are another major source of nosocomial infections. Although most people do not associate influenza specifically with the work environment, the issue should be addressed. Respiratory diseases, such as influenza, are associated with significant morbidity and mortality in older patients, patients with chronic underlying disease, and immunocompromised patients. In other words, patients of all ages seen in a radiation therapy department are at high risk for influenza and other respiratory viral infections.

Respiratory viruses are spread through three major transmission modes: (1) direct contact via large droplets over a short distance; (2) airborne transmission, consisting of small droplet nuclei that can travel long distances; and (3) self-inoculation after contact with contaminated materials (this usually involves the hands transferring the virus to the mucous membranes of the eye or nose).

The common cold, croup, and viral pneumonia are all examples of infections caused by the influenza virus. Influenza is spread mainly by the airborne route via small particle aerosol, thus explaining explosive seasonal outbreaks of the flu. Two major types of influenza are recognized: type A and type B.[11] These two types of influenza are among the most communicable diseases of humans. Shedding of the influenza virus from an infected individual usually lasts 5 to 7 days after the onset of symptoms.[45] Because of the constantly changing nature of these viruses, new subtypes appear at irregular intervals. This translates to the need to develop different influenza vaccinations that will be effective against new mutated subtypes. Prevention of winter influenza outbreaks consists of immunization programs initiated each year before the influenza season. Vaccination programs are typically aimed toward older persons, those with chronic disease states, those with respiratory diseases, and HCWs. Vaccine effectiveness ranges from 60% to 90%.[25] In persons not fully protected the vaccine appears to reduce the severity of symptoms. Adequate serologic response typically takes place a couple of weeks after vaccination.

Unfortunately, HCWs often do not take advantage of free or low-cost vaccinations offered by employers. The workers are apparently reluctant to participate because of misinformation regarding the influenza vaccine's effectiveness and side effects. Famous quotes such as, "The flu shot gave me the flu," and "Flu shots don't work," simply cannot be substantiated. On the other hand, substantial evidence supports the vaccine's effectiveness in preventing and decreasing morbidity.[25] The most commonly reported side effect is soreness at the injection site, which lasts less than 24 hours. Surely this temporary discomfort, which does not occur in all people, is better than a week's sick leave, possible loss of income, and the health risk imposed on patients who are far more likely to develop serious complications, including death. Perhaps with better educational programs, HCWs and the public would participate in greater numbers. In the event that an individual is not inoculated with the influenza vaccine, drugs such as amantadine and rimantadine are 70% to 90% effective in preventing influenza A to the same level of a vaccine or, if administered after the fact, in decreasing the length of illness.[29] Amantadine and rimantadine are not effective against influenza B.[29,86]

EVOLUTION OF ISOLATION PRACTICES

Nosocomial infections have been a serious problem ever since sick patients were placed together in a hospital and a long time before the term *nosocomial* came about. Even in biblical times the need to isolate or quarantine persons with leprosy was recognized. In the early part of this century, HCWs wore special gowns, washed their hands with disinfecting agents, disinfected contaminated equipment, and practiced a wide variety of isolation or quarantine measures to contain contagious diseases such as TB. In 1970 the CDC published its first guidelines for nosocomial infections and isolation techniques.[18] These guidelines recommended the use of seven isolation categories based on the routes of disease transmission. Because all diseases in a given category did not require the same degree of precautions, this approach, although simple to understand and apply, resulted in overisolation for many patients. Over the next decade, it became evident that although this approach helped prevent the spread of classical contagious diseases, it neither addressed new drug-resistant pathogens or new syndromes nor focused on nosocomial infections in special care departments. Thus in 1983 the CDC published new guidelines.[51] In this edition, many infections were moved or placed under new isolation categories. Three new categories were added: contact isolation, acid-fast bacilli (AFB) (another name for TB), and blood and body fluids. The protective isolation category was deleted. These significant changes encouraged the hospital's infection control committee to choose between category-specific and patient-specific isolation categories.

Universal Precautions

Then came AIDS. The onset of the HIV pandemic in the early 1980s drastically altered the way that HCWs practiced overall infection control procedures. For the first time, emphasis was focused on applying blood and body fluid precautions to all persons. According to this new infection control approach now known as *universal precautions* (UP), all human blood and certain body fluids were to be treated as if they were known to be infectious for HIV, HBV, or other bloodborne pathogens.[20-22] UP were intended to supplement rather than replace longstanding recommendations for the control of non-bloodborne pathogens. Although the old blood and body fluids isolation category was negated with the new concept, the earlier CDC category-specific or disease-specific isolation precautions remained intact. Later in 1988 the CDC published an expanded UP guideline that also addressed the prevention of needlesticks and the use of traditional gloves and gowns and that placed new emphasis on masks, eye protection, and other protective equipment and procedures.[21]

Body Substance Isolation

Another system, known as *body substance isolation* (BSI), was proposed in 1987 by two hospitals, one in Seattle and the other in San Diego.[82] As its name implied, BSI concentrated on the isolation of all body fluids for all patients through protective equipment such as gloves. BSI also addressed the transmission of non–body–fluid associated pathogens such as those transmitted exclusively or in part by airborne transmission. In the BSI system, if a patient had an airborne infectious agent, a "stop" sign was placed on the door of the patient's room with further instructions to check with the nurse's station. The decision regarding the type of protective action to be taken was based on the specific patient, with the informed decision being made by the professional practitioners in charge of that patient. Decisions were guided by CDC isolation category–specific or disease-specific recommendations.

Comparison of Universal Precautions and Body Substance Isolation

Overall, many aspects of BSI were identical or extremely similar to the UP concept. BSI differed from UP in that the focus of UP was placed primarily on blood and body fluids implicated in the spread of bloodborne pathogens, whereas BSI focused on the isolation of all moist body substances in all patients. In other words, the term *universal* referred to all patients not to all body fluids or all pathogens. UP did not apply to tears, sweat, saliva, feces, vomit, nasal secretions, or sputum unless visible blood was present.[20,21,23] On the other hand, BSI dealt with all body fluids. One major difference was the guideline for wearing gloves and washing hands. In the BSI system, handwashing was not required after removing gloves unless the glove's integrity had been broken and the hands were visibly soiled. This difference was interpreted by many as a disadvantage of using the BSI concept.

OSHA and Bloodborne Pathogens

On December 6, 1991, OSHA published "29 CFR Part 1910.1030-Occupational Exposure to Bloodborne Pathogens, Final Rule" in the *Federal Register*.[42] For historical perspective, it is interesting to note that this OSHA mandate began in 1986 when various labor unions representing HCWs petitioned OSHA to adopt standards to protect them from what they perceived as dangerous work conditions. Although previous CDC recommendations on UP were not enforceable because they were simply recommendations, the newly published rules and regulations of the U.S. Department of Labor and OSHA were enforceable in terms of occupational exposure. OSHA chose to adopt the UP concept rather than the BSI concept. Major details of these OSHA requirements implemented on July 6, 1992, are addressed in the following text.[42] In late 1999, OSHA published another mandate on enforcement procedures that established policies and provided clarification to ensure that uniform inspection procedures are followed when an OSHA inspection occurs to review records related to bloodborne pathogens.[102]

At minimum, UP must be followed precisely by all HCWs who are at risk of occupational exposure. Enforcement protects the HCW and those for whom they care. In addition, the medical facility can be faced with substantial fines and penalties for failure to comply with OSHA rules and regulations. OSHA requires that employers provide new HCWs with occupational-exposure training at no cost and during working hours before the initial assignment to tasks in which occupational exposure can take place. Employers must also make the hepatitis B vaccine available at no cost to the HCW within 10 working days of the initial assignment. If a HCW declines the hepatitis B vaccine, he or she is required to sign a waiver. If a HCW changes his or her mind later, the employer must make the vaccine available at that time. Annual in-service training of a HCW is required within 1 year of previous training.[42]

The components of UP and their required application under a medical facility's exposure control plan include engineering controls, work-practice controls, personal protective equipment, and housekeeping. Major highlights of OSHA's rules and regulations regarding bloodborne pathogens are shown in Box 10-4.

ISOLATION CHAOS LEADS TO A NEW ISOLATION GUIDELINE

The proponents of UP and BSI continued to argue their individual merits into the early 1990s. Some hospitals had incorporated parts or all of UP, some used parts or all of BSI, and others used various combinations. There was a lot of confusion about what precautions were needed for specific body fluids. Some hospitals stated they practiced UP but in reality were using BSI or vice versa. Hand washing, precautions for airborne and droplet transmission, and implementation of TB

Box 10-4	Major Highlights of the OSHA Rules and Regulations on Occupational Exposure to Bloodborne Pathogens

1. Gloves that meet the FDA standard for medical gloves should be worn in any patient-contact situation in which blood or other specified body fluid contact is possible. Other body fluids defined by OSHA are semen, cerebrospinal fluid, pericardial fluid, peritoneal fluid, pleural fluid, synovial fluid, amniotic fluid, saliva in dental procedures, vaginal secretions, any body fluid visibly contaminated with blood, and all body fluids in situations in which it is difficult or impossible to differentiate between body fluids. Other potentially hazardous materials include any unfixed tissue or organ from a human, cell or tissue cultures, and tissues from experimental animals infected with HIV or HBV. When touching any mucous membrane or broken skin surface, the person should wear gloves. The person should also wear gloves when handling any equipment or surface contaminated with blood or body fluid previously listed when performing any vascular or invasive procedure. Gloves should be changed after each patient and/or procedure. After the gloves are removed, the hands should be washed immediately.
2. Some people are allergic to regular gloves. If this is the case, the employer must provide hypoallergenic gloves, glove liners, powderless gloves, or other suitable alternatives.
3. Employers are required to provide readily accessible hand washing facilities. If this is not feasible, the employer is required to provide an appropriate antiseptic hand cleanser. If such a hand cleanser is used, employees should wash their hands with soap and running water as soon as possible.
4. Hands and any other skin surface should be washed thoroughly and immediately if accidentally contaminated with blood or any of the listed body fluids.

continued

Box 10-4	Major Highlights of the OSHA Rules and Regulations on Occupational Exposure to Bloodborne Pathogens —cont'd

5. Extreme care should be taken when handling needles or any sharp instrument capable of causing injury. Contaminated needles or sharps should not be recapped, bent by hand, or removed from a syringe. Needles, sharps, and associated disposables should be placed in closable, leak-proof, puncture-resistant, specially labeled, or color-coded containers. If reusable needles must be used, recapping or needle removal must be done with a mechanical device that protects the hand or by using a one-handed technique. In general, it is always best to avoid using reusable sharps if possible. Reusable needles and sharps should likewise be placed in closable, leak-proof, puncture-resistant containers for transport to the sterilization department.

6. Masks and protective total-eye shields or whole-face shields must be worn to protect the mucous membranes of the eyes, nose, and mouth in any procedure in which spraying, spattering, or splashing with blood or other potentially infective materials could occur.

7. Personal protective equipment also includes gowns or, preferably, waterproof aprons that should be worn in any procedure in which spraying or splashing with blood or specified body fluid could occur. General work clothes are not considered protective. Surgical caps or hoods and shoe covers or boots must be worn in situations in which gross contamination can be reasonably foreseen.

8. Mouthpieces, resuscitation bags, or other ventilation devices should be available and used in any area in which the need for resuscitation is predictable. HCWs should not perform mouth-to-mouth resuscitation; instead, they should take a moment to get the appropriate equipment. (Note: There is no documentation of transmission following mouth-to-mouth resuscitation.)

9. Eating, drinking, smoking, applying cosmetics or lip balm, and handling contact lenses are prohibited in work areas having potential exposure hazards.

10. Contaminated laundry should be handled as little as possible with no shaking or other forms of agitation and bagged at the location at which it was used. The bag must be labeled or color-coded sufficiently to permit identification of the bag's contents. The bag should be leak-proof if the laundry is wet. Contaminated trash such as used bandages is to be handled with the same general precautions as laundry. The exceptions to labeling and color-coding requirements are when the medical facility takes the BSI approach or considers all laundry and trash to be contaminated.

11. Potential infectious hazards must be communicated to employees through warning signs and labels. OSHA requires that the biohazard label be affixed to containers of regulated waste under specific conditions. The biohazard sign is displayed in Fig. 10-4. The biohazard labels are fluorescent orange or orange-red, with the lettering or symbols in contrasting color. Red bags or red containers are acceptable as substitutes for labels. If the medical facility practices BSI and it is understood that all specimens, used linen, and reusable equipment are treated as if potentially infectious, additional biohazard labeling or colored bags are not necessary.

12. OSHA mandates also address procedures that must be followed if a HCW is exposed.

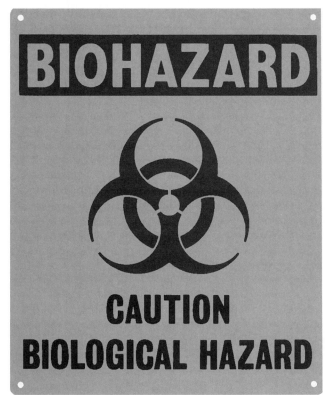

Figure 10-4. The biohazard symbol is used to remind HCWs to be cautious in areas in which the possibility of contamination exists. These reminders can be found anywhere infection control warrants them. The biohazard symbol is orange or orange-red, except in special cases in which white, black, and red combinations are used.

Modified from the Department of Labor, Occupational Safety and Health Administration: Occupational exposure to bloodborne pathogens, final rule, 29 CFR Part 1910.1030, *Federal Register* 56(235):64004, Washington, DC, 1991, The Department of Labor, Occupational Safety and Health Administration.
BSI, Body substance isolation; *FDA,* Food and Drug Administration; *HBV,* hepatitis B virus; *HIV,* human immunodeficiency virus; *OSHA,* Occupational Safety and Health Administration.

transmission procedures were some of the important things lost either through omission or misinterpretation. In reviewing all the problems, it became readily apparent that a change was needed and that a quick fix to any of the existing approaches—UP, BSI, the CDC isolation guideline, or any other isolation system—would not be the answer.

The Hospital Infection Control Practices Advisory Committee (HICPAC) established by the U.S. Department of Health and Human Services (DHHS) issued a *Special Report: Guideline for Isolation Precautions in Hospitals* in January 1996.[68] This new guideline consists of two tiers of precautions. In the first, and most important, tier are precautions designed for the care of all hospital patients regardless of their diagnosis or presumed infection status and are known as *standard precautions*.[68] The second tier known as *transmission-based precautions* are precautions designed only for the care of specific patients.[68]

Standard Precautions

Standard precautions combines the major features of UP and BSI. As expected, standard precautions apply to (1) blood; (2) all body fluids, secretions, and excretions except sweat; (3) nonintact skin; and (4) mucous membranes. Standard precautions are designed to be the primary strategy to control nosocomial infection by reducing transmission risk from both known and unknown sources of infection. The major components of standard precautions are shown in Box 10-5.

Transmission-Based Precautions

Transmission-based precautions are aimed at patients with a confirmed diagnosis or a suspected diagnosis of an epidemiologically important pathogen that warrants additional precautions beyond standard precautions. Table 10-2 lists some of the diseases that would require transmission-based precautions. Airborne, droplet, and contact precautions are the three designated types of transmission-based precautions. Each of the three can be used alone or in combination for a disease that has more than one transmission route. The revised guideline also lists specific clinical syndromes or conditions in both adult and pediatric patients that are associated with a high probability of harboring specific important pathogens. Examples of clinical syndromes and the appropriate transmission precaution approach needed is shown in Table 10-3. This empiric approach to admission and diagnosis is important because often a patient's definitive diagnosis cannot be made until a multitude of tests and procedures have been completed, which may take several hours to several days. In the meanwhile, precautions can be taken to prevent the transmission of the disease if the suspected diagnosis ends up being the definitive diagnosis.

ISOLATION FUNDAMENTALS

Behind any effective isolation program are the basic practices and procedures used around the clock by all HCWs. If the following fundamental infection control measures are routinely observed, the risk of transmitting disease can be greatly diminished.

Hand washing

Hand washing is the single most important way to prevent the spread of infections (Fig. 10-5). To be done properly, routine hand washing includes the use of soap and running water. HCWs should be cautious not to recontaminate their hands when turning off faucets by using several layers of dry paper towels to touch the faucet if foot-operated facilities are not available. The use of special antimicrobial products is not encouraged for routine hand washing because their use has been linked to development of antibiotic-resistant microorganisms, but these kinds of products do provide an extra degree of safety for special circumstances.

Although hand washing continues to be highly desirable, the focus has more recently shifted toward fingernails specifically. In 1973, fingernails were shown to be the primary reservoir of microflora on the hands, even after intense washing.[55] The underside of the nail, the subungual region, has been shown to harbor the highest number of microorganisms.[53] Findings from more recent studies involving the use of fingernail polish and artificial nails have lead to hospital policies forbidding both. In 2000, Hedderwick et al[62] conducted two separate studies. In study 1 HCWs wore artificial nails on one hand and native nails on the other for 15 days, nails on both hands were polished. Results showed that over the 15-day period, pathogens were increasingly likely to be isolated from artificial nails and in greater quantities. Study 2 was composed of HCWs who routinely wore polished acrylic nails and HCWs who did not. Once again, those with artificial nails were more likely to have a pathogen isolated than those with native nails (87% vs. 43%).

Gloving

There are several important reasons for the wearing of gloves. One is to provide the HCW a protective barrier and to keep the hands from becoming grossly contaminated. A second reason is to keep the patient safe from any microorganisms that may be present on the HCW's hands. A third reason is that when gloves are removed immediately after a patient contact and disposed of immediately they cannot serve as a fomite and infect other patients. The wearing of gloves does not guarantee safety, however, because they can have defects too small to be seen, they can be easily torn or punctured by equipment, and hands can be contaminated on glove removal. Hands should always be washed promptly after removing gloves.

Masks, Respiratory Protection, Eye Protection, and Face Shields

The use of masks is intended to prevent or decrease the risk of transmission of infectious agents through the air and applies to large-droplet and small-droplet nuclei. When a cloth or paper mask is worn to protect against infectious large-particle droplets, it gradually becomes damp with

Box 10-5	Synopsis of Standard Precautions*

HAND WASHING

Wash hands after touching blood, body fluids, secretions, or excretions (except sweat) whether gloves are worn or not

Wash hands immediately after gloves are removed, between patients, and when otherwise indicated to prevent the spread of microorganisms

Wash hands between tasks on the same patient to prevent cross-contamination of different body sites

Use a plain (nonantimicrobial) soap for routine hand washing

Use an antimicrobial agent or a waterless antiseptic agent for special circumstances (such as when directed by the infection control department at your hospital to control outbreaks or hyperendemic infections)

GLOVES

Clean, nonsterile gloves are adequate for most procedures

Wear gloves when touching blood, body fluids, secretions, excretions, and any contaminated items

Put on clean gloves just before touching mucous membranes or nonintact skin

Change gloves between tasks and procedures on the same patient after contact with material that may contain a high concentration of microorganisms

Remove gloves promptly and before touching noncontaminated items, equipment, and environmental surfaces and then immediately wash hands

MASK, EYE PROTECTION, AND FACE SHIELD

Wear these devices to protect mucous membranes of your eyes, nose, and mouth during procedures likely to generate splashes or sprays of blood, body fluids, secretions or excretions

GOWN

A clean, nonsterile gown is adequate for most purposes

Wear a gown to protect your skin and to prevent soiling your clothing where splashes or sprays are likely

Select a gown that is appropriate for the amount of fluid likely to be encountered (cloth vs. plastic)

Remove a soiled gown promptly

PATIENT-CARE EQUIPMENT

Handle used equipment in a careful manner to prevent transfer of pathogens

Properly discard single-use items

Ensure that reusable equipment is not used again until it has been reprocessed

ENVIRONMENTAL CONTROL

This pertains to routine care, cleaning and disinfection of environmental surfaces such as treatment couches, treatment equipment, and other frequently touched surfaces

LINEN

Handle, transport, and process used linen soiled with blood, body fluids, secretions, or excretions in a careful manner so as not to spread pathogens

OCUUPATIONAL HEALTH AND BLOODBORNE PATHOGENS

Take care to prevent injuries when using needles, scalpels, and other sharp or heavy instruments or devices

Never recap a used needle, do not manipulate them using both hands, or use any technique that involves directing the point of a needle toward any part of your body

Do use either a one-handed technique or a mechanical device designed for holding the needle sheath

Do not remove used needles from disposable syringes by hand and do not bend, break, or otherwise manipulate used needles by hand

Do place used needles, syringes, and other sharps into puncture-resistant containers, which should be located as close as possible to the area in which such items are used

Use mouthpieces, resuscitation bags, or other ventilation devices as an alternative to mouth-to-mouth resuscitation methods

PATIENT PLACEMENT

Place a patient who contaminates the environment or who does not (or cannot be expected to) assist in maintaining appropriate hygiene or environmental control in a private room or controlled environment

*See Hospital Infection Control Practices Advisory Committee (HICPAC) guidelines for a complete listing of infections requiring precautions.

| Table 10-2 | Diseases requiring transmission-based precautions |

AIRBORNE PRECAUTIONS

Measles
Varicella (including disseminated zoster)*
Tuberculosis

DROPLET PRECAUTIONS

Diphtheria
Pertussis
Pneumonic plague
Mumps
Rubella
Influenza

CONTACT PRECAUTIONS

Multidrug-resistant bacteria in gastrointestinal, respiratory, skin, or wound infections (of special interest to infection control experts at hospital, state, or national level)
Enteric infections with a low infectious dose or prolonged environmental survival including: *Escherichia coli* 0157:H7, *Shigella,* and hepatitis A
Skin infections that are highly contagious or that may occur on dry skin including: herpes simplex virus, impetigo, scabies, zoster (disseminated or in the immunocompromised host)
Viral hemorrhagic infections such as Ebola, Lassa, and Marburg

*Certain infections require more than one type of precaution.
See Centers for Disease Control and Prevention (CDC) tuberculosis guidelines for details.

| Table 10-3 | Clinical syndrome or condition warranting practical precautions until a diagnosis is confirmed* |

Clinical Description	Suspected/Possible Pathogen	Transmission Precautions
Skin or wound infection in which there is draining or an abscess that cannot be covered	*Staphylococcus aureus*	Contact
Diarrhea in an adult with a history of recent antibiotic use	*Clostridium difficile*	Contact
Rash or inflamed skin eruption generalized, cause unknown: maculopapular (reddish flat or raised bumps) with a head cold or inflammation of the nasal mucous membranes and fever	Rubeola (measles)	Airborne
Respiratory: cough, fever, upper lobe infiltrate in a HIV-negative or low risk for HIV patient	*Mycobacterium tuberculosis*	Airborne
Respiratory: sudden, reoccurring attacks or severe persistent cough during periods of pertussis activity	*Bordetella pertussis*	Droplet
Meningitis as characterized by loss of appetite, fever, intense headache, intolerance of light and sound, contracted pupils, delirium, retraction of the head, convulsions, and even coma	*Neisseria meningitides*	Droplet

*Table examples are very limited. See Hospital Infection Control Practices Advisory Committee (HICPAC) guidelines for complete details.

exhalation respiratory moisture. Because transmission risk increases with the degree of wetness, damp masks should be replaced with dry ones as needed. A mask covering the mouth and nose is often combined with goggles or a face shield to protect the eyes. OSHA bloodborne pathogens final rule mandates the wearing of masks, eye protection, and face shields during activities likely to generate splashes or sprays.[42] Particulate respirators are needed to protect against pathogens that consist of small-droplet nuclei.

Gowns and Protective Apparel

Gowns are to be worn as a protective barrier over a HCW's uniform or street clothes. To protect clothing and underlying skin, one should anticipate the amount of fluid contamination

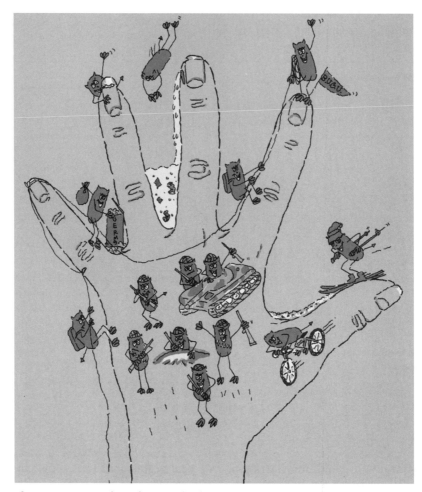

Figure 10-5. Hand washing is the best way to prevent the transmission of disease. *(Courtesy Brevis Co., Salt Lake City, Utah.)*

and choose between ordinary cloth gowns and gowns that are impermeable to liquids. Leg coverings, boots, or shoe coverings are also needed when splashes or large quantities of liquids are present or anticipated. OSHA mandates that such apparel be made available to HCWs as needed and appropriate.[42]

Patient Placement

A vital component of any infection control plan is designating whether it is crucial for a patient to have a private room or not. When direct contact or indirect contact transmission pathogens are involved, a private room is needed when the source patient has poor hygiene practices, contaminates the environment, or cannot be expected to participate in infection control measures. If a private room is not available, then patients infected with the same pathogen can be housed together. A private room with special air handling and ventilation is important in airborne transmission diseases.

Transport of Infected Patients

Patients with epidemiologically significant microorganisms should leave their rooms only for essential procedures to decrease the risk of transmission. For essential procedures, the patient should wear a mask, dressings, or whatever barrier is deemed necessary for the particular pathogen that he or she carries. The personnel in the hospital area performing the essential procedure should be notified in advance so that they can be prepared to receive the patient and the patient should receive instruction on how he or she can help prevent the spread of the pathogen to others.

Patient Care Equipment and Articles

Equipment and articles used for patient care require proper handling once contaminated. Many items are disposable, whereas others may be reused after reprocessing. The method of disposal or reprocessing is determined by the severity of the associated disease, the environmental stability of the pertinent pathogen, and the physical characteristics of the item. If the item is sharp and could cause injury it must be placed in a puncture resistant container to meet OSHA standards.[42] Other items may simply be bagged. Only one bag is needed if the bag is sturdy and the bag remains uncontaminated on the outside; if not, then two bags are used.

Items that can be reprocessed are divided into three categories: critical, semicritical, and noncritical and are covered in a later section of this chapter.

Laundry

Contaminated laundry presents a very low risk of disease transmission provided it is handled, transported, and a laundered in manner that prevents transfer of pathogens. OSHA also addresses how laundry is to be handled.[42] These federal standards state that used laundry is to be handled as little as possible with a minimum of agitation and bagged or placed in a container at the location where it is used. For a radiation therapy department, this translates to a container in every treatment room and every examination room. If contaminated and wet, gloves should be worn and the laundry must be placed in a bag, which prevents soak-through or leakage. Contaminated laundry also has to be placed in labeled or color-coded bags unless the medical facility treats all laundry as if it was contaminated and all employees are aware of the practice.

Routine Cleaning of Environment

Equipment used on patients who have been placed on one or more of the transmission-based precautions should be cleaned in the same manner as patients on standard precautions unless the pathogen or the amount of environmental contamination are such that special procedures are necessary. In addition to routine cleaning, disinfectants may be required for specific pathogens that are capable of surviving in the inanimate environment for prolonged periods of time. Treatment tables and supporting rackets should be cleaned after each patient contact. Guidelines published by the Association for Professionals in Infection Control (APIC) list ethyl or isopropyl alcohol (70% to 90%), sodium hypochlorite (5.2% household bleach), diluted phenolic germicidal detergent solution, and diluted ionosphere germicidal detergent solution as appropriate products for low-level, noncritical items such as tabletops or blood pressure cuffs that come into contact with a patient's intact skin.[95] Method of cleaning and choice of cleaning products and disinfecting products should be determined based on recommendations of the infection care experts at the health care facility.

Blood or Body Fluid Spills

Blood or body fluid spills should be cleaned up immediately. OSHA does not specify a specific procedure or a single specific disinfectant. Either a disinfectant approved by the Environmental Protection Agency (EPA) for hospital use or a 1:10 fresh solution of household bleach (sodium hypochlorite) should be used, with 1 part bleach and 10 parts water.[42] Household bleach has a broad spectrum of antimicrobial activity and is inexpensive and fast acting; however, it is corrosive and is relatively unstable and therefore must be fresh to be effective. It is also inactivated by organic matter, which means that it becomes useless as it kills microorganisms;

thus it does not provide a prolonged effect and must be available in an appropriate quantity for the size of the spill. Disinfectants labeled simply as germicides should not be used unless the germicide also happens to be a tuberculocide (meaning it is capable of killing the TB pathogen) to be in compliance with the OSHA compliance document.[89]

Student Education

Students should receive instruction at the earliest stage of their professional education. Orientation to OSHA rules and regulations and medical facilities' overall infection control programs and hazardous materials programs should take place before active participation in the clinical component of education. In some educational programs, students rotate through multiple health care facilities. These programs must ensure that a student is thoroughly familiar with each facility's specific programs before any active participation occurs.

HANDLING EXPOSURE INCIDENTS RELATED TO HIV

Names such as Rock Hudson, Ryan White, Kimberly Bergalis, Earvin "Magic" Johnson, and Greg Louganis are associated with the most significant epidemic of the twentieth century. The introduction in 1981 of the acronym AIDS and later the acronym HIV struck fear and anxiety in the community and in the health care setting. Since 1983, when the first case of occupational HIV-1 infection was documented, HCWs have been flooded with information and literature about the risk that accompanies caring for HIV-positive patients.[4] Because these patients do not always have obvious characteristics of the disease, the only logical approach that a HCW can use for self-protection is to assume that all patients are HIV positive.

Because HCWs are human, accidents happen. When an exposure incident occurs, the first and most urgent question is, "What actions can be taken to decrease the risk of transmission?" Over the past two decades, the CDC, OSHA, and the scientific community have closely observed exposure incidents in HCWs. Although a multitude of questions and issues have not yet been resolved, these exposure incidents have aided in the development of guidelines for treatment. Before any guidelines and recommendations are addressed, the risk of acquiring HIV should be reviewed.

For perspective, the risk of acquiring HIV is commonly compared with the risk of acquiring HBV. As stated previously in this chapter, before the OSHA-mandated HBV vaccine, approximately 8700 HBV infections occurred annually in U.S. HCWs. These infections also resulted in approximately 200 deaths each year.[42] In contrast, as of December 1994, there were only 42 documented cases of occupationally acquired HIV infections since 1981.[30]

The risk of acquiring HBV has been statistically calculated to be 10 to 100 times greater than the risk of acquiring HIV. The risk of HBV after a needlestick involving blood from an HBV-positive patient has been estimated to be 5% to 43% compared with less than 0.3% (1 in 250) for HIV.[90] These statistics come from an ongoing prospective study of HCWs at the National Institutes of Health (NIH) and other prospective studies.[8,9,30,77] The risk from mucosal and nonintact cutaneous exposure is not zero; however, it is too low to be reasonably calculated at this time. No risk from contamination of normal skin or other types of casual contact exposure has been documented. Other risk factors that may affect transmission include the following: titer of virus in source fluid, volume of material involved, and viral viability.

The type of exposure appears to be highly associated with the risk of acquiring HIV. Percutaneous exposures account for 84% of occupationally acquired HIV cases, followed by mucocutaneous exposure (13%) and combined percutaneous and mucocutaneous exposure (3%).[30] To date, no additional routes of transmission have been proved in occupational HIV exposure, and casual contact that occurs with infected patients apparently poses no risk to the HCW.[9] Also important is whether the infective virus strain is known or suspected to be resistant to antiretroviral drugs.

After an exposure, the type and severity of the exposure must be recorded because this information may eventually provide better epidemiologic data. For example, documenting the type of needle (e.g., hollow-core, surgical), gauge of the needle, depth of penetration, volume of blood or body fluid, and source of fluid (e.g., semen, amniotic fluid) helps provide better analysis.

Some hospitals have defined levels of HIV exposure to be used as guides in counseling the exposed HCW and in initiating prophylactic treatment. See typical exposure levels in Box 10-6.[39]

A true occupational exposure requires that documented seroconversion take place. This means that the HCW tested negative for HIV shortly after an exposure and subsequently developed clinical and/or serologic evidence of HIV infection. This documentation is necessary to sort out HCWs who may have unknowingly been positive for HIV at the time of exposure as a result of nonoccupational factors. In an analysis of 51 HCWs who experienced seroconversion, the average time was 65 days from exposure and 95% had seroconverted within 6 months.[15] In another report, HCWs

tested negative at 6 months but went on to being seropositive by 12 months postexposure.[36]

Although no data are available demonstrating that first aid is effective in preventing the transmission of HIV, the use of first aid procedures is the only logical immediate management strategy. HCWs should be instructed to initiate decontamination procedures immediately if possible. Skin and injured wound sites that have been contaminated with blood or a body fluid should be washed with soap and water. Oral and nasal mucosal surfaces should be rinsed thoroughly with water. Eyes should be thoroughly rinsed with water, saline, or other suitable sterile solutions. The application of an antiseptic is logical even though there is no evidence to show that their use decreases the risk of transmission. There also is no evidence that squeezing or making a wound bleed outwardly decreases risk. The use of a caustic substance such as bleach, injection of an antiseptic, or an application of a disinfectant at a wound site is discouraged.[33] A 1990 article reported a case in which a HCW poured undiluted bleach over a cut that involved blood from an AIDS patient; despite this action the worker still converted to HIV positive.[65]

When an exposure incident occurs, the employer must make immediately available to the HCW confidential medical evaluation and follow-up. Both the source-person and the exposed HCW are evaluated to determine if there is truly a need for HIV postexposure prophylaxis. If the incident involves a source individual, who is defined as any person, living or dead, whose blood or other potentially infectious body materials may be a source of exposure, the identification of the source individual will be made except when doing so is unfeasible or prohibited by law. If the source is known to be HIV positive, information from the medical records can be gathered and used to help plan the HCW's postexposure plan of treatment. If the HIV status is unknown, the source's blood can be tested to determine if the source is positive for HIV, but this can be done in some states only after consent is obtained.[52] Other states have passed legislation that allows HIV testing of the source after occupational exposure even if the source patient refuses to have the test performed.[63] Test results are to be made known to the HCW but the worker also must be advised on laws regarding the confidentiality of the source's identity, if known, and the infectious status.[42]

Box 10-6	**Levels of Typical Human Immunodeficiency Virus (HIV) Exposure**

Massive exposure—example: parenteral exposure to HIV laboratory animals with high viral titers
Definite parenteral exposure—example: intramuscular "deep" injury with needle
Possible parenteral exposure—example: subcutaneous "superficial" needle injury
Doubtful parenteral exposure—example: prior wound or skin lesion contaminated with non–OSHA-specified body fluid
Nonparenteral exposure—example: intact skin contaminated with blood or specified body fluid

OSHA, Occupational Safety and Health Administration.

If the source's HIV status is unknown, testing should be done as soon as possible after consulting laboratory experts who are knowledgeable about the most expeditious methods available. An FDA-approved rapid HIV antibody test kit should be considered, especially if testing by enzyme immunoassay (EIA) cannot be completed within 24 to 48 hours. The enzyme-linked immunosorbent assay (ELISA or EIA) test is performed to detect HIV antibody. Because false-positive results occur, a positive EIA test should be followed with a confirmatory test such as immunofluorescent antibody or the Western blot test.[33,37,42] Early tests for HIV antibody may be negative; however, infection can usually be documented at an early stage by less widely available tests such as measuring p24 antigen, by HIV cultures, or by gene-amplification studies.[52]

The HCW should be evaluated to determine susceptibility to bloodborne pathogen infections. The blood of an exposed HCW should be tested if consent is obtained to establish an HIV baseline. If the source is determined to be negative and has not engaged in behaviors that are associated with a risk for HIV transmission, CDC guidelines state that baseline testing and follow-up is not needed. However, if the HCW is still concerned after counseling, serologic testing should be available. If the source has participated in risky behaviors and is currently testing negative, future testing of the HCW is warranted. The CDC recommends follow-up HIV antibody testing at 6 weeks, 3 months, and 6 months after exposure.[21] Delayed seroconversion, defined as the appearance of the HIV antibody at greater than 6 months, has been documented; thus some institutions test again at 12 months. The rationale for testing after 6 months is that treatment may delay seroconversion. In addition, later testing often reassures the HCW.[52] Symptoms that are compatible with seroconversion include the following: an unexplained fever, lymphadenopathy, a rash, lymphopenia, and a sore throat. OSHA rules further state that if the worker consents to blood collection but not to an HIV test, the sample must be preserved for at least 90 days in case the HCW changes their mind.[42]

If it is determined that postexposure prophylaxis is needed, it should be started in a matter of hours, not days. This urgency of treatment is based on animal studies and the reproductive cycle of the virus. One study involving monkeys infected via a mucosal surface showed that the virus had migrated to regional lymph nodes within 24 to 28 hours and was present in circulating blood within 5 days.[33,97] This combined with the fact that HIV replication is rapid, about 2.5 days, and that 5000 viral particles are created in each replication demands that decision to treat must be implemented without delay.[33] Chemoprophylaxis with zidovudine (ZDV), more commonly known as azidothymidine (AZT), and lamivudine for 28 days is typically recommended for most occupational HIV exposures.[33,64] Both of these drugs fall under a class of drugs known as nucleoside reverse transcriptase inhibitors. AZT is a drug approved by the FDA for use in the treatment of patients with AIDS. Although this drug does not cure AIDS, some evidence exists that AZT delays the progression of AIDS, prolongs survival, and decreases the incidence of opportunistic infections.[5] This evidence and data derived from animal studies and human study form the rationale for using AZT in occupationally exposed HCWs who provide informed consent. AZT has been associated with a decrease in the risk of seroconversion if the drug is administered soon after exposure.[36,79]

An expanded regimen that also includes a protease inhibitor (indinavir or nelfinavir) is recommended for the exposed HCW if there is an increased risk of transmission such a deep bloody needlestick or if the virus is known or suspected to be antiretroviral agent resistant.[32,33] There is no data to directly support the addition of other antiretroviral agents to ZDV to increase postexposure effectiveness, but based on better results in the use of combined drug therapy for HIV patients, the addition of a drug in another class of antiretroviral agents could possibly offer a greater degree of protection.[33]

The efficacy of AZT as a chemoprophylactic is unknown and difficult to determine because of the low risk of transmission. Prospective, randomized trials were attempted in 1988 by Burroughs Wellcome Co., but too few subjects were enrolled to justify continuing the trials.[52] The medical literature also documents cases in which HCWs were given AZT but later experienced positive conversion.[79,81] On the other hand, an encouraging 1991 study documented no seroconversions among 160 HCWs who chose to receive AZT after their occupational exposure.[64] Insufficient data exist to mandate providing AZT or other new drugs or to advise against their use after occupational exposure. The CDC and two pharmaceutical companies have established a confidential registry known as the HIV PEP Registry to assess toxicity, and health care providers are encouraged to enroll exposed HCWs.[33]

Although the use of AZT rarely induces serious toxicity, a wide variety of side effects are associated with its use. Side effects include headaches, nausea, fever, fatigue, gastrointestinal pain, bone marrow suppression, hepatomegaly, muscle weakness, and lactic acidosis.[99] In addition, the optimal AZT time and dose relationship has yet to be determined. HCWs who elect to receive AZT and other agents must be closely monitored. They must also be counseled in regard to issues such as pregnancy and breast feeding, and they must be medically evaluated to rule out conditions such as underlying renal insufficiency, which would contraindicate the use of AZT.[5]

The management of exposed HCWs is extremely sensitive and complex. Workers should be treated on a priority basis in light of the extreme mental anguish associated with an HIV exposure. Psychologic reactions include fear, anxiety, anger, depression, denial, sexual and sleep disturbances, suicide, and psychosis. Counseling must be available immediately and continuously for workers exposed to HIV. Some institutions have even set up 24-hour counseling hotlines for their exposed HCWs.[52]

Counseling of the HCW should also address lifestyle changes that should be made until seroconversion occurs or until enough time has passed (typically 6 months) for the worker to be deemed free of HIV infection. Lifestyle changes include no exchanging of body fluids during sex; deferment of pregnancy; and cessation of breast feeding, intimate kissing, the sharing of razors and tooth brushes; and the donation of blood, sperm, or organs. If the HCW is involved in an accident that results in bleeding, surfaces that are contaminated should be promptly disinfected.

In general, employees should be allowed to perform patient care duties except during times when their condition is infectious through nonbloodborne routes. For example, with infectious diarrhea, skin lesions, and pulmonary infections, work restrictions would be reasonable. In the case of a bloodborne infection status, such as HIV or HBV positive, employers are not allowed to discriminate against the employee. Employees are protected by section 504 of the Rehabilitation Act and the Americans with Disabilities Act, which prohibit discrimination against individuals with disabilities, including persons who are positive for HIV or HBV.[46] Employers must make every effort to maintain the employment of an individual as long as the individual is capable of performing the job and does not pose a reasonable threat of infection to others. At the same time, however, employees and students should take personal responsibility for their actions and not perform any procedure that could be dangerous to their coworkers or patients.

RIGHTS OF THE HEALTH CARE WORKER

Hopefully, today's HCW will never have to wonder what to do if an employer does not provide proper protection equipment, but, if this occurs, HCWs have legal rights. OSHA helps provide job safety and health protection for workers by promoting safe and healthful working conditions throughout the nation. HCWs can lawfully refuse to work in truly unsafe conditions and have the right to insist on wearing protective equipment. However, workers cannot leave their job if they want their rights protected.[40] HCWs must first inform their employer of the unsafe conditions. If an employer does not respond, the worker should contact OSHA to file a complaint and request that an inspection be conducted.[41] OSHA will withhold, on request, the name of the employee filing the complaint.[40] Before complaining, a HCW should be sure that the unsafe condition is indeed serious (i.e., the situation could have caused death or serious harm).

The opposite situation can also occur. On occasion, a HCW may have unreasonable fears and be overly cautious. Examples include the worker who refuses to go anywhere near an AIDS patient or the worker who insists on wearing a full-body space suit. This type of reaction is usually caused by lack of proper education about the risk of transmission and proper protective actions that workers should take. The employer should let the HCW explain fears and perceptions and should then educate the worker with the necessary infor-mation in understandable language. The HCW cannot be discharged or discriminated against in any way just because of a misperception or because of a complaint or a call to OSHA. Workers who believe they have been discriminated against should file a complaint with their nearest OSHA office within 30 days of the alleged discriminatory act.[40] However, if after counseling and if the situation is deemed to be reasonably safe and proper equipment was provided, and the worker still refuses to provide care as in the AIDS patient example, the employer may have the right to dismiss the worker.

HCWs also have legal rights if they develop an occupationally acquired infection. Worker's compensation laws, determined by each state, are in place to protect the employee. To be compensated in a case in which a worker is disabled or killed, the injury must have occurred while the worker was practicing within his or her scope of practice. Bungee jumping off the seventeenth floor of the hospital during lunch hour, for example, would not be covered because it is outside the scope of practice of a radiation therapist. In most cases, workers do not have the right to file a negligence or criminal suit in addition to a worker's compensation claim unless they can prove that their employer intentionally disregarded an infection risk. The worker must also be able to establish that the infection was actually acquired on the job not in the community.

Another extremely important right HCWs have is complete confidentiality. To protect the worker's privacy, most health care facilities take special steps to avoid placing the HCW's "patient" chart where other employees have access to it. In addition, such a diagnosis would not be placed on computerized charting systems.

ROLE OF THE CENTRAL SERVICES DEPARTMENT

In the past, medical supplies and equipment that needed to be sterilized were often sterilized in an autoclave unit housed in the radiation oncology department. With the concerns of bloodborne pathogens and emerging diseases, health care centers have learned that it is far better to leave the reprocessing of medical supplies and equipment in the hands of experts. This area of expertise typically is housed in a department known as central services, or central supply. The central service department (CSD) is accountable for preparing, processing, sorting, and distributing medical supplies and equipment required in patient care. This central location not only is economical but also is subject to stringent levels of quality control according to JCAHO guidelines.[74]

A student or employee tour through a major hospital's CSD can be an extremely enlightening and educational experience. Contaminated equipment is first precleaned and decontaminated by trained, specially clothed workers. This clothing includes items such as waterproof aprons and face shields. Reprocessing may include disassembly and sending equipment through devices that remind a person of a commercial car wash complete with a presoak cycle, wash cycle, and dry cycle. Instruments are then prepared for sterilization by the most appropriate method. Ideally, each package sterilized is labeled with a control number in case any item must be recalled. The labeling process may also identify the sterilizing unit used, its load, the time and date an item was sterilized, the item's expiration date, and sometimes even the individual who packaged the item (Fig. 10-6).

After a package has been disinfected or sterilized, it should be handled as little as possible and stored in a low-traffic, clean, dry, closed area. If an item comes into contact with something and becomes soiled, is exposed to moisture, or is physically penetrated, it is deemed contaminated and should not be used. Sterile items should be stored away from the floor, vents, pipes, doors, and windows. Closed shelves are preferred over drawers because the risk of damaging a sterilized package is greater in opening and closing a drawer than opening the door to a cabinet. If a closed cabinet is not an option, open shelves are a feasible solution. Placing a plastic dust cover over the sterilized packages can decrease the chance of contamination. Each health care facility determines the amount of time that a sterilized item can be stored. Important factors in determining shelf life include packaging material and an open or closed shelf design, both of which combined are more important than time alone. It is further assumed that after the opening of a sterilized package, sterile technique will be used and the date of expiration will be checked.

STERILIZATION AND DISINFECTION TECHNIQUES

Because a radiation therapist must routinely practice infection control techniques, an overview of sterilization and disinfection techniques is desirable and addressed in the following text. Every health care facility should have infection control policies and experts available for consultation. Simple questions regarding whether radiation oncology supplies should be single-use disposables or reprocessed can be answered by these experts. In addition, experts can advise the most economical route and the best method or product for each situation. Expertise is readily available from an institution's CSD and/or epidemiology department. Any policy developed within a radiation oncology department should be reviewed by these experts before the policy's implementation.

In general, medical supplies and equipment can be divided into risk categories based on an item's use. *Critical items* are products or instruments inserted into normally sterile areas of the body or into the bloodstream and must be sterile for use. Items in this category include needles, surgical instruments, urinary catheters, and implants. *Semicritical items* are those that contact mucosal surfaces but do not ordinarily penetrate body mucosal surfaces. These include items such as endoscopes, thermometers, laryngoscopes, and anesthesia equipment. It is preferable to sterilize items in this category, but high-level disinfection may be used. *Noncritical items* do not ordinarily touch the patient or touch only the

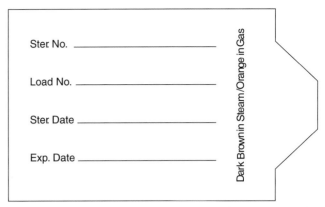

Figure 10-6. Sterilization labels are used as part of the quality-control program in a central services department. If an item must be recalled, it can be tracked by its control number.

patient's intact skin; therefore they do not need to be sterile. This category includes items such as tabletops, stethoscopes, and blood pressure cuffs.[95] The FDA requires that medical devices be sold with instructions stating whether the devices are single-use or reusable items and the way they must be processed if reusable.[47]

Sterilization is a process that destroys all microbial life forms, including resistant spores. Sterilization can be achieved through physical or chemical processes. There are no degrees of sterilization, an item is either sterile or it is not sterile. Processes used for sterilization include steam under pressure, dry heat, low-temperature sterilization (ethylene oxide gas or gas plasma), and specific liquid chemicals.

Disinfection is a process that reduces microbial life forms and can range from *high-level disinfection* to *intermediate-level disinfection* and even *low-level disinfection*.[66] Low-level disinfection is synonymous with *sanitization*. High-level disinfection eliminates all microbial forms except situations in which there are high numbers of bacterial spores (such as anthrax terrorist attacks). Intermediate-level disinfection kills the TB bacterium, most viruses, and most fungi but not most bacterial spores. Low-level disinfection inactivates most bacteria, some viruses, and some fungi but are mostly ineffective against TB bacterium and bacterial spores. There are some microbial life forms that cannot be eliminated by disinfection processes. In the health care setting, disinfection is typically achieved through the use of liquid chemicals or wet pasteurization (hot water).

Antiseptics are different from disinfectants. The term *antiseptic* is reserved for antimicrobial substances applied to skin surfaces. Methods of sterilization and disinfection are addressed in the following text and differ with regard to the biocidal agent, biocidal action, contact between the biocidal agent and microorganism, and severity of treatment.[49] Regardless of whether sterilization or disinfection is appropriate for a given situation, neither process is likely to be successful if meticulous cleaning does not precede the process. Foreign matter that remains after inadequate cleaning and processing generally renders an item unusable.

Heat

The use of heat, moist or dry, is the most reliable, available, and economical method of destroying microorganisms. Boiling water (100° C, 212° F) is probably the oldest method used. Although boiling greatly decreases the number of microorganisms, it does not destroy all microorganisms, such as spores; thus boiling fits into the category of disinfectants rather than sterilants. In fact, temperatures lower than boiling (50° to 70° C, 122° to 158° F) are sufficient to kill most viruses, bacteria, and fungi.[66] HIV is destroyed by moist heat at 60° C (140° F) in 30 minutes, a temperature well below the requirement for boiling water.[38]

Steam under pressure, however, is capable of destroying all life forms, provided that a proper combination of temperature and time is achieved. Older textbooks typically quoted a specific time, temperature, and pressure combination, and the student accepted this combination as an absolute. In reality, steam sterilization works as an inverse relationship and many combinations are equally effective; thus steam sterilization is analogous to the various time-dose relationships used in treating cancer. Simply put, the time required for sterilization decreases as the temperature increases.

With the special exception of an infectious life form known as a *prion* (proteinaceous infectious particle) that cause diseases such as Creutzfeldt-Jakob disease (CJD), no life forms survive if exposed to steam under pressure at 30 pounds per square inch (psi) at 121° C (250° F).[66] An exposure that lasts 15 to 20 minutes at this temperature is adequate for killing most life forms; however, the heat-resistant Creutzfeldt-Jakob agent requires 1 hour of exposure at a temperature of 132° C (270° F).[98]

The term prion, which was introduced in 1982, is used to describe unique, infectious central nervous system agents composed of protein but lacking identifiable nucleic acid. Prions multiply and are extremely resistant to standard sterilization methods.[49] CJD is a progressive, degenerative neurologic disorder and is believed to have a long incubation period. Once active symptoms begin, death follows in a matter of weeks to months. Symptoms are rapidly progressing dementia changing to coma then death, and there is no cure. CJD has been associated with corneal transplants, dura mater graphs, pituitary growth hormone injections, and other neurosurgical procedures. Extreme caution should be taken with brain tissue and central nervous system (CNS) fluids because HCWs have died from an occupational exposure.[85] A better-known prion variant of CJD related disease is bovine spongiform encephalopathy, commonly referred to as mad cow disease, which can be passed on to humans through contaminated beef products.[6] To summarize, sterilization combinations of pressure, temperature, and time are also influenced by the type of microorganism to be destroyed.

Steam sterilizers are commonly referred to as *steam autoclaves* and can be described as closed metal chambers. **Autoclaves** can be grouped into two general categories: gravity-displacement and mechanically evacuated devices. The gravity-displacement type requires a longer exposure time. Steam sterilization is the most commonly used method of sterilization used in health care facilities because of its low cost, its absence of toxic residue, and the fact that it can be used to sterilize an extremely wide assortment of materials. A drying cycle follows exposure to the steam and is often the slowest portion of the autoclave cycle. Another device known as a *flash sterilizer,* or *flash autoclave,* can be used in an emergency situation. This device is operated at a higher temperature, and exposure time is only a few minutes. Flash autoclaving should not routinely be substituted for standard autoclaving procedures.

Cotton fabric and special steam-permeable plastics or paper can be used as packaging materials. Other criteria essential to the selection of appropriate packaging materials for any sterilization method include the resistance to puncture and tears, penetration by microorganisms, and absence of toxic or biologically harmful particles. Care must be exercised in packing items for steam sterilization to ensure that the steam can reach all surfaces and cavities of a specific item. For example, lids must be taken off containers and many items may require disassembly. Items in a package must be arranged loosely because overpacking may lead to *nonsterilization.* Steam sterilization also has its limitations. Instruments with sharp points, such as needles, or cutting edges, such as scalpels, may be dulled. Oxidation and corrosion may also occur with certain metals. Powder and oil products should not be autoclaved because the steam has difficulty in penetrating such substances. Many products such as rubber and synthetic polymers are heat sensitive and could melt or deteriorate. Other products such as injectable solutions may lose their biologic usefulness when subjected to high heat levels.

Because of packing precautions, packaging material differences, product sensitivity to heat, and JCAHO quality-control standards, comprehensive knowledge is required of anyone in charge of steam sterilization or any method of sterilization. For these reasons, sterilization is best done by experts, the employees of the CSD. Unfortunately, some centers operate units without expert advice and without biologic indicators, discussed at the end of this chapter, as a quality control measure.

Dry heat is also used for sterilization. Although its use has sharply declined since the introduction of single-use syringes and needles sterilized by other methods, dry heat is still useful for reusable needles, glass syringes, sharp-cutting instruments and drills, powders and oily products, and metals that oxidize or corrode with exposure to moisture. The advantage of dry heat is its ability to penetrate solids, nonaqueous powders or oils, and closed containers. Its primary disadvantage when compared with steam is that higher temperatures and longer exposure times are required to achieve sterilization. A commonly quoted temperature is 160° C (320° F) with a time of 1 to 3 hours.[66] As with steam sterilization, appropriate time and temperature combinations follow an inverse relationship. Similar to cooking in a home oven, aluminum foil or aluminum containers are commonly used for packaging. As with steam sterilization, items that are heat sensitive should be sterilized by other available techniques.

Incineration, another form of heat, is frequently applied to biohazardous waste materials generated in health care settings. Some incinerators are located on hospital grounds, but most are now located away from hospitals, residential areas, and high-occupancy buildings. Because incinerators are typically located some distance away, designated vehicles are required to transport biohazardous waste to the incinerator site.

Gas

Gas sterilizers are available for medical products that cannot withstand high temperatures. In recent times, the use of gas has become increasingly important in the health care setting and the commercial setting because of the use of a greater number of instruments and products that cannot tolerate high heat exposure. Gas is a more complex and expensive method than dry or wet heat. Ethylene oxide (usually written as ETOX) is the gas used in most gas sterilizers. In the past, ETOX was mixed with Freon, but carbon dioxide (CO_2) is now used because of Freon's harmful effect on the ozone layer. The operation of a gas sterilizer should be attempted only by qualified experts because the gases present fire and explosion hazards. In addition, the gas has a toxic effect on humans, is mutagenic, and is a suspected carcinogen, thus making it subject to OSHA regulations. Gas sterilizers are equipped with special detectors to alert personnel in the event of a gas leak.

Packages sterilized by gas are typically exposed for 4 to 12 hours at temperatures of 25° to 60° C.[49,66] Other time and temperature combinations can be used because the process follows an inverse relationship. Packages are then aerated in special closed cabinets for 12 to 24 hours by heated, high air flows to dissipate any residual ETOX because of its tissue toxicity.[66] If special cabinet aeration is not available, the aeration process may take up to 7 days.[66] Gas should not be used to sterilize products that cannot withstand low heat. To recap, gas is slower, is more expensive, and has the possibility of toxic residue. Very few hospitals have an ethylene oxide sterilizer. Large medical institutions frequently cooperate and provide gas sterilization access to medium and small medical institutions to assist with cost. Gas sterilization is not applied to liquids or products packaged in gas-impervious wrappers. Products can be wrapped in the same packaging materials used for steam sterilization.

Gas plasma, a newer gas alternative, consists of gas in a highly charged vacuum state. Free radicals created then interact with the microorganisms to destroy them. The entire process takes about 75 minutes, and there are no toxic emissions. Very few units exist and there are associated technical problems.[1]

Radiation

Although not routinely used in the health care setting, ionizing radiation is widely applied at commercial industrial sites to heat-sensitive medical products and equipment. Gamma beams from cobalt-60 sources or linear accelerator photon and electron beams are used. Electrons are more limited in use because of their poorer penetration, and photon beams over 10 MV are not used because they can induce significant radioactivity in the sterilized product through artificial nuclide production.[49] Extremely high absorbed doses (kGy) are necessary because microorganisms are far more resistant to the effects of radiation than humans.[76] The time required for sterilization depends on the unit's output rate and the required absorbed dose. Packaging materials and the product contained within are sterilized. Caution must be employed in using radiation as a sterilant for medications because it may induce chemical changes by breaking chemical bonds and thus inactivate or modify some medications. An interesting student project is to check packages for a wide variety of single-use sterile (disposable) products to see how many were irradiated.

Radiation sterilization is used in the autosterilization of a strontium (^{90}Sr) applicator. After a strontium treatment for pterygium of the eye, the radioactive end of the applicator is wiped against a sterile alcohol pad to remove any biologic debris and then rinsed with sterile water. The surface radiation output emitted by a typical 50-mCi ^{90}Sr source is approximately 50 cGy per second, a rate high enough that it sterilizes itself with a dose of over 4 million cGy in a 24-hour period.[71]

Nonionizing radiations such as ultraviolet and infrared light or microwave are also capable of killing microorganisms, but the wavelengths are too low to allow any significant penetration; thus most are not used for sterilization purposes except in a few extremely limited applications.

Chemical Liquids

Using chemicals for sterilization or disinfection is a relatively easy process. Items need only to be placed in a basin deep enough to completely submerge the item, with care taken to ensure that the chemical can reach all inner and outer surfaces and crevices. Caution should also be exercised to ensure that the chemical does not damage the item to be processed or the basin containing the chemical itself. The most difficult part is selecting the best, most appropriate chemical. Therefore a radiation therapist should contact a qualified CSD expert for input in choosing products and protocols for use. The assumption should not be made that oncology physicians or nurses have any more expertise in this subject than a radiation therapist. Chemicals have an extremely wide range of antimicrobial action and are time sensitive. Few can sterilize; most cannot, and those that can are known as chemical sterilants. The FDA has had the responsibility of overseeing the safety and effectiveness of any agent to be labeled and marketed as a liquid chemical sterilant for critical and semicritical medical devices since 1993.[95] The EPA has assumed the main responsibility of overseeing and reviewing agents to be marketed as disinfectants for noncritical items. The FDA also regulates any agent registered and labeled as an antiseptic.[48]

The CDC cannot endorse specific products, but it can provide guidance in choosing products.[50] Other professional groups such as APIC also publish extremely useful guidelines.[93,95] Manufacturers are also responsible for furnishing recommendations on the reprocessing of items that they produce. Thus the chemical to be used on a specific item is based on expert guidelines, scientific literature, and manufacturer product information. Reliance on labels alone is insufficient and at times even misleading. Therefore caution should be used with wording such as, "hospital strength disinfectant." "Hospital disinfectant" is preferred because this term indicates a higher level of disinfection. Many chemical products may have other terminology on their labels that provide useful information about effectiveness. For example, a germicide is capable of killing microorganisms (germs) but does not specify what kind of germs. A bactericide is capable of killing nonsporulating bacteria, fungicides kill fungi and their spores, sporicides are agents that can kill bacterial spores, virucides make viruses noninfective, and tuberculocides kill TB bacteria and other acid-fast bacteria. Commonly used chemicals are addressed in the following text.

Soap's usefulness as a disinfectant is limited because of its feeble antimicrobial action. The main merit of soap is that it aids in the removal of contamination buildup. Chlorine or chlorine compounds are widely used as disinfectants, and, although they are extremely effective against most microorganisms (including HIV and HBV), they are ineffective against spores and have an irritating odor. Alcohol, ethyl or isopropyl, is also ineffective against spores and some viruses. Iodine or iodine compounds may have sporicidal activity. In addition, some people are allergic to it. Hexachlorophene is used for surgical hand disinfection but does not kill all microorganisms. Formaldehyde is effective against all microorganisms, but its vapors are extremely irritating. Alkaline glutaraldehyde (Cidex) can kill spores if they are exposed to it long enough, but it has a pungent odor and is time sensitive, which causes it to eventually lose effectiveness. Some chemicals, when old and/or too diluted, even encourage rather than retard the growth of microorganisms. Some chemical disinfectants are extremely short acting, and others continue to retard the growth of microorganisms for variable lengths of time. Few special-use chemicals are effective as true sterilants. Because of the wide variability in the effectiveness of chemicals and their potential hazardous risks to HCWs, CSD experts should be contacted for advice on each situation to achieve the appropriate degree of asepsis.

A special note of caution is that liquid disinfectants and sterilants should not be used to clean brachytherapy devices such as ovoids. These liquids are known to be capable of corroding the silver brazing that secures the ovoid to the ovoid handle.[78]

STERILITY QUALITY-CONTROL MEASURES

Wide selections of chemical indicators are used externally and/or internally on packages subjected to a sterilization process. The purpose of the indicator is to alert an HCW that something went wrong during the sterilization process. External indicators are commonly used in heat, gas, and radiation sterilization processes and typically consist of an adhesive tape that darkens or changes color if exposed to a sterilization process (Fig. 10-7). External indicators do not guarantee that sterility has been achieved; they indicate only that the package was exposed to the process. Internal indicators are strategically placed inside a package at a site that is least likely to be penetrated by steam or gas (Fig. 10-8). Like external indicators, internal indicators do not guarantee that all microorganisms have been destroyed. Different types of external and internal indicators are commercially available for the different specific sterilization processes.

Biologic indicators are used to determine whether sterilization was achieved. A biologic indicator is a specially prepared strip coated with hard-to-kill microorganisms such as spores and enclosed in a small container placed inside a test package. After the test package has gone through the sterilization process with other packages, a microbiologist or another qualified expert examines the biologic indicator to determine whether all the microorganisms were killed. If not, all packages are recalled by their processing number. Routine use of biologic indicators is required by external accrediting agencies such as JCAHO. These indicators are typically used daily in each sterilization unit cycle and after any repair on a particular unit. Biologic indicators, external and internal indicators, and close attention to proper time and temperature combinations are all needed to ensure that products and equipment are safe for patient use.

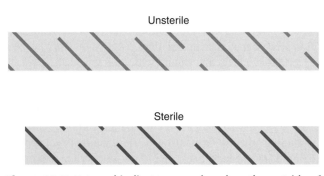

Figure 10-7. External indicators are placed on the outside of a package to be sterilized. After exposed to the sterilization process, the tape darkens or changes color. An external indicator does not guarantee sterility; it indicates only that the package was exposed to the process. Different types of tape are used in different sterilization processes (e.g., gas, steam).

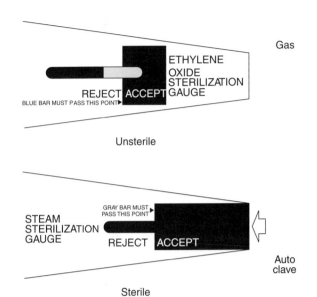

Figure 10-8. Internal indicators are placed inside packages to be sterilized. They are placed in sites least likely to be reached by the sterilization process. Although they provide a higher degree of sterility assurance than do external indicators, internal indicators also do not guarantee sterility.

Review Questions

Multiple Choice

1. Which of the following is a governmental agency that legally oversees job safety and health protection of workers?
   a. CDC
   b. DEA
   c. JSHP
   d. OSHA
2. Which of the following viruses has been shown capable of living on environmentally friendly surfaces for as long as 7 days?
   a. Human immunodeficiency
   b. Hepatitis B
   c. Influenza
   d. Rubeola
3. The term used to describe the number of antibodies present in a blood sample is
   a. Antigen coefficient
   b. Globulin factor
   c. Immune serum level
   d. Titers
4. An employer must provide particulate respirators to HCWs who must interact with a patient diagnosed with active
   a. Human immunodeficiency virus

   b. histoplasmosis
   c. Hepatitis A
   d. Tuberculosis
5. The concept known as universal precautions applied to
   a. All body fluids
   b. All patients
   c. All blood and other certain body fluids in all patients
   d. All patients and all body fluids
6. If an HCW gets stuck by a needle and consents to blood collection but not to an HIV test, the blood sample must be preserved by law for at least
   a. 1 week
   b. 30 days
   c. 90 days
   d. 6 months

Fill in the Blank

7. _____ is the name of the medical science field that studies the incidence, distribution, and determinants of disease.
8. An individual who is colonized but shows no immune response is known as a _____.
9. _____ is the federal agency that oversees safety in the work place.
10. Two nosocomial infectious diseases for which no vaccine is currently available are _____ and _____.
11. The three phases that a susceptible host goes through are _____, _____, and _____.
12. _____ is the gas that is routinely used for gas sterilization.

Questions to Ponder

1. Discuss the differences between universal precautions and body substance isolation.
2. Using documented research, identify 10 infectious diseases that, if caught, result in lifelong immunity.
3. Compare and contrast the differences between killed, toxoid, and attenuated live vaccines.
4. Develop an infection-control protocol for any clinical area task that must be addressed.
5. Compare labels on various liquid chemicals used for infection control in the medical setting and discuss what they can and cannot kill.
6. Compare the major differences between large-droplet and droplet-nuclei transmission.
7. Discuss what actions should be taken when a HCW develops hypersensitivity to latex.
8. Describe the use of sodium hypochlorite in a medical setting.
9. Discuss the significance of delayed seroconversion.

REFERENCES

1. Alfa MJ, DeeGagnee P, Olson N, et al: Comparison of ion plasma, vaporized hydrogen peroxide and 100% ethylene oxide sterilizers to the 12/88 ethylene oxide gas sterilizer, *Infect Control Hosp Epidemiol* 17:92-99, 1996.

2. Alter MJ: The detection, transmission and outcome of hepatitis C virus infection, *Infect Agents Dis* 2:155-156, 1993.

3. Anderson RL: Biological evaluation of carpeting, *Appl Microbiol* 18:180, 1969.

4. Anonymous: Needlestick transmission of HTLV-III from a patient infected in Africa, *Lancet* 2:1376-1377, 1984.

5. Barnhart ER, editor: *Physician's desk reference,* ed 49, Montvale, NJ, 1995, Medical Economics Data Production.

6. Bartholomew A: Mixed up over mad cow: how worried should you really be? Two experts sit down to hash it out, *Reader's Digest* pp 104-109, August 2001.

7. Bartlett JG: *Pocketbook of infectious disease therapy,* Baltimore, 1991, Williams & Wilkins.

8. Beekman SE, Henderson DK: HCWs and hepatitis: risk for infection and management of exposure, *Infect Dis Clin Pract* 1:424-428, 1992.

9. Beekman SE, et al: Risky business: using necessarily imprecise casualty counts to estimate occupational risk of HIV-1 infection, *Infect Control Hosp Epidemiol* 11:371-379, 1990.

10. Beil L: FDA approves vaccine against chickenpox, 70 to 90% effectiveness expected, *Dallas Morning News,* p 1, March 18, 1995.

11. Benenson A, editor: *Control of communicable diseases in man,* ed 13, Washington DC, 1981, American Public Health Association.

12. Bond WW, Favero MS, Petersen NJ et al: Inactivation of hepatitis B virus after drying and storage for one week, *Lancet* 1(8219):550-551, 1981 (letter).

13. Brachman PS: Epidemiology of nosocomial infections. In Bennett JV, Brachman PS, editors: *Hospital infections,* ed 3, Boston, 1992, Little, Brown & Co.

14. Brachman PS: Epidemiology of nosocomial infections. In Bennett JV, Brachman PS, editors: *Hospital infections,* ed 4, Philadelphia, 1998, Lippincott-Raven.

15. Busch MP, Satten GA: Time course of viremia and antibody seroconversion following human immunodeficiency virus exposure, *Am J Med* 102(suppl 5B):117-124, 1997.

16. Campbell CC: Malaria. In Hoeprich PD, Jordan MC, editors: *Infectious diseases,* ed 4, Philadelphia, 1989, JB Lippincott.

17. Cawson RA, et al: *Pathology: the mechanisms of disease,* ed 2, St. Louis, 1989, Mosby.

18. Centers for Disease Control and Prevention: Proceedings of the First International Conference on Nosocomial Infections, American Hospital Association, Atlanta, August 5-8, 1970.

19. Centers for Disease Control and Prevention: Recommendations of the Advisory Committee on Immunization Practices: varicella-zoster immune globulin for the prevention of chickenpox, *MMWR* 33:84-100, 1984.

20. Centers for Disease Control and Prevention: Recommendations for preventing transmission of infection in the human T-lymphotropic virus type III/lymphadenopathy-associated virus in the workplace, *MMWR* 34:681-695, 1985.

21. Centers for Disease Control and Prevention: Recommendations for prevention of HIV transmission in health care settings, *MMWR* 36(suppl 2S):1-19, 1987.

22. Centers for Disease Control and Prevention: Update: human immunodeficiency virus infections in health-care workers exposed to blood of infected patients, *MMWR* 36:285-289, 1987.

23. Centers for Disease Control and Prevention: Update: universal precautions for prevention of transmission of human immunodeficiency virus, hepatitis B virus, and other bloodborne pathogens in health care settings, *MMWR* 37:377-388, 1988.

24. Centers for Disease Control and Prevention: Guidelines for preventing the transmission of tuberculosis in healthcare settings, with special focus on HIV-related issues, *MMWR* 39(Re-17):1, 1990.

25. Centers for Disease Control and Prevention: Recommendations of the Immunization Practices Advisory Committee: prevention and control of influenza, *MMWR* 39(RR-7):1-15, 1990.

26. Centers for Disease Control and Prevention: Hospital Infection Control Practices Advisory Committee: Agenda, *Federal Register* 58:103, 1993.

27. Centers for Disease Control and Prevention: Hospital Infection Control Practices Advisory Committee: Meetings, *Federal Register* 58:204, 1993.

28. Centers for Disease Control and Prevention: Guidelines for preventing the transmission of *Mycobacterium tuberculosis* in health-care facilities, *MMWR* 43(RR-13):69, 78-81, 1994.

29. Centers for Disease Control and Prevention: Prevention and control of influenza: part II. Antiviral agents-recommendations of the Advisory Committee on Immunization Practices (ACIP), *MMWR* 43(RR-15):1-10, 1994.

30. Centers for Disease Control and Prevention: Surveillance for occupationally acquired HIV infection-United States, 1981-1992, *MMWR* 41:823-825, 1992. Personal communication update with CDC National AIDS Clearinghouse, 1995.

31. Centers for Disease Control and Prevention: Tuberculosis morbidity: United States, 1994, *MMWR* 44:387-389, 395, 1995.

32. Centers for Disease Control and Prevention: Guidelines for the use of antiretroviral agents in HIV-infected adults and adolescents, *MMWR* 46(RR-5):43-82, 1997.

33. Centers for Disease Control and Prevention: Public Health Service guidelines for the management of health-care workers exposed to HIV and recommendations for post exposure prophylaxis, *MMWR* 47(RR-7):1-28, 1998.

34. Centers for Disease Control and Prevention: NIOSH TB respiratory protection program in health care facilities—administrator's guide, (DHHS Publication No. 99-143), Cincinnati, Ohio: 1999, National Institute for Occupational Safety and Health, HHS, CDC.

35. Chen SK, Vesley D, Brosseau LM, et al:. Evaluation of single-use masks and respirators for protection of health care workers against mycobacterium aerosols, *Am J Infect Control* 22:65-74, 1994.

36. Ciesielski CA, Metter RP: Duration of time between exposure and seroconversion in health-care workers with occupationally acquired infection with human immunodeficiency virus, *Am J Med* 102(suppl 5B):115-116, 1997.

37. Cooper JS: The role of radiation therapy in the management of patients who have AIDS. In Cox JD, editor: *Moss's radiation oncology: rationale, technique, results,* ed 7, St. Louis, 1994, Mosby.

38. Cuthberton B, et al: Safety of albumin preparations manufactured from plasma not tested for HIV antibody, *Lancet* 2:41, 1987 (letter).

39. Department of Epidemiology, Baylor University Medical Center: Human immunodeficiency virus (HIV) workplace guidelines, Dallas, 1993, The Department of Epidemiology.

40. Department of Labor, Occupational Safety and Health Administration: Title 29, code of federal regulations, part 1903.2, Washington DC, 1989, The Department of Labor, Occupational Safety and Health Administration.

41. Department of Labor, Occupational Safety and Health Administration: Title 29, code of federal regulations, part 1977.12, Washington DC, 1989, The Department of Labor, Occupational Safety and Health Administration.

42. Department of Labor, Occupational Safety and Health Administration: Occupational exposure to bloodborne pathogens, Final rule, 29 CFR Part 1910.1030, *Federal Register* 56(235):64004-64182, 1991.

43. Department of Labor, Occupational Safety and Health Administration: Proposed rules on TB transmission to and among HCWs, *Federal Register* 59(219):58884-58935, 1994.

44. Department of Labor, OSHA, and the Department of Health and Human Services: Joint advisory notice: protection against occupational exposure to hepatitis B virus (HBV) and human immunodeficiency virus, *Federal Register* 54:41818, October 30, 1987.

45. Douglas RG Jr: Influenza in man. In Kilbourne ED, editor: *The influenza virus and influenza,* New York, 1975, Academic.

46. Equal Employment Opportunity Commission: A technical assistance manual on the employment provisions (title 1) of the Americans with Disabilities Act, Washington DC, 1992, Equal Employment Opportunity Commission.

47. Favero MS, Bond WW: Chemical disinfection of medical and surgical materials. In Block SS, editor: *Sterilization and preservation,* ed 4, Philadelphia, 1991, Lea & Febiger.

48. Food and Drug Administration (FDA), Public Health Service (PHS), Environmental Protection Agency (EPA): Memorandum of understanding between the FDA, PHS, and the EPA, Washington DC, June 4, 1993, FDA, PHS, EPA.

49. Gardner JF, Peel MM: *Introduction to sterilization, disinfection and infection control,* ed 2, New York, 1991, Churchill Livingstone.

50. Gardner JS, Favero MS: CDC guidelines for the prevention and control of nosocomial infections: guideline for handwashing and hospital environmental control, *Am J Infect Control* 14:110-129, 1986.

51. Gardner JS, Simmons BP: CDC guidelines for isolation precautions in hospitals, *Infect Control* 4:245-325, 1983.

52. Gerberding JL, Henderson DK: Management of occupational exposure to bloodborne pathogens: hepatitis B virus, hepatitis C virus and human immunodeficiency virus, *Clin Infect Dis* 14:1179-1185, 1992.

53. Gross A, Cutright DE, D'Alessandro SM: Effects of surgical scrub on microbial population under the fingernails, *Am J Surg* 138(3):463-467, 1979.

54. Guvton HG, Decker HM: Respiratory protection by five new contagion masks, *Appl Microbiol* 11:66-68, 1963.

55. Hahn JB: The source of the "resident" flora, *Hand* 5:247-252, 1973.

56. Haley CE: Drug resistant TB, Lecture at Baylor University Medical Center, Dallas, February 25, 1994.

57. Haley CE, McDonald RC, Rossi L, et al: Tuberculosis epidemic among hospital personnel, *Infect Control Hosp Epidemiol* 10:204-210, 1989.

58. Haley RW: *Managing hospital infection control for cost,* Chicago, 1986, American Hospital Publishing.

59. Haley RW: The development of infection surveillance and control programs. In Bennett JV, Brachman PS, editors: *Hospital infections,* ed 3, Boston, 1992, Little, Brown & Co.

60. Haley RW: The development of infection surveillance and control programs in hospital infection. In Bennett JV, Brachman PS, editors: *Hospital infections,* ed 4, Philadelphia, 1998, Lippincott-Raven.

61. Haley RW, Culver DH, White JW et al: The efficacy of infection surveillance and control programs in preventing nosocomial infections in U.S. hospitals, *Am J Epidemiol* 121:182-205, 1985.

62. Hedderwick SA, McNeil SA, Lyons MJ, et al: Pathogenic organisms associated with artificial fingernails worn by healthcare workers, *Inf Control Hosp Epidemiol* 21:8:505-509, 2000.

63. Henderson DK: Zeroing in on the appropriate management of occupational exposure to HIV-1, *Infect Control Hosp Epidemiol* 11:175-177, 1990.

64. Henderson DK: Postexposure chemoprophylaxis for occupational exposure to human immunodeficiency virus type 1: current status and prospects for the future, *Am J Med* 91(suppl 3S):312-319, 1991.

65. Henderson DK, Fahey BJ, Willy M et al: The risk for occupational transmission of human immunodeficiency virus type 1 (HIV-1) associated with clinical procedures: a prospective evaluation, *Ann Intern Med* 113:740-746, 1990.

66. Hoeprich PD, Jordan MC: *Infectious diseases: a modern treatise on infectious processes,* ed 4, 1989, JB Lippincott.

67. Holmberg SD, et al: Health and economic impacts of antimicrobial resistance, *Rev Infect Dis* 9:1065, 1989.

68. Hospital Infection Control Practices Advisory Committee: Guidelines for isolation precautions in hospitals, *Infect Cont Hosp Epidemiol* 17:53-80, 1996.

69. Hughes JM: Hantavirus pulmonary syndrome: an emerging infectious disease, *Science* 262:850-851, 1993.

70. Jacoby GA, Archer GL: New mechanisms of bacterial resistance to antimicrobial agents, *N Engl J Med* 324:601, 1991.

71. James CD: Personal communication, 1995.

72. Jarvas WR: Nosocomial transmission of multidrug-resistant *Mycobacterium tuberculosis, Am J Infect Control* 23:146-151, 1995.

73. Joint Commission on Accreditation of Healthcare Organizations: Standards: infection control. In JCAHO: Accreditation manual for hospitals, Chicago: 1990, Joint Commission on Accreditation of Healthcare Organizations.

74. Joint Commission on Accreditation of Healthcare Organizations: Accreditation manual for hospitals, Chicago, 1995, Joint Commission on Accreditation of Healthcare Organizations.

75. Kates SG, McGinley KJ, Larson EL, et al: Indigenous multiresistant bacteria from flowers in hospital and nonhospital environments, *Am J Infect Control* 19:156, 1991.

76. Kollmorgen GM, Bedford JS: Cellular radiation biology. In Dalrymple GV et al, editors: *Medical radiation biology,* Philadelphia, 1973, WB Saunders.

77. Koziol DE, Henderson DK: Risk analysis and occupational exposure to HIV and HBV, *Curr Opin Infect Dis* 6:506-510, 1993.

78. Kubiatowicz DO: Important safety information (business letter communication), St. Paul, Minn, May 4, 1990, Medical Device Division, 3M Health Care.

79. Lange JMA, et al: Failure of zidovudine prophylaxis after accidental exposure to HIV-1, *N Engl J Med* 322:1375-1377, 1990.

80. Lemonick MD: The killers all around, *Time* pp 183-185, Sept 12, 1994.

81. Looke DFM, Grove DI: Failed prophylactic zidovudine after needlestick injury, *Lancet* 335:1280, 1990 (letter).

82. Lynch P, Jackson MM, Rogers JC: Rethinking the role of isolation precautions in the prevention of nosocomial infections, *Ann Intern Med* 107:243-246, 1987.

83. Mahy BWJ, Centers for Disease Control and Prevention: Overview of infectious diseases in the workplace. Lecture at Baylor University Medical Center, Dallas, February 25, 1994.

84. Matera JR: Sterile tattooing: improving quality of care, *Radiat Ther* 10:2:165-167, 2001.

85. Miller DC: Creutzfeldt-Jakob disease in histopathology technicians, *N Engl J Med* 318:853, 1988.

86. Muldoon RL, Stanley ED, Jackson GG: Use and withdrawal of amantadine chemoprophylaxis during epidemic influenza A, *Am Rev Respir Dis* 133:487-491, 1976.

87. National Institute for Occupational Safety and Health: TB study funding announcement, *Federal Register* 58:148, 1993.

88. Noble RC: Infectiousness of pulmonary tuberculosis after starting chemotherapy: review of the available data on an unresolved question, *Am J Infect Control* 9:6-10, 1981.

89. Occupational Safety and Health Administration: OSHA Instruction CPL 2-2.44C, Washington DC, March 6, 1992, Office of Health Compliance Assistance.

90. Owens DK, Nease RF: Occupational exposure to human immunodeficiency virus and hepatitis B virus: a comparative analysis of risk, *Am J Med* 92:503-512, 1992.

91. Patterson JV, Hierholzer WJ Jr: The hospital epidemiologist. In Bennett JV, Brachman PS, editors: *Hospital infections,* ed 3, Boston, 1992, Little, Brown & Co.

92. Polder JA, Tablan OC, Williams WW: Personnel health services. In Bennett JV, Brachman PS, editors: *Hospital infections,* ed 3, Boston, 1992, Little, Brown & Co.

93. Rhame FS: The inanimate environment. In Bennett JV, Brachman PS, editors: *Hospitals infections,* ed 3, Boston, 1992, Little, Brown & Co.

94. Rhame FS: The inanimate environment. In Bennett JV, Brachman PS, editors: *Hospital infections,* ed 4, Philadelphia, 1998, Lippincott-Raven.

95. Rutala WA: APIC guideline for selection and use of disinfectants, *Am J Infect Control* 24:313-342, 1996.

96. Shaffer JG: Microbiology of hospital carpeting, *Health Lab Sci* 3:73, 1966.

97. Spira AI, Marx PA, Patterson BK, et al: Cellular targets of infection and route of viral dissemination after an intravaginal inoculation of simian immunodeficiency virus into rhesus macaques, *J Exp Med* 183:215-225, 1996.

98. Steelman VM: Creutzfeldt-Jakob disease: recommendations for infection control, *Am J Infect Control* 22:312-318, 1994.

99. Struble KA, Pratt RD, Gitterman SR: Toxicity of antiretroviral agents, *Am J Med* 102(suppl 5B):65-67, 1997.

100. Szuness W, et al: Hepatitis B vaccine: demonstration of efficacy in a controlled clinical trial in a high risk population in the United States, *N Engl J Med* 303:833-841, 1980.

101. Thomas CL, editor: *Taber's cyclopedic medical dictionary,* ed 1, Philadelphia, 1973, FA Davis.

102. US Department of Labor, OSHA: Enforcement procedures for the occupational exposure to bloodborne pathogens, OSHA Directive CPL 2-22.44D, Washington DC, November 5, 1999, Occupational Safety and Health Administration.

103. Williams WW, Centers for Disease Control: CDC guidelines for infection control in hospital personnel, *Infect Control* 4(suppl):326-349, 1983.

11

Assessment

Shirlee E. Maihoff

Outline

Key Terms

Affective
Anemia
Anorexia
Anxiety
Cachexia
Cognitive
Depression
Empathy

Kwashiorkor
Leukopenia
Marasmus
Myelosuppression
Quality of life
Rehabilitation
Thrombocytopenia

ASSESSMENT DEFINED

The assessment of cancer patients and of systems in which they function provides the basis of effective cancer care.[34] The diagnosis of cancer can precipitate significant changes in the lives of the patient and family. These changes can be physiologic, psychologic, and spiritual. To understand the effect of the cancer diagnosis on a patient, significant other, or family, the diagnosis must be considered a process rather than an event. That process is dynamic and continuous and changes over time.

Information obtained through a continuous, systematic assessment allows the health care provider to (1) determine the nature of a problem, (2) select an intervention for that problem, and (3) evaluate the effectiveness of the intervention. The assessment should be continued as long as interventions are needed and wanted by the patient to facilitate an optimal quality of life. Assessment can be accomplished most effectively through a multidisciplinary approach and requires the efforts of the entire oncology team, including surgical oncologists, medical oncologists, radiation oncologists, oncology nurses, radiation therapists, social workers, dietitians, and pastoral counselors.

The Importance of Assessment in Oncology

The assessment of cancer patients serves as the cornerstone for the structure of care. However, patient assessment is much more than obtaining a patient history. Patients come worried and often in pain. They feel extremely vulnerable and in need of help and understanding. Patients are often desperate to put their cancer problems behind them, receive treatment, and get on with their lives. They come hoping that health care providers will listen carefully and know the correct things to do to help them. Most patients want not only physical and psychologic comfort but also another person to firmly stand

<table>
<tr><td colspan="2">**Box 11-1**   **Helpful Behaviors**</td></tr>
</table>

Verbal
- Is nonjudgmental
- Uses understandable words
- Reflects and clarifies patient's statements
- Responds to real messages such as doubt and fear
- Summarizes or synthesizes the words of the patient
- Uses verbal reinforcers such as "I see" and "Yes"
- Approriately gives information
- Uses humor at times to reduce tension

Nonverbal
- Maintains good eye contact
- Touches appropriately
- Nods head occasionally
- Has animated facial expressions
- Smiles occasionally
- Uses occasional hand gestures
- Has moderately calm rate of speech
- Has moderate tone of voice

<table>
<tr><td colspan="2">**Box 11-2**   **Nonhelpful Behaviors**</td></tr>
</table>

Verbal
- Preaches
- Blames
- Placates
- Direct and demands
- Gives advice
- Has patronizing attitude
- Strays from topic
- Talks about self too much
- Overanalyzes or overinterprets
- Intellectualizes
- Uses words patient does not understand
- Probes and questions extensively, especially "why" questions

Nonverbal
- Has poor eye contact
- Frowns
- Has expressionless face
- Has tight mouth
- Yawns
- Shakes pointed finger
- Has unpleasant tone of voice

alongside them with genuine empathy at this vulnerable time. They want someone to resonate with their distress. All this intense emotion is presented after initial contact with the patient. Most people use their coping skills, but few fully reveal the extent of their feelings. Most adults convey varying degrees of ability to remain in control in an environment that appears strange at best and terrifying at worst.

Establishing a Therapeutic Relationship

Health professionals must recognize that the patient feels at a distinct disadvantage and must respect, reassure, and support even those who convey an incredible sense of confidence and comfort. At an initial encounter with a patient, acceptance, interest, and genuineness are imperative to establishing a therapeutic and healing relationship, which is critical to the healing process. Verbal and nonverbal communication between the patient and therapist is the basis of an effective therapeutic relationship. Box 11-1 lists helpful behaviors in working with patients; Box 11-2 lists verbal and nonverbal behaviors that are not helpful.

To be effective in assessment, therapists must use communication skills that involve hearing verbal messages, perceiving nonverbal messages, and responding verbally and nonverbally to both kinds of messages.

Some anthropologists believe that more than two thirds of any communication is transmitted nonverbally. Therefore gestures, facial expressions, posture, personal appearance, and cultural characteristics must be interpreted to understand the patient. Nonverbal behavior provides clues to but not conclusive proofs of underlying feelings. However, research has proved that nonverbal cues (Table 11-1) tend to be more reliable than verbal cues.

Table 11-1	Nonverbal cues in a communicative relationship
Cue	**Example**
Eye contact*	Steady or shifty and avoiding
Eyes	Open, teary, closed, and excessively blinking
Body position	Relaxed, leaning (toward or away), and tense
Mouth	Loose, smiling, tight, and lip biting
Facial expression	Animated, pained, bland, and distant
Arms	Unfolded and folded
Body posture	Relaxed, slouching, and rigid
Voice	Slow, whispering, high-pitched, fast, and cracking
General appearance	Clean, neat, well-groomed, and sloppy

*Eye contact may vary in appropriateness based on cultural differences (e.g., chinese persons do not consider eye contact appropriate with strangers).

Simple phrases to respond to negative nonverbal cues include, "You seem to be upset" and "You appear to be unhappy." Box 11-3 provides an exercise for recognizing nonverbal cues.

Verbal messages are clearer than nonverbal messages. Verbal messages are composed of **cognitive** and **affective** content. Cognitive content comprises the actual facts and

<table><tr><td>

Box 11-3   **Exercise for nonverbal cues**

What do the following gestures mean to you? When you have completed this exercise, compare your answers with those of your classmates. Do you have different perceptions?

1. A patient refuses to talk and avoids eye contact with you.
2. A patient looks directly into your eyes and stretches her hands out with the palms up.
3. The patient with whom you are talking holds one arm behind her back and clenches her hand tightly while using the other hand to make a fist at her side.
4. A patient walks into the examination room for a radiation therapy consultation with the doctor, sits erect, and clasps his folded arms across his chest before saying a word.
5. A patient sits in the waiting room, slouches in his chair, says nothing, and has tears streaming down his cheeks.

</td></tr></table>

words of the message. Affective content may be verbal or nonverbal and comprises feelings, attitudes, and behaviors. The difference in hearing only the obvious cognitive content of a verbal message and hearing the cognitive *and* underlying affective messages is the difference between being an ineffective or effective listener. Affective messages express feelings and emotions. These messages are much more difficult to communicate, hear, and perceive than cognitive messages. Feelings can be grouped into four major categories:

anger, sadness, fear, and happiness. One feeling commonly masks and covers up another. For example, anger may mask fear because fear is at the root of much anger. A cancer patient who appears to be extremely angry may be afraid but not able to honestly show fear. Box 11-4 concerning cognitive and affective responses demonstrates the difference between the two levels of responding to patients.

Identifying underlying feelings in verbal messages is difficult at first and related to a person's comfort level and proficiency in recognizing and expressing personal feelings. The health care professional must listen to patients' messages and identify their feelings rather than project personal feelings onto patients. This ability requires practice and awareness. Different people identify different underlying feelings for the same statement. Careful attention must be given to nonverbal and verbal cues when listening for the true feelings of patients.

Reflective listening involves responding with empathy. **Empathy** is defined as identifying with the feelings, thoughts, or experiences of another person. To arrive at the way the other person feels, the health care provider may ask inwardly, "If I were in this person's position, how would I feel?" A critical part of empathy is sharing feelings about the person's verbal communication. For example, empathic responses include, "Yes, I understand that . . . . I would feel angry too" and "Yes, I'm glad that . . . It would make me feel good too."

People rarely communicate in a direct manner concerning the thoughts and feelings that they are having. Reflective

<table><tr><td>

Box 11-4   **Exercise for cognitive and affective responses**

1. Patient: My skin is getting really red. I think you're burning me up.
Cognitive response: Are you putting that lotion on your skin?
Affective response: I hear your discomfort. It sounds like you're uncomfortable with your skin change. These are normal and temporary, and we're watching it every day.
2. Patient: My throat is getting sore. How much more sore is it going to get? I don't want one of those feeding tubes.
Cognitive response: Are you drinking acidic stuff, smoking, using your magic mouthwash?
Affective response: Sounds like the idea of a feeding tube is really frightening. That's not what happens with sore throats. The worst scenario is if it gets too sore, you'll have a couple days off!
3. Patient: It's only the second day of treatment and I have diarrhea!
Cognitive response: Well, what have you eaten?
Affective response: It's really kind of early for any diarrhea. What else do you think might be causing the diarrhea? Let's see the doctor and ask what she thinks.

4. Patient: I'm still in so much pain! When does this radiation start to work?
Cognitive response: Are you taking your pain medication?
Affective response: I'm sorry you're hurting, but everybody is different and sometimes it takes longer to get pain relief.
5. Patient: I sure am having trouble going to sleep. Is that normal?
Cognitive response: Well, how long is it taking you to go to sleep?
Affective response: Tell me what kinds of things are going through your mind while you're going to sleep.
6. Patient: I have a question and it's probably stupid, but I'm going to ask it anyway.
Cognitive response: No questons are stupid.
Affective response: I always appreciate patients who ask questions. It helps me know the things that are important to you.

</td></tr></table>

listening is a way for a person to listen and communicate effectively. The consequences of good reflective listening are as follows:

- The person becomes aware of small problems and prevents them from developing into major problems.
- The person is perceived by others as genuinely concerned, warm, understanding, and fair.
- The person has more knowledge about others, which helps in relating to them in a real way.

Reflective listening is not the only form of verbal response that radiation therapists can use. Reflective listening is essential to developing verbal responses appropriate for the issues involved. Following are 10 of the most commonly used and helpful verbal responses.

Minimal verbal response. *Minimal responses* are the verbal counterpart to the occasional head nodding. These are verbal clues such as "Yes," "Uh huh," and "I see" and indicate that the health care provider is listening to and understanding the patient.

Reflecting. *Reflecting* refers to health care providers communicating their understanding of the patient's concerns and perspectives. Health care workers can reflect the specific content or implied feelings of their nonverbal observations or communication they feel has been omitted or emphasized. The following are examples of reflecting: "You're feeling uncomfortable about finishing your treatments," "Sounds as if you're really angry at this disease," and "You really resent being treated like you're sick."

Paraphrasing. A *paraphrase* is a verbal statement that is interchangeable with a patient's statement. The words may be synonyms of words the patient has used. Paraphrasing acknowledges to patients that they are really being heard. The following is an example:

Patient: "I had a really bad night last night."
Therapist: "Things didn't go well for you last night."

Probing. *Probing* is an open-ended statement used to obtain more information. It is most effective when using statements such as "I'm wondering about . . . ," "Tell me more about that," and "Could you be saying. . ." in a smooth and flowing style. These statements facilitate much more open conversation than asking how, what, when, where, or who questions.

Clarifying. *Clarifying* is used to obtain more information about vague, ambiguous, or conflicting statements. Examples include the following: "I'm confused about . . . ," "I'm having trouble understanding . . . ," "Is it that . . ." and "Sounds to me like you're saying . . . ."

Interpreting. *Interpreting* occurs when the therapist adds something to the patient's statement or tries to help the patient understand underlying feelings. Health care providers may share their interpretation, the meaning, or the facts, thus providing the patient with an opportunity to confirm, deny, or offer an alternative interpretation. The patient may respond by saying, "Yes, that's it" or "No, not that but . . . ."

Checking out. *Checking out* occurs when therapists are genuinely confused about their perceptions of the patient's verbal or nonverbal behavior or have a hunch that should be examined. Examples are, "Does it seem as if . . ." and "I have a hunch that this feeling is familiar to you, are you saying . . . ." Therapists ask the patient to confirm or correct their perception or understanding of the patient's words.

Informing. *Informing* occurs when the therapist shares objective and factual information. An example is, "Your white blood cell count is extremely low, so it would be safer for you to avoid large crowds where the chances are higher of being exposed to bacteria and viruses."

Confronting. *Confronting* involves therapists making the client aware that their observations are not consistent with the patient's words. This response must be done with respect for the patient and extreme tact so that a defensive response is not elicited. An example of this is, "You say you're angry and depressed, yet you're smiling."

Summarizing. By *summarizing* the therapist condenses and puts in order the information communicated. This is extremely helpful when a patient rambles and has difficulty conveying the sequence of events. An example is, "I hear you saying . . . ."

Box 11-5 is designed to help the individual to learn to recognize and identify the types of major verbal responses just discussed. Box 11-6 is designed to help the individual to listen for feelings.

THE MULTIDISCIPLINARY APPROACH TO THE ASSESSMENT OF CANCER PATIENTS

General Health Assessment

One method of health assessment is the self-report. In a self-report, individuals disclose their perception of what is being measured. Box 11-7 demonstrates a self-assessment tool that is useful in decreasing documentation time by the oncology professional while eliciting comprehensive information.

An alternative assessment method is for the oncology practitioner to do an interview. This often is done by the oncology nurse or radiation oncologist, but a radiation therapist may also conduct the interview. The history includes the collection of data about the past and present health of each patient. A historical and physical evaluation should come from a referring physician, but a verification and current assessment should also be done.

Physical Assessment

Table 11-2 lists physical aspects a therapist is responsible to assess daily and interventions for treatment. Some assessments are relative to the area being treated with radiation therapy. Specific areas in the physical realm in which assessment of the cancer patient is paramount include nutrition, pain, and biochemical balance (blood counts).

Box 11-5 | **Exercise for recognizing and identifying the types of major verbal responses**

Read the following patient and therapist statements, and identify the therapist's response in each case as one of the 10 major verbal responses: minimal verbal response, paraphrasing, probing, reflecting, clarifying, checking out, interpreting, confronting, informing, or summarizing.*

1. Patient: I can't decide what to do. Nothing seems right.
   Caregiver: You're feeling pretty frustrated, and you want me to tell you what to do.
2. Patient: In our family the children don't do any of the work around the house.
   Caregiver: The children in your family don't do any housework.
3. Patient: My wife made me late for treatment today
   Caregiver: Tell me more about that
4. Patient: Do you think this is a good cancer center?
   Caregiver: The XYZ Association has ranked this cancer center number one in the state.
5. Patient: I guess that about covers it.
   Caregiver: Let's see if we can review what we've talked about today . . . . Does this seem right to you?

6. Patient: That's why I'm here. Dr. Jones said you were a good one to talk to.
   Caregiver: Let's see now. You want me to help you decide whether or not you should file for disability. Is that right?
7. Patient: Nobody in this world cares about anyone else.
   Caregiver: It's scary to feel that nobody at all cares about you.
8. Patient: Anyway, I'm unable to do it because it's too expensive. Besides, they won't help me anyway.
   Caregiver: Let me get this straight. You feel the tests will cost too much, and the results won't be worth the cost. Is that it?
9. Patient: I don't want to talk about it.
   Caregiver: You've told me that being open and honest about your illness is important to you, but you aren't willing to do that just now.
10. Patient: I have to go to the grocery store before picking up the children on the way home from my treatment.
    Caregiver: Oh, I see . . .

*See Appendix B for the answers to this exercise.

Box 11-6 | **Exercise for listening for feelings**

For each of the following statement, write what you think the person is really feeling. Ask yourself, "What are the underlying feelings here?"*

1. The doctor told me to come over here and have all these tests. I'll sit over here and wait until you're ready for me.
2. Have you heard anything about the new social worker? I'm supposed to see her at 3 PM.
3. Coming for treatment just doesn't seem to be helping me.
4. Are you going to see me again this week, Doctor?
5. Only 2 more weeks and I'm finished with my treatments.

*Discuss your answers with a small group in your class. Then look at all the possible answers in Appendix B.

Nutritional Assessment

Nutritional assessment involves the multidisciplinary oncology team. Oncology nurses are in an ideal position for the initial assessment of cancer patients and referrals to the nutrition specialist, or dietitian. In addition, therapists' awareness and knowledge in this area enable them to monitor patients under treatment and make appropriate referrals when needed.

Maintaining a good nutritional status is one of the most difficult challenges in treating cancer patients. Nutritional assessment is the critical first step in developing a comprehensive approach to the nutritional management of individuals with cancer. A complete list of components involved in nutritional assessment is outlined in Box 11-8.

After malnutrition is diagnosed, a plan of intervention is developed and implemented based on the information obtained in the nutritional assessment.

Weight loss is often the first physical change that alerts individuals with cancer to seek medical treatment. It is also frequently the first sign of malnutrition.

Specifically, the percent weight change is the most accurate measure of nutritional status. The percent weight change indicates the extent of tissue loss as a result of inadequate nutrition. For this reason, monitoring weight change weekly is imperative for patients who are undergoing radiation therapy. A calculation of a percent weight change is found in Table 11-3.

Nutritional Consequences of Cancer

Anorexia (loss of appetite resulting in weight loss) is a major contributor in the cause of cancer cachexia. **Cachexia** is a state of general ill health and malnutrition with early satiety; electrolyte and water imbalances; and progressive loss of body weight, fat, and muscle. Cachexia affects half to two thirds of patients with cancer.

Anorexia and taste alterations are two of the major causes of protein-calorie malnutrition in patients with cancer. The

Box 11-7	Functional health pattern patient self-assessment*

Health perception and health management
- Who provides your health and dental care?
- How often do you see your doctor and dentist?
- List the medication(s) you take. How much? How often?
- How much alcohol do you drink in a week?
- Do you smoke cigarettes or cigars? If so, how much?
- What allergies do you have? What happens when you have an allergic reaction?
- What other medical probelms do you have?

Nutritional metabolic pattern
- Are you on any special diet?
- What did you eat yesterday (over the last 24 hours)?
- How much fluid do you drink each day?
- List the vitamins you take each day
- Have you noticed any changes in your appetite? If yes, describe.
- Have you noticed any changes in your weight? If yes, describe.
- What foods do you avoid?
- Who cooks your meals
- Do you wear dentures or partial plates?
- How do you take care of your skin? (What creams, lotions, or powders are you using?)
- Do you take baths or showers? How often?

Elimination pattern
- How often do you move your bowels?
- Do you have problems with diarrhea, constipation, or loss of control?
- What foods and medications do you use to regulate your bowels (laxatives, prunes, bran, and others)?
- How many times a day do you urinate?
- Have you had any changes such as loss of control, burning, frequency, or difficulty urinating?

Activity and exercise pattern
- Do you feel tired during the day? Is this new?
- What changes have you noticed in your energy level?
- What exercises do you do? How often?
- What do you do for relaxation and fun?
- Do you need help with ambulating, bathing, toileting, dressing, grooming, feeding, cooking, food shopping, housecleaning, or food preparation?

Sleep and rest pattern
- What time do you go to bed?
- What time do you get up?
- Do you have any problems sleeping?
- How do you feel when you wake up?
- Do you take any medications to help you sleep?

Cognitive and perceptual pattern
- Are you having problems hearing?
- Have you noticed any recent changes in your hearing?
- Do you use any hearing aids?
- Have you noticed any changes in your vision?
- How often do you have your eyes examined?
- Do you wear glasses or contact lenses?
- Are you experiencing any pain? If yes, where is the pain located? Describe it.
- What do you do to manage your pain?
- How does the pain affect your lifestyle?
- What is your occupation?

Roles and relationships pattern
- What is your marital status?
- Do you have children and grandchildren?
- With whom do you live?
- What changes in your family roles or relationships have you noticed since your illness?
- How do you anticipate that the radiation treatment will affect your daily routine?
- What is the best time for your radiation treatment?

Self-perception and conceptual pattern
- How would you describe yourself?
- What are your strengths and weaknesses?

Sexual and reproductive pattern
- Are you sexually active?
- Do you use any form of birth control?
- Have you had any changes in sexual relations?

Coping and stress-management pattern
- How do you handle major problems and stresses in your life?
- How are you coping with your life and diagnosis?
- What do you do to relax?
- What are your concerns regarding your treatment?

Value and belief pattern
- What is important in your life?
- Describe your spiritual needs.
- What part does religion play in your lifestyle?

Life and lifestyle patterns
- Describe your usual day.
- What means of transportation do you have?

Modified from Hirshfield-Batek J, Dow KH, Creaton E: Decreasing documentation time using a patient self-assessment tool, *Oncol Nurs Forum* 17:251-255, 1990. Courtesy Beth Israel Hospital, Boston, Massachusetts.
*In the actual form, space is provided for patients' responses.

Table 11-2	Componets of daily physical assessment
Side effects	**Interventions**

Side effects	Interventions
Skin reactions Erythema (3000-4000) cGy Dry and moist desquamation (4500-6000 cGy)	Instruct the patient to do the following: • Assess and monitor skin integrity and changes • Use a moisturizing lotion after showering, and avoid port marks. • Avoid creams that contain alcohol. • Avoid exposing the treated area to heat, cold, wind, soaps, deodorant, and razor shaving. If skin erythema occurs, do the following: • Use moisturizing lotion according to the physician's orders. • Protect skin from further irritation, and wear loose cotton clothes. If skin breakdown occurs, do the following: • If dry desquamation has occurred, continue to use moisturizing lotion. • If the skin is tender, use cortisone cream as directed. • For moist desquamation, use Burrow's compresses and silver sulfadiazine creams per the physician's prescription. (The physician may consider temporarily stopping further treatment.) Try to aerate areas of skin breakdown, especially in skin folds.
Fatigue	Assess the energy level. Determine periods of increased fatigue. Assist patients to pace activities and listen to their bodies. Ensure adequate nutritional intake.
Sleep	Assess normal sleep patterns and changes. Evaluate the cause of problems.
Mouth changes (3000-4000 cGy)	Inspect the oral cavity. Assess the presence of stomatitis, xerostomia, mucositis, and taste changes. Instruct the patient about a soft, bland diet.
Diarrhea (2000-5000 cGy)	Assess the bowel function. Instruct the patient on a low-residue diet for use as diarrhea occurs. Use antispasmodic medications as prescribed. Instruct the patient on perianal care.
Cystitis (<3000 cGy)	Assess the bladder function. Monitor for urinary retention or hematuria. Use antispasmodic medications as prescribed. Monitor for bladder infections.
Nausea and vomiting (1000-3000 cGy)	Anticipate nausea and vomiting in high-risk patients, and prevent nausea and vomiting by using antiemetics prophylactically before treatment and as needed continuously. Provide fluids to prevent dehydration. Refer or instruct the patient on a low-fat and low-sugar diet. Use nonpharmacologic measures such as relaxation and guided imagery.
Pharyngitis and esophagitis (2000 cGy)	Assess pain during swallowing (dysphagia). Modify the diet to soft, nonspicy, and nonacidic foods. Use topical anesthetics and analgesics as prescribed (lidocaine mixed with Mylanta or Maalox [1:3]).
Alopecia (2000 cGy)	Protect the scalp from heat, cold, and wind. Suggest an appropriate head covering. Do the following to minimize scalp irritation: • Avoid frequent shampooing. • Avoid using blow dryers, hairsprays, gels, or other hair preparations. • Apply moisturizing lotion to the scalp. Explore issues related to body image (e.g., getting a wig or hairpiece at the start of treatment).
Pain	Assess the location and intensity. Instruct the patient on the importance of taking medications regularly.
Skin pallor	Monitor low hemoglobin, white blood cell, and platelet levels with weekly complete blood counts (CBCs).
Weight loss	Monitor once per week, and chart the results. Determine eating problems.

cGy, Centigray.

Box 11-8	Components of the nutritional assessment

Medical history
- Duration and type of malignancy
- Frequency, type, and severity of complications (e.g., infections and draining lesions)
- Type and duration of therapy
- Specific chemotherapeutic agents used
- Radiation sites
- Antibiotics used
- Other drugs used
- Surgical procedures performed (site, type, and date)
- Side effects of therapy (diarrhea, anorexia, nausea, and vomiting)
- Concomitant medical conditions (diabetes, heart disease, liver failure, kidney failure, and infection)

Physical examination
- General appearance
- Condition of hair
- Condition of skin
- Condition of teeth
- Condition of mouth, gums, and throat
- Edema
- Performance status
- Identification of nutritionally related problems (fistula, pain, stomatitis, xerostomia, infection, constipation diarrhea, nausea, vomiting, and obstruction)

Dietary history
- 24-hour recall of foods eaten, including snacks
- Composition of food taken in 24 hours (calories and protein, caffeine, and liquor)
- Income
- Time of day meals and snacks eaten
- Past or current diet modifications
- Self-feeding ability
- Special cancer diet
- Vitamins, minerals, or other supplements
- Modifications of diet or eating habits as a result of treatment or illness
- Foods withheld of given on the basis of personal or religious grounds (e.g., kosher, vegetarian)
- Food preferences
- Food allergies or intolerances

Socioeconomic history
- Number of persons living in the home (ages and relationships)
- Kitchen facilities
- Income
- Food purchased
- Food prepared
- Amount spent on food per month
- Outside provision of meals

Anthropometric data
- Height
- Weight
- Actual weight as percentage of ideal
- Weight change as percentage of usual
- Triceps skinfold measurement
- Actual triceps skinfold as percentage of standard
- Midarm circumference
- Midarm muscle circumference
- Actual midarm muscle circumference as percentage of standard

Biochemical data
- Hematocrit
- Hemoglobin
- Serum albumin
- Serum transferrin
- Creatinine
- Creatinine height index
- Total lymphocyte count
- Delayed hypersensitivity response-skin testing
- Nitrogen balance
- Blood urea nitrogen
- Sodium, potassium, carbon dioxide, chloride
- Glucose

Modified from Groenwald SL et al: *Nutritional disturbances: cancer nursing principles and practice*, ed 3, Boston, 1993, Jones & Bartlett.

three forms of protein-calorie malnutrition are marasmus, kwashiorkor, and marasmus-kwashiorkor mix.

Marasmus, or calorie malnutrition, can be observed in patients who are slender or slightly underweight. It is characterized by weight loss of 7% to 10% and fat and muscle depletion. **Kwashiorkor,** or *protein* malnutrition, is seen in patients with an adequate intake of carbohydrates and fats but an inadequate intake of protein. Kwashiorkor in patients

is often initially overlooked because they appear well nourished. This condition is characterized by retarded growth and development, muscle wasting, depigmentation of the hair and skin, edema, and depression of the cellular immune response. Marasmus-kwashiorkor mix, or protein and calorie malnutrition, is the most life-threatening form of malnutrition because it involves the depletion of fat and muscle stores and visceral protein stores. This condition is most commonly

Table 11-3	Evaluation of weight change*	
Time	Significant Weight Loss	Severe WeightLoss
1 wk	1%-2%	>2%
1 mo	5%	>5%
3 mo	7.5%	>7.5%
6 mo	10%	>10%

From Blackburn GL et al: Nutritional and metabolic assessment of the hospitalized patient, *J Parent Ent Nutr* 1:17, 1977.
*Values charged are for percent weight change.

$$\text{Percent weight change} = \frac{\text{Usual weight} - \text{Actual weight}}{\text{Usual weight}} \times 100$$

found in seriously ill, hospitalized patients who have had inadequate nutritional care throughout their illness. Marasmus-kwashiorkor mix is characterized by weight loss of 10% or greater in a 6-month period, decreased fat and muscle stores, depleted visceral protein stores, and depression of the cellular immune responses.

Pain Assessment

Pain, one of the most feared consequences of cancer, is a complex process that has biologic, social, and spiritual dimensions. All pain is real, regardless of its cause, and most pain is a combination of physiologic and psychogenic factors. This phenomenon is connected to the essence of human existence and often precipitates questions about the meaning of life itself. Pain holds a great deal of power with the cancer patient experiencing it.

A multidimensional conceptualization of cancer pain as defined by Ahles et al[1] aids in understanding the scope of cancer pain. They propose five dimensions to consider in assessing and managing the experience of cancer pain: (1) physiologic (organic cause of pain), (2) sensory (intensity, location, and quality), (3) affective (depression and anxiety), (4) cognitive (the manner in which pain influences a person's thought processes and the way people view themselves or the meaning of pain), and (5) behavioral (pain-related behaviors such as medication intake and activity level).

McGuire[18] proposes a sixth dimension: sociocultural. This dimension involves the effects of cultural, social, and demographical factors that are related to the experience of pain.

Physiologic dimension. Foley[10] described three types of pain (each with a different cause) observed in cancer patients: (1) pain associated with direct tumor involvement, (2) pain associated with cancer therapy, and (3) pain unrelated to the tumor or its treatment.

Two important characteristics of pain are related to the cause of pain: the duration and pattern of pain. Duration refers to whether pain is acute or chronic. Acute pain generally is a sudden onset with an identifiable cause lasting 3 to 6 months and responds to treatment with analgesic drug therapy and treatment of its precipitating cause. Chronic pain is the persistence of pain for more than 3 months with a less well-defined onset. Its cause may not be known. The second characteristic related to the cause of pain (the pattern of pain) has three separate patterns: (1) brief, momentary, or transient; (2) rhythmic, periodic, or intermittent; and (3) continuous, steady, or constant. Melzack[20] first described these patterns in the McGill Pain Questionnaire (MPQ).

Sensory dimension. The second dimension (sensory) as set forth by Ahles et al[1] consists of pain location, intensity, and quality. The first component of establishing the location of pain is extremely important. One of the methods that can be used is to ask the patient to point with one finger to the site of the pain. Another method is to use a picture of the body and ask the patient to mark on the picture the location of the pain.

The second component is the intensity of the pain (i.e., the strength of its feeling). Intensity is the most commonly assessed aspect of pain. The goal is to translate the patient's description of intensity into numbers or words to provide an objective description. Visual analogue scales (VASs) and categorical scales are commonly used to quantify the intensity of pain. A VAS rates 0 (no pain) to 10 (severe pain). A categorical scale also has a numerical system with 0 (no pain), 1 (mild), 2 (discomforting), 3 (distressing), 4 (horrible), and 5 (excruciating). Descriptions of the pain may be helpful in determining its origin and implementing effective measures for its control. For example, burning, hot pain may indicate the involvement of nerve tissue. This type of pain does not do well with narcotic analgesics.

The third component of the sensory dimension is the quality of pain (i.e., the way it actually feels). In the MPQ, some of the most common terms used to describe the quality of pain are as follows: aching, hot-burning, sharp, tender, throbbing, cramping, stabbing, heavy, shooting and gnawing, splitting, tiring-exhausting, sickening, and fearful.

Affective dimension. The third dimension (affective) as defined by Ahles et al[1] consists of depression, anxiety, and other psychologic factors or personality traits associated with pain. Anxiety and depression are critical factors that affect a patient's response to pain and ability to tolerate and cope with pain because anxiety often increases pain. Assessing which measure can be taken to decrease the pain is essential.

Cognitive dimension. The fourth dimension (cognitive) involves the way that pain influences thought processes or the way that people view themselves. A patient can be asked, "Are there any thoughts or images that may make your pain worse?" Some patients experience pain based on faulty logic. The following are examples of problem thinking by patients: "Nothing can be done to control the pain," "Pain is inevitable and should be tolerated," and "Doctors do not want to be bothered with complaints of pain." If undetected, these thoughts impair the assessment and management of pain.

Behavioral dimension. The fifth dimension (behavioral)

includes a variety of observable behaviors related to pain. The assessment of pain behavior can include verbal and nonverbal responses such as moans, grimaces, and complaints. Estimates of physical activity are also important aspects of pain behavior. Factors such as physical exercise, time spent in bed, and ability to do chores have been used to measure pain behavior. An excellent tool for this is the Karnofsky Performance Status[35] (Table 11-4).

The use of analgesics and drugs should also be considered in the assessment of pain behavior. The type and amount of drug and the way the dose is scheduled is important. Patients are often afraid of narcotic pain medications and take them only after they are in pain. Therapists should encourage regular dosing and explain the importance of a stable blood-serum level, which is needed to interrupt the pain cycle. The duration of the effect of the drug and any mood change on administration should be noted.

Sociocultural dimension. The last dimension (proposed by McGuire[18] and added to Ahles et al's five dimensions[1]) consists of a variety of ethnic, cultural, demographical, spiritual, and related factors that influence a person's perception of and response to pain. Cultural and religious practices have a strong influence on the pain experience. Overt actions are accepted in some cultures, whereas other cultures consider such actions weak. A general value held by many Americans is that a good patient does not complain when in pain; a complainer has lost self-control. Unfortunately, health care professionals sometimes directly reinforce these beliefs.

Age, gender, and race may provide different pain experiences. Research shows that females and older individuals have increased verbal expressions of pain.

In considering the six dimensions of cancer pain, a holistic and multidisciplinary approach to assessment and management is essential. As stated, many factors contribute to the pain experience.

The multidimensional concept of cancer pain necessitates the involvement of various health care disciplines in assessment and management. Input is needed from many health caregivers, including oncologists, primary physicians, nurses, radiation therapists, social workers, pharmacists, psychologists, anesthesiologists, and occupational therapists.

Pain assessment has several purposes. First, it establishes a baseline for treatment and interventions. Second, it helps focus which interventions are best for the patient. Third, it enables the evaluation of chosen interventions. Pain assessment should be systematic, organized, and ongoing. In general, certain principles should be followed in evaluating the cancer patient who experiences pain (see Box 11-9).

Tools to assess pain must be simple, short, and relevant for the patient. Pain-assessment tools can be classified according to the number of pain dimensions they assess. Multidimensional tools focus on two or more dimensions of the pain experience. Probably the most well-known and best example is the MPQ.[20]

The MPQ has the ability to assess in the sensory, cognitive, affective, and behavioral dimensions. Specifically, the MPQ elicits information about the location of pain; the intensity and periodicity of the pain; symptoms; effects on sleep, activity, and eating; and patterns of the analgesic used. Two long forms and a short form are used.

A similar multidimensional tool is the Brief Pain Inventory (BPI).[5] The BPI was developed primarily for clinical use with patients in pain who were too ill to be subjected to long and exhausting assessment techniques. The BPI assesses the following dimensions: the history and site of pain; the intensity of pain at its worst, as its usual level, and at its present level; medications and treatments used to relieve the pain; the relief obtained; and the effect of pain on

Table 11-4	Karnofsky performance status
Score (%)	**Status**
100	Normal—no complaints and no evidence of disease
90	Ability to carry on normal activity—minor signs or symptoms of disease
80	Normal activity with effort—some signs or symptoms of disease
70	Self-care—inability to carry on normal activity or do active work
60	Occasional assistance required but ability to care for most needs
50	Considerabe assistance and frequent medical care required
40	Disability—special care and assistance required
30	Severe disability—hospitalization indicated, although death not imminent
20	Extreme sickness—hospitalization and active supportive treatment neccessary
10	Moribund status—fatal processes progressing rapidly
0	Death

Modified from Yates JW, Chalmer B, McKegney FP: Evaluation of patients with advanced cancer using the Karnofsky Performance Status, *CA Cancer J Clin* 45:2220-2224, 1980.

Box 11-9	Evaluating the cancer patient's pain

- Believe the patient's complaint of pain.
- Take a careful history of the patient's pain complaint.
- Evaluate the patient's psychologic state.
- Perform a careful medical and neurologic examination.
- Order and review appropriate diagnostic studies.
- Treat the pain to facilitate the appropriate workup.
- Reassess the patient's response to therapy.
- Individualize the diagnostic and therapeutic approaches.
- Discuss advance directives with the patient and family.

mood, interpersonal relations, walking, sleeping, working, and enjoyment of life. The BPI is a self-administered tool.

A third tool is the Memorial Pain Assessment Card (MPAC).[9] The MPAC consists of three visual analog scales. It is a short, easy-to-administer tool that measures pain intensity, pain relief, and mood by choosing from a list of adjectives describing each. It can distinguish pain from psychologic distress and can be used to study the subtle interaction of these factors.

A sample questionnaire for an initial pain assessment is shown in Box 11-10.

Radiation therapists are vital in the ongoing assessment of a patient's pain. Therapists see patients every day and can evaluate the level of pain and the way the patient is responding. Being aware of personal beliefs and biases about pain, learning how to listen and communicate, and asking key questions are imperative skills for holistic health caregivers.

Accurate assessment of pain is the first step toward understanding the experience as the patient perceives it. Good assessment promotes an essential therapeutic relationship between patient and caregiver. Assessment is the foundation in the process of finding an effective intervention for the devastating experience of pain for the cancer patient.

Blood

Hematologic changes in cancer patients are critical for ongoing assessments because hematopoietic tissue exhibits a rapid rate of cellular proliferation. Hematopoietic tissue is especially vulnerable to cancer treatments (chemotherapy and radiation therapy). A **myelosuppression,** a reduction in bone marrow function, often results. The changes that may occur can result in anemia, leukopenia, and thrombocytopenia.

Anemia is a decrease in the peripheral red blood cell count. Without sufficient red blood cells, the circulatory system's oxygen-carrying capacity is impaired. This is due to a decrease in the hemoglobin level in the red blood cell, which serves as the carrier of oxygen from the lungs to tissues. Patients usually experience pale skin, muscle weakness, and fatigue (probably the most pervasive symptom). Normal blood values are found in Table 11-5.

Leukopenia is a decrease in the white blood cell count, thus increasing the risk of infection for the cancer patient. Because of chemotherapy or the disease process itself, patients may already have compromised immune systems. Therefore monitoring the white blood cell count during treatments is essential. (Normal values can be found in Table 11-5.) Because of patients' inability to fight disease, they need to reduce their exposure risks. Patients should be told to have minimal contact with others, especially if someone is sick. Health care workers also need to keep a distance if sick and at work.

Thrombocytopenia is a reduction in the number of circulating platelets. This decrease may be caused by a failure of the bone marrow to produce megakaryocyte cells, the precursors of platelets. This can be a result of various factors, such as chemotherapy, radiation therapy, the disease, or stress. The most significant factor that determines the risk of bone marrow depression related to radiation therapy is the volume of productive bone marrow in the radiation field. Therefore with large fields, monitoring counts is extremely important. Normal values for platelets can be found in Table 11-5.

Psychosocial Assessment

Quality of life. A growing attention to the quality of life of cancer patients reflects the changing attitude of society and health care personnel. The value of cancer treatments is judged not only on survival but also on the quality of that survival. The term **quality of life** has emerged in recent years to summarize the broad-based assessment of the combined effect of disease and treatment and the tradeoff between the two.

Cancer and its treatment, perhaps more than any other medical condition, becomes a major determinant of a patient's quality of life. The suggestion has been made in the literature that the emotional repercussions of cancer far exceed those of any other disease, and the emotional suffering cancer generates may actually exceed the physical suffering it causes. Therefore good quality-of-life information can make a major contribution in improving the management of cancer patients.

A more general definition of quality of life is a person's subjective sense of well-being derived from personal experience of life as a whole. The areas of life, or domains, most important to individuals resultantly have the most influence on their quality of life.

General agreement exists that the domains of quality of life for assessment should include physical, psychologic, and social factors. In the physical domain the quality of life is affected by loss of function, symptoms, and limited activity as a result of the disease process and physical effects of treatments. In the psychologic domain, five major emotional themes have been identified: (1) fear and anxiety generated by the diagnosis and compounded by inadequate communication with caregivers, (2) loss of personal control associated with the need to be dependent on those administering treatment, (3) uncertainty about the outcome of treatments, (4) the physician's persistent enthusiasm for cure, and (5) the debilitating effect of standard cancer treatments. In addition, loss of self-esteem and feelings of anxiety, depression, resentment, anger, discouragement, helplessness, hopelessness, isolation, and rejection are common.

Assessment. Many measures are available to assess quality of life or health-related quality of life. This is, however, a double-edged sword. Those doing the assessing have choices and can choose tools based on specific characteristics of a particular disease site. However, this divides potential data and makes comparisons of studies and research much more

Box 11-10	Initial Pain Assessment Tool

Patient's Name _____

Diagnosis _____

Date _____

Age _____ Room _____

Physician _____

Therapist/Nurse _____

Location The patient or therapist marks the drawing.

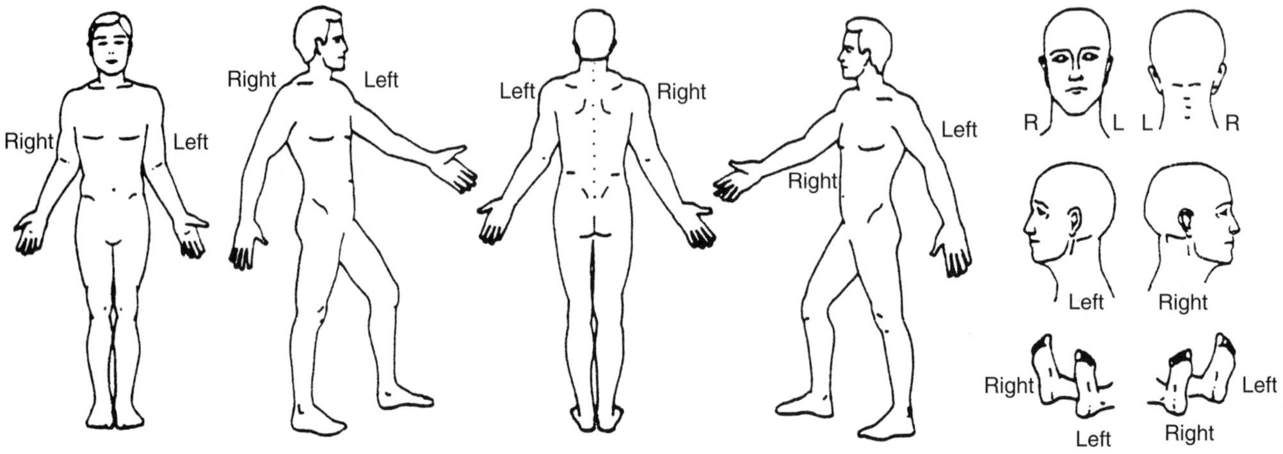

Intensity The patient rates the pain. Scale used: _____

Present level of pain: _____

Worst level of pain: _____

Best level of pain: _____

Acceptable level of pain: _____

Quality Use the patient's own words (e.g., "prick," "ache," "burn," "throb," "pull," "sharp")

_____

Onset, Duration, Variation, and Rhythms _____

Manner of Expressing Pain _____

What Relieves the Pain? _____

What Causes or Increases the Pain? _____

Effects of Pain (Note the decreased function and decreased quality of life)

Accompanying symptoms (e.g., nausea): _____

Sleep: _____

Appetite: _____

Physical activity: _____

Relationship with others (e.g., irritability): _____

Emotions (e.g., angry, suicidal, and crying): _____

Concetration: _____

Other: _____

Other Comments _____

Plan _____

Modified from McCaffery M, Beebe A: *Pain: clinical manual for nursing practice*, St. Louis, 1989, Mosby.

Table 11-5	Normal blood values*	
Level	**Percentage (range)**	
Hematocrit (Hct)		
Men	45 (38-54)	
Women	40 (36-47)	
Hemoglobin (Hgb)[†]		
Men	14-18 g/dl	
Women	12-16 g/dl	
Children	12-14 g/dl	

Blood Counts	Per Cubic Millimeter	Percentage
Erythrocytes (RBCs)		
Men	$5(4.5-6) \times 10$	100
Women	$4.5(4.3-5.5) \times 10$	100
Reticulocytes		0-1
Total leukocytes (WBCs)	5000-10,000	100
Polymorphonuclear leukocytes[‡]	2500-6000	40-60
Bands	0-500	0-5
Lymphocytes	1000-4000	20-40
Eosinophils	50-300	1-3
Basophils	0-100	0-1
Monocytes	200-800	4-8
Platelets	200,000-500,000 (severely low <20,000)	100

*Values may vary slightly according to the laboratory methods used.
[†]Severely low <7.5 g/dl.
[‡]Granulocytes, segmented neutrophils, and polymorphonuclear cells.
RBCs, red blood cells.
WBCs, white blood cells.

difficult. Following are some of the assessment tools* available to examine quality of life.

Quality of Life Index. The Quality of Life Index (QLI)[25] focuses on the present (within the last week) quality of a person's life. It clusters 14 items in 3 groups: general physical condition, normal human quality, and general attitudes as they relate to general quality of life. The patient responds by placing an X on a linear slide. The QLI can be found in Box 11-11.

Normal refers to the normal status before illness. The QLI is easy to use and practical. It has reliability and validity in its statistical components.

Functional Living Index—Cancer. The Functional Living Index—Cancer (FLIC)[29] is a 22-item scale on which patients indicate the effect of cancer on day-to-day living

---

*These tools are several of the cancer-specific, health-related, quality-of-life measures and approaches that are yielding good results.

issues that assess the functional quality of life. It uses a 7-point Likert-type scale. This scale is often used in measuring attitudes and in the following ranges: strongly agree, agree, slightly agree, undecided, slightly disagree, disagree, and strongly disagree. This tool has been used extensively in oncology with predominantly positive results.

Functional Assessment of Cancer Therapy Scales. The Functional Assessment of Cancer Therapy (FACT) Scale[4] has 28 items and specifies subscales that reflect symptoms or problems associated with different diseases (head and neck, breast, bladder, colorectal, and lung cancers). The results yield information on the patient's well-being, social and family well-being, relationship with the physician, emotional well-being, and specific disease concerns. A form of this tool, called the *FACT–G,* can be found in Box 11-12. This tool can also distinguish stages, metastatic from non-metastatic diseases, and inpatients from outpatients.

Coping Strategies and Responses—The Patient. Over the past several decades a great deal of interest has been focused on assessing an individual's psychosocial adjustments to illness. The areas that comprise the realm of psychosocial issues are numerous.

The affective responses that occur most frequently among cancer patients are anxiety and depression. The discussion about tools for assessment focuses on these two major areas.

A working definition for **anxiety** is an individual responding to a perceived threat affectively at an emotional level with an increased level of arousal associated with vague, unpleasant, and uneasy feelings. The instrument used most often to measure anxiety in cancer patients is the State-Trait Anxiety Inventory (STAI).[31] The STAI is composed of two scales: the A-trait and A-state. On the A-state are 20 items with a 4-point scale with the following possible responses: not at all, somewhat, moderately so, and very much. Responses are summed to measure the way the subject feels at a particular moment. Scores demonstrate the level of transitory anxiety characterized by feelings of apprehension, tension, and autonomic nervous system–induced symptoms that are worry, nervousness, and apprehension. The A-trait inventory is designed to measure a general level of arousal and predict anxiety proneness. Construct validity and reliability are established for this tool.

Irwin et al[14] conducted a study of 181 patients receiving external beam radiation and found that all patients (males and females) exhibited higher anxiety scores than nonpatient norms before treatment. In this sample, higher anxiety scores were reported among females over males before treatment began, 1 week after treatment was completed, and 2 months after the completion of therapy. In general, patients showed significantly higher anxiety during rather than after treatment.

Every patient brings a history of coping strategies to the cancer experience. Patients use whatever has worked for them in the past in managing their anxiety. Box 11-13 lists effective and noneffective coping strategies.

Depression is the second most common affective response

Box 11-11	Quality of Life Index

With respect to your general physical condition, please place an X on the line at the pont that best shows what is happening to you at the present time (within the past week):

GENERAL PHYSICAL CONDITION

1. How much *pain* are you feeling?	None	_____	Excruciating
2. How much *nausea* do you experience?	None	_____	Constant nausea
3. How frequently do you *vomit*?	Not at all	_____	Constant vomiting or retching
4. How much *strength* do you feel?	None	_____	Normal for me
5. How much *appetite* do you have?	None	_____	Normal for me

IMPORTANT HUMAN ACTIVITIES

6. Are you able to *work* at your usual tasks (e.g., housework,office work, and gardening)?	Not at all	_____	Normal for me
7. Are you able to *eat*?	Not at all	_____	Normal for me
8. Are you able to obtain *sexual* satisfaction?	Not at all	_____	Normal for me
9. Are you able to *sleep* well?	Not at all	_____	Normal for me

GENERAL QUALITY OF LIFE

10. How good is your quality of life (general QL)?	Extremely poor	_____	Excellent
11. Are you having *fun* (e.g., hobbies, recreation, and social activities)?	Not at all	_____	Normal for me
12. Is your life *satisfying*?	Not at all	_____	Normal for me
13. Do you feel *useful*?	Not at all	_____	Normal for me
14. Do you *worry about the cost* of medical care?	Not at all	_____	A great deal

Modified from Padilla GV et al: Quality of Life Index for patients with cancer, *Res Nurs Health* 6:117-126, 1983.

in cancer patients. **Depression** is defined as the perceived loss of self-esteem resulting in a cluster of affective behavioral (change in appetite, sleep disturbances, lack of energy, withdrawal, and dependency) and cognitive (decreased ability to concentrate, indecisiveness, and suicidal ideas) responses. Depression plays a major role in the quality of life for cancer patients and their families. However, empirical and clinical reports indicate that depression is an underdiagnosed and probably undertreated response among persons with cancer.

Knowing the way to recognize depression is a critical skill for all oncology health caregivers. Instances have been cited in which patients with undiagnosed depression that returned home and committed suicide after receiving a radiation therapy treatment. The physicians, nurses, and therapists thought that the patient who was experiencing severe sequelae in the head and neck radiation treatments was just a "quiet person." The signs of depression were present, and no referral was made to a professional. The criteria for recognizing a depressed condition are the following (usually four of these are present nearly every day for at least 2 weeks):

1. Poor appetite or significant weight loss or increased appetite or significant weight gain
2. Insomnia or hypersomnia (e.g., difficulty with falling asleep, awakening 30 to 90 minutes before time to arise, awakening in the middle of the night with difficulty going back to sleep, increased time of sleep, frequent naps)
3. Psychomotor agitation or retardation (noticeable to others, not just subjective feelings)
4. Loss of interest or pleasure in usual activities or decrease in sexual drive
5. Loss of energy (fatigue)
6. Feelings of worthlessness, self-reproach, or excessive or inappropriate guilt
7. Complaints or evidence of diminished ability to think or concentrate, such as slowed thinking or indecisiveness
8. Recurrent thoughts of death, suicidal ideation, wishes to be dead, or suicide attempt

The radiation therapist who sees and talks to the patient daily is in an excellent position to recognize signs of depression. Questions asked about a patient's eating or sleeping habits or energy level are essential. Therapists must listen and discern carefully the answers to these questions. The danger of routine is to ask how patients are doing and not hear what they are saying, whether through their words or nonverbal cues. Practicing and developing skills discussed in the first part of this chapter is critical for taking care of the whole patient.

Physiologic changes such as sleep disturbance, change in weight, appetite disturbance, and decreased energy are experienced frequently by cancer patients as a result of their

The Fact-G Scale

Fact-G (version 4)

Patient's Name _____ Age _____ Room _____

Diagnosi _____ Physician _____

Below is a list of statements that other people with your illness have said are important. By circling one (1) number per line, please indicate how true each statement has been for you during the past 7 days.

PHYSICAL WELL-BEING	Not at all	A little bit	Some-what	Quite a bit	Very much
GP1 I have a lack of energy	0	1	2	3	4
GP2 I have nausea	0	1	2	3	4
GP3 Because of my physical condition, I have trouble meeting the needs of my family	0	1	2	3	4
GP4 I have pain	0	1	2	3	4
GP5 I am bothered by side effects of treatment	0	1	2	3	4
GP6 I feel ill	0	1	2	3	4
GP7 I am forced to spend time in bed	0	1	2	3	4

SOCIAL/FAMILY WELL-BEING	Not at all	A little bit	Some-what	Quite a bit	Very much
GS1 I feel close to my friends	0	1	2	3	4
GS2 I get emotional support from my family	0	1	2	3	4
GS3 I get support from my friends	0	1	2	3	4
GS4 My family has accepted my illness	0	1	2	3	4
GS5 I am satisfied with family communication about my illness	0	1	2	3	4
GS6 I feel close to my partner (or the person who is my main support)	0	1	2	3	4

Q1 *Regardless of your current level of sexual activity, please answer the following question. If you prefer not to answer it, please check this box ☐ and go to the next section.*

	Not at all	A little bit	Some-what	Quite a bit	Very much
GS7 I am satisfied with my sex life	0	1	2	3	4

By circling one (1) number per line, please indicate how true each statement has been for you during the past 7 days.

EMOTIONAL WELL-BEING	Not at all	A little bit	Some-what	Quite a bit	Very much
GE1 I feel sad	0	1	2	3	4
GE2 I am satisfied with how I am coping with my illness	0	1	2	3	4
GE3 I am losing hope in the fight against my illness	0	1	2	3	4
GE4 I feel nervous	0	1	2	3	4
GE5 I worry about dying	0	1	2	3	4
GE6 I worry that my condition will ge worse	0	1	2	3	4

FUNCTIONAL WELL-BEING	Not at all	A little bit	Some-what	Quite a bit	Very much
GF1 I am able to work (include work at home)	0	1	2	3	4
GF2 My work (include work at home) is fulfilling	0	1	2	3	4
GF3 I am able to enjoy life	0	1	2	3	4
GF4 I have accepted my illness	0	1	2	3	4
GF5 I am sleeping well	0	1	2	3	4
GF6 I am enjoying the things I usually do for fun	0	1	2	3	4
GF7 I am content with the quality of my life right now	0	1	2	3	4

Courtesy Dr. David Cella. Copyright 1987, 1997.

Box 11-13	Effective and noneffective coping strategies

Effective strategies
- Information seeking
- Participation in religious activities
- Distraction
- Expression of emotion and feeling
- Positive thinking
- Conservation of energy
- Maintenance of independence
- Maintenance of control
- Goal setting

Noneffective strategies
- Denial of emotion
- Minimization of symptoms
- Social isolation
- Passive acceptance
- Sleeping
- Substance abuse
- Avoidance of decision making
- Blame of others
- Excessive dependency

Modified from Miller JF: *Coping with chronic illness: overcoming powerlessness*, Philadelphia, 1983, Davis.

disease or treatment. In addition, a level of depression is certainly appropriate because cancer represents to patients a potential loss of not only life but also body parts, image, function, roles, and relationships. The oncology team must assess whether the level of the depression is a change from previous functioning; the way this change occurs; and whether depression is persistent, occurs most of the day, occurs more days than not, and is present for at least a period of 2 weeks.

A variety of instruments are available to assess depression. These tools were designed for psychiatrically ill patients. Therefore the data are limited somewhat with respect to oncology populations.

The first tool is the Beck Depression Inventory (BDI).[3] This is a 21-item self-report scale used to assess symptoms of depression. Each item is composed of a set of statements graduating in severity of symptoms and measured on a scale of 0 to 3 with the higher score representing a more severe symptom. Subjects choose the statement in the tool that best describes their present feelings. The responses are tallied, and a level of depression is assessed.

The second tool is the Hamilton Rating Scale for Depression (HRS-D).[11] It is a 17-item self-report scale used to assess cognitive, behavioral, and physiologic signs and symptoms of typical depression. The scores on each item are totaled to give a level of assessment of the depression.

Another tool is the Psychosocial Adjustment to Illness Scale (PAIS).[23] This tool is explicitly designed to assess a patient's psychosocial adjustment to medical illness in general. The PAIS is composed of 45 questions divided into the following six domains of psychosocial adjustment: health care orientation, vocational environment, domestic environment, sexual relationships, social environment, and psychologic distress. Each of the domains is scored separately and summed. Morrow et al's study reveals that the PAIS indicates an acceptable degree of reliability and initial confidence of validity.

Focusing on systematic and continuous assessment for signs and symptoms of psychosocial responses can improve the quality and quantity of survival for patients who have cancer.

Coping strategies and responses—the family. The dynamics of a diagnosis of cancer reach beyond the patient and extend to the entire family. Responses will vary with respect to economic and psychosocial resources, across developmental stages of the family, and with differing demands of the illness.

Life for families of cancer patients becomes complex. Family members must often learn new roles; self-care skills; and ways of relating to and communicating with each other, friends, and the health care team. To support family members, an assessment of their functioning to reveal problem areas may be necessary.

Instruments for assessing the family include the Family Functioning Index (FFI),[27] the Family APGAR* questionnaire,[30] and the Family Inventory of Resources for Management (FIRM).[17] The FFI is a 15-item self-report instrument designed to assess the dynamics of family interaction in families that contain children. Questions are designed to assess marital satisfaction, frequency of disagreement, communication, problem solving, and feelings of closeness and happiness.

The Family APGAR questionnaire[30] is a screening tool designed to assess the family from the view of the patient. The questionnaire consists of five questions on a 3-point scale. This tool does not assume institutional, structural, or cultural boundaries of a traditional family; therefore it has a wide application to the many configurations of the modern family.

The FIRM is a 69-item self-report questionnaire designed to assess the ability of the family to deal with stressors. This self-report is a 4-point Likert scale evaluating four factors: family strengths (esteem and communication), mastery and health, extended family social support, and financial well-being.

Rehabilitation. In cancer cases the focus is most often on the disease rather than its functional consequences. Cancer and its therapy can produce significant long-term and permanent functional losses, even in cases in which the goal

---

*Adaptability, Partnership, Growth, Affection, and Resolve.

is a cure. Each person with a disability needs opportunities for improving or at least maintaining functional ability, regardless of the cause of the disability. Often, little thought is given to aggressive rehabilitation of the cancer patient compared with patients having other conditions such as cardiac disease, a stroke, or a spinal cord injury. This occurs even though the 5-year survival rate for patients with cancer is currently about 50%. Rehabilitation in cancer is certainly relevant because the number of cancer survivors is growing.

Rehabilitation has been defined as the "dynamic process directed toward the goal of enabling persons to function at their maximum level within the limitations of their disease or disability in terms of their physical, mental, emotional, social and economic potential."[7]

In the early work by Mayer[16] the concept was set forth that cancer rehabilitation should encompass the theme of quality of survival—not just a person's life span but also that individual's ability to live in the constraints of the disease. In their article, "Can life be the same after cancer treatment?" Veroness and Martino[33] stated that rehabilitation is the bridge leading the patient from diversity to normality. Mellette[19] expanded on the idea by suggesting that *prevention*, the initial avoidance of dysfunction, is the key word in discussing rehabilitation.

The National Cancer Rehabilitation Planning Conference, sponsored by the National Cancer Institute, identified four cancer-rehabilitation objectives[7]:
1. Psychologic support after the diagnosis of cancer
2. Optimal physical functioning after the treatment of cancer
3. Early vocational counseling when indicated
4. Optimal social functioning as the ultimate goal of all cancer-control treatment

Probably one of the first major descriptions of a cancer-rehabilitation perspective is that of Dietz[6] in his book *Rehabilitation Oncology.* Dietz considers rehabilitation applicable to all patients who can learn and respond. He stressed readaptation as the synonym for rehabilitation because of widespread reluctance to view rehabilitation as relevant to the cancer patient. He further defined the term as accommodation or adjustment to personal needs for physical, psychologic, financial, and vocational survival. He defined the initial goals of rehabilitation as the elimination, reduction, or alleviation of disability, and he defined the ultimate goal as the reestablishment of patients as functional individuals in their environments. Rehabilitation should begin at the earliest possible time, and it should continue throughout the entire convalescence until maximal benefit can be achieved.

Romassas et al[28] developed a method to be used for assessing the rehabilitation needs of oncology patients. They devised an oncology clinic patient checklist designed to include rehabilitation concepts in the patient-assessment process. The patient was asked information regarding the following areas: fatigue; pain; nutrition; speech and language; respiration; bowel and bladder management; transportation; mobility; self-care and home care; vocational and educa-

tional interests and activities; and emotional, family, and interpersonal relationships.

As in other assessments, the evaluation for rehabilitative purposes is a dynamic event. It should continue as new issues arise or past issues recur and is best accomplished by a multidisciplinary team meeting the specific needs of each patient.

Cultural Assessment

Cultural assessment refers to the systematic appraisal of the cultural beliefs, values, and practices of individuals and communities. Cultural beliefs and individual differences determine health behaviors in families and cultural groups. Many of the problems with health are the result of behavior and lifestyle.

Accepting and respecting patients for who they are is an important attribute of oncology caregivers. Being culturally sensitive is essential in caring for the whole patient. Box 11-14 lists ways to develop cultural sensitivity.

Cultural assessment has several key variables. Fig. 11-1 demonstrates a model of cultural strata useful in examining these variables. In this model, values are the foundation of beliefs that includes attitudes and behaviors. Values, which are most difficult to assess, are established early in childhood through an unconscious process of socialization.

Beliefs that include knowledge, opinions, and faith about life are built on an individual's values. Based on their knowledge, opinions, and faith, cultures view the origin, treatments, and responses to illness differently. Treatment of the whole cancer patient involves evaluating and understanding the patient's values and beliefs. This is especially important when these values and beliefs are different from or in direct

Box 11-14	**Ways to develop cultural sensitivity**

- Recognize that cultural diversity exists.
- Demonstrate respect for persons as unique individuals with culture as one factor that contributes to their uniqueness.
- Respect the unfamiliar.
- Identify and examine your own cultural beliefs.
- Recognize that some cultural groups have definitions of health and illness and practices attempting to promote health and cure illness. (These may differ significantly from the health caregiver's own definitions and practices.)
- Be willing to modify health care delivery in keeping with the client's cultural background.
- Do not expect all members of one cultural group to behave in exactly the same way.
- Appreciate that each person's cultural values are ingrained and therefore extremely difficult to change.

Modified from Stulc P: The family as bearer of culture. In Cookfair JN, editor: *Nursing process and practive in the community,* St. Louis, 1990, Mosby.

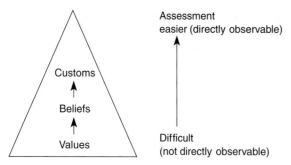

Figure 11-1. A model of cultural strata. *(Modified from Bellack J, Edlund B, editors: Nursing assessment and diagnosis, Boston, 1992, Jones & Bartlett.)*

conflict with those of the health caregiver and may impair the care of the patient.

Customs that are the result of values and beliefs are the most observable and assessable. These customs include dietary habits, religious practices, communication patterns, family structure, and health practices.

An extremely simple and short assessment model is proposed by Kleinman et al.[15] They suggest the following questions; a more thorough cultural assessment tool can be found in Box 11-15:

- What do you think caused your problems?
- Why do you think your sickness started when it did?
- What does your sickness do to you? How does it work?
- How severe is your sickness? Will it have a long or short duration?
- What kind of treatment do you think you should receive?
- What are the most important results you hope to receive from this treatment?
- What are the chief problems your sickness has caused you?
- What do you fear most about your sickness?

Cultural assessment enables the health care provider to develop a solid therapeutic relationship, which is a genuine collaborative effort between the patient and health care provider. This requires the person assessing to use good reflective listening skills and pay careful attention to all the cues. In addition, these cues need to be interpreted in the context of the patient's values, beliefs, and culture to be truly meaningful and helpful in treating and respecting the uniqueness of each cancer patient.

Spiritual assessment. In a holistic approach to care for cancer patients, dimensions of the total person must be recognized and assessed. This includes the patient's spiritual concerns. In a presentation given at the White House Conference for Aging, Moberg[22] defined the *spiritual dimension* as pertaining to "man's inner resources especially his ultimate concern, the basic value around which all other values are focused, the central philosophy of life, which guides a person's conduct, the supernatural and non-material dimensions of human nature." The spiritual dimension encompasses a person's need to find satisfactory answers to questions that revolve around the meaning of life, illness, and death.

To help explore this dimension, Stoll[32] developed guidelines for the spiritual assessment of patients. She suggested the importance of understanding four areas related to this search for meaning and spirituality in patients' lives: (1) patients' concepts of God or deity, (2) their source of hope and strength, (3) the significance of their religious practices, and (4) the relationship between their spiritual beliefs and state of health.

Stoll notes that spiritual topics are emotionally laden and should be handled in the assessment process accordingly. They should probably be introduced late in an interview, perhaps as a continuation of psychosocial assessment. As with all questions asked patients, the basis for inquiry should be explained.

Spiritual support may bring comfort, peace, and, for some, the reason for suffering. To facilitate the essential spiritual aspects of caring, oncology health care providers should do the following:

1. Assist patients to experience their own spirituality.
2. Listen carefully to the patient's expression of belief.
3. If possible, provide an appropriate environment and quiet time for reflection and contemplation.
4. Assist the patient in finding resources for spiritual fulfillment.

The willingness to allow a patient or family to be themselves by being present and supporting them is an essential part of working in oncology. In the spiritual realm, presence implies an unconditional acceptance of persons. To be present with a cancer patient or the family is to listen in the broadest sense to hear the communication clearly. Compassionate presence does not require many words. Sometimes it requires none.

Numerous tools are available for assessing spirituality. They include the Spiritual Well-Being Scale, the Religious Well-Being Scale,[26] the Existential Well-Being Scale,[8] Moberg's Indexes of Spiritual Well-Being,[22] and Hess' Spiritual Needs Survey.[13] Studies indicate a combination of these tools best yields the multifaceted nature of spirituality.

Hope. Hope is the key concept and an essential ingredient in the religious and spiritual aspects of care and a major component in the healing process. Spiritual persons inspire hope more by who they are than by their actions. Giving support with realistic hope is a powerful gift oncology caregivers can offer their patients. For some patients, hope is a major determinant between life and death.

A physician often becomes a symbol of hope. Through the physician's continued interest the patient does not despair. The fear of being abandoned by this person of hope can clearly alter the patient's behavior. Patients may protect their relationships with their physicians by not questioning them, limiting their complaints to them, and treating them as they wish to perceive them, as miracle workers. When this occurs the role of another member of the multidisciplinary team becomes paramount. Establishing a therapeutic relationship and applying good communication skills is essential in caring for this patient.

Box 11-15	Cultural Assessment Guide

Health beliefs and practices
- How does the client define *health* and *illness*?
- Are particular methods such as hygiene and self-care practices used to help maintain health?
- Are particular methods being used by the client for the treatment of illness?
- What is the attitudes toward preventive health measures such as immunizations?
- Do health topics exist to which the client may be partcularly sensitive or that are considered taboo?
- What are the attitudes toward mental illness, pain, handicapping conditions, chronic disease, death, and dying?
- Is a person in the family responsible for various health-related decisions, such as places to go, persons to see, and advice to follow?

Religious influences and special rituals
- Does the client adhere to a particular religion?
- Does the client look to a significant person for guidance and support?
- Do any special religious practices or beliefs affect health care when the client is ill or dying?
- What events, rituals, and ceremonies (birth, baptism, puberty, marriage, and death) are considered important in the life cycle?

Language and communication
- What language is spoken in the home?
- How well does the client undersand English (spoken or written)?
- Do special signs of demonstrating respect or disrespect exist?
- Is touch involved in communication?
- Are there culturally appropriate ways to enter and leave situations (including greetings, farewells, and convenient times to make a home visit)?

Parenting styles and the role of family
- Who makes decisions in the family?
- What is the composition of the family? How many generations are considered a single family? Which relatives comprise the family?
- When the marriage custom is practiced, what is the attitude about separation and divorce?
- What is the role of and attitude toward children in the family?
- When do children need to be disciplined or punished? How is this done? In what way is physical punishment used (if any)?
- Do parents demonstrate physical affection toward their children and each other?
- What major events are important to the family? How are these events celebrated?
- Do special beliefs and practices surround conception, pregnancy, childbirth, lactations, and child rearing?

Dietary practices
- What does the family like to eat? Does everyone in the family have similar tastes in food?
- Who is responsible for food preparation?
- Are any foods forbidden by the culture? Are some foods a cultural requirement in observance of a rite or ceremony?
- How is food prepared and consumed?
- Do specific beliefs or preferences exist concerning food, such as those believed to cause or cure in illness?

From Stulc DM: The family as bearer of culture. In Cookfair JN editor: *Nursing process and practice in the community*, St. Louis, 1990, Mosby.

The literature and published research articles on hope number approximately 20. Of those articles, 10 involve patients with cancer. This suggests that cancer may have a greater effect on hope than other chronic illnesses. Key measurement instruments include the Nowotny Hope Scale,[24] Herth Hope Scale,[12] and Miller Hope Scale.[21]

The Nowotny Hope Scale is a 29-item scale designed to measure hope on six dimensions: confidence in outcomes, relationship to others, possibility of a future, spiritual beliefs, active involvement, and internal origin. This tool is a 4-point Likert-type scale that yields reliable and validated outcomes.

The Herth Hope Scale is a 32-item self-report scale to which patients respond, "does not apply to me" or "applies to me" to each item. A total hope score is attained by adding all the responses on each item. Reliability and validity estimates are determined. Herth's descriptive study investigated the relationship between hope and coping in 120 adult cancer patients receiving chemotherapy in a variety of care settings. A significant relationship was found between the level of hope and level of coping. In addition, patients with a strong religious faith had significantly higher mean scores on the Hearth Hope Scale than subjects with weak, unsure faith.

The Miller Hope Scale is a 40-item scale using a 5-point Likert format. The possible range of scores is 40 to 200, with a high score indicating high hope. Exemplary items include the statement, "I look forward to an enjoyable future." A low score item is, "I feel trapped, pinned down." The strength of this tool is strong reliability and validity.

Hope is a multidimensional construct that is more than goal attainment and has not been easily quantified. Hope is fundamental to meaning and transcendence for humans. For these reasons, including hope in holistic patient assessment is important.

Special Cases in Assessment

Special attention must be given to meet the diverse needs of patients at different stages in life because cancer is a group of diseases that affects individuals across the lifespan.

Children.   To provide holistic care to a child with cancer, assessing the needs and concerns of the child's primary caretakers (usually the parents) is essential. Experiencing a life-threatening diagnosis for their child is an extremely stressful event for parents.

The assessment of children with cancer is a multidimensional task. Areas of functioning that should be considered are depression, withdrawal, anxiety, delinquency, achievement, family relations, and development.

The developmental level of children is directly related to the way they perceive, interpret, and respond to the diagnosis of cancer. A substantial amount of literature in nursing, medicine, psychiatry, psychology, and social work exists detailing the psychologic effect of childhood cancer. The shock of diagnosis, discomfort and inconvenience of treatment, and burden of living with a life-threatening disease are sources of distress and disruption for the child with cancer, patients, siblings, and extended family members.

Those who provide health care to children with cancer have a key role in helping the child and family cope with situations. The study by Armstrong et al[2] suggests that most children with cancer are normally adjusted. This is due in part to the caregivers' concern and help with coping.

Adolescents.   Developmental theory suggests that adolescence is a crucial stage in the process of building self-esteem, forming perceptions about body image, establishing autonomy, and developing social functions. The adolescent with cancer experiences a disruption of these vital processes. As a result, assessment for the adolescent must consider and address these unique areas. The adolescent with cancer may face a loss of self-esteem because of the unfamiliar patient role. This role can cause the adolescent to feel inferior and dependent, thus inhibiting the developmental task of establishing independence.

Relationships with others and self-perception can change as the adolescent goes through treatment and is hospitalized. The unpredictability and uncertainty of cancer can limit the adolescent's sense of control and autonomy. Changes in body image, disruption of activities, and prescribed therapies can have a profound effect on the adolescent's self-image. Rapid changes in physical appearance as a result of treatments, disfigurement caused by the disease or amputation, or reduction in weight can confuse and impair the adolescent's self-perception.

These are complex processes that must be assessed and incorporated into the plan of care for the adolescent. The health care team must promote growth and developmental maturity while recognizing the burden that cancer places on the adolescent in meeting developmental tasks.

Older persons.   As individuals enter the later stages of life, the risk of developing cancer increases. Specific attention to the sociologic issues for older persons are crucial for appropriate assessment and treatment of cancer.

An important problem to assess in older persons is the amount of sensory and cognitive impairment that may be present. Assessing the ability of older patients to hear, see, or understand is paramount in their care. Recognizing any change from normal behaviors, usual routines, and social interactions is extremely important. Loss of physical health, limited economic resources, changes in family structure, and losses of social status greatly affect the quality of life for

---

| **Box 11-16** | **Suggestions for interviewing an older patient** |

- If feasible, gather preliminary data before the appointment. Request previous medical records, or have the patient or family complete a questionnaire at home or by phone.
- Try to avoid making patients tell their story more than once.
- In the review of systems, ask about difficulty sleeping, incontinence, falling, depression, dizziness, or loss of energy.
- Pace the interview. An older patient may need extra time to formulate answers.
- If the patient has difficulty with open-ended questions, use yes-or-no or simple-choice questions.
- Encourage patients and their caregivers to bring a list of their main concerns and questions to help ensure that the issues important to them are discussed.
- Ask patients to bring with them all the medications they are taking (prescription and over-the-counter).
- Ask about the patient's functional status, such as eating, bathing, dressing, cooking, and shopping. Sudden changes in these areas are valuable diagnostic clues.
- Determine whether the patient is a caregiver. Many older women care for spouses, older parents, or grandchildren. Patients' willingness to report symptoms depends on whether they think they can afford to get sick.

Modified from Gastel B: *Working with your older patient: a clinician's handbook*, Bethesda, Md, 1994, National Institute on Aging, National Institute on Health.

older persons. Obtaining a complete medical history that includes medications, the family health experience and history, the functional status, and current concerns is crucial to sound health care. Box 11-16 lists some suggestions for interviewing an older patient.

Ongoing communication is the key to assessing and working effectively with the older patient. The best way to promote ongoing communication is to communicate well from the start and to take time to establish a therapeutic and healing relationship.

Review Questions

1. What is assessment?
2. What is included in the cognitive content of a message? Give an example.
3. What is involved in an empathic response?
4. What are the 10 most common verbal responses in effective communication?
5. What is the assessment responsibility of radiation therapists for daily treatment in the following areas?
   - Skin reactions
   - Diarrhea
   - Alopecia
   - Fatigue
   - Cystitis
   - Pain
   - Sleep
   - Nausea
   - Skin pallor
   - Mouth changes and vomiting
   - Weight loss
   - Pharyngitis and esophagitis
6. What is frequently the first sign of malnutrition?
7. What are two important characteristics related to the cause of pain?
8. What is leukopenia?
9. What are the major symptoms of depression?
10. List five ways to be culturally sensitive.

Questions to Ponder

1. Why is doing an assessment in oncology important?
2. What is the basis of an effective therapeutic (communication) relationship?
3. Why is observing nonverbal communication so important?
4. What are the three purposes of pain assessment?
5. Why is rehabilitation of the cancer patient important?
6. What are four areas related to the search for meaning and spirituality in patients' lives?
7. Describe five helpful methods in interviewing an older patient.

REFERENCES

1. Ahles TA, Blanchard EB, Ruckdeschel JC: The multidimensional nature of cancer-related pain, *Pain* 17:277-288, 1983.
2. Armstrong GD, Wirt RD, Nesbit ME, Martinson IM: Multidimensional assessment of psychological problem in children with cancer, *Res Nurs Health* 5:205-211, 1982.
3. Beck AT, Beamesderfer A: Assessment of depression: the Depression Inventory. In Pichot P, Olivier-Martin R, editors: *Psychological measurements in psychopharmacology: modern problems in pharmopsychiatry,* vol 7, New York, 1974, S. Karger.
4. Cella DF, Tulsky DS, Gray G et al: The Functional Assessment of Cancer Therapy Scale: development and validation of the general measure, *J Clin Oncol* 11:570-579, 1993.
5. Daut RW, Cleeland CS, Flannery RC: Development of the Wisconsin Brief Pain Questionnaire to assess pain in cancer and other disease, *Pain* 17:197-210, 1983.
6. Dietz JH: *Rehabilitation oncology,* New York, 1981, John Wiley & Sons.
7. Dudas S, Carlson CE: Cancer rehabilitation, *Oncol Nurs Forum* 15:183-188, 1988.
8. Ellison CW: Spiritual well-being: conceptualization and measurement, *J Psy Theology* 11:330-340, 1983.
9. Fishman B, Pasternak S, Wallenstein SL et al: The Memorial Pain Assessment Card: a valid instrument for the evaluation of cancer pain, *Cancer* 60:1151-1158, 1987.
10. Foley KN: Pain syndromes in patients with cancer. In Bonica JJ, Ventafridda V, editors: *Advances in pain research and therapy,* vol 2, New York, 1979, Raven Press.
11. Hamilton M: A rating scale for depression, *J Neurol Neurosurg Psychiatry* 23:56-62, 1960.
12. Herth KA: The relationship between level of hope and level of coping response and other variables in patients with cancer, *Oncol Nurs Forum* 16:67-72, 1989.
13. Hess JS: Spiritual Needs Survey. In Fish S, Shelly JA, editors: *Spiritual care: the nurse's role,* Downers Grove, Ill, 1983, Intervarsity Press.
14. Irwin PH, et al: Sex differences in psychological distress during definitive radiation therapy for cancer, *J Psychosoc Oncol* 4:63-75, 1986.
15. Kleinman A, Eisenberg L, Good B: Culture, illness and care: clinical lessons from anthropologic and cross-cultural research, *Am Intern Med* 88:251-258, 1978.
16. Mayer NH: Concepts in cancer rehabilitation, *Semin Oncol* 2:393-398, 1975.
17. McCubbin HI, Comew J: FIRM: Family Inventory of Resources for Management. In McCubbin HI, Thompson AI, editors: *Family assessment inventories for research and practice,* Madison, Wis, 1987, University of Wisconsin-Madison.
18. McGuire DB: Cancer-related pain: a multidimensional approach, *Dissert Abst Int* 48(3):Sec B:705, 1987.
19. Mellette SJ: Rehabilitation issues for cancer survivors: psychosocial challenges, *J Psychosoc Oncol* 7:93-109, 1989.
20. Melzack R: The McGill Pain Questionnaire: major properties and scoring methods, *Pain* 1:277-299, 1975.
21. Miller JF: Development of an instrument to measure hope, *Nurs Res* 37:6-9, 1988.
22. Moberg D: *Spiritual well-being: background and issues,* Washington DC, 1971, White House Conference on Aging.
23. Morrow GR, Chiarell RJ, Derogatis LR: A new scale for assessing patient's psychosocial adjustment to medical illness, *Psychol Med* 8:605-610, 1978.
24. Nowotny ML: Assessment of hope in patients with cancer: development of an instrument, *Oncol Nurs Forum* 16:57-61, 1989.
25. Padilla GV, Presant C, Grant MM et al: Quality of Life Index for patients with cancer, *Res Nurs Health* 6:117-126, 1983.
26. Paloutzian R, Ellison CW: Spiritual well-being and quality of life. In Peplau LA, Perlman D, editors: *Loneliness: a sourcebook of current theory, research, and therapy,* New York, 1982, Wiley Interscience.

27. Pless IB, Satterwhite BB: A measure of family functioning and its application, *Soc Sci Med* 7:613-620, 1973.

28. Romassas ED, et al: A method for assessing the rehabilitation needs of oncology outpatients, *Oncol Nurs Forum* 10:17-21, 1983.

29. Schipper H, Clinch J, McMurray A, Levitt M: Measuring the quality of life of cancer patients: the Functional Living Index–Cancer: development and validation, *J Clin Oncol* 2:472-483, 1984.

30. Smilkstein F: The family APGAR: a proposal for a family function test and its use by physicians, *J Fam Pract* 6:1231-1239, 1978.

31. Spielberger C, Gorusch R, Lushene R: *Manual for the State-Trait Anxiety Inventory,* Palo Alto, Calif, 1970, Consulting Psychologists Press.

32. Stoll RI: Guidelines for spiritual assessment, *Am J Nurs* 79:1574-1577, September 1979.

33. Veroness V, Martino G: Can life be the same after cancer treatment? *Tumori* 64:345-351, 1978.

34. Yasko JM: A model for the assessment of the client with cancer. In Yasko JM, editor: *Guidelines for cancer care symptom management,* Reston, Va, 1983, Reston Publishing.

35. Yates JW, Chalmer B, McKegney FP: Evaluation of patients with advanced cancer using the Karnofsky Performance Status, *CA Cancer J Clin* 45:2220-2224, 1980.

BIBLIOGRAPHY

The American Psychiatric Association: *Diagnostic and statistical manual of mental disorders* (DSM III–R), ed 3, Washington DC, 1987, The American Psychiatric Association.

Blackburn GL, et al: Nutritional and metabolic assessment of the hospitalized patient, *J Parenter Enteral Nutr* 1:17, 1977.

Gastel B: *Working with your older patient: a clinician's handbook,* Bethesda, Md, 1994, National Institute on Aging, National Institute on Health.

Gordon M: *Manual of nursing diagnosis,* New York, 1987, McGraw-Hill.

Groenwald SL, et al: *Nutritional disturbances: cancer nursing principles and practice,* ed 3, Boston, 1993, Jones & Bartlett.

Hirshfield-Bartek J, Dow KH, Creaton E: Decreasing documentation time using a patient self-assessment tool, *Oncol Nurs Forum* 17:251-255, 1990.

McCaffery M, Beebe A: *Pain: clinical manual for nursing practice,* St. Louis, 1989, Mosby.

Miller JF: *Coping with chronic illness: overcoming powerlessness,* Philadelphia, 1983, Davis.

Stulc DM: The family as bearer of culture. In Cookfair JN, editor: *Nursing process and practice in the community,* St. Louis, 1990, Mosby.

Trip-Reimer T: Cultural assessment. In Bellack J, Edlund B, editors: *Nursing assessment and diagnosis,* Boston, 1992, Jones & Bartlett.

12

Pharmacology and Drug Administration

Lynda Reynolds

Outline

Key Terms

The radiation therapist interacts closely with patients in radiation oncology and may be the first to notice adverse reactions or unusual symptoms as they appear. Competent patient care requires that the therapist have a general knowledge of pharmacology and specific details of each patient's medication history. With a basic understanding of medications and their common side effects, the therapist will be able to distinguish an expected side effect from an adverse reaction that requires medical intervention.

Although the administration of drugs is not primarily the role of the radiation therapist, it is a crucial part of overall patient care.[2] The therapist may administer medications specific to radiation therapy, such as contrast media, anesthetics, or intravenous (IV) fluids. The therapist must also be aware of all the drugs that a patient is taking and their purpose to effectively care for the patient.

This chapter discusses general principles of medication administration. Its purpose is not to provide information about specific drugs but to identify the essential prerequisite knowledge the therapist must have to administer drugs safely to patients. Various aspects of assessment, preparation, and administration of medications are discussed. Finally, the legal aspects of medication administration are considered.

DRUG LEGISLATION

The Federal Food, Drug, and Cosmetic Act of 1938 and the Controlled Substance Act of 1971 govern the labeling, availability, and dispensation of all drugs in the United States.[12] Radiation therapists must remain current with information about the drugs in use in their profession. Safer and more effective drugs, such as nonionic contrast media, are continually being developed. Legislation requires extensive testing of all new drugs before they can be used on patients; however, the value and drawbacks of medications are proved through their actual daily use. The therapist administering these drugs plays an important role in providing feedback to the pharmacology community.

DRUG NOMENCLATURE

A **drug** is any substance that alters physiologic function, with the potential for affecting health. A **medication** is a drug administered for its therapeutic effects. All medications are drugs, but not all drugs are medications. **Pharmacology** is the science of drugs, including the sources, chemistry, and actions of drugs. The list of drugs available for medical use changes constantly as new formulas are developed. Each drug has at least four separate names—its chemical name (constituents of the chemical formula), **generic name** (coined by the original manufacturer), official name (usually the same as the generic name), and brand or trade name (the drug's name in official publications).[11,12,16] Several manufacturers may produce the same generic drug but call that drug by different brand names. Radiation therapists and all health professionals need to easily access this drug name information. The most commonly used resources are the *Physicians' Desk Reference (PDR)*, *United States Pharmacopoeia (USP)*, and specific drug packaging.

PHARMACOLOGIC PRINCIPLES

The way in which drugs affect the body is called **pharmacodynamics.** Each drug has a unique molecular structure enabling it to interact with a specific enzyme or a corresponding cell type. The drug attaches itself to a target site in the body called the *receptor site* in the same way that two puzzle pieces interlock. The combined effect alters the behavior of the targeted cells or enzyme and causes physiologic changes in the patient.

The way that drugs travel through the body to their appropriate receptor sites is called **pharmacokinetics.** A drug must be administered so that the body can absorb it, distribute it to the necessary sites, metabolize it, and excrete the excess. Many individual factors cause these steps to vary within each patient; the effectiveness of and reaction to a drug may differ greatly from one patient to another.

Absorption

Every drug must be absorbed into the bloodstream to be effective. The dosage and speed of absorption depend on factors such as the route of entry, the pH of the recipient environment, the solubility of the formula, and the drug's interaction with body chemicals while in transit.[12,16]

Distribution

A drug travels through the circulatory system to its receptor site(s) and then connects with the molecular structure for which it was designed. The drug may need to bind with a certain protein or cross specific membranes to produce the desired response. Many drugs cross the placental villi and affect the fetus. Fewer drugs can cross the blood-brain barrier. Some medications may be stored in the tissues for later use.

Metabolism

"Metabolism, also referred to as biotransformation, is the process by which the body alters the chemical composition of a substance."[12] The liver detoxifies nearly all foreign substances entering the body, including drugs, and changes them into inactive, water-soluble compounds that can be excreted by the kidneys.[12] The breakdown of drugs into waste matter may also involve chemical processes and enzyme reactions in the blood and other organs such as the gallbladder, lungs, and intestines. If drugs accumulate or react synergistically with other substances in the body or the organs are damaged, metabolism and excretion of the drugs may be difficult.[16]

Excretion

The body excretes drugs and their byproducts in a variety of ways. Most drugs leave the body through the kidneys. The lungs sometimes expel those drugs that break down into gases. The sweat glands, tear ducts, salivary glands, intestines, and mammary glands can also eliminate small quantities of drugs. The rate of excretion depends on the body's systems, the drug's half-life, and concentration in the tissues.

VARIABLES AFFECTING PATIENT RESPONSE

The caregiver must consider numerous factors that determine patient response to drugs. The following section discusses several of these factors, which also affect the optimal dose to be prescribed by the physician.

Patient-Related Variables

Age. Young children and older adults generally require smaller than average adult doses to achieve the same results, although for different reasons.

In children and infants the organs are still developing. Children may be hypersensitive to medications, so administration of minimal doses and close monitoring of their responses is the usual process required to decrease the likelihood of an untoward event occurring. Determining dosages by using body weight is safer than using age, but this calculation remains imprecise because of the child's immature metabolism.[15] Getting the prescribed dose into children can be challenging, because they frequently have difficulty swallowing pills, spit out liquid preparations, reject suppositories, and fight injections.

Older adults may require smaller or at times larger doses. Age decreases the efficiency of their organs. Their circulation slows, enzymes are depleted, sensitivities develop, absorption becomes impaired, and the liver and kidneys can no longer detoxify efficiently.[11,12,15,16] In addition, elderly patients frequently take multiple medications that may interact negatively. Elderly patients should be monitored to ensure that the dosage of the medications they are taking is appropriate.

Weight and physical condition. Average doses are based on the median 150-lb, healthy adult. The dose must be adjusted for heavier or lighter patients, and body mass must be taken into account because obesity or excessive thinness affects circulation and organ efficiency. A damaged liver or kidneys, an electrolyte imbalance, poor circulation, nutritional deficiency, infection, and other physiologic disorders should be considered in the determination of the optimal dosage.[12]

Gender. Women have a lower average body weight than men and metabolize drugs differently. Women's hormone profiles and the amount and distribution of their body fat differ greatly from those of men and influence the dosage of medications needed. The difference in fluid balance between the genders is another important factor for figuring dosage. The added complication of pregnancy is critical because many drugs may affect the fetus.

Personal and emotional requirements. Patients react differently to drugs. Caffeine is a common example; some people can drink coffee all day and have no trouble sleeping, whereas others cannot tolerate caffeine. As a result, patients have unique needs and must be evaluated individually. For example, patients with negative attitudes or anxiety require higher levels of sedation than calm patients with positive outlooks. Although some patients prefer to take minimum doses of medication, others see drugs as cure-alls.[15] Health care professionals must relate to patients as individuals and be alert to each patient's emotional response to the drugs administered.

Drug-Related Variables: Nontherapeutic Reactions

An important difference exists between unpleasant but expected side effects and adverse drug responses or complications. Side effects are expected reactions to medication; complications are *unexpected* reactions to medications that range from mild to severe.[12] In radiation therapy the treatment, diagnostic contrast media used, and various medications taken before and after treatment can combine to produce toxicities and discomfort for the patient.

Allergic reactions. **Allergic reactions** result from an immunologic reaction to a drug to which the patient has already been sensitized. In an allergic reaction the drug acts as an antigen, and the body develops antibodies to that drug. The signs and symptoms of such a reaction may range from a light rash to life-threatening **anaphylactic shock.** Once an allergy develops, subsequent exposures to that drug cause increasingly severe symptoms. Penicillin is a common allergenic drug.

Tolerance. **Tolerance** occurs if the body adapts to a particular drug and requires ever-greater doses to achieve the desired effect. For example, the body develops a tolerance for narcotics extremely quickly. If overused, antibiotics become increasingly less effective by killing not only harmful bacteria but also the beneficial ones. Antibiotics may also leave the patient susceptible to further infection. Bacteria that survive antibiotic use can mutate within the patient into strains that are resistant to the antibiotic during subsequent use.[16] The patient may then need to switch to a different drug if the first one loses its effectiveness.

Cumulative effect. A **cumulative effect** develops if the body is unable to detoxify and excrete a drug quickly enough or if too large a dose is taken.[15] Unless the dosage is adjusted, the drug accumulates in the tissues and can become toxic. In some cases the cumulative effect is desirable, such as with medications prescribed to prevent depression.

Idiosyncratic effects. **Idiosyncratic effects** are the inexplicable and unpredictable symptoms caused by a genetic defect within the patient.[15] These symptoms are completely different from the expected symptoms and may even occur the first time a drug is given.

Dependence. Drug dependency can result from extensive exposure to a drug or a compulsion to continue taking a drug to feel good or to avoid feeling bad. Most persons who become drug dependent do so because of physiologic or psychologic problems.

Drug interactions. **Drug interactions** occurring between two or more drugs or a combination of food and drugs can create or produce positive or negative effects in patients. This interaction of drugs may result in synergism, which increases a drug's effects; interaction can also result in antagonism, which decreases a drug's effects. For example, alcohol and sedatives taken together produce a toxic reaction, whereas an antiemetic given with anesthesia can be therapeutic. Older adults commonly take many different medications, and the interactions of these drugs can cause a toxic shock situation. The person administering medications should *never* mix drugs without consulting a drug compatibility chart or checking with a pharmacist.

The therapist should also be familiar with the term **iatrogenic disease.** This disease results from long-term use of a drug that damages organs or causes other disorders over time.

In these nontherapeutic responses, the drugs used to treat disease may also cause disease. The therapist should remain aware of complications caused by drug administration.

PROFESSIONAL DRUG ASSESSMENT AND MANAGEMENT

Assessing the Patient's Medication History

The patient is the managing partner in the business of self-medication. Although the health care professional may educate and evaluate the patient regarding drug use, the patient is ultimately responsible for self-medication. If the patient is forgetful, confused, depressed, or taking several medications simultaneously or has inadequate diet and exercise habits, it may be difficult to differentiate between poor compliance and additional medical needs. For example, impaired liver or kidney function may indicate toxicity from drug overuse, lack of improvement from a prior disease, poor drug distribution because of sluggish circulation, an allergic reaction, damaged organs from alcohol or drug abuse, or a negative response from drug interaction. Assessment is further complicated because the person recording the medical history must rely on the patient's verbal description and inadequate recollection.

Despite these difficulties the therapist must assess the patient's drug use during the patient evaluation by documenting every drug that the patient is taking (including alcohol) and looking especially for overuse and under use of prescribed drugs.* Misuse of drugs can influence the outcome of radiologic diagnosis or treatment. An accurate medication history is essential to proper diagnosis and treatment (see the section on legal aspects).

Applying the Six Rights of Drug Safety

The Five Rights of Drug Safety are as follows: (1) to identify the *right* patient, (2) to select the *right* medication, (3) to give the *right* dose, (4) to give the medication at the *right* time, (5) to give the medication by the *right* route, and (6) to document.† Each of these *rights* is discussed in greater detail later.

To properly identify the right patient, checking the name on the door or looking at the chart in the slot is not enough; the therapist should check the patient's identification bracelet *and* ask patients to give their name if possible. If the patient's name is called and the patient nods or smiles, this doesn't necessarily mean that the name has been called correctly. Other possibilities for such a response include (1) the patient may have nodded or smiled in acknowledgment; (2) a patient may be too young to understand; or (3) he or she may not have a needed hearing aid in place, may not speak English as a primary language, or may be drowsy and misheard. Checking the patient's identification bracelet is *essential.*

The therapist does not bear the primary responsibility for

choosing the correct dose; however, as with all caregivers, the therapist must continually watch for errors. Even if the physician or nurse (in the case of standing orders) has prescribed the drug, the therapist involved should *always* check the dosage.[11,12,15,16] As discussed earlier, extremely old or young patients have special dose requirements, as do people of different weights, genders, physical conditions, allergic statuses, and emotional conditions. The dose should *always* be double-checked.

Although a physician (not a therapist) must prescribe the medications, the therapist may confirm that the physician has ordered the proper drug for the patient and that the drug ordered is also the drug being administered. The patient may be the first to notice if a medication order seems different. A patient's concern can be a "red flag" for a therapist to check for a change in the medication or an error. Every patient deserves to receive the correct medication every time. Therefore the written order should always be checked against the patient's chart and the drug label.

Some drugs can be administered in more than one way; other drugs should only be given by a particular route. If a drug is administered incorrectly, the consequences may range from minor injury to death. In the radiologic sciences profession a drug given by the wrong route can also skew a procedure's results. **Contrast media,** in particular, must be delivered to the proper location by the correct route to enhance the images that facilitate the diagnosis or treatment. Contrast media are any substances introduced into the body to make an organ, the surface of an organ, or materials within the lumen of an organ visible on imaging. The route of entry should *always* be double-checked.

Giving a drug at the wrong time can have serious consequences. Such consequences can include poor absorption, fluctuation of blood or serum levels, increased side effects, or less than optimal diagnostic capability in the case of contrast media. A drug that has been ordered before surgery or before a diagnostic procedure must be administered punctually because the procedure is scheduled for a particular time and depends on the drug's effect. Patients always deserve to receive medications *on time.*

Implementing Proper Emergency Procedures

If a drug emergency occurs, the therapist or another health care professional must follow proper emergency procedures. Each hospital and clinic has its own emergency codes and procedures. At the onset of an emergency the therapist's first duty is to summon help by "calling a code." The therapist should know the location of emergency supplies within the area and the way to administer oxygen and perform cardiopulmonary resuscitation (CPR).

Recognizing symptoms and delivering the appropriate procedure are required skills for therapists.[2] If a reaction develops while a contrast medium is being administered, the therapist must stop the procedure immediately and call the oncologist. The patient must *never* be left alone.

---

*References 3, 5, 11, 12, 16, 17.
†References 5, 7, 11, 12, 15, 16.

Types of emergencies that the radiation therapist is most likely to encounter are as follows:

- Asthma attack, which produces tightness or pressure in the chest, mild to moderate shortness of breath, wheezing, and coughing
- Pulmonary edema, which produces abnormal swelling of tissue in the lungs because of fluid build-up
- Anaphylactic shock produces symptoms such as nausea, vomiting, diarrhea, urticaria, shortness of breath, airway obstruction, and vascular shock
- Cardiac arrest is when the heart stops beating suddenly and respiration and other body functions stop as a result

The ability to handle medical emergencies improves with hands-on experience. All radiation therapists should seek extensive education in this area.

DRUG CATEGORIES RELEVANT TO RADIATION THERAPY

Oncology patients have specific symptoms or indications for certain types of drugs. In radiation therapy, for example, patients may require certain drugs (such as antidiarrheals and antiemetics) to relieve the symptoms of the therapy and other drugs (such as contrast media) to facilitate the pretherapy diagnosis and planning.

Pharmacologists classify drugs in the following ways: according to the effects of the drug on particular receptor sites or body systems, in terms of the symptoms that the drug relieves, or by chemical group[1,5,17] These categories overlap; often a single drug can be used to treat multiple conditions, and several different drugs can be used to treat a single condition. The following categories of drugs contain common medications that are administered to oncology patients for conditions that may precede or relate to the radiation treatment.

Analgesics relieve pain. Narcotic analgesics (such as morphine, codeine and meperidine [Demerol]) are given for moderate to severe pain and are derived from opium. These narcotic analgesics are not only addictive, but they can cause adverse side effects. Nonnarcotic analgesics, such as acetaminophen (Tylenol), propoxyphene (Darvon), and aspirin are not addictive but are also not strong enough to relieve severe pain.

Anesthetics suppress the sensation of feeling by acting on the central nervous system. General anesthetics, such as thiopental (Pentothal), depress the entire central nervous system, thereby rendering the patient unconscious allowing major surgery to be performed. Local anesthetics, such as procaine (Novocain), act only on the nerves in a small area. Lidocaine (Xylocaine), as a viscous solution, is used to treat inflamed mucous membranes in the mouth and pharynx.

Antianxiety drugs are mild tranquilizers that help calm anxious patients and relieve muscle spasms. Lorazepam (Ativan), diazepam (Valium), and chlordiazepoxide (Librium) are antianxiety drugs that may be used concurrently with radiation therapy treatments.

Antibiotics suppress the growth of bacteria. Examples include *erythromycin,* which is usually prescribed for respiratory tract infections, and penicillin and tetracycline, which are broad-spectrum antibiotics, effective against a variety of bacterial infections.

Anticoagulants prevent blood from clotting too quickly in cases of thrombosis or if an IV line must be kept open. The most commonly used drugs in this category are warfarin (Coumadin), which is administered orally, and heparin, which is always administered by injection.

Anticonvulsants inhibit or control seizures. The most commonly used drugs in this category are clonazepam (Klonopin), which is used orally to prevent petit mal seizures, and phenytoin (Dilantin), which is administered orally or parenterally to treat grand mal seizures.

Antidepressants affect communication between cells in the brain. The drugs affect the neurotransmitters, which carry signals from one nerve cell to another and are involved in the control of mood and in other responses and functions, such as eating, sleep, pain, and thinking.

The most commonly used drugs categorized as antidepressants are fluoxetine (Prozac) and sertraline (Zoloft). Other antidepressants, such as amitriptyline (Elavil), act on the serotonin and norepinephrine. Antidepressants generally take a month or longer to work. In addition, they can be addictive, and they frequently react negatively with other drugs.

Antidiarrheal drugs control the gastrointestinal distress that frequently results from bacterial infections, the administration of other medications, or radiation therapy treatments. Two examples of antidiarrheal drugs are diphenoxylate (Lomotil) and loperamide (Imodium).

Antiemetics prevent nausea and vomiting and are most effective when given before symptoms develop. These are frequently used to alleviate side effects of radiation therapy and chemotherapy. Commonly used antiemetics include prochlorperazine (Compazine), promethazine (Phenergan), and ondansetron (Zofran).

Antifungals treat fungal infections, such as yeast or thrush. Ketoconazole (Nizoral) or nystatin may be given to patients with head and neck cancer who have oral thrush.

Antihistamines are usually used to treat allergies but can also be found in cold remedies and motion sickness tablets. Because many drugs trigger allergic reactions in susceptible patients, antihistamines are frequently administered to patients before surgery. Diphenhydramine (Benadryl), promethazine, and chlorpheniramine (Chlor-Trimeton) are common antihistamines.

Antihypertensives lower the blood pressure. Clonidine (Catapres), metoprolol (Lopressor), and reserpine (Serpasil) are all antihypertensives (hypertension can become a factor in many medical procedures).

Antiinflammatory drugs reduce inflammation. Although they do not work as quickly as corticosteroids they may have fewer side effects. Commonly used antiinflammatory drugs include ibuprofen (Motrin), piroxicam (Feldene), and naproxen (Naprosyn).

Antineoplastic drugs are chemotherapeutic agents used by oncologists to treat tumors. Chemotherapy, a treatment modality that uses antineoplastic drugs, can be extremely aggressive and cause adverse side effects.

Contrast media enhance the visibility of internal tissues for diagnostic imaging. Oncologists depend on these agents to pinpoint target areas for radiation therapy treatments.[1,5,9,17]

Corticosteroids reduce inflammation and are sometimes used to treat adrenal deficiency. Common examples of corticosteroids are dexamethasone (Decadron) and hydrocortisone (Solu-Cortef).

Diuretics remove fluid from the cells. They are used to treat edema and are often used with antihypertensives to lower blood pressure. Fluids and electrolytes must be watched closely for imbalance whenever diuretics are used. Commonly used diuretics include acetazolamide (Diamox), chlorothiazide (Diuril), and furosemide (Lasix).

Hormones are used to augment endocrine secretion. Estrogen (Premarin) is given to females; methyltestosterone is given to males. Sex hormones can also be used to treat neoplastic conditions in the opposite sex; that is, estrogens can be given to males and methyltestosterone can be given to females. Other hormone drugs include insulin, which is a hormone commonly used to treat diabetes, and levothyroxine (Synthroid) a hormone used to treat thyroid disorders.

Narcotics are federally controlled substances that relax the central nervous system and relieve pain. Some examples include codeine, meperidine, and morphine.

Radioactive isotopes that are used in nuclear medicine as diagnostic imaging agents include technetium-99m and iodine-131. Radioactive isotopes that are used in radiation therapy for therapeutic purposes include palladium-103, iodine-125, and strontium-89.

Sedatives can calm anxious patients and relax the central nervous system, thereby inducing sleep or unconsciousness. Barbiturates, such as secobarbital (Seconal) and pentobarbital (Nembutal), can be addictive. Examples of nonbarbiturate sedatives include lorazepam, diphenhydramine, and midazolam (Versed). Chloral hydrate is the sedative most often used to sedate children.

Skin agents are used to keep the skin soft and supple while reducing the pain and itching caused by erythema. Some examples include hydrocortisone 1%, Aquaphor, and Eucerin.[6]

Tranquilizers relieve anxiety. Two examples are chlordiazepoxide and diazepam.

Vitamins and other supplements can act as drugs within the body and may have adverse effects if taken in excess or combined with other drugs.

CONTRAST MEDIA

Although some departments do not administer contrast agents, many do, and it often falls within the therapist's scope of practice. The next section focuses on contrast administration.

Contrast agents allow for the enhanced visibility of soft tissue and other areas with low natural contrast. Each diagnostic imaging examination has unique requirements, and every oncology department has its own protocols for the imaging procedures that are performed. The following are fundamental principles that every therapist must understand whenever dealing with radiographic contrast media.

Types of Contrast Agents

The two basic categories of contrast agents are negative (radiolucent) and positive (radiopaque).[1,5,17] Radiolucent agents have low atomic numbers and, as a result, are easily penetrated by x-rays. The spaces containing these compounds (usually in the form of gases) appear dark on the radiographs. Air and carbon dioxide are the most common negative contrast media. Air alone can sometimes provide sufficient contrast for radiography of the larynx or other parts of the upper respiratory system.

Radiopaque agents have high atomic numbers and absorb x-ray photons, so the spaces filled with these agents appear opaque (white) on the film. For some procedures, negative and positive contrast media are given together to demonstrate certain internal structures. For example, diagnostic tests of the stomach and large intestine usually use barium sulfate combined with air or carbon dioxide as the contrast media.

Heavy Metal Salt

Barium sulfate, a heavy metal salt, is the most commonly used contrast agent for gastrointestinal tract examinations.[1,5,17] This contrast agent is delivered orally or rectally in an aqueous (water-based solution) suspension. Barium sulfate coats the lining of the alimentary organs, and because it is radiopaque the contrast is extremely high. Hazards and inconveniences with the use of barium sulfate are that it requires additives to facilitate ingestion and prevent clumping and it must be concentrated to coat the organs. However, if it is too thick, barium sulfate will not flow easily and is difficult to swallow. Barium sulfate can irritate the colon and cause cramping. It can also stimulate the body to absorb too much fluid, thus leading to hypervolemia or pulmonary edema. Barium sulfate can cause constipation or peritonitis if used in patients with a perforation of the colon or vaginal rupture. If preexisting conditions contraindicate the use of barium sulfate, oncologists will prescribe water-soluble iodides instead.

Organic Iodides

As with barium sulfate, iodine atoms have been proven to be one of the best contrast elements for imaging. Iodine atoms attach to water-soluble carrier molecules or oil-based ethyl esters and dispatch to certain areas of the body. These atoms then displace water in the cells and absorb x-ray photons in those regions.

Most of the conventional, older compounds are highly toxic ionic iodine agents. These compounds are called ionic because their molecules split into two particles (i.e., one negatively charged particle and the other positively charged) whenever they come in contact with body fluids. This splitting results in twice as many iodine particles going into solution in the plasma. The chemical structure of these particles pulls water from the cells, and, because so many of the offending particles exist, the fluid balance of the body may be severely affected. The **ionic contrast media** are said to have **high osmolality,** a high number of particles in solution.[1] A large amount of iodine provides greater contrast but also increases toxicity and viscosity. The most common ionic iodides used are meglumine iodine salts and various sodium iodine salts.

The charged ions discussed previously are irritants and can cause allergic reactions. **Nonionic contrast media** have been developed for this reason. Nonionic contrast media have **low osmolality,** the iodides remain intact instead of splitting, and therefore they agitate the cells less. No charged ions are introduced into the body. These agents are equally effective for imaging but cost much more than ionic agents, so some oncology departments reserve them for allergy-prone patients. Three common nonionic contrast agents are iopamidol, iodixanol, and iohexol.

Some contrast agents have characteristics of ionic and nonionic agents (called *ionic dimers*); they have low osmolality because the molecules are larger and do not have an osmotic (water-moving) effect, but they split and are therefore still ionic.[1,17] An example of this type of contrast agent is sodium meglumine ioxaglate.

Iodinated contrast media are generally viscous, especially at room temperature. This causes discomfort to the patient during injection, although the discomfort can be eased somewhat by preheating the solution to body temperature. Some iodinated contrast media are so viscous that they are best injected by a power injector.

The four aforementioned iodides are all aqueous. Iodinated contrast media can also be oil based. Oil-based agents do not dissolve in water and therefore stay in the body longer. They are unstable and decompose if exposed to light or heat. Although historically used for bronchography and myelography, oil-based contrast agents have limited use in modern departments.[8]

ABSORPTION AND DISTRIBUTION OF CONTRAST MEDIA

Each type of radiographic imaging requires specific contrast media and a sophisticated route of delivery. For example, when rapid systemic distribution is desired an IV injection is used. Direct injection of contrast media allows optimal imaging of the organ or joint before the media are absorbed into the bloodstream and later excreted. If the intestinal tract is being imaged, ionic contrast media cause increased fluid in the intestines and increased intestinal contractions (peristalsis), thereby producing a better image.

To increase efficiency and decrease toxicity of contrast media the patient must comply with preparation instructions such as fasting and enemas. Compliance leads to diagnostic-

quality images produced with the least possible contrast media. An accurate patient history helps to determine the optimal dose, prevent unnecessary adverse reactions, and determine the correct route so that the distribution and metabolism of the contrast media illuminate the desired area. Table 12-1 shows some of the common procedures performed with contrast media.

Metabolic Elimination of Contrast Media

When large volumes of foreign materials must be introduced into the body to facilitate imaging, radiation therapy becomes invasive. Unlike drugs in the curative sense, contrast media are nontherapeutic, toxic substances and prompt elimination from the body limits toxic effects.

Excretion through the kidneys is the most common method of elimination; however, a catheter may be used to quickly drain large volumes of aqueous media found in the bladder.

Patient Reactions to Contrast Media

Water displaced by the osmotic action of iodine particles in the plasma is forced into cells or drawn to specific areas. The excess fluid can saturate and distend the blood vessels, inundate the vascular system and cause hypovolemia, or cause shock by withdrawing too much water from the vessels. The osmotic action of ionic molecules can also cause dramatic fluctuations in kidney function. Giving IV fluids can counteract these fluctuations in function.

Nonionic media or water-soluble ionics are toxic to the kidneys. Patients with renal disease, diabetes, allergies, asthma, sickle cell anemia, thyroid disease, pregnancy, old age, hypertension, or coronary disease may suffer life-threatening reactions to contrast agents and should be carefully evaluated. Children and older adults are often unable to tolerate the dehydration caused by ionic contrast media.

Ionic iodine compounds can provoke allergic reactions ranging from **urticaria** (hives) to anaphylactic shock in susceptible patients. If a patient is going to react to contrast media, the reaction usually happens very quickly (i.e., within a few minutes of administration of the compound).

Classifications of the severity of adverse reactions* seen in contrast media administration are as follows:
- Minor reactions are those that usually require no treatment: nausea, retching, mild vomiting
- Moderate reactions are those that require some form of treatment, but there is no serious danger for the patient and response to treatment is usually rapid: fainting, chest or abdominal pain, headache, chills, severe vomiting, **dyspnea,** extensive urticaria, edema of the face and/or larynx
- Severe reactions are those for which there is a fear for the patient's life, and intensive treatment is required: **syncope,** convulsions, pulmonary edema, life-threatening cardiac arrhythmias, cardiac or respiratory arrest
- Death[10]

*Data from American Society of Radiologic Technologists.

Table 12-1	Common diagnostic imaging procedures that use contrast media	
Procedure	**Route of Administration**	**Contrast Agent**
Cardiovascular	Intravascular	Diatrizoate meglumine 60%
		Diatrizoate sodium 50%
		Iopamidol 61.2%
		Iohexol
Arthrography	Direct injection	Diatrizoate meglumine 60%
		Sodium meglumine ioxaglate
		Air
Bronchography	Intratracheal catheter	Propyliodone oil
Cholangiography	IV	Iodipamide meglumine 10.3%
		Diatrizoate sodium 50%
Cholecystography	Oral	Ipodate sodium (500 mg)
		Iopanoic acid (500 mg)
Computed tomography	IV injection or infusion	Ioversol 68%
		Diatrizoate meglumine 60%
		Iohexol
Cystography	Urinary catheter	Iothalamate meglumine 17%
		Iothalamate sodium 17%
		Diatrizoate meglumine 17%
Discography	Direct injection	Diatrizoate meglumine 60%
		Diatrizoate sodium 60%
Esophagraphy	Oral	Barium sulfate 30%-50%
Hysterosalpingography	Cervical injection	Iothalamate meglumine 60%
Lymphography	Direct injection	Ethiodized oil
MRI	IV injection	Gadolinium and derivatives
Myelography	Intrathecal (lumbar puncture)	Iohexol
Pyelography	Instillation via catheter	Diatrizoate meglumine 20%
		Diatrizoate sodium 20%
		Methiodal sodium 20%
Sialography	Catheter	Iohexol
Splenoportography	Percutaneous injection	Diatrizoate meglumine 60%
	Catheter	Diatrizoate sodium 50%
		Sodium meglumine ioxaglate
Upper and lower GI	Oral/rectal	Barium sulfate
Urography and nephrography	IV injection	Diatrizoate meglumine 60%
		Iodamide meglumine 24%
		Sodium meglumine ioxaglate
		Iohexol
Venography	IV injection	Ioxaglate meglumine
		Ioxaglate sodium
		Iohexol

GI, gastrointestinal ; *IV*, intravenous; *MRI*, magnetic resonance imaging.
Note: Some departments prefer to use nonionic contrast media on all of their patients in an effort to reduce patient reactions.

The therapist must be ready to take immediate remedial action if any of the previously mentioned symptoms begin to manifest.

ROUTES OF DRUG ADMINISTRATION

Radiation therapy patients may receive specific medications before or after the radiation treatments. Medications administered before radiation treatments are for sedation, cytoprotective, and diagnostic purposes; medications given after radiation treatments are palliative (i.e., for relief of distress-ing symptoms). Therapists must clearly understand the way to administer medications, whether their knowledge is first hand or a supporting role.

Drugs may be administered via a variety of routes. General information regarding the numerous routes of administration and the effects of each can be found in clinical textbooks.* The following four administration routes are

*References 1, 3, 5, 7, 11, 12, 15-17.

particularly important for radiation therapy and radiologic imaging: oral, mucous membrane, topical, and parenteral. The remainder of this chapter discusses these ways to administer drugs and related patient care issues.

Oral Administration

The oral route of administration is safe, simple, and convenient for both the patient and caregiver. Drugs taken by mouth absorb slowly into the bloodstream and are less potent but longer lasting than drugs given by injection.* The risk of infection is also less from oral administration than from any other route. Some patients are unable to take oral preparations because of vomiting or nausea, unconsciousness, intubation, required fasting before tests or surgery, difficulty swallowing, or refusal to cooperate. The latter two occurrences are especially common with children.

In radiation therapy, some types of contrast media used for pretreatment diagnosis *must* be administered orally such as barium for esophageal or small bowel localization.[1,5,15] Palliative medications administered after the therapy are frequently given by mouth. Whenever oral medications are given, the caregiver should do the following:
1. Wash the hands.
2. Read the label and medication order before and after preparing the dose.
3. Identify the patient.
4. Check for allergies.
5. Assess the patient by checking and recording vital signs.
6. Prepare the medicine accurately without touching it directly.
7. Confirm the order with the physician.
8. Give water or other more palatable liquid, such as ice chips, orange juice, or a strong-tasting chaser, if indicated.
9. Elevate the patient's head if the patient is supine.
10. Observe and ensure that the medicine is swallowed and not aspirated.
11. Discard medication paraphernalia.
12. Rewash the hands.
13. Confirmation of medication administration is required. Record the medication administration in the patient's chart.

Some physicians encourage self-administration of drugs. However, the therapist should be aware that some depressed patients in particular might hide and store drugs for later suicide attempts.

Mucous Membrane Administration

Some drugs cannot be given orally because gastric secretions inactivate the medications or because the drugs have a bad taste or odor, damage teeth, or cause gastric distress. If a drug has one of these potential side effects, it can be given in a suppository form using alternate mucous membranes in the rectum or vagina.

Other methods of introducing drugs through the mucous membrane include the following:
- Inhalation in a medicated mist

- Direct application by swabbing
- Gargling
- Irrigating the target tissue by flushing with sterile or medicated fluid

Medications can also be dissolved under the tongue by sublingual administration. All these methods have a systemic effect, although some affect the system more rapidly than others. Regardless of the route used, the person administering the drug must never compromise sterility by touching the drug directly.

Topical Administration

Topical administration involves placement of the drug directly on the skin. This method is frequently needed after the skin is disturbed by radiation therapy.[6] Topical applications are also used for antiseptics preceding injections, ointments, lotions, and transdermal patches. Such patches can dispense scopolamine, estrogen, or nicotine slowly and at a constant level. If the caregiver is administering topical drugs, gloves should be worn to prevent absorption of the medication and introduction of infectious agents to the patient.

Parenteral Administration

Parenteral administration means that the medication bypasses the gastrointestinal tract. Taken literally, this includes the topical and some mucous membrane routes, but the word *parenteral* colloquially means "by injection."

A drug administered parenterally is absorbed rapidly and efficiently. None of the drug is destroyed by digestive enzymes, so the dose is usually smaller.[15-17] Medications are administered parenterally in the following situations:
- The drug would irritate the alimentary tract too much to be taken orally
- A rapid effect is needed, such as during an emergency
- Drugs need to be dispensed intravenously over time
- The patient is unconscious or otherwise unable to take oral medications

For example, if the patient is fasting before surgery or tests, medication can be given by injection.

Parenteral administration carries with it the danger of infection from piercing the skin and an increased risk of unrecoverable error because of rapid absorption. Injections also cause genuine fear in some patients. Long-term parenteral therapy can also damage injection sites.

Parenteral administration is categorized by the depth of the injection and location of the injection site (Fig. 12-1). The following are the four most common parenteral routes[17]:
- **Intradermal (ID)**—a shallow injection between the layers of the skin
- **Subcutaneous (SQ or SC)**—a 45- or 90-degree injection into the subcutaneous tissue just below the skin
- **Intramuscular (IM)**—a 90-degree injection into the muscle used for larger amounts or a quicker systemic effect
- **Intravenous (IV)**—an injection directly into the bloodstream that provides an immediate effect

The therapist may also become a member of a health care

---

*References 1, 5, 7, 11, 12, 15-17.

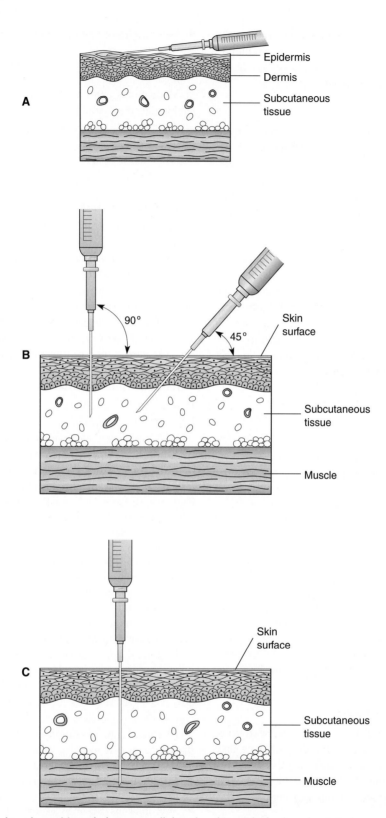

Figure 12-1. A, The syringe is positioned almost parallel to the skin with the bevel pointed upward for intradermal injections. The medication is deposited right under the skin, forming a small, raised area. **B,** The syringe is positioned at a 45- or 90-degree angle to the skin for subcutaneous injections. The medication is deposited in the subcutaneous tissue just below the skin. **C,** The syringe is positioned at a 90-degree angle for intramuscular injections. The medication is deposited in the muscular area just below the subcutaneous tissue.

team that administers drugs by less common parenteral routes as well. Other routes pertaining to radiation oncology include the following:

- Intrathecal administration, in which medications are injected directly into the spinal canal, such as chemotherapeutic agents
- Intratracheal administration, in which medications are administered directly into the trachea
- Intracranial administration, in which medications are administered directly into the brain
- Catheterization, which includes urinary catheterization[6]

The physician or anesthesiologist performs the administration of drugs by these routes with the therapist acting as a support person.

IV ADMINISTRATION

Of the four parenteral routes, therapists most often use the IV route. IV injections, or **venipuncture,** are within the scope of practice for radiation therapists in most states.[2] This technique is best learned by hands-on experience.

When a patient requires ongoing IV therapy, a catheter is inserted into a peripheral vein where it can remain for a number of days. Every therapist should practice error-free preparation, use appropriate equipment and flawless venipuncture technique, and have a caring bedside manner. Even if all these requirements are met, venipuncture is still potentially hazardous. The advantage of having ongoing access is that the vein's integrity is broken only at the time of insertion. This catheter can be used for either intermittent medications, continuous infusions, or a combination of both. If continuous access is not required the caregiver can disconnect the patient from the infusion using a heparin lock. The heparin lock has a self-seal for when it is not in use.

The therapist administering drugs through an IV route must never leave the patient alone during the procedure and must continuously monitor the patient.

Different methods of IV administration serve different purposes. The safest method is continuous infusion, in which the medication is mixed with a large volume of IV solution and given gradually over time. Second, a drug can be piggybacked (added) onto the main IV line by means of a special valve so that the medication can be administered intermittently at prescribed levels.[11,12,15-17] During drug administration the volume of IV fluid administered is lowered. This process usually takes less than an hour after which the volume is restored to the initial level.

A third method of IV injection is a bolus, or push, of a concentrated dose of medication injected by a syringe directly into the vein or through the IV port. This method requires diligent observation of the patient because the effect is rapid and can be irreversible.

Two major types of IV injections pertain to radiation therapists: drugs requiring dilution and drugs requiring delivery by IV bolus. Most contrast media, if not given orally, are injected by bolus. Drugs that are diluted or solutions for the maintenance of fluid levels are administered slowly by IV drip.

Administering Bolus Injections

Certain medications, including contrast media, must be administered at full strength. If the patient has an IV line that is running a continuous infusion, the therapist must temporarily stop the infusion while the bolus is injected to avoid mixing the solutions. The IV line should remain in place because radiopaque materials are highly toxic, and reactions can happen quickly. The IV line allows the patient to receive immediate remedial treatment should a negative reaction occur.

Bolus injection requires the same preliminaries discussed in regard to other routes of administration (i.e., checking the medication, identifying the patient, washing the hands). Proper preparation of the dose of contrast is required. IV contrast medication comes packaged in ampules or vials, each of which has its own specific requirements for use. An ampule contains a single dose of medicine; the tip is snapped off, and the drug is drawn into a syringe through a filter needle (Fig. 12-2, *A*). A vial has a rubber stopper, and the needle is inserted through that stopper to draw out the medicine (Fig. 12-2, *B*) (usually multidose vials are not used because of possible contamination, but if the vial contains more than one dose, a new needle should be used and the stopper of the vial must be wiped with alcohol before every use). The vial should be dated and initialed at the time of use. It should be discarded within 24 hours of initial use.

If the medication is not directly delivered by a vein, an IV port (Fig. 12-3, *A* and *B*) may be used. The injection port of the catheter should be wiped with alcohol or the heparin lock should be flushed with sterile saline, and then the drug may be slowly injected into the port. The correct rate for injecting the drug should be specified on the package or in the medication order. If the medication enters the vein too quickly, the body may go into speed shock, a severe, life-threatening reaction caused by the toxicity of the drug. Following injection, the port should be rewiped with alcohol or the heparin lock should be flushed and refilled with heparin solution. Only then can the IV flow be restored.

Chemotherapy is often administered through a different type of vascular access port such as the Hickman, Groshong, Port-A-Cath, and PAS Port (Fig. 12-3, *C*).[15]

IV Infusion and Venipuncture Equipment

Before the actual venipuncture or injection takes place, the health care professional must gather all the necessary equipment. Interruption of the procedure to find missing equipment is extremely unprofessional and erodes the patient's confidence in the caregiver. The IV equipment can be prepared with the tubing capped and ready to attach before performing the venipuncture or after the IV port is in place. The timing of the preparation depends on institutional policy or the physician's orders.

In the case of an IV drip, required equipment includes IV tubing with a clamp on it, the vacoliter or plastic drip bag, a stand on which to hang the bag of solution, an IV filter, and a meter to measure the flow rate. The most common place for

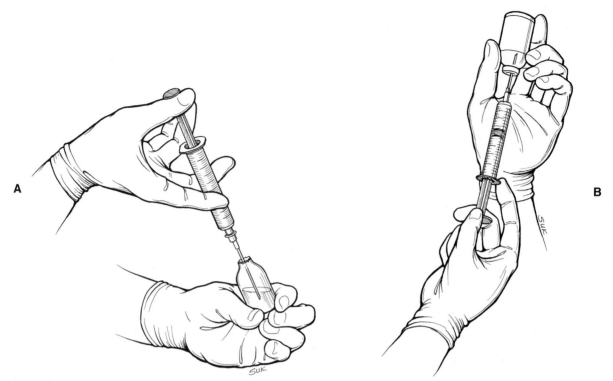

Figure 12-2. A, This drawing shows the way to remove the medication from an ampule. The medication is removed by pulling back on the plunger of the syringe. The therapist should be careful not to contaminate the needle when inserting and removing the needle from the ampule. **B,** This drawing shows the removal of medication from a vial. The rubber stopper must be cleaned with alcohol before the needle is inserted into the vial. The same amount of air must be injected into the vial as will be withdrawn to equalize the pressure in the vial.

sterility to be compromised is in the two ends of the tubing; neither the end going into the sterile solution nor the end connecting with the IV catheter should *ever* be touched, even with gloves.* If either end is inadvertently touched, it must be sterilized before use or discarded and replaced.

IV equipment varies according to the drug and dose. The equipment tray should include a tourniquet, antiseptic swabs, gloves, a syringe, a needle, cotton balls, the correct drug, and adhesive bandages. Any catheters, tubing, drip bottles, poles, and monitors required should also be in place before the procedure begins.

The type of medication and physical characteristics of the patient determine which instrument should be used for IV injection. For a one-time injection of 30 ml or less, a regular needle (i.e., 18 to 20 gauge, depending on the viscosity of the drug and size of the patient's veins) and a syringe should suffice. An infusion that takes place over a longer time requires a butterfly set, which is a special steel needle attached to two plastic "wings" taped to the skin. This butterfly set anchors the needle in the vein.

Whenever the infusion requires a large volume of fluid or

must be administered over an extended period of time, a plastic catheter can be inserted into the vein. Because the tubing is flexible and soft, it allows the patient to move around and it is less irritating than a rigid, metal needle. Two kinds of venous catheters exist; one is a narrow tube inserted through a hollow needle, and the other has the needle through the tube. The through-the-needle catheter is generally longer and thinner and can be inserted deeper into the vein. This type of catheter is commonly used for antineoplastic drugs. After the catheter is in place and taped down, the needle is removed.

Dosage, Dose Calculation, and Dose Response

Medication charts list standard measurements (i.e., metric or apothecary), their abbreviations, and recommended doses for most common medicines. Table 12-2 lists common abbreviations used for prescribing medications.[5,12] Health care personnel must invariably calculate individual doses for their patients if the standard packaging differs from the amount ordered. To calculate the quantity ordered, the therapist or nurse must multiply or divide the dose required by the packaged amount (make sure the two are in the same unit of measurement). The math should *always* be double-checked by a second person.

Doses for children should be calculated according to the

---

*References 1, 5, 7, 11, 13, 16, 17.

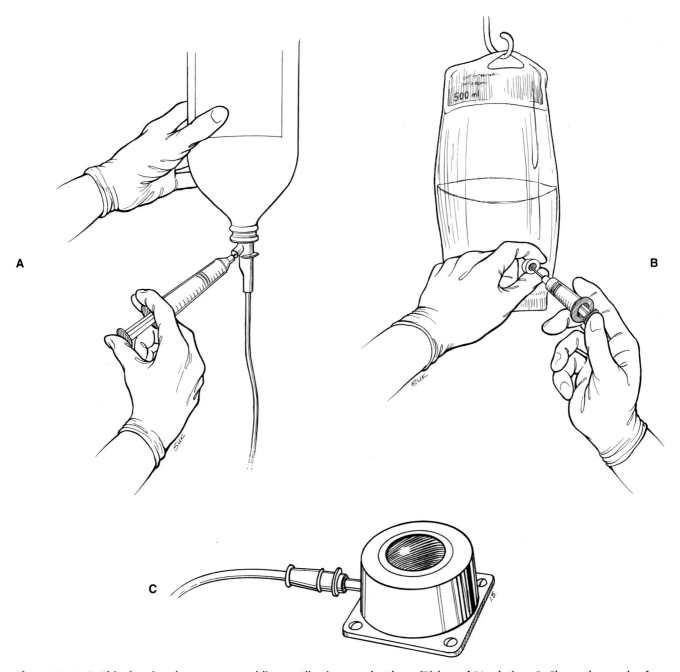

Figure 12-3. A, This drawing demonstrates adding medication to a bottle or **(B)** bag of IV solution. **C,** Chemotherapy is often administered through a vascular access port.

child's weight or body surface area. The latter is more accurate because it also takes into account the child's height and body density.[12,15]

Although the specifics of dose calculation are beyond the scope of this chapter, a good nursing text will explain the way to compute the correct dose.

Whenever drugs are administered by IV, the dosages must be calculated according to the total volume of fluid the patient receives (except in the case of a bolus injection). This calculation must be carefully monitored because flow

and absorption rates can fluctuate. Also, the drug must be given in the correct dilution, at the appropriate rate, and in the correct amount. Controlling the dosage in single injections or piggyback deliveries is easier than in long-term IV treatment.

Many factors can affect the delivery rate of an IV injection. The flow can be interrupted by a kink in the tubing, a clot in the needle or catheter, the needle tip pressing against the vein wall, or a problem at the site of entry. The drip rate may depend on the patient's absorption rate, which always

Table 12-2	Common abbreviations used for prescribing medications
Abbreviation	**Meaning**
a.c.	Before meals
bid	Twice a day
h	Hour
h.s.	At bedtime
IM	Intramuscular
IV	Intravenous
ml	Milliliter
p.c.	After meals
PO	By mouth
p.r.n.	As necessary
q	Every
q3h, q4h, and so on	Every 3 hours, every 4 hours, and so on
qd	Every day
qh	Hourly
qid	Four times each day
qod	Every other day
stat	At once
SQ/SC	Subcutaneous
tid	Three times a day

varies greatly from one person to another. Sudden fluctuations in flow rates happen frequently because of mechanical problems with the equipment or because the patient dislodges the catheter. All these factors influence the accuracy of delivery whenever drugs are infused intravenously.

Initiation of IV Therapy

Patient education. Before any IV drugs are administered, therapists should identify themselves to the patient, assess the patient's condition, and explain the procedure. Assessment involves the following:

- Taking an allergy history (or reading the patient's chart if a history has already been taken)
- Taking the blood pressure for a baseline reading
- Determining whether the patient has had any medication that affects blood clotting
- Asking the patient (not the nurse) whether the patient has been fasting.*

The physician is responsible for explaining the reason the procedure is needed; the therapist can ease any anxiety the patient may have by describing the process and answering questions. Iodinated contrast media can produce adverse reactions within minutes after being administered, so the therapist must ask the patient to report any symptoms that he or she may experience *before* administering the drug. It may

*References 1, 7, 9, 12, 16, 17.

help the patient to know some common sensations related to the medication and whether they are serious or not.

Site Selection for Venipuncture

The site chosen for venipuncture depends on the drug to be administered and the length of time that the IV line will be in place (Fig. 12-4, *A*). The large antecubital vein in the arm is convenient for drawing blood or for injecting a single dose or viscous solution, but this vein is inappropriate for a long-term IV therapy because it hinders the patient's mobility. The best choices for long-term infusion include sites above the anterior wrist (lower cephalic, accessory cephalic, and basilic veins) or veins on the posterior hand (basilic, metacarpal, and cephalic veins) (Fig. 12-4, *B*).[12] If the patient is right-handed, putting the IV line into the left arm allows the patient to maintain use of the dominant arm.

Certain contraindications at a specific venipuncture site mean that a different site should be chosen. These contraindications include scar tissue or hematoma that necessitates injection above this site, infection or skin lesions that could introduce infection into the bloodstream, burns, collapsed veins, or veins too small for the chosen gauge of the needle. Special techniques apply if a patient has rolling veins, has **phlebitis,** is on dialysis, or is extremely obese. If the patient is taking blood thinners, extra compression is needed.

Venipuncture Technique

The venipuncture may be performed after the preliminaries, such as collection of supplies, patient identification, informing the patient of the procedure, and patient assessment, are completed. The procedure[13,17] is as follows:

1. Position the patient. The patient should be sitting or lying down, and the arm should be placed in a relaxed position. The arm may need to be anchored to an arm board if the patient is extremely active.
2. Determine the best site for the venipuncture.
3. Wash the hands and put on gloves. All **standard precautions** should be followed because of potential contact with body fluids. These precautions include wearing gloves, a mask, and protective eyewear; properly handling needles; and disposing of used equipment into containers for biohazardous material.
4. Apply the tourniquet tightly in a way that it can be removed with one hand. The tourniquet should be about 2 to 4 inches above the puncture site. Never leave a tourniquet on for more than 2 minutes.
5. It may be necessary to tap or stroke the vein or to have the patient make a fist to enhance distention of the vein (Fig. 12-5).
6. Cleanse the skin with an antimicrobial solution (tincture of iodine 2%, 10% povidone-iodine, 70% isopropyl alcohol, or chlorhexidine) in small concentric circles outward to a radius of about 2 inches. Do not touch area again with a nonsterile object. If local anesthetic is being used, inject it intradermally at this time.
7. Verify you have the proper medication.
8. Anchor the vein firmly above and below puncture site with

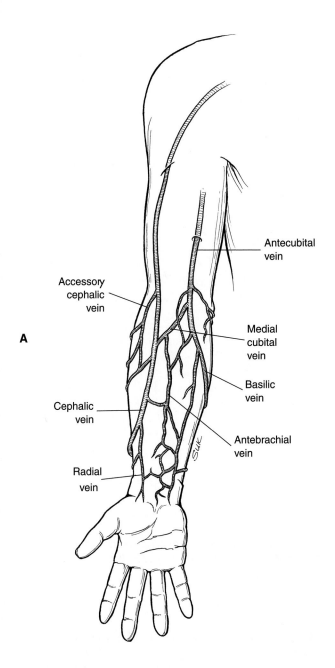

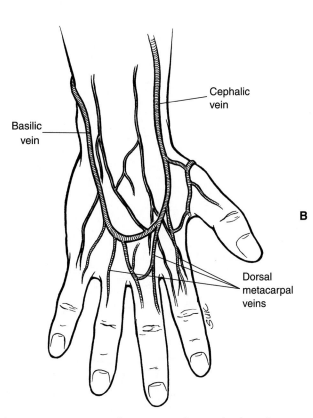

Figure 12-4. A, Venipuncture sites of the forearm. **B,** Venipuncture sites of the wrist and hand.

thumb and index finger of free hand. This will prevent the vein from "rolling."

9. Insert the needle parallel to the vein, bevel side up, at a 30-degree angle, and then flatten the needle to a 10- to 15-degree angle. If the angle is too shallow, the needle will skim between the skin and vein; if the angle is too deep, the needle will penetrate the posterior wall of the vein and cause bleeding into the tissues. When blood flows back into the syringe or hub of the cannula, the needle is in the vein. Allowing the blood to fill the hub before attaching tubing ensures that air bubbles are not trapped in the line.

10. Remove the needle from the catheter. Release the tourniquet and push the catheter deeper into the vein and up to the hub, if possible.

11. Attach IV tubing and place an antiseptic swab or patch over

the puncture site, and fix the catheter in place with adhesive tape or if injecting contrast media with a butterfly and syringe, proceed with the injection after securing the butterfly in place.

12. If the venipuncture is unsuccessful, withdraw the needle or catheter, and immediately apply light pressure to the insertion site.

Infusion of Medication

The procedure* for starting a drip infusion after venipuncture has been performed and an IV line is in place is as follows:

1. Wash the hands.

*References 1, 5, 7, 11, 13, 15, 16.

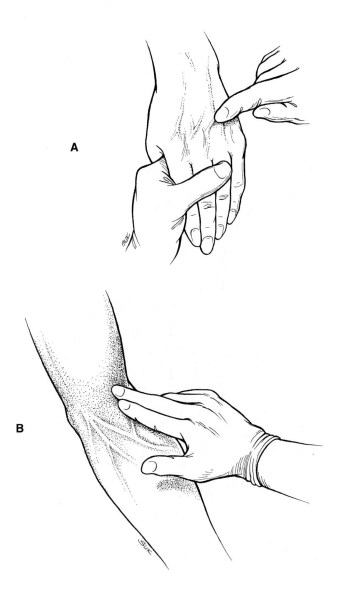

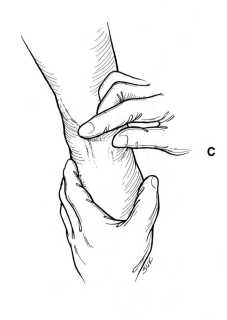

Figure 12-5. Techniques to distend veins include tapping the vein **(A),** gently stroking the vein **(B),** and having the patient make a fist **(C).**

2. Double-check the patient's name. Assess the patient. Ask the patient about allergies to drugs.
3. Triple-check the physician's orders against the solution label.
4. Check the bag or vacoliter for an expiration date, signs of contamination (such as discoloration, cloudiness, or sediment), and cracks or leaks.
5. Put on gloves and follow all standard precautions according to institutional policy.
6. Remove the metal cap and rubber diaphragm from the bottle or bag without touching the rubber stopper.
7. Close the clamp on the tubing, attach the in-line filter, and insert the spike of the drip chamber into the rubber stopper without touching the sterile end.
8. Invert the fluid container and hang it on an IV pole 18 to 24 inches above the vein.
9. Remove the cap covering the lower end of tubing, release the clamp, and allow the fluid to flow through the tube to get rid of air bubbles (if air is left in the tubing, it will be forced into the vein). Close the clamp. Attach the tubing to the IV line.
10. Monitor the flow until the desired rate is established.
11. Monitor the condition of the patient.
12. Discard used materials and gloves according to institutional policy.
13. Rewash hands.
14. Record the medication procedure in the patient's chart.

Many factors can affect the delivery rate of an IV injection. The flow can be interrupted by a kink in the tubing, a clot in the needle or catheter, the needle tip pressing against the vein wall, or a problem at the site of entry. The drip rate may depend on the patient's absorption rate, which always varies greatly from one person to another. Sudden fluctuations in flow rates happen frequently because of mechanical problems with the equipment or because the patient dislodges the catheter. All these factors influence the accuracy of delivery whenever drugs are infused intravenously.

Hazards of IV Fluids

Perhaps the biggest challenge of administering drugs intravenously is to get the drug into the vein without introducing foreign microorganisms that can cause infection. No one should ever touch the fluid ports, needle, ends of tubing, or any other part of the equipment through which germs could pass into the bloodstream. Diligent observation of the venipuncture site allows the caregiver to recognize symptoms of sepsis at its earliest stage.

IV infusion carries unique hazards with it. Any swelling around the injection site accompanied by cool, pale skin and possibly hard patches or localized pain is a sign of **infiltration.**[17] This can occur if the catheter or IV needle has pulled out of the vein and the fluid has seeped into the adjacent subcutaneous tissue. Infiltration can also occur if the IV bottle is hung too high, the hydrostatic pressure is so great that the vein cannot absorb the fluid quickly enough, and the fluid saturates the surrounding tissue. If the therapist mistakenly misses the vein and injects contrast media into the tissues surrounding the vein, the result is a similar condition called **extravasation,** which is not only painful but can cause severe tissue damage.[11,12,15,16]

Other hazards to IV infusion include an allergic reaction to the drug, an air embolism caused by failing to eliminate air bubbles in the equipment, a metabolic or an electrolyte imbalance, edema caused by the dressing being too tight at the site or too much fluid, speed shock from too rapid a delivery, drug incompatibility, thrombus (blood clots), and phlebitis. Phlebitis can be prevented if the needle is a small enough gauge that the blood can flow around it. A "keep vein open" (KVO) drip keeps the blood from clotting at the site; likewise, the heparin in a heparin lock prevents the injection site and bloodstream from developing clots.

Sudden increases in fluid volume introduced by IV equipment can accidentally occur. If the patient is extremely frail or has a head trauma, a sudden overload can be fatal. Any time fluid is infused too quickly, the excess can collect in the lungs, thereby causing pulmonary edema. Rapid infusion can also result in an overdose of the medication. Too little fluid may result in dehydration or an insufficient dose of the required medication. These are only a few of the reasons that monitoring IV lines closely is crucial.

Discontinuation of IV Therapy

Because the potential for contamination is so high in IV therapy, the infusion set should be changed every 24 to 48 hours. If IV therapy must be continued for a longer period of time, changing to a new venipuncture site may be necessary, depending on the condition of the original site. Most of the drugs that therapists administer are infused over a short period of time, through a single site.

To remove the IV line, the therapist must gather the following supplies: sterile gauze pads, gloves, and tape. After the patient has been properly identified and informed of the procedure, these steps should be followed to discontinue IV therapy[1,12]:

1. Wash the hands.
2. Clamp off the IV tubing and remove the tape holding the catheter in place.
3. Put on gloves and follow standard precautions according to institutional policy.
4. Apply a folded gauze sponge over the insertion site and hold it down with your thumb. Grasp the needle or catheter and withdraw in one smooth motion.
5. Before taping the gauze, inspect the site.
6. Tape the gauze pad in place and elevate the patient's arm. Apply direct pressure for 1 to 2 minutes.
7. Dispose of the used IV materials properly.
8. Rewash the hands.
9. Record the appropriate information in the patient's chart.

LEGAL ASPECTS

In considering legal aspects the scope of practice must be reviewed. The scope of practice for radiation therapists includes the delivery of radiation to treat disease. It also requires patient care, including providing comfort, dignity, education, monitoring, and documentation.[2] Increasingly, the practice of venipuncture and the administration of IV medications and contrast media are also included.

The therapist may not legally diagnose, interpret images, reveal test results to patients or family members, prescribe drugs, admit or discharge patients, or order tests. Those duties belong to the physician. The therapist, like every health care professional, is legally required to report incidents or errors and is allowed to act without liability in an emergency if no other care is available (the Good Samaritan laws).

The therapist is legally liable for administering competent treatments and accurately communicating with the patient. The two most common complaints leading to malpractice suits in radiology and oncology are false-negative or false-positive diagnoses of fractures or cancers and the misadministration of contrast media.[4] The oncologist does not bear these risks alone. The radiation therapist is part of the team and on the front line of patient care.

Although radiation oncology team members cannot be held accountable for poor health results, they are liable if they act negligently or cause injury. Because the profession can be so hazardous, it is in everyone's best interest that efforts be taken to communicate *all* risks before any procedure or treatment takes place. Every precaution must be taken in the actual treatment of each patient.

Different states have different laws regulating the radiation therapist's scope of practice. You must adhere to state laws and institutional policies and procedures regarding venipuncture and the administration of medication.

Documentation of Administration

The medical record is a legal document and is evidence for the caregiver and patient in the event of confusion or litigation.[4,9] Therefore it is in the therapist's best interest to make sure the information in the chart is thorough and accurate. For example, if the patient verbally informs the therapist of a sensitivity to iodine and the therapist fails to pass on the information or record it in the chart, the therapist could be held liable for adverse reactions. A previously documented sensitivity should be apparent in the patient's permanent record, and in this situation the therapist is responsible for noticing and making sure the physician is also aware of the sensitivity.[9]

The patient's chart or medical record is often the primary means of communication among the members of a health care team. Each patient is often treated by several different professionals, all of whom need to know the entire medical history to do their jobs effectively.

Accurate documentation protects the patient from errors in treatment; likewise, accurate documentation protects the caregivers from making procedural, ethical, or legal errors. Every medication, every treatment procedure, every diagnostic test, and even verbal communication should be documented in the patient's permanent medical record.

Although each medical institution is allowed to develop its own system of record keeping, certain standard contents are required by the various accrediting bodies in the medical profession; these include the following[14]:
1. Patient identification and demographic information.
2. Medical history, including family history, allergies, and previous illnesses.
3. Nature of the current complaint and a report of examinations and treatments.
4. Orders for and results of any tests or procedures.
5. Record of all medications, whether self-administered, prescribed, or professionally administered. The information should include but is not limited to time, route, dosage, site of administration, and caregiver's signature.
6. Physician's notes, instructions, and conclusions.
7. Informed consent form.

Documentation of any complications or adverse reactions to a medication is especially critical to the medical record of any patient.* A sensitivity to any medication must be prominently displayed in the patient's record. Remedial action taken to counteract the complication must also be recorded.

The therapist bears the responsibility for understanding the way to read the chart accurately and enter information in the record. A written error should not be erased or covered with correction fluid but should have a single line drawn through it and initialed (so that the original information is legible). The information should be rewritten, dated, and initialed.

Medical records are confidential and may not be released without the patient's consent. Orders of any kind *must* be signed by the attending health care professional.

Informed Consent

Radiation therapy and diagnostic imaging require **informed consent** from the patient. In addition to the general consent form the patient signs when entering a health care facility,

each radiation therapy procedure requires a separate form in the patient's record.[17]

Especially in cases of radiation administration and ionic contrast media in which the potential risk is so high, a grey area about what constitutes "informed" consent exists. If a patient agrees in writing to receive ionic contrast media but suffers a reaction, the oncologist could be held liable if that oncologist failed to inform the patient that nonionic agents were available. The issue of cost (e.g., nonionic media costs considerably more than ionic media) should not determine how much the physician tells the patient. Open communication about risk and cost are part of the patient's legal rights.

Informed consent expectations and documentation varies by state and institution. Informed consent forms generally include the name of the authorized physician; a description of the procedure and associated medications; an assurance that the purpose, benefit, risk, and any alternative options have been imparted and understood; an area where patients can write in their words what the procedure entails; and a disclaimer, which does not always hold up in court, releasing the caregiver and facility from liability, if complications develop or the treatment fails.

SUMMARY

The technique of venipuncture and assisting in the administration of IV drugs and contrast media are crucial skills required for the practice of radiation therapy. The descriptions in this chapter do not qualify a radiation therapist to perform those actions but are intended only as an overview. The therapist must study the principles of pharmacology and must have hands-on experience before performing these techniques on patients. The therapist who is knowledgeable in all pertinent aspects of drug administration contributes an invaluable service to the success of the radiation therapy team.

Review Questions

1. List the Six Rights of Drug Safety.

   _____
   _____
   _____
   _____
   _____
   _____

Multiple Choice

2. Which of the following is NOT a patient-related variable affecting response to medications?
   a. Weight
   b. Physical condition
   c. Tolerance
   d. Emotional requirements
   e. Age

---

*References 1, 4, 5, 9, 12, 15.

3. The way in which drugs affect the body is called
   a. Pharmacokinetics
   b. Metabolism
   c. Pharmacodynamics
   d. Drug effectiveness
4. Which of the following is NOT a parenteral route of administration for medications?
   a. Subcutaneous
   b. Instillation
   c. Intravenous
   d. Intramuscular
5. The type of drug given to cancer patients to relieve nausea and vomiting is which of the following?
   a. Antacid
   b. Emetic
   c. Cathartic
   d. Antiemetic
6. The way a drug travels through the body to the appropriate receptor site is known as:
   a. Pharmacodynamics
   b. Excretion
   c. Distribution
   d. Pharmacokinetics
7. The abbreviation "qod" stands for which of the following?
   a. Once daily
   b. Once every other day
   c. Daily
   d. None of the above

Matching

8. Match the following drugs to their drug category.

a. ____ Decadron	I.	Antiseptic
b. ____ Hydrocortisone 1%	II.	Antidiarrheal
c. ____ Dilantin	III.	Sedative
d. ____ Betadine	IV.	Skin agent
e. ____ Xylocaine	V.	Corticosteroid
f. ____ Heparin	VI.	Radioactive isotope
g. ____ Imodium	VII.	Diuretic
	VIII.	Analgesic
	IX.	Anticoagulant
	X.	Anesthetic
	XI.	Anticonvulsant

Essay

9. Define extravasation.
10. Describe the difference between a side effect from a drug and a complication from a drug.

Questions to Ponder

1. You are charting a dose of medication administered in the oncology department. You recorded the wrong route of administration. You "white out" the error and rewrite the appropriate route to correct the record. Is this an acceptable method to correct the record? If not, what is the correct method?
2. Why is following standard precautions during drug administration important?
3. Discuss the importance of parenteral drug administration.
4. Compare the gender differences in the absorption of medications.
5. Analyze the differences between ionic and nonionic contrast media.

REFERENCES

1. Adler AM, Carlton RR, editors: *Introduction to radiography and patient care,* ed 2, Philadelphia, 1999, WB Saunders.
2. American Society of Radiologic Technologists: *Radiation therapist's scope of practice,* Albuquerque, 1993, The American Society of Radiologic Technologists.
3. Beebe RO, Funk DL: *Fundamentals of emergency care,* Albany, NY, 2001, Delmar.
4. Brice J: Imaging and the law: simple tactics minimize exposure to malpractice, *Diagn Imaging* 14(3):43-46, 1992.
5. Ehrlich RA, Daly JA, McCloskey ED: *Patient care in radiography with an introduction to medical imaging,* ed 5, St. Louis, 1999, Mosby.
6. Holleb A, Fink DJ, Murphy GP: *Clinical oncology: a multidisciplinary approach for physicians and students,* Atlanta, 1991, The American Cancer Society.
7. Kemp BB, Pillitteri A, Brown P: *Fundamentals of nursing: a framework for practice,* ed 2, Glenview, Ill, 1989, Scott, Foresman.
8. Kowalczyk N, Donnett KA: *Integrated patient care for the imaging professional,* St. Louis, 1996, Mosby.
9. Lucchese DR, Eikman EA: The medical-legal implications of contrast agent use, *Appl Radiol* 18(12):36-37, 1989.
10. Newman J, Hladik WB: *Pharmacology for the radiologic technologist, Part 3: adverse reactions to radiopaque contrast media,* Albuquerque, 1997, The American Society of Radiologic Technologists.
11. Perry AG, Potter PA: *Clinical nursing skills and techniques,* ed 4, St. Louis, 1998, Mosby.
12. Potter PA, Perry AG: *Fundamentals of nursing,* ed 5, St. Louis, 2001, Mosby.
13. Roberts GH, Carson J: Venipuncture tips for radiologic technologists, *Radiol Technol* 65(2):107-115, 1993.
14. Schwartz HW: *Current concepts in radiology management,* Sudbury, Mass, 1992, American Healthcare Radiology Administrators.
15. Smith SF, Duell DJ: *Clinical nursing skills: nursing process model, basic to advanced skills,* ed 3, Norwalk, Conn, 1992, Appleton & Lange.
16. Taylor C, Lillis C, LeMone P: *Fundamentals of nursing: the art and science of nursing care,* ed 4, Philadelphia, 2001, JB Lippincott.
17. Torres LS: *Basic medical techniques and patient care in imaging technology,* ed 5, Philadelphia, 1997, JB Lippincott.

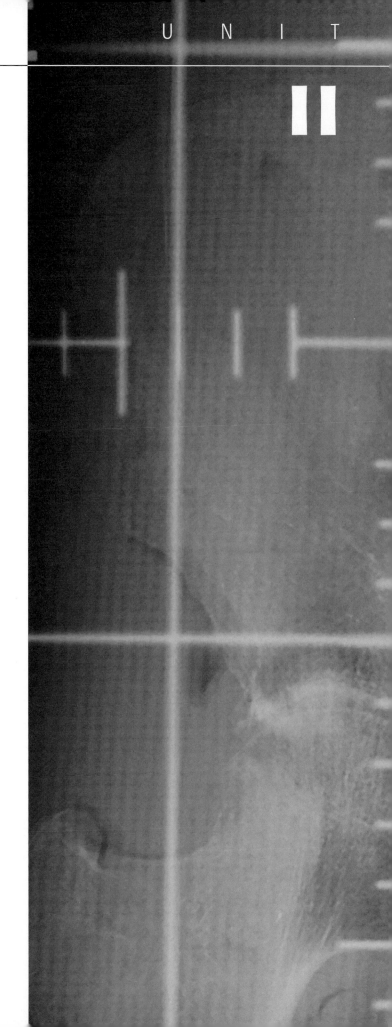

PHYSICS,
SIMULATION,
AND TREATMENT
PLANNING

Applied Mathematics Review

Charles M. Washington, E. Richard Bawiec Jr.

Outline

Key Terms

The practice of radiation therapy requires the use of exact quantitative measurements for the accurate delivery of a therapeutic dose. Patient simulation, treatment planning, and quality assurance have a strong functional dependence on mathematics. Because of this fact, the radiation therapist and the medical dosimetrist must have a good working knowledge of basic as well as advanced mathematical skills to accurately perform their duties. This chapter serves as a review of the principles of the mathematical concepts pertinent to the delivery of ionizing radiation in cancer management. The emphasis is on practical application, not on teaching theoretical principles. This chapter reviews ratios and proportions, exponential functions, logarithms, basic units, uncertainty, and dimensional analysis. Appropriately, practical applications are emphasized. The initial sections are structured as a review and are not intended to "teach" math concepts. The reader is presumed to have a working knowledge of basic entry-level college algebra.

REVIEW OF MATHEMATICAL CONCEPTS

Algebraic Equations with One Unknown

In many situations, an **algebraic equation** is used to describe a physical phenomenon based on the interaction of several factors. For example, the dose to any point from a brachytherapy source requires knowledge of the source activity, source filtration, distance from the source to the point of calculation interest, and several other factors. The ability to solve an equation for the value of an unknown variable is important. The following "rules" of algebra are helpful in remembering how do to this:

- When an unknown is multiplied by some quantity, divide both sides of an equation by that quantity to isolate the unknown.
- When a quantity is added to an unknown, subtract that quantity from both sides of the equation to isolate the unknown. When the quantity is subtracted from the unknown, add it to both sides.
- When an equation appears in fractional form, that is, the unknown is divided by some quantity, cross multiply both sides by that quantity, then solve for the unknown.[3]

Algebraic manipulation is used commonly in radiation therapy so that the radiation therapist and medical dosimetrist should be comfortable solving these types of equations. An example of a typical algebraic manipulation scenario is shown in the practical examples at the end of this chapter.

Ratios and Proportions

A **ratio** is the comparison of two numbers, values, or terms. The ratio denotes a relationship between the two components. Often these relationships allow the radiation therapist to predict trends. The notation for writing a ratio of a value or term, x, to another value or term, y, is most often written as follows:

$$\frac{x}{y} \text{ or } x{:}y$$

One important property of a ratio is that any ratio, x/y, remains unchanged if both terms undergo operations by the same number. For example, the ratio $32/80$ can be simplified to the ratio $2/5$ by dividing both the numerator and the denominator by 16, a common factor of both numbers.

If two ratios are equal, this is known as a **proportion.** A proportion can also be looked at as an equation relating two ratios. This principle can assist in solving for an unknown factor in a proportion. For example, examine the following proportion:

$$5{:}7 = n{:}49$$

This can be rewritten in a more recognizable form as follows:

$$\frac{5}{7} = \frac{n}{49}$$

By cross multiplication, this proportion can be solved for n:

$$(49 \times 5) = 7n \text{ or } 7n = (49 \times 5)$$
$$7n = 245$$
$$n = 35$$

In the clinical radiation therapy environment, inverse and direct proportions can occur in various ways. The concepts of inverse and direct proportionality are pertinent in the management of cancer with ionizing radiation, so a brief review of these concepts is beneficial.

Inverse Proportionality

Consider a hypothetical situation in which a number of aircraft must complete a trip of 1000 miles. Each aircraft travels at a different velocity. The time required for each plane to make the trip depends on that plane's velocity. Table 13-1 lists the times and velocities for each aircraft.

What simple relationship can we determine from these data? By examining the table, the following conclusions can be made:
- As velocity increases, time decreases.
- As velocity is doubled, time is halved.
- As velocity is quadrupled, time decreases by a factor of four.

This example exhibits the concept of **inverse proportionality**. Velocity (V) is inversely proportional to time (t). Mathematically, that is written as follows:

$$v \propto \frac{1}{t} \text{ or } v = \frac{k}{t}$$

where k is a constant of proportionality. We can also relate two different aircraft's velocities and times as an inverse proportion:

$$v_1{:}v_2 = t_2{:}t_1 \text{ or } \frac{v_1}{v_2} = \frac{t_2}{t_1}$$

Example 2 in the practical examples section demonstrates inverse proportionality while solving for an unknown.

Inverse proportionality is commonly seen in radiation therapy. For example, depth and percentage depth dose are inversely related (as depth increases, percentage depth dose decreases) as are beam energy and penumbra width (as energy increases, the width of the beam's penumbra decreases). Another good example of inverse proportionality is the inverse square law, which states that the intensity of radiation from a point source varies inversely with the square of the distance from the source.

Direct Proportionality

The distance traveled by an aircraft moving at a constant velocity depends on the length of time that the aircraft is aloft. Suppose we consider an aircraft traveling at a constant velocity of 400 miles per hour. The time required for this aircraft to travel 100 miles is 0.25 hour, for 200 miles the time is 0.5 hour, and so forth. Table 13-2 lists several distances and the time required by the aircraft to complete each distance.

Table 13-1	Aircraft velocities and times to complete trip	
Aircraft	**Velocity (miles/hr)**	**Time (hr)**
A	500	2.0
B	400	2.5
C	250	4.0
D	200	5.0
E	125	8.0

Table 13-2	Distance and time values for aircraft	
Distance (miles)		**Time (hr)**
0		0.00
100		0.25
200		0.50
300		0.75
500		1.00

Similar to the inverse proportionality example, conclusions can be reached from the data in this table, as follows:
- As time increases, distance increases.
- As time doubles, distance doubles.
- As time triples, distance triples.

Therefore we say that distance (D) is directly proportional to time (t). Mathematically, that is written as follows:

$$D \propto t \text{ or } D = kt$$

where k is the constant of proportionality. We can also relate two different distances and times as a direct proportion:

$$D_1:D_2 = t_1:t_2$$
$$\text{or } \frac{D_1}{D_2} = \frac{t_1}{t_2}$$

Example 3 in the practical examples section demonstrates direct proportionality while solving for an unknown.

Direct proportionality is also commonly seen in radiation therapy. For example, field size and percentage depth dose are directly proportional (as field size increases, percentage depth dose increases) as are beam energy and tissue air ratio (TAR) or tissue maximum ratio (TMR) (as energy increases, TAR and TMR increase). These relationships assume that all other related factors are constant.

Trigonometric Ratios and the Right Angle Triangle

Calculating angles, such as collimator and gantry angles, and depths and lengths that are related to these angles are common in setups during patient simulation and treatment. In many of these cases, a solution is derived by using the properties of a right triangle. A **right triangle** is a three-sided polygon on which one corner measures 90 degrees. The three most common functions associated with the right triangle are the **sine, cosine,** and **tangent.** Fig. 13-1 diagrams these quantities. There are six quantities that describe a right triangle: the three angles (α, β, and the 90-degree angle) and the three lengths (line segments AB, AC, and BC). The sine, cosine, and tangent of an angle on a right triangle are defined mathematically (using the angle a, for example), as follows:

$$\sin(\alpha) = \frac{\text{opposite}}{\text{hypotenuse}} = \frac{AC}{BC}$$

$$\cos(\alpha) = \frac{\text{adjacent}}{\text{hypotenuse}} = \frac{AB}{BC}$$

$$\tan(\alpha) = \frac{\text{opposite}}{\text{adjacent}} = \frac{AC}{AB}$$

In these equations, **opposite** refers to the length of the side of the right triangle that is opposite the specified angle, **hypotenuse** refers to the length of the longest side of the triangle, and **adjacent** refers to the length of the side of the right triangle that is close, or adjacent, to the specified angle.

To solve for any unknown quantity on a right triangle, only specific combinations of two of the five remaining quantities (excluding the 90-degree angle) must be known. One other characteristic of the right triangle is that the angles all add up to 180 degrees. Expressed mathematically, this is simply: $\alpha + \beta + 90 = 180$. Example 4 in the practical example section illustrates how one can determine unknown quantities in a right triangle.

Sine, cosine, and tangent are the primary trigonometric knowledge required of the radiation therapist and is used frequently for specific clinical functions such as matching the divergences of two abutting treatment fields or measuring the angle or thickness of a chest wall. Values of specific trigonometric functions can be determined either by looking them up in tables or by using a handheld scientific calculator. Because of the simplicity and common use of such calculators, this method for calculating the sine, cosine, or tangent of an angle is used here.[1]

Scientific calculators use the SIN, COS, and TAN keys. To obtain the specific trigonometric value desired, enter the known angle into the calculator in degrees and press the desired trigonometric function key. For example, to find the tangent of 30 degrees, type in the following:

$$\boxed{3} \quad \boxed{0} \quad \boxed{\text{TAN}} \quad \boxed{=}$$

The calculator should display 0.57735. This means that the ratio of the opposite side of the 30-degree angle to the side adjacent to the 30 degrees is 0.57735. It is also possible to

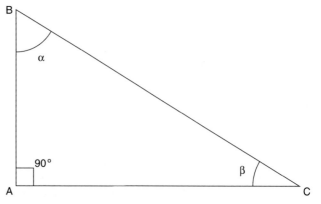

Figure 13-1. A right triangle.

determine the measure of an angle by knowing the ratio between the two sides. If the ratio of the opposite side to the hypotenuse is 0.6, then the angle associated with this ratio can be calculated. Remember that the ratio opposite of hypotenuse defines the sine of the angle. Therefore sin α = 0.6. To calculate the angle, one simply needs the inverse sine of 0.6. This is obtained on most scientific calculators by pressing either the $\boxed{SIN^{-1}}$ button or the $\boxed{INV}$ button followed by the $\boxed{SIN}$ button. For the example, the inverse sine of 0.6 is 36.87 degrees. Therefore α = 36.87 degrees.

Success in understanding trigonometric functions and identities depends, to a large degree, on the clinical application. Trigonometric functions are the most difficult type of mathematical problems for many therapy practitioners. Practice through didactic work or experiencing these problems firsthand can aid the radiation therapist and medical dosimetrist in recognizing these problems and solving them when they occur.

Linear Interpolation

To determine many of the factors that are used often in the practice of radiation therapy, one must be able to find values from tables that contain these needed factors. Field-size dependence factors, TARs, TMRs, percentage-depth doses, and so forth are conveniently listed in easy-to-read tables. For example, a radiation therapist or medical dosimetrist can easily look up the TAR for a 10×10 cm field size at a 10 cm depth. However, the tables only list the factors in incremental values. What happens if the exact depth of calculation and/or field size is not listed in the table or lies between two table values? In this case the radiation therapist or medical dosimetrist can use an approximate evaluation for the intermediate point. The process of calculating unknown values from known values is called **linear interpolation.** Linear interpolation assumes the following[5]:

1. That two particular values are known
2. That the rate of change between the known values is constant
3. That an unknown data point must be found

The rate of change can be assumed as constant between the values typically used when finding the unknown value. To minimize any inherent rate of change and be more precise, it is important to use known values that are close together. In most tables used in radiation therapy dose calculations, algebraic ratios can be employed to assist the radiation therapist and medical dosimetrist in finding the intermediate number. If a desired point is directly between two known points, a simple average of the two factors for the two respective points is all that is required to determine the new value. When the desired point is not directly between the two known points, the new value must be determined by simple ratios. The ratio of the difference between the unknown value and the upper and lower known values equals the ratio of the difference between the desired point and the upper and lower points in the table. In some cases, the number that we need may require a "double-interpolation" where the unknown value is between

known values in two different directions. A TAR may be needed for a field size of 11 cm × 11 cm at a depth of 8.5 cm. In this case, values for the field size and depth needed is not listed in a TAR table and it is necessary to find values for one of the unknowns before the other can be calculated. Example 5 in the practical example section demonstrates how factors are interpolated from a table when the known values lie "above" and "below" the unknown value. Relationships are established between the known values, and these relationships must be maintained through the calculation to arrive at the correct factor.

Working with Exponents

An exponent, or "power," is a shorthand notation that represents the multiplication of a number by itself a given number of times. For example, $4^3 = 4 \times 4 \times 4 = 64$. In this case the superscript 3 represents the **exponent,** and the 4 represents the **base.** The 3 is also said to be the "power." One could verbally express 4^3 as "four raised to the third power." The following simple rules are important to remember when working with exponents:

1. $x^0 = 1$
2. $x^a \times x^b = x^{a+b}$
3. $(x^a)^b = x^{ab}$
4. $(xy)^a = x^a y^a$
5. $\left(\dfrac{x}{y}\right)^a = \dfrac{x^a}{y^a}$
6. $x^{-a} = \left(\dfrac{1}{x^a}\right)$ and $\left(\dfrac{1}{x^{-a}}\right) = x^a$

Scientific notation is a special use of exponents that uses base 10 notation. It is used to represent either very large or very small numbers.[2] Numbers written in scientific notation are written in the following form:

$$n.nnn \times 10^p$$

where n.nnn indicates the first four numerical values of the specified number. The power to which the base of 10 is raised (p) depends on the size of the specified number. For example, 2657.89 can be written in scientific notation as 2.65789×10^3; it can also be written as 26.5789×10^2. However, in the scientific community, placing only one number to the left of the decimal point is the preferred style. Example 6 illustrates the use of exponents.

Significant Figures

All measurements are approximations—no measuring device can give perfect measurements without some experimental uncertainty. In most radiation oncology physics measurements, this uncertainty is typically very small. The number of **significant figures** in a measurement or calculation is simply the number of figures that are known with some degree of reliability. The number 10.2 is said to have 3 significant figures. The number 10.20 is said to have 4 significant figures.

There are several rules for deciding the number of significant figures in a measured quantity:

1. All nonzero digits are significant: 1.234 g has 4 significant figures, 1.2 g has 2 significant figures.
2. Zeroes between nonzero digits are significant: 1002 kg has 4 significant figures, 3.07 ml has 3 significant figures.
3. Zeroes to the left of the first nonzero digits are not significant; such zeroes merely indicate the position of the decimal point: 0.001° C has only 1 significant figure, 0.012 g has 2 significant figures.
4. Zeroes to the right of a decimal point in a number are significant: 0.023 ml has 2 significant figures, 0.200 g has 3 significant figures.[6,7]
5. When a number ends in zeroes that are not to the right of a decimal point, the zeroes are not necessarily significant: 190 miles may be 2 or 3 significant figures, 5,040 centigray may be 3 or 4 significant figures.

The last rule can be made clearer by the use of standard exponential, or scientific, notation. For example, depending on whether 3 or 4 significant figures is correct, we could write 5040 centigray as:

5.04×10^3 centigray (3 significant figures) or
5.040×10^3 centigray (4 significant figures)

When combining measurements with different degrees of accuracy and precision (different number of significant figures), the accuracy of the final answer can be no greater than the least accurate measurement. This principle can be translated into the following rules:

- When measurements are added or subtracted, the answer can contain no more decimal places than the least accurate measurement.
- When measurements are multiplied or divided, the answer can contain no more significant figures than the least accurate measurement.[6,7]

Natural Logarithms and the Exponential Function

A **logarithm** operates as the reverse of exponential notation. Whereas the example 4^3 is considered "four raised to the third power" in exponential notation and equals 64, the logarithm base 4 of 64 equals 3. In mathematical notation the logarithm is written as follows:

$$\log_b(N) = x$$

where b is the base, N is the desired product, and x is the power. In exponential notation, this is written as follows:

$$b^x = N$$

Certain physical processes have been discovered in nature that obey a special type of logarithmic, and thus exponential, behavior. A radioactive substance is said to decay exponentially.[1,3,4,8] This simply means that the physical process that occurs can be described by exponential notation. However, rather than the base being an integer, the base is a special number that was discovered by Euler, a mathematician. This special number is represented by the letter e and is called Euler's constant or the "base of the natural logarithms."

Numerically, e is equal to 2.718272.... Logarithms based on e are called "natural logarithms." Exponential function is the terminology used to describe e raised to a power and is written as follows:

$$e^x = N$$

A special notation is also given to the natural logarithm. The symbol *ln* is shorthand for "(natural) logarithm base e" and can be written as follows:

$$\ln(N) = x$$

These two equations can be combined to yield an important identity:

$$\ln(e^x) = x$$

In other words the natural logarithm and the exponential functions are inverses of each other. The exponential function has a few important properties that can be beneficial to the radiation therapy practitioner:

- If the power (x) is greater than 0 (meaning the power is positive), then the value of e^x is greater than 1.
- If the power is less than 0 (meaning the power is negative), then the value of e^x is a number greater than 0 and less than 1.
- If the power is exactly 0, then the value of e^x is exactly equal to 1.

To summarize:

$$e^x > 1 \text{ if } x > 0$$
$$0 < e^x < 1 \text{ if } x < 0$$
$$e^x = 1 \text{ if } x = 0$$

Example 7 demonstrates how to use the exponential function.

Basic Units

The system of basic units used most commonly in radiation therapy clinics is the metric or International System of Units (SI) system. This system is the world standard for scientific and technical work. The metric system is based on fundamental units of time, distance, mass, and electrical current and several derived units that are combinations of the four fundamental units. In addition, prefixes may be added to the four fundamental units to represent large or small quantities of the fundamental units.[2,3,4,8]

The four fundamental units in the metric system are the second (time), the meter (distance), the kilogram (mass), and the ampere (electrical current). These units are defined internationally by standards kept at a laboratory near Paris, France. However, secondary standards are kept in national laboratories in most countries. In the United States the National Institute of Standards and Technology (NIST) maintains the secondary standards.[2] Commonly used prefixes and their meanings are listed in Table 13-3.

Special units have been defined for the radiologic sciences. The roentgen (r) is the unit of radiation exposure that represents a measure of the amount of ionization created by radiation in the air. A derived unit for exposure is the

Table 13-3	Numerical prefixes used with SI units	
Prefix	**Symbol**	**Multiplier**
pico	p	10^{-12}
nano	n	10^{-9}
micro	m	10^{-6}
milli	m	10^{-3}
centi	c	10^{-2}
deci	d	10^{-1}
kilo	k	10^{3}
mega	M	10^{6}
giga	G	10^{9}

SI, International System of Units.

coulomb/kilogram (C/kg). Thus the relationship between these two quantities is 1 roentgen = 2.58×10^{-4} C/kg.

The accepted unit of absorbed dose is the gray (Gy). Absorbed dose describes the amount of radiation × energy absorbed by a medium. The gray can be expressed in units as joule/kilogram (J/kg). An outdated unit that was replaced by the gray is the rad. A rad is equal to 0.01 gray, or, restated, 100 rads equals 1 gray. Therefore 1 rad equals one **centigray** (cGy).[3]

The accepted unit of energy is the joule (J), which is equal to 1 kilogram-meter^2 per second^2 (1 kgm^2/s^2). A joule of energy is a rather large amount of energy, relative to the energies associated with radiation therapy. Therefore another special "derived" unit is the electron volt (eV). The relationship between the electron volt and the joule is as follows:

$$1 \text{ eV} = 1.602 \times 10^{-19} \text{ J}$$

The kilo-electron volt (keV = 10^3 eV) and the mega-electron volt (MeV = 10 eV) are the most common energy units used in the radiation therapy clinic.[3]

Measurements and Experimental Uncertainty

During the course of a program in radiation therapy a student eventually becomes familiar with certain quantities such as source-to-axis distance (SAD) and source-to-skin distance (SSD) measurements as well as certain units such as absorbed dose (cGy), exposure (roentgen), and activity (millicurie).[2-4,8] Various instruments can be used to measure these and various other quantities. The process of taking a measurement is basically an attempt to determine a value or magnitude of known quantity.

For example, the quantity SSD is a physical measurement of distance. Suppose an SSD of 73.5 cm was measured from the source of radiation to the chest wall of a patient during the treatment simulation process. This indicates that the centimeter was used as a unit of length and that the distance to the skin surface was 73.5 times larger than this unit. Stated differently, a measurement is a comparison of the magnitude

(how large or small) of a quantity to that of an accepted standard. In this measurement and in other measurements such as determining the temperature using a thermometer, the barometric pressure using a barometer, or the exposure rate using an exposure rate meter, an amount of uncertainty is inherent. Therefore the measuring process requires that the person taking the measurement must have the knowledge that this uncertainty exists. Referring to the SSD measurement, the distance of 73.5 cm will contain error that is introduced not only by the measuring device but also by the fact that the patient will most probably be moving as a result of inhalation and exhalation. This inherent or built-in uncertainty in making a measurement is a characteristic of almost all of science. Uncertainties can be grouped into three categories: systematic errors, random errors, and blunders.

Systematic Errors. A systematic error is an error or uncertainty inherent within the measuring device. A systematic error always affects the measurement in the same way: the measurement will either be too large or too small, depending on the device. These errors are commonly obtained, for example, from one or more of the following: human biases such as vision inaccuracies; imperfect techniques that may occur, for example, during experimental setup; and unacceptable instrument calibrations. Stem leakage of an ionization chamber and the inaccuracy of reading an analog temperature meter on an annealing oven are examples of systematic errors.

Random Errors. Random errors, as the name implies, are a result of variations attributed to chance that are unavoidable. Random errors can either increase or decrease the result of a measurement. To correct for this type of error, a common practice is to take several measurements and average them. Random errors can also be reduced by making improvements in the measuring device and/or technique. An uncontrolled rapid change in temperature or barometric pressure, accidental movement of a patient during setup, and electronic noise are all examples of random errors.

Blunders. Blunders during measurement are those errors that occur as a result of human error in algebraic or arithmetic calculations or from improper use of a measuring device. Errors such as these can be avoided by properly educating the individuals who will be making the measurements. They can also be avoided by comparing the measurements being made to previous measurements that are known to be correct or even comparing them to theoretical values. If large discrepancies exist between the correct values and the values that the individual is obtaining, then something must have been done incorrectly, and retracing the setup and procedure can be an easy way to remedy the error.

Accuracy and Precision of Measurements. Another facet of measurements that must be discussed is the importance of and also the difference between the accuracy and precision of a measurement. When measurements are made, the individual must be concerned with how close the measurements are to the "true" value. Although the true value cannot be known exactly, theoretical calculations can define a value that is accepted as a true value. How close a measurement comes to this true value is referred to as accuracy. The precision of a measurement indicates how reproducible a particular measurement is or how consistent the measurement is.

Fig. 13-2 illustrates the difference between accuracy and precision. The bull's eye represents the "true value." The arrows represent measurements. In the first picture the measurements are neither precise nor accurate. The arrows (measurements) did not hit the bull's eye, nor did they land close to each other. In the second picture the arrows were precise but inaccurate. They all hit close to the same location but were not close to the bull's eye. In the third picture the arrows were precise and accurate because they were grouped together close to the bull's eye.

As another example, consider the output measurement of a linear accelerator as performed by three therapists as part of the daily quality assurance program. After setting up the necessary apparatus and following the policy and procedure outline, the following data were gathered. Each therapist made four measurements with the ionization chamber to obtain an average value for the output and thereby eliminate random errors.

	Therapist A	Therapist B	Therapist C
	2.702	2.650	2.738
	2.701	2.660	2.578
	2.702	2.655	2.737
	2.702	2.651	2.579
Average	2.702	2.654	2.657

The accepted value for the output for that accelerator was 2.658. So a number of questions could be asked about the values obtained by the radiation therapists. Which therapist had the most accurate values? Which therapist had the most precise values? Which therapist had the best overall results? The measurements made by Therapist A were more consistent and more precise because values do not differ by more than 0.001 from each other. However, the average results obtained by Therapists B and C were closer to the accepted value. Apparently, Therapists B and C were more accurate than Therapist A, although Therapist A was the most precise. By comparing the individual values that were obtained by Therapists B and C, one can see that Therapist C's values had a large range. Therefore although Therapist C's average value was the closest to the accepted value, it was obtained through imprecise readings. Therefore the values obtained by Therapist B are deemed the most acceptable because they were precise and accurate.

From this example, it is apparent that a measurement can be precise without being accurate and vice versa. Radiation therapy practitioners should be concerned not only with accuracy but also with precision. Discerning between the two is a

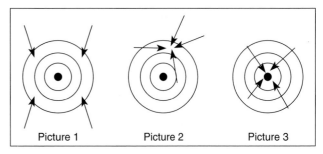

| Picture 1 | Picture 2 | Picture 3 |

Figure 13-2. Representation of the contrast between accuracy and precision. The first picture is neither accurate nor precise. Picture 2 demonstrates precision but not accuracy. Picture 3 illustrates both precision and accuracy.

function of analytical judgment and critical thinking skills, both very important in the practice of radiation therapy.

Experimental Uncertainty. Because it is impossible to eliminate all systematic errors, random errors, and blunders, an absolutely accurate and precise measurement cannot be achieved. Although this seems disheartening to the scientist, there is a method that is accepted by the scientific community to handle this experimental uncertainty. It is common practice to measure the percent relative error in a measurement to discover the degree of accuracy. The percent relative error can be thought of as the percentage of error in a measurement relative to the accepted value. It is calculated by using the following equation:

$$\text{\% Relative certainty} = \left(\frac{\text{Experimental value} - \text{Accepted value}}{\text{Accepted value}} \right) \times 100$$

Look at the measurement result of Therapist A. The percent relative error in that result can be calculated as follows using the previous equation:

$$\text{\% Relative error} = \left(\frac{2.702 - 2.658}{2.658} \right) \times 100 = 1.65\%$$

The percent relative error in the result obtained by Therapist A was +1.65%. This means that the result was 1.65% higher than the accepted value. The percent relative errors in the results obtained by Therapists B and C can be calculated by the reader as 0.15% and 0.04%, respectively. Both of these values were low.

Dimensional Analysis

A technique that can be very useful in radiation therapy (as well as in many other branches of science) is dimensional analysis. **Dimensional analysis** is a process that involves the careful assessment of the units of measurement used in calculating a specific quantity. This technique involves canceling common units that appear in the numerator and denominator of an equation. When one or more quantities are manipulated to obtain a specified quantity, the units of the known quantities when combined must be equivalent to the unit of measurement of that specified quantity. For example, to obtain the specific quantity of velocity, one must divide distance by time. In other words, velocity is measured in meters per second, distance is measured in meters, and time is measured in seconds.[3]

When using an equation, it is important to ensure that all of the units when combined equate to the units desired. There are a few "rules of thumb" that can be used when analyzing the dimensions of an equation. First, any quantity divided by 1 is equal to the quantity itself. Next, any quantity divided by itself is equal to 1. Also, the process of division is equivalent to multiplying the numerator by the inverse of the denominator.[2,3] Using these facts, one can cancel units in any equation until no cancellation possibility remains. The units that remain should be equivalent to the desired units. If this is not true, then an error must have occurred.

PRACTICAL EXAMPLES OF MATHEMATICS IN RADIATION THERAPY

Mathematical theories must be put into practice to really understand the concepts and what it means to radiation therapy practice. Several examples have been used throughout this chapter to help focus the content into useful information. This section of the chapter provides more in-depth analysis of practical application examples of mathematical principles as seen in radiation therapy.

Example 1—algebraic equations: To determine the value of an unknown, it is necessary to use the rules of algebra. For example, if a radiation therapist knows the total dose that a patient is to receive and the dose per fraction, then the number of treatments can be determined. Assume that the total dose is 5000 cGy and the daily dose is 200 cGy. The number of fractions can be determined from the following equation:

$$200 \text{ cGy/fraction} \times N(\text{fractions}) = 5000 \text{ cGy}$$

where N represents the number of fractions. To isolate the unknown (N), the value of 200 can be divided out of both sides of the equation without disturbing the equality:

$$\frac{200 \text{ cGy/fraction}}{200 \text{ cGy/fraction}} \times N = \frac{5000 \text{ cGy}}{200 \text{ cGy/fraction}}$$

The first term in this equation is equal to 1, and any value multiplied by 1 equals that number. Also, because the unit cGy appears in both the numerator and the denominator of the fraction on the right side of the equation, it can be canceled. The resulting equation is thus:

$$N = \frac{5000}{200} \times \frac{1}{1/\text{fraction}}$$

At this point, one other algebraic rule can be applied. Any fraction that appears in the denominator of a fraction can be written as the reciprocal of that fraction. Therefore our final answer becomes the following:

$$N = \frac{5000}{200} \text{ fractions} = 25 \text{ fractions}$$

So the radiation therapist knows that the patient has 25 fractions prescribed.

As already stated, values can be abstracted from both sides of an equation to find an answer. Suppose that a radiation therapist knows that the physician wants to deliver 200 cGy on a particular day and knows that on the previous day the patient received 250 cGy. Therefore the unknown can be determined from the following equation:

$$250 \text{ cGy} - X = 200 \text{ cGy}$$

Obviously, this is a simple problem, but it is used to illustrate a principle. From this point, one can subtract 250 cGy from both sides of the equation, as follows:

$$250 \text{ cGy} - X - 250 \text{ cGy} = 200 \text{ cGy} - 250 \text{ cGy}$$

Subtracting 250 from itself equals 0, and 0 added to any value simply equals that value. Also, one can multiply both sides of an equation by the same value without disturbing the equality. Therefore if both sides of the equation are multiplied by 1, the following results:

$$-X = 200 \text{ cGy} - 250 \text{ cGy} = -50 \text{ cGy}$$
$$(^-1) \times {}^-X = (^-1) \times {}^-50 \text{cGy}$$
$$X = 50 \text{ cGy}$$

So the radiation therapist knows that the daily dose was reduced by 50 cGy.

Example 2—inverse proportionality: A radiation therapist had just learned from a medical physicist that the therapy unit would be running at a dose rate of 400 cGy/min on a given day. The radiation therapist knows that the normal dose rate is 300 cGy/min and wonders how this new dose rate will affect the patient's treatment times. This example illustrates inverse proportionality. If a particular patient's treatments took 1.2 minutes with the normal dose rate of 300 cGy/min, then what would it be with the new dose rate? This can be solved by the following equation:

$$300 \text{ cGy/min} \times 1.2 \text{ min} = 360 \text{ cGy}$$
$$\frac{360 \text{ cGy}}{400 \text{ cGy/min}} = 0.9 \text{ minutes}$$

Therefore as the dose rate increases, the treatment times decrease, which demonstrates the concept of inverse proportionality.

Example 3—direct proportionality: A radiation oncologist wants to increase the dose that a patient receives per fraction but does not want to change the total number of fractions. Assume that, originally, the physician had planned to give 200 cGy per fraction for 25 fractions, then decided that 230 cGy would achieve better results. Initially, the total dose would have been:

$$200 \text{ cGy/fraction} \times 25 \text{ fractions} = 5000 \text{ cGy}$$

But because the dose per fraction was changed to 230 cGy, the total dose would also change:

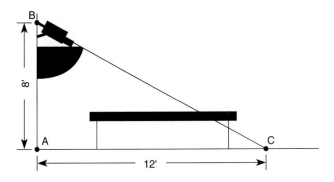

$$230 \text{ cGy/fraction} \times 25 \text{ fractions} = 5750 \text{ cGy}$$

Therefore note that as the dose per fraction increases, the total dose increases. This is an example of direct proportionality.

Example 4—unknown quantities and the right triangle: A medical physicist wants to know at what angle a wall-mounted laser is directed at the floor. Assume that she also wants to know the distance from the laser to its intersection point on the floor. First, she measures the distance from the wall to the intersection point on the floor (segment AC measures 12 ft). Then she measures how far up the wall the laser is mounted (segment AB measures 8 ft).

From the trigonometric identities outlined in the text, the physicist knows that the tangent of the angle is equal to the length of the opposite side divided by the length of the adjacent side. That can be stated in mathematical form as follows:

$$\tan(\beta) = \frac{\text{opposite}}{\text{adjacent}}$$

$$\tan \beta = \frac{\text{Segment AC}}{\text{Segment AB}} = \frac{12 \text{ feet}}{8 \text{ feet}}$$

$$\tan \beta = 1.5$$
$$\beta = \tan^{-1}(1.5)$$
$$\beta = 56°$$

Therefore angle β is equal to 56 degrees. Also, the physicist knows that the sine of β is equal to the length of the opposite side divided by the hypotenuse. This can be written as follows:

$$\sin \beta = \frac{\text{opposite}}{\text{hypotenuse}} = \frac{\text{Segment AC}}{\text{Segment BC}}$$

Because the length of segment BC is desired, the equation can be rewritten and solved for that length:

$$\text{Segment BC} = \frac{\text{Opposite}}{\sin \beta} = \frac{12 \text{ feet}}{\sin(56°)} = \frac{12}{0.829} = 14.5 \text{ feet}$$

Therefore the distance from the laser's position on the beam wall to the point where the beam intersects the floor is 14.5 feet.

Example 5—linear interpolation: A medical dosimetrist wants to determine the output of a cobalt machine for two different field sizes for one specific date from the following output table. The field sizes are 12 cm × 12 cm and 19 cm × 19 cm. The desired date is March 30. Assume that this date is exactly halfway between March 15 and April 15.

Output (cGy/min) for Theratron 780 @ 80 cm in AIR (SAD treatment) 2002 (15th of month)

Field size	Jan 15	Feb 15	Mar 15	Apr 15	May 15
5 cm × 5 cm	210.71	208.41	205.13	203.88	201.66
10 cm × 10 cm	218.58	216.19	213.83	211.50	209.19
12 cm × 12 cm	220.98	218.57	216.18	213.82	211.49
15 cm × 15 cm	224.48	222.03	219.60	217.21	214.83
20 cm × 20 cm	228.19	225.70	223.24	220.80	218.39

Because the 12 × 12 cm field size is listed on the table, the only step required to determine the output for that field size is to determine the intermediate value between the March 15 and April 15 outputs for that field size. The outputs for a 12 × 12 cm field size for March 15 and April 15 are 216.18 and 213.82 cGy/min, respectively. Therefore the output for the 12 × 12 cm field size for March 30 is the simple average of the two outputs:

$$\frac{216.18 + 213.82}{2} = \frac{430.0}{2} = 215.00 \text{ cGy/min}$$

The first step in determining the desired output for the 19 × 19 cm field size is to determine the intermediate values of the output for March 30 for the field sizes nearest to 19 × 19 cm. These would be the 15 × 15 cm and 20 × 20 cm field sizes. The outputs for March 15 and April 15 for the 15 × 15 cm field size are 219.60 and 217.21 cGy/min, respectively, whereas the outputs for March 15 and April 15 for the 20 × 20 cm field size are 223.24 and 220.80 cGy/min, respectively. To determine the intermediate values for March 30 for each field size, the simple averages are calculated and can be shown to be 218.41 cGy/min for the 15 × 15 cm field size and 222.02 cGy/min for the 20 × 20 cm field size. The next step is to determine the ratio of how "far" the 19 × 19 cm field size is from either the smaller or the larger field size. For this example, we will choose the smaller field size. The 19 × 19 cm field size is 4 cm greater than the 15 × 15 cm field size. The difference between the 15 × 15 cm and 20 × 20 cm field sizes is 5 cm. Therefore the 19 × 19 cm field size is four fifths of the "distance" between the two known values, and thus the output for the 19 × 19 cm field size must also be four fifths of the "distance" between the two intermediate outputs that we just determined previously. It should be noted that the direction one would move on the table in going from a 15 cm² field size to a 20 cm² field size will be the same direction one would move on the table to determine the output as well. Now, to calculate the desired output, one must know the distance between the two intermediate values and then multiply that distance by the field size distances ratio. This will give the desired output of 221.30 cGy/min:

$$222.02 \text{ cGy/min} - 214.81 \text{ cGy/min} = 3.61 \text{ cGy}$$
$$3.61 \text{ cGy/min} \times 4/5 = 2.89 \text{ cGy/min}$$
$$218.41 \text{ cGy/min} + 2.89 \text{ cGy/min} = 221.30 \text{ cGy/min}$$

Therefore the output for March 15 for the 19 × 19 cm field size was 221.30 cGy/min.

Example 6—exponents: A brief example of the use of exponents is all that is demonstrated here. The primary use of exponents in the field of radiation therapy is in scientific notation. If one must calculate the product of two numbers that are represented in scientific notation, some of the rules outlined in this chapter can be useful. For example, assume that a radiation physicist desires to determine the total amount of exposure produced by ionizing radiation in a specified mass of air. She knows that 1 roentgen is equal to 2.58×10^{-4} coulombs of charge liberated per kilogram of air present. She measured 3.23×10^{-2} coulombs in 1 kilogram of air mass. Mathematically, this is written:

Exposure (x) =

$$\frac{3.23 \times 10^{-2} \text{ coulombs}}{1 \text{ kilogram of air}} \times \frac{1 \text{ roentgen}}{2.58 \times 10^{-4} \text{ coulombs/1 kg air}}$$

Exposure (x) =

$$\frac{3.23 \times 10^{-2} \text{ coulombs/1 kilogram of air}}{2.58 \times 10^{-4} \text{ coulombs/1 kilogram of air}} \times 1 \text{ roentgen}$$

$$\text{Exposure (x)} = 1.25 \times \frac{10^{-2}}{10^{-4}} \text{ roentgens}$$

If a number with a negative exponent is in the denominator of a fraction, then that is the same as the same number with the equal positive exponent moved to the numerator of the equation:

$$\text{Exposure (x)} = 1.25 \times 10^{-2} \times 10^{4} \text{ roentgens}$$
$$\text{Exposure (x)} = 1.25 \times 10^{(-2+4)} \text{ roentgens}$$
$$\text{Exposure (x)} = 1.25 \times 10^{2} \text{ roentgens} = 125 \text{ roentgens}$$

Example 7—exponential functions: The decay of a radioactive substance behaves in an exponential manner. Therefore if one wishes to calculate the amount of activity of a particular substance that remains after a specific amount of time, the following equation can be used:

$$A_t = A_0 \times e^{-\lambda t}$$

where A_t is the activity after time t, A_0 is the initial activity, and λ is the decay constant that is specific to the particular radioactive substance being used. As an example, assume that the activity of a sample of iridium-131 is known exactly 2 days after it was received from a manufacturer. Assume that we would like to know what the activity was when it arrived. The activity at the present time is 5 curies (Ci). Therefore we know that t = 2 days and A_t = 5 Ci. Also,

the decay constant for iridium-131 is 8.6×10^{-2}/day. So plugging these values into the decay equation gives the following:

$$5 \text{ Ci} = A_0 \times e^{-(8.6 \times 10^{-2}/\text{day}) \times (2 \text{ days})}$$
$$5 \text{ Ci} = A_0 \times e^{-0.172}$$
$$A_0 = 5 \text{ Ci}/e^{-0.172} = \frac{5 \text{ Ci}}{0.842}$$
$$A_0 = 5.94 \text{ Ci}$$

Therefore the activity on arrival 2 days earlier was 5.94 Ci. One can also determine the activity of the substance 2 days after the present date using the same equation. The reader can calculate this independently.

Review Questions

1. $(10^3)^5$ equals
   a. 10^8
   b. 10^2
   c. 10^{15}
   d. 10^{-2}
2. Convert 910,000,000 to scientific notation.
   a. 9.1×10^8
   b. 9.01×10^7
   c. 91.0×10^8
   d. 9×10^7
3. If an instrument positioned 1 m from a point source is moved 50 cm closer to the source, the radiation intensity will be
   a. Increased by a factor of 4
   b. Increased by a factor of 2
   c. Decreased by a factor of 4
   d. Decreased by a factor of 2
4. As the depth in tissue increase, the percentage depth dose values decrease. This is an example of
   a. Inverse proportionality
   b. Direct proportionality
   c. Interpolation
   d. None of the above
5. What is the ratio of 100 cGy to 500 cGy?
   a. 5:1
   b. 1:5
   c. Both a and b
   d. Neither a nor b
6. How many significant figures are there in 780,000,000?
   a. 2
   b. 3
   c. 6
   d. 9
7. How many significant figures are there in 0.0101?
   a. 2
   b. 3
   c. 4
   d. 5

8. Errors that occur as a result of human error in algebraic or arithmetic calculations or from improper use of a measuring device are
   a. Systematic errors
   b. Random errors
   c. Blunders
   d. Precision

9. $\ln(e^x) = x$.
   a. True
   b. False

10. $\frac{10^x}{10^y} = 10^{x+y}$.
    a. True
    b. False

REFERENCES

1. Bernier DR, Christian PE, Langan JK: *Nuclear medicine: technology and techniques,* ed 4, St. Louis, 1997, Mosby
2. Bushong S: *Radiologic science for technologists: physics, biology, and protection,* ed 7, St. Louis, 2001, Mosby.
3. Harris M: *Radiation therapy physics handbook,* The University of Texas MD Anderson Cancer Center, Houston, 1992.
4. Khan FM: *The physics of radiation therapy,* ed 2, Baltimore, 1994, Williams & Wilkins.
5. Linear interpolation: how it works, available at http://www.cs.brown.edu/stc/outrea/greenhouse/nursery/interpolation/itworks.html (accessed October 15, 2001).
6. Significant figures, available at http://learn.chem.vt.edu/tutorials/units/sf.html (accessed October 20, 2001).
7. Significant figures—rules, available at http://chem01.usca.sc.edu/chemistry/genchem/sigfig.htm (accessed October 20, 2001).
8. Stanton R, Stinson D: *Applied physics for radiation oncology,* Madison, Wis, 1996, Medical Physics Publishing.

Introduction to Radiation Therapy Physics

Timothy George Ochran

Outline

Key Terms

Atom
Atomic mass unit
Binding energy per nucleon
Bohr atom model
Bremsstrahlung
Electrical charge
Electron binding energy
Frequency of the wave
Ground state
Half value layer

Mass equivalence
Nuclear binding energy
Nuclear energy level
Nuclear force
Photon
Radioactivity
Rest mass
Wave-particle duality
Wavelength of the wave

Shortly after Roentgen's discovery of x-rays at the University of Wurzberg in Germany, medical applications of x-rays were used worldwide. At that time, x-rays were such a news item that they were discussed in the press. Many physicists began the task of understanding the principles critical to the use and production of x-rays.

Over the past century, great strides have been taken in the area of radiation physics to define the interaction of radiation and matter. Without a basic understanding of this relationship, radiation therapy practitioners would not be able to cure and palliate the multitude of cancer patients treated each year. To that end, this chapter describes the basic principles of radiation therapy physics.

QUANTITIES AND UNITS

Four major quantities that one must know to be versed in radiation physics are as follows: (1) radioactivity, (2) radiation exposure, (3) radiation absorbed dose, and (4) radiation dose equivalent. The original units for each of these quantities can be found in Table 14-1, as well as the new Système Internationale d'Unités (SI units) and conversion factors. These conversion factors compare original units to the SI units that were developed in 1977 to help simplify things worldwide. These quantities are discussed in more detail in following sections.

Units are agreed on standard quantities of measurements such as meters, seconds, and grams. From these fundamental units we can derive the units such as meters per second or

Table 14-1	Radiation activity, exposure, and dose units of measurement		
Measured Property	**Old Unit**	**New SI Unit**	**Conversion Factor**
Radioactivity	curie (Ci) = 3.73×10^{10} dps	becquerel (Bq) = 1 dps	1 Ci = 3.7×10^{10} Bq 1 Bq = 2.7×10^{-11} Ci
Radiation exposure	roentgen (R) = 2.58×10^{-4} C/kg	coulomb/kg (C/kg)	1 R = 2.58×10^{-4} C/kg 1 C/kg = 3.88×10^{3} R
Radiation absorbed dose	rad = 100 erg/g	gray (Gy) = 1 J/kg	1 rad = 0.01 Gy 1 Gy = 100 rad
Radiation dose equivalent	rem = QF × rad	sievert (Sv) = QF × Gy	1 rem = 0.01 Sv Sv = 100 rem

From Bernier DR, Christian PE, Langan JK, editors: *Nuclear medicine: technology and techniques,* ed 3, St. Louis, 1994, Mosby.
QF, quality factor.

even 1 erg (1 g × cm^2/sec^2). There are two different measurement systems: (1) the foot-pound-second and (2) the meter-kilogram-second systems.[1]

It is often necessary to convert between various systems and magnitudes of units:

1. How many minutes are in 2 hours and 14 minutes?

$$2 \text{ hours} \times \frac{60 \text{ minutes}}{1 \text{ hour}} + 14 \text{ min} = 134 \text{ min}$$

2. How many meters are in 5.5 miles?

$$5.5 \text{ miles} \times \frac{5280 \text{ feet}}{1 \text{ mile}} \times \frac{12 \text{ inches}}{1 \text{ foot}} \times \frac{2.54 \text{ cm}}{1 \text{ inch}} \times \frac{1 \text{ meter}}{100 \text{ cm}} = 8851.4 \text{ m}$$

The "trick" is to always multiply by 1. Throughout this chapter and this text you will find the opportunity to convert many types of units.

ATOMIC PHYSICS

Subatomic Particles

The smallest unit of an element that retains the properties of that element is known as an **atom.** Atoms are made up of smaller units called subatomic particles.[1-3] There are many types of subatomic particles that have been discovered or postulated. J.J. Thomson postulated in 1897 that the atom must consist of a tiny cloud of positive charge, with the electrons floating in it.[2] Lenard in 1903 proposed that atoms were made up of "clumps" of positive charge, electrons floating around them, and a relatively large empty space between them. Twentieth-century physicists working with "atom smashers" have been able to break the atom not only into its component parts but also into smaller units, thus discovering the six quarks.

Radiation therapy physics deals with the most basic of the subatomic particles: electrons, neutrons, and protons. Rest mass and electrical charge are the properties of these particles with which we will be concerned. The **rest mass** refers to the mass (weight) of the particle when it is not moving.

Einstein's theory of special relativity states that subatomic particles moving at high speeds will have increased mass. At this point we will not need to concern ourselves with this theory, other than to know of it.

The mass of subatomic particles can be measured in terms of the standard metric system mass unit, the kilogram. For those more familiar with U.S. units of measure, 1 kg is equivalent to about 2.2 lb. Because of the very small masses of these particles, expressing them in kilograms would make these values very cumbersome to handle; therefore a quantity called the atomic mass unit (amu) was defined. The **atomic mass unit** is defined such that the mass of an atom of carbon 12 is exactly 12.000 amu. From this it was determined that the following is true:

$$1 \text{ amu} = 1.66 \times 10^{-27} \text{ kg}$$

This relationship can be used to convert from one mass unit to another.[2]

The mass of a proton is equal to 1.00727 amu. Express this mass in terms of kilograms.

$$(1.00727 \text{ amu}) \times \frac{(1.66 \times 10^{-27} \text{ kg})}{(1 \text{ amu})} = 1.672 \times 10^{-27} \text{ kg}$$

The **electrical charge** is a measure of how strongly the particle is attracted to an electrical field and can be either positive or negative. A positively charged particle is attracted to a negative electrical field, and a negatively charged particle is attracted to a positive electrical field. The electron and the proton have the same amount of electrical charge, 1.6×10^{-19} coulombs (the coulomb is the metric unit of electrical charge), but they differ in that the electron's charge is negative and the proton's is positive. The neutron, as the name implies, carries no electrical charge.

The Bohr Atom

In 1913 Neils Bohr attempted to explain the spectral phenomena of atoms by combining Rutherford's atomic model with the newly postulated quantum theories of Einstein and

Planck. This model, known as the Bohr atom, has since been replaced with complex quantum mechanical models of the atom; however, it is still an excellent way to derive a mental picture of the atom's structure. The **Bohr atom model** stated that the electrons surrounding the nucleus existed only in certain energy states or orbits.[1,4] It further stated that when an electron moved from one orbit to another it needed to gain or lose energy. The lost energy was seen as the spectra that had been observed when atoms were excited by adding energy to them.

The Bohr atom seen in Fig. 14-1 consists of a central core, called the nucleus, and the electron cloud or orbits. The nucleus consists of protons and neutrons tightly bound together by a force known as the strong nuclear force. This force is strong enough at the extremely small distances found within the nucleus that it can hold together the positive charged protons that are trying to repel each other. Outside the nucleus the strong nuclear force quickly becomes ineffective. The number of protons and neutrons within the nucleus defines the physical and chemical properties of the atom. Elements are substances made up entirely of atoms of a single kind. Some familiar substances that are elements include oxygen, carbon, helium, aluminum, and cobalt. All other substances are called compounds and are made up of various combinations of elements. As previously stated, each element contains a unique number of protons in its nucleus: carbon has six, oxygen has eight, and so forth. If a nucleus gains or loses protons, its elemental identity changes. For example, if a carbon atom gains a proton, it becomes an atom of nitrogen (which has seven protons). The number of protons in the nucleus is known as the atomic number of the atom.

Atomic Nomenclature

The symbolism used to identify an atom (X), its atomic number (Z), and atomic mass number (A) is as follows:

$$^A_Z X$$

The periodic table in Fig. 14-2 is a listing of the elements and their symbols.

Nuclear Stability and Isotopes

The total amount of energy that it takes to hold a nucleus together is called the **nuclear binding energy** and is measured in MeV (10^6 electron volts). To compare the binding energy of one atom to another, one must calculate the binding energy per nucleon. The **binding energy per nucleon** is the binding energy divided by the atomic mass number. It should be noted that a peak at an atomic mass number of about 56 represents the most stable state of iron (Fe). A nucleus can have more energy than is required for stability; to illustrate this, one can think of a staircase. The bottom step represents the binding energy of the atom and is called the ground state. The **ground state** is the minimum amount of energy needed to keep the atom together. Higher and higher

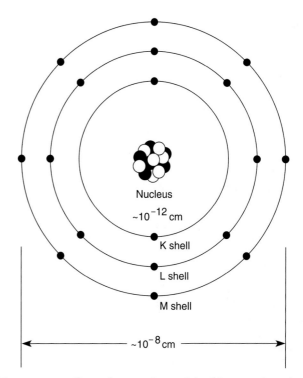

Figure 14-1. The Bohr atomic model with central nucleus surrounded by the electron orbits. *(From Bernier DR, Christian PE, Langan JK, editors: Nuclear medicine: technology and techniques, ed 3, St. Louis, 1994, Mosby.)*

steps of the staircase represent higher and higher energy states of the atom. As in a staircase, the steps have finite levels. The energy levels of an atom do not have transition zones between the steps, so the atom's energy level must be one step or the other, not between. Each of the higher steps is called a **nuclear energy level.** Unstable atoms are those that are not at their ground state. An atom at an energy level different from its ground state tends to try to lose the energy and return to its ground state. This can be achieved in a number of ways, including radioactivity. **Radioactivity** in this case is the emission of energy in the form of electromagnetic (EM) radiation or energetic particles.[4] As you can see, any element can have different nuclear configurations. Atoms with the same atomic number but different atomic mass numbers are called isotopes of that atom.[2,4] Other nuclear configurations, related to the various combinations of atomic number and number of neutrons, are summarized in Table 14-2. An easy way to remember this table is to recall the next to last letter of the configuration—isoto**p**e, isoba**r**, isoto**n**e, and isom**e**r—which tells the value that remains constant (one must assume that e stands for everything). For example, when looking at isotopes, the Z, or atomic number, remains the same. When compared, the number of protons that define the element remains constant. In that case the p (second from the end) becomes a quick reminder. The same is true for the others as well.

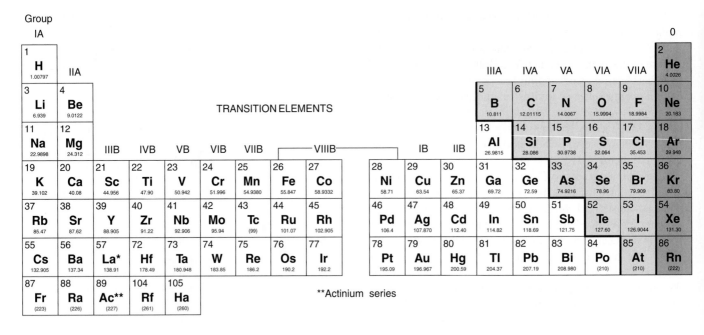

Figure 14-2. Periodic table of elements. *(From Bernier DR, Christian PE, Langan JK, editors: Nuclear medicine: technology and techniques, ed 3, St. Louis, 1994, Mosby.)*

Table 14-2	Nuclear configurations		
Name	**Z**	**A**	**N**
Isotope	Same	Different	Different
Isobar	Different	Same	Different
Isotone	Different	Different	Same
Isomer	Same	Same	Same

A, Atomic mass number; *N*, number of neutrons; *Z*, atomic number.

Atomic Energy Levels

The Bohr atom's other major component, in addition to the nucleus, consists of the electron orbits or shells that surround it. These are not actually orbits, but this term provides a way to imagine the atom. The **electron binding energy** is the amount of energy required to remove that electron from the atom. The binding energy is different for each shell and depends on the makeup of the nucleus. The larger the number of positive charges in the nucleus, the greater the attraction of the electrons toward it, and thus the higher the binding energy.

The electron binding energy has a negative value and is usually measured in kiloelectron volts. It represents the amount of energy that must be added to the electron's total energy before the electron can begin to move away from the atom.

As previously seen in Fig. 14-1, electron shells are numbered and given letter names that represent, in increasing order, their distance from the nucleus. The maximum number of electrons in any shell is determined by the formula $2n^2$, where n is the shell number. As the atomic number increases, the number of electrons needed to keep the atom electrically neutral also increases. The rules by which the electrons fill the shells are as follows:

1. No shell can contain more than its maximum number of electrons.
2. The outermost shell can contain no more than eight electrons.

Describe the electron shell configuration of an atom of stable nitrogen (Z = 7).

The first two electrons will fill the K shell. The five remaining electrons will fill five of the eight electron positions in the L shell.

What is the electron configuration of an atom of electrically neutral cobalt (Z = 27)?

The K and L shells contain 10 electrons. The remaining 17 electrons would be spread between the M and N shells, even though the M shell can hold 18 electrons. This results from the second rule, which states that only 8 electrons can be in the outermost shell. Predicting the exact configuration of the electrons will involve using chemical principles, which we are not concerned with here. The important fact is that the electrons will be in four shells.

Nuclear Forces

To hold a nucleus together, a force must be present. This force must be strong enough to overcome the electrostatic force that is attempting to break up the nucleus. This particular binding force is called the nuclear force. The **nuclear force** comes into play only over very short distances ($\sim10^{-14}$ m). The nature of this force and others within the nucleus to hold it together is complex. This is not discussed in detail here, but the major force that holds the nucleus of an atom together is the nuclear force.

Nuclear Energy Levels

The nucleus possess energy levels similar to the atomic energy levels. The nucleus attempts to remain at a stable or ground state, that is, if the nucleus absorbs energy through rising energy level to an excited state, it will attempt to return to the stable state by giving up the excess energy. This process is discussed later.

Particle Radiation

In 1925 deBroglie hypothesized that photons (EM wave) sometimes act as particles. They exhibit momentum, and particles exhibit wavelike properties. This is important to the definition of particle radiation, because it is the propagated energy that has a definite rest mass, definite momentum (within limits), and a position at any time. This hypothesis is discussed in more detail later.

ELECTROMAGNETIC RADIATION

Radiation is defined as energy that is emitted by an atom and travels through space. This energy can take the form of EM radiation or can be transferred to subatomic particles such as electrons and cause the particles to move away from the atom. This section covers the phenomenon of EM radiation.

Photons

A **photon** is any "packet" of energy traveling through space at the speed of light, 3×10^8 m/sec (in a vacuum). Although a photon can be envisioned as a particle, it has no mass of its own nor does it have an electrical charge. It has only its energy, which is a fixed quantity for that particular photon. Thus high-energy photons can pass through miles of dense material unscathed, because they have no mass to "bump" into atoms with and no electrical charges to attract or repel other particles that might interfere with their travels.

The nature of photons puzzled physicists until early in the twentieth century, when a new branch of physics called quantum mechanics burst into prominence. This field of study was an attempt to explain atomic and nuclear phenomena on their own level rather than trying to make the physics of these extremely small and special bits of matter correspond to the physics of large objects like automobiles or planets. One of the discoveries of the new science was that photons can be viewed in one of two ways, depending on the situation: either as massless particles, as described previously, or, alternatively, as waves, like the movements of a violin string or the human voice. Photons are a special case of a type of wave called an EM wave, which consists of an electrical field and a magnetic field traveling through space at right angles

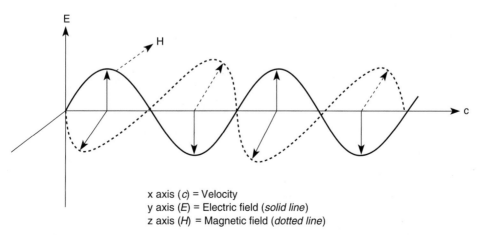

x axis (*c*) = Velocity
y axis (*E*) = Electric field (*solid line*)
z axis (*H*) = Magnetic field (*dotted line*)

Figure 14-3. Electromagnetic wave component energy fields. *(From Bernier DR, Christian PE, Langan JK, editors: Nuclear medicine: technology and techniques, ed 3, St. Louis, 1994, Mosby.)*

to each other (see Fig. 14-3).[1] Thus photons exhibit the characteristics of a particle at times and the characteristics of a wave at other times. This phenomenon is known as **wave-particle duality.** Both of these manifestations of the photon and how they can be related to each other in a single equation are discussed in the following sections.

Physical Characteristics of an EM Wave

An EM wave has three major distinguishing physical characteristics, which are closely interrelated. They are as follows:

1. The **frequency of the wave,** which is represented by the Greek letter nu (υ), is the number of times that the wave oscillates per second and is measured in units of waves per second. Because the term "waves" is not really a unit, but simply a number, the unit for frequency is 1/sec, called the hertz (Hz).
2. The **wavelength of the wave** is the physical distance between peaks of the wave. Wavelength is represented by the Greek letter lambda (λ) and is measured in meters (m). Usually the waves that we will be working with have wavelengths of about one billionth of a meter, so, to avoid having to constantly write very small numbers, we will express wavelengths in terms of the nanometer (nm), which is equal to 10^{-9} meters. Another unit of wavelength seen frequently is the angstrom (Å), equal to 10^{-10} m, or 0.1 nm.
3. The final important wave characteristic is the velocity of the wave as it travels through space. For our purposes, we will assume that all EM waves travel at the same speed, which is the speed of light in a vacuum, represented by the letter c and equal to 3×10^8 m/sec.

The relationship between these three quantities is as follows:

$$c = \upsilon\lambda$$

Note that if you rearrange the variables, there are two other forms of this equation:

$$\upsilon = \frac{c}{\lambda}$$

$$\lambda = \frac{c}{\upsilon}$$

Looking closely at these equations, you can see that the frequency υ and wavelength λ of an EM wave are inversely related. As one gets larger, the other gets smaller. Table 14-3 lists some of the frequencies and wavelengths present in the range of known EM waves.

Calculate the wavelength of an EM wave that has a frequency of 4.5×10^{14} Hz.

To calculate wavelength from frequency, we can use the equation $\lambda = \frac{c}{\upsilon}$:

$$\lambda = \frac{c}{\upsilon} = \frac{3 \times 10^8 \text{ m/s}}{4.5 \times 10^{14} \text{ Hz}} = 6.67 \times 10^{-7} \text{ m}$$

This answer could also be expressed in nanometers and angstroms:

$$(6.67 \times 10^{-7} \text{ m}) (1 \text{ nm}/10^{-9} \text{ m}) = 667 \text{ nm, or } 6670 \text{ Å}$$

An FM radio station broadcasts at a wavelength of 3.125 m.

At what frequency will you find this station on your radio dial?

$$\upsilon = \frac{c}{\lambda} = \frac{3 \times 10^8 \text{ m/s}}{3.125 \text{ m}} = 96,000,000 \text{ Hz, or } 96 \times 10^6 \text{ Hz}$$

This station broadcasts at 96 megahertz (MHz).

Photon Energy

As stated previously, the energy of a photon is its major characteristic, especially from the viewpoint of radiation therapy physics. Fortunately, there are ways to calculate the energy of the wave when its other properties are known. The energy can, for example, be calculated when the frequency (ν) of the wave is known, using the following equation:

$$E = h\upsilon$$

where *E* is the energy of the wave, and *h* is a constant called Planck's constant, which has the value 6.626×10^{-34} J·s; this is equivalent to 4.15×10^{-15} eV·s. Either value can be used, depending on whether you want the resultant energy in joules (J) or electron volts.

A joule (J) is the metric system, or SI, unit of energy and is equivalent to 1 kg m^2/sec^2. This unit is typically used for applications involving "real world" objects, such as billiard balls, cans of light beer, and space shuttles. However, the energies of EM waves are usually much smaller than the energies involved in these situations (with the possible exception of light beer), so another smaller unit is used. This unit is the electron volt and represents the amount of energy that one electron would pick up as it passed through an electrical field whose potential difference was 1 V. This unit will be the standard unit for photon energy in this text and is related to the joule as follows:

$$1 \text{ eV} = 1.6 \times 10^{-19} \text{ J, or } 1 \text{ J} = 6.25 \times 10^{18} \text{ eV}$$

If an EM wave has a frequency of 1.8×10^{20} Hz, what are its wavelength and energy (in eV)?

$$\lambda = \frac{c}{\upsilon} = \frac{3 \times 10^8 \text{ m/s}}{1.8 \times 10^{20} \text{ Hz}} = 1.667 \times 10^{-12} \text{ m}$$

Table 14-3	The electromagnetic spectrum	
Radiation	**Average λ (m)**	**Average ν (Hz)**
Gamma rays	10^{-12}	10^{20}
Ultraviolet light	10^{-8}	10^{17}
Visible light	10^{-6}	10^{14}
Infrared light	10^{-5}	10^{13}
Microwaves	10^{-2}	10^{10}
Radio and television	10^{2}	10^{6}

From Bernier DR, Christian PE, Langan JK, editors: *Nuclear medicine: technology and techniques,* ed 3, St. Louis, 1994, Mosby.

$$E = h\nu = (4.15 \times 10^{-15} \text{ eV} \cdot \text{s}) (1.8 \times 10^{20} \text{ Hz})$$
$$= 747,000 \text{ eV} = 0.747 \text{ MeV}$$

The photon emitted from the decay of the radioisotope ^{99m}Tc has an energy of about 142 keV. What are the frequency and wavelength of this photon?

Because we know that E = 142 keV = 142,000 eV, we can find ν by the following:

$$\upsilon = \frac{E}{h} = \frac{142,000 \text{ eV}}{4.15 \times 10^{-15} \text{ eVs}} = 3.422 \times 10^{19} \text{ Hz}$$

Now λ can be found:

$$\lambda = \frac{c}{\upsilon} = \frac{3 \times 10^8 \text{ m/s}}{3.422 \times 10^{-19} \text{ Hz}} = 8.77 \times 10^{-12} \text{ m}$$

Another interesting fact about photons can be discovered using Einstein's theories of relativity, in which he postulated the famous equation for relating the mass of any object to the amount of energy that it can be converted into:

$$E = mc^2$$

where *E* is the energy, *m* is the mass of the object, and *c* is the speed of light. Note that, because c^2 has units of m^2/sec^2, it is necessary to express the mass of the object in kilograms so that we obtain an answer in joules whenever using this equation.

This equation gave the first indication to the scientific world that matter and energy are really different aspects of the same thing and that one can be directly converted into the other. This discovery has drastically changed the world in which we live by increasing our understanding of the universe and giving us the ability to harness the power of the stars in nuclear fusion reactions, which convert a small amount of matter directly into a huge amount of energy. Unfortunately, the only current use of this knowledge in any viable sense is the stockpile of "hydrogen bombs" present in our defense arsenals.

If you set this equation for E equal to the Planck equation and solve, you find that:

$$m = \frac{h\upsilon}{c^2}$$

With this equation, it is possible to calculate the **mass equivalence** of a photon. Although the photon has no actual mass, the equation allows one to treat the photon as if it actually had mass of its own—the more energy, the greater the mass equivalence. Thus the previous equation neatly combines the particle and wave natures of the photon into a single, tidy equation.

Calculate the mass equivalence of a photon of green light, with a nominal wavelength of 520 nm.

First, calculate the energy of this wave, letting $\upsilon = \frac{c}{\lambda}$

$$E = \frac{hc}{\lambda} = \frac{(6.626 \times 10^{-34} \text{ Js})(3 \times 10^8 \text{ m/s})}{520 \times 10^{-9} \text{ m}} = 3.823 \times 10^{-19} \text{ J}$$

Notice that to keep the units consistent, we have used the

value for Planck's constant that includes joules, so that the SI unit of meters present in the photon wavelength will cancel out. Having found the energy, we can now calculate the mass equivalence by solving Einstein's equation for the mass:

$$m = \frac{E}{c^2} = \frac{(3.823 \times 10^{-19} \text{ J})}{3 \times 10^8 \text{ m/s}} = 4.248 \times 10^{-36} \text{ kg}$$

RADIOACTIVITY

Unstable atomic nuclei tend to seek their ground state, meaning that they tend to give off their excess energy until they reach a point at which the energy in the nucleus is just enough to maintain nuclear stability. The process by which they lose this energy is called radioactivity. Radioactivity may involve the emission of particles, EM radiation (photons), or a combination of the two. This section discusses the processes by which atoms rid themselves of this excess nuclear energy, and the mathematical methods used to describe them.

The Nuclear Stability Curve

The nuclear stability curve is shown in Fig. 14-4. The vertical axis represents the atomic number (Z) of the atom, that is, the number of protons in the nucleus. The horizontal axis represents the number of neutrons (N) in the nucleus. The solid line represents the condition $N/Z = 1$, that is, atoms with the same number of neutrons and protons in the nucleus. The curved line shows the "line of stability"; atoms whose proton/neutron combinations place them on this line are stable and will not undergo radioactive decay, because they have no excess energy. The two curves are coincident at low values of Z, for example, Z less than 20, indicating that these atoms have identical numbers of protons and neutrons. As Z increases, however, the curve begins to diverge from the "ideal" line, curving to the right. This indicates that, as the number of protons grows larger, more neutrons than protons are required to maintain stability and the required neutron/proton ratio increases as Z increases. Atoms that do not meet this criterion appear at other positions on the graph, away from the stability curve; these represent unstable atoms. As these atoms lose energy, they will move closer to the stability curve, finally reaching a stable state.

You may recall that the combinations called isotope, isobar, and isotone refer to different arrangements of nuclear particles. Similarly, the terms isotopic, isobaric, and isotonic refer to types of transformations that change the atom to an isotope, isobar, or isotone of itself. For example, an isotopic transition is one in which the Z of the atom remains constant, but the atomic mass number (A) increases or decreases. Similarly, during an isobaric transition the A of the atom remains the same, and the Z and N change appropriately; during an isotonic transition, the N remains constant and Z (and therefore A) changes. By undergoing as many of these transitions as necessary, atoms can move from an unstable to a stable state.

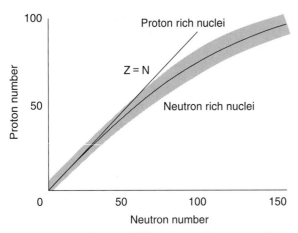

Figure 14-4. Nuclear stability curve. *(From Bernier DR, Christian PE, Langan JK, editors: Nuclear medicine: technology and techniques, ed 3, St. Louis, 1994, Mosby.)*

Types of Radioactive Decay

Alpha decay. An alpha particle, symbolized by the Greek letter a, consists of two neutrons and two protons bound together; this is equivalent to a helium atom (Z = 2) that has been stripped of its two electrons.[1-4] Large, unstable atoms that have a large amount of excess energy tend to undergo radioactive decay by the emission of a particles, which eliminates four nuclear particles and therefore a substantial amount (in nuclear terms) of excess energy. The equation for a decay is as follows:

$$_Z^A X \rightarrow _{Z-2}^{A-4} Y + _2^4 \alpha + Q$$

where Q represents the excess energy shed by the nucleus. This energy frequently appears in the form of photons, which, because of their nuclear origin, are called gamma rays (γ-rays).

Examine this equation carefully. "Reading" it, it says that a nucleus X with a known A and Z decays to a new atom with atomic mass number A-4 and atomic number Z-2; the two missing protons and two missing neutrons appear as an a particle emitted from the nucleus. In addition, a certain amount of energy is given off, either in the form of kinetic energy (i.e., speed of the a particle) or as γ-rays or, more commonly, as a combination of the two. A key feature of this equation is that the numbers of protons, neutrons, and electrical charges on both sides of the arrow are equal. This is a critical feature of all radioactive decay equations: the two sides of the arrow must balance exactly in terms of number of particles, electrical charges, and energy. The most important thing to note, however, is that the original atom has now changed into a new element by the loss of two nuclear protons.

An atom of uranium, $_{92}^{238}U$, undergoes a decay. What is the result?

$$_{92}^{238}U \rightarrow _{90}^{234}Th + _2^4\alpha + \gamma$$

The atom of uranium has been transformed into an atom of thorium.

Alpha decay occurs when the $^N/_Z$ ratio is too low, that is, when the atom falls "underneath" the stability curve on the $^N/_Z$ graph. By eliminating two neutrons and two protons, plus the associated energy, this transition increases the $^N/_Z$ ratio, attempting to correct for the too low $^N/_Z$ ratio that existed before the transition.

The energies of the α particles emitted by a given isotope are fixed and discrete. Even though an isotope may emit more than one α particle energy as the atoms in the sample decay, each α will have one of a selection of fixed energies. This contrasts with β decay, described in the next two sections, in which essentially infinite numbers of particle energies are possible.

Beta-minus decay. Recall that a beta minus (β^-) particle is the same as an electron, the difference in name arising because of the difference in place of origin. An electron is found orbiting in the electron shells, whereas a β^- particle is emitted as the result of a nuclear decay. To understand β^- decay, think of a neutron as a "mixture" of a proton plus an electron:

$$n^\circ \rightarrow p^+ + e^-$$

What essentially happens during a β^- decay is that a neutron in the nucleus "decays" into a proton plus an electron, as shown. The proton remains in the nucleus, and the electron is ejected and leaves the atom; this ejected electron is called the β^- particle. The equation for β^- decay is as follows:

$$_Z^A X \rightarrow _{Z+1}^A Y + _{-1}^0 \beta + \upsilon$$

where the symbol υ stands for the emission of a tiny particle called the antineutrino. This particle carries away the energy that is left over when the β^- does not carry away all of the atom's excess energy. You can see that when undergoing β^- decay, the atom increases its Z by one, while maintaining the same A (having lost a neutron but gained a proton), making this an isobaric transition. Because of this property the ratio of this atom will decrease. (The β^- particle has an "atomic number" of $^-1$, representing its electrical charge relative to the proton.) Usually the daughter nucleus of a β^- decay is itself radioactive and can undergo radioactive decay in many ways, typically by giving off its excess energy as γ-rays. In fact, there are very few isotopes that emit only β^- particles; the majority are accompanied by γ-ray emission from the daughter nucleus.[1-4]

Cobalt-60 decays by β^- decay to an excited state of ^{60}Ni, which then decays by the emission of two high-energy γ-rays as follows:

$$_{27}^{60}Co \rightarrow _{28}^{60}Ni + _{-1}^0\beta + \upsilon \rightarrow _{28}^{60}Ni + 2\gamma$$

Beta-emitting isotopes do not give off β particles of fixed energy as do a emitters. Instead the emitted β^- particles possess energies between 0 and a given maximum (E_{max}), creating what is called a beta spectrum (see Fig. 14-5). The

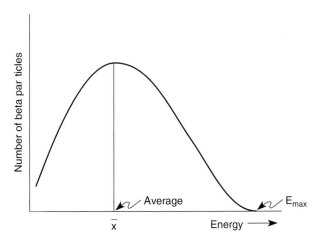

Figure 14-5. Beta particle energy spectrum. *(From Bernier DR, Christian PE, Langan JK, editors: Nuclear medicine: technology and techniques, ed 3, St. Louis, 1994, Mosby.)*

average energy of the beta particle in the spectrum is about one third of E_{max}. The extra energy between E_{max} and the actual energy of the β^- particle is carried away by the antineutrino (υ).

Beta-plus decay. There is a subatomic particle that has exactly the same characteristics as an electron, except that it possesses a positive electrical charge rather than a negative charge. This particle is called a positron and has the symbol β^+. Also, like an electron, it can be ejected from an atomic nucleus; in this case, a nuclear proton decays into a neutron and a positron:

$$p^+ \rightarrow n^0 + \beta^+$$

So the equation for β^+ decay is:

$$^A_Z X \rightarrow ^{\ A}_{Z-1} Y + ^{\ 0}_{+1}\beta + \upsilon$$

Because of the loss of a proton but the gain of a neutron, the atom retains the same A but the Z of the atoms decreases and the $^N/_Z$ ratio of the atom increases, making this an isobaric transition.[1]

Sodium-22 ($^{22}_{11}Na$) is a common radioactive isotope of natural sodium. It decays by β^+ decay to a stable isotope of the gas neon, with the emission of a β^+ particle and a γ-ray, as follows:

$$^{22}_{11}Na \rightarrow ^{22}_{10}Ne^* + ^{\ 0}_{+1}\beta \rightarrow ^{22}_{10}Ne + \gamma$$

As with β^+ decay, a spectrum of energies is emitted, with an average energy of one-third E_{max}; the remainder of the energy is carried off by the neutrino (υ), as in β^- decay.

Electron capture. Although the Bohr model of the atom depicts the electrons as being in fixed orbits outside of the nucleus, the discoveries of quantum mechanics tell us that it is possible that the electrons may, at some time, come very close to the nucleus. An electron that strays too close to the

nucleus may be captured and combined with a proton, reversing the process for β^- decay:

$$p^+ + e^- \rightarrow n^0 + \upsilon$$

This process is known as electron capture and has the same result as β^+ decay; in other words, the Z of the parent nucleus decreases by 1, and the $^N/_Z$—ratio of the atom increases.

Because of the proximity of the K shell to the nucleus, it is most likely that the captured electron will be taken from this shell, although it is possible to capture an electron from the L or M shells. When an electron is taken from one of the electron shells, it leaves a "hole" in the shell; this will place the atom in an unstable configuration in terms of energy, because an inner shell electron has lower energy than an electron from an outer shell. As a result, one of the electrons from an outer shell will "fall" toward the nucleus, moving from a higher energy state to a lower one, and this excess energy, no longer needed to maintain stability, will be given off in the form of an x-ray. This type of radiation is called characteristic radiation and is an important part of many radioactive decay schemes and radiation/matter interactions.

Isomeric transition. An isomer is an atom whose Z and A are identical to another atom's but is currently in what is called a metastable state. This represents a daughter product of some other kind of decay that is itself in an excited state, but, instead of instantly decaying by γ emission (see the example for β^- decay), it remains in this excited state for a given period of time and then decays. Such a nucleus is represented by a small "m" next to its atomic mass number, as in ^{99m}Tc. A nucleus that has no metastable state but decays instantly has a star to the right of its chemical symbol (^{60}Ni*). Metastable isotopes, or isomers, usually decay by emitting the excess energy as a γ-ray.

^{99m}Tc is an isotope used daily in nuclear medicine procedures. It is a daughter product of ^{99}Mo, and the decay equation looks like this:

$$^{99}_{42}Mo \rightarrow ^{99m}_{43}Tc^* + ^{\ 0}_{-1}\beta + \upsilon \rightarrow ^{99}_{43}Tc + \gamma$$

Specification of Radioactivity

To quantify the amount of radioactivity present in a given sample, in the early twentieth century the curie was defined as the activity of 1 g of ^{226}Ra, the most well-known isotope in use at that time. Unfortunately, as measurement techniques improved, disputes arose as to exactly what the activity of 1 g of ^{226}Ra meant in terms of the number of radioactive atoms present. So eventually the unit of radioactivity, the curie, was defined as follows:

$$1 \text{ Ci} = 3.7 \times 10^{10} \text{ dis/sec}$$

where dis/sec stands for nuclear disintegrations per second, that is, the number of atoms that undergo some kind of radioactive decay every second. Because disintegrations is not really a unit but merely a quantity, the curie is numerically equal to 1/s or s^{-1}. In fact, the new proposed unit of radioactivity, the becquerel (Bq), is equal to 1 dis/sec; this unit, however, is rarely used because of the large number of dis/sec present in even a small sample of radioactive material.

For various amounts of radioactive material, multiples of the curie such as the millicurie (mCi, 10^{-3} Ci) and the microcurie (μCi, 10^{-6} Ci) are used. A typical nuclear medicine procedure employs amounts of radioactivity in the range of hundreds of millicuries, whereas a cobalt teletherapy machine uses a source of ^{60}Co of an activity in the range of 5000 to 6000 Ci.

Exponential decay of radioactivity. The amount of radioactivity present in a given sample is never a constant quantity but rather is being reduced continuously by the decay of the radioactive atoms in the sample.[2,4] This decay process follows a mathematical pattern known as exponential behavior. Any value that increases or decreases exponentially will double or halve its value within a certain amount of time; when that time interval passes again, the value will have further reduced by half or increased by two times. Although it is impossible to say exactly which atoms in a radioactive sample will decay at any given time, it is reasonably straightforward to determine what percentage of the atoms will remain after a given amount of time.

The equation of exponential decay of radioactivity is as follows:

$$A_t = A_o e^{-\lambda t}$$

where A_t is the activity at time t, A_0 is the activity at time zero (when the activity was measured), and λ is a value known as the exponential decay constant, which is discussed in more detail later. The symbol e represents the base of the natural logarithms, which governs exponential behavior; it has the value e = 2.718282... .

According to the rules of logarithms, e to any negative power will always be less than 1.000; e to a very small negative number will be very close to 1.000; and many hand calculators will give the value of 1.000 in this case. However, the number should never be greater than 1.000; if this is the case, you have made a mathematical error because radioactive decay will always result in a decrease in the amount of radioactivity present.

To make this point absolutely clear, we will use a little algebra to rearrange the previous equation:

$$\frac{A_t}{A_o} = e^{-\lambda t}$$

This says that the final amount of radioactivity divided by the initial amount is equal to the exponential side of the equation, which will always be between 0 and 1.

Another important principle in working with natural logarithms is that the inverse of the exponential function e is the natural logarithm ln. This means that:

$$\ln (e^{anything}) = Anything$$

or in our case:

$$\ln (e^{-\lambda t}) = -\lambda t$$

A radioactive sample is measured to contain 100 mCi of radioactivity. If the decay constant of this isotope is 0.115 hr^{-1}, how much activity will remain after 24 hours?

$$A_t = A_o e^{-\lambda t} = (100 \text{ mCi})e^{(-0.115)(24)} = 6.329 \text{ mCi}$$

Note the units on λ, which are time^{-1}. Because the units of t are in time and the units of λ are time^{-1}, these must cancel out, leaving the exponent of e with no units. To accomplish this, λl and t must be in the same unit of time, that is, minutes, hours, days, years, and so forth.

λ is a constant for a given isotope, that is, all atoms of a given isotope will decay with the same l, which will not change no matter what environmental conditions persist—you cannot change the λ of an isotope with heat, pressure, or any other known factors.

How can we use the exponential decay equation to derive the useful quantity, known as the half-life of an isotope? The half-life is the time required for the activity of any sample of a particular radioisotope to decay to half of its initial value. So the quantity we seek to solve for is t, the time, which we will give the special symbol t_h to represent half-life.

How do we solve the equation for half-life? We know that the activity after one half-life will be half of the initial activity, by definition. So we can say that:

$$\frac{A_t}{A_o} = 0.5$$

Knowing this, solve for t_h:

$$\frac{A_t}{A_o} = e^{-\lambda t}$$
$$0.5 = e^{-\lambda t_h}$$
$$\ln(0.5) = -\lambda t_h$$
$$-0.693 = -\lambda t_h$$

We now divide and cancel the minus signs to get the final solution:

$$t_h = \frac{0.693}{\lambda}$$

We can, if needed, also rearrange this equation to give:

$$\lambda = \frac{0.693}{t_h}$$

You should go through this derivation several times and try it yourself, so that the method is clear. These equations are used frequently in calculations involving radioactive isotopes.

A sample of an isotope with a half-life of 8.0 days is measured to have an activity of 25.0 mCi on Monday at noon. What would the activity be on Friday of that week, at noon?

electron from the involved shell is ejected from the atom with an energy equal to:

$$E_{electron} = E_{photon} - E_{binding}$$

where $E_{electron}$ is the kinetic energy of the electron leaving the atom (related to its mass and speed), E_{photon} is the energy of the incident photon, and $E_{binding}$ is the binding energy of the involved electron shell. After ejection of the electron, there is a "hole" in the electron shell, which is then filled by outer shell electrons "falling" into it, losing energy in the process. The energy lost by these outer shell electrons usually appears as low-energy x-rays, called characteristic radiation.[1-4]

Whenever characteristic radiation is produced, there is a possibility that the characteristic x-ray photon may be absorbed by an orbital electron rather than leaving the atom. The electron, now having an excess of energy, will be ejected from the atom in place of the photon. An electron that leaves the atom in this manner is called an Auger electron (pronounced "O-zhey") and is capable of causing biologic damage on its own.

Compton (incoherent) scattering. Compton scattering is the most common photon interaction that occurs in the energy range used in radiation therapy.[4] In a Compton interaction, as shown in Fig. 14-7, the incident photon interacts with an outer shell electron, that is, one very loosely bound to the atom (sometimes called a "free" electron). The atom absorbs all of the photon's energy, and the electron is ejected from the outer shell. However, the electron does not carry away all of the remaining energy; instead, a second photon is emitted, which carries off a portion of the leftover energy. This secondary photon has a different energy and wavelength than the incident photon, and this interaction is called "incoherent."

The secondary electron and secondary photon travel away from the atom at different angles, which can be calculated using several complex equations relating the angles and energies of the particles involved both before and after the interaction takes place. Although the mathematics of this situation are complex, a few examples can show the effect of angle on the results of a Compton interaction:

1. *Direct hit on the target atom.* If the incident photon makes a direct hit on the atom, the electron will go straight forward (in the same direction the incident photon was traveling) and carry away most of the energy, whereas the secondary photon will travel backward from the atom and carry away a minimum of energy. This effect is called backscatter. At high photon energies (like those from a typical therapy accelerator), the energy of the secondary photon approaches a maximum value of 0.255 MeV, and the number of photons that scatter directly back is very small.
2. *Grazing hit on the target atom.* A grazing hit on the atom by the incident photon will cause very little energy loss; most of the energy will be carried away by the secondary photon, which as a result will have nearly the same energy as the incident photon.
3. *90-degree scatter.* It is important for radiation protection purposes to look at what takes place when the secondary photon emerges at an angle 90 degrees to the incident photon. It turns out that the energy of this photon reaches a maximum

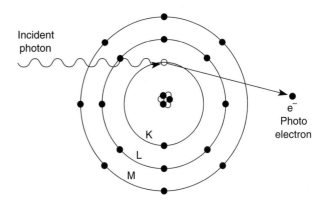

Figure 14-6. In the photoelectric effect, the incident photon is totally absorbed and transfers all of its energy to the resultant photoelectron. *(From Bernier DR, Christian PE, Langan JK, editors: Nuclear medicine: technology and techniques, ed 3, St. Louis, 1994, Mosby.)*

value of 0.511 MeV and is essentially independent of the energy of the incident photon, even at very high photon energies.

Pair production. Pair production interactions occur at high energies; in fact, they are physically impossible below an energy of 1.022 MeV for the incoming photon.[1-4] In the pair production interaction (shown in Fig. 14-8) the incident photon passes close to the nucleus of the atom. When the photon interacts with the EM field of the nucleus, it is absorbed, and instantly the energy is re-emitted as an electron-positron pair (β^-, β^+), which then is ejected from the atom. If you use Einstein's equation $E = mc^2$, letting m equal the mass of an electron, you can calculate that the rest energy of an electron or positron, that is, the energy needed to cre-

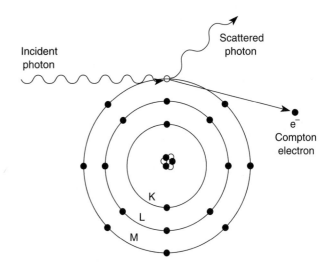

Figure 14-7. Compton scattering occurs in outer electron shells. The atom is left ionized. *(From Bernier DR, Christian PE, Langan JK, editors: Nuclear medicine: technology and techniques, ed 3, St. Louis, 1994, Mosby.)*

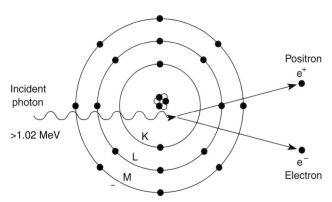

Figure 14-8. In the pair production interaction the incident photon passes close to the nucleus of the atom and creates a positron-electron pair. The positron will undergo annihilation with another electron. *(From Bernier DR, Christian PE, Langan JK, editors: Nuclear medicine: technology and techniques, ed 3, St. Louis, 1994, Mosby.)*

ate one during an interaction, is equal to 0.511 MeV. Because two such particles are created, this explains why you must have at least two times that energy, or 1.022 MeV, for pair production interaction to occur. Whatever energy is left over after the 1.022 MeV has been used is divided between the electron and positron.

The electron created usually begins to interact with other atoms outside of the original atom, until it loses its excess energy and is absorbed. The positron, however, suffers a more interesting fate. When it has undergone several interactions and is moving somewhat more slowly than when it left the atom where the pair production interaction took place, it will collide with a free electron, creating an annihilation reaction. The positron is called an "antimatter" version of the electron, and when the two meet, both are destroyed, with the energy of the two being emitted as two photons of 0.511 MeV each, traveling at 180 degrees to each other (i.e., in opposite directions). Thus following a pair production interaction, two photons as well as the electron-positron pair will be available for further interactions.

Photodisintegration. A photodisintegration reaction is one in which the photon strikes the nucleus of the target atom directly and is absorbed. The sudden absorption of this energy causes the nucleus to emit both neutrons and γ-rays in an attempt to maintain stability. This interaction occurs mainly in high Z materials and at usually higher energies (less than 7 MeV), depending on the material. Thus it is a very unimportant interaction in tissue, where the Z_{eff} is approximately 7.42 (in other words, very low Z). However, it is extremely important when working with high-energy medical accelerators, those with photon or electron beam energies of 10 MeV or greater. Because of the high energies of these beams, combined with the massive amounts of high Z materials like lead and tungsten in the beam production systems of these accelerators, a substantial neutron hazard to patients or personnel can occur. If you look at the inside of the treatment head of a high-energy linear accelerator, you will probably see some neutron shielding in the form of a borated plastic that slows down ("moderates") the neutrons so that they can be captured.

Effects of combined interactions. When a radiation beam interacts with a medium, no single type of photon interaction occurs; instead, the result is usually a combination of two or more of the previous interactions. The factor μ, discussed earlier, actually represents the combined effects of all of the previous interactions for a given energy and material:

$$\mu = \sigma_{coh} + \tau + \sigma_{inc} + \pi + \Pi$$

where σ_{coh} represents Thomson ("coherent") scattering; τ, photoelectric interactions; σ_{inc} the Compton ("incoherent") interactions; π, the pair production interactions; and Π, the photodisintegration and other high-energy reactions that we did not study here. Each of these symbols represents a probability that the photon, when it interacts with the medium, will undergo that type of reaction; μ describes the total probability of an interaction. Table 14-5 shows the relative importance of the three interactions of greatest concern in radiation therapy physics: the photoelectric, Compton, and pair production interactions.

As you can see from the table, at low energies most pho-

Table 14-5	Relative important of photon interactions in water (the number of each type that occurs out of 100 photons)		
Photon Energy (MeV)	**t**	**sinc**	**p**
0.010	95	5	0
0.026	50	50	0
0.060	7	93	0
0.150	0	100	0
4.000	0	94	6
10.00	0	77	23
24.00	0	50	50
100.0	0	16	84

ton interactions taking place are photoelectric (τ) interactions. However, as energy increases, the Compton (σ_{inc}) interaction quickly takes precedence and is itself slowly replaced by the pair production (π) and other interactions as the energy continues to increase. Most radiation therapy energies fall into the range of 1 to 5 MeV, where Compton predominates. You can also see this trend in Table 14-4, especially for lead; the values of μ start at extremely high values, drop to a minimum at energies around 4.0 MeV, then begin to climb again as the pair production interactions begin to produce more and more interactions as energy increases. You should keep this behavior of μ in mind when thinking about exponential attenuation problems.

PARTICLE INTERACTIONS

The interactions of particulate radiation with matter differ considerably from those of photons because of the different nature of particulate radiation. Although photons have no mass and no electrical charge, particles do have mass, and most have some type of electrical charge as well. As a result, interactions between particles and atoms tend to resemble "billiard ball" interactions, familiar to us on an everyday level. This section examines some of the interactions that take place in the cases of two major particle radiations used in radiation therapy: electrons and neutrons.

Elastic and Inelastic Collisions

The collisions of particle radiations can be likened to the collisions between large-scale objects such as billiard balls. Each ball can be described as possessing kinetic energy, that is, energy caused by its motion through space. When the balls collide, their directions and speeds will change depending on the conditions of the collision, and thus each ball may lose or gain kinetic energy; the total kinetic energy, however, may or may not remain the same before and after the collision. If no kinetic energy is lost to the system in the collision, the collision is elastic; if energy is lost from the system, the collision is inelastic.

Two balls with kinetic energies equal to 10 J each collide. After the collision, one ball has a kinetic energy of 15 J, and the other has a kinetic energy of 5 J. Because the total energy in the system has not changed (20 J = 20 J), the collision was elastic.

If, in the same example, the energies of the two balls after the collision had been measured as 12 J and 6 J, this would have been an inelastic collision, because energy was lost during the collision (20 J is greater than 18 J). The remaining 2 J of energy were converted into other forms of energy, such as vibrational energy or heat.

Note that, whether or not kinetic energy is conserved, the total energy of the system (which includes all other forms of energy such as heat) must remain the same. In the second example, the 2 J of kinetic energy lost to the billiard balls did not disappear but rather were converted into another form of energy. This concept is called the principle of conservation of energy and is one of the basic concepts of physics and chemistry.

The interactions between atoms and particle radiations can be classified in the same manner. If the total kinetic energies of the particle and atom are the same after the interaction, then an elastic collision has taken place; if not, the collision was inelastic. We next look at how these definitions apply in the cases of electron and neutron radiations.

Electron Interactions

Electron-electron interactions. When electrons in a medium interact with the electrons in the electron shells of the atoms in the medium, they give up energy to those electrons and are then deflected away from the atom in a new direction. Because they have given up energy to the atomic electron, the original electron is now moving more slowly (and therefore has less kinetic energy). The target electron, in the atomic orbit, may be "kicked up" to a shell farther from the nucleus (call excitation) or may be ejected completely from the atom (ionization) if the energy gained from the incident electron is high enough. Remember that a "collision" between two particles does not necessarily mean that actual physical contact between the particles has occurred; a collision can also result if the EM fields of the two particles come close enough to interact with each other, a distance that may be several times larger than the physical size of the particle itself.

Recall from our study of the Compton interaction that outer shell electrons are considered "free" electrons because their binding energies are very low compared to the energy of the incoming photons. If one of these free electrons is involved in the electron-electron interaction just described, the binding energy of the target electron is so small that it may be ignored; therefore the energy before the collision (incident electron plus target electron), in this case, can be considered elastic. If, however, the interaction involved an electron in a shell close to the nucleus, the binding energy must be taken into account. In this case, because of the principle of conservation of energy already discussed, some of the energy of the original electron will be lost to overcome the binding energy of the target electron before the target electron can change shell or leave the atom, making this an inelastic collision.

When the electron's energy is finally depleted by a series of collisions, it is captured by an atom in the vicinity, exhausted but satisfied.

Elastic electron-nuclei collisions. In materials heavier than hydrogen (Z = 1), electrons with certain energies are more likely to undergo elastic scattering with the nuclei of atoms than with the atomic electrons. Like an electron-electron elastic collision (already described), the incident electrons lose a small amount of energy to the nucleus of the atom and bounce away with reduced energy. Because the nuclei are so much larger than electrons, the electron will

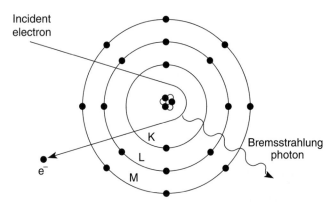

Figure 14-9. Deceleration of charged particle passing near nucleus results in release of energy in the form of bremsstrahlung radiation. *(From Bernier DR, Christian PE, Langan JK, editors: Nuclear medicine: technology and techniques, ed 3, St. Louis, 1994, Mosby.)*

retain a larger percentage of its energy than if it had collided with an electron and is more likely to bounce straight backward from the atom after the collision. This effect diminishes quickly as the energy of the incident electrons is increased, and, at energies in the range usually used in radiation therapy (4 to 25 MeV), the electrons interact mainly by electron-electron scattering (discussed previously) or inelastic nuclear scattering (discussed later).

Inelastic electron-nuclei collisions. High-energy electrons can pass close to the nucleus of a target atom, as seen in Fig. 14-9, and be so strongly attracted by the charges in the nucleus that they will slow down, losing some of their kinetic energy; this energy will be emitted from the atom as a photon with energy (hv) equal to the energy lost by the electron when it slowed down.[1] This process is called **bremsstrahlung** (German, "braking radiation") and is the most important method of producing x-ray beams in therapy units.

The photon created in the bremsstrahlung process can be of any energy from 0 up to the energy of the incident electron and can emerge from the atom in any direction. Thus like β decay, bremsstrahlung produces not a single-energy x-ray but rather a spectrum of x-ray energies ranging from 0 to the energy of the incident electron beam. The average energy of the bremsstrahlung spectrum is about a third of the maximum possible energy (E^{max}).

When the electron beam is in the lower energy range used in therapy (50 to 300 keV), the photons are emitted in a wide range of angles. As the electron beam energy increases, the photons tend to be emitted closer to the direction of the incident electron, a phenomenon known as forward peaking of the photon beam. This effect is very important in the design and use of high-energy photon machines such as linear accelerators and betatrons, because at the high energies used in these machines, the bremsstrahlung photon beam is highly forward peaked.

Bremsstrahlung production is more likely in high Z materials such as lead or tungsten than in a low Z material like water or tissue. For this reason, high Z materials can be bombarded with a beam of high-energy electrons to produce high-energy photon beams in radiation therapy machines.

SUMMARY

To understand the discipline of radiation physics, one must be familiar with the developments, theories, and technologic advances that have taken place since Roentgen discovered the x-ray in 1895. From the Curies who defined the activity of 1 g of radium (^{226}Ra), to Bohr's attempt to explain the atom, to Einstein's work that earned him the Nobel Prize, the area of physics has grown and developed. Using the work of those who have come before us, we are able to understand why an x-ray image taken with photons in the kilovoltage range is superior to one taken with photons in the megavoltage range. The knowledge of the interactions of subatomic particles is critical to understanding these issues.

The inverse square law, linear attenuation, half-life, and exponential decay are a few of the concepts, terms, and tools needed to begin understanding the discipline of radiation physics, providing a solid foundation on which to build.

Review Questions

1. How many seconds are there in 2.54 minutes?
   a. 174.0
   b. 114.0
   c. 152.4
   d. 92.4
   e. 254
2. Calculate the wavelength of an electromagnetic wave that has a frequency of 3.95×10^{14} Hz.
   a. 1.32×10^6 m
   b. 13.2×10^6 m
   c. 7.59×10^{-8} m
   d. 7.59×10^{-7} m
   e. 7.59×10^{-6} m
3. An FM radio station broadcasts at 102.0 MHz on your radio dial. What is the wavelength of the station's signal?
   a. 34.0 m
   b. 3.40 m
   c. 2.941 m
   d. 2.941×10^6 m
   e. 29.41 m
4. An electromagnetic wave has a frequency of 2.1×10^{21} Hz. What is the energy of the wave?
   a. 3.355×10^{54} eV
   b. 1.39×10^{12} eV
   c. 5.060×10^{35} eV
   d. 8.250 MeV
   e. 8.715 MeV

5. If an electromagnetic wave has an energy of 6 MeV, what would its wavelength be?
   a. 50 m
   b. 3.313×10^{-32} m
   c. 2.075×10^{-13} m
   d. 2.075×10^{-12} m
   e. 2.075×10^{-7} m

6. A sample of an isotope has a half-life of 74 days and is measured to have an activity of 8.675 Ci at noon of that day. What will the activity of the isotope be 94 days later at 6 PM?
   a. 4.338 Ci
   b. 3.588 Ci
   c. 3.596 Ci
   d. 5.034 Ci
   e. 2.37 Ci

7. The intensity of a radioactive beam is measured at a distance of 100 cm and found to be 250 mR/min. What will the intensity of this beam be at 105 cm?
   a. 226.8 mR/min
   b. 238.1 mR/min
   c. 205.7 mR/min
   d. 275.6 mR/min
   e. 262.5 mR/min

8. A 6-MeV photon beam is incident on a lead sheet 1.5 cm thick. If the initial dose rate of the beam is 300 cGy/min, what will the dose rate be after passing through the lead sheet if the linear attenuation coefficient for this beam in lead is 0.4911 cm^{-1}?
   a. 79.0 cGy/min
   b. 183.6 cGy/min
   c. 147.33 cGy/min
   d. 143.6 cGy/min
   e. 221.0 cGy/min

9. What is the HVL of the beam in the previous question?
   a. 2.72 cm
   b. 4.07 cm
   c. 0.941 cm
   d. 1.386 cm
   e. 1.411 cm

10. In the problem given in question 8, what minimal thickness of lead is needed to reduce the dose rate to less than 9 cGy/min?
    a. 2 cm
    b. 10 cm
    c. 100 cm
    d. 7.0 cm
    e. 7.5 cm

Questions to Ponder

1. A portal radiograph (port film) is taken with a high-energy photon beam (MeV range). Why is the radiograph inferior in diagnostic quality when compared to a radiograph taken on a simulator (keV range)?

2. Explain the difference between the tenth value layer (TVL) of a material and its linear attenuation coefficient.

3. Explain the reason for using lead as a shielding material for x-ray rooms and/or vaults.

4. Explain the concept of the exponential decay constant and how it relates to half-life.

REFERENCES

1. Bernier DR, Christian PE, Langan JK, editors: *Nuclear medicine: technology and techniques,* ed 3, St. Louis, 1994, Mosby.
2. Hendee WR, Ritenour R: *Medical imaging physics,* ed 3, St. Louis, 1992, Mosby.
3. Johns HE, Cunningham JR: *The physics of radiology,* ed 4, Springfield, Ill, 1983, Charles C Thomas.
4. Khan FM: *The physics of radiation therapy,* ed 2, Baltimore, 1992, Williams & Wilkins.

15

Aspects of Brachytherapy

Charles M. Washington

HISTORICAL OVERVIEW AND PERSPECTIVE

The discovery of x-rays by Roentgen in the late nine-teenth century has proved, more than any other innovation, to have a dramatic impact on modern medicine. Shortly after the discovery of x-rays, Henri Becquerel and Pierre Curie began investigating the existence of similar rays produced by known fluorescent materials. Curie, in his experimentation, deliberately produced an ulcer on his arm and described in detail the various phases of a moist epidermitis and his recovery from it.[1] At that point he gave a small radium tube to a colleague and suggested he insert it into a tumor. Subsequently, several physicians began investigating the effects of these rays on malignant tumors, and the therapeutic use of ionizing radiation began.

The term **brachytherapy** refers to radiation therapy that involves placing radioactive material directly into or immediately adjacent to the tumor, rather than through external beams. *Brachy,* meaning "short," implies therapy at a short distance. Today, brachytherapy is a standard technique in the treatment of a large number of malignancies, including uterus and uterine cervix, lung, prostate, and breast. Brachytherapy use in cancer therapy is increasing and is paralleled by the increasing desire for organ preservation and acceptable cosmetic results. In current oncology practice there are many opportunities for medical dosimetrist and radiation therapist involvement in the practical application of brachytherapy. The scopes of practice for the medical dosimetrist and radiation therapist identify the need for critical thinking skills that involve the application of radiation through these means.

The major advantage of brachytherapy is that very high

doses of radiation can be delivered locally to the tumor in a relatively short time, while very low doses are delivered in the surrounding tissue.[1] As the distance around the source of radiation increases, there is a dramatic reduction of dose absorbed in tissue. This adheres directly to the premise that in radiation therapy, homogeneous tumoricidal doses must be deposited in the tumor while sparing as much normal tissue as possible. Brachytherapy is commonly used to supplement the dose administered by external beam irradiation; this allows additional doses of be delivered to a well-defined volume of tumor tissue. Because the radiation administered in this way does not penetrate through overlying tissues to reach this volume, surrounding tissues are spared from increased doses of radiation.

Brachytherapy can be administered through several types of applications. **Interstitial brachytherapy** is characterized by the placement of radioactive sources directly into a tumor or tumor bed. Rigid needles or flexible tubes may be used in the actual placement of the sources (Fig. 15-1). Interstitial brachytherapy is commonly used in the treatment of neck, breast, soft tissue sarcomas, and skin tumors. **Intracavitary brachytherapy** places radioactive sources within a body cavity for treatment. This type of brachytherapy has been the mainstay in treatment of cervical cancer for more than 50 years.[3] Closely associated with interstitial brachytherapy, **intraluminal brachytherapy** place sources of radiation within body tubes such as the esophagus, uterus, trachea, bronchus, and rectum. **Intravascular brachytherapy** is a rapidly emerging treatment modality with potential applications for peripheral vessel angioplasty, bypass graft anastomoses, and arteriovenous dialysis grafts in addition to its application for coronary vessels. The use of stents and radiation reduce can the rate of restenosis in the vessel. **Topical brachytherapy** places the radioactive sources on top of the area to be treated. Molds of the body part treated may be taken and prepared to place the sources in definite arrangements to deliver the prescribed dose.

REVIEW OF SOURCE STRENGTH SPECIFICATION

Source strength specification plays three roles in brachytherapy. The first is to provide a commonly accepted standard means of describing quantities of emitted radiation. The second allows practitioners to form a basis for *computational dosimetry,* which is the calculation of dose with the aid of a computerized system. Third, source strength specification serves as a prescription parameter in brachytherapy.

The historical term used to describe activity in terms of number of disintegrations per unit time is the curie (Ci). The curie is 3.7×10^{10} disintegrations per second from 1 g of radium. The Système Internationale (SI) unit of activity is the becquerel (Bq). One becquerel equals one disintegration per second. Although the becquerel is the unit recommended for use, the curie is still commonly used in practice. Table 15-1 reviews the conversions commonly used.

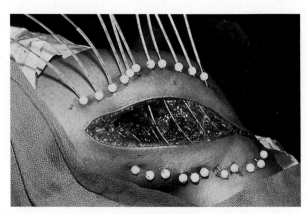

Figure 15-1. Example of interstitial catheters placed along a tumor bed of an extremity. Sources placed inside the catheters will deliver a high dose of radiation to the tumor bed and immediate surrounding area.

Radioactive Decay

The key relationship in understanding radioactivity, which is a statistical process, is:

$$\frac{\Delta N}{\Delta t} \, \alpha \, N$$

where N is the number of atoms and t is the time. The change in the number of atoms per change in unit time is proportional to the number of atoms present. This proportion can be made into an equation by the addition of a constant, l, called the **decay constant:**

$$\frac{\Delta N}{\Delta t} = -\lambda N$$

The negative sign is added because there are fewer atoms present after a given amount of time. The equation can be rearranged to solve for the gamma constant as follows:

$$\lambda = -\frac{\dfrac{\Delta N}{N}}{\Delta t}$$

Table 15-1	Commonly used conversions relating curies to becquerels	
Unit	**Definition**
1 curie (Ci)	3.7×10^{10} disintegration/sec
1 millicurie (mCi)	3.7×10^{7} disintegration/sec
1 microcurie (μCi)	3.7×10^{4} disintegration/sec
1 becquerel (Bq)	1 disintegration/sec
1 megabecquerel (MBq)	1×10^{6} disintegration/sec
1 mCi	37 MBq
1 gigabecquerel (GBq)	1×10^{9} disintegration/sec
1Ci	37 GBq

Therefore the decay constant can be expressed as the total number of atoms that decay per unit time. From this are developed the definition of activity and the formula for exponential decay.

Activity. **Activity**, A, is the rate of decay of a radioactive material or the change in the number of atoms in a certain amount of time and can be written as follows:

$$A = \frac{\Delta N}{\Delta t} = -\lambda N$$

The activity is directly proportional to the decay constant. So, as the decay constant increases, the activity increases.

The previous equation can also be rearranged and integrated to yield the exponential decay equation, as follows:

$$N = N_0 e^{-\lambda t}$$

A (activity) can be substituted for N (the number of atoms) to yield the following:

$$A = A_0 e^{-\lambda t}$$

This formula, as presented in Chapter 14, is commonly used to calculate activity of a radioisotope after some length of time has passed.

Half-life. The concept used to deal with the isotope disintegration is half-life. The **half-life** is the time period in which the activity decays to one half the original value. It is the essential value to employ the decay formula for a particular isotope. Half-life ($T_{1/2}$) is related to the decay constant by the following formula:

$$T_{1/2} = \frac{0.693}{\lambda}$$

The relationship between activity and half-life is given by the formula:

$$A = \lambda N = \frac{0.693}{T_{1/2}}$$

The relationship between half-life and activity is inversely proportional. In other words, as half-life increases, overall activity decreases.

Decay formula. These mathematical expressions can be grouped together and allow the radiation therapist and medical dosimetrist to derive a formula that will relate predict radionuclide decay. This is called the *decay formula*, which is expressed by the following:

$$A = A_0 e^{-\left(\frac{0.693}{T_{1/2}}\right)t}$$

A_0 denotes the originally known activity, A is the current activity, $T_{1/2}$ is the half-life, and t is the length of time passed since time of originally known activity. Table 15-2 lists isotopes commonly used in radiation therapy with their half-lives. The half-life will vary somewhat from different literature sources and from past to present, but these are fairly representative of what is in common use today. A good

way to remember these concepts is to put them into practical use. It is important to make sure that the units used throughout the problem are consistent.

Example 1: Every year a new decayed value must be determined for clinical use of the cesium-137 tubes. The decay is always calculated from the original assayed value obtained when the source was received. One source was received on February 18, 2003; that value was determined to be 69.5 mCi. What would be the activity for this source 365 days later?

$$A = A_0 \times e^{-\left(\frac{0.693}{T_{1/2}}\right) \times t}$$

$$A = A_0 \times e^{-\left(\frac{0.693}{30 \text{ yr}}\right) \times 1 \text{ yr}}$$

$$A = 67.91 \text{ mCi}$$

Mean life. Another concept related to half-life is mean life, which is complicated in explanation but useful and easy in calculation. **Mean life** is the average lifetime for the decay of radioactive atoms. It is the time period for a hypothetical source that decays at a constant rate equal to its initial activity to produce the same number of disintegrations as the exponentially decaying source that decays for an infinite period of time. It is primarily applicable to dose calculations in permanent implants, typically gold-198 and iodine-125. Theoretically, all the dose is delivered over a very long time period because all the activity is not decayed away until the last unstable atom disintegrates. The treatment planning team needs a practical means of calculating a final dose. The relationship between mean life and half-life is as follows:

$$\text{Mean life} = T_{1/2} \times 1.44$$

Example 2: 106 mCi of gold-198 is implanted into a pelvic mass. Determine the emitted radiation.

$$\text{Mean life of gold-198} = 1.44 \times (2.7 \text{ days}) = 3.89 \text{ days}$$
$$\text{Emitted radiation} = 106 \text{ mCi} \times 3.89 \text{ days} = 412.34 \text{ mCi-days}$$

Average energy (E_{ave}). Another property of interest in isotope usage is the average energy of the emitted photons. This is derived from the decay schemes of each isotope. Any beta emission has already been eliminated by filtrating

Table 15-2	Commonly used isotopes	
Isotope	**$T_{1/2}$**
Radium-226	1622 years
Cobalt-60	5.26 years
Cesium-137	30.0 years
Iridium-192	74.1 days
Iodine-125	60.2 days
Gold-198	2.7 days
Radon-222	3.82 days
Copper-64	12.8 hours

Table 15-3	Average energy of isotopes used in brachytherapy
Isotope	E_{ave} (MeV)
Radium-226	0.83
Cobalt-60	1.25
Cesium-137	0.66
Iridium-192	0.38
Iodine-125	0.03
Gold-198	0.41
Radon-222	0.83

encapsulations, because radiation treatment is not accomplished with beta particles. Table 15-3 illustrates a list of the average energy for isotopes commonly used in brachytherapy.

RADIOACTIVE SOURCES USED IN BRACHYTHERAPY

Brachytherapy most commonly uses sealed radioactive sources within or adjacent to a tumor volume. A sealed source is one in which the radioactive material is encapsulated by welded ends. Typically, the isotope is encased within metal casings that serve two main functions: preventing escape of radioactivity and absorption of beta particles. Fig. 15-2 demonstrates a sealed source. The International Organization of Standardization (ISO) classifies sealed sources based on safety requirements. They also specify leak test methods, such as wipe tests, for sealed sources to be carried out at both the manufacturer and user levels.[17]

Most brachytherapy procedures were developed using radium-226, the first radioisotope to be isolated and identified.[11] Other isotopes have come into use when nuclear reac-

tor produced isotopes became readily available. Most of the isotopes used in radiation therapy today have their dosimetry based on the original radium work and are referred to as **radium substitutes.** These substitutes offer several advantages over radium. Both radium and radium substitutes are described later in the chapter.

Radium

Radium ($^{226}_{88}$Ra) decays mainly by alpha emission and is part of a long decay chain that begins with natural uranium ($^{238}_{92}$U) and concludes in an isotope of stable lead ($^{206}_{82}$Pb). The half-life for radium is about 1622 years. As part of the process, radium decays to form radon, a heavy inert gas that further decays down to the stable lead atom. Radon gas has caused concern during home construction in the Midwest to the eastern seaboard. As ore deposits decay, the radioactive gas seeps up into the basements of the homes, causing serious health concerns.

Use of radium was very practical because it has a very high specific activity. **Specific activity** is defined as the activity per unit mass of a radioactive material (Ci/g). The specific activity dictates the total activity that a small source can have. Even though some radionuclides might have some particular advantage for implantation, they may not be suitable because a small size and high activity may not be possible for that particular isotope. The disadvantage of radium concerns itself mainly with radiation hazards.[11,17] Radiation is produced by alpha emission and produces a daughter, radon-222, which is a gas that can possibly leak from the encapsulated sources.

A typical radium source consists of a hollow needle or tube made of a metal such as platinum or stainless steel. Inside the tube, small capsules of radium salt are placed, giving the source a known activity. This activity, together with the thickness of the source capsule (known as the filtration), determines the dosimetric properties of the source and how it can be used in brachytherapy. Note that the area in which the radioactivity is packed is shorter that the total length of the source; the length of the area in which the radioactivity lies in the source is called the **active length** of the source and must be differentiated from the physical length, which it the total length of the source, end-to-end.[11,17]

The gamma (Γ) factor for radium-226 is 8.25 R·cm²/mCi·hr, assuming a filtration of 0.5 mm of platinum. The filtration (shell thickness) of the radium source is very important, because the decay processes of radium-226 result in a large number of low-energy x-rays, which are easily filtered by any additional filtration. In other words, as you increase the filtration of the radium-226 source, the Γ factor will decrease as you eliminate more and more low-energy x-rays. If you have a radium-226 source with more or less than 0.5 mm Pt filtration, the Γ factor from this source will change as follows: increase of 2% for each additional 0.1 mm of platinum added to 0.5 mm, and decrease of 2% for each 0.1 mm of platinum less than 0.5 mm.

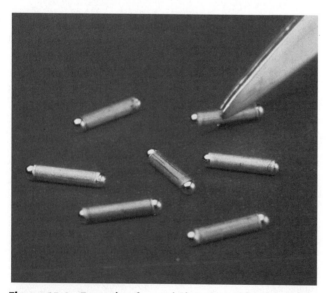

Figure 15-2. Example of a sealed source of ionizing radiation, iodine-125.

Radium sources. The amount of radioactivity in a radium source is expressed in milligrams of radium. In the definition of a curie, it was initially the amount of activity of 1 g of radium. Later, however, the definition of the curie was changed to exactly 3.7×10^{10} disintegrations/sec, whereas $^{226}_{88}$Ra decays with about 3.66×10^{10} disintegrations/sec. Despite this small discrepancy, in clinical situations it is assumed that 1 mg radium has an activity of 1 mCi.

When brachytherapy was becoming a popular treatment method, the manufacturers of radium sources decided on a standard for specifying the ways in which radium can be distributed inside a needle source. A full-strength source is defined as one that has 0.66 mg/cm of activity, and a half-strength source has 0.33 mg/cm of activity.

Example 3: A full-strength radium source has active length of 3 cm. What is the activity of this source in mg?

$$A = (0.66 \text{ mg/cm}) (3.0 \text{ cm}) = 2.0 \text{ mg}$$

Sources that have the same concentration of radioactivity throughout their active length are called *uniform sources.* However, physicians soon found that it is convenient to have available some sources that had a nonuniform distribution of activity in them. Two other types of source were developed: the *Indian club source,* which is heavily loaded with activity at one end, and the *dumbbell source,* which has heavy loading at both ends, with lighter activity concentration in the middle.[11] These types of sources were all *needles;* that is, they were sharply pointed at one end and could be inserted directly into tumor tissue; the other end held an eyelet, to allow the source to be secured with sutures and easily removed (Fig. 15-3).

The use of needle sources presents several problems from medical and radiation safety viewpoints. Because they are stiff, they must be inserted into areas of the body thick enough to accept them without bending them. The possibil-

ity of breakage is always present. Also, the personnel loading the sources are continually exposed to radiation while performing the procedure, which is not in line with the recommended national policy of keeping medical radiation exposure to a minimum for both patients and staff. To avoid these problems, systems were developed to allow devices known as applicators to be inserted into the treatment area first, then loaded with radioactivity quickly and safely when the patient is back in his or her room (Fig. 15-4). This technique, known as **afterloading,** led to the development of tube sources. These are small sources that are rounded on each end, and contain larger amounts of activity than needle sources (up to 50 mg in a single source).

Some isotopes, such as radon-222 and gold-198, have very short half-lives and are implanted permanently rather than temporarily. Such sources are packaged in tiny versions of tube sources called seeds, which are usually about 3 to 5 mm long and the diameter of a pencil lead. These sources are implanted using a gunlike applicator that uses long needles to accurately position the seeds within the tumor during surgery. This type of therapy is used frequently in the case of prostate cancer, as well as other types of solid, localized tumors that can be reached surgically.

Radium Substitutes

The term **radium substitute** is used to indicate any isotope used for brachytherapy whose dosimetry is based on the

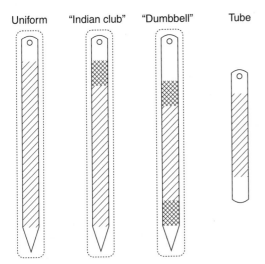

Figure 15-3. Typical radium sources. Note the depiction of the active length and physical length.

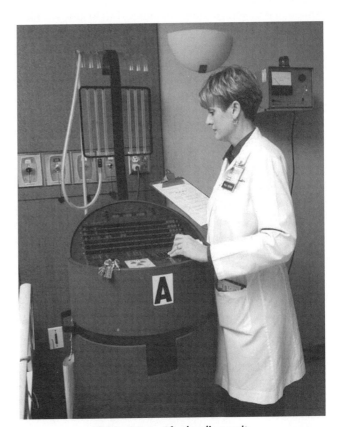

Figure 15-4. Afterloading unit.

original radium work. These include but are not confined to the following: cesium-137, iridium-192, gold-198, and iodine-125. The activities of these isotopes are expressed in millicuries. However, when these isotopes were first introduced, an attempt to correlate the effect of these isotopes with that of radium was made, because all clinical experience up to that time involved the use of radium. A unit was defined, called *radium equivalence,* which is defined as follows:

$$\text{mg Ra eq} = (A_{\text{isotope}}, \text{mCi}) \left(\frac{\Gamma_{\text{isotope}}}{\Gamma_{\text{Ra}}} \right)$$

where A_{isotope} is the activity of the source in millicuries.

Example 4: What is the radium equivalence of a 25.0 mCi source of $^{137}_{55}\text{Cs}$?

$$\text{mg Ra eq} = (25.0 \text{ mCi}) \left(\frac{3.28}{8.25} \right) = 9.939 \text{ mg Ra eq}$$

Cesium-137. Cesium-137 ($^{137}_{55}\text{Cs}$) is one of the most widely used of the radium substitutes and has largely replaced radium as the primary isotope for brachytherapy of the uterus and cervix. It has a primary photon energy of 662 keV, which is comparable to the average photon energy of radium (830 keV). This means that the cesium photon penetrates tissue in about the same manner as radium. This makes the conversion from using radium to using cesium easier for radiation therapy practitioners.

Cesium has some positive advantages over radium. Although the average energy of radium is 830 keV, it emits a spectrum of photon energies (0.047 to 2.45 MeV). Photon energies above 2 MeV result in a radiation safety hazard. The lower energy of cesium and the fact that it has no higher photon energy reduces the radiation safety hazard when using this isotope. This same fact makes storing the isotope less of a problem than with radium. Cesium has a half-life of 30.0 years, so sources can be used for a long time; they decay by only about 2% per year. Because cesium is produced in nuclear reactor fuel as a natural byproduct of nuclear fission, it can be chemically separated from spent nuclear fuel and is therefore widely available. Several manufacturers can provide cesium sources in a wide variety of needle or tube configurations. These facts, plus the wide use of cesium in education institutions, make $^{137}_{55}\text{Cs}$ very popular with hospital-based and privately owned radiation therapy practices.

Iridium-192. Iridium-192 ($^{192}_{77}\text{Ir}$) is supplied in the form of wires of iridium-platinum alloy or as small seeds of this alloy attached to a nylon ribbons with spacing of 1 cm between seeds. This radioisotope undergoes beta decay and has an average energy of 370 keV. The wire form combines flexibility with strength along with filtration characteristics that absorbs the beta particles released. The half-life of 74.2 days is shorter than that of cesium, and it is used for temporary implants of easily reached tumor sites such as the breast and tongue.[17]

The usual technique for iridium wire implants is to insert in the tissue carrier needles that penetrate through the tumor area or alternatively, flexible plastic catheters that can be looped though or around a tumor. Then the iridium wire or seed carrier is threaded into the catheter and left in place for an amount of calculated time. If needed, the wire or seed carrier can be cut to the proper length for insertion into the needles, an operation that requires great care to avoid spreading radioactivity around the work area or patient room. $^{192}_{77}\text{Ir}$ is ordered in batches about every 2 months, and iridium whose activity is too low to use for treatment can be kept until it decays to a low activity level, then returned to the manufacturer. Because $^{192}_{77}\text{Ir}$ is produced in a nuclear reactor, like cobalt, it can be reactivated for future use.

Cobalt-60. Cobalt-60 is a radionuclide that is not commonly used in today's brachytherapy applications. It undergoes a two-tiered beta decay after its neutron activation that produces 1.17 and 1.33 MeV gamma rays, averaging out to the commonly accepted 1.25 MeV. This radionuclide has a half-life of 5.26 years. Cobalt-60 has been typically used as an external beam radiation therapy source, but it has been used for ophthalmic applicators in some countries in needles and tubes. It has also seen some application in high-dose-rate applications. Although there is history of cobalt-60 use in brachytherapy applications, the isotopes main use in radiation therapy treatment delivery has been in external beam applications.

Gold-198. Gold ($^{198}_{79}\text{Au}$) is a popular replacement for $^{222}_{86}\text{Rn}$ in permanent implants. It has a very short half-life of 2.7 days and a monoenergetic (only one energy produced) energy of 412 keV. It is normally supplied in the form of cylindrical grains or seeds encapsulated in platinum.[6,12] Like cesium, the lower photon energy makes radiation safety much less of a problem with gold than with radon, and more of the dose is absorbed locally. Because of the short half-life, gold seeds are shipped with very high activities, and by the time they are ready to be used they have an activity in the range of 5 mCi/seed. Thus gold gives the tissue a very high dose in a short time, a method called high-dose-rate therapy. The prostate can benefit from interstitial implants with permanent gold seeds because other isotopes would require surgical procedures for both insertion and removal of sources.[17]

Iodine-125. The use of iodine-125 ($^{125}_{53}\text{I}$) is becoming more frequent in interstitial seed implants. This radioisotope is produced as a daughter product from the neutron activation of xenon-124 to xenon-125. The activated xenon-125 decays by electron capture to produce the daughter, iodine-125. This isotope decays by electron capture to produce useful 35.5 keV gamma rays. Because of the low energy of the isotope, whose half-life is 60.2 days, shielding requirements are minimal. The dose is deposited very close to the seeds, reducing the dose to structures next to the tumor. In addition, the dose from $^{125}_{53}\text{I}$ is deposited over a longer period of time than a dose from $^{198}_{79}\text{Au}$, making iodine therapy a type of *low dose rate therapy,* which may cause a different biologic reaction than the same dose from gold.[4,5,15] Radiation therapy practitioner education in the use iodine-125 is an important part of any brachytherapy program using this isotope.

These last two isotopes mentioned are used as replacements for radon ($^{222}_{86}$Rn) in seed sources. $^{222}_{86}$Rn is a radioactive gas, making its use very dangerous. If a seed breaks, the radioactivity becomes airborne and can be inhaled, doing great damage to the sensitive tissues of the lung. Because of this very real problem, radon seeds are no longer used.

THE EXPOSURE RATE FROM A RADIOACTIVE SOURCE

Calculation of absorbed dose from radioactive sources can be done using any one of a number of methods, all of which are based on either calculation techniques or tables of measured data. A central component of the calculation techniques is the gamma factor (Γ factor), which can be defined as the exposure rate at 1 meter from a radioactive source of known activity. The units of the Γ factor are as follows:

$$\frac{roentgen \cdot cm^2}{mCi \cdot hr}$$

The actual value of the Γ factor is different for each radioisotope; values for the radioisotopes most commonly used in radiation therapy are given in Table 15-4.

Although the units of the Γ factor may seem complex, they actually make the Γ factor a very useful and easily manipulated quantity. For example, to calculate the exposure rate (roentgen/hr) at some distance from a radioactive source, the Γ factor can be used in the following equation:

$$\dot{X} = (\Gamma\ isotope)(A)(\tfrac{1}{d})^2$$

where $\dot{X}$ is the exposure rate (recall that the dot over the X means "rate" in physics notation), d is the distance from the source to the point of calculation, and A is the activity of the source. Notice that if d is in cm and A is in mCi, the units cancel neatly, leaving roentgens/hr, which is the exposure rate. An example should clarify this process.

Example 5: Calculate the exposure rate at 10 cm from a cesium-137 source with an activity of 10 mCi.

Given that Γ of cesium = 3.226 R $\cdot$ cm^2/mCi $\cdot$ hr, d = 10 cm, and A = 10 mCi:

$$\dot{X} = (3.226\ R \cdot cm^2/mCi \cdot hr)(10\ mCi)(\tfrac{1}{10\ cm})^2$$
$$\dot{X} = 0.3226\ R/hr = 322.6\ mR/hr$$

By arranging the equation, you can find any of the four quantities included in the Γ factor if the other three are known. For example, if you know the total exposure, the distance from the source, and the activity of the source, the total time of exposure in hours could easily be calculated. Another typical use is to find the activity of a source by measuring the exposure rate at some distance, and solving for the activity, as in Example 6.

Example 6: At 15 cm from a ^{192}Ir source, the exposure rate is 305 mR/hr (0.305 roentgen/hr). What is the activity of this source?

With a value of 4.57 R $\cdot$ cm^2/mCi $\cdot$ hr for Γ_{Ir}, solve for A:

$$0.305\ R/hr = (4.57\ R \cdot cm^2/mCi \cdot hr)(A)(\tfrac{1}{15}cm)^2$$

$$A = \frac{(0.305\ R/hr)}{(4.57\ R \cdot cm^2/mCi \cdot hr)(\tfrac{1}{2})^2}$$

$$A = 15.02\ mCi$$

An important limitation to the use of the Γ factor is that it is applicable only to a point source of radiation. A radioactive source can be considered a point source if the distance from the source to the calculation point is at least five times the length of the source. Therefore the size of the source will place a limitation on the distances at which the Γ factor can be applied.

HIGH-DOSE-RATE BRACHYTHERAPY

Brachytherapy is delivered in either a conventional low-dose-rate (LDR) regimen that lasts several days and requires a hospital stay or on an outpatient basis using high-dose-rate (HDR) brachytherapy equipment. Both techniques are practiced in hospital settings today with an increasing use of HDR applications noted.

Although conventional LDR brachytherapy has a long history of use and success in head and neck, gynecologic, breast, and prostate cancers, HDR is also used for management of these same diseases. HDR brachytherapy can be as effective as LDR brachytherapy and have a very low risk of radiation injury. It is suggested that it may be preferable to the LDR treatment because HDR brachytherapy can be given on a fractionated outpatient basis. The actual treatment delivery lasts about 5 to 10 minutes in contrast to a hospital stay that might take several days for LDR brachytherapy.[16]

In the HDR brachytherapy treatment, a device or holder is placed into the area to be treated. The device is connected to an HDR brachytherapy machine (Fig. 15-5), and a small, intense radiation source is loaded into it. A high dose of radiation is given over a short treatment time, with the actual time dependent on the intensity of the source. The radioactive source is withdrawn back into the brachytherapy

Table 15-4	Gamma factors for isotopes
Isotope	**Γ factor** $\left(\dfrac{roentgen \cdot cm^2}{mCi \cdot hr}\right)$
Radium-226	8.25
Radon-222	8.25
Cobalt-60	13.07
Cesium-137	3.226
Iridium-192	4.57
Iodine-125	1.089
Gold-198	2.327

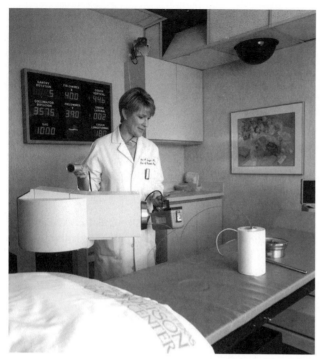

Figure 15-5. High-dose-rate (HDR) unit undergoing quality assurance (QA) tests.

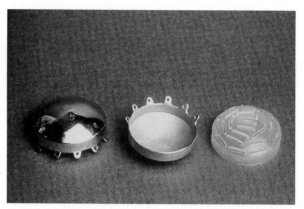

Figure 15-6. Typical plaque used in topical brachytherapy of the eye. The thin gold shielding is sufficient to block neighboring dose-limiting structures from the damaging effects of the low-energy isotope.

machine after the treatment and is then disconnected from applicator in the tumor; the process can then be repeated for any other prescribed fractions. The use of HDR procedures can also be applied to intraoperative applications.[6,16]

The main cited advantages of HDR brachytherapy compared with LDR treatment is that it can be more convenient for the patient and treatment facility in terms of time and space requirements, making it less expensive with similar outcomes.[9-11,15,16]

BRACHYTHERAPY APPLICATORS AND INSTRUMENTS

Just as there are various sources of radioisotope that are used in radiation therapy, there are numerous methods of applying them in clinical practice. It has been apparent since the first uses of brachytherapy that applicator design is important in maintenance of source positioning and radiation safety. As stated earlier, there are several generalized methods of brachytherapy application: external or mold, interstitial, and intracavitary therapy.[11]

External Applicators or Molds

When a patient presents with a well-circumscribed surface lesion that requires a high localized dose, surface molds are commonly used.[1] External applicators usually are molded to fit snugly on the surface of the affected area, with areas specified for radioisotope placement. These molds can be designed to incorporate shielding for adjacent sensitive structures so that they do not receive as high a dose as the lesion. These molds can be designed to fit any shape. Sometimes impressions are made of the body part so that a detailed anatomic template with custom isotope pathways can be designed.

Eye plaques are also a means of using radioisotopes with external application. Iodine-125 is used in the management of uveal melanoma of the eye. Brachytherapy is employed in the management of this disease because of its ability effectively treat tumors near the optic nerve and macula without causing loss of vision secondary to radiation-induced changes. The plaque carrier arranges the sources in appropriate positions so that adequate dose distributions are obtained (Fig. 15-6). The efficacy of this treatment method is often compared with stereotactic and proton therapy procedures, conformal modalities that strive to also deposit high doses of radiation to the tumor while sparing normal and sensitive tissues and structures.

Areas commonly treated with external applicators include any areas on the skin, oral cavity, nasal cavity, hard palate, and orbital cavity, just to name a few. Ingenuity and creative thinking are typically used in creating applicators for treatment of these superficial lesions.

Interstitial Applicators

Interstitial brachytherapy places the radioactive sources directly into or adjacent to the tumor or tumor bed. There are both permanent and temporary applications of interstitial implants used in radiation therapy.

Permanent implants. Permanent implants are performed when the tumor to be treated is inaccessible making the removal of the radioisotope impossible or impractical. Iodine-125 and gold-198 are ideally suited for permanent implants because of their short half-lives. The patient who receives these types of implants does not have to have a second surgical procedure to remove the isotopes. The volumes to be treated commonly require placement of many sources; this requires a rapid and accurate means of application. To accomplish this, gun type applicators with a long, hollow insertion needle is often used. Often, computer tomography (CT) guided, the needle is pushed through the skin into the deep tumor, and the sources are inserted into the tumor. The needle is then withdrawn 5 to 10 mm and the next source is inserted. This is repeated until the desired length and number of sources are applied. Permanent implants using iodine-125 and gold-198 are ideally suited for deep-seated lesions in the pelvis, abdomen, and lung. Fig. 15-7 demonstrates images used in planning a gold-198 colorectal implant to address a recurrence.

Temporary implants. Temporary, removable implants are used in anatomic areas where there is no body cavity or orifice to accept radioactive sources.[1,7] The sources are placed directly into the tumor and tumor bed for a short period of time to deliver a high dose to the area. Radiation therapy boost fields often use of this method of brachytherapy application.

Hollow stainless steel needles can be pushed through the tissues to accommodate catheters holding radioisotopes. Iridium-192 afterloading is used in most applications. The tubes are spaced 1 cm apart; several planes may be used, depending on the tumor size. Catheters are placed in the tubes before removal. When the stainless steel tubes are removed, the catheters are left in place, ready to accommodate dummy sources. Dummy sources are nonradioactive radiopaque seeds that can be seen on a radiographic image. The sources are aligned and spaced just as the radioactive seeds would be. This is done to enable visualization of source placement, to ensure that the implants are positioned correctly, and for treatment planning and dose calculation without unnecessary radiation exposure to the patient and personnel. This is the basic principle of remote afterloading. Table 15-5 outlines the advantages and disadvantages of remote afterloaders.

Once the placement is confirmed, the dummy sources can

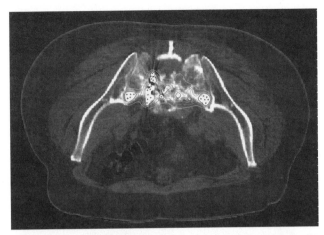

Figure 15-7. Gold-198 permanent seed implant. Note the small size and clustering of the source placement.

be replaced with the radioactive sources and left in place for the desired time. This technique is commonly used in, but not limited to, breast and chest wall irradiation.[1,7,12] Fig. 15-8 demonstrates an iridium-192 breast implant radiograph. Anterior, lateral, and posterior walls of the vagina are also treated with interstitial afterloading techniques (Fig. 15-9).

To improve the accuracy of needle placement and to maintain position during treatment, stabilizers and guides can be used. These are popular in transperineal implants. In these applications, ultrasound as well as radiographic imaging can be used to confirm location and placement of sources. Fig. 15-10 demonstrates a Syed-Neblett template radiograph. Cancers of the rectum, prostate, vagina, and urethra are commonly treated with this applicator.

Intracavitary Applicators

Insertion of radioactive sources into body cavities has been a viable component of radiation therapy for many years.[1,3,7] Several applicators have been designed and used, most for the treatment of gynecologic tumors. The designs used in the newer applicators allow for customized, intricate dose distributions maximizing dose to the tumor and sparing dose to adjacent, sensitive structures (such as the rectum and urinary bladder). Extensive knowledge of physics and anatomy are required to be effective in the dose delivery using this brachytherapy application.

Tandem and ovoids. Gynecologic malignancies are usually treated using standard apparatus; however, standardized applicators typically have room in their design for customized modifications. Gynecologic insertions are done with both LDR and HDR applications today.

A central tandem and a pair of lateral ovoids are commonly used in brachytherapy applications involving the cervix (Fig. 15-11). The **tandem** is a long narrow tube that inserts into the opening of the cervix (cervical os) into the uterus. **Ovoids,** or colpostats, are oval shaped and insert into

Table 15-5	Advantages and disadvantages of remote afterloading systems	
Advantages		**Disadvantages**
Reduction or elimination of exposure to medical personnel		Remote afterloaders are expensive
Treatment techniques are more consistent		Increased maintenance costs
In HDR, allows outpatient treatment thus lowering costs		In HDR, increased room shielding may be needed
In LDR, sources can be retracted in an emergency situation		

HDR, High-dose-rate; *LDR,* low-dose-rate.

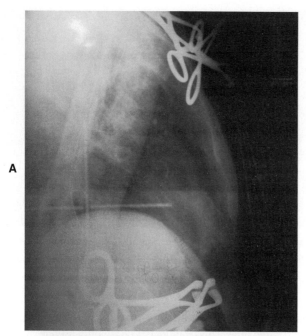

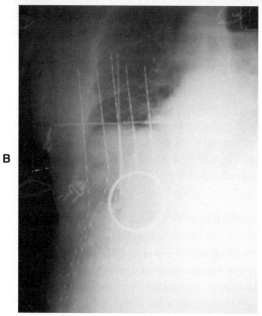

Figure 15-8. Iridium-192 breast implant. Note how the dummy sources can be seen and used for dose calculation. Magnification ring allows for accurate size perspective to be realized. **A,** Anterior. **B,** Lateral.

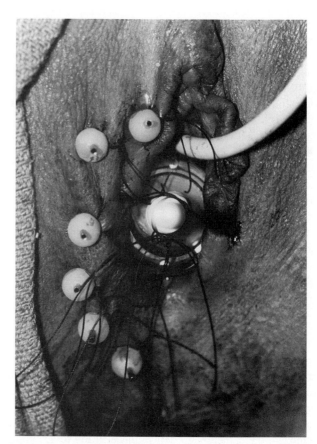

Figure 15-9. Delclos stainless steel needles for afterloading. Iridium implant of the lateral vaginal wall. Note Foley catheter and empty vaginal cylinder.

the lateral fornices of the vagina. Both components are hollow and can accommodate several radioactive sources. The ovoids come in various sizes to accommodate the variances in anatomic structures (wide or narrow vaginas). These ovoids can have shielding that customizes the dose distributions in such a way that dose to the urinary bladder and rectum is minimized. Tandems and ovoids are placed into the female anatomy and stabilized with packing. This packing (sterile gauze) not only stabilizes the apparatus during its 2- to 3-day

placement in the vagina but also serves to displace the rectum and bladder from the sources. Remember that radioisotope emissions adhere to the inverse square law. The farther structures are from the sources, the less dose they will receive.

Location of the applicator is verified with radiographic images and dose calculations can be performed (Fig. 15-12). Once loaded with sources, the tandem and ovoids typically demonstrate a pear-shaped isodose distribution (Fig. 15-13). Currently the standard treatment unit is the cGy to a specific anatomic point or isodose line. The anatomic points used historically for cervical and uterine treatment is points A and B. Point A is located 2 cm superior and 2 cm lateral to the center of the cervical canal (at the cervical os) in the plane of the uterus. Point B was originally 3 cm lateral to point A but is currently noted as being 1 cm lateral to the medial aspect of the pelvic side wall (Fig. 15-14). The dose at point B is typically about one third that at point A. Although these points of dose specification have been used for years, their location is not standard in all patients. Anatomic differences can cause variances. Each case must be considered individually.

Heyman capsules. Heyman capsules allow the uterus to be packed with stainless steel capsules that house cesium sources to treat uterine cancers that are inoperable (Fig. 15-15). Metal

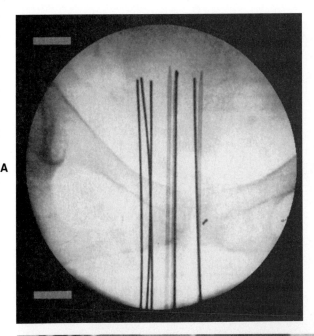

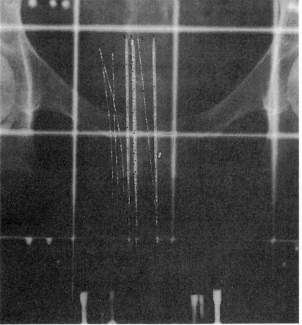

Figure 15-10. Radiograph of a Syed-Neblett template technique for a vaginal carcinoma. **A,** Radiograph of needle placement during surgery. **B,** Radiograph of stylets loaded with dummy iridium-192 sources.

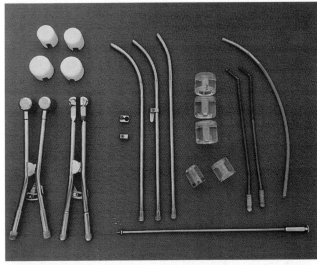

Figure 15-11. Fletcher suit, Delclos Manual Afterloading System. From *left to right:* Small colpostats with additional caps for conversion to medium and large; microcolpostats; intrauterine "tandems"; Delclos and cylindrical colpostats (selected); colpostats carriers; tandem carrier. *Bottom:* (Horizontal) dead seed implanter and seeds. *(From Fletcher GH: Textbook of radiotherapy, Baltimore, 1980, Williams & Wilkins.)*

wires are attached to the capsule (which now can be remote afterloaded) for removal; they protrude through the vagina. Localization of the sources for dose calculation can be done just as in the other applications.

Vaginal cylinders. There are a variety of customized applicators designed to give a high dose to vaginal lesions without giving excessive dose to the urinary bladder or rectum. The applicators are of different lengths, diameters, and

shielding design. In other words, individual application of treatment is optimized. Several designs, like the Delclos uterine-vaginal afterloading system, are designed for simultaneous treatment of the uterine cavity, cervix, and vaginal walls.[1] Vaginal cylinders can be used in conjunction with interstitial implants. The cylinder can not only place sources in proximity to diseased anatomy but it can also assist in the shielding of anatomy from radiation by both shielding material in the applicator as well as the application of the inverse square law.

A specialized type of intracavitary brachytherapy places sources within body tubes such as the esophagus, trachea, and biliary tract. Obstructive lesions can be addresses by placing radioactive sources onto or adjacent to the lesions. Pulsed HDR applications for these types of treatments using cesium-137 and iridium-192 have been done successfully.

Intravascular Stent Applications

There are an increasing number of clinical trials evaluating the role of intravascular brachytherapy radiation following percutaneous transluminal coronary angioplasty (PTCA), an alternative to coronary artery bypass grafts (CABG), to inhibit restenosis in coronary arteries. Although PTCA alone has benefits over CABG surgery, its effectiveness is limited by restenosis occurring in some patients after treatment. It is thought that the addition of radiation may reduce the rate of restenosis in patients receiving the stent therapy. This radiation dose may be delivered with either brachytherapy or external beam. However, because of cardiac motion, external

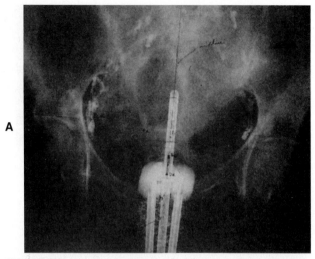

A

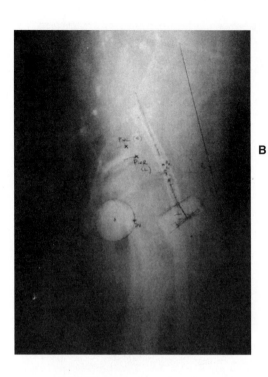

B

Figure 15-12. Orthogonal radiographs of tandem and ovoid location. Note the packing that serves to stabilize the placement of the applicators as well as "push" the urinary bladder and rectum out of the way. **A,** Anterior. **B,** Lateral. *(From Cox JD: Moss' radiation oncology, ed 7, St. Louis, 1994, Mosby.)*

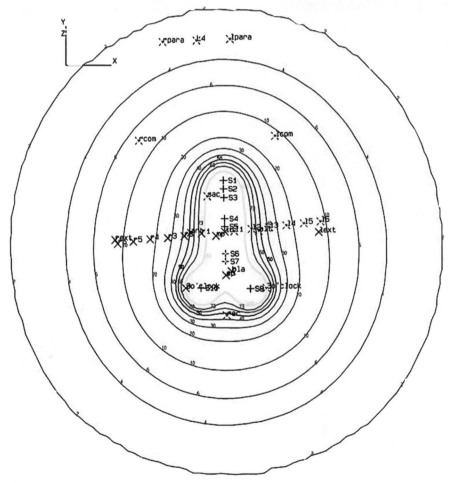

Figure 15-13. Pear-shaped isodose distribution obtained with the use of a tandem and ovoid applicator. Note that the fuller, inferior portion of the distribution can be attributed to the contribution of dose from the location of the ovoids.

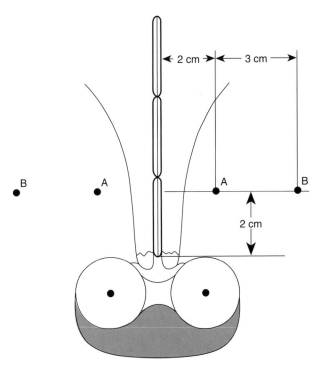

Figure 15-14. Diagram of points *A* and *B*.

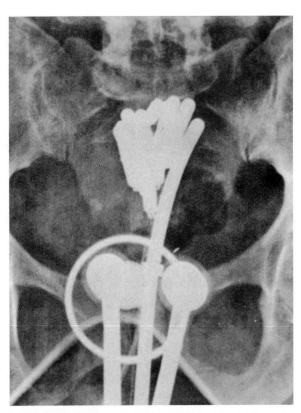

Figure 15-15. Heyman capsules in the endometrium. *(From Fletcher GH: Textbook of radiotherapy, Baltimore, 1980, Williams & Wilkins.)*

beam may be better suited for irradiation of peripheral vessels than coronary vessels.[13,14]

Intravascular brachytherapy may be delivered with either catheter-based systems or radioactive stents. Catheter-based systems consists of a linear array of sources, like ^{192}Ir, attached to a guide wire and inserted into the balloon catheter and pushed into place in the stented area. Other catheter-based systems under development include a number beta sources with phosporus-32 (^{32}P), yttrium-90 (^{90}Y), and strontium-90/yttrium-90 (^{90}Sr/^{90}Y) receiving the most consideration at this time.[8]

BRACHYTHERAPY DOSIMETRY AND DOSE DISTRIBUTION

Dose distribution from radium-226 is the basis of all dose calculations in brachytherapy. As seen earlier, knowing the relationship of radium substitutes and radium allows the radiation therapy practitioner to deliver a dose to a patient accurately. A keen knowledge of anatomy and adherence to a few rules will provide the medical dosimetrist and radiation therapist to develop optimized treatment plans for patients. This section provides basic rules and generalized discussion of dosimetry and dose distribution for interstitial implants. Three systems are discussed: Paterson-Parker, Quimby, and Paris.

The Paterson-Parker (Manchester) System

Using the gamma factor of radium, is it possible to perform radium dosimetry calculations, assuming the point source approximations stated previously. However, for patient dosime-

try a number of sources are typically used, and the accurate calculation of the dose distributions from these implants is a complex procedure. Also, it requires that the radioactive sources be implanted in the patient before the calculations are done, so the physician, medical physicist, and medical dosimetrist have no idea of how the patient is being treated until after the sources are already in place. In the 1930s Ralston Paterson and H.M. Parker at the Manchester Hospital in England developed a series of guidelines and dosimetry methods known as the Paterson-Parker or Manchester system of radium dosimetry to remove these difficulties.

The Paterson-Parker system establishes a set of guidelines that, if followed, will provide a dose of ±10% within the implanted area. Implantation philosophy strives to deliver a uniform dose to a plane or volume. This system uses a nonuniform distribution of radioactive material to produce a uniform distribution of dose. The system assumes the use of linear sources to be implanted in tissue in planes or other geometrical shapes and gives rules for placing the radium sources in each case. Then, the system provides dose tables, which, if distribution rules have been followed, can be used to calculate the dose within the volume. Rules have been established for both planar and volume implants.[2,11]

Planar implants. Planar arrangements of sources can

Table 15-6	Spacing sources in a Paterson-Parker planar implant	
Area	**Activity in periphery/activity over area**	
Area < 25 cm^2	$\frac{2}{3}$	
25 cm^2 < Area < 100 cm^2	$\frac{1}{2}$	
Area > 100 cm^2	$\frac{1}{3}$	

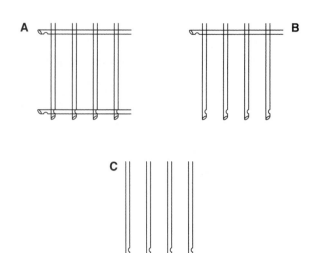

Figure 15-16. Planar implants. **A,** Both ends crossed. **B,** One crossed end (reduce treatment area calculation by 10%). **C,** No crossed ends (reduce treatment area in calculation by 20%).

be summarized in Table 15-6 for square and rectangular implants. In multiple plane implants, the planes should be 1 cm apart and parallel. If there is no crossing source at one or both ends, the area is reduced by 10% for each uncrossed end (Fig. 15-16). If the plane is not square, increase the mg-hr by the appropriate elongation factor for the ratio of long side to short side. Fig. 15-17 depicts a single-plane implant.

For circular and near circular areas the activity should first be placed on the periphery, preferably using more than five sources with spacing no greater than the treatment distance. Then more sources are arranged in an inner circle of half the diameter of the original area. Remaining sources go in the center. The distribution of activity is governed by the ratio of the diameter to the treatment distance.[2] Parameters are outlined in Table 15-7.

Volume implants. If the shape of the implanted volume resembles a three-dimensional shape more than a plane, it is called a volume implant. Shapes defined by the Paterson-Parker system include cylinders, ellipsoids (football-shaped volumes), spheres, and cubes, among others. This type of

Table 15-7	Circular source distribution in Paterson-Parker circular implant				
Diameter/distance (cm)	1-3	3-6	6	7.5	10
Outer circle (%)	100	95	80	75	70
Inner circle (%)	0	0	17	22	27
Center (%)	0	5	3	3	3

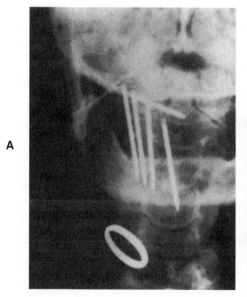
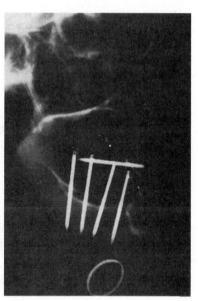

Figure 15-17. Single-plane implant. **A,** Image of a planar implant. **B,** Single-plane implant. *(From Cox JD: Moss' radiation oncology, ed 7, St. Louis, 1994, Mosby.)*

16

Radiation Safety and Protection

Joseph S. Blinick, Elizabeth G. Quate

Outline

Key Terms

Absorbed dose
Activity
Advisory agencies
ALARA
Alpha particle
Beta particle
Dose equivalent
Effective dose equivalent
Exposure
Film badge
Gamma ray
Genetically significant dose

Ionizing radiation
LET
Natural background radiation
Occupancy factor
Photons
Pocket ionization chambers
Regulatory agencies
Thermoluminescent dosimeters
Use factor
Workload
X-ray

The levels of radiation **exposure** in a radiation therapy department can be quite high. Thus it is important to consider the principles of radiation protection to avoid unnecessary exposure to patients, operators, and the general public.

In this chapter we discuss types of radiation and their sources as well as the detection and measurement of levels of radiation in the environment of a therapy department. We also discuss the risks of exposure to **ionizing radiation** (radiation with sufficient energy to separate an electron from its atom), the regulatory requirements for limits of exposure to radiation for various groups, and practical methods for individual radiation protection.

DETECTION AND MEASUREMENT

Types of Radiation

Within a radiation therapy department, there are two major groups of radiation sources. The first comprises external beam therapy machines, such as cobalt teletherapy units or linear accelerators. These use gamma rays, x-rays, and sometimes electrons. The second group comprises brachytherapy sources, which use gamma rays and x-rays from sources such as cesium-137 (^{137}Cs), iridium-192 (^{192}Ir), and iodine-125 (^{125}I). Sources in this group may also emit alpha and beta particles. Table 16-1 summarizes types of ionizing radiation and some of their characteristics.

    Alpha particles. **Alpha particles** consist of two protons and two neutrons and are therefore simply helium nuclei. They are emitted from unstable heavy nuclei such as radium or radon during the decay process. Because of their charge

Table 16-1	Types of ionizing radiation		
Type of Radiation	**Charge**	**Atomic Mass Number**	**Origin**
Alpha particles (α)	+2	4	Nucleus
Beta particles			
Negatron (β⁻)	–1	0	Nucleus
Positron (β⁺)	+1	0	Nucleus
Neutrinos (ν)	0	0	Nucleus
X-rays	0	0	Electron shells
Gamma rays (γ)	0	0	Nucleus

and relatively heavy mass, alpha particles can only travel short distances (most can be stopped by a sheet of paper), but they produce intense ionization and are therefore high linear energy transfer (**LET**) radiation. Thus they are extremely hazardous if ingested or inhaled but are less dangerous if the exposure is external. Alpha particles emitted by radium and radon are easily stopped by the material used to encapsulate the sources. If the integrity of the capsule is compromised, however, exposure to alpha particles is possible.

Beta particles. Beta particles are electrons emitted by the nucleus. They may be either negatively charged (negatron or β⁻) or positively charged (positron or β⁺). Positrons are not stable and may exist for only very short periods of time. Whenever beta particles are emitted, they are accompanied by a small, massless, chargeless particle known as the neutrino (see Chapter 14). Both types of beta particles have the same rest mass as an electron and are usually emitted from the nucleus with high velocities. Beta particles and energetic electrons are more penetrating than alpha particles and may pose both an external and an internal threat. High-energy (1 MeV) beta particles may have a range as long as 2 cm in soft tissue. Metals may be used for shielding, but bremsstrahlung radiation may result. The probability of bremsstrahlung x-ray production is directly proportional to the square of the atomic number of the absorber and inversely proportional to the square of the mass of the incident particle.[1] Thus bremsstrahlung radiation is much more likely to occur with beta particles than with alpha particles. It is often more suitable to shield beta particles with low atomic number materials, such as plastics or glass, than with metals, such as lead or steel.

X-rays and gamma rays. X-rays and gamma rays are both forms of electromagnetic radiation (photons). **Photons** have no mass and no charge. **Gamma rays** are photons emitted from a nucleus. **X-rays** are extranuclear and result from rearrangements within the electron shells or from bremsstrahlung radiation. Except for their origin, there is no difference between x-rays and gamma rays. X-rays and gamma rays may be more penetrating than either alpha or

beta particles, and substantial shielding may be required, depending on the energy of the photon.

Sources of Radiation

People have been exposed to naturally occurring ionizing radiation since the beginning of time. However, it was not until the beginning of the twentieth century that the general public had any exposure to manmade sources of radiation. In fact, even today, it is estimated that 82% of the exposure of the U.S. population to radiation comes from natural background sources[5] (Fig. 16-1).

Natural background radiation. Natural background radiation comes from three sources: cosmic rays that bombard the earth, terrestrial radiation that emanates from radioactive materials naturally occurring in the earth, and internal deposits of radionuclides in our bodies:

1. *Cosmic rays.* Cosmic rays originate from nuclear reactions in space or from our own sun. Although the earth's atmosphere acts as a protective shield against much of the initial bombardment, the primary cosmic rays interact with molecules in the atmosphere to create other reactive agents, known as secondary particles. These include neutrons, protons, and pions (short-lived subnuclear particles), which go on to produce energetic electrons, muons (another subnuclear particle), and photons. The average annual effective dose equivalent at sea level in the United States from cosmic rays is about 0.26 millisieverts (mSv) (26 millirems [mrem]). The exposure from cosmic rays varies with solar sunspot cycles, latitude, and altitude. The magnetic nature of the earth accounts for the variation in dose resulting from latitude. The charged particles incident on the earth are drawn along the magnetic field lines, which are directed toward the poles. Thus exposure is higher at the polar regions than at the equator. Latitude, solar cycles, and other factors may account for a variation of 10% in exposure. The intensity varies even more with increasing elevation. The dose approximately doubles with each 2000-m increase in altitude in the lower atmosphere, because there is less atmosphere to absorb the incident rays. People in Denver (elevation 1600 m) receive about 0.5 mSv (50 mrem) from cosmic rays.[5]

2. *Terrestrial radiation.* The earth is made up of hundreds of materials, many of which are naturally radioactive because of the presence of small amounts of long-lived isotopes of uranium, thorium, and radium, among others. This is the source of terrestrial radiation. The distribution of these materials varies with geographical location and the composition of the soil in the area. In the United States the average annual effective dose equivalent is 0.16 mSv (16 mrem) along the Eastern Seaboard but may be as high as 0.63 mSv (63 mrem) in the Rocky Mountains.[5] Additional exposure to the public occurs because many materials used in construction contain these radioactive elements. The largest exposure to terrestrial radiation involves radon. Radon may be particularly harmful because it is an easily inhaled gas and it and its many progeny emit alpha and beta particles as well as gamma rays. Lung tissue can be damaged as deposited products decay. Radon concentration

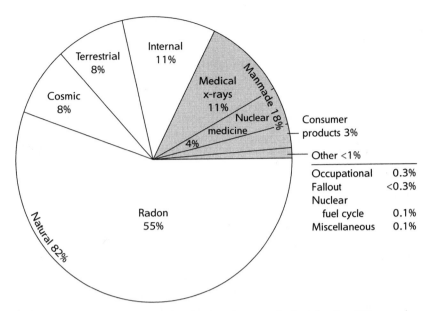

Figure 16-1. The total average effective dose equivalent for the U.S. population results from many sources of both natural and manmade radiation. This diagram illustrates the percentage that each of these sources contributes to the effective dose equivalent. *(From National Council on Radiation Protection and Measurements: Report No. 93, Ionizing radiation exposure of the population of the United States, Bethesda, MD, 1987, NCRP Publications.)*

in houses varies greatly with the makeup of the soil, the design of the building, and the degree to which it is airtight. The average radon concentration in the United States is 37 millibecquerel/L (1 pCi/L), which yields about 2 mSv (200 mrem) to the bronchial epithelium per year.[2] The Environmental Protection Agency (EPA) estimates that radon exposure is the second leading cause of lung cancer in the United States (following smoking).[7]

3. *Internal exposure.* Internal exposure results from the radioactive materials that are normally present in our bodies. These include carbon-14, hydrogen-3, strontium-90, potassium-40, and very small amounts of uranium and thorium. Potassium-40 delivers the highest dose to the body (0.2 mSv/year or 20 mrem/year). Again, concentrations of these radioactive materials in the body depend on geographic location.

The average annual **effective dose equivalent** in the United States resulting from natural background radiation is estimated to be about 1.0 mSv (100 mrem) from all sources except radon. When radon is taken into consideration, the average increases to about 3.0 mSv (300 mrem).[5] These values can vary greatly. In the Kerala region of India, for example, the annual dose may be as great as 13 mSv (1300 mrem).[2]

Manmade sources.   Manmade sources also contribute to the annual dose to individuals. These sources include medical x-rays, nuclear medicine procedures, consumer products such as televisions and tobacco products, nuclear reactors, and the fuel cycle and fallout from above-ground nuclear weapons testing. These sources emit a broad spectrum of alpha and beta particles, electrons, x-rays, and gamma rays. The average

annual effective dose equivalent from these sources to an exposed individual is about 0.60 mSv (60 mrem). Medical procedures contribute about 0.50 mSv (50 mrem) of that total, and consumer products contribute another 0.11 mSv (11 mrem).[5] The other sources together contribute less than 1% of the dose from manmade sources. However, the potential for much higher radiation exposure from these nuclear sources is evident in light of the atomic bomb explosions at Hiroshima and Nagasaki in 1945 and the Chernobyl power plant incident in the Soviet Union in 1986. The other significant dose from manmade sources is from tobacco products. Smokers inhale radioactive materials that are present naturally in tobacco (primarily polonium-210) and may receive an additional annual effective dose equivalent of 13 mSv (1300 mrem).[5]

Most of the radiation to which the general population is exposed comes from natural background radiation, smokers excluded. It is not possible to effectively protect the entire population from these sources. That is why it is important to do all we can to minimize the radiation exposures from manmade sources, and why we strive to develop and implement valid radiation protection practices.

Units

Exposure is defined as the amount of ionization produced by photons in air per unit mass of air. The traditional unit for exposure is the roentgen. One roentgen (R) of exposure creates 2.58×10^{-4} coulomb (C) of charge per kilogram (kg) of air. The Système Internationale (SI) unit for exposure is C/kg of air (see Table 16-2 for conversions between traditional

Table 16-2	Traditional and SI unit equivalents		
Exposure	1 roentgen	=	2.59×10^{-4} C/kg
Absorbed dose	1 rad	=	0.01 Gy
Dose equivalent	1 rem	=	0.01 Sv
Activity	1 Ci	=	3.7×10^{10} Bq

units and SI units). Exposure is only defined for ionization produced by photons interacting with air. For practical reasons, exposure is limited to photons whose energy is less than 3 MeV.

Absorbed dose is defined as the energy absorbed per unit mass of any material. The traditional unit for absorbed dose is the rad, defined as 100 ergs of energy absorbed per gram of absorbing material. The comparable SI unit is the gray (Gy), which is defined as 1 joule of energy absorbed per kilogram of absorbing material (1 Gy = 100 cGy = 100 rad). For interactions between photons and soft tissue (i.e., most tissue besides bone), the numerical values for absorbed dose in rad and the exposure in R will be the same to within 10%. This difference may be ignored for radiation protection purposes but is significant when therapeutic doses to patients are being calculated or measured.

Dose equivalent takes into account the fact that different types of radiation produce different amounts of biologic damage. Alpha particles and neutrons, for example, are high-LET radiation and therefore have a greater biologic effect than x-rays. Thus a 0.2 Gy (20 cGy) absorbed dose of alpha particles would be more damaging to a given mass of human tissue than a 0.2 Gy (20 cGy) absorbed dose of x-rays. To account for these differences in biologic response, each type of radiation is assigned a quality factor (QF). The traditional unit, rem, is defined as the product of the absorbed dose in rads times the QF. The SI unit is the sievert (Sv), and it is defined as the absorbed dose in gray times the QF. For photons and most electrons, the QF is taken to be 1, so that the numerical values of the dose equivalent in Sv or rem and the absorbed dose in Gy are the same.

Effective dose equivalent takes into account the effect of irradiation of only part of the body or the effect of nonuniform irradiation of the body. The dose to each significant organ is multiplied by a weighting factor for that organ and the sum is taken. The resultant value provides a measure of the risk to the individual that a uniform exposure to the entire body of the same value would have. The units for effective dose equivalent are also the sievert and the rem.

Activity is the rate at which a radioactive isotope undergoes nuclear decay. The traditional unit of activity is the curie (Ci), which is defined as 3.7×10^{10} disintegrations per second. The SI unit is the becquerel (Bq), which is 1 disintegration per second.

Measurement Devices

Many instruments and devices can be used to detect radiation, and several find use within the radiation oncology department. An instrument designed to calibrate the radiation output of a therapy machine will not necessarily be suitable for measuring low levels of radioactive contamination. It is important to understand the characteristics of each measuring device and the applications for which each is used.

Gas-filled detectors. One type of device is the gas-filled detector. This instrument has a chamber filled with a gas that is ionized in part or whole when radiation is present. Either the total quantity of electrical charge is measured or the rate at which charge is produced is measured. Two kinds of gas-filled detectors may be found in a radiation therapy department. These are the ionization chamber and the Geiger-Müller (G-M) detector.

The simplest of these, the ionization chamber, consists of two electrodes within a gas-filled chamber, an applied voltage across the electrodes, and electronics and a meter to amplify and measure the electrical signal (Fig. 16-2). The sensitivity of the chamber (smallest amount of radiation detectable) depends on the mass of gas within the chamber (chamber volume). The response of the chamber also depends on the applied voltage (Fig. 16-3). If there is no voltage, the positive and negative ions produced in the gas by the radiation will recombine instead of migrating to either of the electrodes. As the voltage across the electrodes is increased, more and more of the ions produced in the chamber will be collected on the electrodes; positive ions migrate to the cathode and negative ions to the anode. Ideally, ionization chambers should be operated at a voltage at which all of the ion pairs are collected and none recombine. Such a voltage (typically 100 to 300 volts) is said to produce saturation. When a positive ion reaches the cathode, it combines with one of the negative charges to form a neutral atom. This leaves a negative charge vacancy on the cathode, which is filled by a negative charge (electron) from the battery. The electrometer detects either the total charge that flows or the rate of charge flow and displays the value on the meter. The calibration can be set to read mR or mR/hour.

When properly calibrated, the accuracy of ionization chambers approaches 2%, which makes them suitable for measurement of the radiation output of therapy equipment. Ionization chambers with large air volumes are also suitable for environmental surveys around therapy rooms.

A form of ionization chamber, the pocket dosimeter, is used for personnel monitoring (Fig. 16-4). In this chamber the electrodes are arranged concentrically—that is, one electrode is in the form of a thin rod and the other is a cylinder around it. When fully charged, a thin filament within the unit is displaced by static electricity to one end of a scale that can be viewed by holding the dosimeter up to a light. As radiation ionizes the air within the chamber, the ions deplete the charges on the electrodes and the filament is not displaced as far. The instrument is calibrated so that the position of the

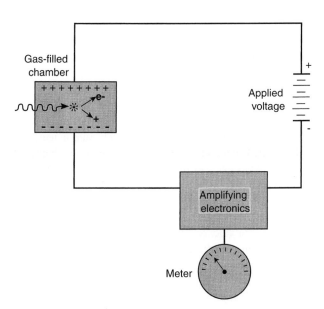

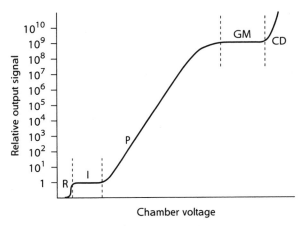

Figure 16-3. The signal output from a gas-filled chamber depends on applied voltage. The stages of the chamber response are R, recombination region; I, ionization region; P, proportional region; GM, Geiger-Müller region; CD, region of continuous discharge. *(From Bushong SC: Radiologic science for technologists—physics, biology and protection, ed 7, St. Louis, 2000, Mosby.)*

Figure 16-2. An ionization chamber that consists of two electrodes within a gas-filled chamber. A voltage is applied across the electrodes. Electronics and a meter are used to amplify and measure the electrical signal.

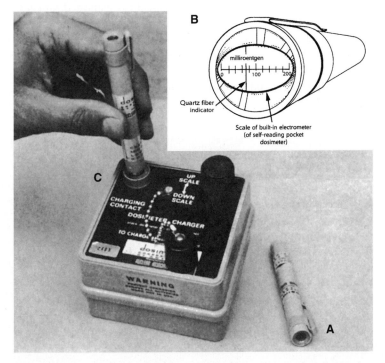

Figure 16-4. Pocket ionization chamber. **A,** The pocket ionization chamber, or pocket dosimeter, resembles a fountain pen. **B,** The quartz fiber indicator of the built-in electrometer of the self-reading pocket dosimeter generally used in radiology indicates exposures of 0 to 5.2×10^{-5} C/kg (0 to 200 milliroentgens). **C,** Before use the pocket dosimeter must be charged to a predetermined voltage by a special charging unit so that the charges of the positive and negative electrodes will be balanced and the quartz fiber indicator reads zero. *(Courtesy Dosimeter Corporation of America, Cincinnati, Ohio.)*

filament indicates the amount of exposure received by the chamber.

Because ionization chambers are not very sensitive, they are not suitable for the detection of very low levels of radiation or radiation contamination.

If the chamber voltage is increased beyond that of the saturation region, the primary ions are energetic enough to produce additional ionizations, or secondary ions, in the gas. The G-M region is reached as the voltage of the chamber is increased even further. An avalanche of secondary ions is produced for each primary ionization that occurs, so that individual events can be detected. This makes the G-M counter a very sensitive instrument and appropriate for detecting low levels of radiation or radioactive contamination (Fig. 16-5). G-M detectors tend to be strongly energy dependent, which means they respond differently to different photon energies. In addition, if a G-M detector is placed in a high-level radiation field, it may produce a reading of zero because of overloading of the gas-filled detector. Increasing the voltage beyond the G-M range causes the gas insulation to break down. Electrical arcing occurs, and a continuous electrical discharge is produced. There is no useful reason for a detector to operate in this range, and damage to the chamber may result.

Thermoluminescent dosimeters.   Because of their small size, **thermoluminescent dosimeters** (TLDs) are widely used to measure radiation in a number of applications (Fig. 16-6). As the name implies, thermoluminescent materials give off light when heated. Whenever a crystalline material is irradiated, electrons are released from bound states in the valence band and become free to migrate in the conduction band. An energy gap separates these two regions, and it is this energy gap that must be overcome by the energy of the incoming radiation. In most materials, electrons immediately drop back from the conduction band to the valence band with the emission of characteristic photons. However, in some materials such as lithium fluoride (LiF) with some impurities deliberately introduced into the crystal structure, traps appear in the energy gap, and some of the electrons that would otherwise drop back to the valence band get caught in the traps. At a later time, if the crystal is heated to 100° to 200° C, the electrons will receive enough thermal energy to move back into the conduction band. Most of them immediately fall back to the valence band with the release of the characteristic photons. In the case of LiF (and other thermoluminescent materials), these characteristic photons are within the visible light range. In general, the more radiation absorbed by the crystal, the more electrons will be in traps, and the more characteristic photons will be released when the crystal is heated later. Thus the amount of light is a measure of the dose received by the crystal.

The atomic number of LiF is close to that of tissue (Li has an atomic number of 3, and F has an atomic number of 9), so LiF mimics tissue closely and is therefore useful as a patient or phantom dosimeter. If proper care is taken, doses can be measured with an accuracy of approximately 5%. TLDs are also used for mailed intercomparison of therapy unit calibration; in ring badges used for personnel monitoring; and for measurements of environmental levels of radiation. In these applications, TLDs have the advantage

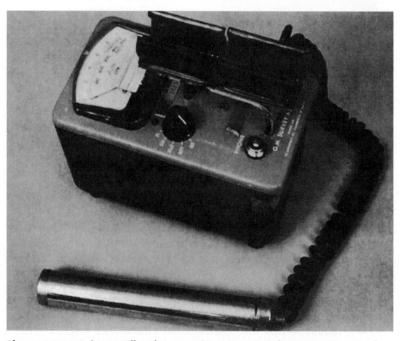

Figure 16-5. Geiger-Müller detector. *(Courtesy Baird Corporation, Nuclear Instruments Division, Bedford, Massachusetts.)*

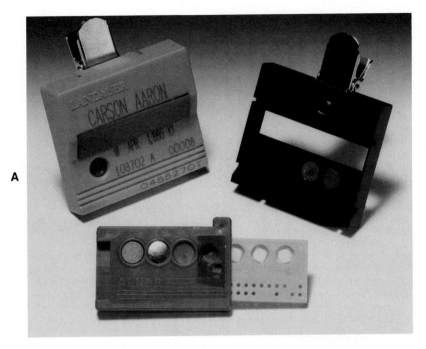

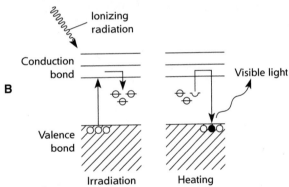

Figure 16-6. Thermoluminescent dosimeters may be used in a number of applications in a radiation therapy department. **A,** A badge containing chips may be used for personnel monitoring. **B,** Electron transitions occurring when thermoluminescent LiF is irradiated and heated. (**A,** *Courtesy Landauer, Inc, Glenwood, Illinois;* **B,** *From Bushong SC: Radiologic science for technologists—physics, biology and protection, ed 7, St. Louis, 2000, Mosby.)*

that the dose information can be stored for hours, days, or even weeks, until the dosimeter is heated. However, the readings may diminish with time because some of the electrons spontaneously leak out of the traps. In addition, if the dosimeter is heated in transit, all the information may be lost. Despite this potential disadvantage, thermoluminescent dosimetry is a well-established technique for the measurement of radiation.

Film. After development, x-ray film exposed to radiation turns black. The amount of blackness is called the optical density, and the optical density is related to the amount of radiation received by the film. The actual relationship is not linear and depends on the type of film, the type and energy of the radiation, and the details of processing the film.

However, once calibrated, film is a convenient and inex-

pensive way to provide information about the doses received by individuals working in or visiting areas where radiation may be present.

A typical **film badge** has a slot in which the film (in its protective paper cover) may be placed and several thin metal filters that surround portions of the film (Fig. 16-7). The filters allow discrimination between different types and energies of radiation. Low-energy radiation will not penetrate any of the filters but can reach the film in the area where no filters are present. Medium-energy radiation will penetrate the no-filter and tin filter areas but will not get through the lead filter. High-energy radiation penetrates all areas. This discrimination is necessary because of the strong energy dependence of film. The response at high energies (1 MeV) may be up to 20 times less than the response at low energies (30 keV).

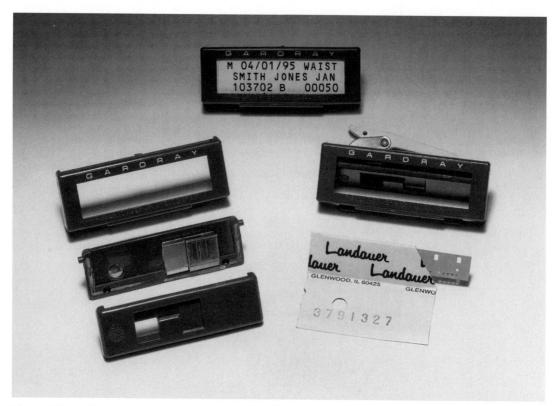

Figure 16-7. Film badge. It consists of sensitive film, several thin metal filters, and a plastic holder. *(Courtesy Landauer, Inc, Glenwood, Illinois.)*

REGULATIONS AND REGULATORY AGENCIES

Advisory and Regulatory Agencies

The primary task of **advisory agencies** is to analyze the existing data related to radiation exposure and to assess the radiobiologic risks associated with those exposures. These agencies can then develop recommendations for dose limits. Some of these agencies include the National Council on Radiation Protection and Measurement (NCRP), the International Commission on Radiation Protection (ICRP), the United Nations Scientific Committee on the Effects of Atomic Radiation (UNSCEAR), and the National Academy of Sciences Advisory Committee on the Biological Effects of Ionizing Radiation (NAS-BEIR). The recommendations may be acted on by Congress or state governments and made into law.

It is the role of the **regulatory agencies** to license users of radioactive materials and radiation-producing equipment, inspect such users, and enforce the appropriate laws. One of the leading federal regulatory agencies in the United States is the Nuclear Regulatory Commission (NRC), which oversees the use of isotopes produced in nuclear reactors. These isotopes are commonly used in nuclear medicine departments, in laboratories, and as sources for teletherapy (external beam radiation) and brachytherapy (internal implants). Many states have entered into agreements concerning licensing, inspection, and enforcement with the NRC and have become "agreement" states. As part of the agreement, states must maintain a certain level of compatibility with NRC regulations.

Transportation of radioactive materials is primarily the concern of the Department of Transportation (DOT) and the NRC. The use of machines that produce ionizing radiation, such as x-ray units and linear accelerators, falls under the jurisdiction of the Food and Drug Administration (FDA) and state agencies. The EPA and the Occupational Safety and Health Administration (OSHA) also have regulations that relate to the use of radiation.

Risk Estimates

Estimating the risks of exposure to ionizing radiation is an extremely complex and difficult process. Although we probably know more about the effects of radiation on humans than is known about any other chemical or biologic hazard, our knowledge is far from complete. Information about the risks of radiation has come from many sources, including victims of the bombs at Hiroshima and Nagasaki, Japan, at the end of World War II; people who received radiation for ankylosing spondylitis; women who received multiple fluoroscopic examinations for tuberculosis; and children treated with radiation for nonmalignant thymus and thyroid diseases.

In all of these cases, individual doses are not known precisely. In addition, individual variations are known to occur for any given radiation dose. Because there are no special effects attributable to ionizing radiation, the many effects that occur at low levels may be indistinguishable from those resulting from normal background levels.

We have a far greater knowledge of the effects of high doses of radiation than those of low doses. In sufficiently high quantities, radiation can be lethal. The lethal dose of whole-body radiation, delivered acutely, to 50% of an exposed human population within 30 days is approximately 4.5 Gy (450 rads). This is known as the $LD_{50/30}$.

Even at levels below the lethal dose there are significant, long-term effects related to exposure to radiation. These fall into two general classifications: nonstochastic and stochastic. Nonstochastic effects are those for which a threshold exists and for which the severity of the effect increases with dose. Examples of such effects are erythema (skin reddening), epilation (loss of hair), cataract formation, and infertility. The threshold doses for these effects are relatively high, which is reflected in the higher permitted doses to the specific organs involved. Stochastic effects are those which have no threshold and for which the probability of occurrence is a function of dose. In this case, the severity of the effect is not a function of the dose. Either the effect occurs or it does not. Examples of stochastic effects are cancer induction, genetic effects, and embryologic and teratogenic effects. Because of the lack of a threshold dose, these effects are of more concern at low levels of radiation exposure. The mechanisms by which these effects occur are discussed in Chapter 4, Radiobiology. Risk estimates for stochastic effects have been compiled by the NCRP in Report No. 115,[6] "Risk Estimates for Radiation Protection." This publication assesses reports prepared by the UNSCEAR (1988), the Committee on the Biological Effects of Ionizing Radiations (BEIR V) (NAS/NRC, 1990), and Publication 60 of the ICRP. These reports discuss in length the methods by which risks associated with radiation exposure are estimated and what those risks are.

Cancer risks. The survivors of the atomic bomb explosions at both Hiroshima and Nagasaki are the primary source for estimating the cancer risks associated with ionizing radiation in NCRP No. 115, although data from other studies were considered. A linear-quadratic response for leukemias and a linear response for solid cancers were used in the estimation process (Fig. 16-8). No distinction was made between high-dose-rate and low-dose-rate exposures. The estimate for lifetime cancer risks for acute whole body exposure to low LET radiation is approximately 8 in 100 per Sv (8 in 10,000 per rem).[6]

Genetic risks. There are large uncertainties in assessing genetic risks. In part the uncertainties occur because the effects mutations have on life-threatening illnesses such as cancer and heart disease are unknown. As a model for radiation protection guidelines, a risk of 1 in 100 per Sv (1 in 10,000 per rem) has been assigned for the occurrence of severe hereditary effects for the general population by the reporting agencies, based only on animal data.[6]

Embryologic and teratogenic effects. The effects of exposure to ionizing radiation on the embryo and fetus are discussed in Chapter 4, Radiobiology. NCRP No. 115 primarily addresses the probability of radiation effects on the fetal brain and the possible induction of childhood cancer. The NCRP assigned an overall risk estimate of 4 in 10 per Gy (4 in 1000 per rem). Both linear and linear-quadratic responses were considered in forming this estimate. In addition, there may be threshold doses below which these effects will not be observed. The thresholds are related to gestational age and are estimated to be 0.12 to 0.23 Gy (12 to 23 rem) for 8 to 16 weeks after conception and 0.23 Gy (230 rem) for 16 to 25 weeks after conception.[6]

The NCRP further estimates that the total detriment from all causes resulting from exposure to low LET radiation is approximately 7 in 100 per Sv (7 in 10,000 per rem) for the general population and about 6 in 100 per Sv (6 in 10,000 per rem) for the working population. This overall risk estimate includes fatal and nonfatal cancers, severe hereditary effects, and nonspecific life shortening.[6] These risks are higher than the previous estimates discussed in NCRP Report No. 91,[4] "Recommendations on Limits for Exposure to Ionizing Radiation," which assigned a nominal lifetime somatic risk of 1 in 100 per Sv (1 in 10,000 per rem) for adults. It is likely that these estimates will change again as more data become available.

There are many uncertainties in assigning risk estimates for the effect of ionizing radiation on humans. These include difficulties in assigning individual doses, choice of appropriate control groups, choice of an appropriate extrapolation model, determination of differences between effects at low dose rates compared to effects at high dose rates, and difficulties with the transfer of risk estimates from one population to another. However, these projections are necessary to develop recommendations for radiation protection standards.

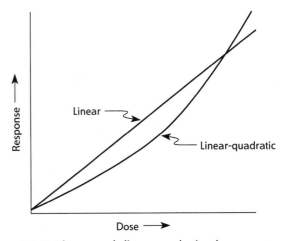

Figure 16-8. Linear and linear-quadratic dose response curves. These are used for estimation of risks from exposure to ionizing radiation. *(From Bushong SC: Radiologic science for technologists—physics, biology and protection, ed 7, St. Louis, 2000, Mosby.)*

Regulatory Concepts

As Low as Reasonably Achievable (ALARA).   Regardless of which models are used to estimate the risks of radiation exposure, it is universally agreed that the less radiation received, the lower the risk. For this reason, it is considered prudent to attempt to maintain exposures as low as reasonably achievable (**ALARA**), in keeping with economic and social factors. In practice, this means that measures should be taken, whenever possible, to reduce individual exposures well below regulatory limits.

Comparable risk.   The NCRP believes that a radiation worker should be at no higher risk of death from his or her employment than a worker in other "safe" industries. A "safe" industry is defined as one in which the annual accidental fatality rate is about 10^{-4} (or 1 in 10,000 per year). The NCRP has made an attempt to compare injuries, illnesses, and accidental death rates in various work places to the risks of ionizing radiation, specifically, cancer induction, and severe hereditary effects. This is a difficult task, in part because of the latent nature of these effects. The effective dose equivalent limits specified by the NCRP reflect the average annual doses received by radiation workers and the risks associated with those doses that we have already discussed.

Genetically significant dose.   The **genetically significant dose** (GSD) is a measure of the genetic risk to a population as a whole from exposure to ionizing radiation of some or all members of that population. It is the effective dose equivalent to the gonads weighted for age and sex distribution. The GSD is the gonadal dose that, if received by every member of the population, would be expected to result in the same total genetic effect on the population as the sum of the individual doses actually received. Everyone does not contribute equally to the GSD. For example, the dose received by a 60-year-old postmenopausal woman would have no impact on the genetic future of a given population. The weighting factor for that person would be zero. The dose received by a teenager would have a much higher impact, because there is a long reproductive life ahead for that person. The weighting factor assigned to the dose for the teenager would reflect the number of children he or she would likely produce. All sources of natural and manmade ionizing radiation contribute some dose to the GSD. NCRP Report No. 93[5] ("Ionizing Radiation Exposure of the Population of the United States") reports the GSD for the United States circa 1980 to 1982 was 1.3 mSv (130 mrem), of which 1.0 mSv (100 mrem) results from natural sources.

Dose Limits

The recommended effective dose equivalent limits for radiation workers and the general public are contained in NCRP Report No. 91 and have been adopted by the NRC and most states. These limits are summarized in Table 16-3.* There are two important points to note about these values: (1) the limits are exclusive of medical exposures for both radiation workers and the general public and (2) the limits are a summation of both internal and external exposures.

Radiation workers.   It can be seen from Table 16-3 that the effective dose equivalent (whole body) limit for radiation workers is more than that for the general public. There are relatively few radiation workers, and it is felt that a slightly increased risk to this group is worth the benefits of radiation to society at large. The same situation occurs in other occupations, such as nursing, driving a truck, or doing construction work, where the amount of risk is similar or even higher.

The effective dose equivalent, which is the limit for stochastic effects, is 50 mSv (5 rem) per year. Nonstochastic limits are set at 150 mSv (15 rem) for the lens of the eye and 500 mSv (50 rem) for all other tissues and organs, including extremities. There are special guidelines for planned special exposures and emergency situations. In general, if the limit for the whole body dose is met by adherence to radiation safety standards at a medical facility, then the nonstochastic limits will also be met.

General public.   The NCRP recommends that the annual effective dose equivalent limit for this population be 1 mSv (0.1 rem) for persons who are exposed continuously or frequently and 5 mSv (0.5 rem) for persons who are infrequently exposed. These limits do not include doses from natural background radiation or medical procedures, which in most cases cannot be controlled.

Embryo/fetus.   The total dose equivalent for an embryo or fetus is 5 mSv (0.5 rem) during the gestational period. It is recommended that the exposure be distributed uniformly with respect to time and should not exceed 0.5 mSv (0.05 rem) in any month.

Personnel Monitoring

Monitoring of the radiation dose received by individual radiation workers serves several purposes: (1) it allows the worker to know how much radiation he or she is receiving (at least in the area where the monitor is kept or worn), (2) it allows the facility safety officer and administration to determine if certain areas or workers are receiving more radiation than expected, and (3) it provides a permanent record of radiation received if questions arise at a later time. The NRC and most state regulatory agencies require individuals to be monitored if it is expected that 10% of the effective dose equivalent limit will be exceeded.

To be effective, devices used for personnel monitoring must be reasonably accurate, inexpensive, and easy to use. Three examples of such devices are the film badge dosimeter, the TLD, and the pocket ionization chamber (pocket

---

*The NCRP has published a more recent report (NCRP No. 116, Limitation of Exposure to Ionizing Radiation, 1993), which has some minor changes in the methodology and recommendations compared to NCRP No. 91.

Table 16-3	Summary of NCRP recommendations*		

A. Occupational exposures (annual)†			
1. Effective dose equivalent limit (stochastic effects)		50 mSv	(5 rem)
2. Dose equivalent limits for tissues and organs (nonstochastic effects)			
a. Lens of eye		150 mSv	(15 rem)
b. All others (e.g., red bone marrow, breast, lung, gonads, skin, and extremities)		500 mSv	(50 rem)
3. Guidance: cumulative exposure		10 mSv × age in years	(1 rem × age in years)
B. Planned special occupational exposure, effective dose equivalent limit†			
C. Guidance for emergency occupational exposure†			
D. Public exposures (annual)			
1. Effective dose equivalent limit, continuous or frequent exposure†		1 mSv	(0.1 rem)
2. Effective dose equivalent limit, infrequent exposure†		5 mSv	(0.5 rem)
3. Remedial action recommended when:			
a. Effective dose equivalent‡		>5 mSv	(>0.5 rem)
b. Exposure to radon and its decay products§		>0.007 Jhm^{-3}	(>2 WLM)
4. Dose equivalent limits for lens of eye, skin, and extremities†		50 mSv	(5 rem)
E. Education and training exposures (annual)†			
1. Effective dose equivalent limit		1 mSv	(0.1 rem)
2. Dose equivalent limit for lens of eye, skin, and extremities		50 mSv	(5 rem)
F. Embryo-fetus exposures†			
1. Total dose equivalent limit		5 mSv	(0.5 rem)
2. Dose equivalent in a month		0.5 mSv	(0.05 rem)
G. Negligible individual risk level (annual)†			
Effective dose equivalent per source or practice		0.01 mSv	(0.001 rem)

From National Council on Radiation Protection and Measurements: Report No. 116. *Limitations of exposure to ionizing radiation*, Bethesda, MD, 1993.
*Excluding medical exposures.
†Sum of external and internal exposures.
‡Including background but excluding internal exposures.
§WLM stands for working level month and refers to a cumulative exposure for a working month (170 hr). As applied to radon and its daughter products, 1 WLM represents the cumulative exposure experienced in a 170-hour period caused by a radon concentration of 100 pCi/L. The occupational limit for miners is 4 WLM/yr, which results in an absorbed dose equivalent of approximately 0.15 Sv (15 rem) per year.

dosimeter). The methods by which these devices work were described earlier in this chapter.

A film badge is the most commonly used personnel monitoring device in medical facilities, especially if only one monitor is to be used. It is relatively inexpensive and is easy to use. The filters within the film holder allow energy discrimination to be made, which in turn allows estimates to be made of the doses received at different tissue depths. In particular, film badge readings may be used to estimate the deep dose equivalent (the dose received at a depth of 1 cm), the eye dose equivalent (that received at the depth of the lens of the eye, taken to be 0.3 cm), and the shallow dose equivalent (that received at a depth of 0.007 cm). The overall accuracy of the film badge is about ±20%, and erroneous readings can result if the badge is not read for a long period of time or if the film is exposed to heat and/or humidity. In addition, for most facilities the film badges cannot be read immediately on site and must be sent out, so there is always a lag between the time of exposure and the receipt of the readings.

TLDs trap electrons in their internal crystal structure when exposed to radiation. When they are heated at a later time, light is given off as the crystals rearrange themselves. The amount of light emitted is proportional to the amount of radiation absorbed. TLDs respond to radiation more like tissue than film does, which results in readings that are potentially more accurate. However, it is not possible to estimate the energy (or energy components) of the radiation beam. The TLD is less susceptible to the effects of temperature and humidity compared to film, but the individual dosimeters are more expensive than film. TLDs are primarily used in ring and wrist badges because of their small size. Like film, TLDs are usually sent out to be read, with a waiting period for receipt of the results.

A new dosimeter, using optimal stimulated luminescence (OSL) technology, has recently been developed that uses laser light to stimulate rearrangement of electrons trapped in aluminum oxide (Al_2O_3) when it is irradiated. This type of dosimeter is more sensitive than film (minimum reading 1 mrem compared to 10 mrem for film) and, through the use of filters, can also distinguish energies allowing determination of deep, eye, and shallow doses. As is the case with both film and TLD, the dosimeters are usually sent out to be read and can be restimulated numerous times to confirm the accuracy of the measurement.

When the dosimeter is analyzed, it is stimulated with laser light at a selected frequency. This causes the aluminum oxide to give off light in direct proportion to the amount of radiation exposure, with accuracy as low as 1 mrem and precision of ± 1 mrem. For pregnant employees and those working in low-level radiation environments, this new degree of sensitivity is an improvement over the film badge system. The Luxel dosimeter, developed by Landauer, is hexagonal in shape, comes preloaded with the aluminum oxide strip, which measures about 1.5 cm × 2.0 cm, and is placed between a plastic holder that incorporates three separate filters. One filter is unique in that it appears as a small metal grid of about 25 small holes, that allow for differentiation of a single exposure or continuous exposure over days or weeks. All of these components are factory sealed within the plastic hexagonal radiation dosimeter used for x-ray, gamma-ray, and beta-ray radiation.

Pocket ionization chambers (pocket dosimeters) can be read immediately, which is a significant benefit, but they are subject to erroneous readings if exposed to humidity or mechanical shock. Their initial cost is high, but once obtained, the operating cost is low, so use of pocket dosimeters over a long period can be cost-effective when compared to the use of film badges.

PRACTICAL RADIATION PROTECTION— EXTERNAL BEAM

The radiation beams produced by radiation therapy equipment, such as linear accelerators, betatrons, and even cobalt-60 units, are much more intense than those produced by conventional x-ray units. In addition, the energy of the beams is much higher, and thus the radiation is more penetrating. For these reasons, extra care must be taken by facility designers and operators to be sure that the radiation exposure to patients, personnel in the department, and the general public is kept ALARA. The time-honored methods of radiation protection are time, distance, and shielding. In addition, there are several safety devices that contribute to the safe operation of radiation therapy facilities.

Time

As expected, the less time one is exposed to radiation, the less dose is acquired. From a practical point of view, there is little opportunity to use this method in a radiation therapy department, because all personnel are outside the therapy room when the equipment is operated. However, cobalt-60 units continuously emit small amounts of radiation even when the source is in the off position (by regulation the maximum level cannot exceed 10 mR/hr at any point 1 m from the source, and the average level cannot exceed 2 mR/hr at 1 m from the source). Therefore it is prudent to spend as little time near the head of a cobalt-60 unit as practicable, con-

sistent with the need to properly position the patient and any accessories. Brachytherapy patients also emit radiation after the sources have been implanted, so that the time spent near such patients should be minimized.

Distance

Increasing the distance from a source of radiation can drastically reduce the radiation exposure. If the source is small, the inverse square law applies, and doubling the distance from the source reduces the exposure to one fourth its original level (Fig. 16-9). If the distance is tripled, the reduction factor is 9. Even if the source is relatively large, the radiation level will fall off with distance. Again, the major applications of this method of protection are around cobalt-60 units and brachytherapy patients, because for all other therapy units the operator will be outside the treatment room during operation of the unit.

Shielding

Shielding is the most important method for protection of operators and members of the general public in a radiation therapy department. The shielding requirements for superficial x-ray therapy units are similar to those for conventional x-ray units, because the energies are similar. However, all other external beam therapy units produce radiation beams of higher energy, and the shielding requirements are consequentially greater. The choice of shielding material depends on the energy of the beam. Lead is the preferred material for superficial units because it is more effective than concrete or steel at stopping photons at these low energies, at which photoelectric collisions dominate. At higher energies, at which Compton interactions dominate (which includes cobalt-60 units, linear accelerators, and betatrons), all materials attenuate radiation equally gram for gram, and the choice of material is usually based on economic and space factors.

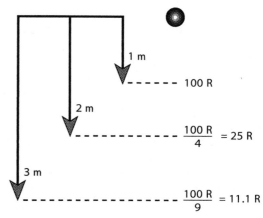

Figure 16-9. Radiation exposure. Radiation exposure from a small source is dependent on the inverse square of the distance from the source. For example, if the distance is doubled, the exposure is reduced to one fourth of its original value.

Table 16-4	Half-value layers: Approximate values obtained at high attenuation for the indicated peak voltage values under broad beam conditions*		
	Attenuation Material HVL		
Peak Voltage (kV)	Lead (mm)	Concrete (cm)	Iron (cm)
50	0.06	0.43	
100	0.27	1.6	
300	1.47	3.1	
500	3.6	3.6	
1000	7.9	4.4	
6000	16.9	10.4	3.0
10,000	16.6	11.9	3.2
Cesium-137	6.5	4.8	1.6
Cobalt-60	12.0	6.2	2.1
Radium	16.6	6.9	2.2

Data obtained from National Council on Radiation Protection and Measurements: Report No. 49, *Structural shielding design and evaluation for medical use of x-rays and gamma rays of energies up to 10 MeV,* Bethesda, Md, 1976, NCRP Publications.
HVL, Half value layer.
*NOTE: With low attenuation, these values will be significantly less.

Stated another way, a given wall may be shielded by equal masses of concrete, steel, or lead. Because of the different densities of these materials, the thickness required will be different for each material. Half-value layers for several materials at different energies are listed in Table 16-4. For cobalt-60 radiation, a 1-m (3.28-ft) thick wall of concrete may be replaced by 0.30 m (1.0 ft) of iron or 0.21 m (8.2 in.) of lead (Fig. 16-10). If space is at a premium (e.g., when an existing room is being upgraded), lead or steel may be preferred, even though they are usually much more expensive than concrete. On the other hand, for new construction, concrete is usually the material of choice because of its relatively low cost.

In calculating the shielding requirements for any radiation-producing machine, several factors must be taken into account. These include the workload (W) of the machine (how many patients will be treated per week and how much radiation will be given to each one), the primary beam use factor (U) for each wall (the fraction of time of use the beam will be aimed at the wall), the occupancy factor (T) for each area adjacent to the therapy room (the fraction of time the area will be occupied), the distance (d) from the source of radiation to the occupied area, and the effective dose equivalent limit (P) for the occupied area (radiation worker or general public). Table 16-5 summarizes the parameters that must be considered in shielding design. Consideration must be given to scatter radiation from the patient and leakage radiation from the head as well as to the primary beam. If the primary beam is intercepted by a beamstopper, the transmission through the beamstopper must be taken into account.

Workload. **Workloads** for superficial and orthovoltage x-ray units are usually specified in mA-min/week and may

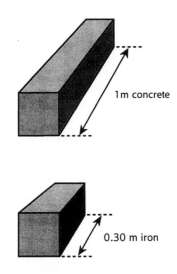

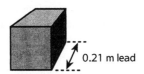

Figure 16-10. Thicknesses of various materials. These thicknesses provide equal attenuation for a cobalt-60 source.

be determined from an estimate of the beam-on time for each patient, the mA used, and the number of treatments per week. For cobalt-60 units and other high-energy units, the workload is usually specified in cGy per week at the isocenter. This number can be determined from the number of treatments given per week and the dose delivered to the isocenter for each one. For a typical linear accelerator, 200 patients may

Table 16-5	Summary of shielding parameters
Workload (W)	Number of patients per week × Amount of radiation for each
Primary beam use factor for each wall (U)	Fraction of time the beam is aimed at a particular wall
Occupancy factor (T)	Fraction of time area will be occupied
Distance (d)	Distance from the source of radiation to occupied area
Effective dose	Limit for occupied area; radiation worker equivalent limit or general public

be treated per week (40 per day) and the isocenter dose may be 300 cGy, which yields a workload figure of 60,000 cGy per week at isocenter.

Use factor. In conventional x-ray rooms the equipment is pointed down most of the time, and, except in chest rooms, the primary beam is rarely aimed at the walls and almost never at the ceiling. Even in fluoroscopy rooms when the beam is aimed up, it must be intercepted by a barrier so that no radiation reaches the ceiling. In radiation therapy rooms, on the other hand, the situation is very different. During anteroposterior or posteroanterior (AP/PA) treatments, for example, the primary beam is alternately aimed down and up. Furthermore, many treatments are given with lateral, oblique, and even rotational beams, so radiation may be aimed at the floor, ceiling, and at least two of the four walls within the room. For these reasons the **use factors** for therapy differ from those used with conventional x-rays. Ideally the use factors (which can range from 0 to 1) should be determined from knowledge about how the equipment is actually used. However, if these values are not known, the use factors recommended by the NCRP in Report No. 49,[3] *Structural Shielding Design and Evaluation for Medical Use of X Rays and Gamma Rays of Energies Up to 10 MeV,* may be used. These are 1 (100%) for the floor, $\frac{1}{4}$ for each wall that may be struck by the primary beam, and $\frac{1}{4}$ for the ceiling, if the beam can be pointed at the ceiling. It can be seen that these figures add up to more than 100%. This overestimate of use is one of many conservative assumptions used in shielding design. It should also be noted that the use factors just discussed apply to the primary beam. Both scatter and leakage radiation strike all surfaces of the room, so the use factor for these sources of radiation is always 1.

Occupancy factor. If the area on the other side of a treatment room wall were totally unoccupied (e.g., if it were below grade and the earth extended for a distance of many meters), no shielding would be required. Similarly, an area that will be occupied all the time the machine is in operation would require considerable shielding. The **occupancy factor** is the fraction of time an area adjacent to the therapy room is occupied. Values can range from 0 to 1. Again, the best occupancy factors are those derived from knowledge about the occupancy of surrounding areas (including allowance for changes in the future). In the absence of such knowledge the

recommendations of NCRP Report No. 49 may be used. These are 1 for offices, laboratories, nurses' stations, and so forth; $\frac{1}{4}$ for corridors, rest rooms, unattended parking lots, and so forth; and $\frac{1}{16}$ for waiting rooms, toilets, stairways, outside pedestrian areas, and so forth.[3]

Distance. As already mentioned, the greater the distance a person is from a source of radiation, the less radiation that is received. Thus adjacent areas that are far from the sources of radiation in a treatment room will receive less radiation than those that are closer, and less shielding will be required. The primary beam distance is measured from the source to the appropriate surface when the machine is pointed toward that surface. For scatter radiation, both the distance from the source to the patient and the distance from the patient to the appropriate surface must be considered. In addition, the fraction of the radiation incident on the patient that is scattered must also be considered. This fraction depends on the incident beam energy and the scatter angle. Values are tabulated in NCRP Report No. 49. For leakage radiation, the most appropriate distance is the distance from the source to the appropriate wall, when the head of the machine is closest to that surface.

Effective dose equivalent limits. As discussed earlier, radiation workers have different effective dose equivalent limits than members of the general public. In general, the shielding requirements for areas that will only be frequented by radiation workers or areas under positive control by a radiation worker (restricted areas) will not require as much shielding as areas accessible to the general public (unrestricted areas). However, in many cases the shielding design for restricted areas is based on the limits for unrestricted areas in the name of ALARA.

The application of the values obtained for each of the factors already discussed to determine actual thicknesses of shielding materials is a complex process for which training, experience, and judgment are required. In the case of shielding designs for cobalt-60 units, the person performing the design must be approved by the NRC or an agreement state. Similarly, shielding designs for linear accelerators must be performed, in most cases, by persons approved by the state.

Partly as a result of the recent reductions in the effective dose equivalent limit for the general public, several groups have reexamined the conservative assumptions that have been made in obtaining values for workloads, use factors, and occupancy factors, and changes in the methodology for performing shielding calculations may be published in the near future.

Safety Equipment

Because of the high levels of radiation that exist within the treatment room, no one but the patient is allowed to be in the room during the treatment. The NRC and virtually all states have additional regulations designed to protect both the operator of the equipment and the patient.

Warning signs. Entrance doors to therapy rooms must be posted with signs to warn anyone about to enter the room that radiation might be present. Because the levels in the room can exceed 1 mSv (100 mrem) in 1 hour, the room must have a sign posted that says "Caution, High Radiation Area." In some cases the radiation levels may be in excess of 5 Gy (500 cGy) in 1 hour, in which case the sign is supposed to read, "Grave Danger, Very High Radiation Area." This wording seems singularly inappropriate for a medical facility.

Warning lights. Beam-on light indicators are required on the control panel, at the entrance door, and on the treatment unit itself. These lights should be illuminated whenever the therapy unit is energized to alert personnel that the beam is on. In the case of cobalt-60 units a mechanical indication that the source is in the on position is also required on the head of the unit.

Door interlocks. Entrance doors to therapy rooms must be equipped with an interlock that will shut off the machine (or in the case of a cobalt-60 unit, return the source to the off position) if the door is opened during treatment. The circuit design must be such that the unit will not produce radiation when the door is closed unless the operator deliberately turns it on. In addition, it is common to have interlocks on access doors to the machine stands so that if someone is working on the unit it cannot be accidentally energized.

Visual and aural communication. It is necessary for the radiation therapist to be able to see the patient throughout the treatment. If the patient moves or shows signs of distress, the therapist can turn the unit off and enter the room. For superficial and orthovoltage units, visual monitoring may be by means of a leaded glass window. However, for high-energy machines the thickness of glass required usually makes this method impractical. In these cases, monitoring is usually done by means of closed circuit television systems. Care must be taken to position the camera so that the patient is in view no matter what the position of the gantry. Frequently, two separate television systems are used. In fact, regulations require that visual communication be available at all times, so that if only one system is used and it fails, the treatment room cannot be used until the television system is repaired. Regulations also require the availability of aural communication between therapist and patient. Again, this is primarily a safety measure for the patient, because it allows the patient to notify the therapist if he or she is in distress.

"Beam-on" monitors. High-energy therapy units are required to have an independent beam-on monitor in the room to alert the therapist if he or she enters the room when the beam is on. This monitor must not be connected to the therapy machine in any way and must have provision for battery operation in the event of an electrical failure.

Emergency off controls. In the unlikely event that a high-energy therapy machine may be energized when an therapist is in the room, emergency push buttons are located at several points within the room and on the machine itself that will remove all power to the unit when pressed. The circuits are designed so that the machine will not be energized when the buttons are released unless the therapist proceeds through the normal start procedure at the control panel. In the case of cobalt-60 units, means and instructions are also provided to therapists so they can mechanically return the source to the off position should it become stuck. This is also an unlikely event. In all cases the therapist must be concerned first with the care of the patient and next with his or her own welfare. The dose received by a therapist standing 1 m to the side of a patient being treated at 300 cGy/min will be approximately 0.5 cGy/min. Although all unnecessary radiation is to be avoided, the few seconds required to move the table to remove the patient from the beam if it cannot be shut off will be unlikely to deliver a dose to the therapist in excess of the effective dose equivalent limit.

Quality assurance. No safety device is effective if it is not working, so frequent testing of the devices on a regular basis is necessary. Such tests are required either by regulation or by recognized protocols. The television and aural communication systems are easy to test daily. Testing of emergency off buttons may cause harm to the treatment unit, so manufacturer's recommendations should be followed carefully. Testing of beam-on monitors can be done either by turning the television camera to visualize the monitor or by using a mirror so that an image of the monitor can be seen by the television camera.

PRACTICAL RADIATION PROTECTION— BRACHYTHERAPY

The sources used for implants require special consideration, because, like cobalt-60, they are always "on." A license from either the NRC or an agreement state is required to receive, possess, and use such sources. Sources may be obtained only from facilities or firms licensed to distribute them. Sources must be stored in heavily shielded "safes" in an area secure from theft or loss.

Written Directives and Inventory

Before an implant is prepared, a written directive must be completed by the requesting physician, and certification must be made that the implant was assembled in accordance with the directive. A careful inventory must be maintained of all sources, and any time sources are removed or returned, a log entry must be made and a complete inventory performed.

Inventories are also required at least weekly, even if no sources have been removed from or returned to the safe.

Transportation

If sources must be transported within the hospital, shielded carriers must be used. In most cases the required shielding makes the carriers too heavy to carry by hand, and wheeled carriers are necessary. Whenever sources are moved within the hospital—either in carriers or already implanted within a patient who is being moved—the route should be chosen to minimize exposure to other hospital personnel or members of the general public.

Patient Rooms

The room used by a patient with a radioactive implant also requires special consideration. A private room with a bath (if the patient will be allowed to use the bath) should be provided. Placement of the patient's bed should be such that a patient in an adjoining room will not receive a dose in excess of the effective dose equivalent limit for the general public. This usually implies that the bed be placed by a wall adjacent to a stairway or other little occupied area. In some cases shielding may be required on the wall. Radiation exposure to the areas above and below the patient's room should also be considered.

Training of Personnel

All personnel who may care for the patient must be thoroughly instructed in radiation safety procedures and the actions to take if the implant is dislodged or other emergencies occur. Nurses should use personnel monitors. Ancillary personnel such as dietary aides, maintenance personnel, and housekeeping personnel also need to receive instruction about radiation safety at a level commensurate with their risk. Personnel monitors are usually not required for such personnel.

Warning Signs and Surveys

The entrance door to the patient's room must be posted with a caution sign, and visiting periods should be limited (typically to 20 minutes per visitor per day), with the visitor remaining behind a line established by the radiation safety officer. Radiation warning signs are also placed on the patient's wrist, bed, and chart to ensure that no one will be inadvertently exposed because he or she was not aware that the patient contained radioactive materials. After the patient returns to his or her room and/or after placement of the radioactive material in the patient, a survey must be performed of the environs of the patient's room. After removal of the implant, a survey must again be performed to ensure that no sources have been inadvertently left behind. Nothing should be removed from the patient's room, nor should the patient be discharged until this survey is done.

Leak Tests

Because it is possible for the material encapsulating the radioactive material in implant sources to sustain damage and leak, brachytherapy sources must be leak tested at intervals not to exceed 6 months. The method used must be sensitive enough to detect removable contamination at a level of 0.005 µCi (11,100 disintegrations per minute [dpm]). Leak tests must also be performed on cobalt-60 units every 6 months. In this case, however, the limit for removable contamination is 0.05 µCi.

High-Dose-Rate Brachytherapy

Conventional low-dose-rate brachytherapy procedures require the patient to be hospitalized for 24 to 72 hours. High-dose-rate units have become available that allow the treatment time to be shortened. The sources in these units have considerably greater activity than those used in low-dose implants (10 Ci iridium-192 vs. 65 mCi cesium-137) and therefore cannot be handled manually. This implies less exposure for those who would normally prepare and insert low-dose-rate implants. However, it also implies the need for computer control of the position and dwell time of the sources and the possibility of error or the loss of control of the source. For these reasons, special procedures are required to ensure the safe operation of such devices.

SUMMARY

Within the radiation therapy department there are two major sources of exposure: megavoltage treatment machines and brachytherapy sources. Regardless of which models are used to estimate the risks of radiation exposure, it is universally agreed that the less radiation received, the lower the risk. This means that in keeping with the ALARA concept, every measure should be taken to reduce individual exposure. Practical radiation protection from external beam radiation should include the time-honored methods of time, distance, and shielding. In addition, a resurgence in the use of brachytherapy sources require the radiation therapy practitioner to be prepared to demonstrate a comprehensive knowledge of its uses in terms of radiation safety and protection.

Review Questions

1. Activity is defined as:
   a. Rest mass is same as an electron, but has a positive charge
   b. Product of absorbed dose and QF
   c. Rate of nuclear decay
   d. Ionization per unit mass of air by photons
2. The source of ionizing radiation that contributes the most to exposure of the general population in the United States is
   a. Medical procedures
   b. Nuclear power plants
   c. Natural background radiation
   d. Above-ground nuclear testing

3. Which type of device is best suited for output measurements of radiation therapy equipment?
   a. TLDs
   b. Ionization chamber
   c. G-M detector
   d. X-ray film
4. Stochastic, or nonthreshold, effects of radiation exposure do not include
   a. Cancer induction
   b. Cataract formation
   c. Genetic effects
   d. Birth defects
5. Exposure of which of the following people would contribute the most to the genetically significant dose?
   a. 50-year-old woman
   b. 70-year-old man
   c. 20-year-old woman
   d. All contribute equally
6. The annual effective dose equivalent limit for radiation workers is
   a. 0.5 mSv
   b. 5 mSv
   c. 50 mSv
   d. 500 mSv
7. A G-M detector is 2 m from a small brachytherapy source and has an exposure rate of 10 milliroentgens/hr. What exposure rate would you expect to measure if the detector were moved to 4 m from the source?
   a. 5 milliroentgens/hr
   b. 20 milliroentgens/hr
   c. 2.5 milliroentgens/hr
   d. 1 milliroentgens/hr
8. Absorbed dose is defined as:
   a. Rest mass of an electron, but has a positive charge
   b. Product of absorbed dose and QF
   c. Ionization per unit mass of air by photons
   d. Energy absorbed per unit mass
9. Exposure is defined as:
   a. Rest mass of an electron, but has a positive charge
   b. Product of absorbed dose and QF
   c. Rate of nuclear decay
   d. Ionization per unit mass of air by photons
10. An alpha particle is best defined as:
    a. Produced by electron rearrangement
    b. Produced during nuclear decay; has no charge or mass
    c. Short range, relatively heavy mass, high-LET particle
    d. Rest mass is same as an electron, but has a positive charge

Questions to Ponder

1. What are some of the sources of natural background radiation? Is it possible or reasonable to attempt to shield or protect the general population from these sources?
2. What are the factors that must be considered in designing the shielding for a linear accelerator facility?
3. Why is it important that regulatory agencies such as the NRC or state agencies oversee the operation of radiation therapy facilities?
4. What are the primary reasons for implementing a radiation protection program? How does the concept of ALARA affect the development of such a program?

REFERENCES

1. Bushberg JT, et al: *The essential physics of medical imaging,* Baltimore, 1994, Williams & Wilkins.
2. Hall EJ: *Radiobiology for the radiologist,* ed 5, Philadelphia, 2000, Lippincott Williams & Wilkins.
3. National Council on Radiation Protection and Measurements (NCRP): Report No. 49, Structural shielding design and evaluation for medical use of x-rays and gamma rays of energies up to 10 MeV, Washington, DC, 1976, NCRP Publications.
4. National Council on Radiation Protection and Measurements (NCRP): Report No. 91, Recommendations on limits for exposure to ionizing radiation, Bethesda, MD, 1987, NCRP Publications.
5. National Council on Radiation Protection and Measurements (NCRP): Report No. 93, Ionizing radiation exposure of the population of the United States, Bethesda, MD, 1987, NCRP Publications.
6. National Council on Radiation Protection and Measurements (NCRP): Report No. 115, Risk estimates for radiation protection, Bethesda, MD, 1993, NCRP Publications.
7. Statkiewicz-Sherer MA, Viscounti PJ, Ritenour ER: *Radiation protection in medical radiography,* ed 2, St. Louis, 1993, Mosby.

17

Quality Improvement in Radiation Oncology

Judith M. Schneider

Outline

Key Terms

Aspect of care
Continuous quality improvement
Customer, external, internal
Flow chart
Health care organizations
Joint Commission on the Accreditation of Healthcare Organizations
Outcomes

Peer review
Quality assessment
Quality assurance
Quality audit
Quality control
Quality improvement
Quality indicators
Radiation oncology team
Total quality management

Q uality improvement (QI) in health care is "an approach to the continuous study and improvement of the processes of providing health care services to meet the needs of patients and others. Synonymous terms include continuous quality improvement (CQI), continuous improvement (CI), and total quality management (TQM)."[17] It is premised on Dr. W.E. Deming's 14 principles of management, which were first introduced in Japan's industry after World War II and into the United States' health care industry in the early 1980s. The Deming principles of management emphasize CQI in a product (service) through proactive employee participation in a "customer-responsive" environment.[19,20,22,29] According to Deming, quality is not only achieved but maintained by the following[20,22]:

1. Delineate the health care organization's mission and goals, so that there is a reason for improving
2. Instead of setting thresholds, which are expected levels of compliance, always strive for improvement no matter how good the product (service)
3. Improve the process rather than "inspect for errors"
4. Plan for the future by analyzing "long-term costs" and "appropriateness of product (service)"
5. Allow the employee to contribute to the improvement process
6. Encourage and support employees through education
7. Ensure qualified leaders for the improvement system
8. Eliminate fear by encouraging employees to offer suggestions
9. Eliminate staffing barriers by helping employees understand the needs of other departments or sections
10. Require management to always keep employees informed of what is happening

11. Emphasize quality first rather than quantity
12. Promote and encourage teamwork versus individual performance
13. Encourage and support an employee's educational and self-improvement program
14. Support and train all employees in the "transformation process"

Today's **health care organizations** are facing the same dilemmas as industry did several years ago involving quality control and cost containment. Appropriate use of CQI assists the health care organization in responding to the problems of "increased competition," "escalating costs," "quality concerns," and "demands for increased accountability."[22] Participation in CQI has been demonstrated to decrease costs, increase customer satisfaction, and ensure quality throughout the health care organization[19,20]

Traditionally, quality assurance activities were used by health care organizations to systematically analyze the quality of health care services rendered and to meet the criteria for accreditation by the **Joint Commission on the Accreditation of Healthcare Organizations** (JCAHO), an independent, not-for-profit organization dedicated to improving the quality of care in health care settings.[17] Quality assurance focuses on performance measurement, which is based on the comparison of processes with **outcomes** to quality indicators, the measurable dimension of quality that defines what is to be monitored.[9,19] It stresses control and assessment of performance,

hence the terms quality control, providing standards of measurement, and quality assessment, involving the systematic collection and review of quality assurance data.

A **continuous quality improvement** (CQI) plan integrates quality assurance, quality control, and assessment into a complex, system-wide improvement program revolving around the health care organization's mission and goals.[19] It eliminates duplication of quality assurance and quality improvement efforts but still provides assurance that services are of high quality.[29]

In recent years, with the increase in complexity of radiation treatment planning and delivery, it has become imperative that a radiation oncology center, regardless of its size, develop and implement a well defined, structured, and functional quality improvement plan. This plan should encompass all aspects of the radiation therapy treatment process from patient consultation through and including follow-up care.

Quality improvement in radiation oncology involves ongoing activities encompassing administrative, clinical, physical, and technical aspects of the radiation oncology process as defined by the American College of Radiology (ACR) and the American Association of Physicists in Medicine (AAPM).[14,18,21] Each of these aspects, which are influenced by their own structure and process, are relevant to the outcomes of the radiation oncology process and should be monitored in a quality improvement plan. (See Fig. 17-1

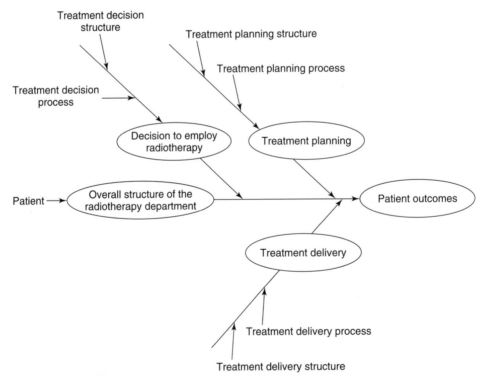

Figure 17-1. A "fishbone" diagram showing the major structure and process elements of the clinical radiation therapy program. *(Used with permission from Brundage MD, Dixon PF, MacKillop WJ et al: A real-time audit of radiation therapy in a regional cancer center, Int J Radiat Oncol Biol Phys 43:121, 1999.)*

for a fishbone diagram indicating the major process and structure elements of the clinical aspects of the radiation therapy process.[8]) The quality improvement plan includes a quality control program to measure the radiation output and mechanical integrity of the treatment and simulation units and brachytherapy sources and equipment, as well as quality assessment programs to measure all aspects of the treatment planning, delivery, and patient care process. A **peer review** and audit mechanism is an integral part of the plan.

EVOLUTION OF QUALITY IMPROVEMENT

Radiation Measurement

Before the process of quality improvement can be implemented, standards must be developed by which one can compare, evaluate, and establish quality control.[33] From the time of the discovery of the x-ray, standards for its measurement have been proposed, starting with the original erythema dose as the unit of measurement and evolving into exact scientific standards for the measurement of the gray (Gy) as specified by national and international agencies. During the Second International Congress of Radiology held in Stockholm, Sweden, in July 1928, several recommendations were made, including that an "international unit of x-radiation" be adopted and that the unit be called the "roentgen" designated by a small "r." The complete recommendations were published in the report entitled "Recommendations of the International X-Ray Unit Committee," published in 1929.[34] This marked the beginning of quality control in radiation measurements, although it was not defined as such. As technology advanced in radiation oncology, the number of governing regulations increased. There is no comparison between this simple two-page document and the volumes of regulations that currently exist. With the advent of the unit of measure came the standardization of equipment performance with an increased emphasis on quality control. Thus quality improvement in radiation oncology was initially focused on the physical aspect of treatment equipment performance.

Hospital Oversight and Accreditation

The oversight of patient care in hospitals began in 1917 when the American College of Surgeons (ACS) established the Hospital Standardization Program, and in 1919 the concept of minimum standards" were developed. From 1917 until 1951 the ACS worked to improve the hospital-based practice of medicine. In 1952 the Joint Commission on Accreditation of Hospitals (JCAH) was formed through the efforts of the ACS, the American Medical Association (AMA), the American Hospital Association (AHA), the American College of Physicians (ACP), and the Canadian Medical Association (CMA). With the passage of Medicare in 1965, JCAH accreditation of hospitals increased in importance when the United States Congress determined that JCAH-accredited facilities would be recognized for purposes of Medicare reimbursement. In 1988 the name of the JCAH was

changed to JCAHO to broaden its scope to include ambulatory centers, group practices, health maintenance organizations, community health centers, emergency and urgent care centers, and hospital-based practices under its accreditation umbrella.

Although the original mission of the JCAH was to ensure plant safety in hospitals, that mission has evolved and expanded to include quality improvement based on the measurement of patient outcomes. Initially, JCAHO standards for radiation oncology were included in those for the radiology departments, because most radiation therapy departments came under the auspices of that department, but rarely were the radiation therapy facilities visited. In 1987, however, the JCAHO developed separate standards for radiation oncology, and a dedicated quality improvement plan is now required for each department. The original emphasis was on the quality control aspects of radiation oncology and concentrated on the treatment units themselves and the process used to deliver patient care. Now the emphasis is on "doing the right thing" and "doing the right thing well" as it relates to the facility's organization-wide performance versus specific departmental performance.[16] Doing the right thing refers to delivering effective and appropriate treatment, and doing the right thing well refers to providing patient care effectively, accurately, in a timely manner, and with respect and caring for the patient.

REGULATING AGENCIES

Today there are a multitude of national, state, and professional agencies with regulations and standards that must be adhered to by the radiation oncology facility to ensure high-quality patient care and safety. These standards and regulations provide the cornerstones for the radiation oncology facility's quality improvement plan. It is imperative that a radiation oncology facility become familiar with all national, state, and professional regulations that affect the facility's operation. This is an ongoing process because along with the development and use of new equipment and treatment techniques comes new guidelines and practice standards that must be followed.

Federal and state government as well as professional and accreditation agencies mandate standards to ensure not only that equipment is functional and operate within acceptable limits but also that operators of this equipment are truly qualified individuals.

Federal Agencies

The U.S. Nuclear Regulatory Commission (NRC) was created in 1974 as a result of Congress passing legislation to divide the Atomic Energy Commission that since 1954 had been managing the nation's atomic energy programs. The Atomic Energy Commission was separated into the Energy Research and Development Administration and the NRC. The mission of the NRC is to "ensure adequate protection of the public health and safety, the common defense and security, and the environment in the use of nuclear materials in the United States." The NRC's scope of responsibility includes regulation of commercial nuclear power reactors; nonpower research, test, and training reactors; fuel cycle facilities; *medical, academic, and industrial uses of nuclear materials; and the transport, storage, and disposal of nuclear materials and waste.* Its regulations are issued under the United States Code of Federal Regulations (CFR) Title 10, Chapter 1.[23,24] Use of radioisotopes in brachytherapy and the cobalt for external treatments falls under the regulation of the NRC.

Although the NRC is the major federal regulating agency for ensuring adequate protection of public health and safety in the use of radioactive materials, other federal agencies assist the NRC in fulfilling its mission. One such agency is the U.S. Environmental Protection Agency (EPA). The EPA was established in 1970 to consolidate into one agency a variety of federal research, monitoring, standard-setting, and enforcement activities to guarantee protection of the environment. The EPA's mission is "to protect human health and safeguard the natural environment—air, water, and land—upon which life depends."[10] Therefore the EPA is involved with regulation of the disposal, storage, and handling of nuclear waste materials as it relates to environmental protection issues.

The transportation of hazardous materials is monitored and regulated through the Department of Transportation (DOT) another federal agency assisting the NRC in carrying out its mission. The DOT's effort is coordinated through the Office of Hazardous Materials (OHM), which is responsible for overseeing a national safety program for transporting hazardous materials by air, rail, highway, and water.[26,32]

In 1968, Congress passed the Radiation Control for Health and Safety Act, which provided for the development and administration of standards that would reduce human exposure to radiation from electronic products. Implementation of this Act was through the Bureau of Radiologic Health (BRH), which is now called the Center for Devices and Radiologic Health (CDRH). This Act is now incorporated into the Federal Food, Drug, and Cosmetic Act (FFDCA), as chapter V, subchapter 3, Electronic Product Radiation Control. This Act regulates both medical and nonmedical electronic products such as diagnostic x-ray or ultrasound imaging devices, microwave or ultrasound diathermy devices, x-ray or electron accelerators, sunlamps, microwave ovens, television receivers and monitors, entertainment lasers, industrial x-ray systems, and cordless and cellular telephones.[11]

Provisions of this Act require the manufacturers' of these products that emit radiation to keep records in reference to quality testing of their products and communications to the dealers, distributors, and purchasers of these products as it relates to radiation safety issues.

Not only does the FFDCA hold the manufacturers responsible in the reporting of safety issues regarding radiation

producing electronic products but also facilities who use these products. The Safety Medical Devices Act of 1991 (SMDA) requires medical facilities to report to the FDA, any medical device that has caused death or injury of a patient or an employee.[11,23] Failure to report such incidences can result in civil penalties to the medical facility as well as to the health care professional.

To ensure safe and healthful working conditions for working men and women, Congress passed the "Occupational Safety and Health Act of 1970." By provisions of this Act, the Occupational Safety and Health Administration (OSHA) was created "to save lives, prevent injuries, and protect the health of America's workers."[6,25]

In the mid-1980s, OSHA mandated a policy on bloodborne pathogens, which stated that an exposure control plan must be in place for all industries in which workers may come in contact with blood and other infectious materials. This plan must contain precautionary procedures, educational programs for employees, and proper disposal procedures.[25,28] The policy on bloodborne pathogens is part of the radiation oncology facilities policy and procedures manual.

OSHA also set standards for exposure to cadmium and lead, which primarily covers industrial work environments, but these standards would apply to mold rooms, where cerrobend (shielding) block is constructed, in radiation oncology facilities.[25] It is important for the personnel working in mold rooms to be aware of and to follow the safety standards outlined by OSHA.

State Agencies

Section 274b of the Atomic Energy Act of 1954, provides a basis for the NRC to relinquish to the states portions of its regulatory authority relating to licensing and regulating by-product materials (radioisotopes), source materials (uranium and thorium), and certain quantities of special nuclear materials. The first agreement state was established in 1962. Currently, a total of 32 states have entered into agreements with the NRC.[27] In such agreements, the NRC provides assistance to the states through reviewing of the agreement request, conducting training courses and workshops, and evaluating technical licensing and inspection issues. The NRC is highly involved with the agreement states keeping all chains of communication open in a variety of areas.

Professional Organizations

Several professional organizations provide practice standards to guide appropriately educated professionals within their organizations. Professional practice standards establish the role of the practitioner and create criteria to be used to evaluate performance. The ACR, with more than 30,000 members, is the primary professional organization of radiologists, radiation oncologists, and clinical medical physicists in the United States. The ACR creates standards in the hopes of producing high-quality radiologic care. It has developed specific standards for brachytherapy and external beam therapy as well.[5]

The AAPM, a professional organization for medical physicists, has been a forerunner in the development of minimum standards to guide medical physicists in the development of a quality assurance program as it relates to treatment planning and delivery. Several reports have been produced by special task groups of the AAPM relating to the development of a comprehensive quality assurance program in radiation oncology such as the AAPM Task Group 40 report and more recently the AAPM Task Group 53 report, which outlined a comprehensive quality assurance program for radiation therapy treatment planning.[1,2,5]

In 1995, the professional organization for radiation therapists, the American Society of Radiologic Technologists (ASRT), developed practice standards for radiation therapists. The professional practice standards are divided into three sections: clinical performance standards, which define activities related to the care of patients and the delivery of procedures and treatments; quality performance standards, which includes the activities of the practitioner in the technical areas of performance involving equipment safety and TQM; professional performance standards, which define activities in the areas of education, interpersonal relationships, personal and professional self-assessment, and ethical behavior.[7] To be effective, the quality improvement plan must incorporate all practice standards for each member of the quality improvement team.

DEFINITIONS

Multiple definitions exist regarding the various components of quality improvement; the definitions used throughout the rest of this chapter are those developed by the International Standards Organization (ISO)[15] and accepted as the American national standard.[1]

Quality, in reference to radiation oncology, is defined as "the totality of features and characteristics of a radiation therapy process that bear on its ability to satisfy stated or implied needs of the patient." To determine whether quality standards are met, each feature or characteristic of the radiation therapy process must be identified and measured and the results analyzed.

Quality assurance is defined as "all those planned or systematic actions necessary to provide adequate confidence that a product or service will satisfy given requirements for quality." The term is used to refer to the planned and systematic actions to ensure that a radiation therapy facility consistently delivers high-quality care in the treatment of patients leading to the best outcomes with the least amount of side effects. All aspects of the radiation therapy process must be routinely and continuously measured, the results analyzed, and corrective action taken as required to ensure quality patient care. This type of review is referred to as a **quality audit.**[9,23]

Quality control is defined as "the operational techniques

and activities used to fulfill requirements of quality." The term is typically used to refer to those procedures and techniques used to monitor or test and maintain the components of the radiation therapy quality improvement program, such as the tests performed to measure the mechanical integrity of the treatment units.

Measurement of patient outcomes is now required by the JCAHO. This measurement includes not only areas such as morbidity, mortality, recurrence of disease, and survival rates but also patient satisfaction and quality of life. As part of its "Agenda for Change," the JCAHO created the Joint Commission's Indicator Measurement System (IM system), which provides a continuous evaluation of performance as part of the accreditation process to help health care organizations measure and improve their quality of care through the use of common **quality indicators.** Every quarter, organizations participating in this system are required to send their data electronically to the system's national database, which then prepares a comparative report for each indicator. The IM system focuses primarily on acute inpatient care, although the indicators may be relevant to some outpatient surgical settings. Currently 130 participants are part of the IM system with the number submitting data steadily increasing.[30] Having an adequate computerized data analysis system is an essential component for CQI.

JCAHO has replaced the term *quality assurance* with terms such as **quality assessment** or *quality improvement,* because the emphasis is now on the ongoing evaluation of all aspects of care for the purpose of determining areas where improvement is needed. The key word is "ongoing"; hence this program is frequently referred to as CQI or **total quality management** (TQM).

COMPONENTS OF QUALITY IMPROVEMENT

Quality Improvement Team

The quality improvement team is composed of all personnel in the radiation oncology department who interact with the patient and family. Each individual makes a contribution to the quality of care and level of patient satisfaction. Only through continuous evaluation of all aspects of the radiation therapy process can the ultimate goal to deliver quality radiation and patient care be achieved. However, this is not accomplished without the cooperative efforts and commitment to quality of each member of the **radiation oncology team.**[12,18]

Common practice is for the medical director of a radiation oncology center to be responsible for the establishment and continuation of a quality improvement program.[12] The director may appoint a quality improvement committee to develop and monitor the program, collect and evaluate the data, determine areas for improvement, implement changes when areas for improvement have been identified, and evaluate the results of the actions taken. Table 17-1 delineates the responsibilities of the quality improvement committee.

Table 17-1	Responsibilities of members of the quality improvement (QI) committee		
QI activity	**Goals**	**Frequency**	**Reporting mechanism**
Develop and monitor a CQI program	Oversee departmental peer review activities	Ongoing	QI committee meeting minutes
Collect and evaluate data	Develop and implement new policies and procedures as needed	Monthly meetings	Chart rounds reports
Determine areas for improvement	Oversee implementation of and adherence to departmental policies and procedures		Policies and procedures
Implement change as necessary Evaluate results of actions taken			Incident reports

It is also the responsibility of the director to ensure that all employees are qualified for their jobs. Job descriptions must clearly state the qualifications, the credentials or license required, continuing education requirements, and the scope of practice for each position. Institutional requirements regarding maintenance of qualifications in cardiopulmonary resuscitation (CPR); attendance at infectious disease, fire, and safety seminars; and observance of all radiation safety standards are to be strictly adhered to.

Staff physicians are required to actively participate in departmental quality improvement activities, and documentation of participation is reviewed as part of the medical staff recredentialing process. The radiation oncologists participate in these activities during chart review, morbidity and mortality conferences, review and development of departmental policies and procedures, portal film review, patient and family education, and the completion and review of incident reports.

Members of the physics division (physicists, dosimetrists, and engineers) develop and carry out the quality control program to meet the needs of the department and to be in compliance with national, state, and professionally accepted or mandated standards. They also conduct weekly and final physics reviews of the treatment records.

The radiation therapists perform warmup procedures on the treatment units, perform quality control tests on the simulation and treatment units, verify the presence of completed and signed prescription and consent forms, review the prescription and treatment plan on each patient before the initiation of treatment, deliver accurate treatment adhering to the prescription, accurately record treatment delivered, take initial and weekly portal films, evaluate the health status of the patient daily before treatment delivery to ensure there are no adverse reactions to treatment or other impending physical or psychologic problems that require assistance, participate in patient and family education, and provide care and comfort to meet the needs of the patient.[3]

The oncology nurses perform a nursing assessment on each new patient to determine overall physical and psychologic status; evaluate the educational needs of each patient and family to determine any barriers to education; develop an educational program to meet the needs of the patient and family; evaluate the effectiveness of the entire educational program, including the education given to the patient by the radiation oncologist, nurses, and radiation therapists; monitor the patient's health status on a routine or as-needed basis throughout the course of treatment; and order, evaluate, and record blood counts and weights according to departmental policy.

The departmental support staff gathers pertinent information and prepares the treatment chart before the patient's initial visit; contacts the patient and/or family to set up appointments and give instructions regarding information or diagnostic studies to be brought with the patient; greets and assists the patient and family daily; informs the radiation oncologists, nurses, and/or radiation therapists of the patient's arrival; answers the patient's questions and gives assistance whenever possible or refers the patient to an individual who can help; completes and files treatment records; and sets the tone for the entire radiation therapy treatment encounter.

Development of a Quality Improvement Plan

A quality improvement plan or program lists the organizational structure, responsibilities, procedures, processes, and resources for implementing a comprehensive quality system. Included in the plan is an audit mechanism to document measurement and evaluation activities to verify that all aspects of the radiation oncology process meet national, state, institutional, and/or departmental quality standards and a mechanism to institute change when quality standards are not met. It requires access to a computerized data acquisition and analysis system.[13]

The plan may be developed and overseen by a departmental quality improvement committee. The objectives of the program are as follows:

1. Establish a program that promotes an ongoing collection of information about important aspects of care
2. Use the information gathered to substantiate that high standards of care are being met or to identify opportunities to improve patient care
3. Implement action as necessary to modify and improve the quality of patient care
4. Assess the effectiveness of actions taken to improve the quality of patient care
5. Report quality assessment activities to the radiation oncology staff, hospital quality improvement department, and other departments or committees as requested

Refer to Box 17-1 for a summary of the elements in a quality improvement plan.

The first step in the development of such a plan is to identify all aspects of departmental activities that affect the patient's care. This process might be facilitated by the use of a **flow chart,** which is a pictorial representation of the steps necessary in a process. Flow charts use ovals to identify the beginning or end of a process, rectangles to indicate an action to be taken, and diamonds to represent a decision. By following the patient's progress, or flow, through the department, areas for improvement can be identified. Quality indicators may then be developed for each important **aspect of care.** As stated previously, indicators are tools used to measure over time a department's performance of functions, processes, and outcomes.[17] Well-defined and measurable indicators help focus attention on opportunities for improved patient care. Please refer to Table 17-2 for some identifiable quality indicators correlated to specific aspects of care in the radiation therapy process.

QUALITY IMPROVEMENT PROCESS

It is the responsibility of each individual radiation oncology center to formulate and implement quality improvement standards, based on its own "strengths and needs, in accordance with previously developed national, state, and professional guidelines."[18,21] Because of the variations in the "strengths and needs" of each individual radiation oncology

center, this chapter does not address the step-by-step technical procedures for specific quality improvement processes but instead refers the reader to reports generated by various professional and national organizations such as the ACR, AAPM, the American College of Medical Physics (ACMP), and the NRC.[1,4,5,18]

Quality Control in Treatment Planning and Delivery

A major component of the quality improvement plan focuses on quality control procedures that are routinely performed, documented, and evaluated on the simulator, image processing equipment, immobilization devices, accessory equipment, treatment planning computer systems, and the treatment units. Safety equipment such as emergency switches, door interlocks, and communication devices are included in the quality control checks.[12,18] This is to ensure that all is in proper working order according to manufacturers', departmental, and national specifications. Instrumentation that is used in performing these quality control checks such as calibration equipment (ionization chamber and electrometer), scanning equipment, dosimetry accessories (solid phantom materials, thermometer, barometer), and miscellaneous dosimetry devices such as the thermoluminescent dosimeter (TLD) system and film must also be periodically tested. Each radiation oncology center determines the frequency of these quality control checks based on the stability of equipment performance. Unstable equipment performance requires more frequent checks until the equipment performance has stabilized and then the frequency may be reduced. Regular intervals such as daily, weekly, monthly, or annually are usually established for the quality control procedures. To reduce the risk of the patient being simulated or treated with faulty equipment it is best to perform the daily quality checks in the morning before the first patient is simulated or treated.[12,18] The quality control procedures and tolerances are established and managed by the physicist; however, the radiation therapist plays a major role in obtaining this information. This is due to the therapist's familiarity and knowledge of the equipment. Therefore it is imperative that the therapist be familiar with

---

Box 17-1	**Components of a Continuous Quality Improvement (CQI) Plan**

Evaluation of both quality and appropriateness of care
Evaluation of patterns or trends
Assessment of individual clinical events
Action to be taken to resolve identified problems
Identification of important aspects of care for assessment
Identification of indicators to monitor and acceptable thresholds
Methods of data collection
Annual review of quality improvement plan for effectiveness

Table 17-2	Quality indicators in the radiation therapy process

Aspect of Care	Indicators
Consultation and informed consent	History and physical report in treatment record
	Pathology report in treatment record
	Consent form signed by patient or legal guardian
	Consent form signed by radiation oncologist
Treatment planning	Quality control program for simulator, imaging processing equipment, immobilization devices, and accessory equipment
	Quality control program for treatment planning computer systems
	Adherence to departmental policies and procedures
	Target volume indicated on planning films
	Setup information, diagrams, and photographs in treatment record
	Calculations and graphic plans double-checked
Treatment delivery	Quality control program for treatment unit, imaging processing equipment, immobilization devices, accessory equipment, and safety equipment
	Written and signed prescription
	Approved treatment plan
	Comparison of portal films with simulation films
	Weekly review of portal films by radiation therapist
	Initial and weekly portal films signed by radiation oncologist
Documentation of treatment delivery	Adherence to the prescription
	Documentation of weekly physics review
	Adherence to professional and departmental standards
	Completeness of treatment record
	Incident/unusual occurrence reports
Patient outcomes	Completion notes/treatment summary filed in chart
	Follow-up notes filed in chart
	Documentation of treatment outcomes, including:
	Morbidity
	Mortality
	Recurrence
	Survival
	Patient satisfaction
	Quality of survival

commonly performed quality control procedures and recommended tolerances for the simulator, cobalt-60 unit, and medical accelerator. Please refer to Tables 17-3, 17-4, and 17-5. Note that the simulator quality control procedures and recommended tolerances are for a conventional simulator not a computed tomography (CT) simulator.

However, quality control procedures and tolerances should be developed for a CT simulator and any other new treatment planning and delivery system that is used in the radiation therapy process. Documentation of quality control testing is an important aspect for determining equipment performance over a period of time. All results should be recorded in a logbook, along with actions that were taken to correct any deviations beyond the tolerance limits and the results of any necessary retesting. This documentation is a legal record and should be kept for the life of the equip-ment or as long as it is used in the radiation therapy process.[12,18]

ASSESSMENT OF THE DATA

An integral part of implementing the quality improvement process in radiation oncology is a continual statistical assessment of the data collected. Having a computerized data analysis system is mandatory.[31]

The JCAHO has developed its own indicator-based performance system (IM system) that organizations may use to provide a continuous evaluation of performance data, which is then used in the accreditation process. Although currently focusing only on acute care hospitals, it is expected that the IM system's scope will be further expanded to include a broader group of health care organization in the future.[30]

Table 17-3	Commonly performed quality control procedures and recommended tolerances for the simulator (as established by the AAPM)[2,13]	
Procedures		**Tolerance (+/−)**
I. DAILY		
Lasers		2 mm
Distance indicator (ODI)		2 mm
II. MONTHLY		
Field size indicator		2 mm
Gantry/collimator angle indicators		1 degree
Cross-hair centering		2 mm diameter
Focal spot-axis indicator		2 mm
Fluoroscopic image quality		Baseline
Emergency/collision avoidance		Functional
Light/radiation field coincidence		2 mm or 1%
Film processor sensitometry		Baseline
III. ANNUALLY		
A. Mechanical checks		
Collimator, gantry, couch rotation isocenter		2 mm diameter
Coincidence of collimator, gantry, couch axes, and isocenter		2 mm diameter
Table top sag		2 mm
Vertical travel of couch		2 mm
B. Radiographic checks		
Exposure rate		Baseline
Table top exposure with fluoroscopy		Baseline
Kilovolt peak and milliamperage calibration		Baseline
High and low contrast resolution		Baseline

From AAPM: Comprehensive QA for radiation oncology: Report of AAPM Radiation Therapy Committee Task Group 40, *Med Phys* 21(4):518-616, 1994; and Khan FM: *The physics of radiation therapy*, ed 2, Baltimore, 1994, Williams & Wilkins.

Each of the aspects of care delineated under the quality improvement process discretely collects data through the use of check sheets, data sheets, and check lists. These data should then be statistically analyzed against **internal** and **external customer** satisfaction and placed in a meaningful format such as charts, graphs and histograms with distribution to all employees.[19,20,22] The selection of the appropriate solution or response should be substantiated by the data analysis. This task may be appropriately delegated to the quality improvement committee. However, in a large health care facility/organization, this might necessitate the procurement of the assistance from other "organization-wide systems such as strategic planning, performance management, measurement, budgetary, and management information." By doing that, the health care organization becomes a true "quality organization which continues to improve."[19]

SUMMARY

A successful quality improvement plan is the end result of total commitment and involvement from all health care providers at all times.[8,18] Linked to cost containment, increased quality of care, professional practice standards, and the JCAHO criteria, CQI has become routine practice in the delivery of health care. It is therefore the responsibility of the radiation therapist and every other radiation oncology team member to become educated about quality improvement. They will undoubtedly be involved in many aspects of CQI in their professional careers with the ultimate benefit going to our customers, especially our patients.

Review Questions

1. What is the recommended frequency of checking audio and video monitors in treatment rooms?
   a. Daily
   b. Weekly
   c. Monthly
   d. Yearly

Table 17-4	Commonly performed quality control procedures and recommended tolerances for the cobalt-60 unit (as established by the AAMP and NRC)	
Procedures		**Tolerance (+/−)**
I. DAILY		
A. *Safety devices*		
Audiovisual monitor (camera, television, intercom)		Functional
Door interlock		Functional
Radiation room monitor		Functional
B. *Mechanical devices*		
Lasers*		2 mm
Distance indicator (ODI)*		2 mm
II. WEEKLY		
Source positioning check		3 mm
III. MONTHLY		
A. *Dosimetry*		
Output constancy		2%
B. *Mechanical checks*		
Light/radiation field coincidence		3 mm
Field size indicator (collimator setting)		2 mm
Gantry and collimator angle indicator		1 degree
Cross-hair centering		1 mm
Latching of wedges, trays		Functional
C. *Safety checks*		
Emergency off buttons		Functional
Wedge interlocks		Functional
Beam orientation restriction interlocks		Functional
Beam condition indicator interlocks		Functional
IV. ANNUAL		
A. *Dosimetry checks*		
Output constancy		2%
Field size dependence and output constancy		2%
Central axis dosimetry parameter constancy		2%
Timer linearity and error*		1%
B. *Safety interlocks*		
Follow test procedures of manufacturer		Functional
Distance indicator (ODI)*		2 mm
C. *Mechanical checks*		
Collimator, gantry, and couch rotation isocenter		2 mm diameter
Coincidence of collimator, gantry, and couch axes with isocenter		2 mm diameter
Table top sag		2 mm
Vertical travel of table		2 mm
Field light intensity		Functional

From AAPM: Comprehensive QA for radiation oncology: Report of AAPM Radiation Therapy Committee Task Group 40, *Med Phys* 21(4):518-616, 1994; and Khan FM: *The physics of radiation therapy*, ed 2, Baltimore, 1994, Williams & Wilkins.
*NRC recommends a monthly check.

2. Quality improvement is specifically:
   a. A proactive means to ensure quality patient care
   b. The operational techniques and activities used to fulfill quality requirements
   c. Both a and b
   d. Neither a nor b

3. Ongoing evaluation of all aspects of care for the purpose of determining areas where improvement is needed is known as:
   a. Total quality management
   b. Quality assessment
   c. Quality assurance
   d. Quality control

Table 17-5	Commonly performed quality control procedures and recommended tolerances for the medical accelerator (as established by the AAMP)			
Procedures	**Tolerance (+/–)**		**Procedures**	**Tolerance (+/–)**
I. DAILY			**III. ANNUAL**	
A. Dosimetry checks			*A. Dosimetry checks*	
X-ray output constancy	3%		X-ray/electron output calibration constancy	2%
Electron output	3%		Field size dependence of x-ray output constancy	2%
B. Mechanical checks			Output factor constancy for electron applicators	2%
Lasers	2 mm		Central axis parameter constancy	2%
Distance indicator	2 mm		Off-axis factor constancy	2%
C. Safety checks			Transmission factor constancy for all treatment accessories	2%
Door interlock	Functional		Wedge transmission factor constancy	2%
Audiovisual monitor (television, cameras, intercom, etc.)	Functional		Monitor chamber linearity	1%
			X-ray output constancy vs. gantry angle	2%
II. MONTHLY			Electron output constancy vs. gantry angle	2%
A. Dosimetry checks			Off-axis factor constancy vs. gantry angle	2%
X-ray and electron output constancy	2%		Arc mode	Manufacturer's specifications
Backup monitor constancy	2%			
X-ray beam flatness constancy	2%		*B. Safety interlocks*	
Electron beam flatness constancy	3%		Follow manufacturer's test procedures	Functional
B. Safety interlocks			*C. Mechanical checks*	
Emergency off buttons	Functional		Collimator, gantry, couch rotation isocenter	2 mm diameter
Wedge, electron cone interlocks	Functional		Coincidence of collimator, gantry, and couch axes with isocenter	2 mm diameter
C. Mechanical checks			Coincidence of radiation and mechanical isocenter	2 mm diameter
Gantry/collimator angle indicators	1 degree		Table top sag	2 mm
Light/radiation field coincidence	2 mm or 1% on side		Vertical travel of table	2 mm
Wedge position	2 mm			
Tray position	2 mm			
Applicator position	2 mm			
Field size indicators	2 mm			
Cross-hair centering	2 mm diameter			
Treatment couch position indicators	2 mm/1 degree			
Latching of wedges, blocking tray	Functional			
Jaw symmetry	2 mm			
Field light intensity	Functional			

From AAPM: Comprehensive QA for radiation oncology: Report of AAPM Radiation Therapy Committee Task Group 40, *Med Phys* 21(4):518-616, 1994 and Khan FM: *The physics of radiation therapy*, ed 2, Baltimore, 1994, Williams & Wilkins.

4. An assessment of an aspect of a plan of action by those with the same job title and responsibilities is known as:
   a. Quality control
   b. Peer review
   c. Quality indicator
   d. Flow charting
5. The operational techniques and activities used to fulfill requirements of quality are called:
   a. Quality audit
   b. Quality control
   c. Quality management
   d. Quality assessment

Questions to Ponder

1. Explain why the phrase "If it ain't broke, don't fix it" cannot be applied in a quality improvement program.
2. An initial step in improving a process is defining those activities used in completing the process. Develop a flow chart outlining the steps necessary to complete a double-exposure portal film in the radiation oncology department.
3. Referring to Deming's principles of management, what suggestions would you give a co-worker who consistently complains about a specific problem relating to the treatment delivery process in radiation oncology?

4. Describe how information collected for quality assessment should be used in a quality management plan.
5. Explain the differences between quality assurance and quality management.

REFERENCES

1. American Association of Physicists in Medicine: Comprehensive QA for radiation oncology: report of AAPM Radiation Therapy Committee Task Group 40, *Med Phys* 21:518-616, 1994.
2. American Association of Physicists in Medicine: Quality assurance for clinical radiotherapy treatment planning: report of AAPM Radiation Therapy Committee Task Group 53, College Park, Maryland, 1998, The American Association of Physicists in Medicine.
3. American Association of Physicists in Medicine: Clinical use of electronic portal imaging: report of AAPM Radiation Therapy Committee Task Group 58, College Park, Maryland, 2001, The American Association of Physicists in Medicine.
4. American College of Medical Physics: Radiation control and quality assurance in radiation oncology: a suggested protocol, Report No. 2, Reston, VA, 1986, American College of Medical Physics.
5. American College of Radiology: Standards, available at http://www.acr.org/departments/stand_accred/standards/standards.html (accessed July 2, 2001).
6. American Society of Radiologic Technologists: Government relations section: OSHA Updates Facility Consultation Regulations, available at http://www.asrt.org/asrt.htm (accessed April 10, 2003).
7. American Society of Radiologic Technologists: Professional Development section: Practice standards for medical imaging and radiation therapy, available at http://www.asrt.org/asrt.htm (accessed April 10, 2003).
8. Brundage MD, Dixon PF, MacKillop WJ et al: A real-time audit of radiation therapy in a regional cancer center, *Int J Radiat Oncol Biol Phys* 43:121, 1999.
9. Earp KA, Gates L: A model QA program in radiation oncology, *Radiol Tech* 61:297-304, 1990.
10. Environmental Protection Agency: Timeline, available at http://www.epa.gov/history/timeline/index.htm (accessed July 3, 2001).
11. Food and Drug Administration: Accidental radiation occurrences and radiation incidents, available at http://www.fda.gov/cdrh/radhlth/aro.html (accessed June 30, 2001).
12. Hendee WR, Ibbott GS: *Radiation therapy physics,* ed 2, St. Louis, 1996, Mosby-Year Book, pp 455-501.
13. Improving organization performance. *Comprehensive accreditation manual for hospitals,* update 3, Oakbrook Terrace, Ill, August 1998, Joint Commission on Accreditation of Healthcare Organizations.
14. ISCRO Subcommittee: Radiation oncology in integrated cancer management, Blue Book, Dec 1991.
15. International Standards Organization: International Standards Organization Report ISO-8402-1986, 1986.
16. Joint Commission on Accreditation of Healthcare Organizations: *1994 accreditation manual for hospitals*.
17. Joint Commission on Accreditation of Healthcare Organizations: *1995 accreditation manual for hospitals*.
18. Khan FM: *The physics of radiation therapy,* ed 2, Baltimore, 1994, Williams & Wilkins.
19. Kirk R: The big picture: total quality management and continuous quality improvement, *J Nurs Admin* 24:37-41, 1994.
20. Lapresti J, Whetstone WR: Total quality management: doing things right, *Nurs Manage* 24:34-36, 1993.
21. Levitte SH, Khan F: Quality assurance in radiation oncology, *Cancer* 74(suppl 9):2642-2646, 1994.
22. Nelson MT: Continuous quality improvement (CQI) in radiology: an overview, *Appl Radiol* 23(7):11-16, 1994.
23. Norris TG: Quality assurance in radiation therapy, *Radiat Ther* 9:161-184, 2000.
24. Nuclear Regulatory Commission: Mission, available at: http://www.ncr.gov/NRC/what is/mission.html # mission (accessed June 11, 2001).
25. Occupational Safety and Health Administration: US Department of Labor, available at http://www.osha-slc.gov/index.html (accessed July 9, 2001).
26. Office of Hazardous Materials: Mission, available at http://hazmat.dot.gov/about.htm (accessed July 3, 2001).
27. Office of State and Tribal Programs: available at http://www.hsrd.orn/gov/nrc/special/about.pdf (accessed July 7, 2001).
28. Papp J: *Quality management in the imaging sciences,* St. Louis, 1998, Mosby, pp 1-12.
29. Sherman J, Malkmus MA: Integrating quality assurance and total quality management/quality improvement, *J Nurs Admin* 24:37-41, 1994.
30. The IM System*: Leading the way to performance measurement. Comprehensive accreditation manual for hospitals,* update 3, Oakbrook Terrace, Ill, August, 1997, Joint Commission on Accreditation of Healthcare Organizations.
31. Thwaites D, Scolliet P, Leer JW: Quality assurance in radiotherapy, *Radiother Oncol* 35:61-73, 1995.
32. US Department of Transportation: Quality assurance home page available at http://www.dot.gov/safety.html (accessed July 3, 2001).
33. Van der Schueren E, Hariot JC, Leunens G: Quality assurance in cancer treatment, *Eur J Cancer* 29A:172-181, 1993.
34. Wambersie A: The role of the ICRU in quality assurance in radiation therapy, *Int J Radiat Oncol Biol Phys* 10(suppl 1):81-86, 1984.

18

Surface and Sectional Anatomy

Charles M. Washington

Outline

Key Terms

Radiation therapy today is a well-established science that requires its practitioners to demonstrate knowledge of human anatomy and physiology. The radiation therapist learns early in the educational curriculum that he or she must have a comprehensive understanding of surface and cross-sectional anatomy. Knowledge of human anatomy is essential in simulation, treatment planning, and accurate daily treatment delivery. This chapter focuses on the surface and sectional anatomy used in simulation and treatment delivery performed by the radiation therapist. Surface anatomy will be related to deep-seated structures within the human body. An overview of the diagnostic tools used to visualize internal structures is presented along with a review of lymphatic physiology. This is included because the lymphatics play a major role in treatment field design and disease management. A brief review of skeletal anatomy is presented to ensure a common basis for understanding important spatial relationships. Surface and sectional along with topographical landmarks are presented in practical radiation therapy applications.

PERSPECTIVE

The primary objective in managing cancer with radiation therapy is to deposit enough dose to result in the cancer cell death while minimizing the effect on the surrounding normal tissues. The challenge is to define a patient-specific therapy plan that entails localizing the tumor and surrounding dose-limiting tissues, such as the spinal cord, kidney, and eyes. In addition, the therapist must maintain the integrity of the plan throughout its administration. The particulars of surface anatomy available to the therapist have changed little during the last 30 years. Clinical application is essential in facilitating the understanding of a disease process on anatomic grounds, corresponding surface location of internal structures, and the appearance of internal imaged structures.[8]

Visual, palpable, and imaged anatomy forms the basis of clinical examination.[9] This is the case in radiation therapy. Surface and sectional anatomy provides the foundation that the therapist needs to be effective in simulation, treatment planning, and the daily administration of therapy treatments. Without this foundation, it would be like traveling from Texas to Maine for the first time, without any planning. We know the general direction of where we want to go, but we would not know the most efficient way to get there. The radiation therapist must have a comprehensive knowledge of imaging modalities that enable tumor visualization, pertinent lymphatic anatomy, and the site-by-site relationship of surface and sectional anatomy. A systematic approach to this information will allow the therapist to link vital classroom information to its clinical application.

RELATED IMAGING MODALITIES USED IN SIMULATION AND TUMOR LOCALIZATION

More than any other innovation, the ability to painlessly visualize the interior of the living human body has governed the practice of medicine during the twentieth century.[2] In recent years new medical imaging techniques allowed for effective ways to diagnose and localize pathologic disorders. The medical imaging modalities used in simulation and tumor localization fit into two categories: ionizing and nonionizing imaging studies. Ionizing imaging studies use ionizing radiation to produce images that demonstrate anatomy. Examples of ionizing imaging studies include conventional radiography, computed tomography (CT), and nuclear medicine imaging. Nonionizing imaging studies use alternative means of imaging the body, such as magnetic fields in magnetic resonance imaging (MRI) and echoed sound waves in ultrasonography.

Conventional Radiography

A radiograph provides a two-dimensional image of the interior of the body. The use of computerized radiography (CR) and digital radiography (DR) can also be used to visualize internal anatomy without exposing a film. In either case, photostimulatable plates or detectors capture the latent images for visualization on computer screens. The latent images produced delineate the obvious differences in tissue densities of the body; however, x-rays do not always distinguish subtle differences in tissue density. Fig. 18-1 demonstrates a conventional chest radiograph produced by a therapy simulator. The pertinent anatomy can be distinguished and outlined for practical application. Any anomaly, a variation from the standard, is recognizable on the image as well as any structure considered to be dose limiting.

Radiation therapy uses an extensive amount of diagnostic imaging in its daily practice. Simulators use specialized diagnostic x-ray equipment to localize the treatment area and reproduce the geometry of the therapeutic beam before treatment. Radiographic localization is the most common method used to localize tumor volumes. Other techniques also aid in visualization of human anatomy. **Lymphangiography,** a specialized technique that uses injected dyes to help visualize the lymphatic system, is still used in some cases. Fig. 18-2 shows a radiograph that employs lymphangiography. The lymphatic channels are the white areas of higher density. Filling defects, lymphatic channels that are not completely visible or appear frothy, can demonstrate the presence of pathologic changes. These all provide valuable information for patient treatment planning. In all, conventional radiology is an essential component in radiation therapy.

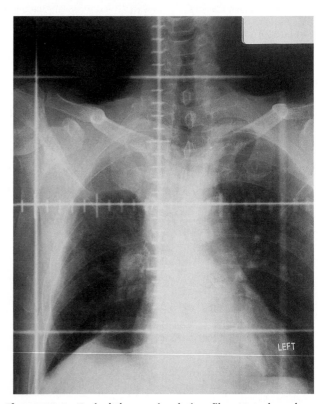

Figure 18-1. Typical thorax simulation film. Note how bony anatomy is distinguishable from cartilage and soft tissue.

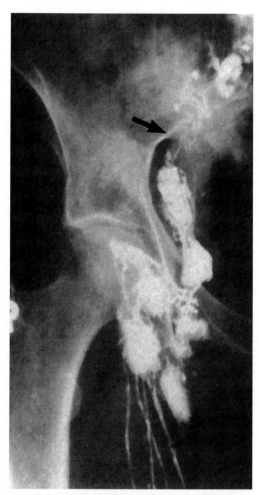

Figure 18-2. Lymphangiogram. The lymphatic channels can be imaged and used to assess the status of the lymphatics.

procedures. The detail of the images produced has about 10 to 20 times the detail of conventional radiography. Display of CT images reflects the differences among four basic densities: air (black), fat (dark/gray), water/blood (gray/light), and bone/metal (white).[1] CT demonstrates bone detail well. Radiation therapy treatment planning commonly uses CT images, particularly with three-dimensional treatment plans and virtual simulation techniques.

Nuclear Medicine Imaging

The branch of medicine that uses radioisotopes in the diagnosis and treatment of disease is known as nuclear medicine. Nuclear medicine imaging uses ionizing radiation to provide information about physiology as well as anatomic structure. This is typically useful in noted abnormalities secondary to tumor activity, specifically metastatic disease.[14] Sensitive radiation detection devices display images of radioactive drugs taken through the body and their uptake in tissues. Although this imaging technique plays an important role in tumor imaging, it detects metastatic disease more than primary tumors. Bone and liver metastases are localized using nuclear medicine scans. These scans are relatively safe and can provide very valuable information. The radionuclide bone scan is the procedure of choice for skeletal scanning. Fig. 18-3 shows a bone scan. Areas of increased uptake, the dark spots, demonstrate high-activity areas that correspond to pathologic changes (uptake in the urinary bladder is normal). The radionuclide liver scan is the initial scan of choice for liver metastasis. Gallium scans localize areas of inflammation and tumor activity in lymphoma patients. They are useful in monitoring changes in tumor size. Radiation safety procedures are important in nuclear medicine scanning. In both intravenous application and ingestion of radioactive isotopes, care in monitoring patient exposure to

Computed Tomography

CT is an ionizing radiation–based technique in which x-rays interact with a scintillation crystal that is more sensitive than x-ray film.[1] CT scanning combines x-ray principles and advanced computer technologies. The x-ray source moves in an arc around the body part being scanned and continually sends out beams of radiation. As the beams pass through the body, the tissues absorb small amounts of radiation, depending on their densities (see Figure 6-31). The beams are converted to signals that are projected onto a television screen. These images look like radiographs of slices through the body. They are typically perpendicular to the long axis of the patient's body. The CT scan provides important anatomic and spatial relationships at a glance. A series of scans allows the examination of section after section of a patient's anatomy.

The entire CT process takes only seconds for each slice, it is completely painless, and the dose of radiation to the patient is typically equal to that of many other diagnostic

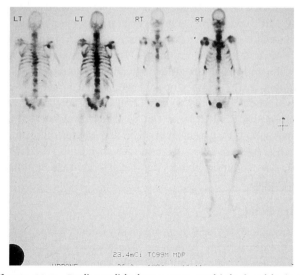

Figure 18-3. Radionuclide bone scan. Multiple focal lesions in bone of patient with prostate cancer.

ionizing radiation is important. The elimination of isotopes that have run through the body (through urination) also requires careful monitoring and precautions.

Positron emission tomography (PET) scanning employs short-lived radioisotopes such as carbon-11, nitrogen-13, or oxygen-15 in a solution commonly injected into a patient. The radioisotope circulates through the body and emits positively charged electrons, called positrons. These positrons collide with conventional electrons in body tissues, causing the release of gamma rays. These rays are detected and recorded. The computer creates a colored PET scan that demonstrates function rather than structure. It can detect blood flow through organs like the brain and heart, diagnose coronary artery disease, and identify the extent of stroke or heart attack damage. PET is useful in diagnosing two types of breast cancer (those with and without estrogen receptors). In that way the physician can prescribe the appropriate treatment regimen early. Also, PET images are being used more and more to outline specific areas of anatomy and are then correlated to other imaging studies like CT and magnetic resonance (MR) in treatment planning.

Magnetic Resonance Imaging

MRI records data that are based on the magnetic properties of the hydrogen nuclei, which can be thought of as tiny magnets spinning in random directions. These hydrogen nuclei (magnets) interact with neighboring atoms and with all applied magnetic fields.[1] In this imaging modality a strong uniform magnetic energy is applied to small magnetic fields that lie parallel to the direction of the external magnet. The patient is pulsed with radiowaves, which cause the nuclei to send out a weak radio signal that is detected and reworked into a planar image of the body. The images, which indicate cellular activity, look similar to a CT scan. Fig. 18-4 shows a sagittal MR scan of the head.

MR has a diagnostic advantage over CT in that it provides information about chemicals in an organ or tissue. In this way, MR can perform a noninvasive (one not involving puncture or incision of the skin or insertion of a foreign object into the body) biopsy on tumors. The disadvantages of MR are the expensive magnetic shielding requirements, low throughput (the number of patients an hour a machine can serve) when compared with CT, and increased cost in comparison to CT. MRI scans can be indexed, registered, and fused with CT scans and used in the treatment planning process. In these cases, the best of both imaging modalities are used to outline tumors for better conformal treatment planning.

Ultrasound

Ultrasound (US) uses high-frequency sound waves, which are not heard by the human ear. These waves travel forward and continue to move until they make contact with an object; at that point, a certain amount of the sound bounces back. Submarines use this principle to find other underwater ves-

sels as well as the depth of the ocean floor. US remains a less expensive and less hazardous alternative to the earlier studies.[14] A transducer, a handheld instrument, generates high-frequency sound waves. It moves over the body part being examined. The transducer also picks up the returning sound waves. Normal and abnormal tissues exhibit varying densities that reflect sound differently. The resultant image is processed onto a screen and is called a sonogram. The images can be a still two-dimensional, cross-sectioned image or a moving image, like the heart of a fetus.

US offers no exposure to ionizing radiation, is noninvasive and painless, and requires no contrast media. However, it does not effectively penetrate bone or air-filled spaces. It is therefore not useful in imaging the skull, lungs, or intestines. In radiation therapy the use of US continues to increase. It is very helpful in noninvasively determining internal organ location as evidenced in the increasing use of US to locate and guide brachytherapy implants, locating tumors within the eye, and increasing positioning efficiency during conformal prostate treatment delivery with intensity modulated radiation therapy applications. Fig. 18-5 shows a radiation therapist obtaining US localization information for a patient about to be treated for prostate cancer.

Modern imaging modalities provide important information to the radiation therapy team for tumor localization. Cross-sectional images are very valuable. They provide views within the patient and display organs with their normal shape and orientation, typically in treatment position. The

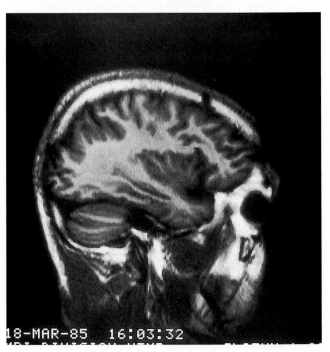

Figure 18-4. Sagittal magnetic resonance image section through the head. *(From Haaga JR: Computed tomography and magnetic resonance imaging of the whole body, St. Louis, 1995, Mosby.)*

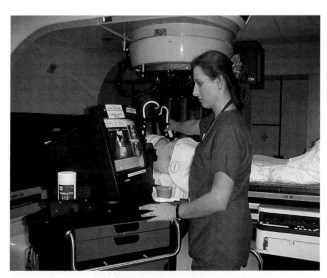

Figure 18-5. Therapist obtaining ultrasound information for intensity modulated radiation therapy (IMRT) prostate treatment.

direct relationships allow for accurate treatment planning. We can relate the patient's surface anatomy to the inner structure. In addition to displaying organs with their normal living shape, normal anatomic relationships can be observed. In particular, the study of sectional images allows the radiation therapy practitioner to develop an excellent three-dimensional concept of anatomy.[10] These modalities provide the basic information necessary to develop critical thinking skills in surface and sectional anatomy that is essential in the role of the radiation therapist.

ANATOMIC POSITIONING

Radiation therapy requires daily reproducible positioning for effective treatment delivery. The radiation therapist uses various terms to describe the relationship of body parts, planes, and sections that serve as the foundation in understanding the body's structural plan.

Definition of Terms

When using terms that reference human body position, it is assumed that the body is in the anatomic position; this allows for clear reference of directional relationships. The **anatomic position** is one in which the subject stands upright, with feet together flat on the floor, toes pointed forward, arms straight down by the sides of the body with palms facing forward, fingers extended, and thumbs pointing away from the body.[9] Fig. 18-6 demonstrates this position.

Directional terms explain the location of various body structures in relation to each other. These terms are precise and avoid the use of unnecessary words and paint a clear picture for the radiation therapist. *Superior* means toward the head; *inferior,* toward the feet; *medial,* toward the midline of the body; and *lateral,* toward one side or the other. Anterior relates to anatomy nearer to the front of the body; posterior, nearer to

or at the back of the body. *Ipsilateral* refers to a body component on the same side of the body, whereas *contralateral* refers to the opposite side of the body. *Supine* means lying face up; *prone* means lying face down. Table 18-1 outlines the directional terms commonly used by the radiation therapy team.

Planes and Sections

The human body may also be examined with respect to planes, which are imaginary flat surfaces that pass through it. Fig. 18-7 illustrates the standard anatomic planes. The *sagittal plane* divides the body vertically into right or left sides. The *median sagittal plane,* also called the midsagittal plane, divides the body into two symmetrical right and left sides. There is only one median sagittal plane. A *parasagittal* plane is a vertical plane that is parallel to the median sagittal plane and divides the body into unequal components, both right and left. A *coronal* or *frontal* plane is perpendicular (at right angles) to the sagittal plane and vertically divides the body into anterior and posterior sections. A *horizontal* or *transverse plane* is perpendicular to the midsagittal, parasagittal, and coronal planes and divides the human body into superior and inferior parts. When a health care professional views a body structure, it is often seen in a sectional view. A sectional view looks at a flat surface resulting from a cut made through the three-dimensional structure.

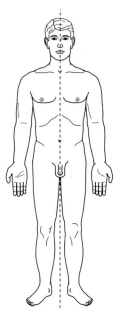

Figure 18-6. Anatomic position and bilateral symmetry. In the anatomic position the body is in an erect, or standing, posture with the arms at the sides and palms forward. The head and feet are also pointing forward. The dotted line shows the body's bilateral symmetry. As a result of this organizational feature, the right and left sides of the body are mirror images of each other. *(From The body as a whole. In Thibodeau GA, Patton KT, editors: Anatomy and physiology, ed 2, St. Louis, 1993, Mosby.)*

Table 18-1	**Directional terms**	
Term	**Definition**	**Example**
Superior	Toward the head or upper part of a structure	The manubrium is superior to the body of the sternum
Inferior	Away from the head or lower part of the structure	The stomach is inferior to the lung
Anterior	Toward or nearer to the front	The trachea is anterior to the esophagus, which is anterior to the spinal cord
Posterior	Nearer to the back	The esophagus is posterior to the trachea
Medial	Nearer to the midline; the midline is an imaginary vertical line that divides the body into equal right and left components	The ulna is on the medial side of the forearm
Lateral	Farther from the midline or to the side	The pleural cavities are lateral to the pericardial cavity
Ipsilateral	On the same side	The ascending colon and appendix are ipsilateral
Contralateral	On the opposite side	The ascending colon and descending colon are contralateral
Proximal	Nearer to the point of origin or attachment	The humerus is proximal to the radius
Distal	Farther from the point of origin or attachment	The phalanges are distal to the carpals
Superficial	On or near the body surface	The skin is superficial to the thoracic viscera
Deep	Away from the body surface	The ribs are deep to the skin of the chest

Modified from Tortora G, Anagnostakos N, editors: *Principles of anatomy and physiology*, ed 6. Copyright © 1990 by Biological Sciences Textbooks, Inc., A & P Textbooks, Inc., and Elia-Sparta, Inc. Reprinted by permission of Harper Collins Publishers, Inc.

Surface and cross-sectional anatomy in radiation therapy are not solely a set of definitions or a listing of body parts. The practitioner must relate the body's physical perspective to its overall function. The standardized anatomic terms presented will assist in accurately realizing those relationships.

BODY HABITUS

Roentgen's discovery of the x-ray allowed scientists at the turn of the nineteenth century to revolutionize the medical field, both diagnostically and therapeutically.[2] These early radiographs showed differences in the location of internal anatomy from one person to the next. Although everyone had the same organs, the organs were not necessarily in the exact same place. It was agreed that humans are a variable species with regard to structural characteristics, and it is evident that variety in general physique corresponds to great variation in visceral form, position, and motility. There is consistency between certain physiques and certain types of visceral form and arrangement. It is obvious that a thorax of certain dimensions can only house lungs of a certain form. The same is true for the abdomen. Knowing this can greatly assist the radiation therapist in relating internal anatomy to varying types.

The physique, or **body habitus**, of an individual can be classified into four groups. The *hypersthenic habitus* represents about 5% of the population. This body type exhibits a short, wide trunk; great body weight; and a heavy skeletal framework. The abdomen is long with great capacity, the alimentary tract is high, and the stomach is almost thoracic. The

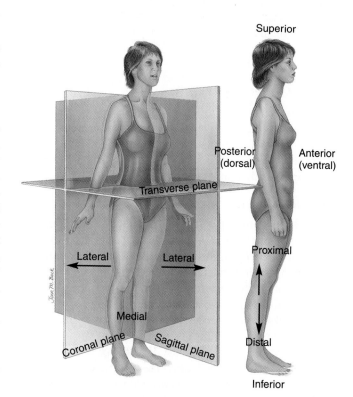

Figure 18-7. Directions and planes of the body. These planes provide a standardized reference for the radiation therapist. *(From Thibodeau GA, Patton KT: Anatomy and physiology, St. Louis, 1994, Mosby.)*

pelvic cavity is small. When taking a chest film of this body type, it may be necessary to turn the cassette sideways to image the entire chest.

The *sthenic habitus* resembles the hypersthenic habitus. These individuals make up close to half (~48%) of the population. They are of considerable weight with a heavy skeletal framework. The alimentary tract is high but not as high as in the hypersthenic habitus. Most stout, well-built persons are sthenics.

The *hyposthenic habitus,* entailing about 35% of the population, has a slender physique. This habitus demonstrates many

of the sthenic characteristics but appears to be frailer. The abdominal cavity falls between the sthenic and the asthenic.

The *asthenic habitus* demonstrates a more slender physique, light body weight, and a lighter skeletal framework. It is found in 10% to 12% of the population. The thorax has long, narrow lung fields with its widest portion in the upper zones. The heart is commonly pendent in form. The asthenic has an abdomen longer than the hypersthenic and is typically accompanied by a pelvis with great capacity. The alimentary tract is lowest of all types mentioned. Fig. 18-8

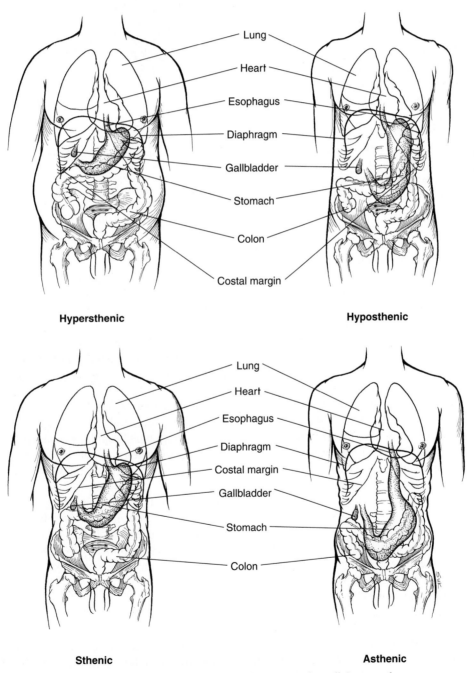

Figure 18-8. Comparison of the four body habiti. Note that all feature the same structures. However, the internal viscera vary in position from one physique to another.

compares the various body habiti. Although the internal components are the same in all body types, the locations vary. These categories can help standardize the variances demonstrated from person to person.

Body Cavities

The spaces within the body that contain internal organs are called **body cavities** (Fig. 18-9). The two main cavities are the posterior, or dorsal, and the anterior, or ventral, cavities. The dorsal cavity can be further divided into the spinal or vertebral cavity, protected by the vertebrae, which contains the spinal cord, and the cranial cavity, which contains the brain.

The anterior cavity is subdivided by a horizontal muscle, called the diaphragm, into the thoracic cavity and the abdominopelvic cavity. The thoracic cavity is further divided into a pericardial cavity, which contains the heart and two pleural cavities, including the right and left lungs.

The abdominopelvic cavity has two sections: the upper abdominal cavity and the lower pelvic cavity. There is no intervening partition between the two. The principal structures located in the abdominal cavity are the peritoneum, liver, gallbladder, pancreas, spleen, stomach, and most of the large and small intestines. The pelvic section contains the rest of the large intestine, rectum, urinary bladder, and internal reproductive system.

The abdominopelvic cavity is large and is divided into four quadrants by placing a transverse plane across the midsagittal plane at the point of the umbilicus (navel). The four quadrants are the right upper, left upper, right lower, and left lower. The abdominal cavity can also be sectioned into a number of regions. Fig. 18-10 shows the quadrants and regions of the abdomen and pelvis. Table 18-2 outlines the regions of the abdominal cavity.

The surface markings and locations of all structures are approximations and generalizations.[8] However, knowledge of the varying body types will provide the radiation therapist with practical information. If the therapist has an idea of where the internal structures are, especially during a simulation, he or she can locate the placement of the treatment portal sooner and more accurately. This equates to less time on the simulation table for the patient and lower fluoroscopic exposure times, since it will not require as much location time.

LYMPHATIC SYSTEM

Knowledge of the **lymphatic system** is very important in radiation therapy. To achieve local and regional control of malignant disease processes, the anatomy of the lymphatic system must be considered. Many tumors spread through this system; often, areas of tumor spread are predicted based solely on that knowledge. For example, in a three-field head and neck treatment plan the supraclavicular fossa (SCF) is commonly treated even if there is no clinical evidence of tumor present (prophylactic treatment). This is important because the lymphatic drainage of the head and neck eventually drains to that area. In any examination of surface and

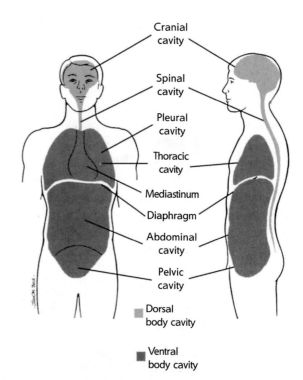

Figure 18-9. Major body cavities. *(From Organization of the body. In Thibodeau GA, Patton KT, editors: Anatomy and physiology, ed 2, St. Louis, 1993, Mosby.)*

cross-sectional anatomy specific to radiation therapy, the lymphatic system should not be overlooked.

The lymphatic system consists of lymphatic vessels, lymphatic organs, and the fluid that circulates through it, called lymph. The system is closely associated with the cardiovascular system and is composed of specialized connective tissue that contains a large quantity of lymphocytes. Lymphatic tissue is found throughout the body.

The lymphatic system has three main functions. First, lymphatic vessels drain tissue spaces of interstitial fluid that escapes from blood capillaries and loose connective tissues, filters it, and returns it to the bloodstream. This is important in maintaining the overall fluid levels in the body. Second, the lymphatic system absorbs fats and transports them to the bloodstream. Third, this intricate system plays a major role in the body's defense and immunity. **Immunity** is the ability of the body to defend itself against infectious organisms and foreign bodies. Specifically, lymphocytes and macrophages protect the body by recognizing and responding to the foreign matter.

Lymphatic Vessels

Lymphatic vessels contain lymph. Lymph is excessive tissue fluid consisting mostly of water and plasma proteins from capillaries. It differs from blood by the absence of formed elements in it. Lymphatic vessels start in spaces between cells; at that point they are referred to as lymphatic capillaries.

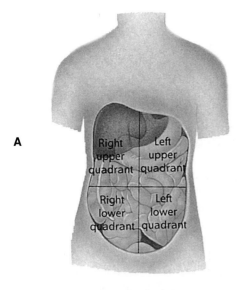

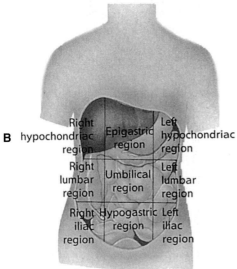

Figure 18-10. Abdomen. **A,** Division of the abdomen into four quarters. Diagram shows relationship of internal organs to the abdominopelvic quadrants; 1, right upper quadrant (RUQ); 2, left upper quadrant (LUQ); 3, right lower quadrant (RLQ); 4, left lower quadrant (LLQ). **B,** Nine regions of abdominopelvic cavity showing the most superficial organs. *(From Seeley RR, Stephens TD, Tate P, editors: Essentials of anatomy and physiology, ed 2, St. Louis, 1996, Mosby.)*

Table 18-2	Regions of the abdominal cavity	
Region	**Description**	
Umbilical	Centrally located around the navel	
Lumbar	Regions to the right and left of the navel; lumbar refers to the lower back, which occurs here	
Epigastric	Central region superior to the umbilical region	
Hypochondriac	Regions to the right and left of the epigastric region and inferior to the cartilage of the rib cage	
Hypogastric	Central region inferior to the umbilical region	
Iliac	Regions to the right and left of the hypogastric region; iliac refers to the hip bones, which occur here	

and transported away for filtration. They start blindly in the interstitial spaces and flow in only one direction.

The lymphatic capillaries join to form larger lymphatic vessels. Lymphatic vessels resemble veins in structure but have thinner walls and more valves that promote the one-way flow. These larger vessels follow veins and arteries and eventually empty into one of two ducts in the upper thorax—the **thoracic duct** or the **right lymphatic duct**—which then flow into the subclavian veins.

Fluid movement in the lymphatic system depends on hydrostatic and osmotic pressures that increase through skeletal muscular contraction. As the muscles around the vessels contract, the lymph is moved past a one-way valve that closes. This prevents the lymph from flowing backward. Respiratory movements create a pressure gradient between two ends of the lymphatic system. Fluid flows from high-pressure areas, like the abdomen, to low-pressure areas, like the thorax where pressure falls as each inhalation occurs.

Lymph Nodes

Along the paths of the lymph vessels are lymph nodes. These nodes vary in size from 1 to 25 mm in length, and they often occur in groups. A lymph node contains both afferent and efferent lymphatic vessels. **Afferent lymphatic vessels** enter the lymph node at several points along the convex surface. They contain one-way valves that open into the node, bringing the lymph into it. On the other side of the node are efferent vessels. The **efferent lymphatic vessels** are typically wider than the afferent vessels; their valves open away from the node, again facilitating one-way flow. There are more afferent vessels coming into a node than efferent vessels coming out of it, slowing the flow through the nodes. Fig. 18-11 demonstrates the components of a typical lymph node. This is similar to driving along a four-lane highway during rush hour and getting to a point of road construction that restricts traffic

These lymphatic vessels are extensive; virtually every region of the body that has a blood supply is richly supplied with these capillaries. It stands to reason that those areas that are avascular do not demonstrate the same number of vessels. Examples of these avascular areas are the central nervous system and bone marrow. These lymphatic capillaries are more permeable than associated blood capillaries for substances to enter. Cellular debris, sloughed off cells, and foreign substances that occur in the intercellular spaces are more readily collected through these lymphatic pathways

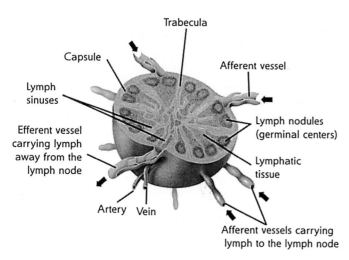

Figure 18-11. Lymph node. Arrows indicate the direction of lymph flow. The germinal centers are sites of lymphocyte production. As lymph moves through the lymph sinuses, macrophages remove foreign substances. *(From The lymphatic system and immunity. In Seeley RR, Stephens TD, Tate P, editors: Essentials of anatomy and physiology, St. Louis, 1991, Mosby.)*

flow to one lane. You can only go in one direction and must wait your turn to move through the area. This slowing of the lymph through the node permits the nodes to effectively filter the lymph, and, through phagocytosis, the endothelial cells of the node engulf, devitalize, and remove contaminants.

The substances are trapped inside the reticular fibers and pathways throughout the node. Edema is an excessive accumulation of fluid in a tissue, producing swelling. This can occur when excessive foreign bodies, lymph, and debris are being engulfed in the node. This is evident when a person has a cold or the flu. The subdigastric nodes, located in the neck just below the angle of the mandible, become swollen and tender because of the heightened phagocytic activity in that area to rid the body of the trapped contaminants. The swelling goes down as the pathogen is devitalized. Edema also occurs when altered lymphatic pathways cause more than normal amounts of lymph filtration. This is commonly seen in postmastectomy patients. The arm on the side of the surgery is often swollen because of the altered natural lymphatic pathways after the operation. The same amount of lymph is redirected through alternate routes, causing the slowdown of lymphatic flow.

Lymphatic Organs

The spleen is the largest mass of lymphatic tissue in the body. It is located posterior and to the left of the stomach in the abdominal cavity, between the fundus of the stomach and the diaphragm. It is roughly 12 cm in length and actively filters blood, removes old red blood cells, manufactures lymphocytes (particularly B cells, which develop into antibody-producing plasma cells) for immunity surveillance, and stores blood. Because the spleen has no afferent lymphatic vessels, it does not filter lymph. However, the spleen is often thought of as a large lymph node for the blood. During a *laparotomy,* which is surgical inspection of the abdominal cavity, in patients with lymphoma, this organ is often removed for biopsy and staging purposes. In this case the bone marrow and liver then assume the functions of the spleen.

The thymus is located along the trachea superior to the heart and posterior to the sternum in the upper thorax. This gland is larger in children than in adults and more active in pediatric immunity. The gland serves as a site where T lymphocytes can mature.

The tonsils are series of lymphatic nodules embedded in a mucous membrane. They are located at the junction of the oral cavity and pharynx. These collections of lymphoid tissue protect against foreign body infiltration by producing lymphocytes. The *pharyngeal tonsils,* or *adenoids,* are in the nasopharynx; the *palatine tonsils* are in the posterior lateral wall of the oropharynx; the *lingual tonsils* are at the base of the tongue in the oropharynx.

The *thoracic duct* is on the left side of the body and is typically larger than the right lymphatic duct. It serves the lower extremities, abdomen, left arm, and left side of the head and neck and drains into the left subclavian vein. This duct is about 35 to 45 cm in length and begins in front of the second lumbar vertebra (L2) where it is called the *cisterna chyli.* As lymph travels through the lower extremities to the cisterna chyli, it continues its upward trek to the thoracic duct. As it passes through the mediastinum, it bypasses many of the mediastinal node stations. Because of this anatomic fact, pedal lymphangiography, a technique used to visualize nodal status by injecting dye into lymphatic outlets in the feet, cannot be used to visualize mediastinal disease. The *right lymphatic duct* serves only the right arm and right side of the head and neck and drains into the right subclavian vein. This duct is about 1 to 2 cm in length. These ducts drain into the right and left subclavian veins, which in turn drain to the heart by way of the superior vena cava. Box 18-1 reviews the flow of lymph through the lymphatic system.

Knowledge of the location of the lymph nodes and direction of lymph flow is important in the diagnosis and prognosis of the spread of metastatic disease. Cancer cells, especially carcinomas from epithelial tissues, often spread through the lymphatic system. Metastatic disease sites are predictable by their lymphatic flow from the primary site.[15] Inadequate knowledge of the lymphatic system often translates into ineffective treatment delivery.

AXIAL SKELETON—SKULL, VERTEBRAL COLUMN, AND THORAX

Most imaging modalities provides valuable information through visualization of differences in anatomic densities. The denser a component, the whiter it appears on a radiograph. The axial skeleton provides the radiation therapist

Tissue fluid leaves the cellular interstitial spaces and becomes

Lymph; as it enters a

Lymphatic capillary, it merges with other capillaries to form an

Afferent lymphatic vessel, which enters a

Lymph node where lymph is filtered. It then leaves the node via an

Efferent lymphatic vessel, which travels to other nodes, then merges with other vessels to form a

Lymphatic trunk, which merges with other trunks and joins a

Collecting duct, either the right lymphatic or the thoracic, which empties into a

Subclavian vein, where lymph is returned to the bloodstream.

with a wealth of information used to reference the location of internal anatomy. The following sections briefly review axial skeleton anatomy and provide the reader with a reference necessary in relating internal structures to surface anatomy.

Skull

There are about 29 bones in the skull, and these are for the most part joined by sutures, joints held together by connective tissue, which limits movement. The mandible and ossicles, which are bones in the middle ear, are the only bones in the skull not joined by sutures.

The frontal, parietal, and occipital bones form the lateral aspect of the skull vault. The first two meet in the midline at the *bregma,* the roof of the skull, often referred to as the "soft spot," and the last two meet at the lambda. The facial skeleton, or visceral cranium, includes the 14 bones of the face. It consists of two maxillary bones, two zygomatic bones, two nasal bones, two lacrimal bones, two palatine bones, two inferior conchae, and one mandible.

Sutures

There are four prominent sutures in the skull. These sutures, or fibrous joints, allow little or no movement between them, which makes the transitions between bones of the skull smooth and stable. The *coronal suture* lies between the frontal bone and the two parietal bones. On either side of the skull, it begins at the bregma and ends at the temporal bone. The *sagittal suture* lies between the two parietal bones and runs from the bregma to the lambda. The *lambdoidal suture* is in the posterior portion of the skull and lies between the parietal and occipital bones. Finally, the *squamosal suture,* one on each side of the skull, is located near the ear and lies between the parietal and temporal

bones. Identification of these sutures radiographically can assist the radiation therapist in locating corresponding underlying structures. Fig. 18-12 shows the bones of the skull and sutures.

Paranasal Sinuses

The bones of the skull and face contain the **paranasal sinuses,** which are air spaces lined by mucous membranes that reduce the weight of the skull and give a resonant sound to the voice. When a person has sinusitis, an inflammation and blockage of the sinus cavities, the voice often has a "stuffed up" tone (loss of resonance). The paired sinuses are formed from each nasal cavity within the frontal, maxillary, sphenoid, and ethmoid bones. They are lined with mucous membranes and are relatively small at birth. They enlarge during development of the permanent teeth and reach adult size shortly after puberty.[8] The paranasal sinuses are easily seen on plain x-ray, CT, and MRI. Cross sections are an excellent tool to study the surface relations in these areas.[13] Fig. 18-13 demonstrates the paranasal sinuses in cross section.

The *maxillary sinus* is a pyramidal-shaped cavity that is enclosed in the maxilla. It is the largest of the paranasal sinuses. The roof of the sinus forms the floor of the orbit. The *frontal sinus* lies in the frontal bone above the orbit. It may be located on the surface by a triangle between the following three points: the nasion, a point 3 cm above the nasion, and the junction of the medial and middle thirds of the superior orbital margin (SOM). The *sphenoid sinus* lies posterior and superior to the nasopharynx enclosed in the body of the sphenoid bone at the level of the zygomatic arch. Superiorly the sinus is related to the sella turcica (which is roughly 2 cm anterior and 2 cm superior to the external auditory meatus) and the pituitary. The pituitary may be surgically removed through a transsphenoidal approach, one that goes through the nasal cavity. The *ethmoid sinus* is bilateral but consists of a honeycomb of air cells lying between the middle wall of the orbit and the upper lateral wall of the nose.

Vertebral Column

The vertebral column, located in the midsagittal plane of the posterior cavity, extends from the skull to the pelvis. It consists of separate bones, the vertebrae, which appear as rectangular densities on radiographs.[8] There are 33 bones in the adult vertebral column, as shown in Fig. 18-14, which also indicates the number of bones in each section. There are 7 cervical, 12 thoracic, 5 lumbar, 5 sacral, and 4 coccygeal vertebrae. At the inferior aspect of the column, the sacrum has 5 fused bones, whereas the coccyx is composed of 4 fused bones.

The sacrum supports the rest of the vertebral column and thus provides the support necessary for the human body's erectness. The vertebrae are separated by radiolucent fibrocartilage called intervertebral disks. In the cervical and thoracic spine the disks are of similar thickness. In the lumbar spine the height increases progressively down the column.[8,11,12]

The vertebral column is also very flexible. Although there

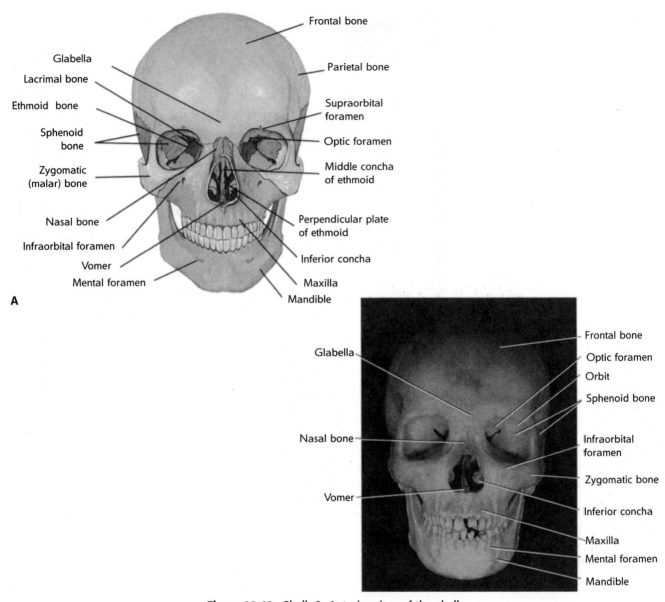

Figure 18-12. Skull. **A,** Anterior view of the skull.

is limited motion between any two neighboring vertebrae, the vertebral column is capable of substantial motion. The column also protects the spinal cord and provides points of attachment for the skull, thorax, and extremities.

Vertebral Characteristics

Most vertebrae share several common characteristics. They have a body that is attached to a posterior vertebral arch. These two components border the *vertebral foramen,* the passage that the spinal cord passes through. There are spinous and transverse processes that allow for muscle attachments. The *spinous process* is posterior and forms where two laminae meet. These laminae are often palpated in aligning spinal treatment fields. The *transverse processes* are lateral projections where a pedicle joins a lamina. Fig. 18-15 exhibits a typical vertebra with its prominent features labeled.

The first two vertebrae, C1 and C2, are atypical from all others. C1, the *atlas,* serves the specialized function of supporting the skull and allowing it to turn. It has no vertebral body. C2, the *axis,* has an odontoid process that extends into the ring of the atlas. When the head turns from side to side, it pivots on this process. These two vertebrae are shown in Fig. 18-16.

Vertebral Column Curvatures

The vertebral column demonstrates several curvatures that develop at different levels.[8] These curvatures can be classified as either primary or compensatory (secondary) curvatures. **Primary vertebral curves** are developed in utero as

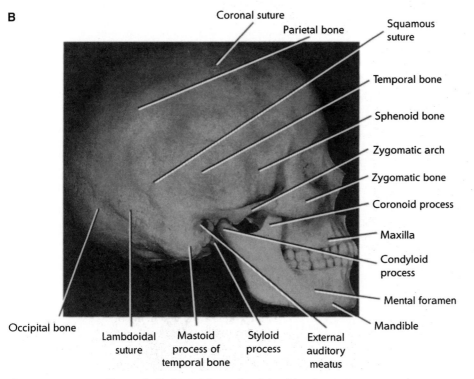

Figure 18-12, cont'd. B, Skull viewed from the right side. *(From Support and movement. In Thibodeau GA, Patton KT, editors: Anatomy and physiology, ed 2, St. Louis, 1993, Mosby.)*

the fetus develops in the C-shaped fetal position, and they are present at birth. **Compensatory** or **secondary vertebral curves** develop after birth as the child learns to sit up and walk. Muscular development and coordination influence the rate of secondary curvature development.

The *cervical curve* extends from the first cervical to the second thoracic vertebrae (C1 to T2). It is convex anteriorly and develops as the child learns to hold his or her head up and sits alone at about 4 months of age. This curve is a secondary curvature. The *thoracic curve* extends from T2 to T12 and is concave anteriorly. This is one of the primary curves of the vertebral column. The *lumbar curve* runs from T12 to

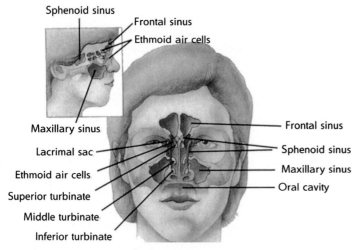

Figure 18-13. The paranasal sinuses. The anterior view shows the anatomic relationship of the paranasal sinuses to each other and to the nasal cavity. The inset is a lateral view of the position of the sinuses. *(From Anatomy of the respiratory system. In Thibodeau GA, Patton KT, editors: Anatomy and physiology, ed 2, St. Louis, 1993, Mosby.)*

the anterior surface of L5. This convex forward curve develops when the child learns to walk at about 1 year of age. The *pelvic curve* is concave anteriorly and inferiorly and extends from the anterior surfaces of the sacrum and coccyx. This is the other primary curve. The thorax can also have a slightly right or left lateral curve that is influenced by the child's predominate use of their right or left hand during childhood and adolescence.

The cervical, thoracic, lumbar, and pelvic curves are demonstrated in the normal human vertebral column. There are also three abnormal curvatures that are present both clinically and radiographically. *Kyphosis* is an excessive curvature of the vertebral column that is convex posteriorly. These curves can develop with degenerative vertebral changes. *Scoliosis* is an abnormal lateral curvature of the vertebral column with excessive right or left curvature in the thoracic region. This abnormal curvature can develop if only one side (half) of the vertebral bodies are irradiated in pediatric patients, as in the case of patients treated for Wilms' tumor. The radiation slows vertebral body growth on one side while the contralateral side grows at a normal rate, thus creating

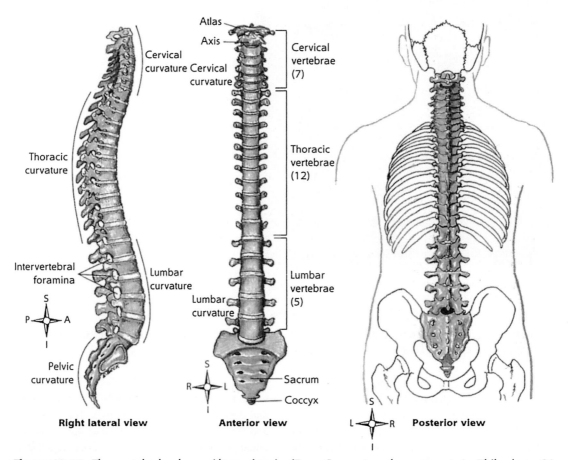

Figure 18-14. The vertebral column (three views). *(From Support and movement. In Thibodeau GA, Patton KT, editors: Anatomy and physiology, ed 2, St. Louis, 1993, Mosby.)*

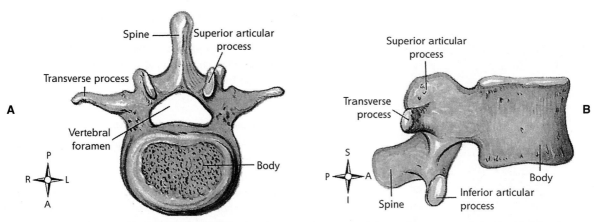

Figure 18-15. Lumbar vertebrae. **A,** Third lumbar vertebra viewed from above (superior). **B,** Third lumbar vertebra viewed from the side (lateral). *(From The skeletal system. In Thibodeau GA, Patton KT, editors: Anatomy and physiology, ed 2, St. Louis, 1993, Mosby.)*

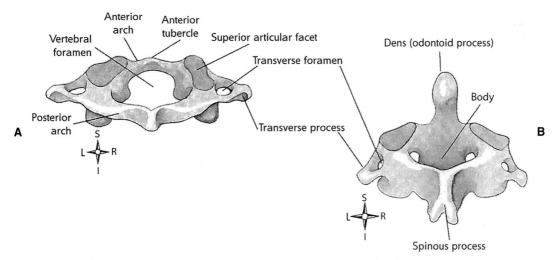

Figure 18-16. Cervical vertebra. **A,** First cervical vertebra (atlas) viewed from behind (posterior). **B,** Second cervical vertebra (axis) viewed from behind (posterior). *(From The skeletal system. In Thibodeau GA, Patton KT, editors: Anatomy and physiology, ed 2, St. Louis, 1993, Mosby.)*

scoliotic changes. *Lordosis* is an excessive convexity of the lumbar curve of the spine.

Thorax

The illustration in Fig 18-17 shows the full thorax made up of the bony cage formed by the sternum, costal cartilage, ribs, and the thoracic vertebrae to which they are attached.[9,15] The *thorax* encloses and protects the organs in the thoracic cavity and upper abdomen. It also provides support for the pectoral girdle and upper extremities.

Sternum and Ribs

The sternum, or breastbone, comprises three parts: the *manubrium,* which is the superior portion; the *body,* the middle and largest portion; and the *xiphoid process,* which is the inferior projection that serves as ligament and muscle attachments. The manubrium has a depression called the **suprasternal notch** (SSN), which occurs at the level of T2 and articulates with the medial ends of the clavicles. This point may be used in measuring the angle of chin tilt in patients with head and neck cancer when thermoplastic immobilization masks are not used. It also serves as a palpable landmark when setting up a SCF field. The manubrium also articulates with the first two ribs. The junction of the manubrium and the body form the *sternal angle,* also called the angle of Louis; it occurs at the level of T4.

The body of the sternum articulates with the second through tenth ribs. There are 12 pairs of ribs, of which the superior 7 pairs are considered true ribs. They are easily seen in the asthenic body habitus and palpable in most others.[9]

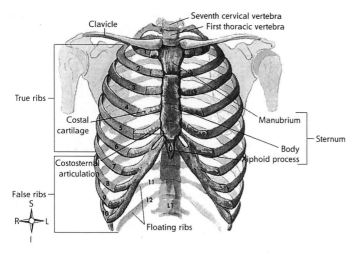

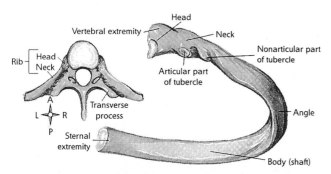

Figure 18-17. The bony framework of the thorax provides many useful landmarks. *(From Support and movement. In Thibodeau GA, Patton KT, editors: Anatomy and physiology, ed 2, St. Louis, 1993, Mosby.)*

They articulate posteriorly with the vertebrae and anteriorly with the sternum directly through a cartilaginous joint. These are known as the vertebrosternal ribs. The next three pairs join with the vertebrae posteriorly and anteriorly with the cartilage of the immediately anterior rib. These ribs are classified as vertebrochondral ribs. The next (last) pairs only articulate with the vertebrae and do not connect with the sternum in any way; they are called floating ribs.

The axial skeleton is easily seen with most imaging techniques used in radiation therapy. A thorough working knowledge of these components serves the radiation therapist in overall daily operations. This information is used in relating the surface and cross-sectional anatomy as well as the palpable bony landmarks that are used in field placement and treatment planning.

SURFACE AND SECTIONAL ANATOMY AND LANDMARKS OF THE HEAD AND NECK

The human head demonstrates various anatomic features that are both interesting and useful to the radiation therapist. These structures are rich in bony, and moveable soft tissue landmarks and lymphatics commonly used in field place-

ment, position locations, and so forth. The bony landmarks are very stable and are typically used as reference points, as in the case of locating a positioning or central axis tattoo. Soft tissue landmarks can also be extremely useful. However, they tend to be more mobile and provide a less reliable reference than the bony landmarks.

Bony Landmarks—Anterior and Lateral Skull

Figs. 18-18 and 18-19 outline the locations of the following anterior and lateral bony structures.

The *frontal bone* is the area of maximum convexity on the forehead and articulates with the frontal process of the maxillary bone on the medial side of the orbit.[8,9] Together with the lacrimal bones, it protects the lacrimal duct and glands.

The *glabella* is the slight elevation directly between the two orbits in the frontal bone. It is just above the base of the nose. This palpable landmark is more prominent in some individuals than in others.

The *nasion* is the central depression at the base of the nose. The point of joining of the frontal and nasal bones forms it.

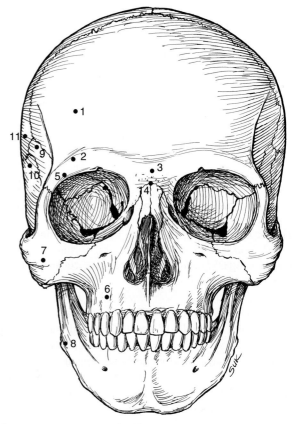

Figure 18-18. Bony landmarks of the anterior skull. *1,* Frontal bone; *2,* superciliary arch; *3,* glabella; *4,* nasion; *5,* superior orbital margin (SOM); *6,* maxilla; *7,* zygomatic bone; *8,* angle of mandible; *9,* sphenoid bone (greater wing); *10,* temporal bone; *11,* parietal bone.

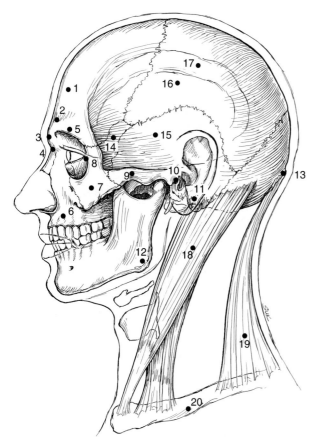

Figure 18-19. Bony landmarks of the lateral skull. *1,* Frontal bone; *2,* superciliary arch; *3,* glabella; *4,* nasion; *5,* superior orbital margin (SOM); *6,* maxilla; *7,* zygomatic bone; *8,* lateral canthus; *9,* mid-zygoma point; *10,* external acoustic meatus (EAM); *11,* mastoid process; *12,* angle of mandible; *13,* external occipital protuberance (EOP) or inion; *14,* greater wing of sphenoid; *15,* temporal bone; *16,* parietal bone; *17,* parietal eminence; *18,* sternocleidomastoid muscle; *19,* trapezius muscle; *20,* clavicle.

The *superciliary arch* starts at the glabella and moves superiorly and laterally above the central portion of the eyebrow. The central part lies superficially to the frontal sinuses on either side and forms the brow of the skull.

The SOM rests just inferior to the eyebrow and is more pronounced on its lateral aspect. The SOM forms the roof of the orbit and serves as one of the points used to delineate the inferior border of whole brain fields (along with the tragus and mastoid tip). By ensuring that part of the SOM is in the treatment field, the frontal part of the brain will also be in the field.

The *maxilla* is the bone felt between the ala (lateral soft tissue prominence) of the nose and the prominence of the cheek. This bone houses the largest of the paranasal sinuses. The inferior alveolar ridge of the maxilla houses the teeth sockets.

The *zygomatic bone* forms part of the lateral aspect of the

orbit and the prominence of the cheek. The articulation between the frontal process of the zygomatic bone and the zygomatic process of the frontal bone can be palpated in the lateral orbital margin (LOM). The *mid-zygoma point,* a point midway between the external auditory meatus (EAM) and the lateral canthus, lies roughly at the floor of the sphenoid sinus and roof of the nasopharynx. One centimeter superior to that point corresponds to the floor of the sella turcica, and 1.5 cm superior to the point corresponds to the pituitary gland.

The *mastoid process* is an extension of the mastoid portion of the temporal bone at the level of the ear lobe. It is commonly used to delineate the posterior point of the inferior whole brain border (imaginary line that extends from the SOM to the mastoid tip, commonly going through the tragus of the ear).

The *external occipital protuberance* (EOP or inion) is the prominence in the posterolateral aspect of the occipital bone of the skull.

The *angle of the mandible* is the point at which the muscles used for chewing are attached. Also, there are several lymph node groups located inferior and medial to that point, and it is also a classic landmark for the tonsils.

Landmarks Around the Eye

Whenever practical, the landmarks used around the eye should be the bony landmarks. They are radiographically visible and are easily checked if a second course of treatment is necessary in the same or neighboring area. The soft tissue landmarks often change with age, weight, and surgical changes. They are open to variable interpretation and misinterpretation because of the extreme flexibility of the skin. Fig. 18-20 illustrates these landmarks. The following outlines the important landmarks about the eye.

The *superior orbital margin* forms the upper border of the orbit.

The *inferior orbital margin* (IOM) forms the lower border of the bony orbit.

The *lateral orbital margin* (LOM) is a bony landmark that forms the lateral border of the bony orbit.

The *medial orbital margin* is extremely difficult to palpate and is therefore not clinically useful as an anatomic landmark. It does have some usefulness radiographically.

The *inner canthus* (IC) is a soft tissue landmark that is formed at the junction of the upper and lower eyelid at the medial aspect of the eye.

The *outer canthus* (OC) is a soft tissue landmark that is formed at the junction of the upper and lower eyelid at the lateral aspect of the eye.

The *punctum lacrimae* is a soft tissue landmark that can be used as a point of reference in the surface anatomy of the eye. This white-appearing section of the eye lies just next to the IC on the lower eyelid. Tears are drained through this duct into the lacrimal duct. This opening can become blocked by fibrotic changes secondary to ionizing radiation administered to the area, causing constant tearing. Extreme

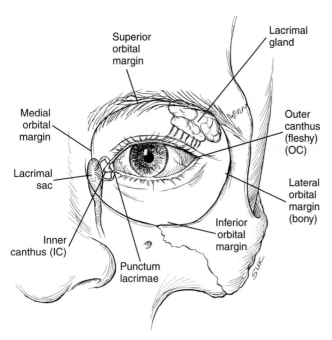

Figure 18-20. Landmarks around the eye and orbit.

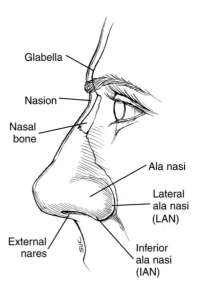

Figure 18-21. Landmarks around the nose.

caution should be exercised to avoid this occurrence, particularly when treating the anterior maxillary sinus field arrangement.

Landmarks Around the Nose

As in the case of the eye, the landmarks used around the nose should be the bony landmarks. Soft tissue landmarks often change with age, weight, and surgical changes and are open to variable interpretation and misinterpretation because of the extreme flexibility of the skin. Fig. 18-21 illustrates these landmarks. The following outlines the landmarks about the nose, some being reiterated from previous sections.

The *lateral ala nasi* (LAN) is a soft tissue landmark formed by the lateral attachment of the ala nasi with the cheek. The *inferior ala nasi* (IAN) is a soft tissue landmark formed by the inferior attachment of the ala nasi with the cheek. Both of these landmarks are prominent in most people and can be very useful landmarks when measuring in any direction, such as superior to inferior, medial to lateral, and anterior to posterior.

The *nasion* is the depression of the nose where it joins the forehead at the level of the SOM. It is a very useful landmark if it is deep and pronounced and coincides with the crease of the nose. If it is shallow, it is more open to variable interpretation.

The *glabella* is the bony prominence in the forehead at the level just superior to the SOM. As in the case of the nasion, it is useful if it is prominent and sharp. It is not very useful if it is flat or extremely curved, where it, too, would be open to misinterpretation.

The ala nasi, dorsum of the nose, and external nares are useful as checkpoints in the surface anatomy of the nose, useful in the positioning of radiation treatment portals.

Landmarks Around the Mouth

Landmarks around the mouth are generally not very accurate because of the extreme flexibility in the area. Every effort should be made to document these landmarks with reference to more stable anatomic points, if possible. If these landmarks are used, it is important to note the position of the mouth as well as any positioning or immobilization devices used, such as a cork, oral stent, or similar devices. Fig. 18-22 illustrates the landmarks around the mouth.

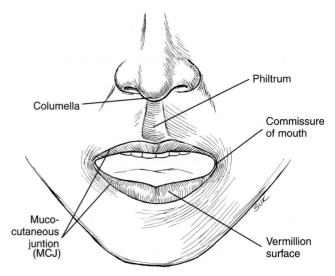

Figure 18-22. Landmarks around the mouth.

The *commissure of the mouth* is formed at the junction of the upper and lower lip. This landmark is extremely mobile.

The *mucocutaneous junction* (MCJ) is located at the junction of the vermilion border of the lip with the skin of the face.

The *columella* is located at the junction of the skin of the nose with the skin of the face at the superior end of the philtrum.

Landmarks Around the Ear

The external ear consists of the auricle or pinna, which is formed from a number of irregularly shaped pieces of fibrocartilage covered by skin. It has a dependent lobule, or ear lobe, and an anterior tragus, commonly used as anatomic references.[7,9,14] Parts of the ear are labeled in Fig. 18-23.

The *tragus* is made up of a fairly stable cartilage that partially covers the external auditory meatus in the external ear and is often used in radiation therapy during initial positioning. A pair of optical lasers, coincident with each other, can be focused on the tragus on both sides of the patient. Doing this places the patient's head in a relatively nontilted position, because their locations are typically symmetrical. Just anterior to the tragus corresponds to the posterior wall of the nasopharynx. The posterior limit of many head and neck off cord fields lies at this point.

The *tragal notch* is the semicircular notch in the ear immediately inferior to the tragus. The *superior tragal notch* (STN) makes up the superior margin of the tragal notch. The *inferior tragal notch* (ITN) defines the inferior margin of the tragal notch. The *anterior tragal notch* (ATN) makes up the anterior margin of the tragal notch.

Landmarks and Anatomy Around the Neck

The boundaries of the anterior aspect of the neck are the body and angles of the mandible superiorly, and the superior border and SSN of the sternum and the clavicles. The posterior aspect of the neck is bound superiorly by the EOP and laterally by the mastoid processes. The posterior inferior border ends at roughly the level of seventh cervical vertebra to the first thoracic vertebra (C7-T1).[8] Fig. 18-24 illustrates the features of the neck anatomy.

The upper cervical vertebrae are not easily palpated; the last cervical and first thoracic vertebrae are the most obvious. The hyoid bone lies opposite the superior border of C4. When the head is in the anatomic position, the hyoid bone may be moved from side to side between the thumb and middle finger, about 1 cm below the level of the angle of the mandible, C2-C3. Table 18-3 relates the location of the cervical bony landmarks to other associated anatomic features.

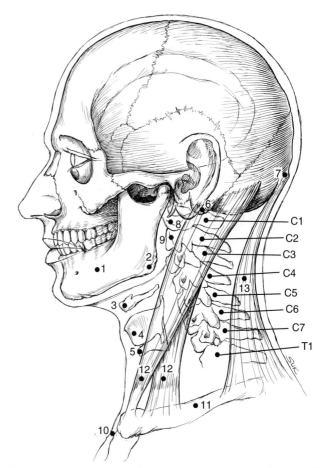

Figure 18-24. The neck demonstrates many useful anatomic landmarks that can assist the radiation therapist. Relating surface structures to deeper anatomy is essential in the practice of radiation therapy. *1,* Body of mandible; *2,* angle of mandible; *3,* hyoid bone; *4,* thyroid cartilage; *5,* cricoid cartilage; *6,* mastoid process; *7,* external occipital protuberance (EOP); *8,* atlas; *9,* axis; *10,* suprasternal notch; *11,* clavicle; *12,* sternocleidomastoid muscle; *13,* trapezius muscle.

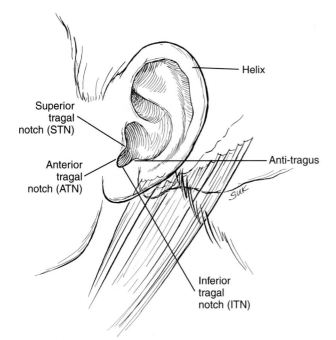

Figure 18-23. Landmarks around the ear.

Table 18-3	Cervical neck landmarks and associated anatomy
Cervical Spine	**Associated Anatomy**
C1	Transverse process lies just inferior to the mastoid process; may be palpated in the hollow inferior to the ear
C2-3	Level with the angle of the mandible; lies 5 to 7 cm below the external occipital protuberance
C4	Located just superior to the hyoid bone of the neck; serves as a point of muscle attachment
C4	Level with the superior portion of the thyroid cartilage and marks the beginning of the larynx
C6	Level with the cricoid cartilage; location of the junction of the larynx to trachea and pharynx to esophagus
C7	First prominent spinous process in the posterior neck

Pharynx

The pharynx is a membranous tube that extends from the base of the skull to the esophagus. It connects the nasal and oral cavities with the larynx and esophagus. It is divided into the nasopharynx, oropharynx, and laryngopharynx, shown in Fig. 18-25. Note that in looking at the low neck in a sectional view, the therapist can easily remember how to distinguish the order of the spinal cord, esophagus, and trachea. If looking from a posterior to anterior perspective, the order is always **SET** up: S—spinal cord, E—esophagus, and T—trachea:

1. The *nasopharynx,* or *epipharynx,* communicates with the nasal cavity and provides a passageway for air during breathing.
2. The *oropharynx,* or *mesopharynx,* opens behind the soft palate into the nasopharynx and functions as a passageway for food moving down from the mouth as well as for air moving in and out of the nasal cavity.
3. The *laryngopharynx,* or *hypopharynx,* is located inferior to the oropharynx and opens into the larynx and esophagus.

Larynx

The larynx connects to the lower portion of the pharynx above it and is connected with the trachea below it. It extends from the tip of the epiglottis at the level of the junction of C3 and C4 to the lower portion of the cricoid cartilage at the level of the C6 vertebra.[7] The larynx is subdivided into three anatomic regions: the supraglottis, glottis, and subglottis. Fig. 18-26 illustrates sectional views of the larynx. The larynx is actually an enlargement in the airway at the top of the trachea and below the pharynx. It serves as a passageway for air moving in and out of the trachea and functions to prevent foreign objects from entering the trachea.

The *thyroid cartilage* forms a midline prominence, the laryngeal prominence or Adam's apple, which is more obvious in the adult male. The vocal cords are attached to the posterior part of this prominence. The *cricoid cartilage* serves as the lower border of the larynx and is the only complete ring of cartilage in the respiratory passage; the others are open posteriorly. It is palpable as a narrow horizontal bar inferior to the thyroid cartilage and is at the level of the C6 vertebra.

Nasal and Oral Cavities

The nasal cavity opens to the external environment through the nostrils. Posteriorly the nostrils are continuous with the nasopharynx and are lined with a ciliated mucous membrane. The oral cavity has a vestibule, which is the space between the cheeks and teeth and the oral cavity proper that opens posteriorly into the oropharynx and houses the soft palate, hard palate, uvula, anterior tongue, and floor of mouth.

Surface Anatomy of the Neck

Anatomic landmarks around the neck are mainly used as checkpoints and reference points that can establish the patient's position or the anatomic position of the treatment field. The most frequently used landmarks of the neck are as follows:
1. Skin profile
2. Sternocleidomastoid muscle—attached to the mastoid and occipital bones superiorly and sternal and clavicular heads inferiorly. These muscles form the V shape in the neck and are associated with a great number of lymph nodes.
3. Clavicle
4. Thyroid notch
5. Mastoid tip
6. EOP
7. Spinous processes

These surface neck landmarks assist the radiation therapist in referencing locations of treatment fields and dose-limiting structures. They are illustrated in Fig. 18-27.

Lymphatic Drainage of the Head and Neck

The lymphatic drainage of the head and neck is through deep and superficial lymphatic channels, around the base of the skull, and deep and superficial lymph chains. The head and neck area is very rich in lymphatics. Enlarged cervical lymph nodes are the most common adenopathy seen in clinical practice.[9] They are typically associated with upper respiratory tract infections but may also be the site of metastatic disease from the head and neck, lungs, or breast or primary lymphoreticular disease such as Hodgkin's disease. The lymph nodes of the head and neck are outlined in the following section. Figs. 18-28 and 18-29 demonstrate the lymphatic chains and nodes in the head and neck.

The *occipital lymph nodes,* typically one to three in number, are located on the back of the head, close to the margin of the trapezius muscle attachment on the occipital bone.

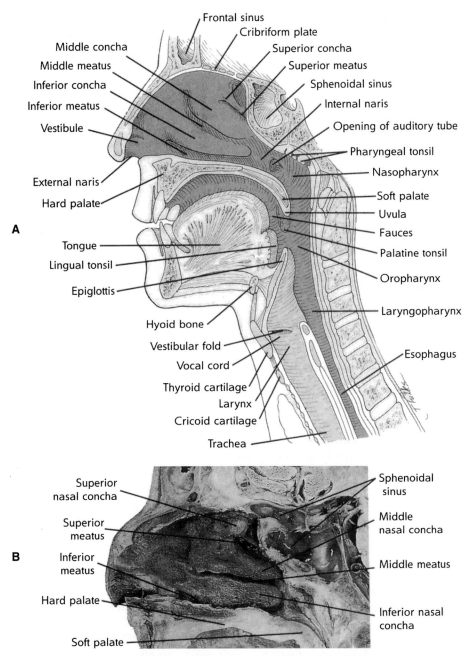

Frontal sinus
Cribriform plate
Middle concha
Superior concha
Middle meatus
Superior meatus
Inferior concha
Sphenoidal sinus
Inferior meatus
Internal naris
Vestibule
Opening of auditory tube
Pharyngeal tonsil
Nasopharynx
External naris
Soft palate
Hard palate
Uvula
Fauces
Tongue
Palatine tonsil
Lingual tonsil
Oropharynx
Epiglottis
Laryngopharynx
Hyoid bone
Vestibular fold
Vocal cord
Esophagus
Thyroid cartilage
Larynx
Cricoid cartilage
Trachea

A

Superior nasal concha
Sphenoidal sinus
Superior meatus
Middle nasal concha
Inferior meatus
Middle meatus
Hard palate
Inferior nasal concha
Soft palate

B

Figure 18-25. Nasal cavity and pharynx. **A,** Sagittal section through the nasal cavity and pharynx viewed from the medial side. **B,** Photograph of a sagittal section of the nasal cavity. *(From The lymphatic system and immunity. In Seeley RR, Stephens TD, Tate P, editors: Essentials of anatomy and physiology, St. Louis, 1991, Mosby.)*

These nodes provide efferent flow to the superior deep cervical nodes.

The *retroauricular lymph nodes,* usually two in number, are situated on the mastoid insertion of the sternocleidomastoid muscle deep to the posterior auricular muscle. They drain the posterior temporooccipital region of the scalp, auricle, and external auditory meatus. They provide efferent drainage to the superior deep cervical nodes.

The *deep parotid lymph nodes* are arranged into two groups. The first group is embedded in the parotid gland, whose superior border is the temporomandibular joint (TMJ); posterior border, the mastoid process; inferior border, the angle of the mandible; and anterior border, the anterior ramus. The second group—the subparotid nodes—are located deep to the gland and lie on the lateral wall of the pharynx. Both drain the nose, eyelid, frontotemporal scalp,

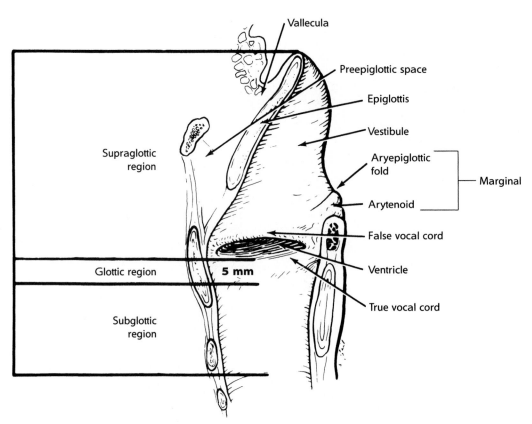

Figure 18-26. Posterior view of the base of the tongue, larynx, and hypopharynx. Note the pyriform sinus, pharyngeal wall, and postcricoid area. *(From Cox JD, editor: Moss' radiation oncology: rationale, technique, results, ed 7, St. Louis, 1994, Mosby.)*

EAM, and palate. They provide efferent flow to the superior deep cervical nodes.

The *submaxillary lymph nodes* are facial nodes that are scattered over the infraorbital region. They span from the groove between the nose and cheek to the zygomatic arch. The *buccal lymph nodes* are scattered over the buccinator muscle. These nodes drain the eyelids, nose, and cheek and supply efferent flow to the submandibular nodes. The *submandibular lymph nodes* lie on the outer surface of the mandible. They drain the scalp; nose; cheek; floor of mouth; anterior two thirds of the tongue; gums; teeth; lips; and the frontal, ethmoid, and maxillary sinuses. They provide efferent drainage to the superior deep cervical nodes.

The *retropharyngeal lymph nodes,* one to three in number, lie in the buccopharyngeal fossa, behind the upper part of the pharynx and anterior to the arch of the atlas. These nodes are commonly involved in nasopharyngeal tumors and subsequently are included in the treatment fields.

The *submental lymph nodes* are found in the submental triangle of the digastric muscles, lower gums and lips, tongue, central floor of mouth, and skin of the chin. These nodes provide efferent drainage to the submandibular nodes.

The *superficial cervical lymph nodes* form a group of nodes located below the hyoid bone and in front of the larynx, trachea, and thyroid gland.

The *deep cervical lymph nodes* form a chain of 20 to 30 nodes along the carotid sheath and around the internal jugular chain along the sternocleidomastoid muscle. The *jugulodigastric lymph node,* at times called the *subdigastric node,* is typically located superior to the angle of the mandible and drains the tonsils and the tongue. Inferiorly, the chain spreads out into the subclavian triangle. One of the nodes in this group lies in the omohyoid tendon and is known as the juguloomohyoid lymph node.[8,9] When these two nodes are enlarged, it may signal carcinoma of the tongue, because enlarged neck nodes may be the only sign of the disease. These vessels supply efferent flow to form the jugular trunk, which drains to the thoracic or right lymphatic duct, both in the SCF. The cervical lymph nodes are typically included in the treatment fields of most head and neck cancers that spread through the lymphatics, which include most of these cancers. The fields that encompass the group are commonly called *posterior cervical strips.*

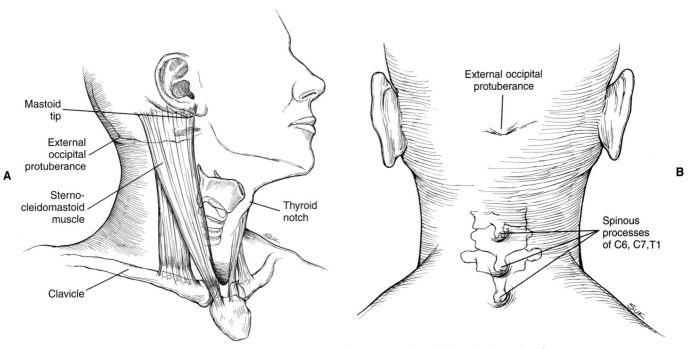

Figure 18-27. Surface anatomy of the neck. **A,** Anterolateral view. **B,** Posterior view.

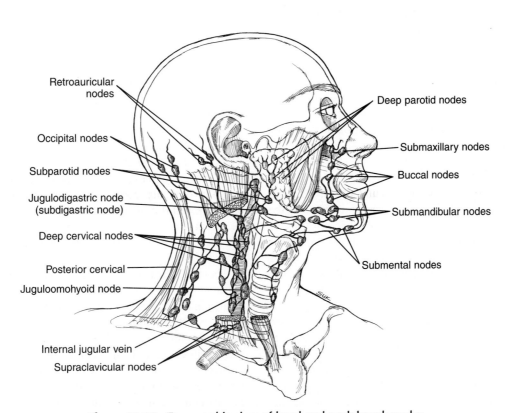

Figure 18-28. Topographic view of head and neck lymph nodes.

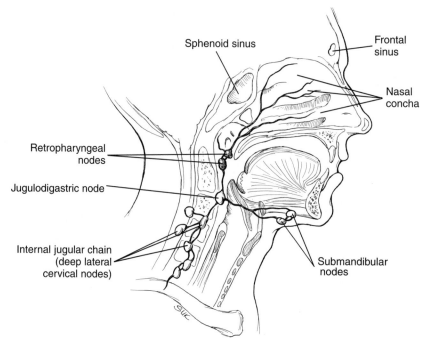

Figure 18-29. Sagittal view of deep lymph nodes in the head and neck in relation to underlying structures.

SURFACE AND SECTIONAL ANATOMY AND LANDMARKS OF THE THORAX AND BREAST

Various malignant diseases manifest themselves in the human thorax. Cancers of the lung, breast, and mediastinal lymphatics require the radiation therapist to have a working knowledge of the surface and sectional anatomy of the thorax. The human thorax demonstrates various anatomic features that are commonly used in field placement, position locations, and so forth. The thorax extends from the clavicles superiorly to the costal margin inferiorly.

Anterior Thoracic Landmarks

The clavicles are visible throughout their entire length in the anterior thorax, especially in the asthenic body habitus. The clavicles are easily palpable. The radiation therapist uses the clavicles when outlining a SCF field to treat the lower neck and upper chest lymphatics. The supraclavicular lymph nodes are located superior to the clavicles; they are often treated prophylactically in head and neck as well as lung cancers. Also, the brachial plexus, a network of nerves located at the medial section of the clavicle and often involved in superior sulcus (Pancoast) tumors of the lung, can be referenced to this point.

The musculature of the anterior chest wall includes the pectoralis major, pectoralis minor, and the deltoid. The pectoralis major is medially attached to the clavicle and superior five costal cartilages. It passes laterally to the axilla. The inferior border of the muscle is not as visible in the female, because it is covered by the breast.[8,9] The pectoralis minor is overlapped by the pectoralis major. The deltoid muscle forms the rounded portion of the shoulder.

The Breast and Its Landmarks

The male breast remains poorly developed throughout life, whereas the female breast develops to a variable degree during puberty. Although the sizes of the female breasts vary, they typically lie between the second rib superiorly and the sixth rib inferiorly. The female breast is shown in Fig. 18-30. The medial border is the lateral aspect of the sternum, and the lateral border would correspond to the midaxilla. The breast tissue is teardrop shaped; the round, drop portion is situated medially, and the upper outer portion, called the tail of Spence, extends into the axilla. The upper limits of tangential treatment fields are typically high near the SSN, to include the entire breast and tail of Spence when the SCF is not treated.

The breast can be divided into quadrants: upper outer, upper inner, lower outer, and lower inner. Most tumors are located in the upper outer quadrant of the breast. Tumor location is important in associating the tumor spread patterns. If the breast tumor is located in an inner quadrant, the medially located nodes, such as the internal mammary nodes, may be involved. If the tumor is located in an outer quadrant, the axillary nodes need to be examined for possible involvement. This information is particularly important to the therapist because tumor location and extension dictate field parameters.

Other surface anatomy of the breast includes the nipple, areola, and inframammary sulcus. The nipple projects just

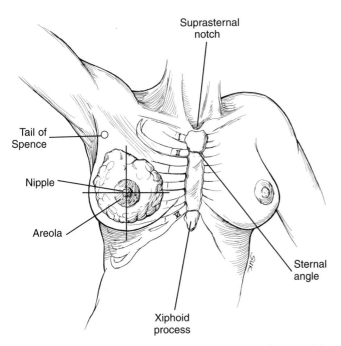

Figure 18-30. Surface anatomy of the female breast. This gland is teardrop shaped with a portion extending from the anterior chest wall into the axilla.

below the center of the breast. In the male the nipple lies over the fourth intercostal space; the location varies in the female. The areola is the area that surrounds the nipple. Its coloration changes with varying hormonal levels, as seen in pregnancy. The inframammary sulcus, the inferior point of breast attachment, varies from person to person. In females with large breasts, the breast overhangs this point of attachment and causes considerable concern during its external beam treatment because the breast can bolus itself in these cases.

Radiographically, the breast produces shadows that are easily seen on conventional radiographs. Fig. 18-31 shows a CT slice through a section of the thorax and breast. Note how the patient's internal anatomy can be related to the contour of the breast. This information is very useful in treatment planning.

Posterior Thoracic Landmarks

The posterior thorax is formed by the structures commonly referred to as the back. On initial inspection, the back is made up of various muscles and bony landmarks. The major musculature includes the trapezius, teres major, and latissimus dorsi. The *trapezius muscle* is a flat triangular muscle that produces a trapezoid shape with the lateral angles at the shoulders and the superior angle at the EOP. The inferior angle is at the level of T12. The *teres major* is a band of muscle between the inferior angle of the scapula and the humerus and forms the posterior wall of the axilla. The *latissimus dorsi* is the broad muscle on either side of the back that spans from the iliac crest of the pelvic bones to the posterior

axilla.[4,5,8,9] Fig. 18-32 demonstrates the surface anatomy of the posterior thorax.

The spines of the thoracic vertebrae slope inferiorly; the tips lie more inferior than the corresponding vertebral bodies and are easily palpable. The scapula, the large posterior bone associated with the pectoral girdle, is easily palpated on the back. The spine of the scapula is located at the level of T3. The inferior angle of the scapula is located at the level of T7.

The lower back has a few bony landmarks that serve the radiation therapist well. The *crest of the ilium* is located at the level of L4. This point is important in locating the subarachnoid space, the point at which lumbar punctures are commonly made. The *posterior superior iliac spine* (PSIS) is roughly 5 cm from midline, is easily palpable, and lies at the level of S2.

Internal and Sectional Anatomy of the Thorax

Bone detail can be visualized sectionally with CT easily. MRI demonstrates soft tissue anatomy not clearly seen with conventional x-ray equipment. Fascial planes are identified, allowing separation of organ systems, vascular supply, muscles, bone, and lymphatic system.[1,3,6] The thorax provides a lot of anatomic information that the radiation therapist uses in the daily administration of ionizing radiation.

The *trachea* is the part of the airway that begins at the inferior cricoid cartilage, at the level of C6. It is about 10 cm long and extends to a point of bifurcation, called the *carina*, at the level of T4-5. Topically, it corresponds to the angle of Louis and is demonstrated in Fig. 18-33. The bifurcation forms the beginning of the right and left main bronchi. This can assist the therapist in locating the initial location of treatment field borders, especially lung cancer fields whose inferior border commonly lies a few centimeters below this anatomic reference point.

The diaphragm is the dome-shaped muscle that separates

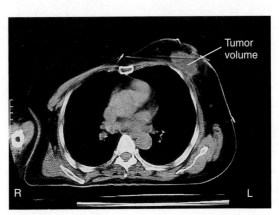

Figure 18-31. Computed tomography view of the female breast and thorax. The contour of the breast and chest wall from images like this greatly enhance accuracy of treatment planning. Note how tumor volume can easily be related to other internal anatomy.

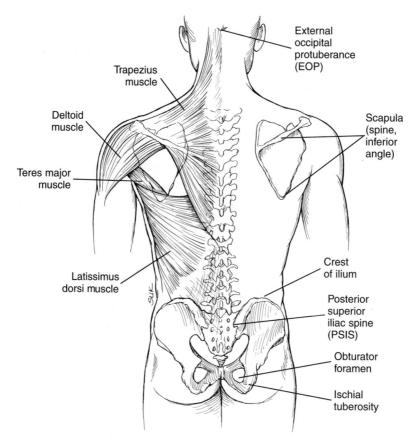

Figure 18-32. Surface anatomy of the posterior thorax.

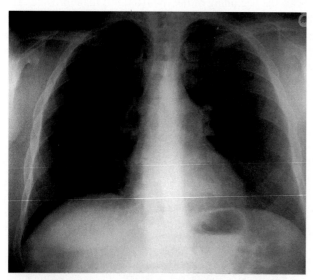

Figure 18-33. This x-ray image demonstrates the trachea and its distal bifurcation, the carina. The branching typically occurs at T3-T4.

the thorax and abdomen. It is important in respiration and lies between T10-T11. The esophagus and inferior vena cava pass through the diaphragm at the level of T8-T9, whereas the descending aorta goes through at the level of T11-T12. These features are shown in cross section in Fig. 18-34.

The pleural cavity extends superiorly 3 cm above the middle third of the clavicle. The anterior border of the pleural cavity reaches the midline of the sternal angle. The pleura is more extensive in the peripheral regions around the outer chest wall. The diaphragm bulges up into each pleural cavity from below. The pleura marks the limit of expansion of the lungs.[8,9]

The lungs correspond closely with the pleura, except in the inferior aspect, where they do not extend down into the lateral recesses. The anterior border of the right lung corresponds to the right junction of the costal and mediastinal pleura down to the level of the sixth chondrosternal joint. The anterior border of the left lung curves away laterally from the line of pleural reflection. The surface projection of the lung and pleura is noted in Fig. 18-35.

The heart rests directly on the diaphragm in the pericardial cavity and is covered anteriorly by the body of the sternum. The base of the heart lies at the level of T4. A cardiac shadow can clearly be seen in a radiograph of the chest.

Associated with the thorax and heart are an abundance of

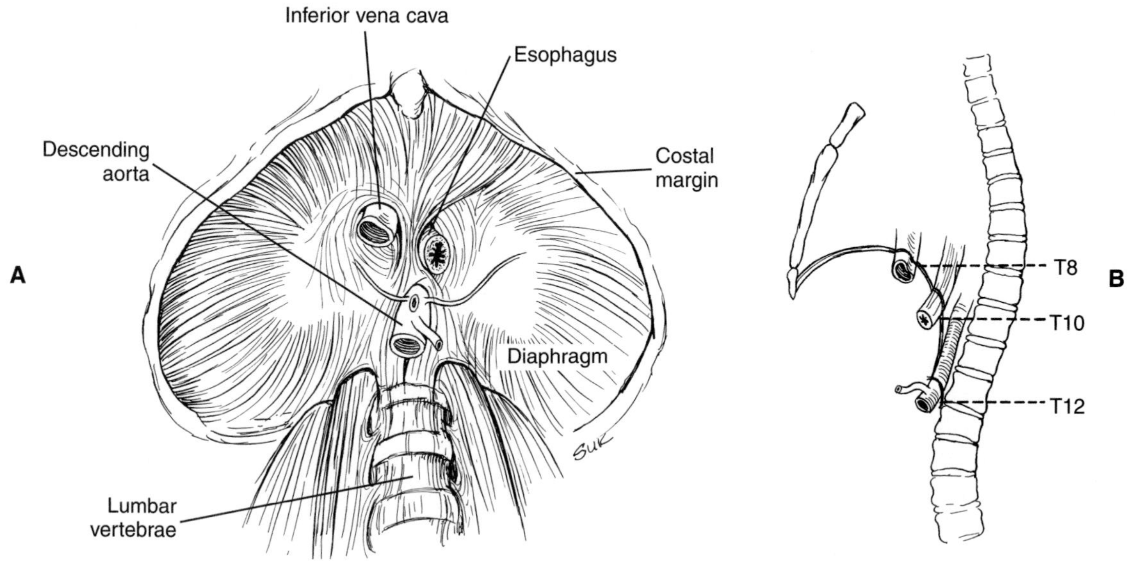

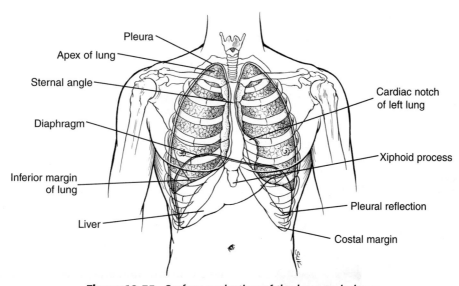

Figure 18-34. Cross section of the lower thorax showing esophagus and inferior vena cava passing through the diaphragm. **A,** Inferior surface of the diaphragm. **B,** Sagittal view of the diaphragm.

Figure 18-35. Surface projection of the lung and pleura.

arteries and veins—the great vessels. The aorta has ascending and descending components. The ascending aorta runs from the aortic orifice at the medial end of the third left intercostal space up to the second right chondrosternal joint. This arch continues above the right side of the sternal angle and then turns down behind the second left costal cartilage. The descending aorta runs down behind this cartilage, gradually moving across to reach a point just to the left of midline, about 9 cm below the xiphisternal joint where it enters the abdomen. This aortic arch has the innominate, left common carotid, and left subclavian arteries extending from it. The superior vena cava is located at the level of T4. It runs down through the pericardium, where it enters the heart. The inferior vena cava does not extend a great distance in the thorax; it lies in the right cardiodiaphragmatic angle and enters the heart behind the sixth right costal cartilage.

Lymphatics of the Breast and Thorax

The lymphatic drainage of the thorax and breast is very important to the radiation therapist. The thorax is very rich in lymphatic vessels. The lymphatics of the axilla, SCF, and mediastinum play a major role in radiation therapy field arrangement of breast, head and neck, lung, and lymphatic cancers. The lymph nodes of the thorax are divided into nodes that drain the thoracic wall and breast and those that drain the thoracic viscera.

Breast lymphatics.   There are three lymphatic pathways associated with the breast: the axillary, transpectoral, and internal mammary pathways. These pathways are the major routes of lymphatic drainage for the breast. There are specific lymph node groups associated with each pathway that are shown in Fig. 18-36.

The **axillary lymphatic pathway** comes from trunks of the upper and lower half of the breast. Lymph is collected in lobules that follow ducts, which anastomose behind the areola of the breast; from that point they drain to the axilla. This pathway is also referred to as the principal pathway. The nodes of this pathway drain the lateral half of the breast. It is important to note these nodes in invasive breast cancers: axillary nodes are commonly biopsied to assess disease spread. The axillary lymph nodes are commonly at the level of the second to third intercostal spaces and can be divided into low-, mid-, and apical axillary nodes.

The **transpectoral lymphatic pathway** passes through the pectoralis major muscle and provides efferent drainage to the supraclavicular and infraclavicular fossa nodes. One of the intermediate nodes in the infraclavicular fossa worth noting is Rotter's node. Nodes of the SCF and low neck, generally 1 to 3 cm deep, are often treated when there is involvement of the transpectoral pathway. The scalene node, found in the low neck/SCF, is often biopsied to note disease spread.

The **internal mammary lymphatic pathway** runs toward the midline and passes through the pectoralis major and intercostal muscles close to the body of the sternum (T4 to T9). Associated with this pathway are the internal mammary nodes. These nodes are more frequently involved with primary breast cancers that are located in the inner breast quadrants and when there are positive axillary nodes. These nodes are generally 2.5 cm from midline (with variations from 0 to 5 cm) and about 2.5 cm deep (with variations from 1 to 5 cm). CT scans are extremely helpful to the radiation oncology team in assessing the location of these nodes. The lateral location and depth assist in determining the field width and treatment energy, respectively.

Breast lymphatic flow is also important from a surgical standpoint. With radical breast surgery, lymphatic flow is often compromised. As the channels of flow are altered because of surgical intervention, the lymph has fewer drainage paths back to the cardiovascular system. This slowed drainage causes edema that is sometimes seen in the arm of patients who have received radical breast surgery. Exercise and elevation of the limb help drain stagnant lymph. This complication has led the cancer management team to use less radical surgery when possible, along with other modalities.

Thoracic lymphatics.   The mediastinum demonstrates a rich intercommunicating network of lymphatics. The most important nodes to note are the lymphatics of the thoracic viscera and pulmonary veins. They are commonly involved in Hodgkin's disease as well as in lung cancers, in which they can be radiographically demonstrated as a widened mediastinum. The lymphatics of the lung and mediastinum are shown in Fig. 18-37.

The *superior mediastinal nodes* are located in the superior mediastinum. They lie anterior to the brachiocephalic veins, the aortic arch, and the large arterial trunks that arise from the aorta. They receive lymphatic vessels from the thymus, heart, pericardium, mediastinal pleura, and anterior hilum. The *tracheal nodes* extend along both sides of the thoracic trachea. They are also called the paratracheal nodes. The *superior tracheobronchial nodes* are located on each side of the trachea. They are superior and lateral to the angle at which the trachea bifurcates into the two primary bronchi.

The *inferior mediastinal nodes* are located in the inferior mediastinum. The inferior tracheobronchial nodes lie in the angle below the bifurcation of the trachea. They are also called the *carinal nodes*. The *bronchopulmonary nodes,* often called the hilar nodes, are found at the hilus of each lung, at the site of the division of the main bronchi and pulmonary vessels into the lobular bronchi and vessels. These nodes are involved in most lung cancer cases. The *pulmonary nodes,* also known as the intrapulmonary nodes, are found in the lung parenchyma along the secondary and tertiary bronchi.

In the right lung, all three lobes drain to the intrapulmonary and hilar nodes. They then flow to the carinal nodes and then to the paratracheal nodes before they reach the brachiocephalic vein through the scalene node and right lymphatic duct. In the left lung the upper lobe drains to the

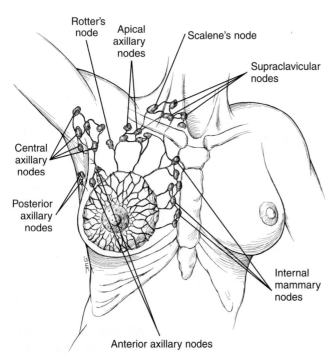

Figure 18-36. The lymphatic pathways associated with the breast: axillary, transpectoral, and internal mammary.

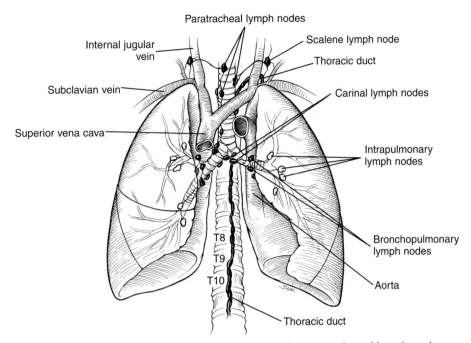

Figure 18-37. The mediastinum demonstrates a large number of lymph nodes.

pulmonary and hilar nodes, carinal nodes, left superior paratracheal nodes, and then the brachiocephalic vein through the thoracic duct. The left lower lobe drains to the pulmonary and hilar nodes, then to the right paratracheal nodes, where it follows the path outlined for the right lung. This is important when designing the treatment field of a lung cancer patient

SURFACE AND SECTIONAL ANATOMY AND LANDMARKS OF THE ABDOMEN AND PELVIS

The abdomen and pelvis house many organs that are treated for malignant disease. Their management presents treatment planning challenges for the radiation therapist and medical dosimetrist because of the abundance of radiosensitive structures within the abdominal and pelvic cavities. Treating a colorectal cancer to a dose of 60+ Gy can be difficult when the neighboring anatomy tolerates much less. Knowledge of surface and cross-sectional anatomy of the abdomen and pelvis is essential in radiation therapy. The radiation therapist must be able to bridge knowledge of surface and sectional anatomy with various body habiti to visualize internal anatomy. However, relating internal structures to the topography of the area is not without certain challenges, particularly in the anterior abdomen. When compared with the head, neck, and thorax, the anterior abdomen does not demonstrate as many bony landmarks to reference. However, there are stable bony landmarks in the pelvis that are commonly referenced.

Anterior Abdominal Wall

The *anterior abdominal wall* is bordered superiorly by the inferior costal margin and inferiorly by the symphysis pubis, inguinal ligament, anterior superior iliac spine (ASIS), and

iliac crest. The anterior aspect of the wall is formed by sheets of interlacing muscles that provide stability and form to the abdomen. The major muscles that help form the anterior abdominal wall include the rectus abdominis, transverse abdominis, internal oblique, and external oblique.

The *external oblique muscle* extends from the lower eight ribs to an insertion point that spans from the iliac crest to the midline aponeurosis, a sheetlike tendon that joins one muscle to another. It extends from the outer lateral body to the midline.

The *internal oblique muscle* spans from the iliac crest and inguinal ligament to the cartilage of the last four ribs. It runs in a midline to an outer, lateral perspective.

The *transverse abdominis muscle* runs from the iliac crest, inguinal ligament, and last six rib cartilages to the xiphoid process, linea alba (a tough fibrous band that extends from the xiphoid process to the pubic symphysis), and pubis on both sides. Thus this muscle runs from side to side.

The *rectus abdominis muscle* is commonly called the "six pack" by sports buffs. This muscle runs from the symphysis pubis to the xiphoid process and has three transverse fibrous bands that separate the muscle into six sections that are prominent in individuals with pronounced muscular tone.

These muscles work together in providing structure to the anterior abdominal wall. Fig. 18-38 shows the interrelated nature of these muscles.

A number of structures can be palpated in the abdomen. The xiphoid process lies in the epigastric region at the level of T9. This bony landmark is very stable. The radiation therapist typically uses this structure and the SSN in making sure that a patient is lying straight on the treatment couch. If both landmarks are in line with the projection of a sagittal laser,

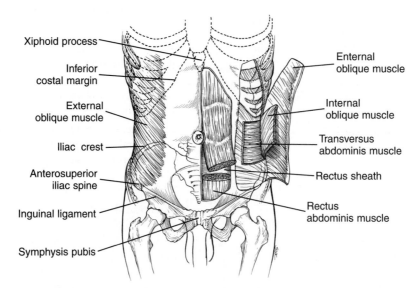

Figure 18-38. The muscles of the anterior and lateral abdominal wall work in unison to provide structure and stability to the torso.

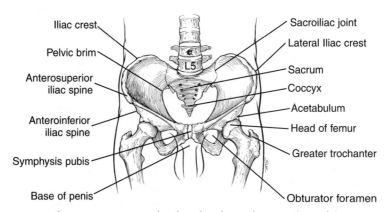

Figure 18-39. Bony landmarks about the anterior pelvis.

the thorax is usually straight. The xiphoid can also be used in conjunction with the pubic symphysis or associated soft tissue landmarks to ensure that the lower body is straight. The cartilages of the seventh to tenth ribs form the costal margin. This forms the inferior border of the rib cage. The umbilicus, also known as the navel or belly button, is an inconsistent, mobile landmark on the anterior abdomen. It is typically at the level of L4 when an individual is in a recumbent position. When standing, in the infant, and in the pendulous abdomen, it lies at a lower level.

Posterior Abdominal Wall (Trunk)

In the posterior wall the lower ribs, lumbar spines, PSIS, and iliac crest are palpable. A line, called the *intercristal line,* can be drawn between the iliac crests.[9] This line will typically pass between the spines of the third and fourth lumbar vertebrae, a location important when performing lumbar punctures.

Landmarks of the Anterior Pelvis

The anterior pelvis exhibits several bony and soft tissue landmarks that are useful to the radiation therapist. They are outlined below and demonstrated in Fig. 18-39.

The *iliac crest* extends from the ASIS to the PSIS. The ASIS is palpable, and measurements may be taken from it in the superoinferior or mediolateral direction. It is frequently used in referencing the location of the femur. The *lateral iliac crest* is also easily palpable and, being on the lateral pelvic wall, may be used as a transverse level on either the anterior or the posterior pelvis. The *lateral iliac crest level* is the line joining the right and left lateral iliac crests. These crests are the most superior margin of the ilium on the lateral pelvic wall. Measurements may be taken from this level in the superoinferior direction.

The head of the femur and greater trochanter, although not direct components of the true pelvis, are important to note when considering the lateral pelvic anatomy. The *head of the femur* articulates with the hip at the acetabulum. If irradiated beyond tolerance, fibrotic changes can occur, causing painful and/or limited motion of the joint. Usually this joint is shielded in moderate to large pelvic portals to limit this occurrence. The *greater trochanter* is the only part of the proximal femur that can be palpated; therefore its relationship to bony points of the hip bone is important.[8] The radiation therapist uses the greater trochanter when aligning patients during simulation to alleviate pelvis rotation. The patient should be horizontally level when the greater trochanters are at the same height from the tabletop. The radiation therapist can measure this using a ruler and optical lasers.

The pubis symphysis appears as the 5-mm midline gap between the inferior parts of the pelvic bones.[8] The *upper border pubis* is the palpable upper border of the midline pubic bone. It is fairly easy to palpate, except in extremely obese patients. When palpating it, care should be taken to allow for overlying tissue. The *lower border pubis* is the palpable lower border of the pubic bone in midline. It is not as easily palpable as the upper border pubis, because it lies more inferiorly and posteriorly. All of these can be accurately located radiographically. The radiation therapist uses these components when setting the anterior border of lateral prostate fields (the prostate lies immediately posterior to the pubis symphysis).

The ischial tuberosities are located in the inferior portion of the pelvis. This corresponds to the lower region of the buttock. When a person sits down, the ischial tuberosities bear the weight of the body. Many radiation oncologists use the ischial tuberosities as the inferior border of the anterior and posterior prostate treatment portals.

When pelvic irradiation is indicated, the radiation therapist can use the anatomy of the perineum, the diamond-shaped area bounded laterally by the ischial tuberosities, anteriorly by the pubic symphysis, and posteriorly by the coccyx, to assist in portal location. Treatment lines in these areas commonly fade because of perspiration and garment rubbing.[8] Knowledge of the area can thus provide a practical means of field verification. Both male and female anatomy demonstrates useful landmarks.

The *anterior commissure of the labia majora* is easily distinguishable in the female. It is an important soft tissue landmark, because it is used as a reference point from which the upper or lower border pubis is measured. Thus checking back to this soft tissue landmark may eliminate variations in the palpation of the pubic bone.

The *base of the penis* is taken as being the line joining the anterior skin of the penis with the skin of the anterior pelvic wall. This level is used as a reference point from which the upper or lower border pubis is measured in the male. A therapist may measure changes in the lateral position of prostate fields by referencing appropriate measurements from the base of the penis.

Landmarks of the Posterior Pelvis

The most commonly used bony surface landmarks of the posterior pelvis are the PSISs, the coccyx, the iliac crests, and the lateral iliac crests. Because the latter two were also mentioned in the previous section, only the PSIS is discussed here. The PSIS are indicated by dimples above and medial to the buttock, about 5 to 6 cm from the midline. They are palpable, and measurements may be taken in the superoinferior or mediolateral direction. The coccyx lies deep to the natal cleft with its inferior end roughly 1 cm from the anus.

Abdominopelvic Viscera

The organs of the abdomen and pelvis can be visualized by various means. Radiographs, CT, MRI, and US are commonly employed to provide information concerning organ location. It is worth noting that the location of any organ in the abdomen and pelvis can vary with respiration, anatomic position, and level of fullness. This is why it is extremely important to place radiation therapy patients in a reproducible position that limits movement daily. As observed earlier, body habitus affects the location of internal organs. This holds true for the abdomen and pelvis as well. This section examines the location of the abdominal and pelvic viscera.

Location of the Alimentary Organs

The esophagus begins at the lower border of the cricoid cartilage in the neck and travels through the diaphragm to the cardiac sphincter, the entrance to the stomach, at the level of T10 about 2 to 3 cm to the left of midline. To visualize the esophagus radiographically the patient commonly is instructed to swallow a radiopaque substance like barium before examination.

The duodenum, a C-shaped section of the small bowel about 25 cm in length, starts to the right of midline at the edge of the epigastric region. The stomach lies between the duodenum and the distal esophagus and is of variable size and location, partly covered by the left rib cage and filling the epigastric region. The root of the small gut mesentery, made up of sections called the jejunum and ileum, extends from the duodenum to the inlet to the large bowel.[8,9]

The start of the large bowel is the cecum. It lies in the right iliac region at the level of L4. The ascending colon (15 cm in length) and hepatic flexure of the colon on the right side and the splenic flexure and descending colon (25 cm in length) on the left side are largely retroperitoneal structures, whereas the transverse and sigmoid colon have a mesentery and vary in their position from one person to the next.[8,9] However, similarities are demonstrated within common body habiti. The rectum starts at the level of S3 and ends about 4 cm from the anus. It is one of the dose-limiting structures when outlining prostate treatment fields. Rectal visualization is thus important during the simulation process.

Fig. 18-40 delineates the surface projections of the alimentary tract in the abdomen and pelvis.

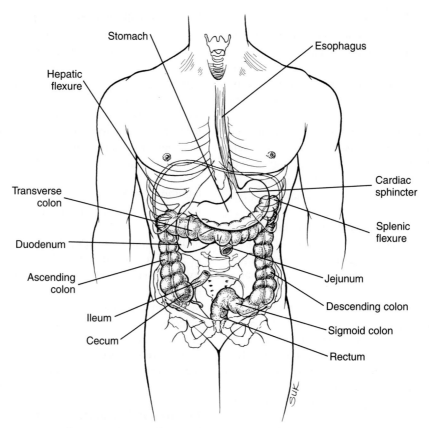

Figure 18-40. Surface projection of the alimentary organs.

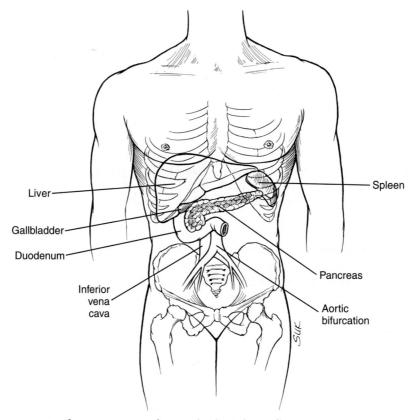

Figure 18-41. Surface projection of nonalimentary organs.

Location of Nonalimentary Organs

The radiation therapist benefits from a working knowledge of the nonalimentary organs of the abdomen and pelvis. Many times these organs are involved in malignant processes and must be included in the patient's treatment scheme. Fig. 18-41 demonstrates the surface projections of the organs outlined here.

The liver is an irregularly shaped organ located in the right hypochondriac region of the abdomen above the costal margin. The superior margin of the liver, which bulges into the diaphragm, is at the level of T7-T8. The liver is commonly imaged with CT, US, and nuclear medicine studies.

The gallbladder is located below the lower border of the liver and contacts the anterior abdominal wall where the right lateral border of the rectus abdominis crosses the ninth costal cartilage. This location is called the transpyloric plane. Again, US is useful in distinguishing biliary obstructions as well as gallstones.

The spleen, mentioned earlier as a lymph node for the blood, is located posteriorly about 5 cm to the left of midline at the level of T10-T11. The normal organ lies beneath the ninth through eleventh ribs on the left side of the body. This organ is often examined surgically in patients with lymphoma to determine disease extension. If the organ is removed for biopsy, the splenic pedicle, the point of attachment of the organ to its vascular and lymphatic connections, is included in the abdominal treatment field for Hodgkin's Disease.

Three components: the head, body, and tail, comprise the pancreas. The head of the pancreas is located in the C section of the duodenum. The body extends slightly superiorly to the left across midline, at the level of L1. The tail of the pancreas passes into the hilum, a concave point of an organ that has vascular inlets and outlets, of the spleen.

Location of the Urinary Tract Organs

The kidneys lie on the posterior abdominal wall in the retroperitoneal space. The hilum of the right kidney is at the level of L2, whereas the hilum of the left is at the level of L1. The right kidney lies lower than the left because of the presence of the adjacent liver. Superior and medial to each kidney are the adrenal glands. The kidneys are generally not fixed to the abdominal wall; they can move as much as 2 cm with respiration. When the radiation therapist outlines the location of these radiation-sensitive structures, it is important to take this into account.

The ureters are tubular structures that transport urine from the kidneys to the urinary bladder. They run anterior to the psoas muscles and enter the pelvis lateral to the sacroiliac (SI) joint. The ureters, as well as the kidneys, are commonly imaged with CT, US, and intravenous and retrograde studies.

The urinary bladder is located in the pelvis. The neck of the bladder lies posterior to the pubis symphysis and anterior to the rectum. This organ also lies immediately superior to the prostate in the male. The urinary bladder is a dose-limiting structure in the treatment of prostatic cancer. It is commonly visualized with contrast agents during the simulation process.

The topographic relations of the urinary tract organs are shown in Fig. 18-42.

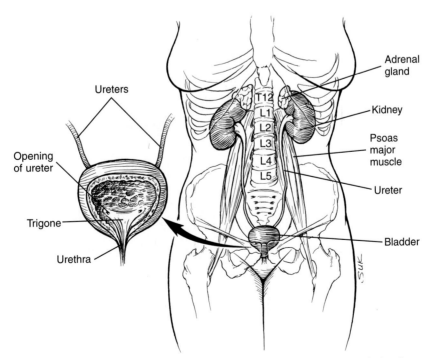

Figure 18-42. Surface projection of the urinary tract and adrenal glands.

Lymphatics of the Abdomen and Pelvis

The lymphatic drainage routes for the abdomen and pelvis are very important to the radiation therapist. There is an abundance of lymphatic vessels in this section of the body. Those of the retroperitoneum and pelvis play a major role in radiation therapy field arrangement of gynecologic, genitourinary, and lymphatic cancers. Figs. 18-43 and 18-44 show the nodes and nodal groups outlined here.

The lymphatic pathways and nodes of the abdomen are frequently referred to as the visceral nodes because they are closely associated with the abdominal organs. The three principal groups of nodes of the abdomen that drain the corresponding viscera before entering the cisterna chyli or the thoracic duct are the celiac, superior mesenteric, and inferior mesenteric groups, also called the preaortic nodes.

The *celiac nodes* include the nodes that drain the stomach, greater omentum, liver, gallbladder, and spleen, as well as most of the lymph from the pancreas and duodenum. The *superior mesenteric nodes* drain part of the head of the pancreas, a portion of the duodenum, the entire jejunum, ileum, appendix, cecum, ascending colon, and most of the transverse colon. The *inferior mesenteric nodes* drain the descending colon, the left side of the mesentery, the sigmoid colon, and the rectum.

The posterior abdominal wall demonstrates a rich network of lymphatic vessels. The paraaortic nodes provide efferent drainage to the cisterna chyli, which is the beginning of the

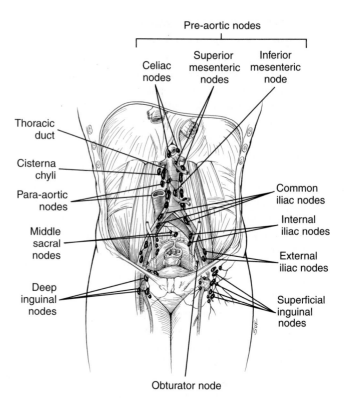

Figure 18-43. Abdominal lymph nodes.

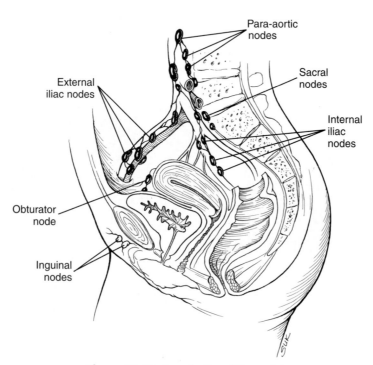

Figure 18-44. Lymphatics of the pelvis.

thoracic duct. These nodes run adjacent to the abdominal aorta from T12 to L4. This major section of the lymphatic system eventually receives lymph from most of the lower regions of the body. The *paraaortics* directly drain the uterus, ovary, kidneys, and testicles. It is interesting to note that embryonically the testes develop near the kidneys and descend into the scrotum after birth. As they descend, they take the vascular and lymphatic vessels with them as direct means for blood and lymph flow.

The *common iliac nodes* lie at the bifurcation of the abdominal aorta at the level of L4. These nodes directly drain the urinary bladder, prostate, cervix, and vagina. This chain moves laterally and breaks up into the external and internal iliac nodes. The *external iliac nodes* drain the urinary bladder, prostate, cervix, testes, vagina, and ovary. The *internal iliac nodes,* also known as the hypogastric nodes, drain the vagina, cervix, prostate, and urinary bladder. These nodes are more medial and posterior to the external iliac nodes previously mentioned.

The *inguinal nodes* are more superficial than the previously mentioned nodes. These nodes directly drain the vulva, uterus, ovary, and vagina. These nodes are commonly treated with electrons because of their superficial location.

APPLIED TECHNOLOGY

Practical application of the material presented in this chapter is very important. To enhance the comprehensive understanding of the relationships presented, the last section of this chapter presents diagrams that relate structures to vertebral body levels and CT scans through the head, neck, thorax, abdomen, and pelvis. The appropriate structures pertinent to the radiation oncology practitioner are demonstrated. Figs. 18-45 through 18-49 show these diagrams and scans.

SUMMARY

Radiation therapy requires its practitioners to demonstrate more than a passing acquaintance with surface and sectional anatomy. The complex simulation procedures and planning used in patient treatment mandates strict attention to detail. The radiation therapist must use information

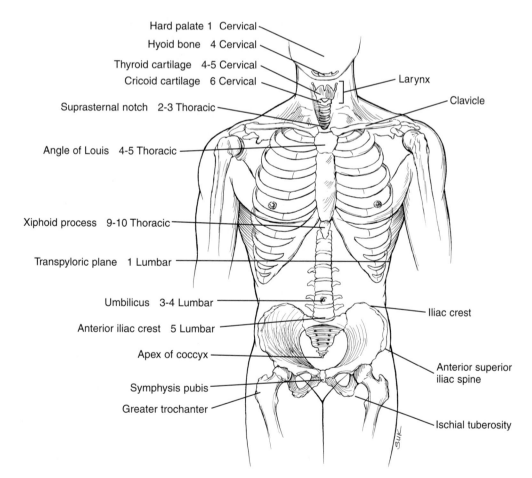

Figure 18-45. Anterior surface projections of selected skeletal anatomy.

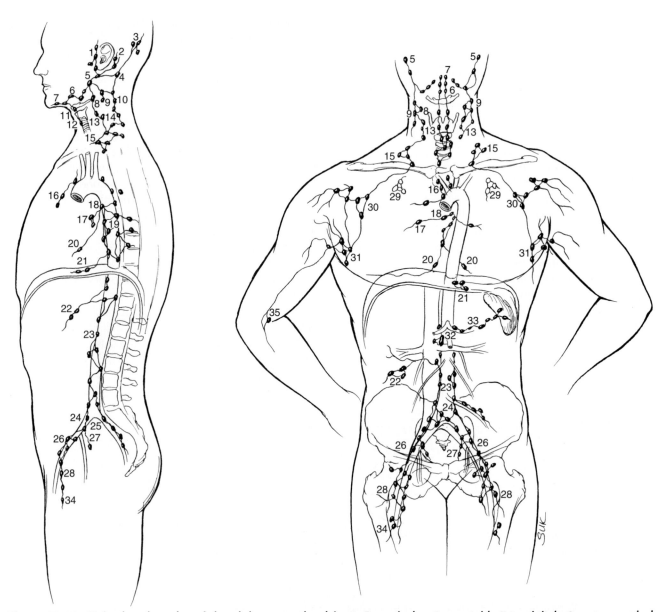

Figure 18-46. Major lymph nodes of the abdomen and pelvis. *1,* Preauricular; *2,* mastoid; *3,* occipital; *4,* upper cervical; *5,* parotid; *6,* submaxillary; *7,* submental; *8,* jugulodigastric; *9,* upper deep cervical; *10,* spinal accessory chain; *11,* infrahyoid; *12,* pretracheal; *13,* juguloomohyoid; *14,* lower deep cervical; *15,* supraclavicular; *16,* mediastinal; *17,* interlobar; *18,* intertracheal; *19,* posterior mediastinal; *20,* lateral pericardial; *21,* diaphragmatic; *22,* mesenteric; *23,* paraaortic; *24,* common iliac; *25,* lateral sacral; *26,* external iliac; *27,* hypogastric; *28,* inguinal; *29,* interpectoral; *30,* axillary apex; *31,* axillary; *32,* cisterna chyli; *33,* splenic; *34,* femoral; *35,* epitrochlear.

provided by several imaging modalities to achieve its ultimate goal: to administer a tumoricidal dose of radiation to the tumor and tumor bed while sparing as much normal tissue as possible. Also, the lymphatic vessels play a major role in treatment field delineation and disease management. To accomplish this goal the radiation therapist must command a comprehensive knowledge of surface and sectional

anatomy. The complexity of radiation therapy requires the radiation therapist to use all available means to function effectively. Without this base the therapist and the technology used are at best mediocre. Each therapist should review his or her practical skills in surface and sectional anatomy, because it is crucial for accurate treatment planning and delivery.

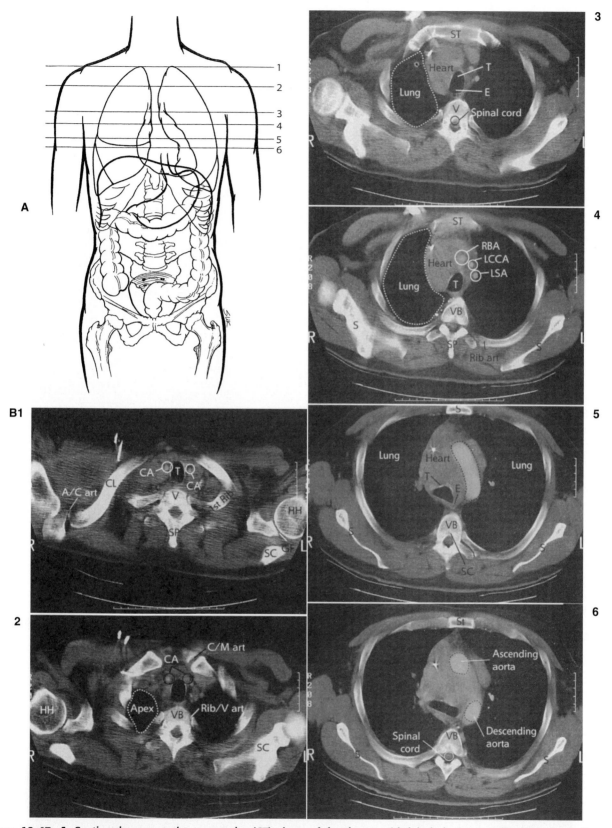

Figure 18-47. A, Sectional computed tomography (CT) views of the thorax with labeled anatomy **(B).** *ACA,* Ascending aorta; *A/C art,* acromial clavicular articulation; *C,* clavicle; *CA,* carotid artery; *C/M art,* Clavicular macrobial articular; *DCA,* descending aorta; *E,* esophagus; *GF,* glenoid fossa; *HH,* humeral head; *LCCA,* left common carotid artery; *LSA,* left subclavian artery; RBA, right bronchocephalic artery; *Rib/V art,* rib/vertebral artery; *S,* sternum; *SC,* scapula; *T,* trachea; *V,* vein; *VB,* vertebral body.

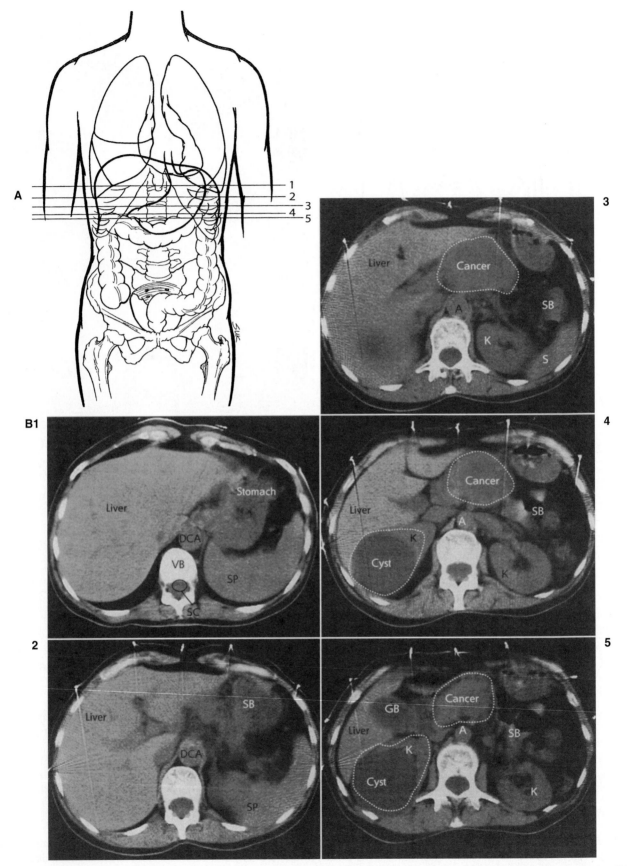

Figure 18-48. A, Sectional computed tomography (CT) views of the abdomen with labeled anatomy **(B).** *A,* Aorta; *DCA,* descending aorta; *GB,* gallbladder; *K,* kidney; *L,* liver; *S,* spleen; *SB,* small bowel; *SC,* spinal cord; *VB,* vertebral body.

Simulator Design

Dennis Leaver, Nora Uricchio, Patton Griggs

Outline

Key Terms

Beam-restricting diaphragms
Central axis
Collimation
Collimator assembly
Controls associated with the
    virtual simulator
    workstation
CT hardware
CT simulation
Fiducial plate
Field-defining wires
Gantry
Grid
Image intensifier
Isocenter

Optical distance indicator
   (ODI)
Orthogonal
Patient marking system
Pendant
Positioning lasers
Protractor
Simulation
Simulator
Simulators with a CT mode
Table top
Tensile strength
Treatment verification
Tumor localization
Virtual simulation

The clinical application of radiation therapy is a complex process requiring the use and involvement of many professionals and high-technology equipment.[7] The effective use of the treatment simulator is important in achieving the goal of delivering a dose of radiation to the cancer tissue and at the same time reducing the dose to the normal surrounding tissue. In most cases this requires a high degree of precision and accuracy. It is the right combination of high-technology equipment, like the simulator, and the involvement of dedicated professionals that can sometimes make the difference between a geographical miss and curing the patient of cancer.

The primary purpose of the **simulator** is to assist the physician and other members of the radiation therapy team in the treatment planning process. It can be assumed that patients treated for cure may have 30 to 40 separate treatments, and those who are treated for palliation may have between 10 and 20 treatments.[35] Therefore reproducibility of treatment is a critical factor for all patients. A modern simulator, which can support up to two or three treatment units in the radiation oncology department, helps to achieve this goal.

There are a number of approaches to the **simulation** process: conventional simulation and computed tomography (CT) simulation. The development of commercially available CT simulators has fused the process of patient scanning, tumor and target localization, treatment planning, and treatment field verification into a single integrated operation.[15] CT simulation differs from conventional simulation in a number of ways. During conventional simulation, patient data is obtained using fluoroscopy, radiographs, and physical measurements of the patient (Fig. 19-1). This information is then entered into the treatment planning computer. With **CT simulation,** patient data is gathered using detailed CT images in the transverse plane. Digitally reconstructed radiographs

(DRRs) and a laser alignment system document the simulation process before patient data is transferred electronically through a computer link to the treatment planning computer (Fig. 19-2). In the following sections, both the conventional and the CT simulator design are discussed along with information related to the historic perspective of the simulation process (Box 19-1).

HISTORICAL PERSPECTIVE

Historically, radiation oncology began as a subsection of diagnostic radiology. The simulation process also has its roots in diagnostic radiology (remember, the conventional simulator uses an x-ray tube as one of its primary components). Before the widespread commercial availability of the simulator, most patients' treatment planning occurred on the cobalt unit, betatron, or linear accelerator. Competition for space and capital budget requests within the radiology department may have contributed to this initial approach (in the early days) of setting up new patients on the treatment unit.

In the past a "simulation time" was scheduled on the treatment unit or a conventional diagnostic x-ray unit to "set up" new patients.[4-6,13,18,22,23] There were several problems associated with this type of procedure. First, it took time away from treating patients. "Room simulations" (treatment room) required a fair amount of time to adequately estimate the target volume and provide some parameters to ensure reproducibility on subsequent days of treatment. Second, the

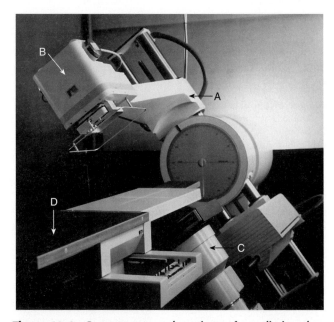

Figure 19-1. Components and motions of a radiation therapy simulator. These include the gantry **(A)** (including the collimator head **[B]** and image intensifier **[C]**) and patient support assembly **(D)** (treatment couch). *(Courtesy Oldelft Corporation, Fairfax, Virginia.)*

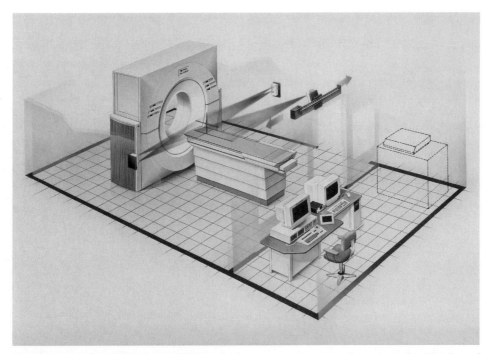

Figure 19-2. Virtual simulation. This technique uses a computed tomography (CT)-based simulator linked into a treatment planning computer. The laser light system delineates field borders once a plan has been completed. *(Used by permission from Picker International, Cleveland, Ohio.)*

quality of the planning radiographs (which were a type of port film) were very poor. High-energy x-rays and gamma rays do not produce good-quality images. In addition, the initial estimates of the target volume (without the aid of fluoroscopy and CT images) depended to a large degree on the radiation therapy team's understanding and application of topographical anatomy. Fig. 19-3 illustrates the difference between a conventional simulation radiograph and a port film. The simulation radiograph (Fig. 19-3, *A*), which is exposed using x-rays in the diagnostic range (70 to 120 kVp), demonstrates overall improved contrast and visibility of detail as compared with the corresponding portal localization radiograph (Fig. 19-3, *B*), which was produced using a 6-MV x-ray beam.

The development of the modern conventional radiation therapy simulator was prompted by the introduction of linear accelerators and other high-energy treatment units.[14] It was thought that if a machine could be built that duplicated the mechanical and geometrical features of a treatment unit, then the treatment unit could be used for its original purpose—to deliver a prescribed dose of radiation to the patient. Initially, it was thought, the cobalt unit, betatron, and linear accelerator deserved most of the credit for curing or effectively palliating a patient's cancer. It was not long before the benefits of the treatment simulator were also established.

Simulator Justification

In the early days of radiation therapy it may have been difficult for a radiation oncologist or radiologist to justify to the radiology administrator the cost effectiveness of a simulator. Many more patients were treated for relief of symptoms such as obstruction, bleeding, and pain than were cured. In the 1960s, only about one in three patients was cured of their cancer. Today, it may be well over 50%.[8] When radiation therapy began, it was considered a small ancillary part of most radiology departments.

It could be argued that the addition of a simulator would increase the number of patients treated on the therapy machine. In addition, the cost to society of serious side effects from less than optimal and sometimes ineffective simulation was also a factor.

The cost effectiveness, increased efficiency, and accuracy of a radiation therapy simulator have been documented.[12,14,16,25] One group of researchers reviewed the records of 97 patients (1970 to 1975) with lung cancer who had survived at least 18 months. All patients were treated with irradiation at one of two Boston hospitals. Three spinal cord injuries were observed in nonsimulated patients, and none were observed in those patients whose treatment planning involved the use of a treatment simulator. This is a small group of patients, but it obviously documents the benefits of a simulator. Spinal cord

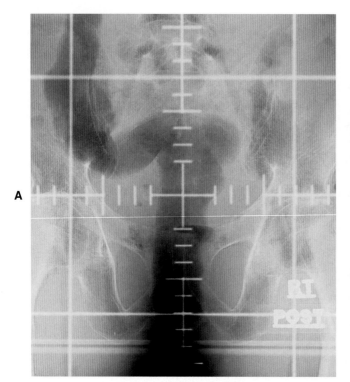
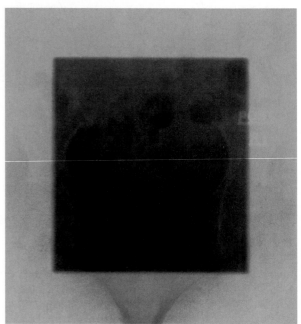

Figure 19-3. Simulation radiograph. **A,** Exposure using x-rays in the diagnostic range (70 to 120 kVp) demonstrates overall improved contrast and visibility of detail as compared with the corresponding portal localization radiograph **(B),** which was produced using a 6-MeV x-ray beam.

injuries not only decrease the quality of life for the patient but also add a considerable financial burden to society.[14]

Increased Simulator Use

If a department had a simulator in the 1950s and 1960s, it was most likely homemade or custom built. Fig. 19-4 illustrates a custom-built simulator first introduced in Newcastle, England in 1955.[17] This unit had a C-shaped **gantry** incorporating the x-ray tube and imaging system. A patient couch pivoted around a magnetic clutch embedded in the floor.[13] This was probably one of the first simulators used; even in the early days of radiation therapy, some understood the simulators' usefulness and importance.

Since the late 1960s, there has been a gradual increase in the application and use of the treatment simulator. Today all radiation therapy facilities should have access to at least one simulator, regardless of the total number of new patients treated each year in the department.[35] Fig. 19-5 documents the increased use of simulation equipment through several studies in radiation facilities throughout the United States from 1978 to 1995.[24,34]

SIMULATION PROCESS

The general responsibility for the patient's clinical progress and proper treatment belongs to the radiation oncologist. The technical aspects of treatment such as simulation, dose delivery, and computerized treatment planning are the responsibility of the radiation therapist, clinical physicist, and dosimetrist. The simulation process, which is an initial step in the treatment planning process and involves several members of the team, is an indispensable element that contributes to the effective and accurate practice of radiation oncology.

As a first step in treatment planning, the simulation process can be simple or complex, depending on the type of cancer, the extent of the tumor, and its proximity to normal surrounding tissue. However, before any planning begins, the diagnosis of a patient's cancer must be established. This is a crucial step. It may involve a complete clinical workup, including histology, staging, grading, and various studies such as x-ray examinations and laboratory work. Fig. 19-6 illustrates the steps, from diagnosis to patient follow-up, involved in the radiation therapy process. Only after a diagnosis has been established does the radiation oncologist discuss with the patient and family (during a consultation) the treatment options, along with the risks and benefits of such treatment. Simulation and treatment planning may follow, if a decision to use radiation therapy alone or in combination with surgery and/or chemotherapy has been made.

Treatment planning consists of **tumor localization** (simulation), computation of dose distribution, and fabrication of treatment aids. Karzmark outlines two setup functions of conventional simulation: (1) tumor localization, which may

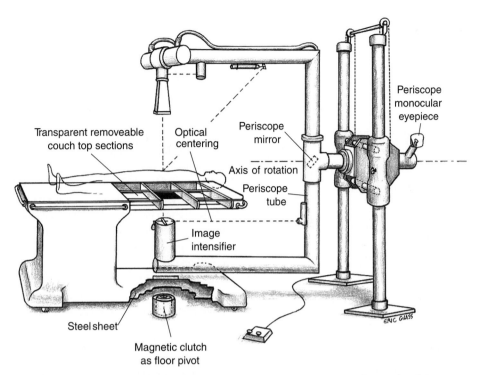

Figure 19-4. Custom-built simulator. This device, used in Newcastle, England, in 1955, shows isocentric capabilities and a periscope system for imaging purposes. *(Redrawn with permission from Farmer ET, Fowler JF, Haggith JW: Megavoltage treatment planning and the use of xeroradiography, Br J Rad 36:426-435, 1963.)*

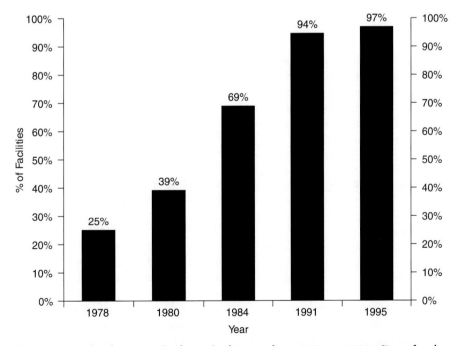

Figure 19-5. Simulator use in the United States from 1978 to 1995. *(Data for the years 1978 to 1984 from Karzmark CJ, Nunan CS, Tanabe E: Medical electron accelerators. Princeton, NJ, 1993, McGraw-Hill. Data for 1991 obtained from Owen J, Coia L, Hanks G: Recent patterns of growth in radiation therapy facilities, poster presentation at the meeting of the American Society of Therapeutic Radiologists and Oncologists, Washington DC, Nov 1991. Data for 1995 were obtained from Owen J at the American College of Radiology, as an estimate from 1995 data on recent patterns of growth in radiation therapy facilities.)*

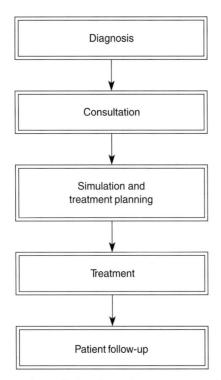

Figure 19-6. The radiation therapy process. Several steps are involved in treating a typical patient with radiation therapy. The process begins with diagnosis and includes consultation, simulation and treatment planning, treatment, and patient follow-up.

involve determining the extent of the tumor and location of critical structures and (2) **treatment verification** using diagnostic quality images of each treatment field from the initial simulation procedure.[3,24] These images, taken during simulation, become the "masters" to compare subsequent port images, which are taken on the treatment unit.

The process of CT simulation differs considerably form conventional simulation. Hunt[20] describes six goals of CT simulation localization and field design, which include the following:

- Aquisition of a patient data set
- Target and normal structure localization
- Definition and marking of a patient coordinate system (triangulation points)
- Transfer of information to the treatment planning system
- Production of an image for treatment verification

The treatment simulator is an important tool in optimizing the radiation therapy process. The following discussion includes the design of both a conventional radiation therapy simulator and CT simulator, its theory, and its operation.

CONVENTIONAL SIMULATOR DESIGN

Conventional simulators are designed to simulate the mechanical, geometrical, and optical conditions of a variety of treatment units.[2,14,16,26,30] This is their basic purpose. It is critical that the mechanical parameters and geometrical characteristics of the simulator match those of the treatment unit. If they do not, a simulator may as well not be used in the treatment planning process.

Simulators have evolved to allow the practice of more aggressive and curative radiation therapy. Design improvements have played a major role in this evolution. Improvements in x-ray characteristics and mechanical performance have contributed greatly to more effective tumor localization and simulation procedures. To ensure that the critical mechanical parameters of the simulator match the geometry of the treatment unit, each department needs a comprehensive quality assurance program. The purpose of a quality assurance program is to objectively and systematically monitor the quality and appropriateness of the simulation process as it relates to patient care.[39] The British Standards Institution, which represents the United Kingdom's view on standards in Europe and at the international level, has published a guide to functional performance values for the radiation therapy simulator.[9] The guide, which is based on International Electrotechnical Commission (IEC) standards for the safety of medical electrical equipment,[†] may be useful in establishing specific elements for a quality assurance program.

The guidelines provided are recommendations both to manufacturers and to users. They provide guidance to manufacturers on the needs of radiation oncologists and radiation therapists in respect to the performance of radiation therapy simulators. They also provide guidelines to users wishing to check the manufacturer's declared performance characteristics. In addition, users can establish and carry out acceptance tests and quality assurance tests to check periodically the performance throughout the life of the equipment.[9]

To create some uniformity in the design of a simulator, certain criteria and specifications should be followed by the manufacturer. Specific design features and performance specifications of the simulator are also outlined in the *British Journal of Radiology* Supplement 23[7] and an assessment by McCullough and Earle.[29] Table 19-1 summarizes the simulator performance specifications in the *British Journal of Radiology* Supplement 23.

Mechanical Components

The mechanical components of the conventional simulator include the gantry, treatment couch, and controls. A number of simulators are on the market today, and the choice depends on the need and budget of the radiation oncology department. Some are highly sophisticated computer-assisted models, and others have more basic functions, including some without fluoroscopy. An introduction to the essential components of the radiation therapy simulator will reveal many similarities,

---

†IEC 601-1: 1988, from BSI Medical electrical equipment-Part 1: General requirements for safety, and Amendment 1, 1991. In addition, IEC 601-1 is supplemented by IEC 1168: 1993, Radiotherapy simulators—Functional performance characteristics.

		Specification	Description
Table 19-1	**A summary of the simulator specifications**		

	Specification	Description
GANTRY		
Height of isocenter above the floor	≤115 cm	
Angle of rotation at ≤100 cm SAD	>360°	0.03-1.0 rpm
Angle of rotation at >100 cm SAD	±90°	
Isocenter accuracy, diameter	2 mm	
Clearance between gantry and isocenter	≤110 cm	
X-RAY HEAD AND COLLIMATOR		
Source-axis distance	80-100 cm*	0.5-5 cm s^{-1}
Beam-limiting diaphragms at 100 cm	50 cm × 50 cm max	
Diaphragm rotation	>220°	0.01 rpm
Beam-delineating wires at 100 cm	50 cm × 50 cm max	
Source-skin distance indicator	60-150 cm	
X-RAY TUBE AND GENERATOR		
Focal spot size	0.3 mm × 0.3 mm	
Target angle	≥20°	
Continuous rating of target	500 HU s^{-1}	
Generator	3 phase	
Radiographic output (minimum)	500 mA, 90 kV	
Fluoroscopic output (minimum)	6 mA, 125 kV	
IMAGING DEVICE		
Film cassette and grid	≥35 cm^2	Manual rotation
Image intensifier	12 inch	
Scanning movements of the image intensifier	±20 cm	3 cm s^{-1}
Radial movements of the image intensifier	210 to 260 cm	3 cm s^{-1}
COUCH		
Couch top	220 cm × 45 cm	
Rotation about couch support	360°	Manual rotation
Rotation about isocenter	±100°	0.003-0.05 rpm
Vertical movement	+2 to 250 cm	0.1-3.0 cm s^{-1}
Minimum couch movement	<50 cm	
Longitudinal movement	230 to +100 cm	Manual, 2 cm s^{-1}
Lateral movement	±20 cm	Manual, 2 cm s^{-1}

Used by permission from Bomford CK et al: *BJR supplement 23: treatment simulators,* London, 1989, British Institute of Radiology.
*Extending to 175 cm source-couch distance when the beam is vertical.

especially in their mechanical functions. This may include the gantry, treatment couch, controls, and other ancillary devices such as the blocking tray and safety features. Each of these components is discussed separately in this section.

Gantry. The gantry arm is the rigid C-shaped structural support of the gantry. It provides support for both the x-ray tube, located within the head of the gantry at one end of the open part of the C, and the image-intensifying/film holder system, located at the opposite end. These components of the gantry should be constructed in such a way that their alignment with the central axis of the beam can be maintained over the life of the simulator.[7] Fig. 19-1 illustrates the three gantry components, including the gantry arm, gantry head,

and image intensifier/film holder. Through 360-degree rotation the gantry can potentially direct the beam toward the patient from any angle. Its speed of rotation is variable and may be from less than 10 degrees/min up to 720 degrees/min.[31] On more basic models, it may be adjusted manually. In addition, the head of the gantry moves in a radial direction, or up and down, much like the periscope on a submarine.

Before looking at each of the components of the gantry in more detail, an explanation and description of the motions of the conventional simulator, as illustrated in Figs. 19-7 and 19-8, may be helpful. Table 19-2 describes each of the motions of the simulator illustrated in Fig. 19-7.

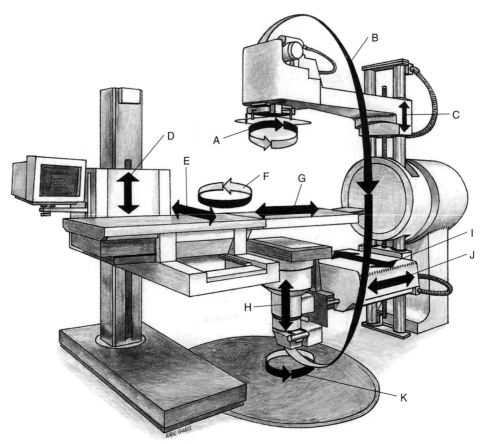

Figure 19-7. Motions of the simulator. Each letter corresponds to one of the 11 motions described in Table 19-2.

Isocenter. The gantry rotates around a fixed point in space, called the isocenter. The isocentric method, proposed by Howard-Flanders and Newbery in 1950, is still used today in radiation oncology.[13] This is an abstract concept. The **isocenter** should be considered as a reference point in space, a fixed distance (80 to 100 cm) from the focal spot on the anode. If the isocenter is placed either on the surface of the patient (fixed source-skin distance [SSD] treatment) or at some location within the patient (isocentric source-axis distance [SAD] treatment) in the simulator room, then it can also be reproduced on or within the patient in the treatment room.

In searching for this invisible point in the simulator or treatment room, it would take some understanding to locate it. It could be measured. The isocenter is generally located 80 to 100 cm from the focal spot and between 100 and 130 cm above the floor, depending on the manufacturer's specifications. The distance from the isocenter to the source of x-ray production (focal spot) is the same from any gantry angle.

The treatment couch, sometimes mounted on a turntable, allows rotation about a fixed axis that passes through the isocenter. Thus there are three axes of rotation—the central axis of the beam, the axis of rotation of the gantry, and the treatment couch axis—that all meet at a point known as the isocenter.[13] The **central axis** is the central portion of the beam emanating from the target. It is the only part of the beam that is not divergent. In a treatment plan with multiple fields, the central axes of each beam are directed toward the isocenter.

Each part of the gantry revolves around the isocenter. It is like the axle of a bicycle wheel. All the spokes of the wheel have a relationship with the axle. The head of the gantry is always, like the spokes of the wheel, the same distance from the isocenter regardless of its position in space.

The **protractor** (gantry angle scale), located at the central point of rotation of the gantry arm, is an instrument in the shape of a graduated circular device. It is used to measure the gantry angle, which may range from 0 degrees to 360 degrees. Because of a lack of agreement among manufacturers of simulators and treatment equipment on the angular specifications of the protractor, some simulators and treatment units do not correspond in this area. One unit may indicate a 0 degree reading when the gantry is in the vertical position, and another may read 360 degrees. The IEC has developed recommendations for linear and angular scale

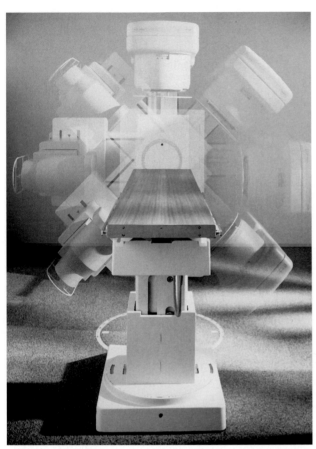

Figure 19-8. Radiation therapy simulator movements. *(Used by permission from Philips Medical Systems, Shelton, Connecticut.)*

placement and 0-degree location on the protractor for treatment units as well as simulators.[21] A conversion chart, located near the simulator work area, may be helpful in matching gantry angle readouts.

Gantry head. The gantry also provides stability for the collimator assembly, optical distance indicator (ODI), x-ray tube, field-defining wires, beam-limiting diaphragm (also called shutters or blades), and accessory holder. Fig. 19-9 illustrates the components of the gantry head. Each of these features are discussed in this section.

Design features of the collimator assembly allow it to provide support for the x-ray tube aperture, field-defining wires, light field indicator, beam-limiting diaphragms, and an accessory holder. Essentially the collimator assembly comprises most of the gantry head, except for an optical beam directing device mounted at the head of the gantry. The **optical distance indicator** (ODI), sometimes called a rangefinder, projects a scale onto the patient's skin, which corresponds to the SSD (Fig. 19-10). This is generally mounted near the collimator. The motorized collimator assembly should rotate around the central axis of the x-ray beam through at least a 220-degree collimator rotation angle.[6,7] For example, this allows a 10 × 10 cm square-shaped field projected on the patient's skin to become a 10 × 10 cm diamond-shaped field, if the collimator is rotated 45 degrees. The **collimator assembly** also directs the path of the x-ray beam toward the patient, after it emerges from the x-ray tube.

Mounting the simulator's x-ray tube onto the diaphragm system is recommended. When or if the x-ray tube must be replaced, the alignment of the geometric axis of the diaphragm system is made easier if it is mounted onto the gantry and not the x-ray tube.[6,7] The x-ray tube used for simulation must have a large and small focal spot; preferably, the small focal spot is no greater than 0.6 mm. To obtain a

Table 19-2	The mechanical motions of the simulator*		
Location	**Motion**	**Major Component**	**Description**
A	Collimator rotation	Gantry head	
B	Gantry rotation	Gantry arm	Variable speed
C	SAD adjustment	Gantry arm	
D	Vertical movement	Patient support assembly	
E	Lateral movement	Patient support assembly	
F	Pedestal rotation	Patient support assembly	Not found on all simulators
G	Longitudinal movement	Patient support assembly	
H	Radial movement	Image intensifier	
I	Lateral movement	Image intensifier	Scanning ability
J	Longitudinal movement	Image intensifier	Scanning ability
K	Rotation about isocenter	Patient support assembly	

SAD, Source-axis distance.
*Each letter (A to J) corresponds to the components illustrated in Fig. 19-7.

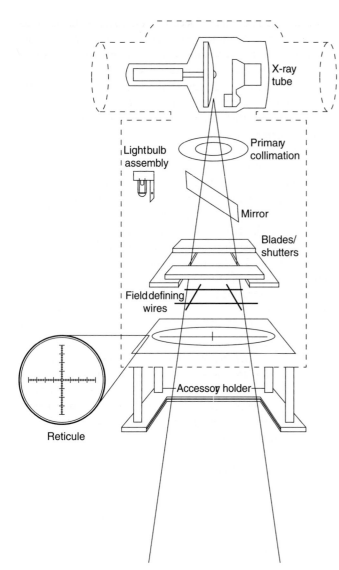

Figure 19-9. Components of the gantry head. These include the port of the x-ray tube housing, the field light mirror, collimator blades (shutters), field-defining wires, central axis crosshairs, and the accessory holder.

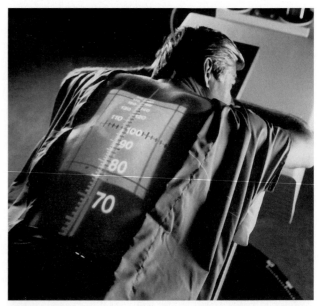

Figure 19-10. Use of the optical distance indicator (ODI). It projects a graduated light beam, in centimeters, on the patient's skin, which allows for accurate measurements of source-skin distance (SSD). (*Courtesy Oldelft Corp, Fairfax, Virginia.*)

sharp image of the 0.5-mm-diameter field-defining wires that are located in the collimator assembly, a small focal spot is necessary. For this reason and others, careful selection of the x-ray tube and generator is significant

Field-defining wires are located in the collimator assembly. It is recommended that the remote and locally controlled field-defining wires (also called delineators) simulate a maximum field size up to 40 × 40 cm at 100 cm SSD on any treatment unit available. The wires represent the edge of the treatment field within the larger image that is defined by the beam-limiting diaphragms (Fig. 19-3, *A*). To simulate a variety of field sizes from zero to 40 × 40 cm (or larger) at 100 cm, the four extremely narrow wires, each representing a field border, must move symmetrically within tolerance. The

scale indicating the range of field sizes at this distance should be displayed accurately within 2 mm inside the simulator room and remotely at the control panel.[7] Some simulators provide independent motorized movement of each of the field-defining wires and beam-limiting diaphragms. This allows for the simulation of half-field blocks and asymmetric beams. One can understand the strict tolerance and routine quality assurance that are necessary if one is to depend on this definition of the beam edge.

Also located within the collimator assembly are the **beam-restricting diaphragms**, which are made of 2 to 3 mm of lead.[32] They are one of the most important parts of the simulator because the diaphragms define both the size and the axis of the x-ray beam.[6,7] Beam-restricting diaphragms (also called x-ray shutters, blades, or collimators) operate much the same way as the field-defining wires. These thin blades of lead define the simulator's x-ray beam during fluoroscopy or during a radiograph by limiting the area exposed. To minimize the amount of unwanted scatter reaching the film or image intensifier, the irradiated field must be kept as small as possible. The diaphragms serve this purpose. Every radiograph should show evidence of **collimation** (restricting the beam with the diaphragms) by displaying a 1 to 2 cm clear border of unexposed film. Primarily, the beam-restricting diaphragms restrict the coverage of the x-ray field.

A secondary purpose of the beam-restricting diaphragms is to optically indicate the coverage of the x-ray field. The field light represents the radiation field, so one can see on the patient's skin where the x-ray field will be directed. It does this much the same way it restricts the x-ray field on a radiograph. In addition to restricting the radiation on a radiograph, it restricts a light field on the patient's skin. A special light bulb (usually a quartz-iodine projector lamp), located within the collimator assembly, is used for this purpose.[13] An angled mirror, located above the field-defining wires and beam-restricting diaphragms, projects an image from the filament of the light bulb through the diaphragms and onto the patient, as demonstrated in Figs. 19-10 and 19-11. Critical care should be taken when replacing this bulb. In fact, each time a field light bulb is replaced (both on the conventional simulator and on the treatment unit), a special test is performed called a light field/radiation field coincidence test. This type of quality assurance test evaluates the maximum distance between the light field edge and the x-ray field edge. At the normal treatment distance for field sizes 5 × 5 cm to 20 × 20 cm the coincidence should be 1 mm or 0.5% for field sizes greater than 20 × 20 cm.[7] It is only through careful evaluation that one can be certain that the light field actually represents the x-ray field.

Fiducial plate. Plexiglas or plastic trays imbedded with lead markers at regular intervals are called **fiducial plates** or beaded trays.[38] These trays, sometimes referred to as a reticule, are positioned in the head of the gantry between the field-defining wires and the accessory holder. Because the lead markers, which may be shaped like BBs or small lines, are spaced to represent the geometry of the field at the treatment

distance, a separate tray is necessary on most simulators to represent 80 and 100 SSD treatments (Fig. 19-12). Other trays are also available from some manufacturers. Tray selection should be checked before each simulation procedure to ensure accurate geometric representation of the treatment unit (if the simulator supports multiple treatment units with different treatment distances). Magnification can be determined using this type of tray system, because the hash marks or lead beads represent 1 or 2 cm at the isocenter. On some simulators the fiducial tray serves a second purpose. The tray not only helps to document the field size on the simulation radiograph, but it also protects the delicate tungsten wire crosshairs (Fig. 19-11), which are located within the collimator assembly and mark the center of the field radiographically.[32]

Accessory holder. On most simulators an adjustable accessory holder is mounted on the collimator or gantry head. It appears to hang down (when the gantry is positioned vertically) from the head of the gantry (Fig. 19-13). The accessory holder may serve two purposes: a block tray holder and an electron cone adapter.

As a block tray holder, a specific block tray distance must be set on the simulator for each treatment unit to provide geometric duplication of shielding blocks. This distance generally ranges from 40 to 60 cm. It is adjustable to accommodate a number of different treatment units within a single department. There are two purposes to the blocking tray. One is to simulate shielded areas during the simulation process. Thin lead foil

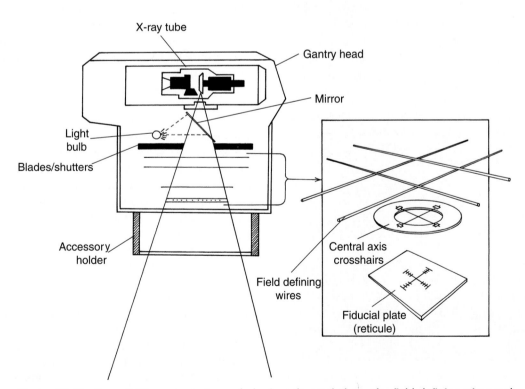

Figure 19-11. X-ray field coverage. An angled mirror, located above the field-defining wires and beam-restricting diaphragms, projects an image from the filament of the light bulb through the diaphragms, field-defining wires, and central axis crosshairs and onto the patient.

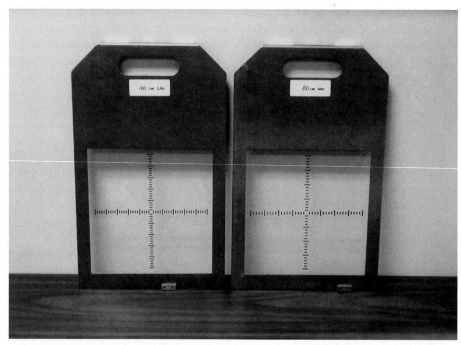

Figure 19-12. Fiducial plates. Sometimes called beaded trays or reticules, these plates are inserted into the head of the gantry to represent various geometries ranging from 80 to 100 source-axis distance (SAD). Notice that the lead marks are embedded in the plastic trays and spaced at regular intervals. They are spaced closer together on the 100 SAD tray as compared with the 80 SAD tray and project 1 cm divisions at either distance.

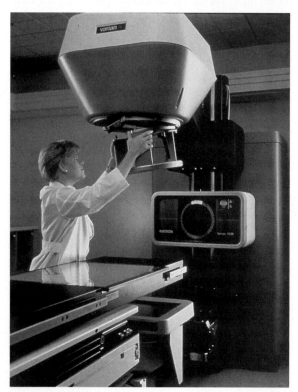

Figure 19-13. Removable accessory holder. This can be mounted on the collimator head of the gantry to accommodate custom blocks or an electron cone. *(Courtesy Varian Medical Systems.)*

blocks or small solder wires can be placed on a Plexiglas tray, which cast a shadow onto the patient's skin. In this way, coverage of any critical external structures such as the lens of the eye or an involved surgical scar is evaluated (otherwise the blocked area can be determined from a scan or drawn directly on the film). A second purpose is to verify the geometry of individualized custom shielding blocks on the simulator before they are used during an actual treatment. Some individual shielding blocks, which are constructed after the initial simulation procedure, can weigh up to 35 to 45 pounds. The average weight of a set of custom blocks realistically averages around 10 to 15 pounds. If actual block verification is performed on the simulator, the blocking tray should rotate with the collimator head and support this amount of weight. With the introduction of multi-leaf collimators, custom blocks are used less frequently than they were in the past.

An accessory holder should also support the weight of various electron cones because it may be necessary to simulate electron setups for the treatment unit. This can easily be accomplished on the simulator if the accessory holder can support the weight of an electron cone and reproduce the geometry of the desired treatment field.

Image intensifier system.   Another valuable component, located at the opposite end of the gantry arm, is the **image intensifier.** This complex device receives and processes the created image, which is a result of radiation interacting with the patient, field-defining wires, beam-restricting diaphragms, crosshairs, and accessory holder.

A typical image intensifier system contains four major components: the film holder, the image intensifier, television camera, and video monitor. As illustrated in Fig. 19-14, the image intensifier system can scan in several directions. Besides its scanning design during fluoroscopy, the image intensifier also provides mechanical support as a film holder in the radiography mode.

The image intensifier has a frame mounted onto it, which can accommodate a 35 × 43 cm radiographic cassette. The cassette slides into a groove in the film holder, which supports it at right angles to the central axis of the x-ray beam, regardless of the gantry position. This is an important feature that reduces distortion (elongation and foreshortening) in the production of radiographs. Some film holders provide 180-degree rotation of the 35 × 43 cm (14 × 17 inch) cassette. This is a feature found on some simulators, so the cassette may be positioned crosswise instead of lengthwise, if necessary, during a radiographic exposure. In most European countries, 35 × 35 cm cassettes are commonly used.

Some film holders also provide a slot for positioning an optional grid in front of the cassette to help control scatter radiation. As a rule of thumb, any time the thickness of the body part exceeds 10 to 12 cm, a grid should be employed. All tissues of the foot, hand, lower leg, forearm, and elbow can be adequately demonstrated without the use of a grid. In many cases the knee and upper arm may also be examined using only screen-type radiographic techniques. Beyond this, a grid should be employed both to absorb the scattered radiation emitted from the thicker body parts and to allow the use of beam energies needed to maximize differential absorption between similar tissues.

The image intensifier also reduces object-film distance (OFD). It should be remembered that the image intensifier can move radially (closer to and away from the gantry head). In doing so, OFD is reduced to a minimum during fluoroscopy or for a radiographic exposure. Fig. 19-15 illustrates two radiographs, taken at 100 SSD and the same radiographic exposure technique. However, the source-film distance (SFD), thus the OFD, has been increased for radiograph B. Note two things as a result. The image in radiograph B is somewhat larger because of magnification from the increased OFD. Also, note the overall density of radiograph B is decreased because of the inverse square law (the same amount of radiation has been spread out over a larger area).

The image intensifier is a useful tool during fluoroscopy because it converts an x-ray image into a light image. There are several design components that enable it to accomplish this task. Structurally, it is made up of a glass envelope containing an input screen, photocathode, electrostatic lenses, anode, and output screen, as shown in Fig. 19-14. It amplifies the brightness of an image, usually between 500 and 8000 times.[11] The ultimate purpose of an image intensifier is to convert the x-ray image into a video image, which is then viewed on a television monitor. Let us examine that process in more detail.

The primary x-ray beam exiting the patient passes through the table top and strikes the input screen of the image intensifier. A fluorescent screen, which is built into the image intensifier as the input screen, absorbs x-ray photons. It can range in size from 12.5 to 35 cm in diameter.[39] The larger the diameter, the less scanning that is required during fluoroscopy. During fluoroscopy, light photons, emitted by the input screen (much like the photons emitted from an intensifying screen in a radiographic cassette) are then absorbed by the photocathode. Electrostatic lenses, positioned inside the perimeter of the unit, focus and accelerate the converted electrons. As the electrons are focused, they gain more speed as they near the end of their journey through this vacuum tube containing the cathode and anode. The focusing lens helps direct the electrons toward the anode at the opposite end of the image intensifier tube. As the electrons accelerate and focus toward the anode, they increase in their energy and their ability to emit light at the output screen. The output is significantly greater than the input. For example, one 50 keV photon striking the input screen may produce 200,000 light photons at the output screen.[11] Light photons produced at the output screen are then processed electronically through a video system. Located in a small shielded area of the simulator room, the video image appears on a television monitor. The image intensification process simply changes the quantity of photons and electrons, representing the image, at each stage of the process.

During fluoroscopy the x-ray tube current is usually less than 10 mA. This is in contrast to the 100 to 500 mA used for producing radiographs. The kilovoltage (or kVp) used during fluoroscopy depends on the body section examined. Most

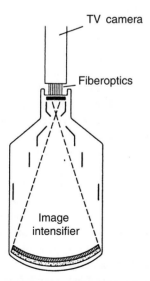

Figure 19-14. Image intensifier. This device is made up of a glass envelope containing an input screen, photocathode, electrostatic lenses, anode, and output screen. *(From Bushong S: Radiologic science for technologists: physics, biology and protection, ed 5, St. Louis, 1993, Mosby.)*

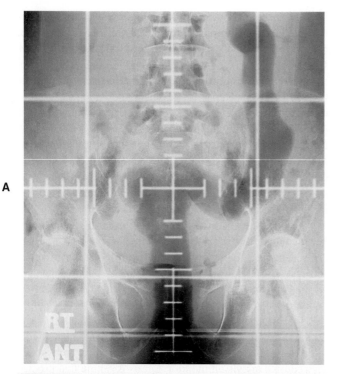

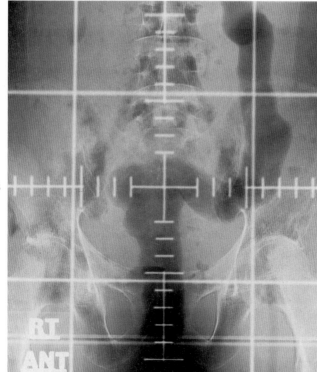

Figure 19-15. Effect of increasing object-film distance (OFD). These two radiographs A and B were taken at 100 source-skin distance (SSD) and with the same radiographic exposure technique. The source-film distance (SFD), thus the OFD, has been increased for radiograph B from 140 to 155 cm SSD. Note two things as a result. The image in radiograph B is considerably larger because of magnification from the increased OFD. Also note the overall density of radiograph B is decreased as a result of the inverse square law (the same amount of radiation has been spread out over a larger area).

image intensifiers have an automatic brightness system maintained by varying the kilovoltage (kVp) or milliamperes (mA) automatically during fluoroscopy. Such features may be referred to by different names, such as automatic brightness control (ABC), automatic brightness stabilization (ABS), automatic exposure control (AEC), or automatic gain control (AGC).[10]

Storage of a still fluoroscopic image is possible with some systems. This allows the members of the treatment planning team to study and evaluate an image without continuous exposure to the patient. Some systems also allow the electronic image, available for video display, to be digitized through computer enhancement and stored for later use. Digitized images may then be available for treatment planning purposes involving dosimetric calculation. They may also be available at the treatment unit for verification and comparison to portal images created on the therapy machine. The storage and retrieval of electronic images may open the door to even more efficient and accurate treatment of the patient in the future.

The image intensifying system must have a collision avoidance system. This may take the form of a mechanical touchbar/microswitch system, which will prevent the image intensifier from colliding with the patient or treatment couch.[25] A combination of electronic position sensors and some type of computer logic may accomplish the same objective. A computer, integrated with the simulator, can prevent the collision of gantry or image intensifier with the floor or treatment couch by plotting and constantly evaluating the position of each component. Some simulators also come equipped with audio alarms as part of their collision avoidance system.

Patient table top.   The device in which a patient is positioned during treatment or simulation may be called a treatment couch or patient **table top** (Fig. 19-1). It is essential that the patient table top on the simulator provide support identical to that of the patient table top on the treatment unit to maintain reproducibility. Many table tops support up to 182 kg (400 lb) and range in width from 45 to 50 cm. If the couch width in the simulator is not similar to that of the treatment unit, then reproducibility may become a problem, especially with larger patients.

It is desirable for the table top to be a hard flat surface that minimally attenuates the x-ray beam. Part of the table should enable the therapist to view the patient through the table top when the beam is directed up vertically through the table. This is important in recording posterior and posterior oblique SSDs. Some simulators provide a table top with a segment that can be removed and a section of more supportive transparent material substituted in its place. This may be a square or rectangular section of plastic or a frame with strings, similar to a tennis or racquetball racquet woven tightly together (Fig. 19-16). After extended use this tennis racquet section should be restrung to provide more patient support and reduce the amount of sag during simulation. The tennis racquet insert, if used on the simulator, may more accurately represent the potential for sag during actual treatment conditions, when a similar insert can be used. This process may reduce the number of discrepancies between simulation and treatment. Table top manufacturers have developed some models that are hard, flat, and radiolucent and come without metal supports. These table tops are mostly constructed out of a carbon fiber material.

What is carbon fiber material? The material used for radiologic purposes, such as table tops and cassettes, is made by binding a fabric of pure carbon fiber with a resin. The result is a material that is extremely supportive with a low density and low x-ray absorption. It also has a high **tensile strength** (resistance in lengthwise stress, measured in weight per unit area). Carbon fiber is used in table tops as the outside support around a plastic foam center.[19]

There are several unique features of the simulator couch, which allows the table top its mobility. A standard feature allows the table top to mechanically move in a horizontal and lengthwise direction. It must do this smoothly and accurately with a patient in the treatment position. This permits the precise and exact positioning of the isocenter during simulation. Some table tops may provide the opportunity through rotation of the couch for patient positioning in two additional directions. One direction allows the table top to be rotated horizontally (laterally) 90° in either direction. For example, if the table top were the big hand of a watch at the 6 o'clock position, it could be rotated to either the 3 or the 9 o'clock position, while maintaining the same isocenter. This type of positioning limits gantry rotation to about 30 degrees from vertical because of the possible collision of the image intensifier with the couch. The amount of gantry rotation depends on the thickness of the patient and the level of the isocenter. A second motion on some models also allows the couch to extract the patient from the C-shaped opening in the gantry by rotating the patient on another axis. This other axis is located several meters from the isocenter within the couch. Experimenting with the various motions of the couch will demonstrate its versatility and range of motion.

In addition, a set of local controls may be located on the couch. These can mimic those of the treatment units as a **pendant** (handheld control) suspended from the ceiling or attached to the treatment couch through a telephone-like cord. In some models the control panel can also be located on one side of the couch. In either case, these controls should allow access to the mechanical movements and optical features of the simulator.

Simulator controls. Control of simulator movements should be possible through local control within the simulator room and through remote control, usually located behind a separately shielded area. Local and remote control of the mechanical simulator functions should provide for all motor-driven motions, specifically, the field-defining wires, beam-restricting diaphragms, collimator rotation, radial movement of the gantry head, and linear and rotation movements of the couch. Scanning and radial movements of the image intensifier should also be located within the simulator room. Activation of the optical features of the simulator, such as the field light, ODI, positional lasers, and room lights, should be available along with several emergency off switches, positioned strategically throughout the simulator room.

Remote controls, located in the shielded control room, should duplicate those within the simulator room. This includes all of the optical features and motor-driven movements of the simulator along with digital indicators for field size, SAD, SSD, gantry, and collimator angle. Familiarity with all of the simulator's features will allow for efficient and accurate treatment planning. This can become more critical, especially when simulating certain palliative cases in which the patient is experiencing severe pain.

Control area. Within the shielded control area, several components are strategically positioned (Fig. 19-17). This includes the x-ray generator (along with a circuit breaker for the incoming voltage), a television monitor, the remote control panel, and an observation window. It is important that this

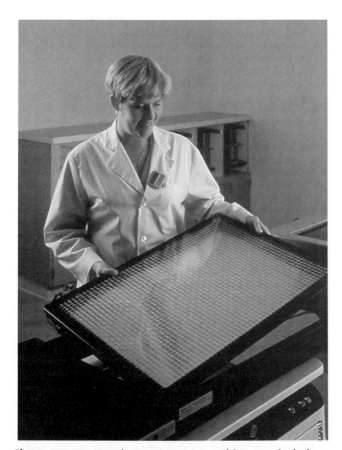

Figure 19-16. Couch top accessory. This may include a square or rectangular frame with strings, similar to a tennis or racquetball racquet, woven tightly together. After extended use, the tennis racquet section should be restrung to provide more patient support and reduce the amount of sag during simulation. *(Courtesy Varian Medical Systems.)*

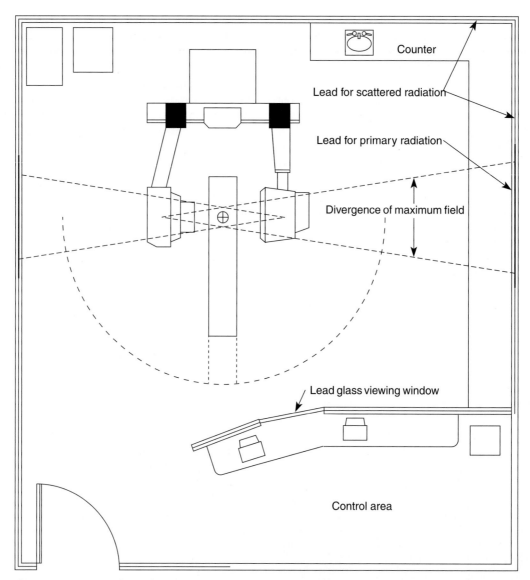

Figure 19-17. Typical simulator room design. Note the location of the simulator in relationship to the primary barriers and control area with lead glass window.

room be large enough to hold several members of the radiation therapy team, students, and other interested observers.

An observation window, installed along the wall facing the simulator, allows the radiation therapist and others involved in the simulation process to view the patient and the mechanical motions of the equipment. Whether the window is made of thick plate glass or lead glass depends on the distance it is located from the simulator and/or whether it is inclined to be irradiated by the primary beam. A 0.7 × 1.5 m (2.3 × 5 ft) size is recommended.[7] Usually, larger sizes can adapt to additional staff and students without overcrowding. The control panel should be located close enough to the observation window so the radiation therapist can observe the patient while the simulator is moving.

In addition, a video monitor positioned near the control

panel provides ready access to the fluoroscopic image during the simulation process. A dimmer switch, which can control the lighting level in the simulator and control area, is also necessary. Monitoring a fluoroscopic video image without the distraction of overhead lighting is more efficient. It might be compared with watching television in a dark room (sometimes while watching television, the image may appear sharper and more detailed when the room lighting is kept low or turned off). X-ray view boxes mounted in the control room are helpful in comparing radiographs or scans during the simulation process. In addition, other video monitors may be used for patient data storage and retrieval.

The x-ray generator is another important component, which provides radiographic and fluoroscopic control of the simulator. Exposure reproducibility, which should be maintained within 5%, is an important consideration for guaranteeing radiographic image quality.[40] The *British Journal of Radiology* Supplement 23[7] recommends that the tube and generator ratings be 8 to 10 times greater than for general diagnostic radiography. In part, this may be because of the increased distance used in radiation therapy simulation (70 cm in diagnostic imaging to between 130 and 200 cm on the simulator). A three-phase generator is recommended. It should be capable of radiographic outputs of up to 500 mA at 90 kVp, 300 mA at 150 kVp, and 6 mA at 125 kVp for fluoroscopy.[7] A single-phase generator may limit the higher exposure factors needed for some examinations, especially a large lateral pelvis—a most challenging body part to image effectively.

Kilovoltage and milliamperage exposure factors are controlled by the radiation therapist at the operating console. By adjusting the voltage and current of the x-ray generator, exposure factors can be selected. It may appear intimidating to the novice at first, with its many buttons and control knobs, although some systems are equipped with anatomically programmed radiography (APR). Bushong[10] describes the process from a diagnostic radiography perspective: "Rather than have the radiologic technologist select a desired kVp and mAs, graphics on the control panel guide the technologist. To produce an image the technologist simply touches a picture or a written description of the anatomy to be imaged and another indication of body habitus. The microprocessor selects the appropriate kVp and mAs automatically. The whole process is phototimed, resulting in near-flawless radiographs. . . ."

In more conventional radiation therapy settings, the therapist must select the appropriate kilovoltage, milliamperage, and time manually. Most x-ray control panels provide a range of steps (buttons) for the selection of each of the radiographic controlling factors. Technique charts, with suggested exposure factors, are required by some state and local laws. Additional features located on the x-ray control panel include the exposure switch, a possible digital heat unit display, and fluoroscopic specifications. Fluoroscopic specifications may include zoom modes, ABC, and a mandatory 5-minute timer. The timer is a carryover from diagnostic radiology. It is set at the start of each fluoroscopic procedure and attempts to limit patient exposure (when an audible alarm sounds at the end of 5 minutes) during lengthy fluoroscopy procedures.

It is easy to see why the control room should be large enough to accommodate several members of the radiation therapy team along with students and other interested observers. Field size, gantry angle, exposure technique, and several other important parameters can be manipulated from within the shielded walls of the control room. If the components within the control room are well positioned and accessible, the entire simulation process is more efficient. Detail to room design is a wise investment that will provide many dividends, especially during peak times of the simulator's use.

ROOM DESIGN

The design of a simulator room is a process that must involve the expertise of numerous professionals, including an architect, an engineer, and a radiologic physicist. Input should also be encouraged from the therapists and the radiation oncologists in the department. Before designing the room, the site must be chosen. The ideal location is close to the treatment machines. This facilitates communication among all parties involved in the patient's treatment.

Space Allocations

The simulator room should be of sufficient size to accommodate not only the machine and all of its components but also its full range of motions. The equipment will have a longer life if enough space is provided to avoid collisions, such as bumping into walls and countertops with the table. It will also be a more pleasant work area if personnel have enough room to comfortably perform their duties. It is recommended that a minimum size be approximately 400 sq ft.[7]

Space must also be allocated for a good-sized counter that should include a sink and a work space and writing area. The work space should be of sufficient size to allow for the manufacture of various immobilization devices used in radiation therapy. Cabinets and drawer space for the storage of simulation equipment, contour-taking devices, and spare simulator parts are necessary in any simulator room. In addition, storage space should be available for routine immobilization devices and other related equipment such as a breast board and especially a hot water tank used in the construction of thermoplastic immobilization devices.

The control area is normally set in one corner of the room, usually near the entrance. This area is designed to protect the operators from radiation and to house the simulator's controls and x-ray generator. It must be large enough for several pieces of equipment, which might include a record and verify system, work area, and numerous personnel. It is important that the operator have full visual and aural contact with the patient at all times. A lead glass window may be installed for patient visualization. Fig. 19-17 illustrates a typical simulator room design.

If space allows, a film processing area should be included in the area. This could be in the form of an adjacent darkroom or a daylight film system. The daylight system eliminates the need for additional walls.

Other Considerations

There are several other considerations worth mentioning concerning the simulator. Simulator manufacturers have very specific requirements for ventilation of the room. They reserve the right to negate the warranty if these requirements are not met. The lighting system is also important. The intensity must be adjustable, with independent control of the room and the control area. Visualization of the light field is easier in low light, as is the fluoroscopy image. On the other hand, certain simulation duties need maximum light, such as recording pertinent information, preparing contrast materials, or designing an immobilization device. Task lighting in certain areas, as under cabinets, is very beneficial.

Positioning lasers, which project a small red or green beam of light toward the patient during the simulation process, must be installed. There are several types available, and the department personnel must choose the style they believe best suits their needs. Side lasers are more stable if they are recessed in the wall to prevent inadvertent collisions. A third overhead laser is installed and represents the anterior central axis or midsagittal plane when the gantry is rotated from its vertical position. These lasers provide the therapist several external reference points in relationship to the position of the isocenter. Daily checks, which provide strict quality control of the positional lasers, are a must.

Shielding Requirements

As with all radiation equipment, room shielding is an important consideration. Shielding radiation rooms is done most commonly with lead or concrete or a combination of the two. Lead is the denser of the two, and less is needed to stop an equal amount of radiation. Lead is also more expensive than concrete and very difficult to support structurally. This is the reason one finds many diagnostic and radiation therapy departments in the basements of hospitals. Shielding costs are reduced significantly by the surrounding earth, and precious space is gained when thick concrete walls need not be built.

All walls may not have the same amount of shielding. Primary walls are those that the radiation will aim at directly and therefore need more shielding than secondary walls, which have only scattered radiation impinging on them.

Several factors are taken into consideration in determining the required wall thickness. The time the machine is normally aimed at a wall or ceiling is called the use factor (U). A standard use factor for a simulator's primary walls and ceilings is $1/4$. Floors are usually 1 because more exposures are made with the simulator in the vertical position. An occupancy factor (T) takes into consideration how an area on the other side of an irradiated wall is going to be used. An office where someone could be sitting for 40 hours a week would require more shielding in the wall than a storage closet where workers would spend 10 minutes once or twice a week.

Another important factor is workload. Workload (W) for a simulator is defined as the current (mA) times the time (min) a department expects to run the machine in a normal week. These estimates are always on the high side to calculate the largest possible scenario. A value in units of mA-mins is used to describe workloads of diagnostic machines.

The weekly permissible dose (P) is 10 times higher (under normal conditions) for people who have chosen a career in the radiation field (radiation workers) compared with members of the general public. The most recent recommendations are 1 mSv/week for the occupationally exposed and 0.02 mSv/week for the general public.[33] Controlled areas are made off-limits to members of the general public for this reason. Uncontrolled areas (areas where access is not limited) will have a lower P value and therefore need more shielding.

The calculation of barrier thickness is much more complicated than is shown here, but the following formula is the basis of most shielding calculations:

$$B = P(d)^2/WUT$$

The distance (in meters) from the source to the opposite side of the barrier is symbolized by *d*. The transmission of radiation through the barrier required to meet the weekly permissible dose is shown as B. This value is then used as a reference (to a graph or chart) to determine the barrier thickness relative to the maximum photon energy and the type of shielding that will be used. See Fig. 19-18 for a sample graph using 125-kVp x-rays.

Many of the factors used in consideration of the simulator room design, such as space allocations, equipment motions, and shielding design, provide for more efficient use of this essential piece of equipment. Because the time invested during the simulation process can seriously affect the outcome of a patient's treatment plan, a thorough knowledge of the simulator, its use, and its limitations is necessary if the simulator's maximum potential is to be reached.

Simulators with CT Mode

When referring to CT simulation, two types of machines may actually produce CT images; one may be an actual CT scanner adapted for simulation and the other a conventional **simulator with a CT mode.** They both can provide an external contour of the patient and additional information on the location, size, and thickness of internal structures. This advanced method of simulation, using CT images, has replaced conventional simulation in some instances and will continue to grow in popularity. CT provides the most useful information for treatment planning purposes because the scans can produce a three-dimensional representation of the patient and external structures.[27] In the following section, both simulators with a CT mode and CT simulators are discussed.

Simulators with a CT mode incorporate the conventional benefits of a simulator with the added benefits of cross-sectional information obtained during the simulation process. In contrast, conventional simulators provide information from **orthogonal** projections (two radiographs taken at right angles). To produce a reconstructed image similar to a conventional CT image, the imaging device (x-ray tube and receptor) on the simulator must record information while the gantry rotates.[8] This recorded information consists of transmitted beam intensities that correspond to tissue densities (Fig. 19-19).

The cost, compared with purchasing a conventional CT scanner for this purpose, is an advantage with this type of simulator. Disadvantages include poor image quality compared with that of a conventional CT scanner, increased amount of time to simulate a patient, and the limitation that

Transmission 125 kVp

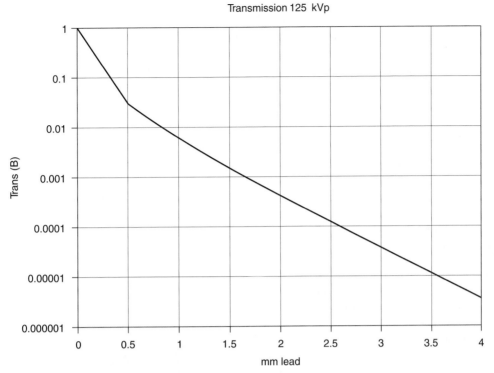

Figure 19-18. Barrier thickness. This graph shows the thickness of lead (in mm) needed for 125-kVp x-rays using a transmission factor (B) in the workload formula.

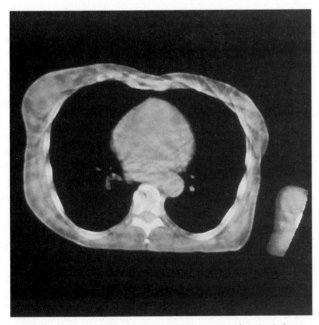

Figure 19-19. Planning computed tomography (CT) image. This CT image of the thorax, generated by a simulator, is used for treatment planning purposes. *(Courtesy Varian Medical Systems.)*

the x-ray tube can only tolerate a specific amount of heat (each scan generates more heat units than a conventional x-ray, so delays may be encountered waiting for the tube to cool down). The differences in image quality between a conventional CT scanner and a simulator with a CT mode are very noticeable. However, the geometry produced with a simulator using a CT mode is not restricted by the conventional CT aperture opening (the opening through which the patient passes through the scanner) and is more representative of the treatment unit geometry.

CT Simulator

CT and magnetic resonance imaging (MRI) scans provide the most useful data for treatment planning purposes. As was mentioned, if the conventional simulator is equipped with a CT mode, scans can be performed before, during, or after the simulation process using the same equipment. In addition, treatment planning CT scans can be performed on a dedicated scanner in the radiation oncology department or scheduled on a CT scanner in the radiology department shortly after the initial conventional simulation, always with the patient in the treatment position.

With CT simulation, a **virtual simulation** workstation

(Fig. 19-2) equipped with a CT scanner, software to perform target volume definition/treatment planning dose calculation, and the production of DRRs can be used in the simulation process. CT hardware configuration, the controls associated with the virtual simulator workstation, and patient marking system are part of the CT simulator.

Gantry

The gantry of a CT scanner is essentially the circular "doughnut" in which the patient is inserted during the scan (Fig. 19-20). On the periphery of the doughnut there may be as many as 2400 scintillation or gas-filled detectors, designed to receive and measure the attenuated beam from a rotating x-ray tube. Scintillation detectors contain crystal photodiode assemblies. The crystal of choice is cadmium tungstate ($CdWO_4$). Spacing of the detectors varies depending on the design; however, generally 1 to 8 detectors/cm or 1 to 5 detectors/degree are available. Ninety percent of the incident x-ray is absorbed and contributes to the output. Because of the spacing of the detectors the net output is near 50%. Gas detectors are constructed of large metallic chamber with baffles spaced at 1-mm intervals. The baffles are like grid strips, which divide the large chamber into many small chambers. The small chamber functions as a detector, in which the detector array is sealed and filled under pressure with a high atomic number material such as xenon. This type of detector is about 45% efficient.[10]

During an axial scan, the patient is positioned at a fixed point and the x-ray tube rotates 360 degrees around the patient (translation). With spiral CT, the patient is positioned at a fixed point, and, while the x-ray tube is rotating, the patient moves into the aperture to create a scan pattern that resembles a "slinky" or coiled spring (Fig. 19-21). Aperture size (the diameter of the hole the patient is positioned into) is an important factor in radiation oncology. Ideally the aperture would be 80 cm or greater to accommodate a variety of patient setups, especially breast simulations and wide body sections such as the pelvis.[15,27] However, as aperture size increases, so does the number of detectors, the patient dose, and time to scan the patient. The exact treatment position may not always be produced on a scanner with a small aperture that is found on some units.[15]

Spiral CT

Spiral CT places larger demands on the x-ray tube than conventional CT. Conventional CT is energized for one rotation

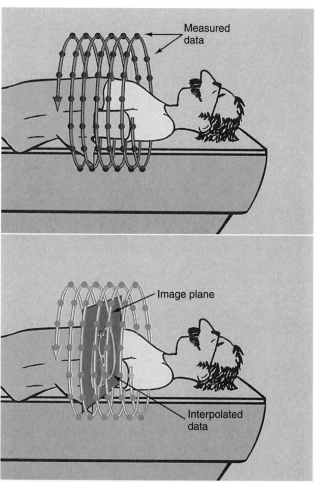

Figure 19-21. A, During spiral computed tomography (CT), image data are continuously sampled. **B,** Interpolation of data is performed to reconstruct the image in any transverse plane. *(Used by permission from Bushong SC: Radiologic science for technologists: physics, biology, and protection, ed 7, St. Louis, 2001, Mosby.)*

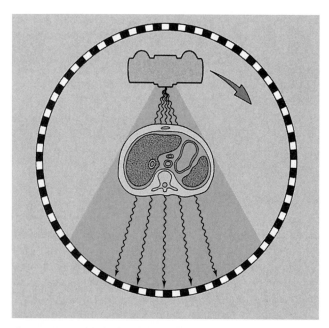

Figure 19-20. Computed tomography (CT) scanners operate with a rotating x-ray source and stationary detectors. *(Used by permission from Bushong SC: Radiologic science for technologists: physics, biology, and protection, ed 7, St. Louis, 2001, Mosby.)*

(translation) for approximately 1 second every 6 to 10 seconds. This time allows the tube to cool. The spiral CT tube has a high thermal demand. It is continuously energized up to 30 seconds. High power levels must be sustained. Thus x-ray tubes must be larger and have a high heat capacity and high cooling rates. Spiral CT uses solid-state detectors, which are approximately 80% efficient. Efficient detectors reduce patient dose, improves image quality, and allows for faster scan times.[27] There are advantages and disadvantages to using spiral CT. Patients can be scanned in a shorter amount of time, which results in reduced motion artifacts. In addition, slices can be obtained in any position at various thicknesses in the scanned volume.[27] Limitations for the spiral CT include increased processing time, increased axis resolution, and increased image noise (unwanted artifacts that appear on the monitor or image).

Patient Treatment Couch

The **couch** (Fig. 19-22) is similar to that of a conventional simulator in that it is capable of translation and made of low Z material such as carbon fiber. If the scanner has a curved couch top, an insert should be purchased to provide a flat surface for scanning patients in the treatment position. Some couches come with predrilled holes along the lateral edge of the couch to provide a suitable locking location to register immobilization devices such as headholders and breast boards. This becomes an important feature with the increased use of three-dimensional conformal therapy and intensity-modulated radiation therapy.

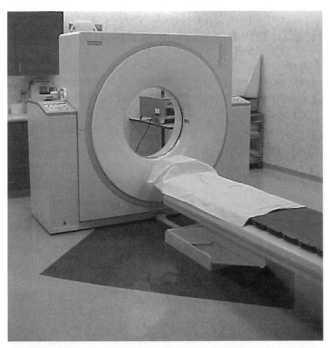

Figure 19-22. Spiral computed tomography (CT) imaging system showing the circular gantry and patient couch.

Computer Control Station

As computer technology increases with faster processors and larger memory, scan time and image reconstruction time is reduced. Depending on the image format, as many as 30,000 equations must be solved simultaneously, requiring a large capacity computer to process the images.[10] Reconstruction time, the time it takes the computer to analyze and process the information received from the detectors and display it on a TV monitor, is an important variable in the application of CT simulation. With the use of special array processors, image reconstruction can be accomplished in less than 1 second.[10] The results are seen at the control station on one or more video monitors and can also be copied on x-ray film as a DRR.

Variable slice thickness and spacing are extremely important criteria in obtaining CT studies beneficial to producing high-quality DRRs. Some scanners provide limited slice thickness settings (e.g., 2 mm or 5 mm) and slice spacing (e.g., 2 mm, 3 mm, or 5 mm) during the actual scan.[27] For optimal image reconstruction in producing a high-quality DRR, slice thickness and slice spacing should be evaluated for each anatomic region. Gerbi[15] recommends thin CT scans with no more than 5 mm spacing to reduce the problem of volume averaging while accurately representing the target in three-dimensional space. To maximize the useful resolution on the DRR when performing CT simulation of the head and neck, Martin[27] recommends acquiring 1-mm slices at 1-mm spacing through the region containing tumor and 3-mm slices at 3-mm spacing through peripheral areas of the treatment volume. Slice thickness and spacing are important in producing useful DRRs and also affect storage and communication components within the computer system. Variable slice thickness and spacing, along with other important variables, are selected at the time of the scan at the control console.

Controls Associated with the Virtual Simulator Workstation

The workstation associated with CT simulation may appear complex and cumbersome with multiple monitors, controls for the CT console, hardware necessary to produce high-quality DRRs, and a virtual simulation workstation to perform target volume definition and dose calculation. Learning to use the equipment properly takes time and patience. Numerous hardware configurations are possible, depending on the type of equipment and needs of the department. Fig. 19-2 demonstrates the physical layout and possible hardware configuration of a virtual simulation room.

Two main components of a CT simulator workstation are a target localization routine that allows the target to be defined and transfers the appropriate marks to the patient skin surface and a virtual simulation package that generates DRRs, which are used to evaluate and simulate the case.[15] The DRRs become the "master" to compare subsequent portal images to during the treatment verification process (Fig. 19-23).

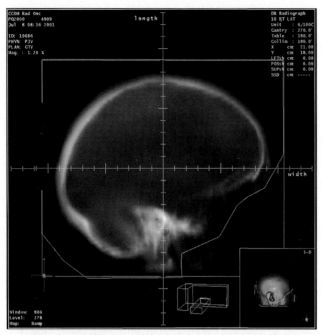

Figure 19-23. This is an example of a digitally reconstructed radiograph (DRR) taken with the virtual simulation workstation and used in place of a conventional simulation film.

Located within a properly shielded environment and with viewing access to the patient, the CT console allow for the selection of radiographic technical factors (such as kVp, mA, and scan time); mechanical movements of the gantry and couch; and computer commands for manipulating, reconstructing, and storage of the CT slices. The operator's console usually has two monitors. One to indicate patient data and provide information for each scan (number and thickness of slices, radiographic technique, and couch position) and the other to view and manipulate the reconstructed images before storing or transfer to external devices, such as a virtual simulation workstation.

The virtual simulation workstation is essentially a computer and monitor with huge amounts of storage capacity, memory, and processing capability. With conventional simulation, the field locations are determined first, the target is defined, and then the fields are shaped to treat the target. In virtual simulation, the target is defined first, and then the fields are shaped to conform to the target.[15] To accomplish this goal, the virtual simulation workstation needs access to vast amount of data, which may include the following[27]:

- CT study
- DRRs
- Field parameters
- Patient information
- Treatment plan information
- Estimated dose grids

If the virtual simulation workstation is used to perform tar-

get volume definition, virtual simulation, DRR production, and treatment planning, a single station may easily become overused. Additional virtual simulation stations should be considered in the design of a CT simulation system.[27] Just as a busy retail store may need numerous computer terminals to adequately process customer purchases, additional virtual simulation workstations may help streamline treatment planning in a busy radiation therapy department.

Patient Marking System

Either isocenter or field edge marking systems are available for CT simulation. In conventional simulation, side lasers and an overhead laser are used to triangulate three reference points on the patient. After the target is defined and the fields are shaped to treat the target, the patient's isocenter is tattooed or otherwise marked. With CT simulation, the patient is temporarily marked with reference points before scanning. After the target volume has been determined, the computer calculates the isocenter, with reference to the temporary marks and the lasers and/or couch adjusted automatically. Movable lasers can be used for all three reference points. Field edge marking systems are available with some CT scanners used to control the position of lasers that identify on the patient's skin the superior, inferior, and lateral field borders and/or isocenter.[37]

SUMMARY

The use of the simulator is important in achieving maximum use of the treatment planning process in radiation therapy. To adequately deliver a precise dose to the tumor volume and at the same time spare as much normal tissue as possible requires the use of a simulator, with few exceptions. It is important to determine appropriate fields and adequate shielding for each case in which a prescribed dose of radiation therapy is delivered.

Several equipment options exist to simulate a planned course of radiation therapy. Conventional simulators, simulators with a CT mode, and CT simulators should be considered based on departments needs, such as types of treatment (radical or palliative) and number of patients and fields treated each day, with special consideration given to the type and complexity of treatment (conventional, three-dimensional conformal, or intensity modulated radiation therapy [IMRT]).

With the evolution of the simulator design from more conventional simulators using radiography and fluoroscopy to applications of CT simulation and DRRs, there has been a shift in responsibility and effort from the simulator equipment to the dosimetry computer. Simulation times on a conventional simulator are often longer than the CT counterpart! The educational community is in a state of flux as to how CT simulation education must evolve as therapists are physically required to do less in the planning progress and more dosimetry work. The role of the CT simulator will probably expand as the demand for conventional simulation decreases. However, it must be remembered that not all cases requiring radiation therapy are suitable for CT simulation. The conventional simulator may actually be more suitable in some cases.

Review Questions

1. The device that projects a scale onto the patient's skin, corresponding to the SSD, is called a(n)
   a. Couch
   b. Gantry
   c. ODI
   d. Collimator assembly
2. To control scatter radiation during fluoroscopy, the _____ should be adjusted.
   a. Isocenter
   b. PSA
   c. Field-defining wires
   d. Beam-restricting diaphragms
3. All of the following are optical devices used during the conventional simulation process except
   a. Patient table top
   b. ODI
   c. Light field
   d. Lasers
4. The accessory holder on the simulator may serve which of the following purposes?
   I. Function as an electron cone adapter
   II. Simulate custom block verification
   III. Absorb scatter radiation from thicker body parts
   IV. Provide scanning movements for the imaging system
   a. I and II only
   b. I and III only
   c. II and IV only
   d. I, II, III, and IV
5. Which of the following factors are NOT taken into consideration when determining shielding requirements for a simulator?
   a. Use factor (U)
   b. Occupancy factor (T)
   c. Workload (W)
   d. Inverse scattering intensity (I)
6. Which of the following involve three-dimensional treatment planning?
   I. Virtual simulation
   II. AP images
   III. CT simulators
   IV. Portal images
   a. I and II only
   b. I and III only
   c. II and III only
   d. II and IV only

7. Computed tomography and MRI scans provide the most useful information for treatment planning purposes because
   a. They are most cost-effective method
   b. They are least cost-effective method
   c. The scans can produce a three-dimensional representation of the patient and external structures
   d. The image are essential in comparing to port film taken during treatment
8. Which of the following is NOT considered a drawback to CT simulation?
   a. The size of the aperture may be too small to accommodate all treatment positions
   b. The verification and use of certain beam-shaping devices and treatment accessories is limited
   c. Simulation of mechanical clearance of the treatment machine is normally NOT a problem on the CT simulator
   d. The digitally reconstructed radiographs (DRR), which are used as "masters" to compare with the portal images, are of poor quality compared with conventional simulation radiographs
9. Which of the following steps in the radiation therapy process immediately proceeds the actual treatment of a patient?
   a. Simulation and treatment planning
   b. Diagnosis
   c. Consultation
   d. Biopsy of the tumor
10. The major difference between a conventional simulator and a CT simulator is
    a. The image intensifier
    b. The collection of anatomic patient data
    c. The room shielding requirements
    d. The production of scatter radiation

Questions to Ponder

1. Discuss the importance of tumor localization.
2. Describe, as though you were educating an interested patient, the purpose of the isocenter.
3. Explain the purpose of each of the components within the head of the gantry.
4. How do the couch and the additional movements of the simulator provide an accurate representation of the treatment plan?
5. Discuss the process of tumor localization and treatment planning using CT simulation.
6. What are the advantages and disadvantages of CT simulation versus conventional simulation?

REFERENCES

1. American College of Radiology: *ACR standards for radiation oncology,* Reston, Va, 1999, American College of Radiology, pp 1-6.
2. Bentel CG: *Radiation therapy planning,* New York, 1993, McGraw-Hill.

3. Bleehen NM, Glastein E, Haybittle JL, editors: *Radiation therapy planning,* New York, 1983, Marcel Dekker.

4. Bomford CK: Do simulators simulate? *Br J Rad* 43:583, 1970.

5. Bomford CK, Craig LM, Hanna FA et al: Treatment simulators, special report No 10, *Br J Rad* (special report no 10), 1976.

6. Bomford CK, Craig LM, Hanna FA et al: Treatment simulators, *Br J Rad* (suppl 16), 1981.

7. Bomford CK, Dawes PJDK, Lillicrap SC et al: Treatment simulators, *Br J Rad* (suppl 23), 1989.

8. Boring CC, Squires TS, Tong T et al: Cancer statistics, 1994, *Cancer J Clin* 44:7-26, 1994.

9. British Standard Institution: Medical electrical equipment; part 3. Particular requirements for performance, section 3.129. Methods of declaring functional performance characteristics of radiotherapy simulators, Supplement 1. Guide to functional performance values, London, 1994, 1-14.

10. Bushong SC: *Radiologic science for technologists: physics, biology, and protection,* ed 7, St. Louis, 2001, Mosby.

11. Carlton RR, McKenna-Adler A: *Principles of radiographic imaging,* Albany, NY, 2000, Delmar Publishing.

12. Conners SG, Battista JJ, Bertin RJ: On technical specifications of radiotherapy simulators, *Med Phys* 11:341-343, 1984.

13. Day MJ, Harrison RM: Cross-sectional information/treatment simulation. In Bleehen NM, Glatstein E, Haybittle JL, editors: *Radiation therapy planning,* New York, 1983, Marcel Dekker.

14. Dritschilo A, Sherman D, Emami B et al: The cost effectiveness of a radiation therapy simulator: a model for determination of need, *Int J Radiat Oncol Biol Phys* 5:243, 1979.

15. Gerbi B: The simulation process in determination and definition of the treatment volume and treatment planning. In Levitt SH, Khan FM, Potish RA et al, editors: *Technological basis of radiation therapy,* ed 3, Philadelphia, 1999, Lippincott Williams & Wilkins.

16. Glasgow GP, Purdy JA: External beam dosimetry and treatment planning. In DeVita Jr VT, Hellman SE, Rosenberg SA, editors: *Cancer: principles and practice of oncology,* Philadelphia, 1985, JB Lippincott.

17. Farmer ET, Fowler JF, Haggith JW: Megavoltage treatment planning and the use of xeroradiography, *Br J Rad* 36:426-435, 1963.

18. Hendrickson FR, Ovadia J: Radiation treatment simulators, *Radiology* 100:701, 1971.

19. Hufton AP, Crosthwaite CM, Davies JM et al: Low attenuation material for table tops, cassettes, and grids: a review, *Radiography* 53:17-18, 1987.

20. Hunt M: Localization and field design using a CT simulator. In Purdy JA, Starkschallg G, editors: *3D planning and conformal radiation therapy,* Madison, Wisc, 1999, Advanced Medical Publishers.

21. International Electrotechnical Commission: *CEI/IEC 976 medical electron accelerators in the range 1-50 MeV—functional performance characteristics,* Geneva, 1989.

22. Jung B, Larsson B, Rosengren B et al: Roentgen stand for field positioning in high-energy radiotherapy, *Acta Radiol* 7:282, 1968.

23. Karzmark CJ: Radiotherapy simulators—a case for special v. general purpose designs, *Br J Rad* 44:558, 1971.

24. Karzmark CJ, Nunan CS, Tanabe E: *Medical linear accelerators,* Princeton, NJ, 1993, McGraw-Hill.

25. Karzmark CJ, Rust DC: Radiotherapy treatment simulators and automation, *Radiology* 105:157, 1972.

26. Kereiakes JG, Elson HR, Born CG, editors: *Radiation oncology physics—1986,* New York, 1987, American Institute of Physics.

27. Martin EE: CT simulation hardware. In Purdy JA, Starkschallg G, editors: *3D planning and conformal radiation therapy,* Madison, Wisc, 1999, Advanced Medical Publishers.

28. McCullough E: Radiotherapy treatment simulators. In Purdy JA, editor: *Advances in radiation oncology, physics, dosimetry, treatment planning, and brachytherapy,* New York, 1992, American Institute of Physics.

29. McCullough EC, Earle JD: The selection, acceptance, testing, and quality control of radiotherapy treatment simulators, *Radiology* 131:226, 1979.

30. Meetens H, Bijhold J, Strachee J: A method for the measurement of field placement errors in digital portal images, *Phys Med Biol* 35:299, 1990.

31. Mizer S, Scheller RR, Deye JA: *Radiation therapy simulation workbook,* New York, 1986, Pergammon Press.

32. Myles J: Personal communication, Varian Oncology Systems, March, 1994.

33. National Council of Radiation Protection and Measurements: NCRP Report #16: limitation of exposure to ionizing radiation, Bethesda, Md, 1993, NCRP.

34. Owen J, Coia L, Hanks G: Recent patterns of growth in radiation therapy facilities. Poster presentation at the meeting of the American Society of Therapeutic Radiology and Oncology, Washington, DC, November, 1991.

35. Parker RG, Bogardus CR, Hanks GE et al: *Radiation oncology in integrated cancer management,* Philadelphia, 1991, American College of Radiology.

36. Smith L, Picker International, Inc.: Personal communication, April, 1995.

37. Ragan DP, He T, Mesina CF et al: CT-based simulation with laser patient marking, *Med Phys* 20:379-380. 1993.

38. Stanton R, Stinson D, Shahabi S: *An introduction to radiation oncology physics,* Madison, Wisc, 1992, Medical Physics Publishing.

39. Taylor J: *Imaging in radiotherapy,* Kent, England, 1988, Croom Helm.

40. Van Dyk J, Mah K: Simulation and imaging for radiation therapy planning. In Williams JR, Thaites DI, editors: *Radiotherapy physics in practice,* Oxford, 2000, Oxford University Press.

20

Simulation Procedures

Dennis Leaver, Rosann Keller, Nora Uricchio,
Charles M. Washington

Outline

Key Terms

Patients treated with radiation therapy, either for cure or for palliation, will be involved in numerous procedures ranging from diagnosis to ongoing patient follow-up. Fig. 20-1 lists the various steps that a patient may experience as part of the entire process of external beam radiation therapy. The actual delivery of a prescribed dose of radiation, although important, is a small part of the whole process. Before therapy can begin, a simulation procedure is necessary. The ultimate success of treatment is directly related to the effectiveness of the simulation procedure. This procedure helps in determining the location and extent of disease relative to adjacent critical normal tissues.[5,34] Each step in the radiation therapy process may not be needed for every patient nor will the steps occur in sequence. The process varies for each patient, depending on the patient's condition and the type and extent of disease.

DIAGNOSIS
- tumour pathobiology
- staging

THERAPEUTIC DECISIONS
- cure/palliation
- treatment modalities

TARGET VOLUME LOCALIZATION
- tumour/nor mal tissue definition
- patient measurements
- field shaping

TREATMENT PLANNING
- selection of technique
- computation of dose distribution
- optimization

SIMULATION
- treatment
- confirmation of measurements
- confirmation of shields

FABRICATION OF TREATMENT AIDS
- blocks/shields
- compensators/bolus
- immobilization devices

TREATMENT
- verification of set-up
- verification of equipment performance
- dosimetry checks
- record keeping

PATIENT EVALUATION DURING TREATMENT
- treatment tolerance
- tumour response

PATIENT FOLLOW-UP
- tumour control
- normal tissue response

Figure 20-1. The various steps involved in the process of external beam radiation therapy. *(From Van Dyk J, Mah K: Simulators and CT scanners. In Williams JR, Thwaites DI, editors: Radiotherapy physics in practice, Oxford, 2000, Oxford University Press.)*

Table 20-1	Key staff functions in the radiation therapy process	
Function	**Team member(s)**
Diagnosis	Pathologist
	Referring physician
	Radiation oncologist
Therapeutic decisions	Radiation oncologist
	Referring physician
Target volume localization	Radiation oncologist
	Radiation therapist
	Dosimetrist
	Physicist
Treatment planning	Radiation oncologist
	Physicist
	Dosimetrist
Simulation	Radiation therapist
	Radiation oncologist
	Dosimetrist
	Physicist
Fabrication of treatment aids	Dosimetrist
	Radiation therapist
	Mold room technologist
Treatment	Radiation therapist
	Physicist
	Dosimetrist
	Radiation oncologist
Patient evaluation during treatment	Radiation oncologist
	Radiation therapist
	Oncology nurse
Patient follow-up	Radiation oncologist
	Oncology nurse
	Radiation therapist

The simulation process involves the participation of several team members, each with a variety of unique skills. Both simulation and treatment require a solid foundation in the theory and application of radiation oncology techniques. In addition, patient care skills are necessary. It is the team approach, involving each member, that can provide effective planning as well as localization and documentation of the patient's disease in relationship to normal tissue structures. Table 20-1 identifies key staff functions in the radiation therapy process.

A simulator can take various forms, ranging from a simple diagnostic radiographic unit attached to a treatment machine to a complicated isocentric unit with fluoroscopy and/or computed tomography (CT) capabilities. In each case the outcome should define the anatomic area so that it is reproducible for daily treatment. An elaborate and complicated simulation is of no value unless it is reproducible on the treatment unit.

In this chapter the complexities of simulation and target volume localization are discussed. This includes some nomenclature (definitions) and the importance of patient assessment and education before the simulation procedure. A description of tumor and normal tissue localization methods and an outline of the steps involved in the simulation procedure and treatment verification process are also included. In addition, a practical application section is presented to help provide an appreciation of the importance of the simulation process.

NOMENCLATURE

Before a discussion of exactly what simulation is, a review of several key definitions and acronyms, designed to provide a foundation in simulation procedures, will be helpful.

Simulation (which may be a one- or a two-step process)

is carried out by the radiation therapist under the supervision of the radiation oncologist. It is the precise mockup of a patient treatment with radiographic documentation of the treatment portals.[14] The term simulation may take on different meanings, depending on the institution and the individual. First, it is a general term describing the mockup process, which can also include the selection of immobilization devices, radiographic documentation of treatment ports, measurement of the patient, construction of patient contours, and shaping of fields.[14] Second, it may be a more specific term in which the simulator artificially duplicates the actual treatment conditions (verification) by confirming measurements, verifying treatment, and confirming shields.[34] Third, it may involve a virtual simulation workstation, equipped with a CT scanner, software to perform target volume definition and treatment planning dose calculation, and the production of digitally reconstructed radiograph (DRRs).

Localization means geometrical definition of the position and extent of the tumor or anatomic structures by reference of surface marks that can be used for treatment setup purposes.[4] The radiation oncologist and radiation therapist, along with other team members, localize the tumor volume and critical normal structures using clinical, radiographic, and/or CT image information.

Verification is a final check that each of the planned treatment beams does cover the tumor or **target volume** and does not irradiate critical normal structures.[4] This is usually done as the second part of a two-step process on the simulator or treatment unit. It involves taking radiographic images or portal images of each of the treatment beams using external marks and other immobilization devices intended for treatment reproducibility.

Radiopaque marker refers to a material with a high atomic number. It is usually made of lead, copper, or solder wire. Frequently it is used on the surface of a patient or appropriately placed in a body cavity. This is done to delineate special points of interest for calculation purposes or to mark critical structures requiring visualization during treatment planning. Radiopaque markers are often used to mark specific points on a patient during the CT acquisition phase of the simulation procedure.

Separation refers to the measurement of the thickness of a patient along the central axis (CA) or at any other specified point within the irradiated volume. Separations are helpful in calculating the amount of tissue in front of, behind, or around a tumor. A **caliper,** which is a graduated ruled instrument with one sliding leg and one that is stationary, is used to determine the patient's thickness. A patient's separation is also referred to as the intrafield distance, or sometimes the innerfield distance (IFD).

Field size involves the dimensions of a treatment field at the isocenter, which are represented by width × length. This measurement, determined by the field-defining wires on the conventional simulator and collimator opening on the treatment unit, defines the dimensions of the treatment portal.

There are several definitions related to the patient planning process provided by the International Commission on Radiation Units and Measurements in an effort to standardize radiation therapy terminology.[13] Fig. 20-2 illustrates several target volumes described by the International Commission on Radiation Units and Measurements Report #50. Uniform application of these terms when radiation treatments are prescribed, recorded, and reported helps with the comparison of treatment results from different centers.[3]

Three specific target volumes are further defined (Fig. 20-3); gross tumor volume (GTV), clinical target volume (CTV), and planning target volume (PTV).[13]

Gross tumor volume (GTV) indicates the gross palpable or visible tumor.

Clinical target volume (CTV) indicates the gross palpable or visible tumor (GTV) and a surrounding volume of tissue that may contain subclinical or microscopic disease.

Planning target volume (PTV) indicates the CTV plus margins for geometric uncertainties, such as patient motion, beam penumbra, and treatment setup differences.

Acronyms

Acronyms are commonly used in any highly technical work environment. A common language evolves in communicating thoughts and ideas between team members. An introduction to several more important acronyms used during simulation procedures will be helpful. Many of the useful acronyms are illustrated in Fig. 20-4, *A* and *B.* In trying to standardize radiation therapy terminology, the American Registry of Radiologic Technologists (ARRT) has also provided a list of terms or abbreviations listed in the ARRT *Conventions Specific to Radiation Therapy Technology Examinations*[1] (Table 20-2).

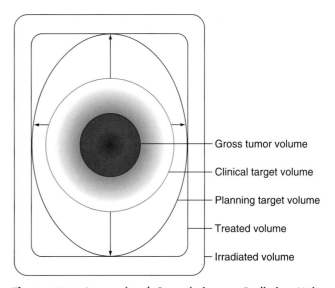

Figure 20-2. International Commission on Radiation Units (ICRU) Report #50 defining target volumes used in radiation therapy. *(From Cox JD, Ang KK, editors: Radiation Oncology: Rationale, Technique, Results, ed 8, St Louis, 2003, Mosby.)*

- Gross tumor volume
- Clinical target volume
- Planning target volume
- Treated volume
- Irradiated volume

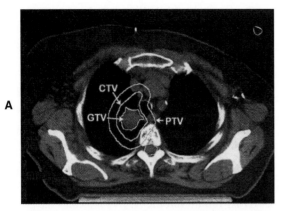
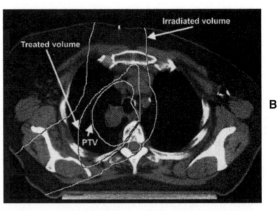

Figure 20-3. A, CT image of the mid-thorax showing a cancer of the lung. The obvious tumor mass is outlined as the GTV. The CTV and PTV are also shown. **B,** The same CT image as in **A,** showing the PTV, the treated volume, and the irradiated volume. A two-field technique was used, with anterior and posterior oblique fields of 6-MV x-rays. *(Used by permission from Van Dyk JV, Mah K: Simulation and imaging for radiation therapy planning. In Williams JR, Thwaites DI, editors: Radiotherapy physics in practice, Oxford, 2000, Oxford University Press.)*

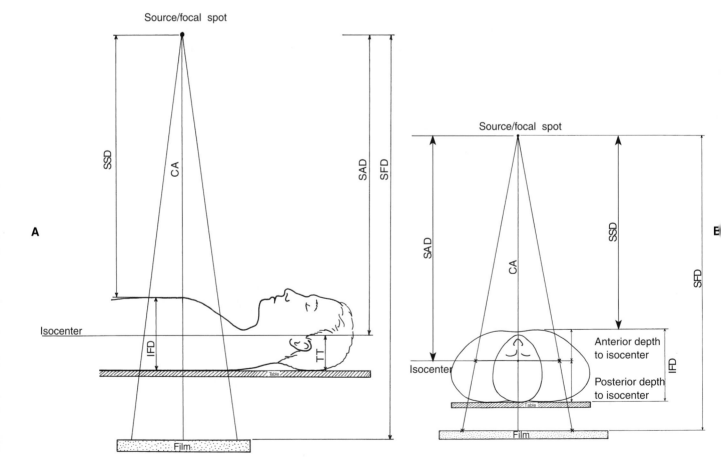

Figure 20-4. A list of common acronyms used in radiation therapy; **(A)** a lateral view and **(B)** a superior view illustrating terms in a transverse plane.

Table 20-2	American Registry of Radiologic Technologists (ARRT) conventions

Anteroposterior (AP)*	The central axis is directed from anterior to posterior.
Central axis (CA, CAX)	The central axis, which is an imaginary ray perpendicular to the cross section of the simulation or treatment field.
Film*	Refer to "film" if it is truly film (i.e., unexposed); otherwise, use "radiograph."
Intrafield distance (IFD)	The measurement of the thickness of the patient along the central axis of the beam (or along a line parallel to the central axis) from the entrance point to the exit point. Also referred to as the patient's "separation."[18]
Left anterior oblique (LAO)*	The central axis is directed from the left anterior aspect of the patient.
Left posterior oblique (LPO)*	The central axis is directed from the left posterior aspect of the patient.
Parallel opposed (POP)	Two treatment fields planned 180 degrees apart.
Patient support assembly (PSA)	Also referred to as the table or couch.
Right anterior oblique (RAO)*	The central axis is directed from the right anterior aspect of the patient.
Right posterior oblique (RPO)*	The central axis is directed from the right posterior aspect of the patient.
Optical distance indicator (ODI)	A device mounted on or near the collimator head that optically displays the SSD on the patient's skin.
Source-axis distance (SAD)*	The distance from the source of radiation to the axis of the radiation beam or isocenter.
Source-to-collimator distance (SCD)*	The distance between the source of radiation and the heavy metal collimators.
Source-to-diaphragm distance (SDD)*	The distance between the source of radiation and the collimators; used interchangeably with SCD.
Source-film distance (SFD)*	The distance from the source of radiation to the film. It replaces target-film distance (TFD) and focal-film distance (FFD).
Source-skin distance (SSD)*	The distance from the source of radiation to the skin or surface of the patient (either x-ray or radionuclide). It replaces target-skin distance (TSD) and focal-skin distance (FSD).
Source-tray distance (STD)*	The distance from the source of radiation to the blocking tray.
Table top distance (TT)	The distance from the tabletop to the isocenter.

*Indicates those terms or abbreviations described in the *ARRT Conventions Specific to Radiation Therapy Technology Examination.* Used with permission from the ARRT, St. Paul, Minn.

TUMOR AND NORMAL TISSUE LOCALIZATION

The primary function of the simulator is to localize the tumor volume in three dimensions. The simulator is not used exclusively or in total isolation for the localization of most tumors but together with other imaging modalities such as CT, magnetic resonance imaging (MRI), positron emission tomography (PET), and single photon emission computed tomography (SPECT).[5] However, some simulation procedures may be done exclusively on the simulator radiographically, fluoroscopically, or using a CT scanner with or without the aid of contrast media. In this section, several aspects of tumor localization are discussed. These include anatomic body planes, CT, source-skin distance/source-axis distance (SSD/SAD) localization methods, fluoroscopy and radiography, and the use of contrast media in tumor and normal tissue localization.

One of the greatest challenges that faces the medical-physics community is the ability to combine imaging modalities such as CT, MRI, PET, and SPECT so that data can be intercompared accurately in the planning and verification stages of radiation therapy.[34] This process of overlaying one image study onto another provides more information during the planning process and enhances the strength of each indi-vidual imaging modality through a synergistic effect. More research is needed to study and examine computerized image correlation.

Anatomic Body Planes

A review of the three major body planes helps in understanding the nature of three-dimensional localization. As illustrated in Fig. 20-5, the body can be described in three planes: the coronal, sagittal, and axial planes. An anteroposterior (AP) radiograph displays anatomy in the coronal plane, showing structures in the inferior/superior and left/right direction (two dimensions only). This radiographic view provides information for planning purposes in only one plane. The depth of the tumor volume cannot be found on a conventional simulator without the aid of a lateral radiograph (Fig. 20-6). This view shows anatomic information in the sagittal plane, displaying structures in the inferior/superior and AP direction. Axial images can only be obtained through CT and MRI modalities.

CT Imaging

Applications and advantages of CT and MRI in radiation therapy treatment planning have been documented.[9-12,25,34]

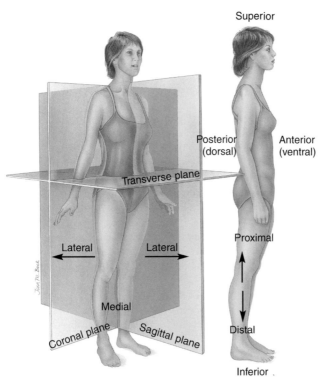

Figure 20-5. The body described in three planes: the coronal, sagittal, and axial planes. *(From Thibodeau GA, Patton KT: Anatomy and physiology, St. Louis, 1994, Mosby.)*

Radiation therapy CT planning procedures are distinctly different from conventional diagnostic procedures. For example, unlike CT scans done for diagnostic purposes, in which a curved couch top is used, a flat insert is required when scanning for radiation therapy planning purposes, unless it is a CT simulator used exclusively for radiation therapy. It is important to scan the patient in the treatment position. If the treatment position is supine on a flat couch, then the patient should be scanned supine on a flat surface. In addition, positional lasers incorporated into the design of the CT scanner will aid in the reproducibility of the simulation process.[34]

Some studies have shown modifications in 30% to 80% of a select number of conventional non-CT treatment plans because of the additional information provided by CT. In addition, some 10% to 40% of all radiation therapy patients might benefit from CT scanning for radiation therapy treatment planning. Cross-sectional information provided by MRI and CT imaging contributes considerable information to the radiation oncologist in four major areas: diagnosis, tumor and normal tissue localization, tissue density data for dose calculations, and follow-up treatment monitoring.[34]

There are two types of applications involving CT imaging in radiation therapy. One provides detailed diagnostic information used by the radiologist and radiation oncologist to evaluate the extent of the disease. This is conventional CT (usually performed outside the radiation therapy department). The second is designed solely for radiation therapy

treatment planning. Concerning the second application, some manufacturers have introduced simulators that can reconstruct information analogous to conventional CT images. Others have developed software in which the radiation therapy beam can be displayed in coronal, sagittal, and axial planes. A CT simulator can provide several advanced image manipulation and viewing advantages such as beams eye view display, which allows the anatomy to be viewed from the perspective of the radiation beams and allows field shaping electronically at the computer work station.[25] A beams eye view allows the possibility of virtual simulation. By outlining target volumes on each image, irregular field shapes can be determined and a special laser device used to outline this field shape directly on the patient's skin.[19,34] Some authors predict that conventional simulators will soon be rendered obsolete by the CT simulator. Although some developmental work still remains, such as larger scan tunnel, improved image segmentation, and correlation software.[25]

Conventional Simulation and CT Simulation

A CT scanner operates much differently than the conventional simulation method of recording an image with fluoroscopy or a radiograph. There is no image receptor such as film or image intensifier. A collimated x-ray beam is directed at the patient, and the attenuated beam is measured by a detector whose response is transmitted to a computer. The computer analyzes the signal from the detector, reconstructs the image, and then stores and/or displays the image. The microprocessor and primary memory of the computer determine the reconstruction time, which is the time between the end of scanning and the appearance of an image.[6] Two main components of a CT simulator workstation are a target localization routine that allows the target to be defined and transfers the appropriate marks to the patient skin surface and a virtual simulation package that generates DRRs used to evaluate and simulate the case.[18] The virtual simulation package is essentially a computer and monitor with huge amounts of storage capacity, memory, and processing capability.

With conventional simulation, the field locations are determined first, the target is defined, and then the fields are shaped to treat the target. In virtual simulation, the target is defined first, and then the fields are shaped to conform to the target.[25] To accomplish this goal, the virtual simulation workstation needs access to vast amount of data. Two methods of simulation are discussed in this chapter: conventional simulation and CT simulation. Specific details of each approach to treatment planning are discussed in detail.

Conventional Simulation Localization Methods

Most treatment planning on the conventional simulator is divided into two types of procedures: SAD and SSD setups. Both methods may use fluoroscopy to initially view the area. In each case, radiographs document what has been done during the simulation process. These radiographs are considered part of the patient's medical record. They are routinely used

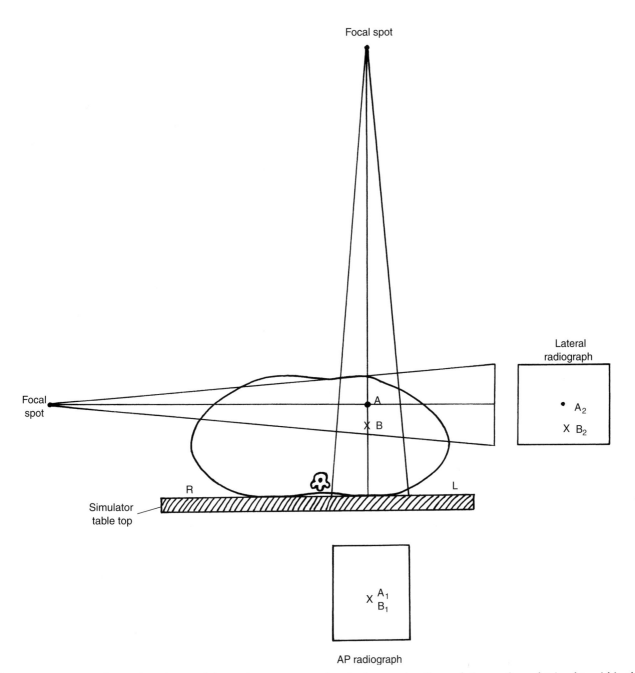

Figure 20-6. Two radiographs taken at right angles to one another (orthogonal radiographs) are often obtained to aid in the treatment planning process. Note in this schematic that points *A* and *B* cannot be distinguished from one another, except on the lateral radiograph.

as "masters" when comparing subsequent port films from the treatment unit.

The decision to use one setup method over the other may be decided by many factors. They include the nature and extent of the patient's disease and the goals and expected outcome of the treatment (cure or palliation). Other factors that are considered include the type of equipment available and the philosophy and education of the radiation therapy team.

The SSD approach positions a fixed treatment distance of 80 or 100 cm on the patient's skin for each field (Fig. 20-7, *A*). This method requires repositioning the patient for each field before treatment. Usually this approach uses a single field, two laterals or an AP/posteroanterior (PA) treatment approach (sometimes called parallel opposed [POP] fields because the central axes of each field oppose each other). This field arrangement requires tumor localization in two dimensions only, because all tissues within these fields are treated and the exact depth of the tumor is not critical.[3] Note that in Fig. 20-7, *A,* the field size is defined (at 100 cm) on the patient's skin.

The SAD approach is also called the **isocentric technique** (Fig. 20-7, *B*). It provides tumor localization in three dimensions. With the SAD strategy the isocenter is placed within the target volume with the aid of fluoroscopy and other imaging modalities. Here, as illustrated in Fig. 20-7, *B,* the field size is defined at the isocenter within the patient (100 cm). In both situations the field size is defined at 100 cm. The only

difference is where that distance is located (on the skin surface or within the patient). Once the isocenter has been located, orthogonal films may be taken. **Orthogonal films** are two radiographs taken at right angles to one another. They are often obtained to aid in the treatment planning process (see Fig. 20-6). In simulating a four-field pelvis, for example, some departments may take one radiograph to represent the anterior and posterior fields and one radiograph to represent the right and left lateral fields.

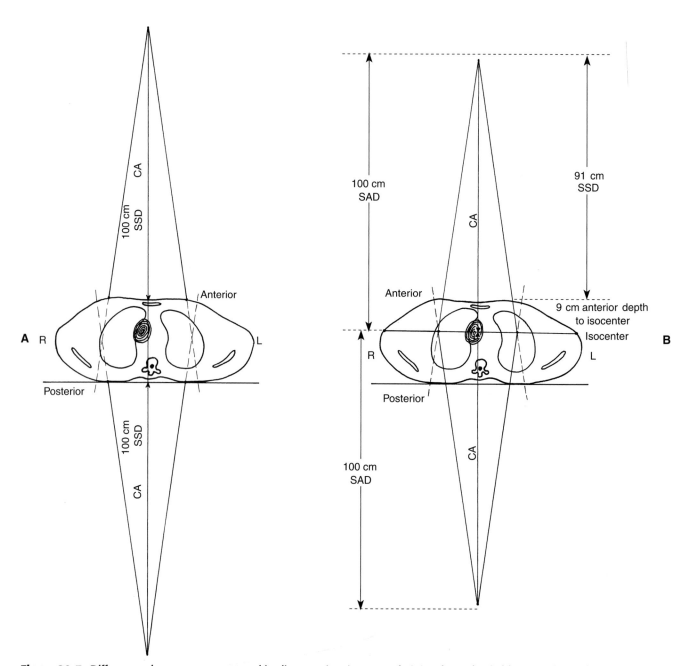

Figure 20-7. Differences between an source-skin distance (SSD) approach **(A),** where the field size is defined on the surface, and source-axis distance (SAD) **(B)** approach, where the field size is defined at a depth calculated within the patient, are demonstrated. Both methods used in the planning and delivery of a prescribed course of radiation therapy require careful documentation.

With the isocentric approach, the reading on the patient's skin varies from field to field. It depends on several factors. It will not be 80 or 100 cm, as happens with the SSD approach. Rather, the distance will vary for each field (Fig. 20-8), depending on the thickness or separation of the patient. It may also depend on the depth of the tumor from the AP, PA, oblique, or lateral skin surface.

Contrast media. To help in localizing the tumor volume and normal critical structures, contrast media may be needed during the simulation procedure. Contrast media, used in radiographic or fluoroscopic studies, visually enhance anatomic structures that would normally be more difficult to see. Commonly used contrast media include: barium sulfate, iodinated contrast materials, and negative contrast agents. Fig. 20-9, a lateral radiograph of the pelvis, illustrates both barium and iodine contrast agents used to localize the prostate.

Before the administration of any contrast medium, a careful evaluation of the patient should be performed. Severe allergic reactions to some contrast agents, requiring emergency intervention, have been observed. In addition, barium sulfate, for example, may be contraindicated with a suspected bowel perforation or obstruction. The proper selection and administration of the contrast medium should be evaluated before the simulation procedure.

Barium sulfate, which is not absorbed by the gastrointestinal (GI) tract when administered, outlines the GI tract. Before its administration either orally or rectally, it is prepared as a suspension in water to obtain the desired concentration or consistency. It is commonly used to visualize the esophagus, stomach, small bowel, colon, or oral cavity. Depending on the patient's condition, amount of barium, and its application, the patient should be advised as to the use of a laxative. Patients who had a small dab of barium paste inside the cheek to help localize a tonsillar lesion would be advised differently than someone who drank a 12-oz cup of barium to evaluate the amount of small bowel in a pelvic treatment field.

Iodinated contrast materials used in radiation therapy are usually of two types: aqueous ionic contrast medium and nonionic contrast medium.[35] Although their actions are different, both provide positive contrast (a white area on the radiograph) of a vessel or organ. Iodinated contrast materials are commonly used to help localize the kidneys, bladder, and prostate, and they are sometimes used in the GI tract when barium is contraindicated. Except for the GI tract, sterile procedures must be followed when administering iodinated contrast material. For example, contrast medium may be used intravenously to document the location of the kidneys (for Hodgkin's disease or seminoma) or through a bladder catheterization to localize the prostate.

Negative contrast agents, which include substances such as carbon dioxide, oxygen, and air, have a low atomic number and appear as dark areas on a radiograph. Examples of their use include a small amount of air introduced (with or without barium) into the rectum to help define its location or the use of normal gas exchange in the thorax, which helps define some lung tumors. Another example might include a Foley catheter balloon filled with 5 to 10 cc of air within the bladder. This is used to define the inferior extent of the bladder in reference to the prostate gland.

The primary function of the conventional simulator is to localize the tumor volume relative to normal tissue structures. The use of contrast agents, fluoroscopy, and radiography together with other imaging modalities, such as CT and MRI, greatly enhances the ability to localize and pinpoint the tumor volume. Many of these tools are available to the radiation oncologist and radiation therapist. However, their use and application may vary from patient to patient and institution to institution. The actual process of simulating a patient

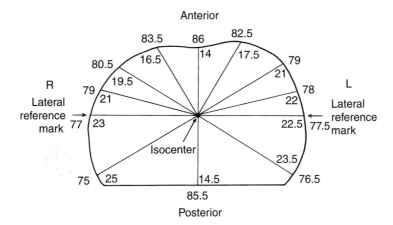

Figure 20-8. Source-skin distance (SSD) varies with the patient's separation when using an isocentric technique. Note that using a combination of SSD measurements, a patient's IFD can be calculated. In this example, the anterior SSD through the central axis (CA) is 86 cm (depth of 14 cm) and the posterior SSD is 85.5 (depth of 14.5 cm). The IFD can be calculated by adding the two depths (14 + 14.5 = 28.5).

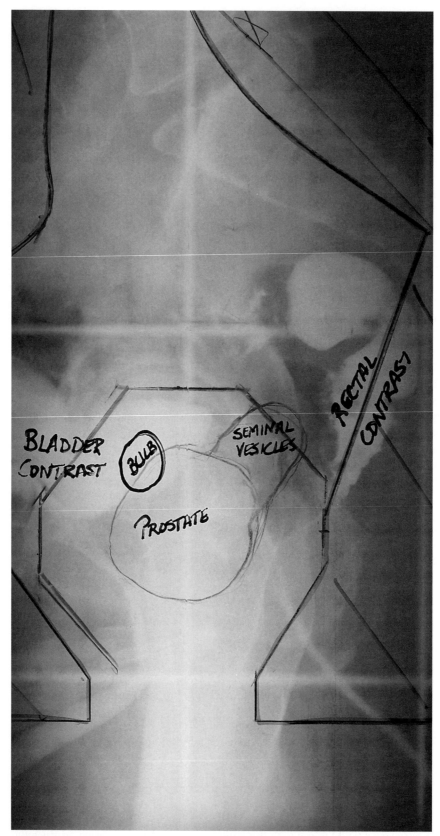

Figure 20-9. A lateral radiograph of the pelvis with contrast medium used to localize the prostate. In this example, barium is used to visualize the rectum and an iodinated contrast medium helps to localize the bladder.

on a conventional simulator, which is discussed in the next section, varies less.

CONVENTIONAL SIMULATION PROCEDURE

The use of treatment simulators during tumor and normal tissue localization is well documented.[*] The localization of a treatment field during simulation must reflect precisely what will happen in the treatment room. Patient position, beam alignment, and field size must be the same at the end of simulation and the beginning of treatment.[27] In this section the simulation procedure is discussed in detail. Box 20-1 outlines the common components involved in a conventional simulation procedure.

Presimulation Planning

An assessment of all relevant patient information and an evaluation of possible treatment approaches before the patient arrives are ideal. This is especially true for difficult cases, involving patients who have had previous treatment or have extensive disease.[9] In many institutions this may be done as part of a morning conference, where the discussion of specific cases occurs among the radiation therapy team members. The discussion during these meetings should relate to treatment planning, simulation, and concerns for those patients under treatment, although, because of busy schedules or a late addition to the day's schedule, this is not always possible. Minimally, the patient's history and physical examination notes should be reviewed by the radiation oncologist and radiation therapist, using other available pertinent information such as radiographs, CT and MRI scans, pathology reports, and operating reports.

The importance of the therapist and physician consultation before the actual simulation cannot be overemphasized. Radiation oncologists, even within the same institution, vary in their approach to simulation and treatment. For example, one physician may prefer to use a small amount of barium in the rectum for all endometrial cases, whereas another physician may use flexible beaded tubing to identify the rectum radiographically. In addition, the physician may be called away from the simulation area during the procedure and may not be immediately available to answer questions. So a plan should be established before beginning the simulation procedure if at all possible.

Additional attention in the presimulation planning process may involve the preparation of specialized immobilization devices. Certain accommodations for unique cases and an assessment of whether the simulation procedure is simple, intermediate, or complex should also be made. It is important to consider the patient's fears and anxieties, especially when doing simulations for small children and others with special needs (Box 20-2). For all cases, if a clear treatment approach is known at the beginning of the simulation, the procedure

Box 20-1	Procedure Outline for Conventional Simulation

1. Presimulation planning
2. Room preparation
3. Explanation of procedure
4. Patient positioning and immobilization
5. Operation of simulator controls
6. Setting field size parameters
7. Selecting exposure techniques
8. Radiographic exposure
9. Documenting pertinent data
10. Final procedures

will go more efficiently and accurately, enhancing the patient's confidence in the entire process and reducing the time needed to complete it.[9]

Preparing the Room

Effective use of time on the simulator is essential. Proper room preparation can aid in the effective use of that time. A review of all the pertinent information needed for the simulation procedure allows the therapist to prepare the simulation room in advance. The time demands on the simulator can be pressing, bearing in mind that one simulator can serve two or three treatment units.[3] A typical simulation day involves simulating 3 to 12 cases, depending on the number of treatment units in the department, the total number of new patients seen at the institution each year, and other factors. To explain the specific needs concerning the simulator's room preparation, two examples are provided.

Head and neck. The room is first cleaned from the simulation previous to this patient. If a thermoplastic mask is used, the heating element in the water tank is turned on low. This is done so that the water will be warm as the patient walks through the door. A clean sheet or piece of paper is placed on the simulator couch. The head rest (which can range from A to F and will be either transparent plastic or a solid foamlike material) selected for the simulation procedure is related to the patient's anatomy. For this simulation, a C or D headrest is selected. This should elevate the chin and isolate the treatment area (neck). The gantry head is positioned to the appropriate SSD for this patient's treatment machine. For example, some departments may have a 6-MV treatment unit with 100 SSD and an 80 SSD cobalt-60 unit.

If the patient requires a stent or special mouthpiece, this is made before the simulation begins. Wires help to visualize a surgical scar or any other pertinent anatomic areas. Pull straps or some kind of mechanism should be available (if needed) to pull the top of the shoulders down inferiorly and out of the treatment field. Tape is placed at the head of the couch. This is handy for drawing the marks on the

---

*References 4, 9, 16, 22, 27, 34.

Box 20-2	Helpful Hints in Patient Positioning During Simulation Procedures

1. If possible, one position should be established for all treatment fields, including boost fields. Internal structures can change dramatically if the patient's position is changed (e.g., from supine for one field to a prone position for the other).[3,16] The supine position should be used whenever possible because it is more comfortable for the patient and easier to document reproducibility.

   Exceptions: May include mantle irradiation on a treatment unit with which large fields are not possible, except at extended distances. This requires the patient to be treated in both supine and prone positions to adequately cover the treatment volume. It may not always be possible to treat breast and head and neck patients in the same position for their boost treatment, especially if electrons are used. Here, small fields are generally used for the boost, and electron cones do not offer the physical flexibility that photon fields offer.

2. Spending time before the simulation procedure educating, informing, and answering patient questions allows the patient to participate and cooperate more in maintaining a comfortable and reproducible treatment position.

   Exceptions: May include infants, small children, and severely handicapped individuals. In some situations premedication or anesthetics may be helpful in immobilizing the patient during the simulation procedure.

3. Consistent preparation of the treatment area should be carried out on a daily basis. Asking the patient to remove certain articles of clothing; dress in comfortable, loose-fitting clothing; or change into a specific type of hospital gown will add to consistent and reproducible positioning. Use of a bed sheet or suitable material prevents the shifting of skin marks when sliding a patient along the couch top.

   Exceptions: Include treatment areas that are not normally covered by clothing, such as the head and neck region and portions of the extremities. Patients requiring hospitalization may need special care and communication with the nursing staff regarding clothing or bandages that may interfere with visualizing external ink marks, tattoos, or anatomic landmarks.

4. Clinical considerations and medical conditions may restrict or inhibit patient positioning. Patient pain and discomfort or physical disabilities might result in very limited positioning.[3] For example, a breast cancer patient recovering from a lumpectomy or axillary node dissection may have limited arm movement. Special accommodations or a delay in initiating the simulation procedure may be considered.

   Exceptions: Include certain patients treated for palliation. Perez and Brady[24] define the palliative aim of therapy as one in which there is no hope of the patient surviving for extended periods. However, symptoms that produce discomfort, impair the self-sufficiency of the patient, or cause severe pain require treatment. It must be remembered that in curative therapy, a certain probability of side effects, even though undesirable, may be acceptable. The same is not generally true in palliative treatment. For example, a patient with metastatic breast cancer requiring treatment to the lumbar spine should not be denied a comfortable pad to lie on during treatment at the expense of a hard treatment couch and a small amount of skin sparing.

5. Accurate and complete setup instructions are necessary. The use of additional skin marks, reference to topographic anatomy, or special instructions for unusual patient positioning can be critical in the daily reproducibility of the treatment position. This requires accurate record keeping and careful documentation of the simulation procedure. A conventional or digital photograph of the setup, whenever possible, is helpful.

   Exceptions: None.

6. Sometimes it is necessary to move normal critical tissues out of the field or away from the edge of the beam. Examples include rotating the eye to spare the lens and moving the testicle(s) or ovaries to reduce the gonadal dose. A surgical procedure called an oophoropexy can relocate the ovaries to the midline of the body, where they may be more easily shielded.[3]

   Exceptions: Include critical structures that may be involved with tumor. In addition, many normal tissue structures can be shielded with custom blocking, multileaf collimation, or special shielding devices. Radiographic documentation of the lens with the aid of a radiopaque BB or arrow provides the physician information regarding the construction of customized blocks. Special shielding devices are available to reduce the dose to the testes.

7. Simulation or CT scanning of patients on solid couch tops while treating them on flexible "tennis racquet" type windows can result in discrepancies between the planned volume and the irradiated volume.[3]

   Exceptions: Rare. Kahn[18] recommends, for lateral portal exposure of the pelvis, that the Mylar section of the couch or tennis racquet be removed. The patient can be placed on a solid surface to avoid sag during positioning, reserving the tennis racquet for parallel opposed anteroposterior treatments in which skin sparing is of concern. Setup discrepancies in the pelvic area from the simulator to the treatment couch, especially with larger patients, can be as much as 1 to 1.5 cm. Part of this discrepancy may result from the inconsistent use of couch top surfaces between the simulator and treatment unit. For example, a solid couch top may be used during the simulation of a four-field pelvic procedure. Discrepancies may result if the patient is positioned on a tennis racquet couch top during treatment.

CT, Computed tomography.

thermoplastic mask (if used) or securing a wire on the patient's skin. A cloth or paper towels should be available to dry the excess water from the thermoplastic mask. The **treatment volume** may have already been decided during the presimulation session with the physician, making the simulation more accurate and time efficient.

Thorax. Because the patient will receive part of the treatment through the treatment couch from a direct posterior field or posterior oblique portal, a table pad is not recommended. The simulation must duplicate the treatment setup in all aspects. A cushion on the table may interfere with reproducibility. If the patient is in severe pain, accommodations required for a pad or cushion during treatment and simulation can be calculated. The B headrest may be appropriate when the treatment portal will not cover the cervical lymph nodes. If the cervical lymph nodes must be encompassed in the treatment volume, a C headrest may be used to elevate the chin more, thus isolating the neck lymph nodes.

Depending on the patient's arm position, an alpha cradle can be constructed or the **Vac-lok** (a type of cushion constructed of thin plastic film with a fill material of tiny polystyrene spheres) used to provide patient **immobilization.** This increases the stability of the patient's arms (especially if they are positioned above the head) and increases reproducibility during treatment. An appropriate field size is set, positioning the collimator with no rotation.

If a CT scan is needed for treatment planning purposes, the therapist must arrange this ahead of time. This will involve additional time for the patient and therapist. This may be performed on the simulator if it is equipped with a CT mode or may be scheduled on a conventional CT scanner either in the radiation therapy department or in the radiology department. If the scan is performed on a conventional CT scanner, the therapist must accompany the patient to ensure the patient is in the same treatment position when scanned. Radiopaque markers may also be needed to obtain accurate CT data for treatment planning purposes. BBs, wires, arrows, or another type of radiopaque material is necessary to visualize specific points of interest on a radiograph and/or CT scan. This is done to help the dosimetrist transfer these anatomic points to the treatment planning computer. For example, a cross-table lateral film may be taken to provide data for a dose calculation to the spinal cord. A chain or wire is taped to the patient's posterior surface before the simulation begins.

Details concerning the preparation of the room become more important with a busy schedule. Establishing a definite treatment approach at the beginning of the simulation procedure allows the process to proceed more efficiently and accurately. The patient gains confidence in the radiation therapy staff if one of the first impressions of the department is a positive one. This can be enhanced if the simulation procedure is accurate, organized, and not rushed. It also provides an opportunity to educate the patient and answer questions concerning the treatment process, side effects, and skin care.

Explanation of Simulation Procedure

Assessment. Our entire health care system is based on effective communication. Miscommunication can have a major impact on the patient's care. The therapist must assess the patient's needs, recognize cultural differences, respond to nonverbal communication, and then attempt to communicate therapeutically and effectively with the patient.[35]

In the simulator, the therapist should assess the patient's physical condition and emotional state. The therapist should determine if the patient is nervous, fearful, or withdrawn. If a patient requires oxygen or medications or has difficulty standing, sitting, or walking, the therapist can try to make the patient more comfortable. If a patient has difficulty hearing or speaking, provisions can also be made. Good observation and listening skills are essential to proper patient assessment.

Communication. The therapist should also establish an environment conducive to communication. If there are distractions in the area, such as unwanted noises or the usual distractions of a radiation oncology department, it may be preferable to retreat to a private area to communicate with the patient (the simulator room is much better for this than a busy waiting room). Therapists must establish an environment where they can facilitate the communication clearly, effectively, and therapeutically.[35]

A health care professional should make a conscious effort to speak clearly, confidently, and at a rate and tone conducive to listening. With practice a therapist can increase listening skills by not only listening to what the patient is saying but also hearing what he or she is not saying.[26,35] For example, if during a conversation a patient cannot say the word "cancer," this could indicate this patient has not accepted the disease, which in turn can cause the therapist to communicate differently than with someone who talks freely about the disease diagnosed.

Observation is also an important skill in effective communication. The therapist should observe the patient at all times during a conversation, noting facial expressions, body gestures, space relations, and contradictions in the patient's communication. If a patient explains that he or she is in great pain but then is laughing and smiling, the therapist should pay close attention to the patient's nonverbal communication. Any barriers to communication may affect the patient's health care.

Nonverbal communication not only includes what the therapist and patient can observe but also includes what the therapist and patient hear in the speech, what is felt as the person is touched, and what each person smells (e.g., a lack of good personal hygiene or overuse of perfume or cologne) as they get closer to each other.[26,35] If a patient hears lack of interest and/or monotony in the therapist's voice, frequently because the same speech has already been made many times that day, the patient may feel that the therapist is disinterested in the situation. As the therapist touches the patient and the patient retreats back, the therapist should know the patient is anxious and refrain from touching him or her or ask before touching the patient again.

Cultural diversity. The therapist must be aware of cultural differences in both verbal and nonverbal communication to avoid being misunderstood, offending someone, or being offended by someone during communication.[26,35] This is especially important in culturally diverse areas and in teaching hospitals, where a larger percentage of patients may be foreign or from different parts of the country. Gestures displayed in the United States do not always have the same meaning in every culture. For example, in the United States, people tend to be more protective of their "personal space," whereas in other countries, it is considered rude to stand far away from a person while communicating. Language barriers can be overcome through an interpreter provided by the hospital or a local church group. This should be planned in advance if possible. A family member may also serve as an interpreter for a patient. In addition, the family member can be a source of support for the patient and may hear something the patient does not.

Therapeutic communication. Therapeutic communication enables the patient to feel part of the team or a partner in the situation. The caregiver should not just repeat orders but rather establish a relationship with the patient. This takes some time and effort on the part of the caregiver. For a radiation therapist, this realm of communication is the most valuable because once a relationship with a patient is established, he or she trusts the caregiver and allows help to be given throughout the disease process (especially during the administration of the treatment). A therapist should first establish the basis for the communication by introducing the staff and explaining the simulation procedure in detail. Therapists should always face the patient and maintain eye contact whenever possible. A therapeutic communicator listens while the patient is speaking and never interrupts. It is inappropriate to be busy planning a response rather than listening while the patient is speaking.

During communication the therapist should also check for understanding, restating or repeating statements made by the patient is very useful. This lets the patient know you understand what he or she is saying verbally or nonverbally and also affirms to the patient that he or she is being heard. This can help a patient in making decisions because the same information is repeated back in another form, providing the opportunity to look at the problem from a different perspective and facilitating understanding. If at any time during communication the therapist does not understand the patient, clarification should be sought.

The main objective of therapeutic communication is to keep the conversation directed toward the patient. The therapist should avoid close-ended sentences, which are sentences answered with a "yes" or "no" response. The patient should be involved and the communication focused on him or her—not on the therapist. Therapeutic communication is kept short with open-ended questions, always directing the communication to the patient.

Educating the patient and family. Using therapeutic communication is also a vital process when educating the patient. Professionally the therapist is obligated to educate the patient not only about the physical aspects of radiation therapy that the patient can see and feel but also about the emotional aspects of radiation therapy. The simulation treatment procedure should be explained in detail. This explanation should be done slowly and clearly, using all therapeutic communication techniques. The equipment must be explained to the patient. It is helpful to mention that the simulation is not an actual treatment and that the simulator is an x-ray machine not a therapeutic treatment machine. The patient should be shown where he or she will lie on the table, which way the head should be placed, whether the patient will be supine or prone, and whether he or she will be on a belly board or with the arms above the head. Basic patient positioning should be communicated along with an explanation of why that position is needed. This facilitates patient cooperation.

The patient should also be given an explanation of what procedures to follow after the simulation. The patient should receive instructions on how to take care of the skin marks as well as the skin itself before the treatments begin and while under treatment. When special orders are needed before the patient is to receive treatment, such as arriving for treatment with a full or empty bladder, this should be communicated at this time. When barium is used during the simulation, follow-up instructions are needed. An appointment time for the first treatment should be discussed, providing the therapist's name and department number in case communication is necessary before the next appointment.

Patient Positioning and Immobilization

One of the weakest links in treatment planning is patient positioning.[2,11,34] If the patient is not comfortable and does not remain still during treatment administration, then sophisticated treatment plans and elaborate immobilization devices are not as effective. If a stable position cannot be maintained and reproduced daily, the result is either a geometric miss of the target volume or irradiation of greater amounts of uninvolved normal tissue.[9,11]

For most simulation procedures the patient is positioned supine or prone. Occasionally other positions are used. On rare occasions, a sitting position may be necessary because of the patient's medical condition. For example, a patient may need to be positioned in an erect or semierect position (sitting on the end of the treatment table) because of an advanced lung mass that has compromised the patient's breathing and the return of blood through the superior vena cava. Helpful hints regarding patient positioning and immobilization are listed in Box 20-2. These suggestions and recommendations can be considered in an effort to improve patient positioning and reproducibility.

Daily reproducibility is essential. The positioning of the patient for treatment is usually depicted by a patient alignment system (Fig. 20-10, *A* and *B*). Three-directional lasers

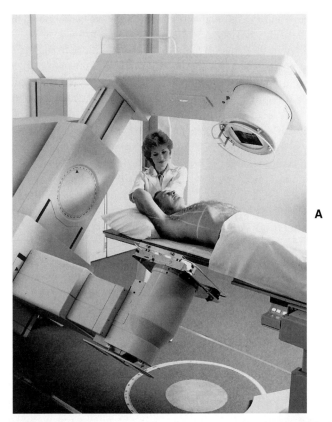

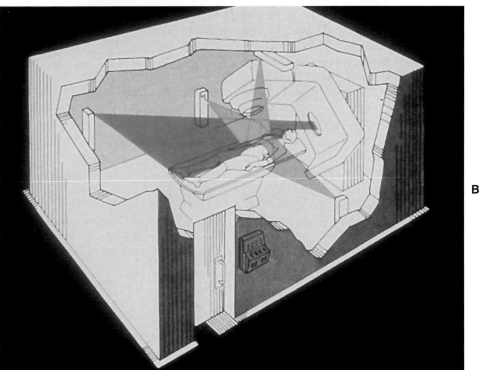

Figure 20-10. Usually two side lasers and an overhead laser are used to accurately define the location of the isocenter during simulation **(A),** which demonstrates an oblique setup on a Philips SLS Simulator and **(B)** treatment delivery, which shows the THER-A-CROSS system. The directional lasers correspond to external reference marks on the patient. *(**A,** Courtesy Philips Medical Systems, Shelton, Connecticut. **B,** Courtesy Gammex RMI, Milwaukee, Wisconsin.)*

accomplish this through the transverse and sagittal planes. A patient's age, weight, and general health as well as the anatomic area to be simulated can affect the patient's position. Usually India ink tattoos, visual skin marks, or references to topographic anatomy are used to delineate the treatment area. Immobilization devices improve the accuracy and reproducibility of a planned course of treatment. To achieve this, the integrity of a patient's position must be maintained throughout the course of treatment. As little as one or two patient positioning errors can increase the possibility of missing the treatment volume. This can reduce the dose to the tumor volume by 10% or greater as well as treat areas that do not need treatment.[11] Thus daily reproduction of the prescribed, planned, and simulated treatment is essential to its outcome. Also important is prohibiting patient movement during simulation, treatment setup, and treatment delivery.[17,33] Effective immobilization is essential to achieving this goal.

Patient immobilization. Patient positioning and immobilization must be used to achieve true reproducibility and accuracy in setup. In a study conducted by Byhardt et al.,[7] field placement errors occurred in 15% of the patients treated. The most common sites of field placement error were the pelvis, chest, and abdomen areas. These are sites where immobilization has traditionally not been considered as important as the head and neck area. A later study by Soffen et al.[33] evaluated the use of rigid immobilization for the pelvic regions of early stage prostate cancer patients. The 10% of daily positioning errors representing the greatest movements (anterior/posterior and superior/inferior) were eliminated by the use of immobilization. It was reported that for these patients, daily setup variation could be diminished by 67%.

Accuracy and reproducibility of daily setup is essential to reducing possible treatment complications. Once the threshold dose for tumor response has been reached, small increases in the absorbed dose may make large differences in tumor control. In a similar manner, once the threshold for normal tissue injury has been reached, small increases in dose may greatly increase the risk of complications.[23] Thus the need for accurate patient positioning and the maintenance of that positioning by immobilization is evident.

Although the need for immobilization is apparent, achieving it is not always simple or easy. Effective immobilization devices constrain the patient from moving during treatment and do the following[30]:
- Aid in daily treatment setup and provide reproducibility
- Ensure that immobilization of the patient or treatment area is done with a minimum of discomfort to the patient
- Achieve the conditions prescribed in the treatment plan
- Enhance precision of treatment with minimal additional setup time

It is also important that immobilization devices provide the following benefits:
- Are rigid and durable enough to withstand an entire course of treatment

- Take into consideration the patient's condition and treatment unit limitations

In addition, immobilization and positioning aids that can be adapted for many patients with minimal modification and that are cost effective are desirable. They can usually be broadly divided into three categories: positioning aids, simple immobilization, and complex immobilization.[34] **Patient positioning aids** are devices designed to place the patient in a particular position for treatment. There is generally very little structure in these devices to ensure that the patient does not move. Simple immobilization devices restrict some movement but usually require the patient's voluntary cooperation. **Complex immobilization devices** are individualized immobilizers that restrict patient movement and ensure reproducibility in positioning.

Positioning aids are the most commonly used devices in patient setup. Generally speaking, they are widely available, easy to use, and may be used for more than one patient, thus making them convenient and inexpensive. Head holders are probably the most widely used positioning aids. They are usually made of formed plastic or molded polyurethane foam. They come in a variety of heights and neck contours. The different heights and contours allow for the desired head and neck angulation to achieve the best treatment position. Patients who must be treated in prone position may use different versions of a support device, which elevates the face from the table top and supports the head or chin (Fig. 20-11). There are also devices that support the patient's chin while in the prone position (Fig. 20-12). This device typically may be

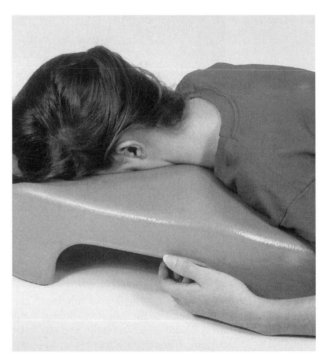

Figure 20-11. Prone pillow. *(Courtesy Radiation Products Design, Inc., Albertville, Minnesota.)*

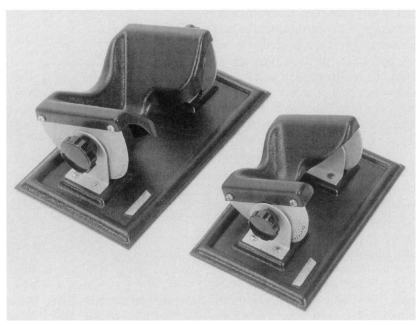

Figure 20-12. Chin support. *(Courtesy Radiation Products Design, Inc., Albertville, Minnesota.)*

angled to have the patient in the desired position but face and forehead are left virtually free from pressure.

A variety of sponge pillows and foam cushions are available. Various sizes and shapes are useful in different treatment positions. Foam neck rolls assist in proper chin extension, and other shapes and sizes are particularly useful in positioning extremities. Foam cushions and pillows also tend to make patients more comfortable on hard treatment and simulation tables. Comfortable patients are more likely to be cooperative and are better able to maintain treatment position, both of which contribute to setup reproducibility and treatment accuracy.

Sandbags are another commonly used positioning device. A well-placed sandbag helps to prevent movement or rotation of a body part during treatment. They are especially helpful in treating extremities.

To position the arm, particularly for breast treatment, the L-shaped arm board is still used in some radiation oncology centers. More recent styles of arm boards are contoured to the shape of the arm and allow the arm to rest comfortably above the patient's head. They also tend to allow for more flexibility in achieving greater arm tilt and extension (Fig. 20-13).

The positioning devices mentioned in this chapter are widely used in radiation oncology departments. They assist the therapist in positioning the patient for treatment. Most are designed to be comfortable for the patient, which encourages him or her to maintain proper treatment position. These devices will not, however, prevent patient movement during treatment. The patient must be cooperative and fully under-

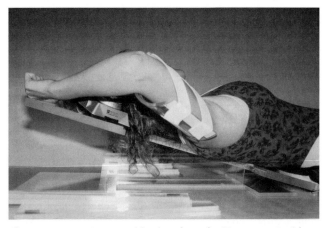

Figure 20-13. Arm positioning board. *(Courtesy Smithers Medical Products, Inc., Akron, Ohio.)*

stand the importance of not moving during setup or treatment in order for the devices to be effective.

Simple immobilization devices are commonly used in addition to positioning aids. They typically provide some restriction of movement and stability of treatment position in cooperative patients. However, patients who insist on moving will not be entirely deterred by these devices.

The least complex and most readily available simple immobilization tool is tape. Masking tape or paper tape is a standard supply in almost every treatment room. Plastic or cloth straps with Velcro at the ends can sometimes be substituted for tape.

Another very simple and accessible immobilization device is the rubber band. Large rubber bands, approximately 2 cm in thickness, can be used to bind the patient's feet together when he or she is in supine position. This helps to ensure that the legs and feet are consistently in a reproducible position by limiting hip motion.

There are a number of devices available to restrict patient movement for treatment of the head and neck area. With some slight variation, most consist of a head frame and a bite block (Fig. 20-14). The head frame can be used for many different patients. Each patient will require his or her own bite block. The **bite block** serves two purposes. It helps the patient maintain the position of the chin, and it moves the tongue out of the treatment area. These can be made of cork, Aquaplast pellets, or dental wax.

Immobilization of the shoulders, arms, and legs can be accomplished by using arm to foot straps. There are several versions of these (Fig. 20-15) that are commercially available. The primary purpose is to pull the patient's shoulders out of lateral head and neck fields. As the patient grasps the straps, the tension of the straps running the length of the patient's body and around the soles of the feet provides traction to move the shoulders inferiorly and out of the lateral treatment field.

Simple immobilization devices are easy to use and generally cost effective. Items such as tape and rubber bands are inexpensive. Some devices may be used by several patients over time, which reduces costs. In choosing to use any simple immobilization device, the radiation therapist must keep the patient in mind. Patients must understand the importance of holding still during treatment and must cooperate with the radiation therapist, otherwise any simple immobilization device will be ineffective.

Complex immobilization devices are becoming more and more popular because there are many new products available to quickly produce immobilization for individual patients. Because each device is individualized, they tend to be more costly. However, the advantages are that unusual patient positions can be achieved, and, in many cases, portal markings can be made on the device, thus alleviating the need for patients to keep skin markings. Complex immobilization devices can be made of a number of different products, such as plaster, plastic, and Styrofoam. The materials used will depend on the treatment area, availability of materials, and individual practitioner preference.

The earliest complex immobilization devices were constructed of plaster of paris. Plaster is still used today in some radiation oncology centers. The plaster is used to make a cast of the body part to be treated. Preparing a plaster cast is fairly easy. A thin piece of cloth or plastic wrap is placed over the part to be immobilized. Plaster of paris strips are prepared and applied. A number of strips must be used in order for the cast to be thick and strong enough so that it will maintain its shape and not break during the course of treatment. Care must also be taken to allow the strips to dry thoroughly before remov-

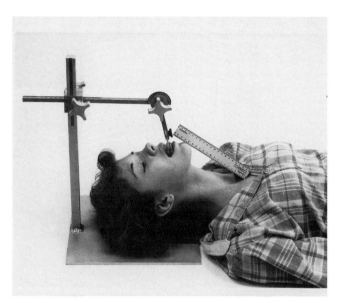

Figure 20-14. Bite block system. *(Courtesy Radiation Products Design, Inc., Albertville, Minnesota.)*

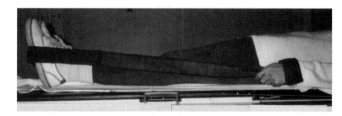

Figure 20-15. Arm to foot straps.

ing the cast because failure to do so will jeopardize the cast's integrity. Plaster masks of the head and neck area can be secured to a head frame, which is placed on the treatment table. This device must be used when the mask is made. Once the cast is thoroughly dry, the treatment portal can be cut out if necessary. Field markings may also be made on the cast.

Foaming agents have become a widely used immobilization device (Fig. 20-16). It is becoming popular because it can be used to immobilize practically any anatomic part, such as the head and neck area, the thorax, and the extremities. Before being made for the individualized patient, a shell with a plastic bag or other protective sheeting and a set of foam agents is set aside. When the foaming agents are combined and placed in the plastic-covered shell, they begin to expand. When a patient is positioned in the shell, the foam contours or molds around the patient. After approximately 10 minutes, the foam will have hardened and the cradle is complete and ready to use. Making the cradle takes very little time on the therapist's part. The chemical reaction of the foaming agents produces a small amount of heat, which most patients do not find uncomfortable. One concern in the making this type of immobilization device is the safe use of the

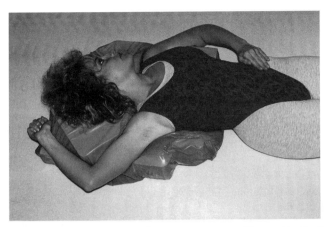

Figure 20-16. Alpha cradle. *(Courtesy Smithers Medical Products, Inc, Akron, Ohio.)*

foaming agents. Inappropriate use of the agents and inaccurate disposal of their containers after use could lead to environmental problems and/or hazardous situations.[32]

Another immobilization device that is currently available is called Vac-lok (MED-TEC, Inc.) (Fig. 20-17). This device consists of a cushion and a vacuum compression pump. The patient is placed into treatment position on a partially inflated cushion. The cushion is partially evacuated until it is semirigid and the therapist molds it around the area to be immobilized. Once the shape is established, the vacuum procedure is completed until the cushion is completely rigid. Cushions are available in several shapes and sizes to accommodate most anatomic sites. The advantage to using this system is that the cushions can be deflated, cleaned, and reused after a patient has completed his or her treatment course.[21]

Aquaplast (WFR Aquaplast Corporation) is yet another commonly used immobilization device (Fig. 20-18). It is a thermoplastic that becomes pliable when warmed in a hot water bath. When pliable, it can be molded around the patient. The material comes in sheets, perforated or unperforated. It is lightweight and easy to use in making immobilization devices and is very popular for immobilization for head and neck treatment. Using an Aquaplast mask requires the addition of a headrest and some type of frame to secure the mask on the patient and to the table during setup and treatment. Although Aquaplast has traditionally been used for immobilization of the head, newer uses include pelvic immobilization, full body molds, and supports for large breasts (Fig. 20-19).

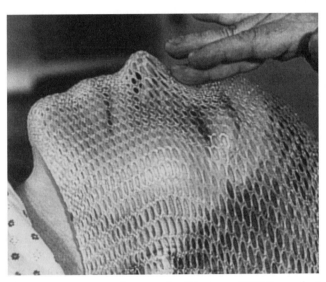

Figure 20-18. Aquaplast mask. *(Courtesy WFR/Aquaplast Corp, Wyckoff, New Jersey.)*

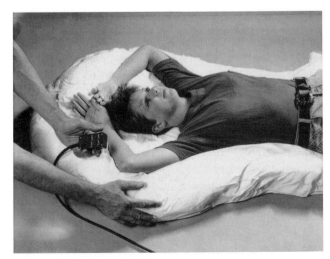

Figure 20-17. Vac-lok. *(Courtesy MED-TEC, Inc, Orange City, Iowa.)*

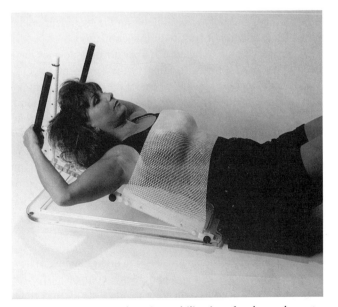

Figure 20-19. Aquaplast immobilization for large breasts. *(Courtesy WFR/Aquaplast Corp, Wyckoff, New Jersey.)*

There are several advantages to using a thermoplastic immobilizer. Patient markings can be made right on the mask. The perforated plastic also helps patients feel more comfortable because they can breath and see through the perforations.[36] The casts may be cut to further increase patient comfort, especially if the mask is tight around the eyes and forehead or if a patient feels claustrophobic. The treatment field may also be cut out to reduce beam attenuation, thus minimizing possibility of skin reactions. It should be noted, however, that excessive cutting reduces the integrity of this immobilizer. In addition, modifications in the mask to accommodate weight loss or reduction in swelling can be made on a completed mask at any time during the course of treatment. A heat gun may be used to heat the problem area until it is pliable and then changes may be made.

Although complex immobilization devices are somewhat time consuming and costly to make, they allow for unique patient positioning options. They typically provide more stability and prevent more patient movement and are usually time saving in daily treatment procedures, thus justifying the cost for many practitioners.

With the advent of record and verify systems, tolerances may be set on many of the treatment unit's positions, such as couch height and couch positions in the left/right and inferior/superior direction. If this is a consideration, indexing complex immobilization devices, such as thermoplastic immobilization devices and foaming agent devices to the treatment couch, may provide for "tighter" tolerance settings. Specific points may be marked during the simulation process on the immobilization device and will correspond to the relative position of the device located on the treatment couch. In some situations, the immobilization device is secured to the same spot, through perhaps predrilled holes along the lateral length of the table top, on both the simulator and treatment couch. During the treatment setup process the immobilization device is indexed or positioned on the treatment couch in the same position it was in during simulation.

Over the years, a number of immobilization devices have been developed and used to improve the treatment outcome for radiation therapy patients. Some of the devices are simple yet effective in immobilizing the patient. Others are more complex and are made individually for the particular patient. The choice of immobilization devices depends on many considerations, including the condition of the patient, the area to treated, and the availability and cost of materials. Radiation therapists must be prepared to recommend and use the appropriate device for a particular patient to ensure the best possible treatment outcome for that patient.

Operating Conventional Simulator Controls

Accurate patient positioning requires an understanding of how the mechanical, optical, and radiographic components of the simulator work. An understanding of their use is important. Mechanical components of the simulator include the motions of gantry rotation, collimator movements, and treatment couch. Optical components may include the laser system, optical distance indicator (ODI), and field light indicator.

Previous background in radiography and CT is helpful, but not essential, in understanding the radiographic components of the simulator. State regulations may require the use of technique charts, which include guidelines for selecting kVp, mA, and time factors used in deciding radiographic exposure techniques. In some institutions, in an attempt to increase familiarity with simulation procedures, certain therapists will perform most of the simulation procedures. This means they rotate less frequently, if at all, through other (treatment) areas of the department.

It is also important to know the limits of the mechanical, optical, and radiographic components. For example, it is important to know the limits of gantry rotation with the use of specific immobilization devices or table angles. This is helpful in avoiding possible collisions on the treatment unit. In addition, it is important to know how to handle a burned-out ODI light bulb partway through a simulation procedure. Can the simulation procedure be completed or should it be interrupted? This will depend on when during the simulation process the ODI fails.

Radiographically, obtaining good quality lateral pelvic radiographs may require the use of a double-exposure technique with some x-ray generators. This may be caused by heat limits on the x-ray tube. Two shorter exposures, instead of one longer one, may produce a better-quality radiograph. A lateral view of the pelvis can be a most challenging radiograph to produce for the radiation therapist.

Setting Field Parameters

Familiarity with both the controls in the simulator room and those located on the control console is essential for a smooth, accurate, and efficient simulation procedure. Once the patient has been oriented to the simulation procedure and positioned on the simulator couch, the actual localization process can begin.

Establishing the field parameters may be done in one or more sessions, depending on the complexity of the case. It is the complex cases that often require more than one session. In these situations the target volume may not be visible on routine radiographs. It may be close to sensitive structures. Sometimes previous diagnostic studies identifying the location of the target volume were obtained with the patient in a different position than that of the simulation. In those cases the primary purpose of the first simulation is to establish a frame of reference between the data obtained during simulation and previously obtained diagnostic information, such as a CT scan.[9]

Field parameters such as width, length, gantry angle, collimator angle, and position of the isocenter should be established for both the SSD and SAD (isocentric) setup. Initially an estimate of the tumor volume may be established before fluoroscopy. This may be done by positioning the isocenter and setting a field width and length. The isocenter is positioned at the CA (middle of the treatment field) on the patient's skin for an SSD approach and within the patient for a SAD technique. The locations of the CA and field edges are then more accurately localized, usually with the aid of fluoroscopy.

Orthogonal films, which provide three-dimensional information, may be used with the isocentric technique. An example may help clarify the use of these radiographs in tumor localization. Small fields treated to high doses are often used to control prostate cancer. Here the patient's isocenter may be established using contrast medium and documented with an orthogonal pair of radiographs. At this point, two radiographs have been taken to document the position of the isocenter. The primary purpose of the first simulation is to establish a frame of reference. A CT scan is then performed with the patient in the treatment position (perhaps in the radiology department). A shift in the isocenter may be necessary based on information about the tumor volume obtained from the CT scan. Any shifts can be measured from the original isocenter (first simulation) on the first day of treatment or verified on the simulator during a second session.

There is no one universally accepted approach to establishing the field parameters. For simple parallel opposed treatment fields a short simulation session may be all that is necessary. More complex cases can be simulated using various approaches. A longer single simulation session can be used to document the isocenter, field width, and length along with other setup parameters in more complex cases. Multiple simulation sessions can also be used, incorporating orthogonal films and/or CT treatment planning. Even longer sessions may be required if using a virtual simulation technique.[19] Whatever approach is used, it is necessary to document the treatment fields with radiographs. Whenever possible, a radiograph should be taken for each treatment portal.

PRODUCING QUALITY RADIOGRAPHIC IMAGES

Radiographic images taken at the time of simulation document the treatment portals. Not only do they serve as part of the patient's medical record but also they are used as masters to compare with portal images (taken on the treatment unit). Quality is important. Several aspects of producing good-quality radiographs are discussed in this section, including selecting exposure techniques, orienting the film, processing the film, and documenting the radiographic images.

Selecting appropriate radiographic exposure techniques is a complex process. Several important details contribute to choosing the best technical factors. The use of critical thinking skills is the secret to producing good-quality radiographs. This happens especially when those skills are applied to the four main technical factors (kVp, mA, time, and distance) in the right combination. Students should also be aware that exposure techniques will vary from one clinical site to the next and from one simulator to another.

Categorizing patients into a specific **body habitus** (general physical appearance and body build; see Chapter 18) is

helpful in selecting adequate exposure factors. Attenuation of the x-rays will vary, depending on the patient's thickness and, to a lesser degree, the body's composition. The composition of the patient's tissues can also change because of a specific disease process. For example, it is easier to penetrate the chest without the presence of pneumonia or congestive heart failure. Both pathologic conditions result in increased radiation absorption. Knowing when to deviate from average exposure factors displays evidence of good critical thinking skills and is often necessary to producing useful images, especially in systems without phototiming.

Before the technical factors are selected, several elements concerning the type and orientation of the film must be considered. Will a grid be used? Some departments may have the option of using a grid or various cassettes with different screen and film combinations. The use of a fast screen and film combination may provide the extra edge in obtaining a good-quality lateral radiograph of the pelvis. Other factors to consider before exposure include centering the film, reducing the size of the diaphragm opening, and setting an appropriate source-film distance. Some simulators will not allow an exposure unless the image intensifier is centered in relationship to the CA. Evidence of collimation, by reducing the diaphragm opening on the radiograph, should appear as a clear 1 to 2 cm border on the processed film. This not only makes it easier to visualize the **irradiated volume** and some surrounding anatomy but also reduces the amount of unwanted scatter radiation from reaching the film. Reducing scatter radiation generally improves radiographic contrast and the visibility of detail. Source-film distance should be recorded to document the magnification factor. This information may be needed for calculations or fabricating custom shielding blocks.

Phototiming is a form of automatic exposure control (AEC) in which one or more ionization cells automatically stop the exposure. With phototiming, the operator can preselect the desired density. Anatomically programmed radiography is also available. These systems are simply computerized technique charts. For example, a button representing an anatomic site is selected and then correlated to a small, medium, or large patient. They provide more consistency in the production of radiographs with appropriate contrast and density.

Quality control experts agree that the radiographic film processor is the most sensitive variable factor in the production of a radiograph.[8] It may be the therapist's responsibility, especially in smaller satellite facilities and freestanding clinics, to monitor the quality control of the processor. This may be done through film sensitometry using a densitometer. The whole process adds a few minutes to the morning warm-up procedure on the simulator. For the sake of convenience, a darkroom should be located near the simulator. One processor should adequately serve two simulators and several treatment units.

All radiographs should be documented with pertinent

patient information. Part of this process may occur in the darkroom, where information such as the patient's name, date, and identification number are permanently "stamped" on the film. Additional information, such as field size, gantry and collimator angle, SSD/SAD, source-film distance (SFD), treatment unit, and sometimes a reference to the radiation oncologist caring for the patient, is written on the radiograph after processing. Additional information included on the radiograph is helpful to someone comparing the port film (especially without the treatment chart or other details of the patient's history nearby) and includes the patient's diagnosis, incisions and palpable nodes, and other important reference points.[2] This can be done with a waxed pencil, felt-tipped marker, preglued simulation labels, or other suitable means. Each film should be identified for further reference and as part of the patient's legal medical record.

Documenting Pertinent Data

Information gathered during the simulation procedure needs accurate documentation. This information is essential to accurately reproduce the geometry of the setup on the treatment unit (Box 20-3). It is also used to maintain accurate medical records and to aid in the treatment planning and dose calculation processes. Documentation of pertinent information involves both marking the patient and documenting information in the patient's chart. Some institutions make use of a simulation worksheet designed to guide the therapist in documenting all of the patient's field parameters and measurements.

One of the most important measurements obtained during the conventional simulation process is the patient's intrafield distance (IFD) or separation. This measurement directly influences the dose to both the tumor and other, normal tissues. Therefore it is important to use a caliper correctly in determining the patient's IFD. If the treatment area is relatively flat, then one IFD measurement is generally taken at the CA. If the treatment area is sloped, as is often the case in the thorax, then multiple IFD measurements are obtained (superior, center, and inferior field edge). Caution must be used when obtaining an IFD value in an area where there may be an air gap, as is common in the cervical and lumbar regions. Here the lordotic curve is more pronounced. Accurate IFD measurements translate into accurate dose calculations.

There are two schools of thought in documenting and communicating the location of treatment fields. One method involves establishing marks on the patient's skin. The other method references bony landmarks in and around the treatment area.

Using bony landmarks the treatment field's CA and field edge(s) are referenced to specific anatomic landmarks. For example, in the treatment of head and neck cancer, the patient's CA might be referenced 2 cm inferior and 1.3 cm posterior to the external auditory meatus. Gerbi,[9] in describing the location of the treatment field using bony landmarks,

lists several advantages over the use of skin marks: (1) skin marks are highly mobile, especially for obese patients, whereas the location of the target volume remains essentially constant with respect to bony structures; (2) a resimulation is not required if the skin marks are lost; and (3) the treatment field can be easily reconstructed long after the current course of therapy.

External skin marks or permanent tattoos can also be used to reference the patient's treatment position. Small tattoos on the patient's skin may be used to reference the position of the treatment field's CA or field edges. They are applied at the time of simulation using India ink with a small gauge needle. Semipermanent marks, applied with felt-tipped markers or carfusion (a silver nitrate–based solution effective in "staining" the skin), also help to reference the treatment

Box 20-3	Documentation of Treatment Field Location

Machine parameters
Treatment SSD
Table top to isocenter distance
Collimator width
Collimator length
Gantry angle
Couch angle
Collimator angle
Multileaf collimator
Electron cone
Block tray
Patient's position
Supine/prone/other
Arm position
Leg position
Head support
Spirit level
Table pad/egg crate
Immobilization devices
Other special devices
Shifts from isocenter
Diagram of the field arrangement
Schematic diagram for field arrangement
Blocked field diagram
Location of central axis
Location of field edges
Location of tattoos
Reference to bony anatomy
Wedge orientation
Other pertinent data
Bolus
Wedges
Tissue compensator
Special instructions
Setup photographs

SSD, Source-skin distance.

area on the patient's skin but is less accurate. A small tattoo less than 1 mm in size provides more accuracy than skin marks for laser alignment. However, tattoos must be used with caution in certain circumstances, especially in cases of obesity, weight loss, and change in tumor size, in which the skin can shift in relation to the internal anatomy.[3] Some institutions employ a combination of both methods, depending on the individual case.

Information documented in the treatment chart to aid in the daily setup of the patient may be organized in several ways and is usually institutionally dependent. Fig. 20-20, *A* and *B*, illustrates treatment setup sheets in which pertinent data gathered

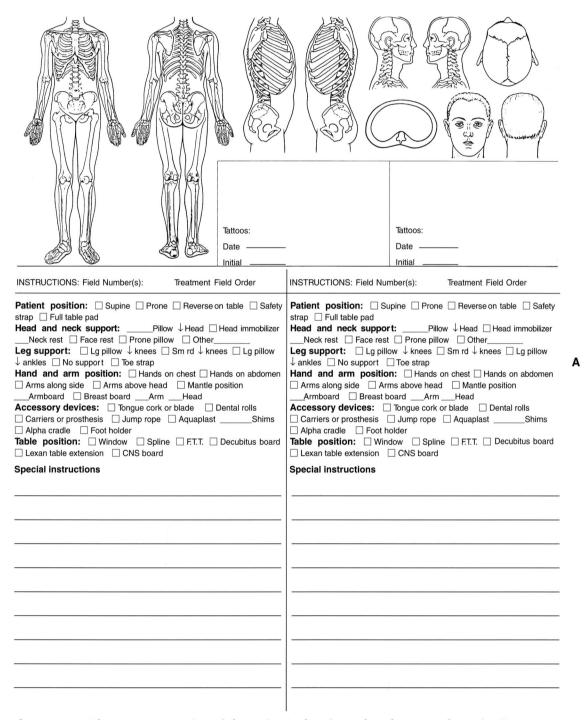

Tattoos:

Date ———

Initial ———

Tattoos:

Date ———

Initial ———

INSTRUCTIONS: Field Number(s):   Treatment Field Order

Patient position: ☐ Supine ☐ Prone ☐ Reverse on table ☐ Safety strap ☐ Full table pad
Head and neck support: _____ Pillow ↓ Head ☐ Head immobilizer ___ Neck rest ☐ Face rest ☐ Prone pillow ☐ Other_____
Leg support: ☐ Lg pillow ↓ knees ☐ Sm rd ↓ knees ☐ Lg pillow ↓ ankles ☐ No support ☐ Toe strap
Hand and arm position: ☐ Hands on chest ☐ Hands on abdomen ☐ Arms along side ☐ Arms above head ☐ Mantle position ___ Armboard ☐ Breast board ___ Arm ___ Head
Accessory devices: ☐ Tongue cork or blade ☐ Dental rolls ☐ Carriers or prosthesis ☐ Jump rope ☐ Aquaplast _____ Shims ☐ Alpha cradle ☐ Foot holder
Table position: ☐ Window ☐ Spline ☐ F.T.T. ☐ Decubitus board ☐ Lexan table extension ☐ CNS board

Special instructions

INSTRUCTIONS: Field Number(s):   Treatment Field Order

Patient position: ☐ Supine ☐ Prone ☐ Reverse on table ☐ Safety strap ☐ Full table pad
Head and neck support: _____ Pillow ↓ Head ☐ Head immobilizer ___ Neck rest ☐ Face rest ☐ Prone pillow ☐ Other_____
Leg support: ☐ Lg pillow ↓ knees ☐ Sm rd ↓ knees ☐ Lg pillow ↓ ankles ☐ No support ☐ Toe strap
Hand and arm position: ☐ Hands on chest ☐ Hands on abdomen ☐ Arms along side ☐ Arms above head ☐ Mantle position ___ Armboard ☐ Breast board ___ Arm ___ Head
Accessory devices: ☐ Tongue cork or blade ☐ Dental rolls ☐ Carriers or prosthesis ☐ Jump rope ☐ Aquaplast _____ Shims ☐ Alpha cradle ☐ Foot holder
Table position: ☐ Window ☐ Spline ☐ F.T.T. ☐ Decubitus board ☐ Lexan table extension ☐ CNS board

A

Special instructions

Figure 20-20. The treatment portion of the patient's chart is used to document the patient's setup parameters. Note institutional differences between **A** (Mayo Clinic, Rochester, Minnesota) and **B** (Central Maine Medical Center, Lewiston, Maine). Both provide documentation of pertinent patient data.

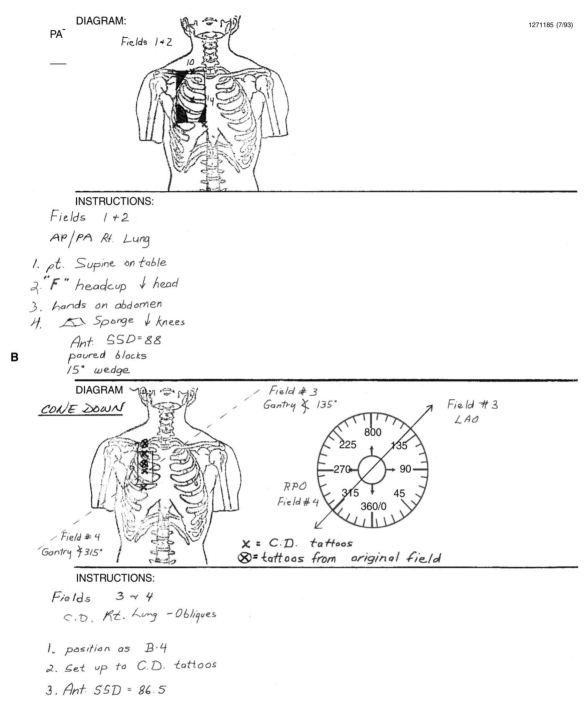

DIAGRAM:

PA⁻

Fields 1+2

1271185 (7/93)

INSTRUCTIONS:

Fields 1+2

AP/PA Rt. Lung

1. pt. Supine on table
2. "F" headcup ↓ head
3. hands on abdomen
4. ◁▷ Sponge ↓ knees
   Ant. SSD = 88
   poured blocks
   15° wedge

B

DIAGRAM

CONE DOWN

Field #3
Gantry ∡ 135°

Field #3
LAO

RPO
Field #4

Field #4
Gantry ∡ 315°

X = C.D. tattoos
⊗ = tattoos from original field

INSTRUCTIONS:

Fields 3 & 4

C.D. Rt. Lung – Obliques

1. position as B·4
2. Set up to C.D. tattoos
3. Ant. SSD = 86.5

Figure 20-20, cont'd.

from the simulation procedure are documented at two different clinical sites. Pertinent information should include machine parameters such as SSD; table top to isocenter distance; collimator width and length (field size); and gantry, couch, and collimator angles. Any indicated shifts from the isocenter should also be documented. A description of the patient's position along with any immobilization and support devices used in reproducing the patient's position should be documented. Included in the setup instructions is a schematic diagram of the field arrangement. Also included is a blocked diagram. This is helpful in orienting the therapist to the position of shielding blocks, location of the CA, and field edges. There should also be an area for setup photographs (if used); a face photo; and an area describing bolus, wedges, and tissue compensator.

CONTOUR DEVICES

A **contour** is a reproduction of an external body shape, usually taken through the transverse plane of the CA of the treatment beam (or center of the treatment volume).[2,35] Contours may be taken through other planes of interest in the treatment volume to provide more information about the overall dose distribution. A contour is usually taken at the end of the conventional simulation and treatment planning procedure when the treatment volume has been defined and verified with radiographic images and setup or alignment marks have been placed on the patient.

The purpose of a contour is to provide the therapist and dosimetrist with the most precise replica of the patient's body shape so that accurate information may be gathered concerning the dose distribution within the patient. The treatment volume and internal structures (tumor volume, critical organs) are transposed within the contour using data from the simulation images and/or CT or MRI films. Fig. 20-21 shows a typical patient contour taken with a conventional technique. The representation provides information essential to accurate treatment planning. At that point, isodose distributions from all treatment beams may be superimposed over the contour and summarized to produce the treatment plan.

Another purpose of a contour is to assist in repositioning the patient. A therapist or dosimetrist can check the location of field edges and treatment marks, the CA location, and separations at a glance. It is important to realize, however, that the information will only be as accurate as the data recorded.

Production of an accurate contour takes time. Often the contour is the last step in the simulation procedure, and accuracy may be compromised by the pressure to hurry and fin-ish as a result of patient physical or department schedule concerns.[28] If a contour is inaccurate, adequate treatment planning may be compromised. The setup distances may not correspond to the actual treatment distances encountered during patient positioning. This could translate into taking the patient back to simulation for a new contour, which in turn would require a new treatment plan and possibly a delay in the delivery of treatment.

Types of Contours

The most common type of contour is usually taken through one transverse plane of the body through the CA of the beam, typically within the treatment volume.[3,35] This type of contour runs across the patient, from left to right, and sections the patient into the upper and lower halves. The planes of the body are shown in Fig. 20-5. In treating an area with few variances in topography, it is reasonable to view the dose distribution through only one plane. However, when the patient's contour within the treatment volume varies more than a few centimeters, the dose distribution will not be the same as calculated through the CA transverse contour. In this case, off-axis contours should be taken to verify the dose distribution in these areas. An off-axis contour is any contour parallel to the CA transverse plane, in the inferior or superior directions. Fig. 20-22 demonstrates examples of sites where off-axis contours should be taken in the treatment of the chest (through anterior, posterior, or oblique fields) and in the treatment of the pelvis of an obese patient (through anterior and posterior fields).[3]

Another site where the patient contour varies considerably is in the head and neck area. This is true for both the transverse and the coronal planes. The lateral diameter of the patient's neck may differ significantly in the superior and inferior regions of the lateral treatment volume, as demonstrated in Fig. 20-23. When treating the head and neck with

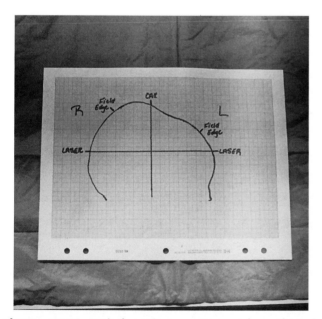

Figure 20-21. Typical patient contour taken through mechanical means. Note the common points of interest that are labeled for accurate use.

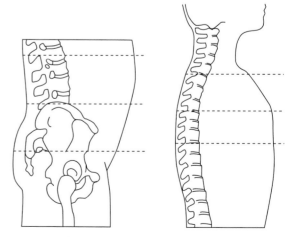

Figure 20-22. Examples of sites where off-axis contours are typically taken. Contours at different levels through the body provide information that is essential in treatment planning.

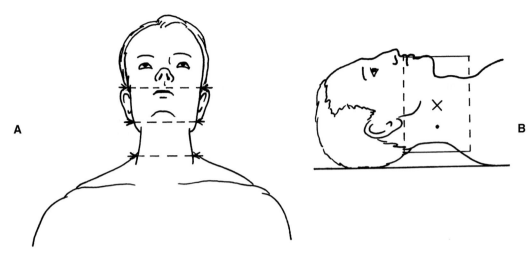

Figure 20-23. Lateral diameter of patient's neck **(A)** is significantly different in superior, central, and inferior regions **(B)** of the lateral treatment volume.

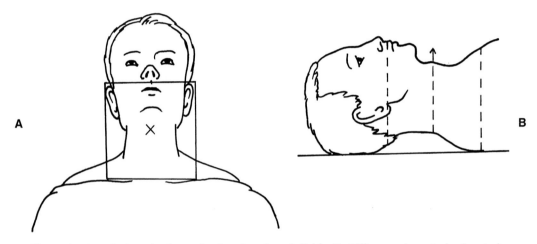

Figure 20-24. A, Anterior/posterior head and neck fields. **B,** Difference in anterior/posterior diameter within superior, central, and inferior regions of treatment volume.

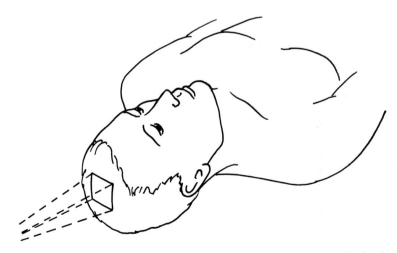

Figure 20-25. Coronal contour taken along lateral aspect of the body and through vertex of the head.

anteroposterior/posteroposterior (AP/PA) fields, the AP/PA diameter varies significantly from the superior to the inferior region of the treatment volume. Fig. 20-24 demonstrates this.

A coronal contour is one taken along the coronal plane of the body, cutting the patient in half from front to back. It is most likely to be used when parallel opposed beams enter the patient laterally or when a beam enters through the vertex of the head (Fig. 20-25). A coronal contour must include both the left and right sides of the body or it will not provide enough information to be useful.

A sagittal contour is taken along the median sagittal plane of the body, cutting the body into left and right halves, and is useful when there is a need to verify the dose distribution along the length of the body. Examples of sites where a sagittal contour may be useful are in AP/PA treatment of the head and neck and in the posterior spinal axis, as shown in Fig. 20-26. Additional measurements are needed to complete the anterior to posterior part of the contour.

It is evident that various contours can provide much needed information to the radiation therapy practitioner. Body topography must be taken into account when planning a patient's treatment regimen.[35]

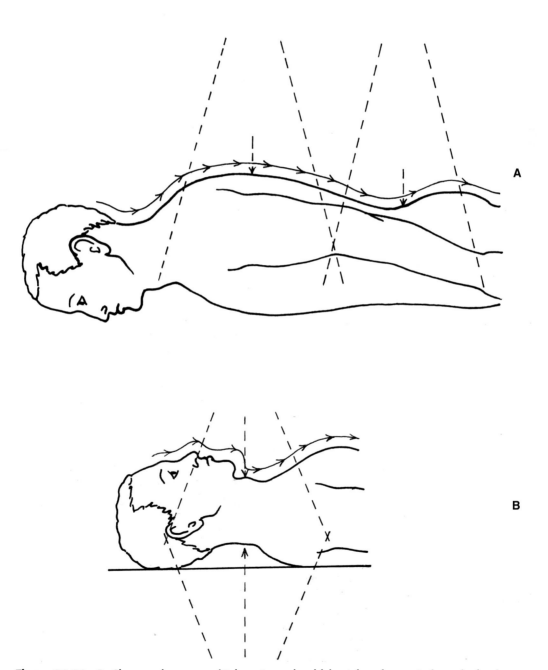

Figure 20-26. A, Shows where a sagittal contour should be taken for posterior spinal axis fields. **B,** Identifies where a sagittal contour should be taken for anterior/posterior neck fields.

Box 20-4	Contouring with Solder Wire: Points to Remember

1. The solder wire end may be rounded by holding a match under it for a few seconds after being measured out and before patient use. This lowers the opportunity to accidentally stick the patient.
2. An "R" and an "L" can be formed onto the ends of the wire to aid in remembering the corresponding side of the patient.
3. The solder wire should be cleaned with alcohol between uses. This eliminates confusion with old marks and achieves asepsis.

Most radiation therapy departments have preferences regarding the one or two contouring methods that fit their needs and will adhere to those methods for consistency.

Hand-molded Materials

Solder wire is a commonly used type of contouring material and is suitable for all body sites. It is inexpensive and readily available. Solder comes in various thicknesses; the thinner variety is more useful in the head and neck regions, whereas the thicker wire works well in areas that have large separations.

The advantages of using solder wire in contouring include the ability to cut it to any size needed, its pliability, and its reuse capacity. The major disadvantage is its pliability, which means the shape can be easily distorted. Extreme care must be taken when removing the molded solder wire from the patient so as to retain the exact shape. Sometimes it is difficult to mold the thicker solder wire around structures like the nose, lips, eyes, and ears. A slight amount of pressure must be applied when molding the solder wire, which can cause some patient discomfort and distortion. Box 20-4 notes points of interest that may be useful to the practitioner using this medium.

A plaster strip is another contouring material that can be used in any body site. These are the same type of strips used to make plaster immobilization devices. When determining the length of plaster strip to use, enough material should be used to span from the table top on one side of the patient to that on the other. Plaster strips work best when folded to approximately 2.5 cm wide and 6 to 8 layers thick. Although this thickness makes molding more difficult, the contour's shape will be easily retained. Use of hot water reduces the plaster drying time. Caution should be exercised so that the water temperature does not cause undue patient discomfort. As the plaster dries, it will give off some heat of its own. This is called an exothermic reaction, and patients should be made aware of this before contouring. Also, if the strip is to be made over any body hair, a layer of plastic wrap should cover the hair to avoid epilation on removal.[35] Fig. 20-27 demonstrates a contour being taken using a plaster strip.

Plaster is fairly inexpensive and is very easy to apply; very little pressure is needed to form an accurate shape. It is good for areas where there is a lot of detail, and it retains its shape very well. If the points on the patient have been marked with a dark ink, the marks will usually transpose right onto the plaster with very little distortion. This eliminates one step in the general process, that of having to remember to transpose the points onto the contour material. There are a few disadvantages when using plaster strip contouring. It can be messy. It also requires substantial drying time before it can be removed from the patient. Although there are fast-setting plaster strips with a drying time of 2 to 4 minutes, because of the thickness required of the strip it usually takes at least 5 to 6 minutes to dry adequately. If a patient is very uncomfortable or tired, this might not be the best method to use. It is also difficult to get an accurate contour around an area with a lot of hair.[35]

W.R. Aquaplast makes inexpensive 4.8-mm-diameter contour tubes in 3-ft lengths that can be used in most sites of the body. The tubes are hollow and made of a low-temperature thermoplastic that molds very easily. The shape of the contour is maintained very well, and the material can be used several times by reheating. Fig. 20-28 demonstrates a contour being taken with a thermoplastic tube. There are some disadvantages when using this product. It requires proper facilities for heating the water to the proper temperature (160° F) to make the tube pliable. The drying time of 2 to 5 minutes is similar to that for the plaster strip method. Although it is pliable, it is not pliable enough for very detailed areas, such as the ears, nose, lips, and eyes. There is also some shrinkage as the material hardens, which may produce contour inaccuracies.

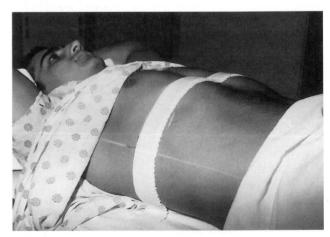

Figure 20-27. Contour being taken using a plaster strip.

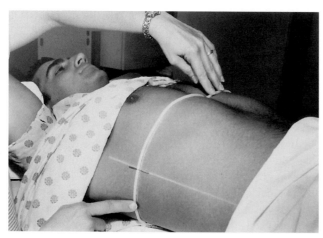

Figure 20-28. Contour being taken using a thermoplastic tube.

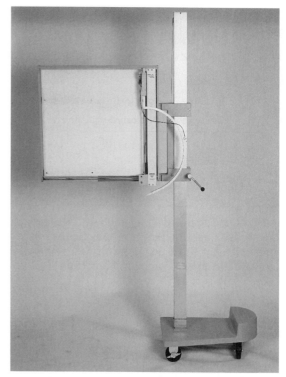

Figure 20-29. Pantograph contouring device on a rolling stand. *(Courtesy Radiation Products Design, Inc., Albertville, Minnesota.)*

Mechanical Contouring Device

Although there are many different types of mechanical devices used for contouring, two types are commonly used.

The most widely used and most accurate mechanical contouring device is the **pantograph** contour plotter. The physical contour of the patient is traced with a stylus, and the device transfers the body's transverse contour to an overhead drawing board by way of a pen attached to the arm of the stylus. There are several types of pantographs available; some can be mounted to a wall, and some are mounted on a rolling stand as shown in Fig. 20-29. These devices save a lot of time in that the contour is immediately transferred to the paper and only one person is required to use the device to obtain an accurate contour. Pantographs can be very good for tracing detailed areas of the body, such as the ears, nose, lips, and eyes (as long as the plotted points are close together). A major disadvantage is the cost of these devices. Also, they tend to be bulky and require adequate room for storage when not in use. Occasionally the lines may not be accurate if the patient is ticklish and moves while the therapist is tracing the stylus over the body.[3]

The second type of mechanical device consists of an array of low-friction nylon or aluminum rods, the tips of which are pulled down to touch the patient's skin surface in a 180-degree cross section, as shown in Fig. 20-30. The rods are locked into place, removed, and placed on a sheet of paper where the shape of the patient is traced. It is fairly easy to use devices of this type for any transverse contour site, and it requires only one person to operate. One disadvantage is that the size of the area to be contoured is limited by the size of the device. Also, these devices tend to be large and bulky, which could cause concern if used with an uncooperative patient. Translation of the information is also time consuming.

CT-generated contours are probably the most accurate of all transverse contouring methods, because there is no hand

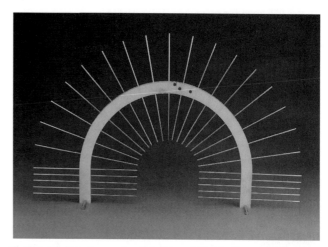

Figure 20-30. An example of a mechanical contour maker. The tips of the rods touch the skin surface and are locked in place to give a rendering of the patient's contour. *(Courtesy Radiation Products Design, Inc., Albertville, Minnesota.)*

molding or manipulation to introduce significant error. An important point to note is that the patient must be in the exact treatment position on the scanner with a flat table top comparable to the simulator and treatment tables. Because most scanners have concave table tops, a flat surface insert must be used.[35] Also, a large-diameter CT aperture (85 cm) should be

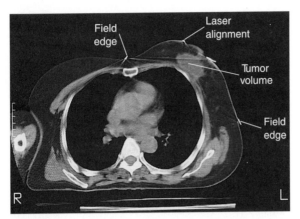

Figure 20-31. Computed tomography (CT) slice used for treatment planning. Note how the radiopaque markers on this breast patient show up. This provides useful information for the treatment planning team (tumor volume is marked).

used to allow patient positioning in the CT scanner that exactly matches simulation and treatment. Patient immobilization devices should be used that will not cause image artifacts.[18] Sometimes the total contour of the patient is missing from the field of view, especially on large patients, which would cause errors in the accuracy of the information. The external alignment marks on the patient should be marked with plastic, radiopaque catheters so they can be delineated on the CT scan for reference (Fig. 20-31).

MRI has versatility in producing contours in transverse, sagittal, and coronal planes. The same considerations for contouring should be followed as outlined for CT scanning.

Ultrasound imaging for delineating patient contours has been widely used in radiation therapy, although the image quality is not as good as CT. Deeply seated anatomic structures are not as easily defined as in CT and MRI. This being the case, the advantage of visualizing intricate anatomic detail is lost in the process.

Many different materials and devices are used in the production of contours, each having both advantages and disad-

vantages. Each department must assess its own needs in deciding which means are to be employed. Although CT is becoming the mainstay of patient contouring, any of the materials and methods described can be used effectively. Table 20-3 summarizes the advantages and disadvantages of each method.

TREATMENT VERIFICATION

As discussed earlier in the chapter, simulation can have more than one meaning. First, it is a general term describing the mockup process. This can include the selection of immobilization devices, radiographic documentation of treatment ports, measurement of the patient, construction of patient contours, and shaping of fields.[14] For most cases in most institutions, the word *simulation* is applied to this type of procedure. However, it can also refer to a type of treatment verification. This may be a more specific term, in which the simulator artificially duplicates the actual treatment conditions by confirming measurements, verifying treatment, and checking custom blocks.[34]

Verification simulation is a final check that each of the planned treatment beams covers the tumor or target volume and does not irradiate critical normal structures.[4] This is usually done as the second part of a two-step process on the simulator (it may also be performed on the treatment unit during the first day of treatment using portal images). It involves taking radiographic images or portal images of each of the treatment beams using external marks and other immobilization devices intended for treatment reproducibility. An example might help further explain this idea.

A patient with cancer involving the head of the pancreas might benefit from external beam radiation therapy. Two simulation procedures might be necessary. The first simulation is done to establish a point of reference for the radiation oncologist and treatment planning staff. This is accomplished through orthogonal films. An isocenter is located in the patient and then documented by reference to external landmarks or tattoos. At the end of the first simulation, a target volume has not been established. A field size may not have been selected. Before the second simulation (in this case

Table 20-3	Advantages and disadvantages of contouring materials/methods	
Material/Method	**Advantage**	**Disadvantage**
Solder wire	Reusability, pliability	Pliability (distortions)
Plaster strips	Inexpensive, transferability of surface ink markings	Drying time, messy, not reusable
Aquaplast contour tubes	Inexpensive, reusable, shapes well	Drying time, not well-suited for intricate areas
Pantograph contouring device	Time-saving operation, reproduces detail well	Cost, size, storage space required
CT	Accurate transverse views	Cost of interface
MRI	Accurate transverse, coronal, and sagittal contours	Cost of interface
Ultrasound	Discernible transverse correlation of internal structures	Poor quality of imaged deep structures

CT, Computed tomography; *MRI,* magnetic resonance imaging.

called treatment verification), additional treatment planning must be done.

Often the patient's tumor volume is drawn on the contour or planned with the aid of a CT or MRI scan with the patient in the treatment position. The information from the CT scan or contour is transferred to the treatment planning computer, where a new isocenter may be determined based on the extent of disease. Usually only a slight shift, if any, from the original isocenter is needed. The second simulation or verification is done as a final check. Does each of the treatment beams cover the target volume? Are any critical structures such as the spinal cord affected? Radiographic images of each of the treatment beams using external marks and other immobilization devices are taken to complete the verification process.

Verification of custom blocks is also done on the simulator. This is done to correct block cutting and mounting errors before the patient is treated. Small adjustments to custom blocks are not uncommon. Several potential causes for error exist in the use and fabrication of custom blocks. For example, setting incorrect SFD and source-tray-distance (STD) marks before cutting the blocks or orienting the blocks incorrectly on the tray can result in a misadministration of the treatment. An error of approximately ±3 mm in the size of the finished blocks can result if either too little or too much tension is applied to the hot cutting wire during the cutting procedure.[9] Johnson and Gerbi[15] describe a three-step block-checking procedure designed to eliminate blocking errors and increase treatment precision. The steps involve (1) a static light check on the simulator using the custom blocks and the original simulation radiograph, (2) a parallel opposed film check to check for block misalignment, and (3) a final block check with the patient on the simulator. Block verification can improve the precision, accuracy, and eventual outcome of the treatment.

Treatment verification, using portal images produced in the radiation therapy treatment room, on the first day of treatment provides additional assurance that the correct area is irradiated. Ideally, portal images of each treatment are compared with the simulation images before treatment. Greater differences between the simulation images and portal images as compared with differences between one portal image and the next have been documented.[24] Extra time should be scheduled the first day of treatment to evaluate the patient's position and verify the treatment plan. Errors and setup inaccuracies are more common during the transfer of information from the simulator to the treatment unit. This stresses the importance of verification on the first day of treatment.

SIMULATION USING A CT SIMULATOR

The use of CT simulators during tumor and normal tissue localization is fairly new. Pfizer in the 1970s and early 1980s attempted to market a type of CT simulation scanner. This failed for two reasons: the lack of high-quality DRRs and a limited treatment planning system that did not allow for inter-active definition of target volumes and dose calculations.[12] Four developments occurred in the early 1990s, which greatly affected radiation treatment planning:

1. Virtual simulation was introduced, which provide the ability to use a diagnostic-type scanner to take multiple images.
2. CT images on a standard treatment simulator were dramatically improved, which allowed them to be used for planning purposes.
3. Treatment panning computers were developed that could carry out three-dimensional treatment planning.
4. A true virtual simulator provided the ability to generate high-resolution DRRs.

A state-of-the-art CT simulator, specifically designed for the radiation therapy department, may include a high-performance CT scanner with laser and patient marking systems and a virtual simulator.[12] The localization and verification of a treatment field during CT simulation must reflect precisely what will happen in the treatment room. Patient position, beam alignment, and planning volume must be the same at the end of treatment planning and the beginning of treatment[27] (Table 20-4).

Policies and procedures should be developed within the radiation therapy department related to the unique issues involved in CT and virtual simulation procedures. Before introducing the many steps (Box 20-5) involved in the CT simulation process, some of the benefits, considerations, and limitations are discussed.[12,25,34]

Benefits of CT Simulation

1. CT simulation provides the ability to outline critical structures and view an up-to-date image of the potential target volume and lymph nodes.
2. CT simulation allows for unconventional beam orientations with ease.
3. Cone down or boost fields can be accomplished without the patient present.
4. Beams eye view display allows anatomy to be viewed from the perspective of the radiation beam.
5. CT simulation allows field shaping electronically at the graphic display station.
6. Virtual simulation allows comparison of beams and construction of DRRs without the patient present.

Considerations and Limitations of CT Simulation

1. The size of the aperture of the CT scanner must be large enough to accommodate patients in the treatment position with immobilization devices.
2. Patient couch must simulate treatment couch including the width and shape of the couch.
3. Laser system to localize isocenter must be present.
4. The time between the start of CT acquisition and patient marking must be minimized to avoid potential patient movement.
5. Careful consideration must be taken when using CT numbers for dose inhomogeneity corrections.
6. Certain beam-shaping devices and treatment accessories such as block verification have limited use.

In the following section, CT simulation procedures are

Table 20-4	Summary of CT simulation major steps	
With a Dedicated CT Simulator	**Without a Dedicated CT Simulator**

• Explanation of procedure • Straighten patient • Immobilization and positioning • Administration of contrast ↓ • Mark reference point on patient using laser system ↓ • Scout or Pilot film (preliminary image) • Physician selects area to scan ↓ • CT scan completed using appropriate scan as designed by the specific department protocol • Transfer reconstructed image to virtual simulation station ↓ Virtual simulation station • Contouring • Localize tumor and target volumes and normal structures ↓ • Determination of target isocenter and transfer to patient using laser system • Patient is marked, patient leaves ↓ • Transfer CT scan to treatment planning system	• Explanation of procedure • Strighten patient • Immobilization and positioning • Administration of contrast ↓ • Localize are of interest • Take orthogonal films • Mark reference point on patient using laser system ↓ • Patient gets a CT • The patient is aligned to reference points • Patient marks are the beginning point for CT scan. CT is "zeroed out" • CT scan is transferred to TP system to optimize plan ↓ • If no DRRs can be created, the patient is brought to the conventional simulator to document treatment portals

CT, Computed tomography; *DRR*, digitally reconstructed radiographs; *TP*, treatment planning.

Box 20-5	Procedure Outline for Computed Tomography (CT) Simulation

1. Presimulation planning
2. Room preparation
3. Explanation of procedure
4. Patient positioning and immobilization
5. CT data acquisition
6. Target and normal tissue localization
7. Virtual simulation of treatment fields
8. Generation of dose distributions
9. Documenting pertinent data
10. Final procedures

discussed in detail. The CT simulation process consists of consultation with the patient, fabrication, and registration of immobilization devices, CT data acquisition, target and normal tissue localization, virtual simulation of treatment fields, generation of dose distributions, marking of the patient with planned fields, and production of images for treatment verification (DRRs).[35] Consultation of the patient occurs in the same manner as in conventional simulation. Tumor localization, isodose planning, and block design take on new dimensions with CT simulation. These occur using virtual simulation.

Virtual simulation simulates fluoroscopy in conventional simulation. Once scans are completed through the area of interest, it is transferred to the virtual simulator via local area network. At this station, physicians working with dosimetrists and/or radiation therapists can delineate tumor and critical structures. After the target volume is delineated, the patient is marked. Virtual simulation can generate DRRs once the treatment planning is finalized. Without the ability to create DRRs, the patient may need to return for a conventional simulation, which incurs additional time and cost and provides a greater chance for error.[12]

Presimulation Planning

The presimulation planning for CT simulation is the same as conventional simulation. The physician and therapist need to be aware of the limitations of the CT scanner especially with regard to immobilization and patient positioning. Discussion with the patient should also include the time involved for the procedure. Will the acquisition of data and generation of dose distribution occur in one session or divided into two sessions? Will this be a simple or complex simulation? Who will be present during the simulation?

Room Preparation

The room preparation for CT simulation is similar to conventional simulation. In addition, contrast agents used in conventional simulation or in diagnostic CT scanning can also be considered in the CT simulation process. Special attention to the fabrication and registration of immobilization devices should be given careful thought because of the aperture (bore) size of the scanner.

Explanation of Procedure

As with conventional simulation, patients are told to hold still and breath normally. This may be in contrast to diagnostic CT in which patients may be asked to hold their breath. The simulation time may also vary, depending on the institution and the needs of the patient. It is possible to complete the patient portion of the simulation (data acquisition and temporary marking) in 10 to 15 minutes. If the CT simulation session encompasses all facets of planning while the patient remains on the scanner couch for the duration, the session will generally exceed 30 minutes, require additional staff, and possibly require a further verification simulation on a conventional simulator.[12]

Patient Positioning and Immobilization

Many of the same considerations used with conventional simulation are appropriate for CT simulation. Optimizing the patient position and immobilization device depends on several factors including the patient medical condition and treatment technique.[12] The transfer of information, such as the exact location of immobilization devices, from simulation to the treatment machine is improved when devices are referenced or indexed to the treatment table (Fig. 20-32). The patient and immobilization device are then "locked" into place on the treatment table using a system of numbered or lettered holes, or notches, along the lateral edge of the carbon fiber table top. This should reduce the possibility of movement and increase daily reproducibility of the treatment setup.[37] Initially, the patient should be clinically straightened and marked before scanning. This may provide documentation related to patient movement during the data acquisition phase of the simulation. It also provides temporary reference marks that may be used later in the simulation process. A scout scan may be performed to simulate fluoroscopy on the conventional simulator and check patient alignment.

Immobilization devices are also fabricated as in conventional simulation. The CT scanner may have limitations on

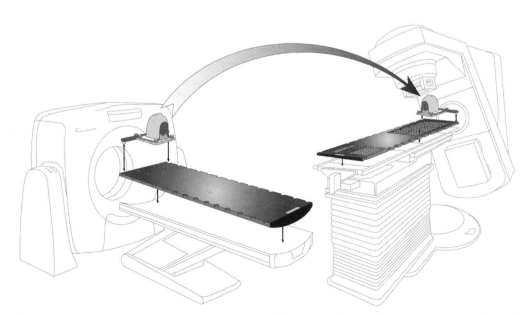

Figure 20-32. This drawing of a CT simulator and linear accelerator shows a thermoplastic mask used primarily to immobilize the head and neck area, indexed to both the simulator and treatment couch. (*Artwork courtesy MED-TEC, Orange City, Iowa.*)

the number and type of immobilization device, depending on the size of the aperture. Before beginning the scan, the therapist should be sure that the devices and the patient will fit into the CT scanner. For example, a patient treated for breast cancer with a steep slope may need an angle board for treatment. Depending on the type and angle of breast board, the patient and device may not fit into the scanner.

CT Data Acquisition

Spiral scanners are especially applicable to CT simulation. They transport the patient through the gantry aperture while continuously rotating the x-ray source.[12] The CT process begins with a scout or pilot image. This is accomplished by scanning the patient quickly in the inferior/superior dimension to obtain data used to reconstruct an image that looks similar to a radiograph (Fig. 20-33). The image is used to select the area to be scanned. Departmental protocol may identify the number of cuts, thickness of the cuts, and in some circumstances the space between cuts. Often in the newer scanners these protocols are preset.

The therapist must select an inferior and superior reference border on the patient indicating to the computer the volume of tissue to be scanned in the craniocaudal direction. Less is best, because data acquisition generates huge volumes of data and heat units on the x-ray tube. If heat units can be minimized during the scan, it will extend the life of the x-ray tube, depending on the type of scan used with spiral CT and thickness of slice, the actual scan time may be only 2 to 3 minutes. Slice thickness and spacing are important criteria in obtaining CT studies beneficial to producing high-quality DRRs. Some scanners provide limited slice thickness settings (e.g., 2 mm or 5 mm) and slice spacing (e.g., 2 mm, 3 mm, or 5 mm) during the actual scan.[20] For optimal image reconstruction needed to produce a high-quality DRR, slice thickness and slice spacing should be evaluated for each anatomic region. Gerbi[9] recommends thin CT scans with no more than 5-mm spacing to reduce the problem of volume averaging while accurately representing the target in three-dimensional space. To maximize the useful resolution on the DRR when performing CT simulation of the head and neck, Martin[20] recommends acquiring 1-mm slices at 1-mm spacing through the region containing tumor and 3-mm slices at 3-mm spacing through peripheral areas of the treatment volume. Not only are slice thickness and spacing important in producing useful DRRs but also they affect storage and communication components within the computer system.

Target and Normal Tissue Localization

Once data generated from the CT scanner has been reconstructed and transferred to the virtual simulation workstation, target and normal tissue localization can begin. The virtual simulation workstation may consist of a second computer with a monitor and keyboard located adjacent to the CT simulator workstation. In addition, other monitors and keyboards may be located in other work areas within the radiation ther-

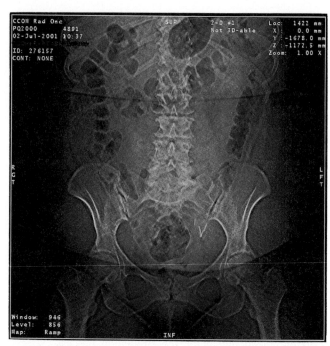

Figure 20-33. The computed tomography (CT) process begins with a scout or pilot image, sometimes referred to as a "topogram." This is accomplished by scanning the patient quickly in the inferior/superior dimension to obtain information needed to reconstruct a digitally reconstructed radiograph (DRR) image that looks similar to a radiograph.

apy department. If the intent is to mark and plan the patient during a single CT simulation session, simultaneous and fast network transfer of data between the CT console and the virtual simulation workstation is essential to help minimize patient motion between scanning and field marking.[20] The physician must localize the target volume and identify critical normal tissue structures on each of the high-resolution two-dimensional CT images obtained during the scanning process. This is probably the most labor-intensive step in CT simulation. Attention to detail is a must. The software must be easy to use and provide a number of options for the user to localize and draw volumes on each scan. Van Dyk and Mah[34] describe six important recommendations for accurate, flexible, and fast localization of normal and critical structures:

1. The tools for entering outlines on each scan include keyboard, mouse, trackball, light-pens, and others. Although individuals will have preferences, response time and accuracy should be considered priorities.
2. Manual localization options should include point and click and continuous modes to "draw" on the scan. Interpolation between slices and the ability to copy an outline to other images can aid in this process.
3. Semiautomatic or automatic localization options should be available to outline normal structures demonstrating high contrast with adjacent tissues such as skin, lung, spinal cord, and bone.

4. The ability to automatically add uniform and nonuniform margins around localized volumes will aid in the implementation of tissue and tumor volumes described in *ICRU Report 50* (Figs. 20-2 and 20-3).
5. Editing functions such as erase, stretch, translate, scale, and rotate, as well as the ability to edit CT numbers, should be applicable to single-slice outlines or to entire structures.
6. Measuring functions of the virtual simulation workstation should include rulers, statistics, voxel values, and CT histograms.

Virtual Simulation of Treatment Fields

The field size for each treatment field is established at the virtual simulation station after the target and normal tissue localization process has been competed. Unlike conventional simulation, the fields can be designed, if desired, after the patient has left the CT scanner.

Hunt and Coia[12] describe three levels of complexity in the virtual simulation process. A simple level, in which the fields are based on anatomic landmarks. In this case, a scan would be completed and DRRs would be constructed. No other planning would be necessary. The next level uses CT to localize target volumes and normal tissue structures; however, little isodose planning would be necessary. The most complex field design involve cases in which beams are determined by graphical isodose planning. The physician must communicate preferences for beam arrangements to the treatment planner. The virtual simulation process determines the isocenter in reference to marks placed on the patient earlier in the simulation process.

Generation of Dose Distributions

Dose distributions, calculated by the treatment planning system, are based on the target drawings on each CT slice transferred to the system. Dose distribution is based on information gained from the patient's external contour, the outlined targets to be irradiated, and any internal organs of interest.[29] Treatment planning systems allow dose computation from CT numbers. A CT number, which corresponds to the electron density of a specific tissue such as lung, soft tissue, and bone, is set at −1000 for air (zero density), 0 for water (unit density), 15 for cerebrospinal fluid (CSF), 20 for blood, 40 for gray matter, 50 for muscle, and 1000 for dense bone.[12,25] The dose calculation algorithms that use electron density values derived from CT images are complex and require computer processing. One type of algorithm, which can produce greater accuracy at the expense of increased computational time, is the Monte Carlo technique. This calculation technique predicts dose distribution from a beam of radiation passing through a patient by simulating the behavior of a large number of photons that make up the beam.[29]

DOCUMENTING DATA

Information documented in the treatment chart to aid in the daily setup of the patient may be organized in several ways and is usually institutionally dependent. Patient position and immobilization devices must be documented. A digital camera can capture the patient's position and immobilization devices as they appeared during the simulation process. This information can then be transferred to the verification and record system for use during treatment. With CT simulation, the exact field size, gantry position, and shielding are often completed after the treatment plan is completed. Otherwise, either isocenter or field edge marking systems, available with the CT simulator, can be used to mark the patient. Recall that with CT simulation, the patient is temporarily marked with reference points before scanning. Thus after the target volume has been determined, the computer calculates the isocenter, with reference to the temporary marks, and the lasers and/or couch are adjusted automatically. Movable lasers can be used for all three reference points. Field edge marking systems are available with some CT scanners used to control the position of lasers that identify on the patient's skin the superior, inferior, and lateral field borders and/or isocenter.[31] If the treatment unit is equipped with a verification and record system, patient setup data can be captured and transferred.

EMERGENCY PROCEDURES

Any sudden, unexpected situation requiring immediate attention is an emergency. Fortunately the radiation oncology department generally does not experience this often. There are, of course, emergencies in which a patient may need immediate treatment because of the sudden onset of symptoms. Examples of this include treatment for spinal cord compression, excessive bleeding, or a life-threatening obstruction caused by the unchecked growth of the tumor. Even in these situations there is some time for planning. The simulation procedure can be discussed and a plan developed for the patient's treatment. This plan may be as simple as several large fractions of radiation to a single field.

There are other situations arising during a simulation procedure that may require immediate attention. Certification in cardiopulmonary resuscitation equips the therapist to respond to specific medical conditions involving an obstructed airway or heart attack. In addition, a "crash cart" should be available. Usually the cart contains specific drugs and equipment needed to respond to certain emergencies, such as cardiac arrest or anaphylactic shock. The most common cause of anaphylactic shock during a simulation procedure is an allergic reaction to the contrast medium.

In any case there should be access to a nearby phone to initiate a response. Many hospitals have specific procedures to initiate a rapid response, such as "code 99" or "code blue." Knowing what to do before an emergency occurs can sometimes make the difference.

The mechanical operations of the simulator equipment can create a potential hazard to the patient and medical personnel. Knowing the location of "emergency off" switches is vital. These switches, which cut the power to the mechanical motions of the gantry and treatment couch, are generally incorporated into the room design and strategically located on the walls. It is also important to know the location of the main circuit breaker for the simulator. The circuit breaker generally controls power to both the mechanical components and the x-ray generator. Emergency switches are also incorporated into the simulator controls, both in the room and remotely in the shielded control area. An observation window allows the radiation therapist and others involved in the simulation process to view the patient and mechanical motions of the equipment. It is made of thick plate glass or leaded glass and installed in the control area along the wall facing the simulator. Anticollision devices, mounted on the collimator head and image intensifier of a conventional simulator, may prevent a potential collision by terminating the power and/or sounding an audio alarm. Some CT simulators are equipped with an integrated computer circuitry that prevents collisions by monitoring each component through a type of internal surveillance. In addition, some simulation rooms are equipped with cameras and monitors similar to those found in the treatment rooms.

The response to any sudden, unexpected situation requiring immediate attention during the simulation procedure should be well thought out in advance. Many potential emergency situations are minimized through careful planning of the procedure and observation of the equipment.

SUMMARY OF SIMULATION PROCEDURES

Patients treated with radiation therapy, either for cure or for palliation, will be involved in various procedures, including simulation. It helps in figuring out the location and extent of the patient's disease. The simulation process may include presimulation planning, room preparation, patient positioning and immobilization, operation of controls, setting field parameters, radiographic exposure, documenting pertinent data, treatment verification, and emergency procedures.

The outcome of the simulation procedure should define the anatomic area so that it is reproducible for daily treatment. Landmarks may be used to document and position the CA and field edges during a simulation procedure (Table 20-5). A complicated simulation is of little value unless it is reproducible. This means the ultimate success or failure of treatment may be directly related to the effectiveness of the simulation process.

Achieving ideal results in radiation therapy depends on delivering an appropriate dose to a well-defined region and at the same time reducing the dose to normal critical structures. Accomplishing this task demands a high degree of precision and accuracy in delivering the dose. In addition, a systematic and logical approach to the treatment of the particular disease is necessary. The use of the simulator is essential in achieving this goal.[9]

Table 20-5	Anatomic landmarks of the head and neck region
Landmark	**Description**
Superior orbital margin (SOM)	The roof of the of the orbit
Inferior orbital margin (IOM)	Forms the lateral margin of the bony orbit
External occipital protuberance (EOP)	The central prominence in the occipital bone
Mastoid process	The most lateral and inferior extension of the temporal bone
Zygomatic arch	The bony prominence of the cheek
Glabella	Located between the orbits
Nasion	The depression at the base of the nose
Inner canthus (IC)	Located at the medial aspect of the eye where the upper and lower eyelids meet
Outer canthus (OC)	Located at the outer aspect of the eye where the upper and lower eyelids meet
Tragus	Located near the external auditory meatus
Commissure of the mouth	Located at the junction of the upper and lower lip
C1	Lies inferior to the mastoid process
C2	Located at the level of the angle of the mandible
C3-4	Lies at the level of the hyoid bone
C4	Corresponds to the level of the thyroid cartilage
C6	Located at the level of the cricoid cartilage
C7	The first prominent process of the cervical vertebrae
Sternocleidomastoid muscle	A thick band of muscle in the neck, originating at the level of sternum and clavicle and inserting at the mastoid process of the temporal bone

Review Questions

1. A patient's separation = 25 cm. If the posterior SSD = 89 cm, what will the anterior SSD measure be?
   a. 87.5 cm
   b. 89 cm
   c. 88.25 cm
   d. 86 cm
2. Mr. Carson has metastatic cancer originating from the prostate. He has been coming to the radiation oncology department for months and is about to be simulated for the third time. Before you bring him into the room Mr. Carson says, "I don't know why I am here today. These treatments are not doing any good. This is my third time back to see you." Your best response would be
   a. "Now, now, Mr. Carson. You know these treatments will make you feel better."
   b. "Once you start the treatments you will feel better— just wait and see."
   c. "It seems you feel discouraged because these treatments are not working, Mr. Carson."
   d. "Now, what do you expect, Mr. Carson? You do have metastatic disease."
3. The GTV treatment volume will contain
   a. Tumor
   b. Involved lymphatics
   c. Normal tissue
   d. All of the above
4. _____ is the initial phase of treatment planning in which actual visualization of the treatment volume is documented before treatment.
   a. Initial consultation
   b. Simulation
   c. Brachytherapy
   d. Radiation treatment
5. The distance from a source of radiation to a radiograph is
   a. SAD
   b. SFD
   c. SSD
   d. All of the above
6. The distance from a source of radiation to the patient's skin is
   a. SAD
   b. SSD
   c. SDD
   d. SFD
7. Traits of a therapeutic listener are
   a. Desire to listen, respond, and solve the patient's problems
   b. Partially listen so you can prepare your response ahead of time
   c. Listen while you work as quickly as possible, so you do not fall behind schedule
   d. All of the above

8. When simulating the chest, which major landmark(s) can be used to straighten the patient?
   a. Suprasternal notch
   b. Xiphoid
   c. Vertebrae
   d. All of the above
9. Which of the following is not a desirable quality of an effective and useful immobilization device?
   a. Ensures immobilization with minimal patient discomfort
   b. Requires additional setup time
   c. Is durable enough to withstand the entire treatment plan
   d. Achieves conditions prescribed in treatment plan
10. Patient immobilization is important because
   a. Sophisticated treatment planning techniques allow more accurate delivery of treatment
   b. Missing the tumor once or twice in a treatment course can reduce planned dose by 10% or more
   c. Daily reproduction of the planned treatment is essential to treatment outcomes
   d. All of the above

Questions to Ponder

1. Discuss the importance of the presimulation consultation among radiation team members.
2. Explain the differences between GTV, CTV, and PTV.
3. While in the middle of a simulation the SAD is inadvertently changed from 100 cm to 110 cm. Will the size field change? If so, how can the simulation therapist detect this change?
4. Discuss several ways that you can check a patient's separation and SSDs while simulating the patient.
5. Write out an appropriate explanation for a patient about to have a simulation for lung cancer.
6. Describe at least six treatment parameters documented during a simulation procedure and discuss their importance.
7. Describe the importance of immobilization devices in radiation therapy.
8. Describe the differences between patient positioning and immobilization devices.
9. Compare and contrast the differences between conventional and CT simulation.

REFERENCES
1. American Registry of Radiologic Technologists: *Conventions specific to the radiation therapy technology examination,* St. Paul, Minn, 1995, American Registry of Radiologic Technologists
2. Bentel GC: *Radiation therapy planning,* New York, 1993, McGraw-Hill.
3. Bentel GC: *Patient positioning and immobilization in radiation oncology,* New York, 1999, McGraw-Hill.
4. Bleehen NM, Glatstein E, Haybittle JL: *Radiation therapy planning,* New York, 1983, Marcel Dekker.

5. Bomford CK, et al: Treatment simulators, *Br J Radiol* (suppl 23):17-22, 1989.

6. Bushong SC: *Radiologic science for technologists: physics, biology, and protection,* ed 8, St. Louis, 2001, Mosby.

7. Byhart R.W, Cox JD, Hornburg A, et al: Weekly localization films and detection of field placement errors, *Int J Radiat Oncol Biol Phys* 4:881-887, 1978.

8. Carlton RR, McKenna-Adler A: *Principles of radiographic imaging,* Albany, NY, 2000, Delmar.

9. Gerbi B J: The simulation process in the determination and definition of treatment volume and treatment planning. In Levitt SH, Khan FM, Potish, RA, Perez CA, editors: *Levitt and Tapley's technological basis of radiation therapy: clinical application,* ed 3, Philadelphia, 1999, Lippincott Williams & Wilkins.

10. Goitein M: Applications of computed tomography in radiotherapy treatment planning. In Orton CG, editor: *Progress in medical radiation physics,* New York, 1982, Plenum.

11. Hendrickson FR: Precision in radiation oncology, *Int J Radiat Oncol Biol Phys* 8:311-312, 1982.

12. Hunt M, Coia L: The treatment planning process. In Purdy JA, Starkschall G, editors: *3D planning and conformal radiation therapy,* Madison, Wisc, 1999, Advanced Medical Publishers.

13. ICRU Report 50. Prescribing, recording, and reporting photon beam therapy, Bethesda, Md, 1993, International Commission on Radiation Units and Measurements.

14. Inter-Society Council for Radiation Oncology: *Radiation oncology in integrated cancer management,* Philadelphia, 1991, American College of Radiology.

15. Johnson JM, Gerbi BJ: Quality control of custom block-making in radiation therapy, *Med Dosimetry* 14:199, 1989.

16. Karzmark CJ, Nunan CS, Tanabe E: *Medical linear accelerators,* New York, 1993, McGraw-Hill.

17. Keller R: Immobilization devices. In Washington CM, Leaver DT, editors: *Principles and practice of radiation therapy,* St. Louis, 1996, Mosby.

18. Khan FM: *The physics of radiation therapy,* ed 2, Baltimore, 1994, Williams & Wilkins.

19. Manolis J: Personal communication, St. Louis, May 1994, The Mallinckrodt Institute of Radiology, Washington University School of Medicine.

20. Martin EE: CT simulation hardware. In Purdy JA, Starkschall G, editors: *3D planning and conformal radiation therapy,* Madison, Wisc, 1999, Advanced Medical Publishers.

21. Med-Tec, Inc, Orange City, Iowa. Personal communication, March 2002.

22. Mizer S, Scheller RR, Deye JA: *Radiation therapy simulation workbook,* New York, 1986, Pergamon.

23. O'Connor-Hartsell S, Hartsell W: Minimizing errors in patient positioning, *Radiat Ther* 3:15-19, 1994.

24. Perez CA, Brady LW: *Principles and practice of radiation oncology,* ed 3, Philadelphia, 1998, Lippincott-Raven.

25. Purdy JA: Principles of radiologic physics, dosimetry and treatment planning. In Perez CA, Brady LW, editors: *Principles and practice of radiation oncology,* ed 3, Philadelphia, 1998, Lippincott-Raven.

26. Purtilo R: *Ethical dimensions in the health professions,* Philadelphia, 1981, WB Saunders.

27. Rabinowitz I, et al: Accuracy of radiation field alignment in clinical practice, *Int J Radiat Biol Phys* 11:1857, 1985.

28. Rathe JC, Elliott P: *Radiographic tumor localization,* St. Louis, 1982, Warren H Green.

29. Redpath AT, McNee SG: Treatment planning for external beam therapy: advanced techniques. In Williams JR, Thwaites DI, editors: *Radiotherapy physics in practice,* Oxford, UK, 2000, Oxford University Press.

30. Sampiere VA, Khan FM, Delclos L: Treatment aids for external-beam radiotherapy. In: Levitt SH, Tapley N, editors: *Technological basis of radiation therapy: practical clinical applications,* Philadelphia, 1984, Lea & Febiger.

31. Smith L: Picker International, Inc, personal communication, April, 1995.

32. Smithers Medical Products, Inc, Tallmadge, Ohio. Personal communication, March 2002

33. Soffen EM, et al: Conformal static field therapy for low volume prostate cancer with rigid immobilization. *Int J Radiat Oncol Biol Phys* 20:141-146, 1991

34. Van Dyk JV, Mah K: Simulation and imaging for radiation therapy planning. In Williams JR, Thwaites DI, editors: *Radiotherapy physics in practice,* Oxford, UK, 2000, Oxford University Press.

35. Washington CM, Taylor F: Contours. In Washington CM, Leaver DT, editors: *Principles and practice of radiation therapy,* St. Louis, 1996, Mosby.

36. WFR/Aquaplast Corp, Wyckoff, NJ. Personal communication, April 2003.

37. Leaver DT: IMRT: Part 2. *Radiat Ther* 11:17-32, 2003.

BIBLIOGRAPHY

Leaver DT: IMRT: Part 1, *Radiat Ther* 11:106-124, 2002.
Leaver DT: IMRT: Part 2, *Radiat Ther* 11:17-32, 2003.

Photon Dosimetry Concepts and Calculations

Charles M. Washington, Julius Armstrong

Outline

Key Terms

INTRODUCTION AND PERSPECTIVE

The administration of ionizing radiation for cancer treatment requires knowledge of anatomy, physics, and biologic responses. The success or failure of a radiation therapy course depends on adequate and accurate delivery of radiation to a localized site outlined by a radiation oncologist. The treatment planning team has to quantify the overall prescribed dose of radiation and determine how much dose will be delivered over the time frame outlined. There are many parameters of photon beam dose calculation that must be addressed; the radiation therapist and medical dosimetrist must be able to determine treatment machine settings to deliver the prescribed dose through manual and computerized methods.

Today, more and more emphasis is placed on determining dose delivery to volumes of tissues. Understanding volumetric dose concepts require a basic understanding of the factors that affect dose delivery and a comfort level with **monitor unit** (MU), a measure of output for linear accelerators, and point-dose calculations. It is not possible to cover every established method of performing dose calculation, as most clinical settings have site-specific methods for calculating dose, normally determined by a medical radiation physicist. This chapter provides clinical examples of dose calculations, both MU and time, examples that encompass components used in treatment planning. This will allow the treatment planning and delivery team to use the principles presented with the calculation methods employed in any radiation therapy center.

It is important to mention that this chapter was written with the beginning practitioner in mind. A brief review of basic terminology and concepts provides a basic overview, starting with basic calculations and then moving toward the more advanced calculations.

RADIATION THERAPY PRESCRIPTION

When a patient requires medicine to address an ailment, the physician writes a medical prescription. That prescription is a communication tool between the physician and the pharmacist. The medical prescription provides the pharmacist the name of the medication as well as its dose, route, and quantity and must also state how often and how long the patient should take the medicine. The pharmacist must also be familiar with the effects of the drug or combination of drugs prescribed.

The **radiation therapy prescription** is a communication tool between the radiation oncologist and the treatment planning and delivery team, particularly the radiation therapist and medical dosimetrist. The prescription provides the information required to deliver the appropriate radiation treatment. This legal document defines the treatment volume, intended tumor dose (TD), number of treatments, dose per treatment, and frequency of treatment.[2] The prescription also states the type and energy of radiation, beam-shaping devices such as wedges and compensators, and any other appropriate factors. The radiation therapist must be able to discuss with the patient the treatment procedure, function of the devices, and treatment side effects. In practice, there is no standard radiation therapy prescription. The organization and detail of prescriptions vary from one radiation therapy center to another. It is very important that the radiation prescription be clear, precise, and complete. For example, if a thorax is to be treated using anterior and posterior opposed fields, the prescription commonly sets a spinal cord limit not to exceed 4500 cGy. This instruction should be clear and exact; there should be no instruction that is open to interpretation. Every parameter and phase of the treatment must be clearly defined in the radiation therapy prescription.

The radiation oncologist will commonly define the region to be treated, technique, treatment machine, energy, fractionation, and daily and total doses within a radiation prescription form, either in an electronic record or on a paper format. All of the necessary parameters may be located in another area of the treatment record. The field sizes and gantry, collimator, and couch angles may be in the patient setup instructions, on a simulation sheet, or on the treatment plan. Often a computerized isodose or three-dimensional treatment plan are part of the patient's record. The isodose plan may show field sizes, machine angles, doses, beam weighting, wedges, compensators, or blocks. The isodose plan is considered part of the radiation therapy prescription and should always be signed by the radiation oncologist.

The radiation therapist and medical dosimetrist must make sure that all parts of the prescription match before treatment. For example, the doses, treatment machines, and so forth should be the same on the prescription form and the isodose plan.

CONCEPTS USED IN PHOTON BEAM DOSE CALCULATIONS

When ionizing radiation is administered to a patient, many factors must be accounted for. As noted earlier, beam energy, distance from the source of radiation, and field size are just a few of the variables that must be addressed to accurately calculate a **treatment time** (length of time a unit is physically left on to deliver a measured dose) or MU setting. The radiation physicist uses mathematics, computers, and specialized equipment to develop dose calculation data used by the medical dosimetrist and radiation therapist. Many of the data are organized in tables to provide quick reference for these calculations. Before any attempt at performing a dose calculation is made, a number of terms used must be defined. It is important to be consistent in the use and understanding of these terms. The nomenclature used outlines the parameters necessary for accurate treatment delivery. It is important to remember that there are different approaches, methods, and terms used for dose and MU calculations. The radiation therapist and medical dosimetrist must ensure that the appropriate information for each individual application is used.

Dose

Everyone involved with treatment planning and delivery must have a clear idea of what is meant by dose. The *dose,* or **absorbed dose,** is measured at a specific point in a medium (typically a patient or phantom) and refers to the energy deposited at that point. Dose is commonly measured in gray (Gy), which is defined so that 1 Gy equals 1 J/kg.[1,2]

Depth

Depth is the distance beneath the skin surface where the prescribed dose is to be delivered. Sometimes the radiation oncologist will specify the depth of calculation. For example, when an area is treated with a single treatment field, the radiation oncologist will state the exact point, or depth, for the calculation. Using a posterior field for treatment of vertebral body metastasis, the radiation therapy prescription may state that 3 Gy are to be delivered per fraction to a depth of 5.0 cm. For opposed fields the patient's midplane is often used for the depth of calculation. Most multiple field arrangements use the isocenter, or intersection of the beams, for the calculation depth. Plain radiographic images and computed tomography (CT) scans are useful in determining the point of calculation. It is necessary to take measurements of the patient's thickness or separation. Depth affects measurements of dose attenuation.

Separation

Separation is a measurement of the patient's thickness from the point of beam entry to the point of beam exit. When calculating a treatment time or MU setting, the separation is normally measured along the beam's central axis. The separation can be measured directly using calipers, indirectly using the readings supplied by optical distance indicators (ODIs) located on the treatment units, or measuring it from the treatment plan. It is important to know the patient's separation when performing dose calculations. Often, for parallel opposed treatment fields (two fields focused at a point of specification directed 180 degrees apart), the calculation is done to deliver the prescribed dose at the patient's midplane or midseparation. To find the midseparation, the total separation is divided by two. For example, if the treatment prescription requires delivery of 2 Gy per fraction at midseparation using opposed fields, the patient's separation at the central axis would be measured. If the separation were measured as 20 cm, the midseparation would be 10 cm. In that case, a depth of 10 cm would be used for the MU calculation.

Source-skin Distance

Source-skin distance (SSD) is the distance from the source or target of the treatment machine to the surface of the patient or phantom (a volume of tissue equivalent material). The SSD is normally measured using an ODI. This device projects a distance scale onto the patient's skin (Fig. 21-1, A). The number read is the distance from the source of photons to the patient's skin surface.

Isocenter

The **isocenter** is the intersection of the axis of rotation of the gantry and the axis of rotation of the collimator for the treatment unit. This is usually a point in space at a specified distance from the source or target that the gantry rotates around. Cobalt-60 treatment machines typically have a source-axis distance (SAD) of 80 cm, whereas the SAD for most modern linear accelerators is 100 cm.

Source-axis Distance

SAD is the distance from the source of photons to the isocenter of the treatment machine (Fig. 21-1, B). Each isocentric machine has its own SAD. When the gantry rotates around

the patient, the SSD will continually change; however, the SAD and isocenter are at a fixed distance and therefore do not change. In an isocentric setup the isocenter is established inside the patient. The treatment machines are designed so that the gantry will rotate around this reference point.

Field Size

Field size refers to the physical size set on the collimators of the therapy unit that determines size of the treatment field at a reference distance. The field size is defined at the machine's isocenter. For example, when a field size of 10 × 10 cm is set on the treatment unit collimator, the square treatment field measures 10 × 10 cm at that particular machine's isocentric distance. On a cobalt-60 machine, it would be at 80 cm; on most linear accelerators, it would be at 100 cm.

Field size changes with distance from the source of radiation because of divergence. The 10 × 10 cm field size would measure smaller at distances shorter than the isocentric distance and larger at distances greater than the isocentric distance. In an isocentric patient setup, the field size set would be inside the patient at the isocenter. This is called an SAD treatment setup. The physical size measured on the patient's surface at that point would be smaller, because it would be at a distance shorter than the isocenter. In the nonisocentric (SSD) patient setup, the field size set on the collimator would be the same as measured on the skin surface, because the isocentric distance is set at the skin surface in this instance.

Scatter

The radiation treatment beam is composed of both primary and scatter radiation. Any interaction of the primary radiation may result in scatter. When the primary beam interacts with matter, the result is scatter radiation made up of photons or

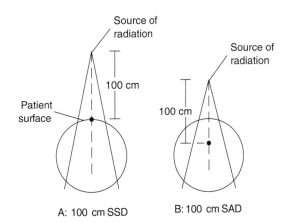

Figure 21-1. These diagrams graphically define source-skin distance (SSD) and source-axis distance (SAD). **A,** SSD is the distance from the source of radiation to the surface of the patient or phantom for a linear accelerator (100 cm to surface). **B,** SAD is the distance from the source of radiation to the isocenter of the treatment unit. The isocenter is typically placed within the patient.

electrons. Usually there is a change of direction associated with scatter radiation. When an electron interacts with the target in the linear accelerator, photons are produced. These photons are the primary beam. As the primary photons travel to the patient, some of them will interact with the collimator. When the primary photon interacts with the collimator, an electron from the collimator may be ejected and travel toward the patient. The primary photon beam may also be deflected back toward the patient. Both the electron and the deflected photon are considered scatter radiation. Radiation that is scattered back toward the surface of the patient is called *backscatter*. The absorbed dose received by the patient results from secondary radiation caused by interactions where the photon imparts energy to an electron. Then the electron undergoes tens of thousands of collisions while giving up some energy at each collision. Most of the absorbed dose received by the patient results from the collisions of the scattered electrons.

D_{max}

D_{max}, also known as the depth of maximum equilibrium, is the depth at which electronic equilibrium occurs for photon beams. D_{max} is the point where the maximum absorbed dose occurs for single field photon beams and mainly depends on the energy of the beam. The depth of maximum ionization increases as the energy of the photon beam increases. D_{max} occurs at the surface for low-energy photon beams and beneath the surface for megavoltage photon beams. Other factors such as field size and distance may influence the depth at which maximum ionization occurs. Table 21-1 lists the approximate depth of D_{max} for various photon beam energies.

There are times when it is important to know what the dose is at D_{max}. When a patient is treated using a single field, the dose at D_{max} should be calculated and recorded because the dose at D_{max} will be higher than the prescribed dose. The dose at D_{max} is also greater than the prescribed dose when opposed treatment fields are used to treat the patient and will be greater than the dose delivered to the patient's midplane. The dose at D_{max} will be slightly greater than the midplane dose for high-energy treatment beams and for patients with a small separation. When low-energy treatment beams (cobalt-

60, 4 MV, and 6 MV) are used, the dose at D_{max} can be significantly higher than the midplane dose. This is especially true for large patient separations. When using megavoltage photon beams, it may not be necessary to calculate the dose at D_{max} when using multiple field arrangements to treat the patient. By using many fields, the dose at D_{max} will normally be less than the prescribed dose.

Output

The **output** can be referred to as the dose rate of the machine and is measured in the absence of a scattering phantom and in tissue equivalent material.[1] It is the amount of radiation exposure produced by a treatment machine or source as specified at a reference field size and at a specified reference distance. The reference field size and distance are used so that we may relate standardized measurements to those that vary from the standards. Changing the field size, distance, or attenuating medium will change the dose rate. **Dose rate** increases with increased field size. Remember that a therapeutic beam of radiation is made up of primary and scatter and measured at a point of reference. If the field size is increased on a treatment machine, the primary component would remain the same. However, the increased area would cause increased scatter, which would add to the output (all other parameters remaining constant). If the distance from the source of radiation to the point of measurement increases, the dose rate would decrease because of the inverse square law. An example of output on a cobalt-60 unit may be 150 cGy/min, whereas a linear accelerator output may be 1 cGy/mu at reference field size and distance.

Output Factor

The **output factor** is the ratio of the dose rate of a given field size to the dose rate of the reference field size. The output factor allows for the change in scatter as the collimator setting changes. The output factor is usually normalized or referenced to a 10 × 10 cm field size. This means that the output factor for a 10 × 10 cm field size is 1.00 for the linear accelerator or cobalt-60 unit. The output factor will be greater than 1.00 for field sizes larger than 10 × 10 cm because of an increase in scatter as the collimator setting is increased. The output factor will be less than 1.00 for field sizes smaller than 10 × 10 cm because of a decrease in scatter as the collimator setting is decreased.

The term output factor may be a generic term. Many institutions use other terminology, such as relative output factor, collimator scatter factor, field size correction factor, and phantom scatter factor. Khan[4] defines measured values for collimator scatter factor and total scatter factors and a derived value for phantom scatter factor.

Output factors relate the dose rate of a given collimator setting to the dose rate of the reference field size and are very useful and practical for calculations involving cobalt-60 treatment machines. The reference dose rate for the cobalt-60 treatment machine is constantly changing. Usually the refer-

Table 21-1	Approximate depths of D_{max}	
Beam Energy		**Depth of D_{max} (cm)**
200 kV		0.0
1.25 MV		0.5
4 MV		1.0
6 MV		1.5
10 MV		2.5
18 MV		3.5
24 MV		4.0

ence dose rate is updated monthly. Even though the reference dose rate is changed every month, the output factors do not change. Therefore by using output factors, only the reference dose rate must be changed. Normally the reference dose rate is 1.0 cGy per MU for linear accelerators. The reference dose rate does not normally change for linear accelerators. This means that in some centers the output factor is the dose rate for that field size (any number multiplied by 1 does not change). For example, let us say that the reference dose rate is 1.0 cGy per MU for a 10×10 cm field size measured at 100 cm from the target in free space. Let us also say that the output factor for the 15×15 cm collimator setting is 1.02 (larger than 1.00 because the field size is greater than the reference). The dose rate for the 15×15 cm collimator setting can be calculated as follows:

$$\text{Dose rate}_{\text{(Given field size)}} = \text{Dose rate}_{\text{(Reference field size)}} \times \text{Output factor}_{\text{(Given field size)}}$$
$$\text{Dose rate}_{\text{(Given field size)}} = 1.0 \text{ cGy/MU} \times 1.02$$
$$\text{Dose rate}_{\text{(Given field size)}} = 1.02 \text{ cGy/MU}$$

Today some treatment centers use more than one output factor. For example, some calculation models require the use of a collimator output factor (COF) and a phantom scatter factor (PSF). The COF is used to determine the scatter, usually measured in air, from the collimators. The PSF is used to determine the scatter from the patient.

Inverse Square Law

The inverse square law is a mathematical relationship that describes the change in beam intensity caused by the divergence of the beam. As the beam of radiation diverges or spreads out, there is a decrease in the intensity. Therefore as the distance from the source of radiation increases, the intensity will decrease. For example, a photon beam that is made up of 400 photons is administered in a field size of 10×10 cm at a distance of 100 cm. The area of the beam is 100 cm^2 (given by the formula, width × length). If the photon coverage is uniform, there is an intensity of 4 photons/cm^2. At a distance of 200 cm, the field size will double to dimensions of 20×20 cm. The area of this field would then be 400 cm^2. There are still only 400 photons to cover this larger area. Now if the photon coverage is uniform, there will be 1 photon/cm^2. By doubling the distance, the intensity or number of photons per square centimeter has decreased by one fourth.

One practical application of the inverse square law is its effect on the output or dose rate of the treatment machine. The dose rate is commonly measured at the isocenter of the treatment machine. For linear accelerators, the dose rate at the isocenter for a 10×10 cm field is often 1.0 cGy/MU. When the MUs are calculated for setup at distances greater than the standard, the inverse square law is used to account for the decrease in dose rate at distances beyond the isocenter. The dose rate of the beam is inversely proportional to the square of the distance. This means that even a small change in distance can have a large effect on the dose rate. For exam-

ple, if the dose rate is 1.0 cGy/MU at 100 cm, then the dose rate is 0.64 cGy/MU at 125 cm. The equation commonly used for the inverse square law is as follows:

$$\frac{I_1}{I_2} = \frac{(d_2)^2}{(d_1)^2}$$

This equation may be used to find the change in dose rate with a change in distance:

$$\frac{\text{Dose rate at distance}_1}{\text{Dose rate at distance}_2} = \frac{(\text{Distance}_2)^2}{(\text{Distance}_1)^2}$$

Distance$_1$ is defined as 125 cm for this example. Rearranging the previous equation, we get the following:

$$\text{Dose rate at distance}_1 = \text{Dose rate at distance}_2 = \frac{(\text{Distance}_2)^2}{(\text{Distance}_1)^2}$$

Substituting the values in our example we have the following:

$$\text{Dose rate at 125 cm} = \text{Dose rate at 100 cm} \times \frac{(100 \text{ cm})^2}{(125 \text{ cm})^2}$$

$$\text{Dose rate at 125 cm} = 1.0 \text{ cGy/MU} \times \frac{(100 \text{ cm})^2}{(125 \text{ cm})^2}$$

$$\text{Dose rate at 125 cm} = 0.64 \text{ cGy/MU}$$

Equivalent Squares of Rectangular Fields (ESRF)

A square field is a field that has equal dimensions for the field width and length, such as a 10×10 cm field. A rectangular field has a field width and length that are different, as is the case with a 10×15 cm field. In a clinical setting, most patients are treated with rectangular fields of different sizes. Treatment calculation tables use field size as a qualifying parameter. Using different rectangular field sizes would require extensive tables with thousands of number combinations. Because of this, a method was needed to make the amount of data and number of tables manageable. The method devised was to take different rectangular field sizes and compare them to square fields that demonstrate the same measurable scattering and attenuation characteristics, known as an **equivalent square.**

A formula may be used to calculate the equivalent square of a rectangular field. One formula is commonly called the $4 \times \text{Area} \div \text{perimeter}$ method. Using this formula the area and perimeter of the rectangular field are calculated. The area is divided by the perimeter, and the result is then multiplied by four. The number derived would be one side of the square field that has approximately the same measurable scattering and attenuation characteristics as the original rectangular field. This essentially takes field shape into account. This formula is an approximation and should be used when an ESRF table is not available. In general, if the ratio of width or length exceeds 2, the use of standardized tables of equivalent squares are recommended. Table 21-2 demonstrates an example of a chart showing ESRF.

ESRF are used to find the output, output factor, and tissue absorption factors. Most radiation beam data tables are con-

Table 21-2	Sample equivalent squares of rectangular fields chart												
Long Axis (cm)	**0.5**	**1.0**	**2.0**	**3.0**	**4.0**	**5.0**	**6.0**	**7.0**	**8.0**	**9.0**	**10.0**	**11.0**	**12.0**
0.5	**0.5**												
1	0.7	**1.0**											
2	0.9	1.4	**2.0**										
3	1.0	1.6	2.4	**3.0**									
4	1.1	1.7	2.7	3.4	**4.0**								
5	1.2	1.8	2.9	3.8	4.5	**5.0**							
6	1.2	1.9	3.1	4.1	4.8	5.5	**6.0**						
7	1.2	2.0	3.3	4.3	5.1	5.8	6.5	**7.0**					
8	1.2	2.1	3.4	4.5	5.4	6.2	6.9	7.5	**8.0**				
9	1.2	2.1	3.5	4.6	5.6	6.5	7.2	7.9	8.5	**9.0**			
10	1.3	2.2	3.6	4.8	5.8	6.7	7.5	8.2	8.9	9.5	**10.0**		
11	1.3	2.2	3.7	4.9	6.0	6.9	7.8	8.5	9.3	9.9	10.5	**11.0**	
12	1.3	2.2	3.7	5.0	6.1	7.1	8.0	8.8	9.6	10.3	10.9	11.5	**12.0**
13	1.3	2.2	3.8	5.1	6.2	7.2	8.2	9.1	9.9	10.6	11.3	11.9	12.5
14	1.3	2.3	3.8	5.1	6.3	7.4	8.4	9.3	10.1	10.9	11.6	12.3	12.9
15	1.3	2.3	3.9	5.2	6.4	7.5	8.5	9.5	10.3	11.2	11.9	12.6	13.3
16	1.3	2.3	3.9	5.3	6.5	7.6	8.6	9.6	10.5	11.4	12.2	12.9	13.7
17	1.3	2.3	3.9	5.3	6.5	7.7	8.8	9.8	10.7	11.6	12.4	13.2	14.0
18	1.3	2.3	3.9	5.3	6.6	7.8	8.9	9.9	10.9	11.8	12.6	13.5	14.3
19	1.4	2.3	4.0	5.4	6.6	7.8	8.9	10.0	11.0	11.9	12.8	13.7	14.5
20	1.4	2.3	4.0	5.4	6.7	7.9	9.0	10.1	11.1	12.1	13.0	13.9	14.7

structed so that the equivalent square of the rectangular field must be known to use the table. For example, to look up the output factor for a collimator setting of 7 × 19 cm, converting the rectangular field to a square one is required. Its equivalent square is found to be 10 × 10 cm.[8] The output factor for a 10 × 10 cm field would be used, because it is effectively the same as that of a 7 × 19 cm field, all other parameters remaining unchanged. The output factor for a 10 × 10 cm field is 1.000. Therefore the output factor for a 7 × 19 cm field is 1.000.

When blocks are used to customize the shape of the treatment area, two portions of the field are created. The first is the area being shielded, and the second is the area being treated. When looking at the area being treated, its dimensions must be determined. This derived field size is called the blocked field size (BFS) or **effective field size** (EFS), which is the equivalent rectangular field dimension of the open or treated area within the collimator field dimensions. Usually some method of approximation is used to determine the EFS (a square or rectangular field that approximates the same physical volume as the blocked shape). The EFS is normally smaller than the collimator field size, although it may be larger for some extended distance setups. The general rules for measuring EFS are as follows:

1. Basic field shape should be maintained for the effective field (a field that looks like an elongated rectangle should retain a rectangular shape after measurement).

2. One should visualize the closest rectangular area that can be adapted to the irregular field. Total area should approximate the area of the treatment field.

3. The rectangular field is converted to an equivalent square.

The unblocked equivalent square may be used to determine the output factor. The EFS equivalent square is normally used to determine the **tissue absorption factors,** such as the percentage depth dose (PDD), tissue-air ratio (TAR), tissue-phantom ratio (TPR), or tissue-maximum ratio (TMR), which are discussed in the following section.

TISSUE ABSORPTION FACTORS

As the beam of radiation travels through the body, it gives up energy. The more tissue the beam traverses, the more it is attenuated (the more energy it gives up). There are a number of different methods for measuring the attenuation of the beam as it travels through tissue. These are **percentage depth dose** (PDD), **tissue-air ratio** (TAR), tissue-phantom ratio (TPR), and **tissue-maximum ratio** (TMR). The first of these methods used in a treatment setting was PDD. It may be helpful to remember that in the early days of radiation therapy the patients were treated using an SSD technique. PDD was primarily developed for SSD setups. Using appropriate corrections, any of the four methods (PDD, TAR, TPR, and TMR) may be used for SSD or SAD setups. However, PDD works best with SSD (nonisocentric) treatments, whereas TAR, TPR, and TMR work very well with SAD (isocentric) treatments.

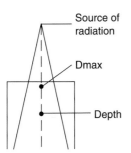

Figure 21-2. Diagram of percentage depth dose (PDD). PDD measures the dose along the central ray at depth as it compares to the dose at maximum equilibrium (D_{max}).

Percentage Depth Dose (PDD)

PDD is the ratio, expressed as a percentage, of the absorbed dose at a given depth to the absorbed dose at a fixed reference depth usually D_{max}[7,8] (Fig. 21-2) as follows:

$$PDD = \frac{\text{Absorbed dose at depth}}{\text{Absorbed dose at } D_{max}} \times 100\%$$

Normally the depth of D_{max} is used for the fixed reference depth. PDD is dependent on four factors: energy, depth, field size, and SSD. PDD increases as the energy, field size, and SSD increase. This is a direct relationship. Higher energies are more penetrating, so a greater percentage is available at a specific depth when compared with a lower energy. As field size increases, more scatter is added to the deposited beam, thus increasing PDD. PDD decreases as the depth increases (inverse relationship); because dose is deposited in tissue as it traverses it, a smaller percentage is available at greater depths.

Tissue-air Ratio (TAR)

TAR is the ratio of the absorbed dose at a given depth in phantom to the absorbed dose at the same point in free space (Fig. 21-3):

$$TAR = \frac{\text{Dose in tissue}}{\text{Dose in air}}$$

Free space (in air) is a term used for measurements using a build-up cap or miniphantom. It may not be possible to do a true air measurement. A build-up cap is a device made of acrylic or other phantom material that is placed over an ionization chamber to produce conditions of electronic equilibrium. The miniphantom is a sphere of tissue-equivalent material surrounding a point of interest. There is just enough material to produce build-up at the center (depth of D_{max}).[4] The ionization chamber then measures the flow of electrons and eventually the dose rate of the treatment machine (Fig. 21-4).

When determining the TAR, the dose is measured at a reference distance from the target but within two sets of conditions. The first measurement is in air or free space, and the second measurement is in phantom (the point of measurement does not change between the two measurements). The amount of phantom material used for the second measurement corresponds to the depth of interest.

TAR depends on energy, field size, and depth.[4] TAR increases as the energy and field size increase and decreases as the depth increases. These characteristics are consistent with PDD. However, TAR is independent of SSD (distance). TAR is normally used to perform calculations for SAD treatments involving low-energy treatment units such as a cobalt-60 or 4-MV linear accelerators. Some treatment centers use TAR for energies greater than 4 MV.

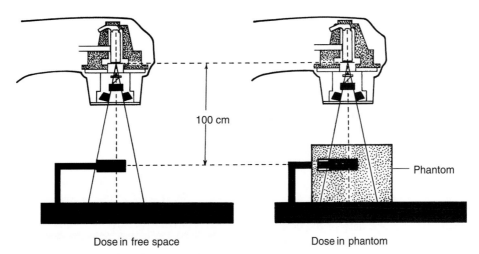

Dose in free space   Dose in phantom

Figure 21-3. Diagram of tissue-air ratio (TAR). TAR compares the dose in tissue at a specific depth to the dose in air at the same distance from the source (at the isocenter). When the depth in tissue corresponds to the level of D_{max}, the TAR is known as the backscatter or peak/phantom scatter factor.

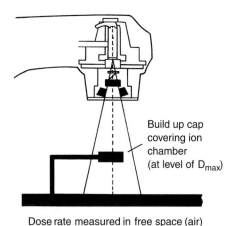

Build up cap
covering ion
chamber
(at level of D_{max})

Dose rate measured in free space (air)

Figure 21-4. Dose rate measured in air. There is a build-up cap over the ionization measuring chamber to allow for maximum scatter component to be accounted for.

Scatter Air Ratio (SAR)

The absorbed dose of radiation used to treat cancer are made up of two distinct components as it is measured along the central ray of the beam at the point of calculation: primary radiation that is emitted from the treatment unit and scatter radiation from the surrounding irradiated tissue. Several noted physicists (Clarkson, Cunningham, etc.) contributed greatly to this concept of primary and scatter making up the therapeutic beam. The primary part of total absorbed dose is represented by the zero-area tissue-air ratio (TAR). This zero-area TAR cannot be measured directly. The difference between the TAR for a field of definite area and that for a zero area would be a measure of the contribution from scattered radiation. The contribution of scatter to points of calculation in the irradiated tissue, along the central ray and points off axis, is particularly important as the irregular shape of the treatment fields are considered.

Off-axis point doses can also be calculated to good approximation by entering the appropriate SSD and depth, with allowance for off-axis output profile in determining the primary dose contribution. In their use they are added back to adjusted SAR values to calculate an effective TAR for a specific field geometry, so the result is not sensitive to what model was used provided the same one is used to derive SAR. Virtually all modern treatment planning computer systems include the SAR data tables and irregular field algorithms to accurately calculate treatment doses.[3,5]

Backscatter Factor (BSF)

The **backscatter factor** (BSF) is the ratio of the dose rate with a scattering medium (water or phantom) to the dose rate at the same point without a scattering medium (air) at the level of maximum equilibrium.[1-4,6,7] Backscatter is then a TAR at the level of D_{max}. The BSF is measured at the surface for orthovoltage and other low-energy x-ray treatment machines (energies less than 400 kV) (Fig. 21-5). The BSF is measured at the depth of D_{max} for megavoltage photon beams. Therefore the BSF is also a PSF for megavoltage radiation. The PSF is sometimes normalized to a reference field size, usually 10×10 cm, for energies of 4 MV and higher.[1] In the applications section of this chapter, the term PSF is used in a number of the calculations. However, many tables still use BSF for both low-energy and megavoltage photon beams.

Tissue-phantom Ratio and Tissue-maximum Ratio

TPR is the ratio of the absorbed dose at a given depth in phantom to the absorbed dose at the same point at a reference depth in phantom as follows:

$$TPR = \frac{Dose\ in\ tissue}{Dose\ in\ phantom}$$

The reference depth may be any depth but 5.0 cm is commonly chosen. If the reference depth is chosen to be the depth of D_{max}, then the TPR is referred to as the **tissue-maximum ratio** (TMR), as seen in Fig. 21-6:

$$TMR = \frac{Dose\ in\ tissue}{Dose\ in\ phantom\ (D_{max})}$$

The TMR is related to the TAR by the formula: TAR = TMR $\times$ BSF for low-energy beam, or TAR = TMR $\times$ PSF for high-energy beams.

TMR and TPR were developed because of difficulties in measuring the TAR for high-energy beams. TAR is measured using some form of a build-up cap. With high-energy beams a large build-up cap would be required to accurately measure it. As the build-up cap becomes increasingly larger, phantom scatter is introduced into the "in-air measurement" of the TAR. A build-up cap is not needed for measuring TMR,

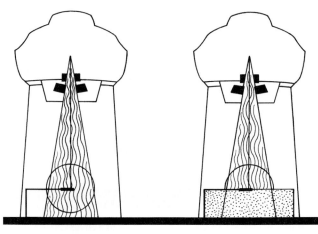

Dose measured in air   Dose measured in tissue at level of D_{max}

Figure 21-5. Backscatter or peak/phantom scatter factor relates dose in tissue to dose in air at the level of maximum equilibrium.

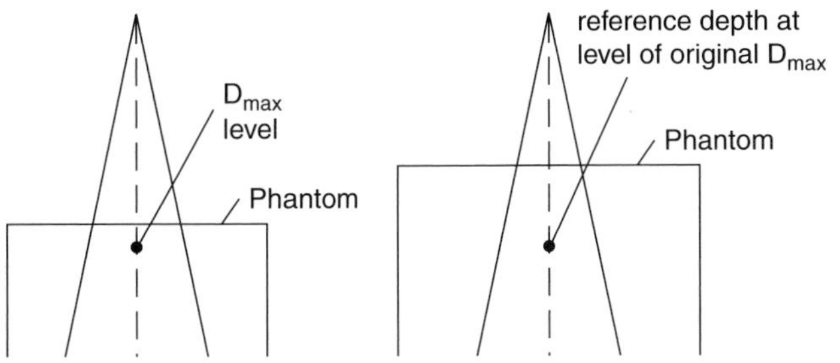

Figure 21-6. Tissue-maximum ratio compares dose at the depth of D_{max} to dose at depth where the distance from the source to each point is the same. If another point of reference is used instead of D_{max}, the relationship is known as tissue-phantom ratio.

because both measurements are done in phantom. Thus TMR overcame the problem of getting a true in-air measurement.

Because the depth of D_{max} depends on field size, the reference depths for TMR change accordingly. One advantage of a TPR over a TMR is that the reference depth will not change with field size. By using a reference depth of 5 cm for the 10×10 cm field size, the dependence of the depth of D_{max} with field size has been eliminated with TPR.

When determining the TMR and TPR, the dose is measured at one distance from the target but at two different depths under phantom-specific conditions. The first measurement is at the depth of D_{max} or another established standard, and the second measurement is at the desired depth. The point of measurement does not change between the two measurements. The amount of phantom material used for the second measurement is determined by the depth of interest. The value of TMR is never greater than 1.00, and the value of TPR has no upper limit. The deeper the reference depth, the greater the TPR.[7]

Dose Rate Modification Factors

Any device placed in the path of the radiation beam will attenuate some of it. The transmission factor is the ratio of the radiation dose with the device to the radiation dose without the device and accounts for the material in the beam's path. Examples of such factors would include tray transmission, wedge, and compensating filter factors.

Tray Transmission Factor

The *tray transmission factor (tray factor)* defines how much of the radiation is transmitted through a block tray. Most block trays are made of a plastic derivative. When the beam of radiation hits the tray, some amount of the radiation beam will be attenuated by the tray. The radiation not attenuated by the tray will pass through and continue to the patient. To correctly calculate an MU or time setting, the amount of radiation transmitted through the tray must be measured and accounted for. The medical physicist takes two measure-

ments: the first measurement is with the tray in the path of the beam, and the second measurement is without the tray in the path of the beam. The ratio of these two measurements is known as the tray transmission factor. For example, if a dose with the tray in place is measured as 97 cGy and the dose without the tray is 100 cGy, the ratio of the two doses, $^{97}/_{100}$, will yield a tray transmission factor of 0.97. This means that 97% of the radiation is transmitted through the tray, and 3% of the radiation is attenuated. Tray factors vary with beam energy. As energy increases, the effect of the material in the beam's path is lessened because of the increased penetrating power of the higher energy. Thus departments may use the same trays on different treatment units (Fig. 21-7) and simply use an appropriate tray factor for the energy with which it is used.

To deliver the correct dose to the patient, the radiation attenuated by the tray must be taken into consideration. This is normally done by having the tray transmission factor as a dose rate modifier. When the tray transmission factor is handled in this manner, it should always be represented by a number less than 1.00. Although this is the method used in this chapter, some therapy departments may multiply the MU or time setting by a tray factor that is greater than 1.00. For example, if the calculated MU setting before taking the tray into account is 100 MU and the tray factor is 1.03 (denoting a 3% attenuation), by multiplying the 100 MU by 1.03, a corrected MU setting of 103 would be obtained. When the tray factor is greater than 1.00, it is not a tray transmission factor and cannot be multiplied by the dose rate to account for the attenuation. In these cases, the machine setting must be increased by this factor.

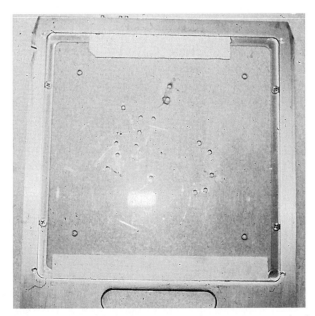

Figure 21-7. Typical blocking tray used to support standardized or custom shielding blocks.

Wedge and Compensator Filter Transmission Factors

The wedge transmission factor (wedge factor) depicts the amount of the radiation transmitted through a physical wedge placed in the beam to shape the beam delivery. A wedge is made of a dense material, usually lead or steel, which attenuates the radiation beam progressively across a field. The thinner side of the wedge attenuates less of the beam than the thicker side, resulting in an alteration of the beam isodose patterns.[1,2] The physicist takes several measurements and defines the wedge transmission factor, which is specific for each beam energy with which it is used. If a wedge has a wedge transmission factor of 0.67, this means that 67% of the radiation is transmitted through the wedge and 33% of the radiation is attenuated. To deliver the correct dose to the patient, a correction must be made for this amount of beam attenuation.

The compensator filter transmission factor is measured in the same manner as the wedge transmission factor. A compensator filter alters the isodose patterns just as in the wedge (Fig. 21-8). However, the compensator filter is individually produced for each patient and alters the patterns so that they are at maximum efficiency for that patient. Both factors are normally multiplied into the dose rate when doing a treatment unit calculation. Examples of treatment unit calculations involving physical wedges and compensators can be found in the section on applications.

PRACTICAL APPLICATIONS OF PHOTON BEAM DOSE CALCULATIONS

Having a clear understanding of the factors that affect radiation treatment delivery is extremely important to the radiation oncology team. Small changes in parameters can change the dose administered to the patient. A field size set incorrectly will change the machine output in reference to the patient. A sagging tabletop that inaccurately sets the patient at a wrong distance can have the same effect. With all this in mind and continuing to focus on the relationships presented, this section presents practical applications of treatment unit calculations. Tables needed for the calculations are located at the end of the chapter.

Calculating the Given Dose for an SSD Setup Using PDD

Often it is important to know the dose to points other than the prescription point. Dose-limiting and critical structures are anatomic sites that cannot withstand the same amount of exposure as neighboring tissues without damage. The spinal cord, bowel, and lens of the eye are examples of dose-limiting structures that are commonly monitored. The anatomy be monitored will be determined chiefly by the region of the body being irradiated.

Often SSD calculations are done at D_{max}. When a single field is used to treat a patient, such as a posterior spine field, the dose at D_{max} is known as the given dose. Other names for the given dose are applied dose, entrance dose, peak absorbed dose, or D_{max} dose. This is the point where the PDD is equal to 100%. As the depth increases from that point, the PDD will decrease. If a prescription calls for the administration of 300 cGy to a certain depth below D_{max} through a single field, the given dose will have to be more than the 300 cGy based on these concepts The dose at depth is also called the TD. This is done for cobalt-60 as well as linear accelerators.

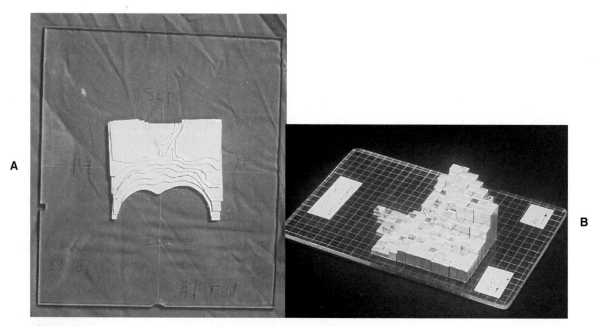

Figure 21-8. Compensating filters. **A,** Lead sheet comp filter. **B,** Aluminum cube comp filter. These filters attenuate the beam so that topographic variances are accounted for. Through this process, the distribution of dose at depths below the surface is even.

Each treatment field has its own given dose. Calculating the given dose can be accomplished by using the ratio of the prescribed dose for the field and the PDD at the depth of the prescribed dose as follows:

$$\text{Given dose} = \frac{\text{TD}}{\text{PDD}} \times 100$$

When writing the PDD, the following convention will be used: PDD (d,s,SSD), indicating that this refers to the PDD at depth (d), for equivalent square (s), at the setup distance (SSD). If the PDD at a depth of 5 cm for 10×10 cm field setup is 80 cm, the PDD is 78.3%; the convention for writing this information is PDD (5,10,80) = 78.3%.

There is a direct relationship between the dose and the PDD at a point. Thus a ratio or direct proportion can be established as follows:

$$\frac{\text{Dose at point A}}{\text{PDD at point A}} = \frac{\text{Dose at point B}}{\text{PDD at point B}}$$

The following example calculates the given dose.

Example 1: A patient is treated on the cobalt-60 treatment machine at 80 cm SSD. The collimator setting is 10×10 cm. There is no blocking used for this treatment. The prescription states that a dose of 3000 cGy is to be delivered to a depth of 5 cm in 10 fractions (the dose per fraction is 300 cGy). Calculate the given or applied dose:

$$\text{Given dose} = \frac{\text{TD}}{\text{PDD}} \times 100$$

$$\text{Given dose} = \frac{300\ \text{cGy}}{78.3} \times 100$$

$$\text{Given dose} = 383.1\ \text{cGy}$$

Again it should be noted that in this case to deliver 300 cGy to a depth of 5 cm with a 10×10 cm field at 80 cm SSD, a dose of 383.1 cGy is delivered to D_{max}. This calculation would be done exactly the same for any linear accelerator.

The given dose formula can be rearranged to solve for the TD if the given dose is known. The following example demonstrates this. Before any calculations, it should be noted that the TD should be less than the given dose in a single field calculation because the TD will be located at a depth greater than the level of D_{max}.

Example 2: A patient is treated on the 6-MV linear accelerator at 100 cm SSD. The collimator setting is 15×15 cm. There is no blocking used for this treatment. The prescription states that a dose of 300 cGy per fraction is to be delivered at D_{max}. What is the dose delivered at a depth of 5 cm?

$$\text{TD} = \text{Given dose} \times \frac{\text{PDD (5,15,100)}}{100}$$

$$\text{TD} = 300\ \text{cGy} \times \frac{87.9}{100}$$

$$\text{TD} = 263.7\ \text{cGy}$$

As expected, the TD is lower than the given dose.

Any other point along the central axis can be found if the depth and PDD are known. If a dose at a depth of 3 cm was sought in the preceding example, it would be somewhere between the dose at D_{max} and the dose at 5 cm. By looking up the PDD at the desired depth, the information can be derived.

In earlier years of radiation therapy the higher given doses presented problems. To treat tumors at depth, it was necessary to give the superficial tissues higher doses. Coupled with the use of lower-energy therapy machines that had a shallower D_{max}, heightened skin reactions were common and sometimes limited the administration of radiation therapy.

There are times when nonisocentric treatments are done for parallel opposed fields. At those times, it may be beneficial to the radiation oncology team to note the total dose at D_{max}. In this case, the given dose is added to the exit dose. The exit dose is the dose absorbed by a point that is located at the depth of D_{max} at the exit of the beam. For example, the depth of D_{max} for a 6-MV photon beam is approximately 1.5 cm. If a patient is treated using parallel opposed anterior and posterior photon beams and the patient's central axis separation is 20 cm, the total D_{max} dose can be calculated. The given dose would be calculated at a depth of 1.5 cm and the exit dose at a depth of 18.5 cm (20 cm − 1.5 cm). The following example calculates the total D_{max} dose and cord dose using a linear accelerator. Each field contributes to the total dose of each.

Example 3: A patient is treated on the 6-MV linear accelerator at 100 cm SSD. The collimator setting is 15×15 cm. The field is blocked to an 8×8 blocked equivalent square. A 5-mm solid plastic tray is used to hold the blocks. The prescription states that a dose of 4000 cGy is to be delivered to a depth of 10 cm in 20 fractions using an anterior and posterior (AP:PA) treatment field arrangement. The patient's central axis separation is 20 cm. The cord lies 3.0 cm beneath the posterior skin surface. Calculate the total D_{max} dose and the cord dose.

We see that in this arrangement, the calculation point lies 3.0 cm from the posterior surface and 17.0 cm from the anterior surface. It is important to note here that all points of calculation are along the central axis. To obtain the anterior depth of the cord, the posterior depth of the cord should be subtracted from the patient's total separation (20.0 cm − 3.0 cm = 17.0 cm). The depth of D_{max} for the 6-MV linear accelerator is 1.5 cm. The depth of the posterior field exit point is 18.5 cm (20.0 cm − 1.5 cm).

The factors required for this calculation are as follows:

$$\text{PDD (1.5,8,100)} = 100.0$$
$$\text{PDD (3,8,100)} = 95.0$$
$$\text{PDD (10,8,100)} = 66.7$$
$$\text{PDD (17,8,100)} = 45.2$$
$$\text{PDD (18.5,8,100)} = 41.6$$
$$\text{PSF (15} \times \text{15 cm)} = 1.039$$
$$\text{PSF (8} \times \text{8 cm)} = 1.016$$

Determining Total D_{max} Dose

A. Calculate the anterior dose contribution to D_{max} (given dose)
In this problem, the direct proportion formula is used as follows:

$$\frac{\text{Dose at point A}}{\text{PDD at point A}} = \frac{\text{Dose at point B}}{\text{PDD at point B}}$$

$$\frac{\text{Dose}_{1.5\,cm}}{\text{PDD}_{1.5\,cm}} = \frac{\text{Dose}_{10\,cm}}{\text{PDD}_{10\,cm}}$$

$$\frac{\text{Dose}_{1.5\,cm}}{100} = \frac{100\ \text{cGy}}{66.7}$$

$$\text{Dose}_{1.5\,cm} = 149.9\ \text{cGy}$$

B. Calculate the posterior dose contribution to D_{max} (exit dose)
Using the exit point (A) and D_{max} point (B), we have depths of 18.5 cm and 1.5 cm, respectively:

$$\frac{\text{Dose}_{1.5\,cm}}{\text{PDD}_{1.5\,cm}} = \frac{\text{Dose}_{18.5\,cm}}{\text{PDD}_{18.5\,cm}}$$

$$\frac{149.9\ \text{cGy}}{100} = \frac{\text{Dose}_{18.5}}{41.6}$$

$$\text{Dose}_{18.5} = 62.4\ \text{cGy}$$

C. Add the anterior and posterior dose contributions to obtain total D_{max} dose

$$D_{max}\ \text{dose (total)} = D_{max}\ \text{dose (anterior)} + D_{max}\ \text{dose (posterior)}$$
$$D_{max}\ \text{dose (total)} = 149.9\ \text{cGy} + 62.4\ \text{cGy}$$
$$D_{max}\ \text{dose (total)} = 212.3\ \text{cGy}$$

Determining Cord Dose (Contribution from Both Fields)

A. Calculate the anterior dose contribution to the cord
Using the cord point (A) and D_{max} (B), we have depths of 17.0 cm and 1.5 cm, respectively:

$$\frac{\text{Dose}_{1.5\,cm}}{\text{PDD}_{1.5\,cm}} = \frac{\text{Dose}_{17\,cm}}{\text{PDD}_{17\,cm}}$$

$$\frac{\text{Dose}_{17\,cm}}{45.2} = \frac{149.9\ \text{cGy}}{100}$$

$$\text{Dose}_{17\,cm} = 67.8\ \text{cGy}$$

B. Calculate the posterior dose contribution to the cord
Using the cord point (A) and D_{max} point (B), we have depths of 3.0 cm and 1.5 cm, respectively:

$$\frac{\text{Dose}_{1.5\,cm}}{\text{PDD}_{1.5\,cm}} = \frac{\text{Dose}_{3\,cm}}{\text{PDD}_{3\,cm}}$$

$$\frac{\text{Dose}_{3\,cm}}{95.0} = \frac{149.9\ \text{cGy}}{100}$$

$$\text{Dose}_{3\,cm} = 142.4\ \text{cGy}$$

C. Add the anterior and posterior dose contributions to obtain the total cord dose

$$\text{Cord dose (total)} = \text{Cord dose (anterior)} + \text{Cord dose (posterior)}$$
$$\text{Cord dose (total)} = 67.8\ \text{cGy} + 142.4\ \text{cGy}$$
$$\text{Cord dose (total)} = 210.2\ \text{cGy}$$

If this calculation were done on a cobalt-60 treatment machine (1.25 MeV) and compared with the preceding calculation, the following chart could be built:

Point of Calculation	Cobalt-60	6 MV	% Difference
Total dose at D_{max}	232.5	212.3	9.5%
Total cord dose	218.9	211.2	3.7%
Total dose to midplane	200.0	200.0	0.0%

Although the midplane dose is constant in both cases, the total doses to D_{max} and the cord are different for the two energies. The data demonstrate that the total dose at D_{max} and the cord dose are less for higher treatment energies. One of the advantages of using higher energy beams, especially for parallel opposed treatment field arrangements, is that the total dose at D_{max} will be significantly less. In this case the patient will receive approximately 3.7% less dose to the cord if a 6-MV beam is used instead of the cobalt-60 beam.

Treatment Unit Calculations General Equation

When attempting to perform treatment unit calculations, a number of variables must be accounted for. Field size variations, energy changes, and modifiers in the beam's path can alter the amount of radiation received by a patient, as either an underdose or an overdose. Although the complexity of each calculation varies within these parameters, there is one basic equation that addresses virtually every scenario. The general equation for performing MU or treatment time calculation can be represented as follows:

$$\text{unit/ time setting} = \frac{\text{Dose at a point}}{\text{Dose rate at that point}}$$

The MU setting represents the setting to be used on a linear accelerator, and the time setting represents the minutes for a cobalt-60 treatment unit. The dose at a point represents the prescribed dose as determined by the radiation oncologist. The dose rate at that point represents the dose rate of the treatment unit at the point of calculation. There are three general points necessary when performing a treatment calculation: (1) one must know the dose at a point, (2) one must know the dose rate at that point, and (3) the dose and dose rate must be in the same medium.

Normally the dose and dose rate will be expressed in air or tissue. If the dose is expressed in tissue and the dose rate in air, then we have an "apple and orange" situation. As a rule for simplifying these calculations, it is desirable to have the dose rate expressed in air when using TAR for the megavoltage setting calculation. It is also desirable to have the dose rate expressed in tissue when using PDD, TPR, or TMR for the MU setting calculation.

SOURCE-SKIN DISTANCE (SSD) CALCULATIONS

An SSD setup occurs when the patient's skin surface is set up at the reference distance or isocenter distance. Therefore in an SSD setup the field size is defined on the patient's skin. It is important to know the reference isocenter distance because they can vary between treatment unit type; cobalt-60 is typically 80 cm and linear accelerators are 100 cm. The output or dose rate of the machine for SSD setups should be expressed at the depth of D_{max}; the field size will be defined at the skin surface, and the dose rate will be measured in tissue at the depth of D_{max}.

To perform nonisocentric SSD calculations, a five-step process can be employed:

Step 1. Find the equivalent square of the collimator setting (used for output factor).
Step 2. Find the equivalent square of the BFS (used for PDD) if applicable.
Step 3. Using the appropriate tables, determine the PDD.
Step 4. Determine the prescribed dose.
Step 5. Use the appropriate equation for determining the treatment unit setting.

Example 4: A patient is treated on the cobalt-60 treatment machine at 80 cm SSD to his thoracic spine. The patient is prone and will be treated through a single treatment field. The collimator setting is 10×10 cm. There is no blocking used for this treatment. The prescription states that a dose of 3000 cGy is to be delivered to a depth of 5 cm in 10 fractions. Calculate the treatment time.

This is the most basic calculation and involves only the reference dose rate, output factor, and PDD. Because there is no blocking used, the equivalent square for the collimator setting or actual field size is used to look up the output factor and PDD.

Step 1. Find the equivalent square of the collimator setting

The equivalent square of a 10×10 cm field is 10×10 cm.

Step 2. Find the equivalent square of the BSF

There is no blocking in this field. Therefore the BSF is the same as the collimator equivalent square.

Step 3. Using the appropriate tables, look up the dose rate factors

The factors for the dose rate at a point are reference dose rate, output factor, and tissue absorption factor, in this case, PDD. The following information can be obtained in the data table located at the end of the chapter (Tables 21-4 through 21-12):

Reference dose rate = 51.7 cGy/min
Output factor (10×10 cm) = 1.000
PDD (5,10,80) = 78.3

Step 4. Determine the prescribed dose

From the prescription, the total prescribed dose to a depth of 5 cm is 3000 cGy. This dose is to be delivered in 10 fractions.

Therefore the dose per fraction is 300 cGy. To obtain the dose per fraction, you divide the total dose by the number of fractions as follows:

$$\text{Dose per fraction} = \frac{\text{Total prescribed dose}}{\text{Number of fractions}}$$

$$\text{Dose per fraction} = \frac{3000 \text{ cGy}}{10 \text{ fraction}}$$

$$\text{Dose per fraction} = 300 \text{ cGy}$$

$$\text{Dose per treatment field} = \frac{\text{Dose per fraction}}{\text{Number of field}}$$

$$\text{Dose per treatment field} = \frac{300 \text{ cGy}}{1}$$

$$\text{Dose per treatment field} = 300 \text{ cGy}$$

Step 5. Use the appropriate equation for determining the treatment setting

$$\text{Time setting} = \frac{\text{Dose at a point}}{\text{Dose rate at that point}}, \text{ so}$$

$$\text{Time setting} = \frac{\text{Prescribed dose}}{\text{Output} \times \text{Output factor} \times \frac{\text{PDD}}{100}}$$

$$\text{Time setting} = \frac{300 \text{ cGy}}{51.7 \text{ cGy/min} \times 1.00 \times \frac{78.3}{100}}$$

$$\text{Time setting} = \frac{300 \text{ cGy}}{40.4811 \text{ cGy/min}}$$

$$\text{Time setting} = 7.41 \text{ min}$$

The treatment unit would have to be set for 7.41 minutes to treat a 10×10 cm field size at 80 cm SSD to deliver 300 cGy to a depth of 5 cm.

Example 5: A patient is treated on the cobalt-60 treatment machine at 80 cm SSD to his thoracic spine. The patient is prone and will be treated through a single treatment field. The collimator setting is 15×15 cm. There is no blocking used for this treatment. The prescription states that a dose of 3000 cGy is to be delivered to a depth of 5 cm in 10 fractions.

Example 5 is essentially the same setup as Example 4. The only difference is that the collimator setting has changed. In this setting, the output factor and PDD will change because of the different field size.

Step 1. Find the equivalent square of the collimator setting

The equivalent square of a 15×15 cm field is 15×15 cm.

Step 2. Find the equivalent square of the BSF

There is no blocking in this field. Therefore the BSF is the same as the collimator equivalent square, that is, 15×15 cm.

Step 3. Using the appropriate tables, look up the dose rate factors

The factors for the dose rate at a point are reference dose rate, output factor, and PDD as follows:

Reference dose rate = 51.7 cGy/min
Output factor (15 × 15 cm) = 1.046
PDD (5,15,80) = 80.7

Note that the reference dose rate is the same in both examples. This is because the reference dose rate is always the dose rate for the 10 × 10 cm collimator setting. The reference dose rate is multiplied by the output factor of the actual collimator setting to correct for the variance from the standard. This takes the different amount of scatter into account. Also note that both the output factor and the PDD have increased in Example 5 because of increased scatter from the larger collimator surface and larger volume of tissue treated.

Step 4. Determine the prescribed dose

The dose per fraction is 300 cGy.

Step 5. Use the appropriate equation for determining the treatment setting

$$\text{Time setting} = \frac{\text{Prescribed dose}}{\text{Output} \times \text{Output factor} \times \frac{\text{PDD}}{100}}$$

$$\text{Time setting} = \frac{300 \text{ cGy}}{51.7 \text{ cGy/min} \times 1.046 \times \frac{80.7}{100}}$$

$$\text{Time setting} = \frac{300 \text{ cGy}}{40.6411 \text{ cGy/min}}$$

$$\text{Time setting} = 6.87 \text{ min}$$

The time setting has decreased from Example 4 because of the increased scatter raising the dose rate at the point of calculation. Because the dose rate has increased, the time necessary to deliver the dose will decrease. This is similar to driving a car. If a person must travel 300 miles and drives at 50 miles per hour, the trip will take 6 hours. However, if the driving speed is increased to 60 miles/hr, the driving time will be reduced to 5 hours.

Example 6: A patient is treated on the cobalt-60 treatment machine at 80 cm SSD to his thoracic spine. The patient is prone and will be treated through a single treatment field. The collimator setting is 15 × 15 cm. The field is blocked to an 8 × 8 cm blocked equivalent square. A 5-mm solid plastic tray is used to hold the blocks. The prescription states that a dose of 3000 cGy is to be delivered to a depth of 5 cm in 10 fractions. Calculate the treatment time.

In example 6, blocks are added to the treatment field. This makes the calculation slightly more complex. The reference dose rate will remain unchanged. The output factor is a combination of the scatter from the collimator and the scatter from the phantom or patient. Although the blocking has little effect on the collimator scatter, it does affect the phantom scatter. One approach for correcting the measured output factors is to take out the phantom scatter for the collimator setting and then put back in the phantom scatter for the BSF. To accomplish this, the output factor is multiplied by the ratio of the BSF. The output factor for the equivalent square of the collimator setting (15 × 15 cm) is multiplied by the BSF (or PSF) of the blocked equivalent square and divided by the BSF of the collimator setting equivalent square. There are other solutions to this problem of handling the effect of blocking on the output factor. There is also a change in the PDD because the blocks have affected the area or amount of tissue being treated. In this case the area of tissue treated has been reduced to less than the 15 × 15 cm collimator setting. If less tissue is irradiated, then there will be a decrease in scatter. Therefore the PDD will be decreased. The equivalent square of the BSF is used to look up the PDD.

Step 1. Find the equivalent square of the collimator setting

The equivalent square of a 15 × 15 cm field is 15 × 15 cm.

Step 2. Find the equivalent square of the BSF

There is blocking in this field. Therefore the BSF equivalent square is 8 × 8 cm.

Step 3. Using the appropriate tables, look up the dose rate factors

The factors for the dose rate at a point are reference dose rate, output factor, PDD, and tray factor. Because there is blocking, a PSF is needed:

Reference dose rate = 51.7 cGy/min
Output factor (15 × 15 cm) = 1.046
PDD (5,8,80) = 76.9
PSF (8 × 8 cm) = 1.028
PSF (15 × 15 cm) = 1.051
Tray factor = 0.96

Step 4. Determine the prescribed dose

The dose per fraction is 300 cGy.

Step 5. Use the appropriate equation for determining the treatment setting

Note that the basic equation has been modified to account for tray factor and PSF, because both are needed to accurately calculate the time setting in the following example:

$$\text{Time setting} = \frac{\text{Prescribed dose}}{\text{Output} \times \text{Output factor} \times \frac{\text{PSF}_{(EFS)}}{\text{PSF}_{(CS)}} \times \frac{\text{PDD}}{100} \times \text{Tray factor}}$$

$$\text{Time setting} = \frac{300 \text{ cGy}}{51.7 \text{ cGy/min} \times 1.046 \times \frac{1.028}{1.051} \times \frac{76.9}{100} \times 0.96}$$

$$\text{Time setting} = \frac{300 \text{ cGy}}{39.049 \text{ cGy/min}}$$

$$\text{Time setting} = 7.68 \text{ min}$$

The treatment time has increased because the dose rate is decreasing. The decrease in dose rate was caused by two factors. First, the PDD was decreased because of the BSF and therefore less scatter radiation reaching the point of calculation. Second, the blocking tray attenuated some of the radiation. To compensate for the attenuation by the blocking tray, the time setting had to increase. A tray factor of 0.96 means that there is approximately 4% attenuation caused by the tray. Another way to look at this tray factor is that the time setting will need to be increased by approximately 4% to compensate for the radiation attenuated by the tray.

Example 7: A patient is treated on the cobalt-60 treatment machine at 80 cm SSD. The collimator setting is 15×15 cm. The field is blocked to an 8×8 cm blocked equivalent square. A 5-mm solid plastic tray is used to hold the blocks. The prescription states that a dose of 4000 cGy is to be delivered to a depth of 10 cm in 20 fractions using an anterior and posterior (AP:PA) treatment field arrangement.

Example 7 is similar to Example 6; however, in Example 7 the patient is going to be treated using more than one treatment field. The fields are equally weighted, meaning that the same dosage is administered through each portal. The treatment setting for each treatment field should be done individually.

Step 1. Find the equivalent square of the collimator setting

The equivalent square of a 15×15 cm field is 15×15 cm.

Step 2. Find the equivalent square of the BSF

There is blocking in this field. Therefore the BSF equivalent square is 8×8 cm.

Step 3. Using the appropriate tables, look up the dose rate factors

The factors for the dose rate at a point are reference dose rate, output factor, PDD, and tray factor:

$$
\begin{aligned}
\text{Reference dose rate} &= 51.7 \text{ cGy/min} \\
\text{Output factor } (15 \times 15 \text{ cm}) &= 1.046 \\
\text{PDD } (10,8,80) &= 54.5 \\
\text{PSF } (8 \times 8 \text{ cm}) &= 1.028 \\
\text{PSF } (15 \times 15 \text{ cm}) &= 1.051 \\
\text{Tray factor (TF)} &= 0.96
\end{aligned}
$$

Step 4. Determine the prescribed dose

From the prescription, the total prescribed dose to a depth of 10 cm is 4000 cGy. This dose is to be delivered in 20 fractions. Therefore the dose per fraction is 200 cGy. Because there are two treatment fields that will get the same dose, the dose per treatment field is 100 cGy.

Step 5. Use the appropriate equation for determining the treatment setting

$$
\text{Time setting} = \frac{\text{Prescribed dose}}{\text{Output} \times \text{Output factor} \times \frac{\text{PSF}_{(EFS)}}{\text{PSF}_{(CS)}} \times \frac{\text{PDD}}{100} \times \text{Tray factor}}
$$

$$
\text{Time setting} = \frac{100 \text{ cGy}}{51.7 \text{ cGy/min} \times 1.046 \times \frac{1.028}{1.051} \times \frac{54.5}{100} \times 0.96}
$$

$$
\text{Time setting} = \frac{100 \text{ cGy}}{27.6745 \text{ cGy/min}}
$$

$$
\text{Time setting} = 3.61 \text{ min}
$$

The time setting will be 3.61 minutes for the anterior field and 3.61 minutes for the posterior field.

The treatment time for the cobalt-60 machine is given in real-time (i.e., minutes). The dose rate for the cobalt-60 machine is defined in centigray per minute. Real-time is used with the cobalt-60 machine because the dose rate is caused by the radioactive decay of the isotope source. The half-life of cobalt-60 is approximately 5.3 years. This means that after 5.3 years, the dose rate of the unit will be half of its original dose rate. For example, if the dose rate is 50 cGy/min today, then the dose rate will be 25 cGy/min 5.3 years from today. As the dose rate decreases, the time it takes to deliver the prescribed dose increases.

Because the rate of decay for the cobalt-60 machine is relatively slow, it can be assumed that the dose rate is constant over a short period of time. The time frame for this constant dose rate is 1 month. This means that every month the minute settings used to treat the patient with the cobalt-60 machine must be adjusted. The rate of adjustment is approximately 1.1% each month. The following equation can be used to make the monthly adjustment in the minute setting for patients who are already on treatment:

$$
\text{New minute setting} = \text{Old minute setting} \times 1.01
$$

If it takes 2.00 minutes to deliver 100 cGy on January 1, then it will take 2.02 minutes to deliver 100 cGy on February 1. Also, because of the slow decay or long half-life, the dose rate of the cobalt-60 machine is considered constant for a given treatment.

LINEAR ACCELERATOR NONISOCENTRIC MONITOR UNIT (MU) SETTING CALCULATIONS

The major difference in the time setting calculation for the cobalt-60 machine and the MU setting calculation for the linear accelerator is in the measurement of the reference dose rate. The reference dose rate for the cobalt-60 treatment machine is measured in centigray per minute, whereas the reference dose rate for the linear accelerator is measured in centigray per MU.

In looking at the dose rate for the linear accelerator, it might be helpful to look at a simple time, distance, and speed calculation. The following formula can be used to calculate the time it takes to drive a given distance:

$$
\text{Time} = \frac{\text{Distance}}{\text{Speed}}
$$

If a driver makes a 450-mile trip, driving the entire distance at exactly 50 miles per hour, it will take exactly 9 hours to complete the trip:

$$
\text{Time} = \frac{450 \text{ miles}}{50 \text{ miles/hr}}
$$

$$
\text{Time} = 9 \text{ hours}
$$

No matter how many times this trip is made, it will take 9 hours as long as a constant speed of 50 miles/hr is maintained. This type of constant speed (dose rate) happens in the cobalt-60 machine and is the principle behind the time setting calculation. In the linear accelerator, the dose rate varies slightly from one moment to the next. If the dose from the linear accelerator were measured using real-time, the dose could be different each time. Therefore real-time cannot be used to deliver the prescribed dose with a linear accelerator. Instead, a different system of time called MU is used. Normally the dose rate for the linear accelerator is 1.0 cGy/MU for a 10×10 cm field size defined at the isocenter.

Linear Accelerator Nonisocentric Calculations

The parameters for examples of cobalt-60 will be repeated for the linear accelerator. The same trends seen between the cobalt-60 calculations will be noted in the linear accelerator calculations.

Example 8: A patient is treated on the 6-MV linear accelerator at 100 cm SSD. The collimator setting is 10×10 cm. There is no blocking used for this treatment. The prescription states that a dose of 3000 cGy is to be delivered to a depth of 5 cm in 10 fractions. Calculate the MU setting.

The factors for the dose rate at a point are reference dose rate, output factor, and PDD:

$$\text{Reference dose rate} = 0.993 \text{ cGy/MU}$$
$$\text{Output factor } (10 \times 10 \text{ cm}) = 1.000$$
$$\text{PDD } (5,10,100) = 87.1$$

$$\text{MU setting} = \frac{\text{Prescribed dose}}{\text{Output} \times \text{Output factor} \times \frac{\text{PDD}}{100}}$$

$$\text{MU setting} = \frac{300 \text{ cGy}}{0.993 \text{ cGy/MU} \times 1.00 \times \frac{87.1}{100}}$$

$$\text{MU setting} = \frac{300 \text{ cGy}}{0.8649 \text{ cGy/MU}}$$

$$\text{MU setting} = 347 \text{ MU}$$

Example 9: A patient is treated on the 6-MV linear accelerator at 100 cm SSD. The collimator setting is 15×15 cm. There is no blocking used for this treatment. The prescription states that a dose of 3000 cGy is to be delivered to a depth of 5 cm in 10 fractions. Calculate the MU setting.

The factors for the dose rate at a point are reference dose rate, output factor, and PDD:

$$\text{Reference dose rate} = 0.993 \text{ cGy/MU}$$
$$\text{Output factor } (15 \times 15 \text{ cm}) = 1.035$$
$$\text{PDD } (5,15,100) = 87.9$$

$$\text{MU setting} = \frac{\text{Prescribed dose}}{\text{Output} \times \text{Output factor} \times \frac{\text{PDD}}{100}}$$

$$\text{MU setting} = \frac{300 \text{ cGy}}{0.993 \text{ cGy/MU} \times 1.035 \times \frac{87.9}{100}}$$

$$\text{MU setting} = \frac{300 \text{ cGy}}{0.9034 \text{ cGy/MU}}$$

$$\text{MU setting} = 332 \text{ MU}$$

Note that the MU setting is lower in Example 9 when compared with Example 8. This change is caused by the increase in field size and scatter component.

Example 10: A patient is treated on the 6-MV linear accelerator at 100 cm SSD. The collimator setting is 15×15 cm. The field is blocked to an 8×8 cm blocked equivalent square. A 5-mm solid plastic tray is used to hold the blocks. The prescription states that a dose of 3000 cGy is to be delivered to a depth of 5 cm in 10 fractions.

The factors for the dose rate at a point are reference dose rate, output factor, PSF, and PDD:

$$\text{Reference dose rate} = 0.993 \text{ cGy/MU}$$
$$\text{Output factor } (15 \times 15 \text{ cm}) = 1.035$$
$$\text{PDD } (5,8,100) = 86.8$$
$$\text{PSF } (15 \times 15 \text{ cm}) = 1.039$$
$$\text{PSF } (8 \times 8 \text{ cm}) = 1.016$$
$$\text{Tray factor} = 0.97$$

$$\text{MU setting} = \frac{\text{Prescribed dose}}{\text{Output} \times \text{Output factor} \times \frac{\text{PSF}_{(EFS)}}{\text{PSF}_{(CS)}} \times \frac{\text{PDD}}{100} \times \text{Tray factor}}$$

$$\text{MU setting} = \frac{300 \text{ cGy}}{0.993 \text{ cGy/MU} \times 1.035 \times \frac{1.016}{1.039} \times \frac{86.8}{100} \times 0.97}$$

$$\text{MU setting} = \frac{300 \text{ cGy}}{0.8462 \text{ cGy/MU}}$$

$$\text{MU setting} = 355 \text{ MU}$$

Example 11: A patient is treated on the 6-MV linear accelerator at 100 cm SSD. The collimator setting is 15×15 cm. The field is blocked to an 8×8 cm blocked equivalent square. A 5-mm solid plastic tray is used to hold the blocks. The prescription states that a dose of 4000 cGy is to be delivered to a depth of 10 cm in 20 fractions using an anterior and posterior (AP:PA) treatment field arrangement.

The factors for the dose rate at a point are reference dose rate, output factor, PSF, PDD, and tray factor:

$$\text{Reference dose rate} = 0.993 \text{ cGy per MU}$$
$$\text{Output factor } (15 \times 15 \text{ cm}) = 1.035$$
$$\text{PDD } (10,8,100) = 66.7$$
$$\text{PSF } (15 \times 15 \text{ cm}) = 1.039$$
$$\text{PSF } (8 \times 8 \text{ cm}) = 1.016$$
$$\text{Tray factor} = 0.97$$

$$\text{MU setting} = \frac{\text{Prescribed dose}}{\text{Output} \times \text{Output factor} \times \frac{\text{PSF}_{(EFS)}}{\text{PSF}_{(CS)}} \times \frac{\text{PDD}}{100} \times \text{Tray factor}}$$

$$\text{MU setting} = \frac{100 \text{ cGy}}{0.993 \text{ cGy/MU} \times 1.035 \times \frac{1.016}{1.039} \times \frac{66.7}{100} \times 0.97}$$

$$\text{MU setting} = \frac{100 \text{ cGy}}{0.6502 \text{ cGy/MU}}$$

$$\text{MU setting} = 154 \text{ MU for each port}$$

EXTENDED DISTANCE CALCULATIONS USING PDD AND SSD SETUP

There are occasions when large areas of a patient's body must be treated that are larger than the collimator areas achievable by conventional radiation therapy treatment units. This is the case in total body and total skin irradiation techniques and some mantle field arrangements. In these cases, larger field areas are possible by extending the distance of the treatment area. Because of divergence, as the distance from the source increases, the field size increases. In this manner, very large areas can be treated in a single field. The alternative would be to split the treatment fields up into areas that could be accommodated at conventional distances with the challenge of accurately matching divergent fields. To avoid this challenge, extended distances are commonly used. For example, the isocenter on a linear accelerator is 100 cm. In a standard SSD setup the patient is treated at 100 cm SSD. However, to set up a larger field, the patient may be set up at 125 cm SSD. To reiterate, an extended distance setup is one in which the patient is set up at a distance beyond the isocenter or reference distance.[7]

In performing this type of calculation, several points must be considered. PDD is used for the calculation because its arrangement is nonisocentric. PDD depends on four factors: energy, field size, depth, and SSD. If any of these factors change, the PDD changes. If the energy is increased from cobalt-60 (1.25 MeV) to 6 MV, the PDD increases because of increased penetrating power. If the field size, at a given energy, changes from 10×10 cm to 15×15 cm, the PDD increases because of an increase in scatter. If the depth is increased from 6 cm to 10 cm, the PDD will decrease, because more attenuation and beam absorption occur. As the SSD is increased the PDD will increase because of a change in the inverse square law with a change in distance and because of an increase in scatter. As a result of these changes, special considerations must be employed to calculate treatment times and MUs at extended distances.

Mayneord's Factor

Mayneord's factor is a special application of the inverse square law. There are many forms of Mayneord's factor cited by different authorities. If it is understood where the numbers for Mayneord's factor are derived from, the likelihood of applying the numbers correctly is increased, resulting in no real need to memorize what appears to be a complex equation.

Reference or standard distance PDD values are determined from direct measurement. When patients are treated at an extended distance, the distance from the source of radiation to the depth of D_{max} and the depth of the calculation point changes. Note that the distances change and not the specified depth of treatment. If a patient is treated on a 6-MV linear accelerator with a 10×10 cm field size at 100 SSD to a depth of 8 cm and the distance is extended to 125 SSD, the level of D_{max} and the point of calculation remain the same; the depths are 1.5 cm and 8 cm, respectively. However, the

distance to these points for a 125-cm SSD setup will be 126.5 cm and 133 cm, respectively.

There are other factors to consider. The energy of the treatment machine is the same in the standard and extended distance setup. A 6-MV accelerator has the same energy at 125 cm as it does at 100 cm. If the field size was 10×10 cm in both cases and the depth of calculation is 8 cm for both setups, these factors should have little or no effect on the calculation. Because the 10×10 cm field was defined on the skin in both setups, the field size at the calculation point will be slightly different because of divergence. This would slightly change the amount of scatter. The major change will result from the change in distance. The original distances from source to D_{max} and depth were 101.5 and 108 cm, respectively. These distances should be removed from the measured PDD by multiplying by the inverse as follows:

$$\frac{(108)^2}{(101.5)^2}$$

Then the correct distance is used in the calculation by multiplying by the square of the ratio of the new distances:

$$\frac{(126.5)^2}{(133)^2}$$

This allows for the correct attenuation of the beam for the new distances. These derived correction factors are then multiplied by the PDD referenced from the table, the result being the new PDD for the extended distances.

Mayneord's factor can be calculated using these distances. Note that the depth of D_{max} is 1.5 cm for a 6-MV linear accelerator and is reflected in the numbers. The PDD (8,10,100) is 75.1%.

The original distances were 101.5 cm and 108 cm. The new distances are 126.5 cm and 133 cm:

$$\text{New PDD}_{(8,10,125)} = 75.1\% \times \frac{(108)^2}{(101.5)^2} \times \frac{(126.5)^2}{(133)^2}$$

$$\text{New PDD} = 76.9\%$$

Again, Mayneord's factor is an inverse square correction of the PDD. It can also be used in shortened treatment distances. It should be noted that Mayneord's factor does not account for changes in scatter because of a change in beam divergence. Therefore Mayneord's factor gives us the approximate value for the new PDD. To obtain the exact value for the new PDD, actual beam measurements using an ionization chamber or other appropriate devices would be necessary.

The following example uses the Mayneord's factor in the calculation of a MU setting for a 6-MV accelerator.

Example 12: A patient is treated on the 6-MV treatment unit at an extended distance of 125 cm. The collimator setting is 20×20 cm, and the field size on the patient's skin is 25×25 cm. The prescription states that a dose of 3000 cGy is to be delivered to a depth of 5 cm in 10 fractions using a single posterior treatment field arrangement. Calculate the MU setting.

We can use a similar process for extended distance calculations. We will use the same five steps discussed earlier and add a sixth step for Mayneord's factor.

Step 1. Find the equivalent square of the collimator setting (used for output factor)

The collimator setting is 20×20 cm, which is conveniently the equivalent square.

Step 2. Find the equivalent square of the BFS (used for PDD)

The field size at the setup SSD of 125 cm is 25×25 cm. The equivalent square of a 25×25 cm field is 25×25 cm.

Step 3. Using the appropriate tables, look up the dose rate factors

$$\text{Reference dose rate} = 0.993 \text{ cGy/MU}$$
$$\text{Output factor } (20 \times 20 \text{ cm}) = 1.058$$
$$\text{PDD } (5,25,100) = 88.9$$
$$\text{PSF } (20 \times 20 \text{ cm}) = 1.045$$
$$\text{PSF } (25 \times 25 \text{ cm}) = 1.0525$$

Step 4. Determine the prescribed dose

The prescribed dose is 3000 cGy in 10 fractions. Therefore the daily prescribed dose is 300 cGy/fraction.

Step 5. Calculate the new PDDs using Mayneord's factor

Determine the PDD at a depth of 5 cm:

$$\text{New PDD}_{(5,25,125)} = 88.9\% \times \frac{(105)^2}{(101.5)^2} \times \frac{(126.5)^2}{(130)^2}$$

$$\text{New PDD}_{(5,25,125)} = 90.1\%$$

Step 6. Use the appropriate equation for determining the time setting

The equation to be used is again a variation of dose divided by dose rate. The dose rate is affected by the factors mentioned in the problem. Because the treatment is at an extended distance, the intensity of the beam is affected by the inverse square law, just as the PDD was. Although the PDD increased because of increased scatter, the intensity of the beam would decrease because of the increased distance. The correction relates the distance from the source to the point of treatment unit calibration (where referenced data were measured) and the treatment SSD plus D_{max}. The inverse square correction would then be included as a dose rate correction in the denominator of the equation. It may be written as follows:

$$\text{Inverse square correction} = \frac{(\text{Reference source calibration distance})^2}{(\text{Treatment SSD} + D_{max})^2}$$

The treatment time can now be calculated, as follows:

$$\text{MU setting} =$$
$$\frac{\text{Prescribed dose}}{\text{Output} \times \text{Output factor} \times \text{Inverse square correction} \times \frac{\text{PSF}_{(EFS)}}{\text{PSF}_{(CS)}} \times \frac{\text{PDD}}{100}}$$

$$\text{MU setting} = \frac{300 \text{ cGy}}{0.993 \text{ cGy/MU} \times 1.058 \times \frac{(101.5)^2}{(126.5)^2} \times \frac{1.0525}{1.045} \times \frac{90.1}{100}}$$

$$\text{MU setting} = \frac{300 \text{ cGy}}{0.6138 \text{ cGy/MU}}$$

$$\text{MU setting} = 488.77 \text{ MU}$$

SOURCE-AXIS DISTANCE (SAD) CALCULATIONS

An SAD treatment occurs when the treatment machine's isocenter is established at some reference point within the patient. When this is established, it can also be referred to as an isocentric technique. Because the field size is defined at the isocenter, the collimated field matches the field size setting inside the patient and not on the skin surface as seen in the nonisocentric, SSD treatment setup.

One advantage that SAD treatment techniques have over SSD techniques is that when the patient has been properly positioned and the isocenter for the treatment has been established, there is usually no movement of the patient relative to the treatment isocenter for each of the subsequent treatment field. For example, a patient treated using an anterior and posterior treatment field arrangement on a 6-MV, 100-cm isocentric linear accelerator. The patient's central axis separation is 20 cm, and the dose is calculated at the patient's midplane (equal distance established from both anterior and posterior skin surfaces). If we were to treat this arrangement with an SSD technique, the anterior field would be established at 100 cm to the anterior skin surface. After treating the anterior field, the gantry would be rotated 180 degree to treat the posterior field. However, the treatment table would have to be raised until the ODI reads 100 cm on the patient's posterior skin surface.

In treating the same patient with an SAD (isocentric) technique, the anterior SSD would be established at 90 cm. The isocenter is positioned 10 cm beneath the anterior skin surface and 10 cm beneath the posterior skin surface, making it midplane as prescribed. (Note that the 10-cm anterior depth and 10-cm posterior depth add up to the 20-cm central axis separation.) The SAD is 100 cm (90 cm SSD plus 10 cm depth). After treating the anterior field the gantry would be rotated 180 degrees to treat the posterior field. However, in an isocentric technique, the gantry is rotating about the isocenter, which has been established inside the patient. Therefore the patient is at the correct posterior SSD of 90 cm without raising or lowering the treatment table. Less movement between treatment fields lowers the chance of having treatment errors because of positioning variations that occur during patient movement.

TAR, TMR, and TPR work very well with isocentric techniques. PDD can also be used for isocentric treatment techniques. There are two main differences from PDD that will affect calculations using TAR, both caused by the way PDD and TAR are calculated. PDD is calculated from two measurements at two different points in space. TAR is calculated using two measurements at the same point in space. This affects the beam geometry, field divergence, and application of the inverse square law.

First, when using TAR for calculations, the field size at the point of calculation must be used. Under some conditions the field size at the point of interest must be determined. One example would be when trying to determine a dose delivered to points other than the isocenter along the central axis. In this case the treatment field size at the alternate point would change because of beam divergence and would need to be calculated. Another effect on the calculation involves the application of the inverse square law. There will be an inverse square correction needed when calculating the dose to a point other than the isocenter. These points are covered in greater detail in the example problems.

ISOCENTRIC CALCULATION PROCESS

The same basic five-step process described earlier in the section on nonisocentric calculations involving PDD will be used with these isocentric technique calculations:

Step 1. Find the equivalent square of the collimator setting (used for output factor).
Step 2. Find the equivalent square of the BFS (used for TAR, TMR, or TPR).
Step 3. Using the appropriate tables, look up the dose rate factors.
Step 4. Determine the prescribed dose.
Step 5. Use the appropriate equation for determining the time setting.

Several examples are performed using both cobalt-60 and linear accelerator treatment units.

Example 13: A patient is treated on the cobalt-60 treatment machine at 80 cm SAD. A single field is used with the collimator setting of 15×15 cm. There is no blocking used for this treatment. The prescription states that a dose of 3000 cGy is to be delivered to a depth of 5 cm in 10 fractions. Calculate the treatment time.

Step 1. Find the equivalent square of the collimator setting

The equivalent square of a 15×15 cm field is 15×15 cm.

Step 2. Find the equivalent square of the BFS

There is no blocking in this field so the BFS equivalent square is the same as the collimator equivalent square.

Step 3. Using the appropriate tables, look up the dose rate factors

The factors for the dose rate at a point are reference dose rate, output factor, and TAR (TAR is commonly used in lower therapeutic isocentric calculations):

$$\text{Reference dose rate} = 50.6 \text{ cGy/min}$$
$$\text{Output factor } (15 \times 15 \text{ cm}) = 1.030$$
$$\text{TAR } (5,15) = 0.941$$

(The reference dose rate is modified by multiplying it by the output factor of the actual collimator setting.)

Step 4. Determine the prescribed dose

From the prescription the total prescribed dose to a depth of 5 cm is 3000 cGy. This dose is to be delivered in 10 fractions. Therefore the dose per fraction is 300 cGy.

Step 5. Use the appropriate equation for determining the time setting

$$\text{Time setting} = \frac{\text{Dose at a point}}{\text{Dose rate at that point}}, \text{ so}$$

$$\text{Time setting} = \frac{\text{Prescribed dose}}{\text{Output} \times \text{Output factor}_{(CS)} \times \text{TAR}_{(EFS)}}$$

$$\text{Time setting} = \frac{300 \text{ cGy}}{50.6 \text{ cGy/min} \times 1.03 \times 0.941}$$

$$\text{Time setting} = \frac{300 \text{ cGy}}{49.043 \text{ cGy/min}}$$

$$\text{Time setting} = 6.12 \text{ min}$$

Example 14: A patient is treated on the 6-MV linear accelerator treatment machine at 100 cm SAD. The setup SSD is 95 cm. The collimator setting is 15×15 cm. The field is blocked to an 8×8 cm blocked equivalent square. A 5-mm solid plastic tray is used to hold the blocks. The prescription states that a dose of 3000 cGy is to be delivered to a depth of 5 cm in 10 fractions through a single field. Calculate the MU setting using TAR.

The factors for the dose rate at a point are reference dose rate, output factor, TAR, and tray factor:

$$\text{Reference dose rate} = 1.0 \text{ cGy/MU}$$
$$\text{Output factor } (15 \times 15 \text{ cm}) = 1.021$$
$$\text{TAR } (5,8) = 0.941$$
$$\text{Tray factor} = 0.97$$

$$\text{MU setting} = \frac{\text{Prescribed dose}}{\text{Output} \times \text{Output factor}_{(CS)} \times \text{TAR}_{(EFS)} \times \text{TF}}$$

$$\text{MU setting} = \frac{300 \text{ cGy}}{1.0 \text{ cGy/MU} \times 1.021 \times 0.941 \times 0.97}$$

$$\text{MU setting} = \frac{300 \text{ cGy}}{0.9319 \text{ cGy/MU}}$$

$$\text{MU setting} = 322 \text{ MU}$$

In Example 14, shielding blocks are added to the treatment field, making the MU calculation slightly more complex. The reference dose and output factor rate would be the same if there were no blocking. However, there will be a change in the TAR. The area of tissue treated has been reduced to less than the 15×15 cm collimator setting, decreasing the scatter.

The factors for the dose rate at a point are reference dose rate, output factor, TAR, and tray factor.

Example 15: A patient is treated on the cobalt-60 treatment machine at 80 cm SAD. The collimator setting is 15×15 cm. The field is blocked to an 8×8 cm blocked equivalent square. A 5-mm solid plastic tray is used to hold the blocks. The prescription states that a dose of 4000 cGy is to be delivered to a depth of 10 cm in 20 fractions using an anterior and posterior (AP:PA) equally weighted treatment field arrangement. Calculate the time setting.

The factors for the dose rate at a point are reference dose rate, output factor, TAR, and tray factor:

$$\text{Reference dose rate} = 50.6 \text{ cGy/min}$$
$$\text{Output factor } (15 \times 15 \text{ cm}) = 1.030$$
$$\text{TAR } (10,8) = 0.687$$
$$\text{Tray factor} = 0.96$$

$$\text{Time setting} = \frac{\text{Prescribed dose}}{\text{Output} \times \text{Output factor}_{(CS)} \times \text{TAR}_{(EFS)} \times \text{TF}}$$

$$\text{Time setting} = \frac{100 \text{ cGy}}{50.6 \text{ cGy/min} \times 1.03 \times 0.687 \times 0.96}$$

$$\text{Time setting} = \frac{100 \text{ cGy}}{34.373 \text{ cGy/min}}$$

$$\text{Time setting} = 2.91 \text{ min}$$

Example 16: A patient is treated on the 6-MV linear accelerator treatment machine at 100 cm SAD. The setup SSD is 90 cm. The collimator setting is 15×15 cm. The field is blocked to an 8×8 cm blocked equivalent square. A 5-mm solid plastic tray is used to hold the blocks. The prescription states that a dose of 4000 cGy is to be delivered to a depth of 10 cm in 20 fractions using an anterior and posterior (AP:PA) treatment field arrangement. Calculate the MU setting using TAR.

The factors for the dose rate at a point are reference dose rate, output factor, TAR, and tray factor:

$$\text{Reference dose rate} = 1.0 \text{ cGy/MU}$$
$$\text{Output factor } (15 \times 15 \text{ cm}) = 1.021$$
$$\text{TAR } (10,8) = 0.787$$
$$\text{Tray factor} = 0.97$$
$$\text{Prescribed dose} = 100 \text{ cGy/field}$$

$$\text{MU setting} = \frac{\text{Prescribed dose}}{\text{Output} \times \text{Output factor}_{(CS)} \times \text{TAR}_{(EFS)} \times \text{TF}}$$

$$\text{MU setting} = \frac{100 \text{ cGy}}{1.0 \text{ cGy/MU} \times 1.021 \times 0.787 \times 0.97}$$

$$\text{MU setting} = \frac{100 \text{ cGy}}{0.7794 \text{ cGy/MU}}$$

$$\text{MU setting} = 128 \text{ MU/field}$$

When high-energy linear accelerators are used (energies above 10 MV), TMR and TPR are commonly used in the isocentric MU calculations as opposed to TAR.

When TMR or TPR is used for dose calculation, the output for the 10 cm $\times$ 10 cm field size is normally 1.0 cGy/MU.

In the TMR calculations presented in this chapter, two output factors are used. One of the output factors corrects for collimator scatter and is commonly referred to as the COF. The other output factor corrects for patient scatter and is often called the phantom scatter factor (PSF). The total output factor is obtained by multiplying the COF by the PSF.

Example 17: A patient is treated on the 6-MV linear accelerator treatment machine at 100 cm SAD. The setup SSD is 95 cm. The collimator setting is 15×15 cm. There is no blocking used for this treatment. The prescription states that a dose of 3000 cGy is to be delivered to a depth of 5 cm in 10 fractions through a single field. Calculate the MU setting using TMR.

The factors for the dose rate at a point are reference dose rate, output factor, and TMR:

$$\text{Reference dose rate} = 1.0 \text{ cGy/MU}$$
$$\text{COF } (15 \times 15 \text{ cm}) = 1.021$$
$$\text{PSF } (15 \times 15 \text{ cm}) = 1.014$$
$$\text{TMR } (5,15) = 0.937$$
$$\text{Prescribed dose} = 300 \text{ cGy}$$

$$\text{MU setting} = \frac{\text{Prescribed dose}}{\text{Output} \times \text{COF}_{(CS)} \times \text{PSF}_{(EFS)} \times \text{TMR}_{(EFS)}}$$

$$\text{MU setting} = \frac{300 \text{ cGy}}{1.0 \text{ cGy/MU} \times 1.021 \times 1.014 \times 0.937}$$

$$\text{MU setting} = \frac{100 \text{ cGy}}{0.9701 \text{ cGy/MU}}$$

$$\text{MU setting} = 309 \text{ MU}$$

Example 18: A patient is treated on the 6-MV linear accelerator treatment machine at 100 cm SAD. The setup SSD is 90 cm. The collimator setting is 15×15 cm. The field is blocked to an 8×8 cm blocked equivalent square. A 5-mm solid plastic tray is used to hold the blocks. The prescription states that a dose of 4000 cGy is to be delivered to a depth of 10 cm in 20 fractions using an anterior and posterior (AP:PA) treatment field arrangement. Calculate the MU setting using TMR.

The factors for the dose rate at a point are reference dose rate, output factor, and tissue absorption factor:

$$\text{Reference dose rate} = 1.0 \text{ cGy/MU}$$
$$\text{COF } (15 \times 15 \text{ cm}) = 1.021$$
$$\text{PSF } (8 \times 8 \text{ cm}) = 0.992$$
$$\text{TMR } (10,8) = 0.775$$
$$\text{Tray factor} = 0.97$$
$$\text{Prescribed dose} = 100 \text{ cGy/port}$$

$$\text{MU setting} = \frac{\text{Prescribed dose}}{\text{Output} \times \text{COF}_{(CS)} \times \text{PSF}_{(EFS)} \times \text{TMR}_{(EFS)} \times \text{TF}}$$

$$\text{MU setting} = \frac{100 \text{ cGy}}{1.0 \text{ cGy/MU} \times 1.021 \times 0.992 \times 0.775 \times 0.97}$$

$$\text{MU setting} = \frac{100 \text{ cGy}}{0.76141 \text{ cGy/MU}}$$

$$\text{MU setting} = 131 \text{ MU}$$

The next example is similar to the previous one except that TPR will be used.

Example 19: A patient is treated on the 10-MV linear accelerator treatment machine at 100 cm SAD. The setup SSD is 90 cm. The collimator setting is 15×15 cm. The field is blocked to an 8×8 cm blocked equivalent square. A 5-mm solid plastic tray is used to hold the blocks. The prescription states that a dose of 4000 cGy is to be delivered to a depth of 10 cm in 20 fractions using an anterior and posterior (AP:PA) treatment field arrangement. Calculate the MU setting, the total dose to the depth of D_{max}, and the total dose to the cord. For this example, the cord lies at a depth of 5 cm beneath the patient's posterior skin surface.

MU Setting Using TPR

The factors for the dose rate at a point are reference dose rate, output factor, and TPR:

$$Reference\ dose\ rate = 1.0\ cGy/MU$$
$$COF\ (15 \times 15\ cm) = 1.021$$
$$PSF\ (8 \times 8\ cm) = 0.992$$
$$TPR\ (10,8) = 0.8740$$
$$Tray\ factor = 0.97$$
$$Prescribed\ dose = 100\ cGy/port$$

$$MU\ setting = \frac{Prescribed\ dose}{Output \times COF_{(CS)} \times PSF_{(EFS)} \times TPR_{(EFS)} \times TF}$$

$$MU\ setting = \frac{100\ cGy}{1.0\ cGy/MU \times 1.021 \times 0.992 \times 0.874 \times 0.97}$$

$$MU\ setting = \frac{100\ cGy}{0.8587\ cGy/MU}$$

$$MU\ setting = 116\ MU$$

In the next part of the problem, the total dose delivered to two points, at D_{max} and at the level of the spinal cord, must be calculated. There is a dose contributed to each point from both the anterior and posterior treatment fields (obtained by adding the dose delivered by the anterior field to the dose delivered by the posterior field). Deriving this information is explained in the next series of steps. It should be noted that deriving this information can be done with TPR, TMR, and TAR.

Deriving Given Dose in Isocentric Problems

The given dose is the dose delivered at the depth of D_{max} for a single treatment field. In this example problem, each treatment field has its own given dose. Calculating the given dose using TAR, TMR, or TPR is more complex than when using PDD. To calculate the given dose using TPR for this example, the prescribed dose for the field, the source to calculation point distance, and the TPR at the depth of the prescribed dose must be known.

As discussed earlier, both measurements for the TPR are made at the same distance from the source. The field size increases because of divergence as the distance from the source increases. Therefore when using TPR (or either TAR

or TMR) the field size at the point of calculation must be known. To find the field size at any distance, the following relationship can be used:

$$\frac{Field\ size\ at\ distance_1}{Distance_1} = \frac{Field\ size\ at\ distance_2}{Distance_2}$$

In practice the equivalent square of the rectangular field is used in place of the actual field size. For example, if the field size is 20×10 cm, the equivalent square of 13.0 would be used for the field size. To calculate the given dose using TPR, the following equation is used:

$$Dose_A = \frac{Dose_B}{TPR_B} \times \frac{(SCPD_B)^2}{(SCPD_A)^2} \times TPR_A$$

Where:
$Dose_A$ = Dose at point A
$Dose_B$ = Dose at point B
TPR_A = TPR at point A
TPR_B = TPR at point B
$SCPD_A$ = Source to calculation point distance for point A
$SCPD_B$ = Source to calculation point distance for point B

Note that the ratio of $SCPD_B$ and $SCPD_A$ is the application of the inverse square law. SCPD is found by adding the depth to the SSD for that point. The following table assists in the organization of data when calculating the dose to points using TAR, TMR, and TPR.

Point	SSD	Depth	SCPD	Equivalent square	TPR	Dose
A						
B						
C						

Part 1. Calculate the dose to points from the anterior field

Point A represents the depth of D_{max} beneath the skin surface. Point B represents the isocentric point, in this case at a depth of 10 cm at midplane. Point C represents the depth of the cord beneath the anterior skin surface. The cord depth below the skin surface is found by subtracting the depth of the cord beneath the posterior surface (5 cm) from the patient's total central axis separation. With that we have the following.

Point	SSD	Depth	SCPD	Equivalent square	TPR	Dose
A	90	2.5	92.5			
B	90	10	100	8.0	0.874	100
C	90	15	105			

With this the equivalent square and TPR for points A and C can be found:

Field size at point A:

$$\frac{Field\ size\ at\ distance_A}{92.5\ cm} = \frac{8.0\ cm}{100\ cm},\ therefore\ 7.4\ cm$$

$$\frac{Field\ size\ at\ distance_A}{92.5\ cm} = \frac{8.0\ cm}{100\ cm},\ therefore\ 7.4\ cm$$

Now the TPR (2.5, 7.4) can be found. Note that the exact numbers are not directly listed in the tables. Interpolation, as discussed in the Chapter 13, can be used to derive the exact numbers. In this case, TPR (2.5, 7.4) = 1.0426.

Field size at point C:

$$\frac{\text{Field size at distance}_C}{105 \text{ cm}} = \frac{8.0 \text{ cm}}{100 \text{ cm}}, \text{ therefore } 8.4 \text{ cm};$$

So, TPR (15, 8.4) = 0.7486.

At this point there is enough information to calculate the dose from the anterior field to points A and C.

Dose to point A (from anterior):

$$\text{Dose}_A = \frac{\text{Dose}_B}{\text{TPR}_B} \times \frac{(\text{SCPD}_B)^2}{(\text{SCPD}_A)^2} \times \text{TPR}_A$$

$$\text{Dose}_A = \frac{100 \text{ cGy}}{0.8740} \times \frac{(100 \text{ cm})^2}{(92.5 \text{ cm})^2} \times 1.0426$$

$$\text{Dose}_A = 139.4 \text{ cGy}$$

Dose to point C (from anterior):

$$\text{Dose}_C = \frac{\text{Dose}_B}{\text{TPR}_B} \times \frac{(\text{SCPD}_B)^2}{(\text{SCPD}_C)^2} \times \text{TPR}_C$$

$$\text{Dose}_C = \frac{100 \text{ cGy}}{0.8740} \times \frac{(100 \text{ cm})^2}{(105 \text{ cm})^2} \times 0.7486$$

$$\text{Dose}_C = 77.7 \text{ cGy}$$

At this point the table for the anterior perspective can be completed.

Point	SSD	Depth	SCPD	Equivalent square	TPR	Dose
A	90	2.5	92.5	7.4	1.0426	139.4
B	90	10	100	8.0	0.8740	100
C	90	15	105	8.4	0.7486	77.7

At this point, note the confirmation of trends discussed earlier in the chapter. As the depth of calculation increases, the TPR decreases (because of more attenuation). Also, the dose is greater closer to the skin surface.

Part 2. Calculate the dose to points from the posterior field

Again, point A represents the depth of D_{max} beneath the anterior skin surface. Point B represents the isocentric point, in this case at a depth of 10 cm at midplane. Point C represents the depth of the cord beneath the anterior skin surface. However, these points are now measured with respect to the posterior surface. Another grid can be produced.

Point	SSD	Depth	SCPD	Equivalent square	TPR	Dose
A	90	17.5	107.5			
B	90	10	100	8.0	0.8740	100
C	90	5	95			

With this the equivalent square and TPR for points A and C can be found:

Field size at point A (from posterior):

$$\frac{\text{Field size at distance}_A}{107.5 \text{ cm}} = \frac{8.0 \text{ cm}}{100 \text{ cm}}, \text{ therefore } 8.6 \text{ cm}$$

TPR (17.5, 8.6) = 0.6914.

Field size at point C (from posterior):

$$\frac{\text{Field size at distance}_C}{95 \text{ cm}} = \frac{8.0 \text{ cm}}{100 \text{ cm}}, \text{ therefore } 7.6 \text{ cm}$$

TPR (5, 7.6) = 1.00.

At this point there is enough information to calculate the dose from the posterior field to points A and C.

Dose to point A (from posterior):

$$\text{Dose}_A = \frac{100 \text{ cGy}}{0.8740} \times \frac{(100 \text{ cm})^2}{(10.5 \text{ cm})^2} \times 0.6914$$

$$\text{Dose}_A = 68.5 \text{ cGy}$$

Dose to point C (from posterior):

$$\text{Dose}_C = \frac{100 \text{ cGy}}{0.8740} \times \frac{(100 \text{ cm})^2}{(95 \text{ cm})^2} \times 1.00$$

$$\text{Dose}_C = 125.8 \text{ cGy}$$

At this point the grid from the posterior perspective can be completed.

Point	SSD	Depth	SCPD	Equivalent square	TPR	Dose
A	90	17.5	107.5	8.6	0.6914	68.5
B	90	10	100	8.0	0.8740	100
C	90	5	95	7.6	1.00	126.8

Part 3. Add the doses to the points from the anterior and posterior fields to finalize the problem

Point	Anterior	Posterior	Total
A	139.4	68.5	207.9
B	100	100	200
C	77.7	126.8	204.5

This technique gives a perspective of the doses received at points other than the isocenter for SAD calculations. If calculations for several energies were performed for the parameters just given, a pattern would definitely be noted. Lower energies would deposit a higher dose at the outer aspects of the treatment volume. In other words, the D_{max} doses would be higher for the lower energies, all other parameters remaining the same. Conversely, as energy increases, the superficial doses would be lower. In all cases the dose to isocenter would be the same. The higher energy beams exhibit more skin sparing (less superficial dose) and are therefore deemed to be better suited for treatment of deep-seated tumors.

UNEQUAL BEAM WEIGHTING

Some radiation therapy cases use parallel opposed or multiple beam arrangements, with different doses delivered to the treatment portals. This is commonly done when the tumor volume lies closer to the skin surface but would still benefit from multiportal treatment. The result is a greater dose near the entrance of the favored field and a lower dose in the tissue near the entrance of the opposing field.[1,2] Although uneven doses are administered in the outer tissues, the doses to the point of specification should remain consistent with the prescription. In other words, the isocenter in an SAD technique still receives the overall prescribed dose.

Look at the basic dose calculation equation:

$$\text{Treatment setting} = \frac{\text{Dose}}{\text{Dose rate}}$$

The component that is affected directly by the field weighting is the prescribed dose per port. If a prescription is written to deliver 200 cGy through two ports and the fields are equally weighted, each port would deliver 100 cGy to the prescription point. However, if the prescription describes a treatment to be delivered from an AP:PA perspective and specifies that the AP field is to receive twice the amount of the PA field (written as 2 to 1 or 2:1), a different dose must be delivered through each field.

The total dose to be delivered through all ports (in this case two) should be divided by the sum of the weighting. In this case, the weighting sum is three (2 + 1) and the total dose is divided by this number: 200 cGy/3 = 66.7 cGy. This defines the amount of each dose component. Then this component is multiplied by the weighting for each port; this provides the appropriate dosage to be delivered through each port as follows:

$$\text{AP dose} = 66.7 \text{ cGy} \times 2 = 133.4 \text{ cGy}$$
$$\text{PA dose} = 66.7 \text{ cGy} \times 1 = 66.7 \text{ cGy}$$

These numbers would be used in the dose calculation to find the time or MU setting for each treatment portal. A quick check for accuracy would be to add the individual port doses; they should equal (or be less because of rounding off numbers) to the original dose prescribed.

This method can be used for any number of treatment ports and beam arrangements and can be used in all treatment calculations. Weighting does not affect the dose rate, only the dose to be administered through each port.

SEPARATION OF ADJACENT FIELDS

Many treatment techniques involve the junction of fields with the adjoining margins either abutted or separated depending on various circumstances. This may be due to the need to break what would be a very large, irregularly shaped field into two or more that would be better managed. It may also be needed because of the need to use different beam energies over a large area that need to also be continuous. Because of rapid "fall off" of the dose near the edge of each field, a small change in the relative spacing of the field borders can produce a large change in the dose distribution in the junction volume.

The hazard of having a "gap" or junction area may be a dose that (1) exceeds normal tissue tolerance or (2) is inadequate to therapeutically treat the tumor.

Fields may be abutted or have a gap between them:

1. *Abutted fields*—If the adjacent fields are abutted on the surface, the fields overlap to an increasing degree with depth because of divergence.
2. *Separated fields*—The theory behind this is that one can abut the field edges at depth as opposed to on the skin surface. In this way one can spare a tissue at depth an overdose because of overlapping fields. One would have them abut at a desired depth leaving a gap on the skin surface.

Examples of abutting fields would include lateral head and neck and supraclavicular fossa fields or tangential breast and supraclavicular fossa arrangements. Examples of separated fields are evident in craniospinal irradiation or mantle and para-aortic fields in lymphoma cases. In either case of abutting or separated fields, the medical dosimetrist and radiation therapist must be able to make sure that the area of overlap (or non-overlap) occurs where it is intended.

There are several common methods of obtaining dose uniformity across field junctions. These include dosimetric isodose matching, junction shifts, half-beam blocking, and geometric matching:

Dosimetric isodose matching—With the availability of modern treatment planning computers, separation of fields can easily be calculated and plotted for maximum dose uniformity. The hot and cold spots can easily be seen and compensated for. The accuracy of dosimetric isodose matching depends on the accuracy of the individual field isodose curves.

Junction shift—Fields that abut on the skin surface can be moved during the course of treatment so that any hot or cold spot inherently present can be spread, or feathered, over a distance. This technique calls for a shift in field sizes for the abutting fields. The fields are shifted one or more times during the course the patient's treatment to move the areas of overlap. In this way, the overall dose in any areas of overlap is spread out over a greater volume and allows for a better opportunity of lowering side effects in that area.

Half-beam blocking—Specific shielding blocks can be designed to block out one side of a treatment field to produce a field that has no divergence along one side, most commonly along the central ray of the beam where there is no divergence. Two abutting fields can then be used to match field borders on the phantom surface and have no divergence at depth. Asymmetric jawed fields or multileaf collimators can also accomplish this on modern treatment units.

Geometric matching—It is possible to achieve dose uniformity at the junction of two fields at depth through geometric means (Fig. 21-9). This is possible because the geometric boundary of each abutting field is defined by the 50% decrement line (at the edge of all fields, the dose to the very edge falls off to 50% of the dose at the central ray). By knowing the field sizes of adjacent fields, the treatment SSD, and the depths, the size of the gap on the patient can be calculated to ensure that the fields abut at the correct depth. Note that it is possible to have fields at different depths; the important aspect is that the fields abut at a depth and that the gap measurement on the skin surface can be calculated with the following equation:

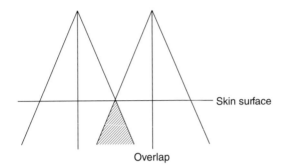

- Skin surface

Overlap

Figure 21-9. Geometric matching at depth. Because of divergence, a gap on the patient's skin between two adjacent fields converges at a depth within the patient.

$$\text{Gap} = \left(\frac{L_1}{2} \times \frac{d}{SSD_1} \right) + \left(\frac{L_2}{2} \times \frac{d}{SSD_2} \right)$$

Where:
Length$_1$ = Length of the first field
SSD$_1$ = Treatment source to skin distance of the first field
Length$_2$ = Length of the second field
SSD$_2$ = Treatment source to skin distance of the second field
Depth = Depth of abutment

The following example demonstrated the calculation of a field gap.

Example 20: A patient is treated using two adjacent fields. The collimator setting for Field 1 is 8 cm width × 12 cm length. The collimator setting for Field 2 is 10 cm width × 20 cm length. Both fields are set up at 100 cm SSD. Calculate the gap on the skin surface for the fields to abut at 5 cm depth.

The geometric gap calculation is based on the principles of similar triangles. A very important consideration when performing a gap calculation is to make sure that the field size (L) is corrected for the SSD. In this example, the field size is defined at the skin surface that is 100 cm SSD. Therefore the field size is the same as the collimator setting. A second consideration is that the depth must be the same for both fields:

$$\text{Gap} = \frac{12 \text{ cm}}{2} \times \frac{5 \text{ cm}}{100 \text{ cm}} + \frac{20 \text{ cm}}{2} \times \frac{5 \text{ cm}}{100}$$
$$\text{Gap} = 0.3 \text{ cm} + 0.5 \text{ cm}$$
$$\text{Gap} = 0.8 \text{ cm}$$

The 0.8 cm calculated is the minimal skin gap between the two fields. This means that the distance between the inferior border of Field 1 and superior border of Field 2 must be at least 0.8 cm. Often the gap is made slightly larger to allow for variations in the day-to-day setup.

Example 21: A patient is treated using two adjacent fields. The collimator setting for Field 1 is 8 cm width × 16 cm length. The collimator setting for Field 2 is 10 cm width × 26 cm length. Field 1 is set up at 95 cm SSD and Field 2 is set up at 90 cm SSD. Calculate the gap on the skin surface for the fields to abut at 5 cm depth.

Because the collimator setting is the field size at 100 cm, we must adjust the field sizes to the appropriate SSD. For Field 1 this is 15.2 cm and for Field 2 it is 23.4 cm:

$$\text{Gap} = \frac{15.2 \text{ cm}}{2} \times \frac{5 \text{ cm}}{92.0 \text{ cm}} + \frac{23.4 \text{ cm}}{2} \times \frac{5 \text{ cm}}{90.0 \text{ cm}}$$
$$\text{Gap} = 0.413 \text{ cm} + 0.65 \text{ cm}$$
$$\text{Gap} = 1.063 \text{ cm}$$

Again, 1.063 cm is the minimum gap and the treatment team would probably round up and measure 1.07 on the skin.

Table 21-3	Reference dose rate	
Treatment Machine	**Dose Rate Specified for**	**Reference Dose Rate for a 10 × 10 cm Collimator Setting**
Cobalt-60	SSD/PDD	51.7 cGy/min at depth of D$_{max}$
Cobalt-60	SAD/TAR	50.6 cGy/min in air at 80 cm
6 MV	SSD/PDD	0.993 cGy/MU at depth of D$_{max}$
6 MV	SAD/TAR	1.000 cGy/MU in air at 100 cm
10 MV	SSD/PDD	0.968 cGy/MU at depth of D$_{max}$
10 MV	SAD/TAR	1.000 cGy/MU in air at 100 cm
10 MV	SAD/TMR	1.015 cGy/MU at 100 cm at depth D$_{max}$
18 MV	SSD/PDD	0.944 cGy/MU at depth of D$_{max}$
18 MV	SAD/TAR	1.000 cGy/MU in air at 100 cm
10 MV	SAD/TPR	1.000 cGy/MU in air at 100 cm

PDD, Percentage depth dose; *SAD*, source-axis distance; *SSD*, source-skin distance; *TAR*, tissue-air ratio; *TMR*, tissue-maximum ratio; *TPR*, tissue-phantom ratio.

Table 21-4 Output factors

Output factor for PDD calculations (Sc, Sp)

Mach/Eq Sq	4.0	5.0	6.0	7.0	8.0	9.0	10.0	11.0	12.0	13.0	14.0	15.0	16.0	17.0	18.0	19.0	20.0	22.0	24.0	26.0	28.0	30.0	32.0	35.0
Cobalt-60	0.928	0.945	0.962	0.971	0.980	0.990	1.000	1.009	1.019	1.028	1.037	1.046	1.053	1.060	1.067	1.074	1.081	1.089	1.096	1.102	1.105	1.109		
6 MV	0.927	0.940	0.954	0.967	0.979	0.990	1.000	1.007	1.014	1.021	1.028	1.035	1.039	1.044	1.049	1.053	1.058	1.065	1.072	1.079	1.084	1.088	1.092	1.098
10 MV	0.925	0.938	0.953	0.967	0.979	0.990	1.000	1.005	1.011	1.016	1.022	1.027	1.032	1.037	1.041	1.046	1.051	1.058	1.065	1.069	1.071	1.073	1.077	1.081
18 MV	0.904	0.922	0.941	0.961	0.976	0.988	1.000	1.007	1.014	1.021	1.028	1.036	1.041	1.046	1.051	1.056	1.060	1.067	1.073	1.079	1.084	1.087	1.090	1.093

PDD, Percentage depth dose; *TAR*, tissue-air ratio.

Output factor for TAR calculations (Sc)

Mach/Eq Sq	4.0	5.0	6.0	7.0	8.0	9.0	10.0	11.0	12.0	13.0	14.0	15.0	16.0	17.0	18.0	19.0	20.0	22.0	24.0	26.0	28.0	30.0	32.0	35.0
Cobalt-60	0.946	0.961	0.975	0.981	0.987	0.993	1.000	1.006	1.012	1.018	1.024	1.030	1.035	1.039	1.044	1.048	1.053	1.057	1.061	1.063	1.063	1.063		
6 MV	0.948	0.961	0.970	0.979	0.987	0.994	1.000	1.004	1.008	1.013	1.017	1.021	1.024	1.028	1.031	1.035	1.038	1.041	1.045	1.048	1.051	1.052	1.053	1.055
10 MV	0.938	0.951	0.962	0.973	0.982	0.991	1.000	1.005	1.009	1.014	1.018	1.023	1.026	1.030	1.033	1.037	1.040	1.044	1.048	1.051	1.052	1.054	1.057	1.061
18 MV	0.914	0.931	0.948	0.965	0.978	0.989	1.000	1.006	1.012	1.017	1.023	1.029	1.032	1.036	1.039	1.043	1.046	1.052	1.057	1.063	1.066	1.067	1.069	1.070

Table 21-5 Output factors

Phantom scatter factor for TMR and TPR calculations (Sp)

Mach/Eq Sq	4.0	5.0	6.0	7.0	8.0	9.0	10.0	11.0	12.0	13.0	14.0	15.0	16.0	17.0	18.0	19.0	20.0	22.0	24.0	26.0	28.0	30.0	32.0	35.0
Cobalt-60	0.981	0.983	0.987	0.990	0.993	0.997	1.000	1.003	1.007	1.010	1.013	1.016	1.017	1.020	1.022	1.025	1.027	1.030	1.033	1.037	1.040	1.043		
6 MV	0.978	0.978	0.984	0.988	0.992	0.996	1.000	1.003	1.006	1.008	1.011	1.014	1.015	1.016	1.017	1.017	1.019	1.023	1.026	1.030	1.031	1.034	1.037	1.041
10 MV	0.986	0.986	0.991	0.994	0.997	0.999	1.000	1.000	1.002	1.002	1.004	1.004	1.006	1.007	1.008	1.009	1.011	1.013	1.016	1.017	1.018	1.018	1.019	1.019
18 MV	0.989	0.990	0.993	0.996	0.998	0.999	1.000	1.001	1.002	1.004	1.005	1.007	1.009	1.010	1.012	1.012	1.013	1.014	1.015	1.015	1.017	1.019	1.020	1.021

TMR, Tissue-maximum ratio; TPR, tissue-phantom ratio.

Table 21-6   Percentage depth dose table cobalt-60 at 80 cm SSD

Eq Sq Depth (cm)	0.0	4.0	5.0	6.0	7.0	8.0	9.0	10.0	11.0	12.0	13.0	14.0	15.0	16.0	17.0	18.0	19.0	20.0	22.0	24.0	26.0	28.0	30.0
0.0	14.9	15.0	17.4	19.8	21.7	23.6	25.5	27.4	28.1	28.8	29.5	30.1	30.8	32.3	33.7	35.2	36.7	38.1	41.2	44.3	47.4	50.4	53.4
0.5	100.0	100.0	100.0	100.0	100.0	100.0	100.0	100.0	100.0	100.0	100.0	100.0	100.0	100.0	100.0	100.0	100.0	100.0	100.0	100.0	100.0	100.0	100.0
1.0	95.6	96.4	96.6	96.8	96.9	97.0	97.0	97.1	97.1	97.1	97.2	97.2	97.2	97.3	97.3	97.4	97.4	97.5	97.7	97.8	98.0	98.1	98.2
2.0	87.4	90.2	90.7	91.3	91.6	92.0	92.3	92.6	92.8	92.9	93.1	93.3	93.5	93.6	93.7	93.8	93.9	94.0	94.1	94.2	94.3	94.4	94.4
3.0	80.1	84.2	85.1	85.8	86.4	87.0	87.4	87.8	88.1	88.5	88.8	89.1	89.3	89.5	89.7	89.9	90.1	90.1	90.2	90.3	90.4	90.5	90.4
4.0	73.2	78.4	79.4	80.4	81.2	81.9	82.6	83.1	83.5	84.0	84.4	84.8	85.1	85.3	85.5	85.8	86.0	86.0	86.1	86.2	86.4	86.5	86.3
5.0	67.1	72.9	74.0	75.1	76.0	76.9	77.7	78.3	78.8	79.4	79.9	80.4	80.7	81.0	81.3	81.6	81.9	81.9	82.0	82.1	82.2	82.3	82.1
6.0	61.4	67.7	68.9	70.1	71.1	72.0	72.9	73.6	74.2	74.8	75.4	76.0	76.3	76.7	77.0	77.3	77.5	77.6	77.7	77.9	78.1	78.2	78.0
7.0	56.2	62.7	64.0	65.3	66.4	67.4	68.3	69.0	69.7	70.3	71.0	71.6	71.9	72.3	72.7	73.1	73.3	73.4	73.6	73.7	73.9	74.0	73.8
8.0	51.5	58.0	59.4	60.7	61.9	62.9	63.9	64.6	65.3	66.1	66.8	67.4	67.8	68.2	68.6	69.1	69.2	69.3	69.5	69.7	69.9	69.9	69.7
9.0	47.3	53.7	55.1	56.4	57.5	58.6	59.6	60.4	61.1	61.9	62.6	63.2	63.6	64.1	64.5	65.0	65.1	65.2	65.4	65.7	65.9	65.9	65.8
10.0	43.3	49.7	51.0	52.3	53.5	54.5	55.6	56.3	57.1	57.9	58.6	59.2	59.7	60.2	60.6	61.1	61.2	61.3	61.6	61.9	62.1	62.1	61.9
11.0	39.8	45.9	47.2	48.5	49.7	50.7	51.7	52.5	53.3	54.1	54.9	55.4	55.9	56.4	56.9	57.3	57.4	57.5	57.8	58.1	58.4	58.4	58.2
12.0	36.4	42.4	43.7	45.0	46.2	47.2	48.1	48.9	49.7	50.5	51.3	51.8	52.3	52.8	53.3	53.6	53.8	53.9	54.3	54.6	55.0	54.8	54.7
13.0	33.4	39.2	40.5	41.6	42.8	43.8	44.7	45.5	46.3	47.1	47.8	48.3	48.8	49.4	49.9	50.1	50.3	50.5	50.9	51.2	51.6	51.4	51.3
14.0	30.7	36.1	37.4	38.6	39.6	40.6	41.5	42.3	43.1	43.9	44.6	45.1	45.6	46.1	46.7	46.8	47.0	47.2	47.6	48.0	48.3	48.1	48.0
15.0	28.1	33.4	34.6	35.7	36.7	37.7	38.5	39.3	40.0	40.8	41.5	42.0	42.5	43.1	43.6	43.8	43.9	44.1	44.6	45.0	45.2	45.1	44.9
16.0	25.9	30.8	31.9	33.0	34.0	34.9	35.7	36.4	37.2	38.0	38.6	39.1	39.6	40.2	40.6	40.8	41.0	41.2	41.6	42.1	42.2	42.1	42.0
17.0	23.8	28.4	29.5	30.5	31.4	32.3	33.1	33.8	34.6	35.3	35.9	36.4	36.9	37.5	37.8	38.0	38.3	38.5	38.9	39.4	39.5	39.3	39.2
18.0	21.8	26.2	27.2	28.2	29.1	30.0	30.7	31.4	32.1	32.8	33.4	33.9	34.4	34.9	35.2	35.4	35.6	35.9	36.3	36.8	36.8	36.7	36.6
19.0	20.0	24.2	25.1	26.0	26.9	27.7	28.4	29.1	29.8	30.5	31.0	31.5	32.0	32.5	32.8	33.0	33.2	33.5	33.9	34.4	34.4	34.3	34.2
20.0	18.4	22.3	23.2	24.1	24.9	25.7	26.3	27.0	27.6	28.3	28.8	29.3	29.8	30.3	30.5	30.7	30.9	31.2	31.7	32.2	32.1	32.0	31.9
21.0	17.0	20.6	21.5	22.3	23.1	23.8	24.4	25.0	25.7	26.3	26.8	27.2	27.7	28.1	28.4	28.6	28.8	29.1	29.6	30.0	29.9	29.8	29.7
22.0	15.6	19.0	19.8	20.6	21.3	22.0	22.6	23.2	23.8	24.3	24.8	25.3	25.7	26.1	26.3	26.6	26.8	27.0	27.5	27.9	27.8	27.7	27.6
23.0	14.3	17.5	18.3	19.0	19.7	20.4	20.9	21.5	22.1	22.6	23.1	23.5	23.9	24.3	24.5	24.7	25.0	25.2	25.7	26.0	25.9	25.8	25.7
24.0	13.1	16.1	16.8	17.5	18.2	18.8	19.3	19.9	20.4	20.9	21.4	21.8	22.2	22.5	22.7	23.0	23.2	23.4	23.9	24.1	24.1	24.0	23.9
25.0	12.1	14.9	15.6	16.2	16.8	17.4	17.9	18.5	19.0	19.5	19.9	20.3	20.7	20.9	21.2	21.4	21.6	21.8	22.3	22.5	22.4	22.3	22.3
26.0	11.1	13.7	14.3	14.9	15.5	16.1	16.6	17.1	17.6	18.0	18.4	18.8	19.2	19.4	19.6	19.8	20.1	20.3	20.8	20.9	20.8	20.7	20.7
27.0	10.2	12.7	13.3	13.8	14.4	14.9	15.4	15.8	16.3	16.7	17.1	17.5	17.8	18.1	18.3	18.5	18.7	18.9	19.4	19.4	19.4	19.3	19.2
28.0	9.4	11.7	12.2	12.8	13.3	13.7	14.2	14.6	15.1	15.5	15.8	16.2	16.5	16.7	17.0	17.2	17.4	17.6	18.0	18.0	18.0	17.9	17.9
29.0	8.7	10.8	11.3	11.8	12.3	12.7	13.1	13.6	14.0	14.4	14.7	15.1	15.4	15.6	15.8	16.0	16.2	16.4	16.8	16.7	16.7	16.6	16.6
30.0	8.0	9.9	10.4	10.9	11.3	11.7	12.1	12.5	12.9	13.3	13.6	13.9	14.2	14.4	14.6	14.8	15.0	15.2	15.6	15.5	15.5	15.4	15.4
BSF/PSF	1.000	1.015	1.018	1.021	1.025	1.028	1.032	1.035	1.038	1.041	1.045	1.048	1.051	1.053	1.056	1.058	1.061	1.063	1.066	1.070	1.073	1.077	1.080

PDD COBLT

BSF, Backscatter factor; *PDD*, percentage depth dose.

Table 21-7 6 MV percentage depth dose at 100 cm SSD

Eq Sq Depth (cm)	0.0	4.0	5.0	6.0	7.0	8.0	9.0	10.0	11.0	12.0	13.0	14.0	15.0	16.0	17.0	18.0	19.0	20.0	22.0	24.0	26.0	28.0	30.0	32.0	35.0
0.0	19.2	19.2	19.2	20.5	21.8	23.0	24.3	25.6	26.7	27.9	29.1	30.2	31.4	32.6	33.8	35.1	36.3	37.5	39.0	40.4	41.9	43.2	44.5	45.7	47.6
1.0	96.8	96.9	96.9	97.0	97.0	97.0	97.1	97.1	97.2	97.2	97.3	97.3	97.4	97.4	97.5	97.5	97.6	97.6	97.7	97.8	98.0	98.1	98.1	98.2	98.3
1.5	100.0	100.0	100.0	100.0	100.0	100.0	100.0	100.0	100.0	100.0	100.0	100.0	100.0	100.0	100.0	100.0	100.0	100.0	100.0	100.0	100.0	100.0	100.0	100.0	100.0
2.0	97.4	98.2	98.4	98.4	98.5	98.5	98.6	98.6	98.6	98.6	98.6	98.6	98.6	98.6	98.6	98.7	98.7	98.7	98.7	98.7	98.7	98.7	98.7	98.7	98.7
3.0	91.1	93.8	94.4	94.7	94.9	95.0	95.0	95.1	95.1	95.1	95.2	95.2	95.2	95.3	95.3	95.4	95.4	95.5	95.5	95.6	95.6	95.6	95.6	95.6	95.5
4.0	85.3	89.6	90.6	90.9	91.3	91.4	91.5	91.5	91.5	91.6	91.6	91.7	91.7	91.8	91.9	92.0	92.1	92.2	92.2	92.3	92.4	92.3	92.3	92.3	92.2
5.0	79.9	84.5	85.6	86.1	86.6	86.8	87.0	87.1	87.3	87.5	87.7	87.8	87.9	88.1	88.2	88.3	88.5	88.6	88.7	88.8	89.0	89.0	89.0	89.0	88.9
6.0	74.8	79.7	80.9	81.5	82.1	82.4	82.7	83.0	83.2	83.5	83.8	84.0	84.1	84.3	84.5	84.7	84.8	85.0	85.2	85.4	85.6	85.6	85.7	85.8	85.7
7.0	70.1	75.1	76.3	77.1	77.8	78.3	78.7	79.0	79.3	79.6	79.9	80.3	80.4	80.6	80.8	81.0	81.2	81.4	81.7	82.0	82.2	82.3	82.4	82.5	82.3
8.0	65.7	70.8	72.1	72.9	73.7	74.2	74.7	75.1	75.5	75.9	76.2	76.6	76.8	77.0	77.3	77.5	77.8	77.9	78.3	78.6	78.8	78.9	79.0	79.1	79.0
9.0	61.5	66.7	68.0	68.9	69.8	70.4	71.0	71.4	71.8	72.2	72.6	73.0	73.2	73.5	73.8	74.1	74.3	74.5	74.9	75.3	75.5	75.6	75.8	76.0	75.7
10.0	57.7	62.8	64.1	65.1	66.1	66.7	67.4	67.8	68.3	68.8	69.2	69.6	69.8	70.1	70.5	70.8	71.0	71.2	71.6	72.0	72.3	72.5	72.7	72.8	72.6
11.0	54.0	59.2	60.4	61.5	62.4	63.1	63.8	64.2	64.8	65.3	65.8	66.1	66.4	66.8	67.1	67.5	67.7	67.9	68.4	68.8	69.0	69.2	69.4	69.6	69.3
12.0	50.7	55.7	57.0	58.0	58.9	59.7	60.4	60.9	61.4	61.9	62.4	62.8	63.1	63.5	63.9	64.3	64.5	64.8	65.3	65.8	66.0	66.2	66.4	66.5	66.2
13.0	47.5	52.4	53.6	54.6	55.6	56.4	57.2	57.7	58.2	58.8	59.3	59.7	60.0	60.4	60.8	61.2	61.5	61.7	62.2	62.7	63.0	63.2	63.4	63.5	63.3
14.0	44.6	49.4	50.6	51.6	52.5	53.3	54.1	54.6	55.1	55.7	56.3	56.6	57.0	57.4	57.8	58.2	58.5	58.8	59.4	59.9	60.1	60.3	60.6	60.6	60.4
15.0	41.8	46.6	47.8	48.7	49.6	50.5	51.2	51.7	52.3	52.9	53.5	53.9	54.2	54.7	55.1	55.5	55.8	56.1	56.6	57.1	57.4	57.6	57.9	57.8	57.6
16.0	39.2	43.9	45.1	46.0	46.9	47.8	48.5	49.1	49.7	50.3	50.9	51.2	51.6	52.0	52.5	52.8	53.1	53.4	54.0	54.5	54.8	55.1	55.4	55.2	55.1
17.0	36.8	41.4	42.5	43.5	44.3	45.2	45.9	46.4	47.1	47.7	48.2	48.6	49.0	49.4	49.9	50.2	50.6	50.9	51.5	52.0	52.3	52.6	52.9	52.7	52.6
18.0	34.5	39.0	40.1	41.0	41.9	42.7	43.4	44.0	44.6	45.3	45.8	46.2	46.6	47.0	47.5	47.8	48.2	48.5	49.1	49.6	49.9	50.2	50.5	50.3	50.2
19.0	32.4	36.8	37.8	38.7	39.6	40.5	41.1	41.7	42.3	43.0	43.5	43.9	44.3	44.7	45.1	45.5	45.8	46.1	46.8	47.2	47.6	48.0	48.2	48.0	47.9
20.0	30.4	34.6	35.7	36.6	37.4	38.2	38.9	39.5	40.1	40.7	41.2	41.6	42.0	42.5	42.9	43.2	43.6	43.9	44.6	45.0	45.4	45.7	45.9	45.8	45.6
21.0	28.6	32.7	33.7	34.5	35.3	36.1	36.8	37.4	38.0	38.6	39.1	39.5	39.9	40.3	40.7	41.1	41.4	41.8	42.4	42.9	43.2	43.6	43.7	43.6	43.5
22.0	26.8	30.8	31.8	32.6	33.4	34.2	34.8	35.4	36.0	36.9	37.1	37.5	37.9	38.3	38.7	39.1	39.4	39.8	40.4	40.8	41.2	41.6	41.7	41.6	41.5
23.0	25.2	29.1	30.0	30.8	31.6	32.4	33.0	33.6	34.2	34.8	35.2	35.6	36.0	36.4	36.8	37.2	37.5	37.9	38.5	38.9	39.3	39.7	39.8	39.6	39.5
24.0	23.6	27.5	28.4	29.1	29.9	30.6	31.2	31.8	32.4	32.9	33.4	33.7	34.1	34.6	35.0	35.3	35.7	36.0	36.7	37.1	37.5	37.9	37.8	37.7	37.6
25.0	22.2	26.0	26.8	27.6	28.3	29.0	29.6	30.1	30.7	31.3	31.7	32.0	32.4	32.9	33.2	33.6	33.9	34.3	34.9	35.3	35.7	36.1	36.0	35.9	35.8
26.0	20.9	24.5	25.3	26.0	26.7	27.4	27.9	28.5	29.1	29.6	30.0	30.4	30.8	31.2	31.5	31.9	32.2	32.6	33.2	33.6	34.0	34.4	34.3	34.2	34.1
27.0	19.6	23.2	24.0	24.7	25.3	26.0	26.5	27.0	27.6	28.1	28.4	28.8	29.2	29.6	30.0	30.3	30.7	31.0	31.6	32.0	32.4	32.7	32.6	32.6	32.4
28.0	18.4	21.9	22.6	23.3	24.0	24.6	25.1	25.6	26.1	26.6	26.9	27.3	27.7	28.1	28.4	28.8	29.2	29.5	30.1	30.5	30.9	31.1	31.1	31.0	30.9
29.0	17.3	20.7	21.4	22.0	22.7	23.3	23.7	24.2	24.7	25.2	25.6	25.9	26.3	26.7	27.0	27.4	27.7	28.1	28.6	29.0	29.4	29.6	29.5	29.5	29.4
30.0	16.2	19.5	20.2	20.8	21.4	22.0	22.4	22.9	23.4	23.8	24.2	24.6	24.9	25.3	25.7	26.0	26.4	26.7	27.2	27.6	28.0	28.1	28.0	28.0	27.9
																									PDD 6 MV
PSF	1.000	1.002	1.003	1.007	1.012	1.016	1.021	1.025	1.028	1.031	1.033	1.036	1.039	1.040	1.041	1.043	1.044	1.045	1.048	1.051	1.054	1.057	1.060	1.063	1.067

PDD, Percentage depth dose.

| Table 21-8 | 18 MV percentage depth dose at 100 cm SSD | | | | | | | | | | | | | | | | | | | | | | |

Eq Sq	0.0	4.0	5.0	6.0	7.0	8.0	9.0	10.0	11.0	12.0	13.0	14.0	15.0	16.0	17.0	18.0	19.0	20.0	22.0	24.0	26.0	28.0	30.0	32.0
0.0	10.0	10.0	10.1	11.7	13.4	15.4	17.6	19.8	21.3	22.8	24.3	25.8	27.3	28.7	30.1	31.5	32.9	34.4	36.2	38.0	39.3	41.2	42.0	42.9
1.0	77.8	77.8	77.8	78.3	78.7	79.3	80.0	80.6	80.9	81.2	81.6	81.9	82.2	82.7	83.2	83.7	84.2	84.7	85.2	85.7	86.2	86.5	86.8	87.0
2.0	95.4	95.5	95.5	95.6	95.7	95.8	96.0	96.2	96.2	96.2	96.2	96.2	96.3	96.5	96.7	96.9	97.2	97.4	97.5	97.7	97.8	97.9	98.0	98.0
3.0	98.3	98.4	98.4	98.4	98.4	98.5	98.6	98.6	98.6	98.6	98.6	98.6	98.7	98.7	98.8	98.9	99.0	99.0	99.1	99.1	99.2	99.2	99.3	99.3
3.5	100.0	100.0	100.0	100.0	100.0	100.0	100.0	100.0	100.0	100.0	100.0	100.0	100.0	100.0	100.0	100.0	100.0	100.0	100.0	100.0	100.0	100.0	100.0	100.0
4.0	98.1	98.8	98.9	98.9	98.9	98.9	98.9	98.9	98.9	98.8	98.8	98.8	98.8	98.8	98.8	98.8	98.8	98.8	98.8	98.7	98.7	98.8	98.8	98.8
5.0	93.5	95.8	96.3	96.3	96.2	96.2	96.1	96.1	96.1	96.0	96.0	96.0	95.9	95.9	95.8	95.8	95.8	95.7	95.7	95.7	95.7	95.7	95.7	95.8
6.0	89.0	92.8	93.4	93.4	93.4	93.3	93.3	93.3	93.2	93.2	93.2	93.1	93.1	93.0	93.0	92.9	92.9	92.8	92.8	92.8	92.8	92.9	92.9	93.0
7.0	84.9	89.0	89.8	89.9	89.9	89.8	89.8	89.8	89.8	89.8	89.8	89.8	89.8	89.8	89.7	89.7	89.6	89.6	89.6	89.6	89.6	89.7	89.8	89.8
8.0	81.0	85.4	86.2	86.3	86.4	86.4	86.4	86.5	86.5	86.6	86.6	86.7	86.6	86.6	86.5	86.5	86.4	86.4	86.4	86.4	86.5	86.6	86.7	86.8
9.0	77.2	81.8	82.6	82.9	83.1	83.0	83.0	83.1	83.2	83.2	83.3	83.4	83.4	83.4	83.3	83.3	83.3	83.3	83.3	83.4	83.6	83.7	83.8	83.9
10.0	73.6	78.3	79.1	79.5	79.7	79.9	79.7	79.9	80.0	80.1	80.3	80.3	80.3	80.3	80.3	80.3	80.2	80.3	80.3	80.4	80.6	80.8	81.0	81.1
11.0	70.2	74.9	75.7	76.1	76.4	76.5	76.6	76.7	76.9	77.0	77.1	77.2	77.3	77.3	77.3	77.3	77.3	77.3	77.4	77.5	77.7	77.9	78.0	78.1
12.0	67.0	71.7	72.5	72.9	73.2	73.3	73.5	73.6	73.8	73.9	74.1	74.2	74.3	74.3	74.4	74.4	74.4	74.4	74.5	74.6	74.9	75.0	75.2	75.2
13.0	64.0	68.7	69.4	69.8	70.1	70.3	70.5	70.7	70.9	71.0	71.2	71.3	71.4	71.5	71.6	71.6	71.6	71.6	71.7	71.9	72.1	72.3	72.4	72.5
14.0	61.0	65.7	66.4	66.8	67.1	67.4	67.7	67.9	68.0	68.2	68.3	68.5	68.6	68.8	68.9	68.9	68.9	69.0	69.1	69.3	69.5	69.7	69.8	69.8
15.0	58.3	62.8	63.6	64.0	64.4	64.7	64.9	65.1	65.3	65.5	65.7	65.9	66.0	66.2	66.3	66.3	66.3	66.4	66.6	66.8	67.0	67.2	67.4	67.4
16.0	55.6	60.2	60.9	61.4	61.7	62.1	62.4	62.6	62.8	63.0	63.2	63.4	63.5	63.7	63.7	63.8	63.9	64.0	64.2	64.4	64.7	64.9	65.0	65.0
17.0	53.1	57.6	58.3	58.8	59.1	59.5	59.8	60.0	60.3	60.5	60.8	61.0	61.1	61.3	61.4	61.5	61.5	61.6	61.8	62.1	62.3	62.5	62.8	62.7
18.0	50.7	55.1	55.8	56.4	56.7	57.1	57.4	57.7	58.0	58.2	58.5	58.7	58.8	58.9	59.1	59.1	59.2	59.3	59.6	59.8	60.1	60.3	60.5	60.4
19.0	48.4	52.8	53.5	54.0	54.4	54.7	55.0	55.3	55.6	56.0	56.2	56.4	56.6	56.7	56.8	56.9	57.0	57.1	57.3	57.6	57.9	58.2	58.3	58.2
20.0	46.3	50.5	51.2	51.7	52.1	52.4	52.8	53.1	53.4	53.7	54.0	54.2	54.3	54.5	54.6	54.7	54.8	54.9	55.2	55.5	55.9	56.1	56.2	56.1
21.0	44.2	48.3	49.0	49.6	49.9	50.3	50.6	51.0	51.3	51.7	51.9	52.1	52.2	52.4	52.5	52.6	52.7	52.9	53.2	53.5	53.9	54.1	54.2	54.1
22.0	42.3	46.3	46.9	47.5	47.8	48.2	48.6	48.9	49.3	49.6	49.9	50.0	50.2	50.4	50.5	50.6	50.7	50.9	51.3	51.6	51.9	52.2	52.3	52.2
23.0	40.4	44.3	45.0	45.5	45.9	46.3	46.6	47.0	47.3	47.7	47.9	48.1	48.3	48.4	48.5	48.7	48.8	49.0	49.4	49.7	50.0	50.3	50.3	50.2
24.0	38.6	42.4	43.1	43.7	44.0	44.4	44.7	45.1	45.4	45.8	46.0	46.2	46.4	46.6	46.8	46.9	47.0	47.2	47.5	47.8	48.2	48.5	48.4	48.4
25.0	36.9	40.7	41.3	41.9	42.2	42.6	42.9	43.3	43.6	44.0	44.2	44.4	44.6	44.9	45.0	45.1	45.2	45.4	45.8	46.1	46.4	46.7	46.6	46.6
26.0	35.3	38.9	39.6	40.2	40.5	40.9	41.2	41.6	41.9	42.2	42.5	42.7	42.9	43.1	43.2	43.4	43.5	43.7	44.0	44.4	44.7	44.9	44.9	44.8
27.0	33.7	37.3	38.0	38.5	38.9	39.2	39.6	39.9	40.3	40.6	40.8	41.0	41.3	41.5	41.6	41.7	41.9	42.0	42.4	42.7	43.0	43.3	43.2	43.1
28.0	32.2	35.7	36.4	36.9	37.3	37.7	38.0	38.3	38.7	39.0	39.2	39.5	39.7	39.9	40.0	40.1	40.3	40.4	40.8	41.1	41.5	41.6	41.6	41.5
29.0	30.9	34.3	34.9	35.4	35.8	36.1	36.5	36.8	37.1	37.4	37.7	37.9	38.2	38.4	38.5	38.6	38.7	38.7	39.3	39.6	39.9	40.1	40.0	40.0
30.0	29.5	32.9	33.5	34.0	34.3	34.7	35.0	35.3	35.6	35.9	36.2	36.4	36.7	36.9	37.0	37.1	37.3	37.4	37.8	38.1	38.5	38.6	38.5	38.5
PSF	1.000	1.002	1.003	1.006	1.009	1.011	1.012	1.013	1.014	1.015	1.017	1.018	1.019	1.021	1.022	1.024	1.025	1.027	1.028	1.028	1.029	1.030	1.031	1.033

PDD 18 MV

PDD, Percentage depth dose; *PSF*, phantom scatter factor.

Table 21-9 6 MV tissue-air ratio

Eq Sq / Depth (cm)	0.0	4.0	5.0	6.0	7.0	8.0	9.0	10.0	11.0	12.0	13.0	14.0	15.0	16.0	17.0	18.0	19.0	20.0	22.0	24.0	26.0	28.0	30.0	32.0	35.0
0.0	0.186	0.187	0.187	0.200	0.213	0.227	0.240	0.254	0.266	0.279	0.291	0.304	0.316	0.329	0.342	0.354	0.367	0.380	0.396	0.412	0.428	0.443	0.457	0.471	0.492
1.0	0.957	0.960	0.961	0.965	0.970	0.974	0.979	0.984	0.987	0.990	0.994	0.997	1.000	1.002	1.003	1.005	1.006	1.008	1.012	1.017	1.021	1.025	1.028	1.032	1.037
1.5	1.000	1.002	1.003	1.007	1.012	1.016	1.021	1.025	1.028	1.031	1.033	1.036	1.039	1.040	1.041	1.043	1.044	1.045	1.048	1.051	1.054	1.057	1.060	1.063	1.067
2.0	0.982	0.992	0.994	0.999	1.004	1.009	1.014	1.018	1.021	1.024	1.027	1.030	1.032	1.034	1.035	1.037	1.038	1.039	1.043	1.046	1.049	1.052	1.055	1.057	1.061
3.0	0.936	0.966	0.973	0.979	0.986	0.991	0.996	1.001	1.004	1.007	1.010	1.013	1.016	1.018	1.020	1.021	1.023	1.025	1.028	1.032	1.035	1.038	1.041	1.043	1.047
4.0	0.894	0.940	0.951	0.959	0.966	0.972	0.977	0.982	0.985	0.988	0.991	0.994	0.997	0.999	1.001	1.004	1.006	1.008	1.012	1.015	1.019	1.022	1.025	1.027	1.031
5.0	0.853	0.903	0.915	0.924	0.933	0.941	0.946	0.952	0.956	0.961	0.965	0.970	0.974	0.977	0.979	0.982	0.984	0.987	0.991	0.996	1.000	1.003	1.006	1.009	1.013
6.0	0.814	0.867	0.880	0.890	0.900	0.909	0.916	0.923	0.928	0.933	0.939	0.944	0.949	0.952	0.955	0.958	0.961	0.964	0.969	0.974	0.979	0.984	0.987	0.990	0.995
7.0	0.777	0.831	0.845	0.857	0.868	0.878	0.886	0.894	0.900	0.906	0.911	0.917	0.923	0.926	0.930	0.933	0.937	0.940	0.946	0.951	0.957	0.962	0.965	0.969	0.974
8.0	0.742	0.798	0.812	0.824	0.837	0.847	0.856	0.865	0.871	0.878	0.884	0.891	0.897	0.901	0.905	0.908	0.912	0.916	0.922	0.928	0.934	0.939	0.943	0.946	0.952
9.0	0.708	0.765	0.779	0.792	0.805	0.817	0.826	0.836	0.843	0.850	0.856	0.863	0.870	0.874	0.878	0.883	0.887	0.891	0.898	0.904	0.911	0.916	0.920	0.924	0.930
10.0	0.676	0.733	0.747	0.761	0.775	0.787	0.798	0.808	0.815	0.822	0.830	0.837	0.844	0.848	0.853	0.857	0.862	0.866	0.873	0.880	0.887	0.892	0.897	0.901	0.908
11.0	0.645	0.702	0.716	0.730	0.744	0.756	0.767	0.778	0.786	0.793	0.801	0.808	0.816	0.821	0.826	0.830	0.835	0.840	0.847	0.854	0.861	0.867	0.872	0.876	0.883
12.0	0.616	0.672	0.686	0.700	0.714	0.727	0.738	0.749	0.757	0.765	0.772	0.780	0.788	0.793	0.798	0.804	0.809	0.814	0.822	0.829	0.837	0.843	0.848	0.852	0.859
13.0	0.588	0.643	0.657	0.671	0.684	0.697	0.709	0.721	0.729	0.737	0.745	0.753	0.761	0.766	0.772	0.777	0.783	0.788	0.796	0.804	0.812	0.818	0.823	0.828	0.835
14.0	0.561	0.616	0.630	0.643	0.656	0.669	0.681	0.693	0.701	0.709	0.718	0.726	0.734	0.740	0.745	0.751	0.756	0.762	0.771	0.779	0.788	0.794	0.799	0.804	0.811
15.0	0.536	0.590	0.604	0.617	0.630	0.642	0.655	0.667	0.675	0.684	0.692	0.701	0.709	0.715	0.721	0.726	0.732	0.738	0.747	0.755	0.764	0.771	0.776	0.781	0.788
16.0	0.511	0.565	0.579	0.592	0.605	0.617	0.630	0.642	0.651	0.659	0.668	0.676	0.685	0.691	0.697	0.702	0.708	0.714	0.723	0.732	0.741	0.748	0.753	0.758	0.766
17.0	0.488	0.542	0.555	0.568	0.581	0.593	0.605	0.617	0.626	0.634	0.643	0.651	0.660	0.666	0.672	0.678	0.684	0.690	0.699	0.708	0.717	0.725	0.730	0.736	0.744
18.0	0.466	0.518	0.531	0.544	0.557	0.569	0.581	0.593	0.602	0.611	0.619	0.628	0.637	0.643	0.649	0.655	0.661	0.667	0.676	0.686	0.695	0.703	0.708	0.714	0.722
19.0	0.445	0.496	0.509	0.521	0.534	0.546	0.558	0.570	0.579	0.588	0.596	0.605	0.614	0.620	0.626	0.632	0.638	0.644	0.653	0.663	0.672	0.680	0.686	0.692	0.701
20.0	0.424	0.474	0.478	0.499	0.512	0.524	0.535	0.547	0.556	0.565	0.573	0.582	0.591	0.597	0.603	0.609	0.615	0.621	0.631	0.640	0.650	0.658	0.664	0.670	0.679
21.0	0.405	0.455	0.467	0.479	0.490	0.502	0.513	0.525	0.534	0.543	0.551	0.560	0.569	0.575	0.581	0.587	0.593	0.599	0.609	0.618	0.628	0.636	0.642	0.649	0.658
22.0	0.387	0.435	0.447	0.459	0.470	0.482	0.493	0.504	0.513	0.522	0.530	0.539	0.548	0.554	0.560	0.566	0.572	0.578	0.588	0.597	0.607	0.615	0.622	0.628	0.638
23.0	0.370	0.417	0.429	0.440	0.451	0.463	0.474	0.485	0.493	0.502	0.510	0.519	0.528	0.534	0.539	0.546	0.552	0.558	0.567	0.577	0.587	0.595	0.602	0.608	0.618
24.0	0.352	0.399	0.411	0.422	0.433	0.443	0.454	0.465	0.473	0.482	0.490	0.499	0.507	0.513	0.519	0.525	0.531	0.537	0.547	0.557	0.567	0.575	0.582	0.588	0.598
25.0	0.337	0.383	0.394	0.405	0.415	0.426	0.436	0.447	0.455	0.463	0.471	0.480	0.488	0.494	0.500	0.506	0.512	0.518	0.528	0.538	0.548	0.556	0.562	0.569	0.579
26.0	0.321	0.366	0.377	0.387	0.398	0.408	0.418	0.428	0.436	0.444	0.453	0.461	0.469	0.475	0.481	0.486	0.492	0.498	0.508	0.518	0.528	0.536	0.543	0.549	0.559
27.0	0.307	0.351	0.362	0.372	0.382	0.392	0.402	0.412	0.419	0.427	0.435	0.443	0.451	0.457	0.462	0.468	0.474	0.480	0.490	0.500	0.510	0.518	0.525	0.531	0.541
28.0	0.292	0.336	0.347	0.357	0.366	0.376	0.385	0.395	0.403	0.410	0.418	0.425	0.433	0.439	0.444	0.450	0.455	0.461	0.471	0.482	0.492	0.500	0.507	0.513	0.523
29.0	0.279	0.322	0.333	0.342	0.351	0.361	0.370	0.379	0.386	0.394	0.401	0.409	0.416	0.422	0.427	0.433	0.438	0.444	0.454	0.464	0.474	0.483	0.489	0.495	0.505
30.0	0.266	0.308	0.318	0.327	0.336	0.345	0.354	0.363	0.370	0.377	0.385	0.392	0.399	0.405	0.410	0.416	0.421	0.427	0.437	0.447	0.457	0.465	0.471	0.478	0.487

6 MV TAR

TAR, Tissue-air ratio.

Table 21-10   18 MV tissue-air ratio

Eq Sq Depth (cm)	0.0	4.0	5.0	6.0	7.0	8.0	9.0	10.0	11.0	12.0	13.0	14.0	15.0	16.0	17.0	18.0	19.0	20.0	22.0	24.0	26.0	28.0	30.0	32.0	35.0
0.0	0.093	0.094	0.094	0.110	0.126	0.145	0.166	0.187	0.201	0.216	0.230	0.245	0.259	0.273	0.287	0.301	0.315	0.329	0.347	0.364	0.382	0.395	0.404	0.413	0.426
1.0	0.739	0.741	0.742	0.748	0.755	0.762	0.769	0.776	0.780	0.784	0.788	0.792	0.796	0.802	0.808	0.814	0.820	0.826	0.831	0.837	0.842	0.847	0.851	0.854	0.860
2.0	0.925	0.928	0.929	0.932	0.935	0.939	0.942	0.945	0.946	0.947	0.949	0.950	0.951	0.955	0.958	0.962	0.965	0.969	0.971	0.975	0.977	0.979	0.982	0.985	0.985
3.0	0.972	0.975	0.975	0.978	0.981	0.984	0.986	0.988	0.989	0.990	0.991	0.992	0.994	0.996	0.998	1.001	1.003	1.005	1.006	1.007	1.009	1.010	1.012	1.014	1.016
3.5	1.000	1.002	1.003	1.006	1.009	1.011	1.012	1.013	1.014	1.015	1.017	1.018	1.019	1.021	1.022	1.024	1.025	1.027	1.028	1.029	1.030	1.030	1.031	1.033	1.035
4.0	0.989	0.998	1.000	1.003	1.005	1.007	1.008	1.009	1.010	1.011	1.013	1.014	1.015	1.016	1.018	1.019	1.021	1.022	1.023	1.024	1.025	1.025	1.026	1.028	1.030
5.0	0.960	0.986	0.992	0.994	0.997	0.998	0.999	1.000	1.001	1.002	1.002	1.003	1.004	1.005	1.006	1.008	1.009	1.010	1.010	1.011	1.011	1.012	1.014	1.015	1.018
6.0	0.932	0.971	0.981	0.983	0.986	0.987	0.988	0.990	0.990	0.991	0.991	0.992	0.993	0.994	0.995	0.996	0.997	0.998	0.998	0.999	0.999	1.000	1.002	1.004	1.007
7.0	0.906	0.949	0.960	0.963	0.966	0.968	0.969	0.970	0.971	0.972	0.974	0.975	0.976	0.977	0.978	0.979	0.980	0.981	0.982	0.982	0.983	0.984	0.986	0.988	0.991
8.0	0.880	0.926	0.938	0.942	0.946	0.949	0.950	0.951	0.953	0.954	0.956	0.957	0.959	0.960	0.961	0.962	0.963	0.964	0.965	0.965	0.966	0.967	0.970	0.972	0.976
9.0	0.855	0.903	0.915	0.920	0.925	0.928	0.929	0.930	0.932	0.934	0.936	0.938	0.940	0.941	0.942	0.944	0.945	0.946	0.947	0.948	0.949	0.951	0.954	0.956	0.960
10.0	0.830	0.880	0.892	0.898	0.904	0.908	0.909	0.910	0.912	0.915	0.917	0.920	0.922	0.923	0.924	0.926	0.927	0.928	0.929	0.931	0.932	0.935	0.938	0.941	0.945
11.0	0.806	0.856	0.869	0.875	0.881	0.885	0.888	0.890	0.892	0.895	0.897	0.900	0.902	0.904	0.905	0.907	0.908	0.910	0.911	0.913	0.914	0.917	0.920	0.923	0.927
12.0	0.783	0.834	0.847	0.853	0.859	0.863	0.866	0.869	0.872	0.874	0.877	0.879	0.882	0.884	0.886	0.887	0.889	0.891	0.893	0.894	0.896	0.899	0.902	0.905	0.909
13.0	0.761	0.812	0.825	0.831	0.837	0.842	0.845	0.849	0.852	0.854	0.857	0.859	0.862	0.864	0.866	0.869	0.871	0.873	0.875	0.876	0.878	0.881	0.884	0.887	0.891
14.0	0.739	0.790	0.803	0.809	0.815	0.820	0.825	0.829	0.832	0.834	0.837	0.839	0.842	0.845	0.847	0.850	0.852	0.855	0.857	0.859	0.861	0.864	0.867	0.870	0.874
15.0	0.718	0.768	0.781	0.788	0.795	0.800	0.805	0.809	0.812	0.815	0.818	0.821	0.824	0.827	0.829	0.832	0.834	0.837	0.839	0.842	0.844	0.847	0.850	0.853	0.858
16.0	0.697	0.748	0.761	0.768	0.775	0.780	0.785	0.790	0.793	0.796	0.800	0.803	0.806	0.809	0.811	0.814	0.816	0.819	0.822	0.825	0.828	0.831	0.834	0.837	0.842
17.0	0.677	0.727	0.740	0.747	0.754	0.760	0.765	0.770	0.774	0.777	0.781	0.784	0.788	0.791	0.794	0.796	0.799	0.802	0.805	0.808	0.811	0.814	0.817	0.821	0.826
18.0	0.658	0.708	0.720	0.728	0.735	0.741	0.746	0.751	0.755	0.759	0.763	0.767	0.771	0.774	0.776	0.779	0.781	0.784	0.787	0.791	0.794	0.798	0.801	0.805	0.810
19.0	0.639	0.689	0.701	0.709	0.716	0.722	0.727	0.732	0.736	0.740	0.745	0.749	0.753	0.756	0.759	0.761	0.764	0.767	0.770	0.774	0.777	0.781	0.785	0.788	0.794
20.0	0.621	0.670	0.682	0.690	0.697	0.703	0.708	0.713	0.717	0.722	0.726	0.731	0.735	0.738	0.741	0.743	0.746	0.749	0.753	0.757	0.761	0.765	0.769	0.772	0.778
21.0	0.603	0.651	0.663	0.671	0.679	0.685	0.690	0.695	0.700	0.704	0.709	0.713	0.718	0.721	0.724	0.726	0.729	0.732	0.736	0.741	0.745	0.749	0.753	0.757	0.763
22.0	0.586	0.633	0.645	0.653	0.660	0.667	0.672	0.677	0.682	0.687	0.691	0.696	0.701	0.704	0.707	0.709	0.712	0.715	0.720	0.724	0.729	0.733	0.737	0.742	0.748
23.0	0.569	0.605	0.627	0.635	0.643	0.650	0.655	0.660	0.665	0.670	0.674	0.679	0.684	0.687	0.690	0.692	0.695	0.698	0.703	0.708	0.713	0.717	0.721	0.726	0.732
24.0	0.553	0.599	0.610	0.618	0.626	0.633	0.638	0.643	0.648	0.653	0.657	0.662	0.667	0.670	0.673	0.677	0.680	0.683	0.688	0.692	0.697	0.701	0.705	0.710	0.716
25.0	0.538	0.582	0.594	0.602	0.610	0.617	0.622	0.627	0.632	0.636	0.641	0.646	0.651	0.654	0.657	0.660	0.664	0.667	0.672	0.676	0.681	0.686	0.690	0.694	0.701
26.0	0.522	0.556	0.577	0.585	0.594	0.601	0.606	0.611	0.616	0.620	0.625	0.629	0.634	0.637	0.641	0.644	0.648	0.651	0.656	0.661	0.666	0.670	0.674	0.679	0.685
27.0	0.507	0.551	0.565	0.570	0.578	0.585	0.590	0.596	0.600	0.605	0.609	0.614	0.619	0.622	0.626	0.629	0.633	0.636	0.641	0.645	0.650	0.655	0.659	0.663	0.670
28.0	0.492	0.535	0.546	0.554	0.562	0.569	0.574	0.580	0.585	0.589	0.594	0.598	0.603	0.607	0.610	0.614	0.617	0.621	0.626	0.630	0.635	0.639	0.644	0.648	0.655
29.0	0.479	0.521	0.532	0.540	0.548	0.554	0.560	0.565	0.570	0.574	0.579	0.583	0.588	0.591	0.595	0.599	0.602	0.606	0.611	0.615	0.620	0.625	0.629	0.634	0.641
30.0	0.465	0.507	0.517	0.525	0.533	0.540	0.545	0.550	0.554	0.559	0.563	0.568	0.572	0.576	0.580	0.583	0.587	0.591	0.596	0.601	0.606	0.610	0.615	0.619	0.626

Table 21-11 6 MV tissue maximum ratio

Depth (cm)	Eq Sq 0.0	4.0	5.0	6.0	7.0	8.0	9.0	10.0	11.0	12.0	13.0	14.0	15.0	16.0	17.0	18.0	19.0	20.0	22.0	24.0	26.0	28.0	30.0	32.0	35.0
0.0	0.186	0.187	0.186	0.199	0.210	0.223	0.235	0.248	0.259	0.271	0.282	0.293	0.304	0.316	0.329	0.339	0.352	0.364	0.378	0.392	0.406	0.419	0.431	0.443	0.461
1.0	0.957	0.958	0.958	0.958	0.958	0.959	0.959	0.960	0.960	0.960	0.962	0.962	0.962	0.963	0.963	0.964	0.964	0.965	0.966	0.968	0.969	0.970	0.970	0.971	0.972
1.5	1.000	1.000	1.000	1.000	1.000	1.000	1.000	1.000	1.000	1.000	1.000	1.000	1.000	1.000	1.000	1.000	1.000	1.000	1.000	1.000	1.000	1.000	1.000	1.000	1.000
2.0	0.982	0.990	0.991	0.992	0.992	0.993	0.993	0.993	0.993	0.993	0.994	0.994	0.993	7.692	0.994	0.994	0.994	0.994	0.995	0.995	0.995	0.995	0.995	0.994	0.994
3.0	0.936	0.964	0.970	0.972	0.974	0.975	0.976	0.977	0.977	0.977	0.978	0.978	0.978	7.692	0.980	0.979	0.980	0.981	0.981	0.982	0.982	0.982	0.982	0.981	0.981
4.0	0.894	0.938	0.948	0.952	0.955	0.957	0.957	0.958	0.958	0.958	0.959	0.959	0.960	7.692	0.962	0.963	0.964	0.965	0.966	0.966	0.967	0.967	0.967	0.966	0.966
5.0	0.853	0.901	0.912	0.918	0.922	0.926	0.927	0.929	0.930	0.932	0.934	0.936	0.937	7.692	0.940	0.942	0.943	0.944	0.946	0.948	0.949	0.949	0.949	0.949	0.949
6.0	0.814	0.865	0.877	0.884	0.889	0.895	0.897	0.900	0.903	0.905	0.909	0.911	0.913	7.692	0.917	0.556	0.920	0.922	0.925	0.927	0.929	0.931	0.931	0.931	0.933
7.0	0.777	0.829	0.842	0.851	0.858	0.864	0.868	0.872	0.875	0.879	0.882	0.885	0.888	7.692	0.893	0.895	0.898	0.900	0.903	0.905	0.908	0.910	0.910	0.912	0.913
8.0	0.742	0.796	0.810	0.818	0.827	0.834	0.838	0.844	0.847	0.852	0.856	0.860	0.863	7.692	0.869	0.871	0.874	0.877	0.880	0.883	0.886	0.888	0.890	0.890	0.892
9.0	0.708	0.763	0.777	0.786	0.795	0.804	0.809	0.816	0.820	0.824	0.829	0.833	0.837	7.692	0.843	0.847	0.850	0.853	0.857	0.860	0.864	0.867	0.868	0.869	0.872
10.0	0.676	0.732	0.745	0.756	0.766	0.775	0.782	0.788	0.793	0.797	0.803	0.808	0.812	7.692	0.819	0.822	0.826	0.829	0.833	0.837	0.842	0.844	0.846	0.848	0.851
11.0	0.645	0.701	0.714	0.725	0.735	0.744	0.751	0.759	0.765	0.769	0.775	0.780	0.785	7.692	0.793	0.796	0.800	0.804	0.808	0.813	0.817	0.820	0.823	0.824	0.828
12.0	0.616	0.671	0.684	0.695	0.706	0.716	0.723	0.731	0.736	0.742	0.747	0.753	0.758	7.692	0.767	0.771	0.775	0.779	0.784	0.789	0.794	0.798	0.800	0.802	0.805
13.0	0.588	0.642	0.655	0.666	0.676	0.686	0.694	0.703	0.709	0.715	0.721	0.727	0.732	7.692	0.742	0.745	0.750	0.754	0.760	0.765	0.770	0.774	0.776	0.779	0.783
14.0	0.561	0.615	0.628	0.639	0.648	0.658	0.667	0.676	0.682	0.688	0.695	0.701	0.706	7.692	0.716	0.720	0.724	0.729	0.736	0.741	0.748	0.751	0.754	0.756	0.760
15.0	0.536	0.589	0.602	0.613	0.623	0.620	0.642	0.651	0.657	0.663	0.670	0.677	0.682	7.692	0.693	0.696	0.701	0.706	0.713	0.718	0.725	0.729	0.732	0.735	0.739
16.0	0.511	0.564	0.577	0.588	0.598	0.607	0.617	0.626	0.633	0.639	0.647	0.653	0.659	7.692	0.670	0.673	0.678	0.683	0.690	0.696	0.703	0.708	0.710	0.713	0.718
17.0	0.488	0.541	0.553	0.564	0.574	0.584	0.593	0.602	0.609	0.615	0.622	0.628	0.635	7.692	0.646	0.650	0.655	0.660	0.667	0.674	0.680	0.686	0.689	0.692	0.697
18.0	0.466	0.517	0.529	0.540	0.550	0.560	0.569	0.579	0.586	0.593	0.599	0.606	0.613	7.692	0.623	0.628	0.633	0.638	0.645	0.653	0.659	0.665	0.668	0.672	0.677
19.0	0.445	0.495	0.507	0.517	0.528	0.537	0.547	0.556	0.563	0.570	0.577	0.584	0.591	7.692	0.601	0.606	0.611	0.616	0.623	0.631	0.638	0.643	0.647	0.651	0.657
20.0	0.424	0.473	0.486	0.496	0.506	0.516	0.524	0.534	0.541	0.548	0.555	0.562	0.569	7.692	0.579	0.584	0.589	0.594	0.602	0.609	0.617	0.623	0.626	0.630	0.636
21.0	0.405	0.454	0.466	0.476	0.484	0.494	0.502	0.512	0.519	0.527	0.533	0.541	0.548	7.692	0.558	0.563	0.568	0.573	0.581	0.588	0.596	0.602	0.606	0.611	0.616
22.0	0.387	0.434	0.446	0.456	0.464	0.474	0.483	0.492	0.499	0.506	0.513	0.520	0.527	7.692	0.538	0.543	0.548	0.553	0.561	0.568	0.576	0.582	0.587	0.591	0.598
23.0	0.370	0.416	0.428	0.437	0.446	0.456	0.464	0.473	0.480	0.487	0.494	0.501	0.508	7.692	0.518	0.523	0.529	0.534	0.541	0.549	0.557	0.563	0.568	0.572	0.579
24.0	0.352	0.398	0.410	0.419	0.428	0.436	0.445	0.454	0.460	0.468	0.474	0.482	0.488	7.692	0.499	0.503	0.509	0.514	0.522	0.530	0.538	0.544	0.549	0.553	0.560
25.0	0.337	0.382	0.393	0.402	0.410	0.419	0.427	0.436	0.443	0.449	0.456	0.463	0.470	7.692	0.480	0.485	0.490	0.496	0.504	0.512	0.520	0.526	0.530	0.535	0.543
26.0	0.321	0.365	0.376	0.384	0.393	0.402	0.409	0.418	0.424	0.431	0.439	0.445	0.451	7.692	0.462	0.466	0.471	0.477	0.485	0.493	0.501	0.507	0.512	0.516	0.524
27.0	0.307	0.350	0.361	0.369	0.377	0.386	0.394	0.402	0.408	0.414	0.421	0.428	0.434	7.692	0.444	0.449	0.454	0.459	0.468	0.476	0.484	0.490	0.495	0.500	0.507
28.0	0.292	0.335	0.346	0.355	0.362	0.370	0.377	0.385	0.392	0.398	0.405	0.410	0.417	7.692	0.427	0.431	0.436	0.441	0.449	0.459	0.467	0.473	0.478	0.483	0.490
29.0	0.279	0.321	0.332	0.340	0.344	0.355	0.362	0.370	0.375	0.382	0.388	0.395	0.400	7.692	0.410	0.415	0.420	0.425	0.433	0.441	0.450	0.457	0.461	0.466	0.473
30.0	0.266	0.307	0.317	0.325	0.332	0.340	0.347	0.354	0.360	0.366	0.373	0.378	0.384	7.692	0.394	0.399	0.403	0.409	0.417	0.425	0.434	0.440	0.444	0.450	0.456

Table 21-12	Tray wedge and compensator factors					
	Tray	Factor	Wedge	Factor	Brass Compensator	Factor
Cobalt-60	5 mm solid	0.96	15 degree	0.828	1 mm	0.956
	5 mm slotted	0.97	30 degree	0.744	2 mm	0.914
			45 degree	0.653	3 mm	0.874
			60 degree	0.424	4 mm	0.835
6 MV	5 mm solid	0.97	15 degree	0.828	1 mm	0.965
	5 mm slotted	0.98	30 degree	0.714	2 mm	0.931
			45 degree	0.580	3 mm	0.899
			60 degree	0.424	4 mm	0.867
10 MV	5 mm solid	0.97	15 degree	0.895	1 mm	0.971
	5 mm slotted	0.98	30 degree	0.802	2 mm	0.943
			45 degree	0.702	3 mm	0.916
			60 degree	0.513	4 mm	0.889
18 MV	5 mm solid	0.98	15 degree	0.866	1 mm	0.927
	5 mm slotted	0.99	30 degree	0.775	2 mm	0.945
			45 degree	0.656	3 mm	0.918
			60 degree	0.449	4 mm	0.892

SUMMARY

This chapter has introduced the concepts that affect dose delivery along with some basic methods of performing photon beam dose calculations. The methods used in most therapy centers will reflect that treatment team's philosophy, as developed by the medical physics team and the radiation oncologists. The calculations presented here represent only a limited perspective of photon beam dose calculations. This material should provide the radiation therapist and medical dosimetrist with a good basis on which to further explore dosage treatment factors and concepts of treatment planning in radiation therapy.

Review Questions

1. Percentage depth dose increases with increasing
   I.   Energy
   II. Depth
   III. Field size
   a. I and II
   b. I and III
   c. II and III
   d. I, II, and III
2. Tissue-air ratio decreases with decreasing
   I.   Field size
   II. Depth
   III. SSD

   a. I
   b. II
   c. III
   d. I, II, and III
3. When blocking is used in a treatment calculation, the area of the collimator is used in determining
   I.   TMR
   II. OF
   III. PDD
   a. I
   b. II
   c. III
   d. I, II, and III
4. Which of the following central axis depth dose quantities would most likely be used to compute an accurate monitor unit setting on an 18-MV unit for an isocentric treatment?
   a. Percentage depth dose
   b. Backscatter factor
   c. Tissue-maximum ratio
   d. All of the above
5. Two parallel opposed equally weighted cobalt-60 fields are separated by 20 cm of tissue and treated with an SSD technique. The maximum dose will occur
   a. Directly on the skin surface
   b. At the midline of the patient
   c. 0.5 cm under skin surface
   d. 5 cm under the skin surface

6. The advantages of using parallel opposed isocentric fields for treatment delivery are (compared with non-isocentric)
   a. Less opportunity for movement error
   b. Less overall dose to the skin surface
   c. Both A and B
   d. Neither A nor B

7. A wedge filter _____ the output of the beam and must thus be taken into account in the treatment calculations.
   a. Increases
   b. Decreases
   c. Does not affect
   d. Not enough information given

8. Mayneord's factor is used to convert
   a. PDD with a change in SSD from the standard
   b. TAR with a change in SSD from the standard
   c. Exposure rate with a change in SSD from the standard
   d. An exposure in roentgens to cGy

9. Any time an object is placed in the path of a therapeutic beam of radiation, it must be corrected for in the dose calculation to account for beam absorption.
   a. True
   b. False

10. A therapeutic radiation beam is composed of the TAR for a 20 × 10 cm field size plus the scatter component.
    a. True
    b. False

Questions to Ponder

1. Analyze how the collimator or field size can affect the output of a linear accelerator.

2. Describe how the source-skin distance causes percentage depth dose to vary.

3. A patient's larynx is to be treated using an isocentric technique on a linear accelerator; the patient's separation at the central axis (CAX) is 9 cm and will be treated to midplane. The treatment will use parallel opposed right and left lateral fields. The isocenter of the machine is established at 100 cm.
   a. What is the SSD on the patient's skin?
   b. If a field size of 6 × 6 cm is set on the collimator, what is the field size on the skin surface?

4. Explain the relationship between beam quality (energy) and TMR.

5. A 20-cm thick patient is to be treated on a cobalt-60 unit at 80 cm SAD. Two opposed 15 × 15 cm ports are used to deliver a treatment dose of 180 cGy per day to the midline (midplane). Determine the treatment time per port.

6. A patient is to receive 5040 cGy to his lung in 28 fractions. The treatment will use 15 × 11 cm opposed 6-MV photons to midplane at 100 cm SAD. The separation is 21 cm. The field is blocked to a 11 × 11 cm equivalent field. A 5-mm solid tray is used to support the blocks. Find the MU for each port each day.

7. Calculate the MU setting to deliver 300 cGy to a depth of 12 cm on a 6-MV unit using a single beam at 100 cm SSD using a field size of 15 × 8 cm. Using this information, determine what the dose would be at a depth of 6 cm.

8. Compare and contrast the factors that influence percentage depth dose and tissue-phantom ratio.

9. Look up the percentage depth dose at 80 cm SSD and 7 cm depth for a cobalt-60 unit with a 10 × 10 cm field size. Determine the percentage depth dose for the same field size and depth at 100 cm SSD.

10. Two opposing 10 × 10 cm cobalt-60 fields at an SSD of 80 cm are used with a separation of 20 cm. If the given dose is 100 cGy from each field, what is the dose at midline?

REFERENCES

1. Bentel GC: *Radiation therapy planning,* ed 2, New York, 1996, McGraw-Hill.
2. Bentel GC, Nelson CE, Noell KT: *Treatment planning and dose calculations in radiation oncology,* ed 4, Elmsford, NY, 1989, Pergamon Press.
3. Johns H, Cunningham J: *The physics of radiology,* ed 4, Springfield, Ill, 1983, Charles C Thomas.
4. Khan FM: *The physics of radiation therapy,* ed 2, Baltimore, 1997, Williams & Wilkins.
5. *Medicalibration,* available at http://www.medicalibration.com/our-products/oc3d-expert-system/glossary.doc/odyframe.htm (accessed 1 August 2002).
6. Selman J: *The basic physics of radiation therapy,* ed 3, Springfield, Ill, 1990, Charles C Thomas.
7. Shahabi S: *Blackburn's introduction to clinical radiation therapy physics,* Madison, Wisc, 1989, Medical Physics Publishing.
8. Stanton R, Stinson D: *Applied physics for radiation oncology,* Madison, Wisc, 1996, Medical Physics Publishing.

22

Dose Distributions

Karl L. Prado, Charlotte Prado

Outline

Key Terms

"The patient will benefit from a course of radiation therapy."

Thus begins the treatment-planning process. Radiation will be used to treat the patient. How is the patient best treated? What are the goals and constraints of treatment? How will these goals be achieved? **Treatment planning** can be defined as the process by which dose delivery is optimized for a given patient and clinical situation. The radiation therapy planning and delivery process is intricate. Radiation dose deposition methods must be properly understood and planned to ensure disease is treated and normal structures are spared. The clinical picture is often variable and decision making is complex. The treatment-planning method must be an effective tool in the decision-making process. It should simplify the definition of specific treatment goals and facilitate their implementation. In this chapter, clinical radiation dose distributions produced by external beams of photons are discussed and photon-beam treatment-planning methods are reviewed.

PHOTON DOSE DISTRIBUTIONS

Isodose Distributions

Dose distributions are spatial representations of the magnitude of the dose produced by a source of radiation. They describe the variation of dose with position within an irradiated volume. The percentage depth dose (PDD) curve (Fig. 22-1) is an example of a one-dimensional representation of the variation of dose. Percent depth dose curves, explained in a previous chapter, describe dose variation with depth along the central axis of a beam. **Isodose distributions,** on the other hand, are two-dimensional (2D) spatial representations of dose. Typical isodose distributions illustrate dose variation both along as well as across the direction of a beam of radiation. These are illustrated in greater detail in later sections of the chapter.

Treatment planning attempts dose distribution optimization for a given clinical goal in a given clinical situation. Treatment fields are used in ways that produce adequate tumor dose and minimal normal-tissue dose. It is, hence, nec-

essary to understand how dose distributions are both produced and then used. The discussion begins with simple, single fields and then progresses to more complex multiple field arrangements.

Open-fields: profiles. A beam profile is another one-dimensional spatial representation of the variation of beam intensity. A **profile** describes radiation intensity as a function of position across the beam at a given depth. It depicts the beam's intensity in a direction perpendicular to the beam's direction. The concept of beam-intensity variation as a function of position within the beam is best understood if one thinks about the response of a small radiation detector moving within a tank of water that is being irradiated. Fig. 22-2 illustrates this process—a common method of measuring clinical beam data. As the radiation detector moves across the beam at some depth in the phantom, beam intensity (detector response) is plotted as a function of position within the beam. The resulting intensity curve as a function of position within the beam is called a profile. The intensity curves shown in Fig. 22-2 are typical of photon field profiles. They are characterized by a rapid increase in intensity (as the radiation detector enters the beam), followed by a region of relatively uniform intensity (characterizing the central portion of the beam), then ending with a rapid decrease in intensity (as the detector exits the beam).

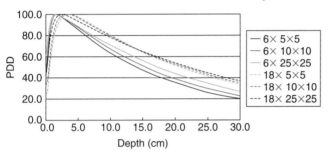

Figure 22-1. Percentage depth dose (PDD) curves are typically plotted as a function of depth and are normalized to the PDD at the depth of maximum dose. Here are shown 6-MV and 18-MV x-ray depth-dose curves. Note the variation of PDD with energy and field size. Note also the shift of the depth of maximum dose and the difference in PDD field-size variation between 6 -and 18-MV x-rays.

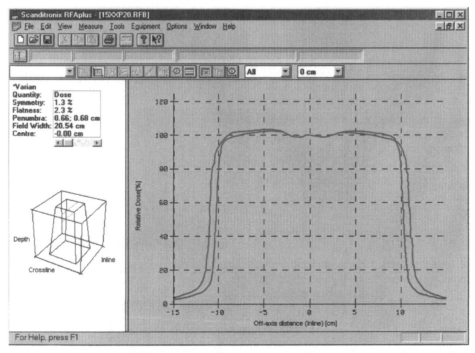

Figure 22-2. Beam profiles are normally measured with a computerized beam-data acquisition system that includes a water tank, radiation detector, and specialized software designed for radiation beam measurement and analysis. Note the beam-data acquisition geometry shown on the bottom-left portion of the screen showing the direction of ionization-chamber travel within the water tank. Two "in-plane" scans were acquired and the resulting profiles are displayed.

The shape of a beam's profile is a function of depth. At shallow depths, because scatter is less of a contributor to the total intensity of the beam than it is at deeper depths, the beam's profile better characterizes the beam's "primary" intensity. The D_{max} profile, shown in Fig. 22-3, illustrates the influence of the accelerator's flattening filter on the beam. Flattening filters are introduced into photon beams to reduce the increased photon intensity existing in the center of the

beam. Evidence for this effect is the somewhat reduced intensity shown in the center of the beam compared with that existing away from the central axis. The flattening filter is designed to produce a "flat" intensity pattern at some predefined depth (normally 10 cm). Box 22-1 expands on this thought. Note the flatter shape of the 10-cm depth profile of Fig. 22-3 compared with the D_{max} profile. At deeper depths, scatter becomes a more significant component of dose and a greater amount of scattered radiation exists along the center of the beam than along the periphery. This offsets the shape of the beam's primary profile producing a relatively flat dose distribution.

Open-fields: isodose distributions. Isodose distributions consist of a series of isodose curves. The traditional **isodose curve** is a 2D representation of how dose varies with position within a beam along directions both parallel and perpendicular to the beam's direction. It is a collection of points, all having the same dose (hence the term *iso*dose). Fig. 22-4 presents typical isodose distributions produced by photon beams of different energies.[9] The numerical values of the lines represent percentages of the dose existing at a point along the central axis at the depth of D_{max}. Thus the 90% isodose contains all points within the plane of presentation where the dose is equal to 90% of the dose at D_{max}. The dose at points between isodose curves will lie between the dose represented by the curves.

Isodose distributions combine both the depth-dose and off-axis-profile characteristics of the beam. The numerical value of the isodose line along the central (depth) axis of the isodose curves is equal to the PDD at that depth. The shape

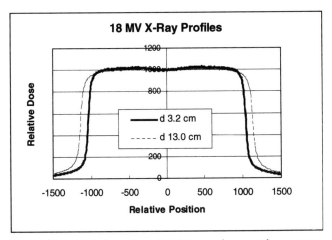

Figure 22-3. Profiles of an 18-MV x-ray beam taken at two depths, D_{max} and 13.0 cm. Note the differences in shape and size. The deeper profile is wider because the field diverges and its size increases with depth. The deeper profile is also "flatter" than the shallower profile because the accelerator's beams are designed to produce flat beams at a depth of approximately 10 cm (see Box 22-1).

Box 22-1	**Photon-Beam Shape Specifications**

It is often necessary to analyze profiles quantitatively to characterize the shape of photon beams. When profiles are measured along a direction parallel to the direction of electron motion along the accelerator's waveguide (parallel to the treatment couch), the profile is often termed a radial or "in-plane" profile. A profile measured along a direction perpendicular to the direction of the electron travel (perpendicular to the treatment couch), is often called a transverse or "cross-plane" profile.

Accelerator manufacturers provide specifications of the flatness and symmetry of photon beams. These specifications ensure that the accelerator produces beams possessing characteristics suitable for clinical use. The flatness and symmetry of clinical beams are checked periodically as a part of the accelerator's ongoing quality control. A common way to define **flatness** is by noting the difference between the maximum and minimum intensity of the central 80% of the profile and specifying this difference as a percentage of the central axis intensity:

$$\text{Flatness}_{(\%)} = 100 \times [(I_{Max} - I_{Min})/I_{CAX}]$$

In the previous equation, I_{max} and I_{min} are the maximum and minimum intensities of the central 80% of the profile, and I_{CAX} is the intensity of the profile on its central axis. **Symmetry** can also be quantified in a similar fashion by noting profile intensities on either side of the central axis:

$$\text{Symmetry}_{(\%)} = 100 \times [(I_{+x} - I_{-x})_{max}/I_{xo}]$$

In this equation, I_{+X} and I_{-X} are corresponding profile intensities at a distance x on either side of the profile's central axis, and I_{X0} is the central-axis intensity. A common definition of symmetry specifies the maximum point-to-point difference. As before, symmetry is defined in the central 80% of the profile.

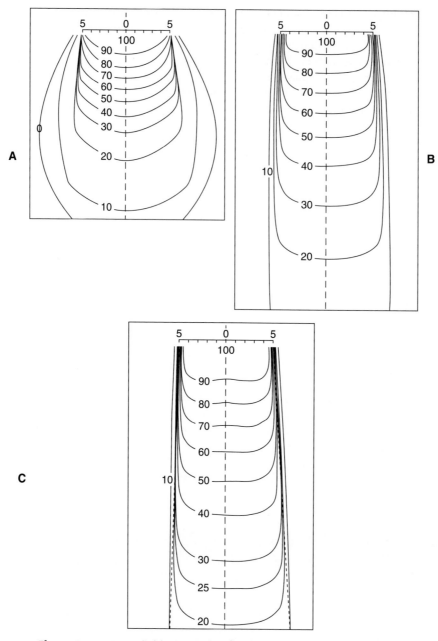

Figure 22-4. Open-field, 10 × 10 cm² field size, isodose distributions for an 80-cm source-skin distance (SSD) cobalt-60 **(A)**, and 100-cm SSD 4-MV **(B)**, and 10-MV **(C)** treatment beam. Note the difference in isodose shape, particularly at the shallower depths. *(Redrawn from Khan FM: The physics of radiation therapy, ed 2, Baltimore, 1994, Williams & Wilkins.)*

of the isodose curve along a direction perpendicular to the central axis describes the off-axis characteristics of the beam. Isodose distributions will vary with beam energy, source-skin distance (SSD), and field size. Note also from Fig. 22-4 that beams produced by accelerators are, in general, flatter than cobalt-60 or low-energy x-ray beams. As mentioned previously, this is due to the introduction of flattening filters used in linear accelerators. Note the shape of the 90% isodose

curve of the 4-MV beam shown in Fig. 22-4, *C.* The flattening filter causes the "dip" in the central region of the curve.

Wedged-fields: isodose distributions.   It is often desirable to produce beams of nonuniform intensity across the field. Introducing an attenuator of varying thickness in the beam can produce the desired difference in intensity. As a consequence of its shape, this variable-thickness attenuator is called a **wedge.** When a wedge is introduced into a beam, differential attenuation along the varying thickness of the wedge produces a dose gradient along the wedged dimension of the beam; that is, less dose exists under thicker portions of the wedge than exists along less thick portions. At a given depth within a wedged beam, and in a direction toward the toe or thinner portion of the wedge, the dose increases with distance from the central axis of the beam. Similarly, the values of isodoses toward the heel or thicker portion of the wedge, decrease with increasing distance from the central axis.

Examples of wedged-field isodose distributions are shown in Fig. 22-5.[3] Note that wedged-field isodose lines are now "tilted"—a given-valued isodose penetrates to a greater depth along thinner portions of the wedge. The amount of incline of the isodose curves depends on the shape of the wedge. Wedges with a greater variation in thickness from heel to toe will produce more inclined isodoses. The angle between the slanted isodose line and a line perpendicular to the central axis of the beam is called the **wedge angle.** Wedges are designed to produce certain discrete wedge angles. Traditionally, wedges supplied with the treatment machine are fabricated to produce discrete wedge angles of 15 degrees, 30 degrees, 45 degrees, and 60 degrees. Because, for any given wedge, the tilt of isodose lines varies slightly with depth (again because of the relative influence of scatter), either the depth of the 80% depth dose or a depth of 10 cm is often chosen for wedge-angle measurement and subsequent wedge attenuator design.[6,8]

Wedged-field isodoses demonstrate similar dependencies on beam energy, SSD, and field size as do open-field isodoses. Because of the presence of the wedge attenuator in the beam, on the other hand, the energy spectrum of wedged fields differs slightly from that of its nonwedged counterpart. This results in slight differences between open- and wedged-field PDD. The effect is more pronounced at lower beam energies and larger wedge angles. Table 22-1 shows data that illustrate this effect. The PDD at 20 cm depth in a 6-MV, 15×15 cm photon field increases by 4% when a 45-degree wedge is introduced; an 18-MV photon beam shows a 2% increase in depth dose under similar circumstances.

Wedged-field isodose distributions can be produced also without the use of wedge attenuators. If a collimator jaw is allowed to move across the beam during irradiation, a variation in intensity across the beam similar to that produced by a wedge can be achieved. The use of a moving collimator jaw to produce a wedged field is often termed **dynamic wedge.** Frequently, jaw movements during production of dynamic wedge fields are controlled to produce only fields equivalent to those produced by conventional wedges—15-degree, 30-degree, 45-degree, and 60-degree wedged fields. More recently, dynamic wedge capability has been extended to produce a wider range of wedged fields not limited to the conventional wedge angles. This capability has been called "enhanced" dynamic wedge.[16]

Clinical use of dynamic wedges has far-reaching dosimetric consequences beyond the scope of this chapter. The tradi-

tional "wedge attenuation factor" no longer exists as such because the wedging function is no longer produced by differential attenuation through an attenuator. Dynamic wedge factors are more related to field-size dependent output factors because wedging is now a function of collimator jaw positions. Also because wedge attenuators are not used, the PDD of dynamic wedge fields is the same as that of their open-field counterparts.

Combined-field isodose distributions: open fields. Except for a few clinical situations in which the treatment depth is shallow, such as the treatment of supraclavicular nodes or portions of the spinal column, single photon fields are rarely used solely. Very often, multiple fields are used in combination to take advantage of the improved dose distribution that results from aiming multiple fields from different directions at a common target area. Multiple fields convergent on a shared target result in a concentrated dose in the common target area.

The most common combined-field geometry is the **parallel-opposed field set.** In this field geometry, two treatment fields share common central axes, 180 degrees apart. A second field equal in size and mirrored in shape but opposite in direction compensates for the fall-off in dose with depth from the first field. Parallel-opposed fields are often used to treat regions near the middle of the treatment area. Examples of clinical parallel-opposed fields are anteroposterior (AP) and posteroanterior (PA) thoracic fields and right- and left-lateral head and neck fields.

Parallel-opposed fields work best in situations in which beam energy and patient thickness can be matched to allow for a uniform dose within the irradiated volume. With proper selection of energy and under favorable patient-thickness conditions, parallel-opposed fields can be used to deliver reasonably uniform doses. This can be seen in Fig. 22-6.[9] In this figure, the doses at all points along the central axes of parallel-opposed beams 25 cm apart are shown for beams of different energies. (This figure is best understood if one thinks of the parallel-opposed beams as entering from the left and right of the figure.) Note that as beam energy increases, the dose along the central axes of the beams becomes more uniform. Lower-energy beams, because of their decreased penetrating ability, produce higher doses at their respective entrance depths producing a less uniform dose distribution as a function of depth. A similar situation occurs as patient thickness increases and the entrance-to-midline dose ratio becomes unacceptably high. This is shown in Fig. 22-7 where, for example, 15% more dose exists at the entrance of 4-MV beams in 25-cm thick patient than at the patient's midline.[9] Under these circumstances, other beam combinations may be more appropriate.

Multiple convergent beams are often used in situations in which parallel-opposed beams cannot produce acceptable dose distributions or when it may be desirable to further restrict the high-dose region of the dose distribution. This is demonstrated in Fig. 22-8 where the dose distributions

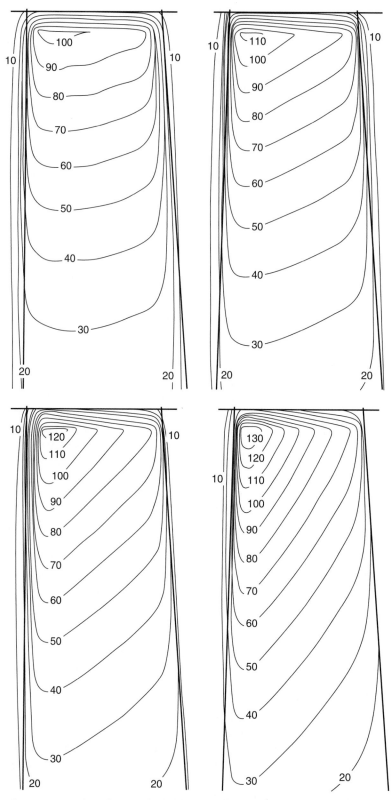

Figure 22-5. The tilt of wedged field isodose curves are dependent on the particular wedge filter used. This figure shows typical isodose distributions produced by conventional 15-degree, 30-degree, 45-degree, and 60-degree conventional wedge filters. *(Redrawn from Bentel GC: Radiation therapy planning, ed 2, New York, 1996, McGraw-Hill.)*

Table 22-1	6- and 18-MV open- and wedged-field percent depth dose data*			
Percentage Depth Dose	6-MV Open	6-MV 45-degree Wedge	18-MV Open	18-MV 45-degree Wedge
Depth 10 cm	69.3	70.5	79.1	80.7
Depth 20 cm	41.8	43.5	53.7	54.7

*Data for a Varian Clinac 2100C, 15 × 15 cm fields, 100 cm source-skin distance (SSD).

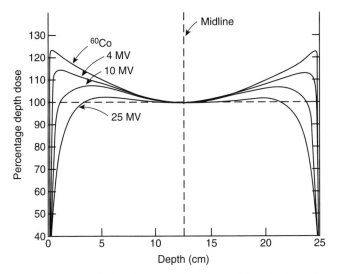

Figure 22-6. Relative dose as a function of depth along the central axis of parallel-opposed fields incident on a patient 25-cm thick. Curves, showing dose relative to the dose existing at mid-depth, are representative of the dose produced by 10 × 10 cm² treatment fields of energies cobalt-60, 4 MV, 10 MV, and 25 MV. *(Redrawn from Khan FM: The physics of radiation therapy, ed 2, Baltimore, 1994, Williams & Wilkins.)*

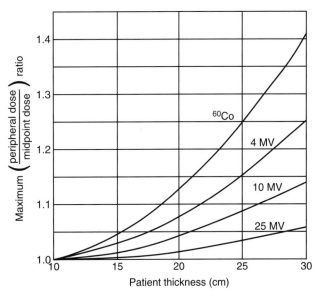

Figure 22-7. A patient is treated with parallel-opposed fields. This figure shows the maximum dose along the central axes of the fields expressed as a ratio of dose at the patient's midline. The curves, plotted as a function of patient thickness, are representative of cobalt-60, 4-MV, 10-MV, and 25-MV 10 × 10 cm², 100-cm source-skin distance (SSD) fields. Note that, for a patient 25-cm thick, parallel-opposed cobalt-60 fields produce a maximum dose along the central axis 25% greater than that produced at the patient's midline. *(Redrawn from Khan FM: The physics of radiation therapy, ed 2, Baltimore, 1994, Williams & Wilkins.)*

resulting from the use of a parallel-opposed field set, a three-field arrangement, and a four-field arrangement are contrasted. Note that as supplementary fields are added, the high-dose region conforms to the intersection of the beams and that the relative dose outside the beams' intersection decreases. Note also that, as a consequence of the equal angles between the fields, the dose distribution is relatively uniform within the region of the beams' intersection.

Combined-field isodose distributions: wedged fields. Not uncommonly, there are clinical situations in which parallel-opposed or equally angled beams are not appropriate for the particular treatment scenario. An example is the treatment of disease in one side of the brain where sparing of the opposite hemisphere is desired. In this situation, a pair of wedged beams can be used to produce a region of reasonably uniform dose. Recall that the isodoses of wedged fields are tilted at an

angle characterized by the wedge angle. A region of uniform dose can be achieved in the area common to two wedged fields if the angles of the central axes of the fields bear an appropriate relationship to the wedge angles if the beams. If ϕ is the angle between the beams' central axes, called the **hinge angle,** and θ is the wedge angle of the beams, then the relationship between the hinge and wedge angles that produces a uniform dose distribution is as follows:

$$\phi = 180° - 2\theta \text{ or } \theta = 90° = \phi/2$$

The previous relationship applies to pairs of wedged fields. The hinge angle can be adjusted slightly to accommodate clinical restraints such as protection of normal structures for instance. Wedged-field combinations are not limited to only pairs of wedged fields. Wedged fields can be used with open or other wedged fields in other fashions. Fig. 22-9 shows examples of the use of wedged fields to achieve more uniform dose distributions under normal-structure sparing constraints.

Corrections to Isodose Distributions

Beam data for treatment-planning systems are almost always obtained from measurements acquired in water phantoms. The data represent dose distributions obtained when flat-

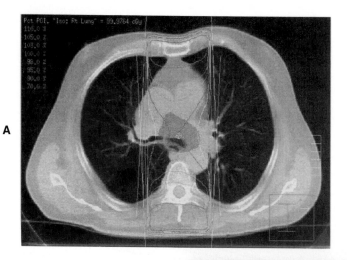

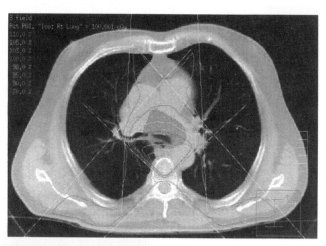

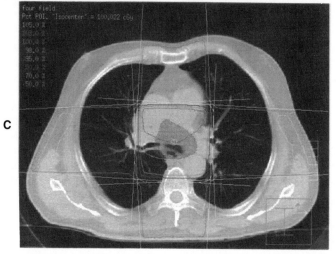

Figure 22-8. Thorax isodose distributions produced by a parallel-opposed field arrangement **(A)**, a three-field arrangement **(B)**, and a four-field arrangement **(C)**. The shaded area in the center of the computed tomography (CT) image represents the "target" volume. The numeric values of the isodoses represent percentages of the dose at the isocenter of the fields.

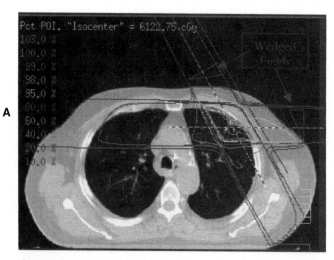

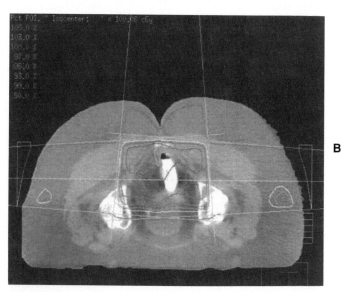

Figure 22-9. Isodose distributions produced by combinations of fields with wedges. **A,** An angled wedge pair. **B,** A combination of a posterior open field with two lateral wedged field.

surfaced homogenous (water) media is irradiated. When actual irradiation conditions differ from those under which standard isodose distributions were obtained, corrections must be applied. Corrections for beam for beam incidence onto surfaces other than flat surfaces and for angles of incidence other than 90 degrees ("normal" incidence) are called **obliquity** or **contour corrections.** Corrections that account for the presence of irradiated media other than water are called **heterogeneity corrections.**

Obliquity/contour corrections. The effective SSD method is a graphical contour-correction method that employs an isodose chart (a set of isodose curves). It entails "sliding" the isodose chart along the irregular contour such that its surface line is at the contour surface at a vertical line above the given point of interest. The PDD value at the point of interest is read and then corrected using an inverse-square correction. Referring to Fig. 22-10, the isodose chart is shifted from its position at the central axis (surface $S'' - S''$) to a position on the contour above the point A.[9] The PDD value (P) at point A is read off the chart and is then corrected by multiplying it by an inverse square factor to give the corrected PDD value (P'). The inverse square correction factor (CF) to be applied is as follows:

$$P' = P \times \left(\frac{SSD + d_m}{SSD + d_m + h} \right)^2$$

Where, in the previous equation, h is the tissue deficit or excess (either plus or minus) above the point of interest relative to the central axis.

For example, suppose that (in Fig. 22-10) point A was located at a depth of 5 cm in a 10×10 cm field and that the gap above point A was 3 cm. A 10×10 cm isodose curve would be slid down until the horizontal line representing the surface intersects the surface of the contour directly above the point of interest (i.e., point A). Suppose the isodose value now read *(solid line)* at P is 78%. This isodose value is corrected using the previously shown inverse square correction to yield the resultant depth dose:

$$P' = P \times \left(\frac{SSD + d_m}{SSD + d_m + h} \right)^2 = 78\% \times \left(\frac{100 + 1.5}{100 + 1.5 + 3} \right)^2 = 73.6\%$$

The dose at point A is 73.6% of the dose at the (preshift) D_{max} point.

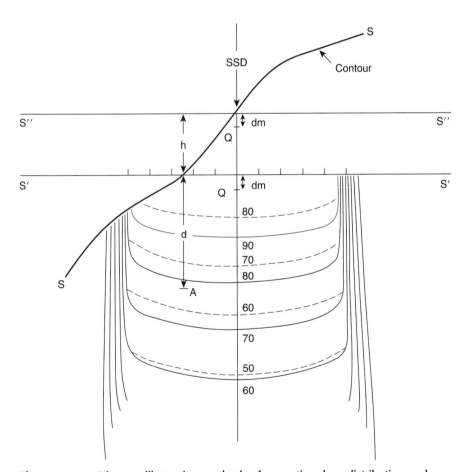

Figure 22-10. Diagram illustrating methods of correcting dose distribution under an irregular surface such as $S - S$. The solid curves are from an isodose chart that assumes a flat surface located at $S' - S'$. The dashed isodose curves assume a flat surface at $S'' - S''$ without any air gap. *(From Khan FM: The physics of radiation therapy, ed 2, Baltimore, 1994, Williams & Wilkins.)*

The tissue-air ratio (TAR) (or tissue-maximum ratio [TMR]) method assumes that the tissue deficit (h) mentioned previously is filled with tissue-like material. In this method, again using Fig. 22-10, the isodose curve is placed on the central axis at the surface $S'' - S''$ and the (dashed curve) isodose value (P) at A is read as if a flat surface existed at $S'' - S''$. Because the isodose value has been underestimated by assuming that a depth of $h + d$ rather than d exists at point A, the isodose value P is corrected using the TAR (or TMR) ratio:

$$P' = P \times (TAR(d)/TAR(d + h))$$

The TAR method can be illustrated, again using Fig. 22-10 and the numerical assumptions of the previous example. Suppose that the PDD value at point A (when the isodose chart is placed at $S'' - S''$) is 64.0%. Because this value assumes a depth of $5 + 3 = 8$ cm, it is corrected using the TAR ratio:

$$\left(\frac{TAR(5)}{TAR(8)}\right) = \left(\frac{0.905}{0.787}\right) = 1.15$$

$$P' = 64.0\% \times 1.15 = 73.6\%$$

Heterogeneity corrections.   Standard isodose charts and depth dose tables assume homogeneous, unit density (water) medium. However, within a patient are fat, bone, muscle, and air, which attenuate and scatter the beam differently than does water. Boundary interfaces can present additional (transitional zone) problems (i.e., near bone, air cavities, metal prostheses, and so forth).

In the megavoltage range of x-ray energies, common in radiation oncology, the Compton effect is the predominant mode of interaction[5,6] and thus the attenuation of the beam in any medium is a function, mostly, of the electron density of the medium (number of electrons per cm^3). To explain some of the methods used to account for the presence of some material that is not water equivalent we use the schematic representation shown in Fig. 22-11.[9]

Assume that dose is to be calculated at a point P at a depth d in a heterogeneous phantom. The radiation beam traverses first a depth d_1 of water equivalent material, then through some other material (inhomogeneity) having a depth d_2, and then again through a depth d_3 of water equivalent material. If ρ_e represents the density of the heterogeneous material relative to water, then the total (uncorrected) depth d, and the effective (corrected) depth d_{eff} are each given by the following equations:

$$d = d_1 + d_2 + d_3$$
$$d_{eff} = d_1 + \rho_e d_2 + d_3$$

The effective SSD method assumes that the corrected PDD is equal to the PDD for the effective depth d_{eff} multiplied by an inverse square correction. The effective depth is the equivalent radiologic path length, d_{eff} previously:

$$PDD \; (FS, SSD, d) \; corrected = PDD \; (F, SSD, d_{eff}) \; x$$
$$(SSD + d_{eff} / SSD + d)^2$$

The TAR or TMR method applies an attenuation correction to the use of a TAR (or TMR) that is based on the physical depth as opposed to the effective or radiologic depth:

$$CF = \frac{TAR(d_{eff}, r_d)}{TAR(d, r_d)} \; or \; \frac{TMR(d_{eff}, r_d)}{TMR(d, r_d)}$$

In the previous expression, d is the actual, physical depth to the point P; d_{eff} is the effective water depth taking into account the relative electron densities of the materials ($d_{eff} = d_1 + \rho_e d_2 + d_3$); and r_d is the field size at the depth of calculation. The dose at point P (achieved assuming water equivalent depths) is multiplied by the CF to get the inhomogeneity-corrected dose. Note that TMRs can also be used in the same fashion as TARs.

Consider the following example as an illustration of the TAR method for heterogeneity corrections and refer to Fig. 22-11. Assume the phantom of Fig. 22-11 is irradiated with a 10×10 cm, 80 cm SSD, cobalt-60 field. Further assume that $d_1 = 5$ cm, $d_2 = 10$ cm, and $d_3 = 3$ cm and that the density ρ_e of the 10-cm thick medium relative to water is 0.3. Under those assumptions, $d_{actual} = 5 + 10 + 3 = 18$ cm, and $d_{eff} = (5 \times 1) + (10 \times 0.3) + (3 \times 1) = 11$ cm. The distance to the point P is $80 + 18 = 98$ cm, and the field size at P is $(98/80) \times 10 = 12.25 \times 12.25$ cm. The CF to be applied is as follows:

$$CF = TAR \; (11, 12.25)/TAR \; (18, 12.25) = 0.704/0.487 = 1.45$$

The dose at P, considering the presence of the heterogeneity, is 1.45 times the dose computed ignoring the presence of the

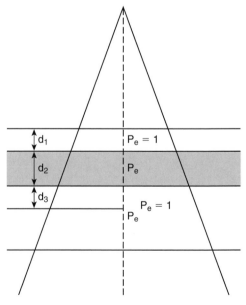

Figure 22-11. Schematic diagram showing a water equivalent phantom containing an inhomogeneity of electron density P_e relative to that of water. P is the point of dose calculation. *(From Khan FM: The physics of radiation therapy, ed 2, Baltimore, 1994, Williams & Wilkins.)*

heterogeneity. (Note that the previous correction produces the "effective" TAR that results as a consequence of the presence of the heterogeneity. The effective TAR at P = 0.487 × 1.45 = 0.487 × (0.704/0.487) = 0.704.)

The heterogeneity correction methods explained up to this point assume infinite slabs of heterogeneous media and do not take into account the relative location of the heterogeneity with respect to the point of calculation. As such, these methods yield only rough approximations of the effects of heterogeneities on dose calculations performed under assumptions of homogeneous media. More sophisticated calculations take these effects into account to varying degrees of accuracy.[18] Some of these methods are as follows:

1. *Power law TAR method:* a TAR correction method that accounts for the relative location of the point of calculation with respect to the inhomogeneity.
2. *Generalized Batho correction:* a generalization of the power law method to allow for dose calculations at points within the heterogeneity.
3. *Equivalent TAR method:* a method that considers the effects of heterogeneities on scatter as well as on primary. In this method, both the field size and the depth are "scaled" to account for the presence of heterogeneities.
4. *Delta volume method:* In this method, primary and scatter are separated. The irradiated volume is broken into volume elements and scatter is computed from a weighted summation of the scatter from each of the volume elements. This scatter is then added to the primary.

Typical heterogeneity corrections. Tables 22-2 and 22-3, modified from reference 1, can be useful in estimating the dose or correction to the dose beyond a given inhomogeneity.

Example (refer again to Fig. 22-11): Assume that this phantom is irradiated with a single beam of 4-MV photons and that the dose is calculated at a point P assuming homogeneous media. The point P is located at a total physical depth of 6 cm. It is located beyond an inhomogeneity 2-cm thick. The homogenous dose at P from the single 4-MV beam is 100 cGy. If the inhomogeneity has a relative density of healthy lung (0.25), what is the radiologic depth and what is the heterogeneity-corrected dose at P? If the inhomogeneity has a relative density of bone (1.65), what is the radiologic depth and what is the heterogeneity-corrected dose at P?

The physical depth is 6 cm of which 2 cm consists of the inhomogeneity. Thus the radiologic (or effective) depth of the point P is: 4 + (0.25 × 2.0) = 4.5 cm (assuming healthy lung), and is 4 + (1.65 × 2.0) = 7.3 cm (assuming bone). The dose at P assuming a lung heterogeneity is approximately: 100 cGy + (100 × 0.03 × 2) = 106 cGy (an increase in dose of 3% per cm of lung). The dose at P assuming a bone heterogeneity is approximately: 100 cGy − (100 × 0.03 × 2) = 94 cGy (a decrease in dose of 3% per cm of bone).

TREATMENT-PLANNING ESSENTIALS

The treatment-planning process has changed significantly over the last few years. Treatment-planning systems, capable of handling large three-dimensional (3D) anatomy data sets, accurately modeling treatment unit capabilities, and offering very useful visualization tools, have now taken on the role of virtual patient simulators. Treatment-planning tools allow for greater dose delivery precision. The accuracy of dose calculations has increased considerably. Optimization techniques permit more homogenous tumor volume irradiation while providing increased normal tissue protection.

This section provides an overview of current treatment-planning capabilities and methods. Although both three-dimensional conformal radiation therapy (3DCRT) and intensity-modulated radiation therapy are addressed, the characteristics common to both techniques are pointed out. Treatment-planning fundamentals including basic concepts, treatment-planning algorithms, and the treatment-planning process are emphasized.

Rationale for 3D Conformal Radiation Therapy

It is well known in radiation oncology that radiation dose affects both tumor-bearing as well as normal tissues. The degree of biologic effect is dependent on several factors, among them the magnitude of the dose and the radiosensitivity of the tissue. The desired outcome in radiation oncology is a high degree of tumor control with very little deleterious side effects. This is often achievable only to a certain degree.

Fig. 22-12 is often used to explain the compromise between probability of tumor control and the incidence of normal-tissue complications.[13] Both tumor control probability and

Table 22-2	Increase in dose to tissues beyond healthy lung*	
Beam Quality		**Correction Factor**
Orthovoltage		+10%/cm of lung
Cobalt-60		+4%/cm of lung
4 MV		+3%/cm of lung
10 MV		+2%/cm of lung
25 MV		+1%/cm of lung

*TAR Method and $\rho_{e\ lung}$ = 0.25.

Table 22-3	Reduction of dose beyond 1 cm of hard bone*
Beam Quality	**Correction Factor (%)**
1 mm Cu HVL	−15%
3 mm Cu HVL	−7%
Cobalt-60	−3.5%
4 MV	−3%
10 MV	−2%

Cu, Copper; *HVL,* half value layer.
*TAR Method and $\rho_{e\ bone}$ = 1.65.

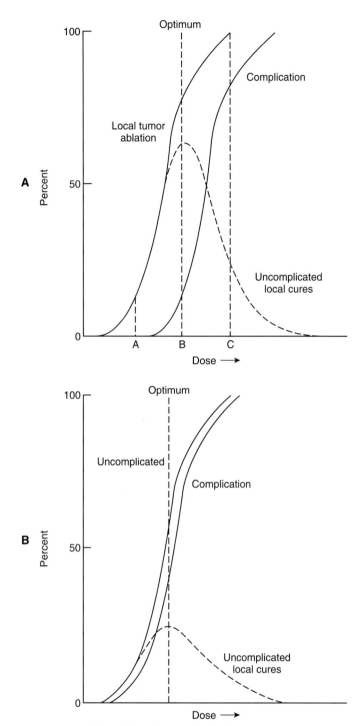

Figure 22-12. Probability of tumor control and of complication incidence as a function of dose. In the first scenario **(A)**, local tumor control is achieved at doses lower than those producing local normal-tissue complications. In the second scenario **(B)**, local tumor control probability and normal tissue complication rates follow essentially the same dose response curves. In both scenarios, however, greater tumor control and less complication probability can be achieved simultaneously if tumor doses and normal-tissue doses are kept at different levels. *(Redrawn from Perez CA, and Brady LW: Principles and practice of radiation oncology, ed 2, Philadelphia, 1992, J.B. Lippincott.)*

normal-tissue complication incidence increase with dose. When tumors are more radiosensitive than their surrounding normal tissues, a relatively high degree of tumor control may be achievable, at some given dose, with a reasonably low normal-tissue complication probability. This is the case shown in Fig. 22-12, *A*. When tissues of equivalent radiosensitivity surround tumors, any dose producing a reasonable tumor control probability will also induce normal-tissue complications with a high probability. This is the case illustrated by Fig. 22-12, *B*, where the dose producing a reasonable tumor-control probability also produces a high complication rate.

Under either of the relative radiosensitivity scenarios explained previously, both greater tumor control probability and lower normal-tissue complication probability can be achieved simultaneously if tumor doses are maximized while normal tissue doses are maintained at a minimum. This is the rationale for conformal radiation therapy. In **3D conformal radiation therapy (3DCRT)**, 3D image visualization and treatment-planning tools are used to conform isodose distributions to only target volumes while excluding normal tissues as much as possible. This section discusses the tools and processes used during 3DCRT.

3D treatment-planning and delivery methods. Three-dimensional treatment planning (3DTP) is the process by which 3D visualization, dose calculation, and plan evaluation tools are used to produce optimized treatment-field arrangements. Planning is image based and patient anatomy is represented by computed tomography (CT) data sets. Tumor volumes and critical structures are identified using image contouring tools that enhance their visualization. Margins are established around tumor volumes to include disease microinvasion and allow for tumor volume motion. Beams are arranged to target tumor volumes and avoid critical structures. Treatment plans are then objectively evaluated on the basis of their volume-dose relationships.

Current 3DTP methods include both conventional 3DCRT and intensity modulated radiation therapy (IMRT). In both methods, target volumes and critical structures are defined and beams are arranged in an attempt to maximize the dose to targets while minimizing the dose to critical structures. Intensity modulation techniques allow for the modification of the distribution of intensity within a treatment beam to achieve the stated goal.

There are several types of IMRT delivery systems; most use multileaf collimators (MLCs). A "step-and-shoot" system will have the gantry in a fixed position with an initial MLC pattern. A portion of the dose is delivered through this leaf pattern or segment. (Beam is delivered *after* the MLC has achieved the shape corresponding to it appropriate segment.) With the gantry in the same position, the beam is automatically interrupted and the leaf pattern changes to that corresponding to the second segment. The beam is then turned on for the second segment This may occur several times to produce the desired intensity map. During dynamic

MLC (DMLC) treatment delivery techniques, the leaves of the MLC move during the delivery of the dose ("sliding window" technique). After the dose of the first beam is delivered for either of these two types of IMRT techniques (segmental MLC and dynamic MLC), the gantry is moved to the next position and the treatment is delivered in the same way for the next beam.

Some treatment units are able to deliver IMRT using arc therapy. This capability has been termed "tomotherapy," which means slice therapy. In one type of tomotherapy, a specialized rectangular, computer-controlled device is positioned on the head of the linear acceleraor. Radiation is delivered through a narrow slit opening in the collimator device as the gantry rotates. The process is repeated for each slice. Because small positioning errors in matching fields can result in large dose errors, a special indexing table is used to achieve accurate positioning of the patient between slices.

Robotic IMRT, a futuristic method of delivering IMRT treatment has been used in some institutions. The concept is similar to radiosurgery, in which small beams are delivered to the tumor volume through multiple angles. This method of IMRT requires the purchase of a separate dedicated treatment unit to provide treatment verification and dose delivery with the pencil-like beams of radiation.

IMRT is often "inverse planned." IMRT **inverse planning** systems calculate dose distributions and create MLC patterns based on initial dose delivery and avoidance parameters. The intensity of the beams are then altered, by opening and closing the MLC, to achieve the requested doses. Beam arrangements are set up by the planner. The planning system then computes alternative intensity patterns until the best possible solution is determined.

3DCRT uses conventional **forward planning.** Forward planning requires that dose altering parameters and beam modifiers be entered into the treatment plan by the planner. After the initial dose calculation is completed, the planner evaluates the dose distribution and edits the modifiers or other parameters to produce an improved plan. This process is repeated until an acceptable plan is achieved.

Treatment-planning Algorithms

Treatment-planning algorithms are the planning-systems' dose calculation processes. They consist of a series of mathematical equations, and their associated input parameters, that produce values of dose as a function of position within the **dose calculation matrix**—a grid of points at which dose is computed and subsequently displayed.

Treatment-planning algorithms can be categorized on the basis of their dose calculation methodology.[14] Data-driven algorithms compute dose mainly from interpolations between measured beam data—depth dose data, off-axis profiles, and so forth. CFs are applied to account for differences between the measurement geometry and the geometry of the patient. Examples of data-driven algorithms are the Bently-Milan algorithm (used in the GE Target treatment-planning

system) and the scatter integration algorithm (used in the ROCS treatment-planning system).

Model-driven algorithms mainly use equations, "fit" to measured data, that are intended to predict the variation of dose with changes in parameters such as depth, distance off-axis, and proximity to field edges. Patient dose is computed by simulating the actual physics of the radiation transport process—the beam is produced in the target of the accelerator, is transported through the head of the machine, and is incident on the patient where it is attenuated and absorbed. An example of a modern model-driven algorithm is the convolution algorithm (such as the one employed by the ADAC Pinnacle[3] treatment-planning system).

Treatment-planning algorithms can be classified also according to the dimensionality of the calculation methodology. A common classification is 2D and 3D algorithms. Although descriptions of 2D and 3D algorithms oftentimes differ, several distinguishing traits are salient. Some of the features of 2D and 3D systems are shown in Table 22-4. 3D algorithms make use of entire CT data sets that are treated as one, comprehensive CT volume; 2D algorithms often treat CT data as a series of independent CT planar contours. This is of particular importance during the dose calculation phase. 3D algorithms use the entire data set when estimating scatter to each point in the volume; 2D algorithms assume that all CT-image planes are of equal size, shape, and composition as the current calculation plane and compute scatter under that (inaccurate) presumption. Because if the availability of volume information, 3D algorithms also permit evaluations of plan quality using a tool called the dose-volume histogram (DVH). The DVH is discussed later in the chapter.

Treatment-planning algorithms can be evaluated based on several criteria. Algorithms differ in their ability to properly model beam intensities under different irradiation conditions. An ideal algorithm will properly represent a beam's depth dose and off-axis intensity. It will properly characterize the irradiation geometry (gantry, collimator, and couch angles) and the effects of beam modifiers such as independent jaws, MLCs, wedges, compensators, and bolus. Treatment-planning algorithms should also properly model patient data sets such as CT and magnetic resonance imaging (MRI) data. Dose calculation accuracy and speed are yet other considerations.

Table 22-4	Characteristics of 2D versus 3D calculation algorithms	
3D Algorithms	**2D Algorithms**	
3D data set	Independent contours	
Comprehensive anatomy	Limited anatomy	
3D dose corrections	In-plane corrections only	
Volumetric evaluation (DVH)	Limited evaluation tools	

DVH, Dose-volume histogram; *3D,* three-dimensional; *2D,* two-dimensional.

Calculation algorithms—scatter integration. To simplify the explanation of the dose calculation process, it is often useful to consider dose as consisting of primary and scatter components.[1] In basic terms, at all points in the irradiated volume, dose from primary radiation is computed first, then the dose from scattered radiation is added. A scatter-integration-like algorithm may use an equation similar to the schematic formula that is shown in the following:

$$D(f,r,d,x) = D_{ref} \times OF_{pri} \times ISF(f+d) \times OAF(x,d) \times T(r) \times OF_{scat}(r) \times [TPR(0,d) + SPR_{avg}(r,d)]$$

Where:

$D(f,r,d,x)$ = dose at some point P at a depth d, source-surface distance f, field size r, and off-axis distance x

D_{ref} = a known reference dose, for example, dose at D_{max}, 100 cm SSD, 10×10 cm field

OF_{pri} = an output factor describing the change in primary output as a function of collimator setting (akin to Khan's S_c)[9]

$ISF(f+d)$ = an inverse-square correction

$OAF(x,d)$ = an off-axis factor that models the beam's profile

$T(r)$ = beam transmission through wedges, trays, and other possible beam modifiers

OF_{scat} = an output factor describing the change in scatter contribution as a function of field size and shape (akin to Khan's S_p)

$TPR(0,d)$ = the primary (0×0 field) TPR or TMR

$SPR_{avg}(r,d)$ = the average scatter-phantom (or scatter-maximum) ratio, a function of field size and shape, that is added to the primary TPR (or TMR) to produce an effective TPR (or TMR)

The product of $D_{ref} \times OF_{pri} \times ISF(f+d) \times OAF(x,d) \times T(r)$ describes the primary radiation intensity that is available at P. The remaining parameters OF_{scat}, $TPR(0,d)$, and $SPR_{avg}(r,d)$ are a function of the conditions within the attenuating media.

The previous equation may seem complex but in reality it is not. The perceived complexity is due to the large number of variables and parameters that require definition. To illustrate the calculation method, consider the following situation: Suppose that a phantom is irradiated with a 12×12 cm field; the SSD is 90 cm and dose is to be computed to a point P which is 10-cm deep. If the accelerator is calibrated so that 1 cGy/MU (D_{ref}) exists at D_{max}, 100-cm SSD, for a 10×10 cm field, then the dose at P is 1 cGy/MU × the output factors for a 12×12 cm field (OF_{pri}) and (OF_{scat}) × an inverse-square correction for possible differences between calibration and calculation distances ($ISF(f+d)$) × the appropriate TMR ($TPR(r,d)$) and tray transmission factors ($T(r)$). Remaining variables (such as $SPR_{avg}(r,d)$ and $OAF(x,d)$) are used when needed to account for situations such as irregular blocking or dose to points away from the central axis.

Calculation algorithms—convolution algorithm. Newer algorithms, such as the convolution algorithms used in 3D planning systems, work in a similar way. Primary and scatter contributions are computed separately and then are summed. A 3D convolution algorithm[11] may use a calculation methodology described by the following:

$$D(r) = \int \frac{\mu}{\rho}(r) \times \Psi(r) \times K(r' \to r) dV$$

Here, $D(r)$ represents the dose at some point r. The primary fluence, $\Psi(r)$, describes the primary dose that exists at the point r. It is the in-air fluence that exits the head of the treatment unit, is moderated by beam modifiers, and is then attenuated by the patient. The $\Psi(r)$ term contains all primary radiation output, inverse-square, off-axis, and beam modifier corrections. (It is analogous to the product $D_{ref} \times OF_{pri} \times ISF(f+d) \times OAF(x,d) \times T(r) \times TPR(0,d)$ used in the description of the scatter-integration algorithm.)

The product of $\Psi(r)$ and $\mu/\rho(r)$ produces a quantity that represents the total radiation energy released at the point r. The incident fluence is projected onto the patient's CT data set and is attenuated.

The result is a matrix of radiation energy that is available for dose deposition.

The dose-spread kernel, $K(r' \to r)$, represents the energy distribution from the primary interaction site throughout the irradiated volume. $K(r' \to r)$ is a description of how dose is deposited in the vicinity of a primary interaction site. $K(r' \to r)$ can be thought of as describing the dose at r that is produced at all contributing interaction sites r'. (It is, in some ways, analogous to the terms OF_{scat} and $SPR_{avg}(r,d)$ used to compute scattered dose in the scatter integration algorithm.)

Because the total dose at the point r is dependent on the total radiation energy released at all points r', the total dose at r is the "superposition" (a "fluence and attenuation coefficient-weighted summation") of the function $\Psi(\rho) \times \mu/\rho(r)$ and the dose-spread function $K(r' \to r)$. The integration sign, $\int$, represents the summation process.

Treatment-planning Concepts and Tools

Treatment-planning algorithms constitute the calculation engine of the treatment-planning process. Calculation algorithms are only one piece of the entire 3D-planning process. Before dose is calculated, treatment beams must be established in a way that achieves the intent of radiation therapy—maximization of tumor, or target, dose, and minimization of normal-tissue dose.

Planning volume and margin concepts. Because the 3DCRT process seeks to conform dose to specific target volumes, it is imperative that these volumes be accurately defined. The International Commission on Radiation Units and Measurements (ICRU) has recommended the use of specifically defined volumes[7]:

Gross tumor volume (GTV) is the gross palpable, visible, and/or demonstrable extent and location of malignant growth. It is the volume of known disease. Disease that is visible on CT is a common example of a GTV.

Clinical target volume (CTV) is a tissue volume containing the GTV and/or subclinical microscopic malignant disease. The CTV includes gross visible or palpable disease *plus* any possible microscopic extensions of disease that may not be visible or palpable. The CTV is the volume that must always be enclosed by the treatment isodose. Untreated portions of the CTV could lead to local failure of therapy.

Planning target volume (PTV) is a geometrical volume; it has dimensions believed to always contain the CTV, taking into account all possible geometric uncertainties such as setup uncertainties and patient and/or organ motion.

Treated volume is the volume enclosed by the isodose surface selected as being appropriate to achieve the purpose of treatment (i.e., the volume enclosed by the prescription isodose surface).

These volumes are shown schematically in Fig. 22-13.[7]

The PTV includes a margin around the CTV to ensure that the CTV is always contained within the PTV. The margin of the PTV around the CTV is designed to make certain that the CTV is always contained within the treated volume. Note that the PTV margin around the CTV is not necessarily symmetric. The PTV allows for target motion and uncertainty in positioning.[17] Greater spatial uncertainties in the position of the target volume may exist in one dimension than in another. For example, it is generally believed that prostate motion in the anterior-posterior direction may exceed lateral prostate motion.[2] Thus the PTV margin around the CTV should be designed to account for these types of uncertainties.

Prescriptions are commonly formulated based on isodose surfaces, generated by the treatment-planning system, relative to the PTV. The PTV should be enclosed by an isodose surface within an accepted percent range of the prescribed dose. (For example, dose could be prescribed to the isocenter based on the fact that the PTV is enclosed by a 95% to 98% isodose surface.) This process will ensure that the CTV will always receive a dose that has been deemed adequate within an acceptable dose range.

Treatment fields are often designed from **beam's eye views (BEVs)** of PTVs. (BEVs are images reconstructed from CT data that represent the patient's anatomy and defined volumes from the perspective of the treatment beam. BEVs are discussed in more detail in the next section). BEV-designed treatment fields should include a margin that allows for full dose coverage of the PTV and accounts for beam

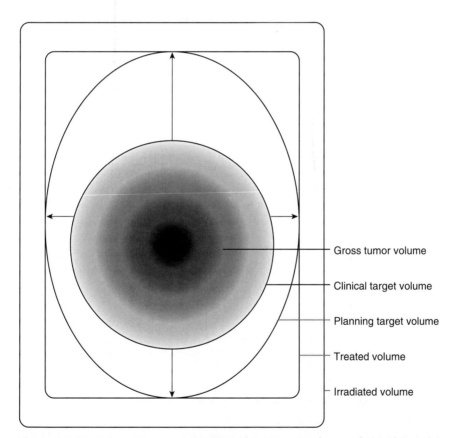

- Gross tumor volume
- Clinical target volume
- Planning target volume
- Treated volume
- Irradiated volume

Figure 22-13. Schematic representation of treatment-volume relationships. The clinical target volume contains the gross tumor volume and also volumes with possible (subclinical) disease. The planning target volume is designed to always contain the clinical target volume under all treatment conditions. See text for details. *(Reprinted with permission from International Commission on Radiation Units and Measurements: Prescribing, recording, and reporting photon beam therapy, ICRU Report 50. Bethesda, Md, 1993.)*

penumbral effects—the distance from the 50% to the 90% profile level. Although this margin will account, primarily, for possible lateral radiation-transport equilibrium losses, it should also allow for exclusion of critical structures as well.[12] Fig. 22-14 illustrates the volume and margin concepts that have just been discussed.

Treatment-planning tools.   Virtual simulation is a process by which treatment fields are defined using patient CT image data and treatment-unit geometric information.[4] Specialized software is used to contour patient anatomy, set up the treatment beam arrangement, identify the location of patient markings, and design blocking for the treatment fields (Fig. 22-15). Most of the simulation process is completed without the presence of the patient. Because the virtual simulator software contains treatment machine parameters, the limitations of conventional simulators, such as the presence of image intensifiers and possible differences between simulator and treatment-unit geometry, do not interfere with the field arrangements. Clinicians are better able to make decisions on the field arrangement. He or she also has more information available to use in virtual simulation. The patient's cross-sectional CT anatomy can be used to view the path of the beam through possible sensitive structures. Field shape and position can be edited to avoid critical structures.

Treatment-planning systems have drawing tools that allow the planner to outline structures and planning volumes. The process of identifying structures, target volumes or normal tissues, by creating contours around them is often called **organ segmentation.** Segmented structures can be displayed graphically either as outlines surrounding the structure or can be filled to create a solid volume. Segmented structures are commonly used to assist in field shaping and positioning and also in isodose evaluation.

Anatomy that is to be identified for treatment planning may be better defined using other imaging modalities in addition to CT. Because of the physical principles underlying their image production, MRI and positron emission tomography (PET) scans show anatomy differently than does CT. Both MRI and PET incorporate physiology in the production of images. This can be used to better differentiate between diseased and normal tissues. Treatment-planning systems are often capable of combining the images from the different modalities with the CT image. The process of combining the images is called **image fusion.** Properly fused images combine the enhanced imaging capabilities of MRI and/or PET with the spatial accuracy of CT. Anatomy can be defined on any of the image data sets and can then be displayed on the CT image (Fig. 22-16).

Once a beam has been created, it is possible to view the patient as seen through the opening of the beam. As stated previously, this particular view of the patient anatomy from the perspective of the treatment field is called a BEV. The BEV changes in shape and size the same way the radiation beam diverges through the patient. Field size and blocking can be demonstrated according to their size and shape in relation to the plane of the body being viewed. When a BEV is reconstructed such that diverge-corrected patient anatomy from the CT data set is also included in an image that

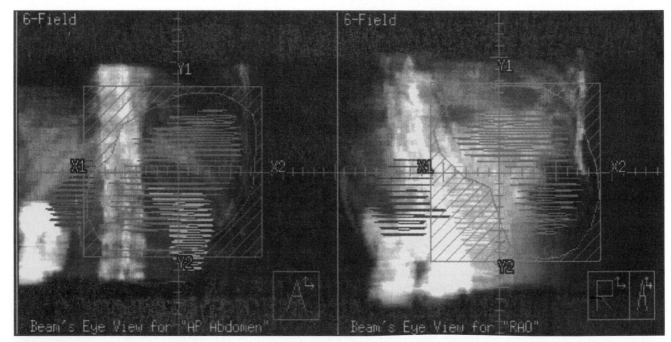

Figure 22-14. Use of the BEV tool for treatment-field design and placement. Note the differences between the anteroposterior (AP) and right anterior oblique (RAO) fields. The shape and spatial relationships of the tumor and the kidney volumes change as function of gantry angle allowing more favorable tumor-volume targeting.

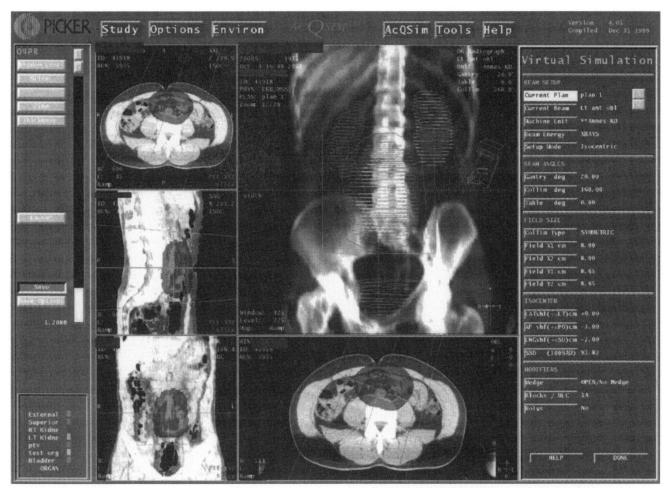

Figure 22-15. Virtual simulation software sample screen. A "virtual" patient is created from computed tomography (CT) data. The software supports normal-tissue and target volume definition and identification; treatment fields can then be designed and placed.

imitates a radiograph, the resulting image is called a **digitally reconstructed radiograph (DRR).** A typical DRR is shown in Fig. 22-17.

A **room's eye view** demonstrates the geometric relationship of the treatment machine to the patient. The room's eye view allows clear visualization of the entrance and exit of the beam through the patient. This view may also help prevent possible orientations of the equipment that could result in collisions with the patient.

Other image rendering techniques allow visualization of anatomic structures that have been highlighted. The skeleton of the body or the skin can be distinguished by choosing image-visualization techniques that display the specific ranges of CT density. Skin rendering allows the planner to see markers that were placed on the skin during the CT scan. Room lasers, field and block outlines can be displayed on the patient's skin (Fig. 22-18). This technique is similar to looking at the field light on the patient in a conventional simulator.

3D treatment plans can be objectively evaluated using dose and volume information. An extremely useful evalua-

tion tool is the **dose-volume histogram (DVH).** Lawrence et al.[10] have explained the fundamentals of DVHs and their clinical interpretations in detail. The DVH is a plot of target or normal structure volume as a function of dose. It is, in essence, a frequency distribution of the number of target or normal-structure voxels (volume elements) receiving a certain dose. In its most common form (the "cumulative" DVH), it is a plot of volume versus the minimum dose absorbed within that volume. Fig. 22-19 presents a cumulative DVH for a hypothetical PTV, CTV, and GTV. The characteristics of an optimal target-volume DVH are (1) high percentage volume at prescribed target dose (adequate target volume coverage) and (2) rapid decrease in volume beyond the prescribed dose (dose uniformity within target).

Interpretation of normal-tissue DVHs is somewhat more complex. Clearly, a desired trait of a normal-tissue DVH is large volumes maintained at lower doses. This is often not attainable and DVHs such as those shown in Fig. 22-20 result.[15] Depending on their response to radiation, tissues can be characterized as either serial response tissues or parallel

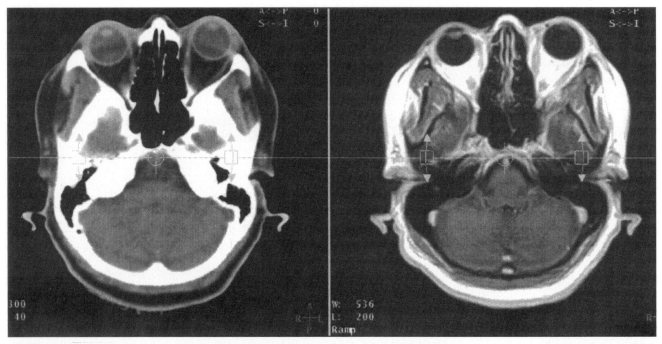

Figure 22-16. Computed tomography (CT) and magnetic resonance imaging (MRI)-image fusion. The superior soft-tissue imaging ability of the MRI image of the right can be combined with the superior spatial accuracy of the CT image on the left, to produce a composite, correlated image. In the fusion process, common anatomic features are identified in each image, and these common features are then used to "link" the data sets so that they form a composite set. From that point on, features identified on an image of one modality are shown on its corresponding second-modality image.

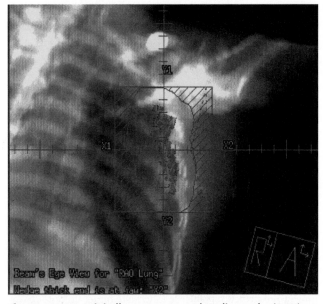

Figure 22-17. Digitally reconstructed radiograph (DRR). A DRR is a two-dimensional radiograph-like image that is reconstructed from a computed tomography (CT) data set. The image of this figure was reconstructed from a thoracic data set to produce a view equivalent to that obtained if a radiographic image were obtained from the patient's right-anterior side. Superimposed on the image is the projection of the contoured clinical target volume and of the treatment field designed to cover the volume with a 2-cm margin.

response tissues. The overall function of organs consisting of **serial response tissues** can be affected by the incapacitation of only one element. The spinal cord is such an organ. The high-dose region of a serial-tissue DVH is of particular importance. The overall function of organs consisting of **parallel response tissues,** on the other hand, is affected by the injury of a number of elements of that organ above a certain minimum "reserve." The liver is an example of such an organ. Interpretation of DVHs of organs of parallel-response tissue is less clear.

The 3D Treatment-planning Process

Imaging and anatomy differentiation. The treatment-planning process begins at the time of patient CT imaging. The area to be imaged is identified. It is important to include enough anatomy to identify anatomic landmarks for treatment setup confirmation. Setting the CT slice thickness and table indexing to small increments will increase the quality of radiographs created from the CT data sets. The patient is set up on the CT scanner in treatment position. Immobilization devices are made and used during the scan. Once the patient is positioned on the table, the center of the volume to be scanned is placed at the intersection of the transverse, sagittal, and coronal positioning lasers. Preliminary marks are made on the patient, and radiopaque markers are placed to identify the location of patient marks on the CT images. These marks will

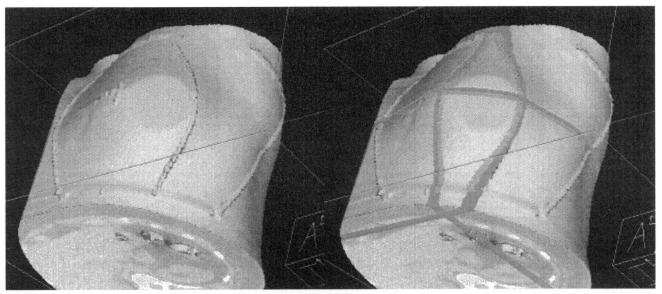

Figure 22-18. Use of image-visualization tools to aid in treatment-field placement during virtual simulation and treatment planning. The computed tomography (CT) data set can be visualized using an image-rendering technique that emphasizes the patient's skin and any markers placed on the skin. In this figure, beams have been placed such that the lasers that indicate their isocenter coincide with catheters placed on the patient before CT.

be used later as the reference position for final isocenter localization following the virtual simulation (Fig. 22-21).

CT images are reconstructed and sent to the planning system. The images in the planning system can be viewed either three dimensionally or through different anatomic planes, the most common being transverse, sagittal, and coronal views. Important anatomic areas are defined in the course of organ segmentation. Target areas are identified on the patient's CT data set. Tumor bearing regions classified and contoured as GTVs, CTVs, and PTVs are defined. The minimum dose acceptable for target structures is identified, as well as the acceptable homogeneity of the dose throughout the target. Within the volume to be irradiated, there may be critical structures requiring that a specified volume be limited to a certain maximum dose. These significant anatomic structures are outlined in the treatment-planning system as well. Normal-tissue volumes and their dose limits are generally determined by clinical criteria.

Treatment-field definition. After target and anatomy definition, the orientation of treatment beams are arranged. Beam location is referenced to the marks previously made on the patient. In the planning system, the location of patient marks becomes the origin or starting point of the plan. To identify the origin, the transverse CT image containing the radiopaque markers is used. Alignment tools are used to find the point where lines through the markers would intersect. The origin point is placed at this intersection. Beam coordinates can now be referenced to this point to define the isocenter position. The center of the PTV is a recommended starting point for the placement of isocenter. Some treatment-planning

systems can automatically set the isocenter to the center of the PTV. If manual means are necessary for isocenter positioning, coronal, transverse, and sagittal views can be used to set the position of the isocenter to the center of the PTV.

Using both 2D and 3D viewing techniques, the angles of the gantry and couch are adjusted to include the PTV in the beam while excluding critical structures out of the path of the beam. The collimator size and rotation can be adjusted also to exclude structures from the beam. The shape of the treatment field can be fashioned using an MLC or conventional blocking. Autofielding, a technique used to set an open area around the PTV from the perspective of the BEV, can be used to shape the field following the contour of the PTV. The autofield should include a margin around the PTV that allows for beam penumbra and block edge effects. The margin should be sufficient to allow isodose lines of 90% or greater to cover the PTV. A blocking technique called autoblocking can be used to create a block or an MLC shield to decrease dose to critical structures. These structures can be covered with the block plus a margin of extra blocking if deemed necessary.

Several beams are commonly created to deliver dose to the PTV. Once the beams have been set up, the amount of dose to be delivered from each beam is determined. Beam weighting is used to set dose limits for each beam. A point inside of the area to be treated is chosen to receive 100% of the dose. This normalization point is usually the beams' isocenter. If the isocenter of any of the beams is close to a block or near the surface of the patient, another point of normalization can be chosen. Each beam is then assigned a percentage of the total dose to be delivered.

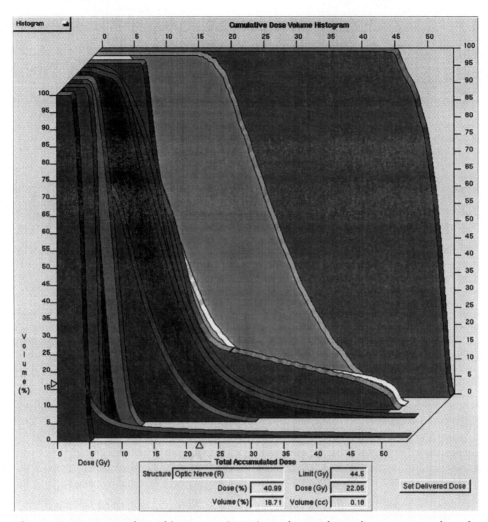

Figure 22-19. Dose-volume histograms (DVHs) used to evaluate the treatment plan of a patient. This figure shows a composite plot of the DVHs of the target volume and of critical structures within the irradiated volume. Dose is represented on the x-axis of the plots, and the y-axis represents percent of total volume enclosed by that dose level. To illustrate, note the x,y value of the target DVH on the upper-right corner of the figure. It appears that 100% of the target volume will be receiving a dose of 45 Gy or greater. Moving a little further to the right on the target DVH shows that approximately 80% of the target volume will be receiving a dose of about 50 Gy or greater.

When the plan is "normalized," numerical values of isodoses are equal to fractions of the dose existing at the point of normalization.

Treatment plan evaluation and implementation. The plan is evaluated after the dose calculations are completed. Each treatment plan is assessed to decide if it can be used to deliver the prescribed dose within target dose homogeneity and normal tissue protection constraints that have been established. Multiple plans can be compared using DVHs as bases for the comparison. Dose distributions can be displayed as isodose lines on 2D planes or as clouds of dose for 3D viewing (Fig. 22-22). 3D isodose clouds allow the planner to select an isodose value and than rotate the 3D image of the PTV to view the distribution of dose around it. This technique will show if any portion of the PTV extends outside of the isodose cloud and is not covered properly.

The complexity of the treatment plan is also reviewed. The number of fields used and the viability of the field arrangement is considered. Time of treatment delivery, setup reproducibility and complexity, and plan-verification feasibility are important plan evaluation criteria as well.

Once the plan is approved, documentation is produced and filed in the patient's treatment record to clearly communicate plan parameters. Isodose distributions in transverse, coronal, and sagittal planes are printed. These should show the approved isodose distribution and the magnitude and

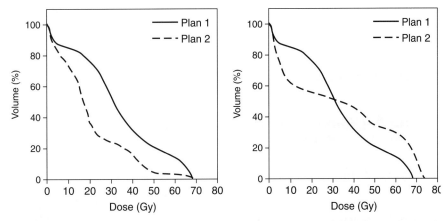

Figure 22-20. Cumulative normal tissue DVHs for two rival treatment plans. *Left panel,* plan 2 superior over complete dose range; *right panel,* superior plan will depend upon how organ responds to radiation damage. *(From Purdy JA and Starkschall G, editors: A practical guide to 3-D planning and conformal radiation therapy, Madison, Wisc, 1999, Advanced Medical Publishing.)*

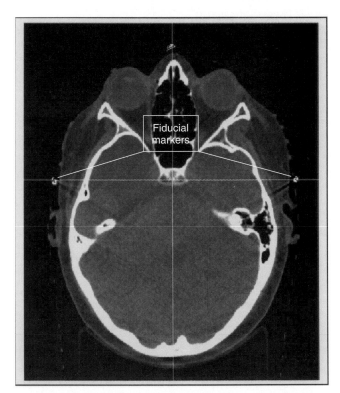

Figure 22-21. Establishment of treatment-plan coordinate-system origin. External radiopaque markers, placed on the patient before computed tomography (CT), are routinely used to register the origin of the coordinate system of the treatment plan. This origin corresponds with the skin marks made on the patient. In this figure, markers placed on the immobilization mask of a patient are used to register the position of the plan origin. Any possible isocenter displacement from this point is noted as an "isocenter shift."

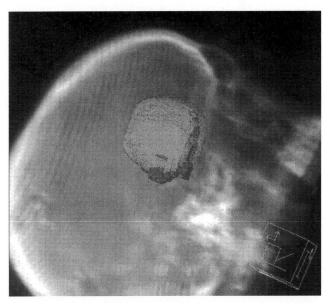

Figure 22-22. An isodose "cloud" enclosing a target volume. The prescription isodose level can be demonstrated in a three-dimensional (3D) visualization called "an isodose cloud." If the cloud is shown semitransparent, the coverage of the target volume can be assessed. In this figure, a semitransparent isodose cloud produced by a three-field beam arrangement is superimposed on a hypothetical pituitary target volume. Shown are target areas not covered by the prescribed dose.

location of hot spots. The use of heterogeneity corrections is documented. BEVs or, preferably, DRRs for each field are printed along with the corresponding MLC information if applicable. An orthogonal pair of DRRs can be printed to be used as a reference of the location of isocenter. Applicable DVHs should also be included in the documentation. Patient setup instructions should be clearly documented so that the position of the beams' isocenter and its relationship to patient markings are evident. If the patient is to be set up to original markings and the isocenter is to be shifted to a new position, shift instructions should be clearly specified and properly verified. It is highly recommended that a record and verify system be used because 3D treatment plans are often complex and commonly have multiple beams with varying combinations of couch, gantry, and collimator positions.

The treatment plans of new patients should be verified as they are implemented clinically for the first time. Treatment initiation is an extremely important last step of the planning process. Before delivery of the treatment, each field should be checked to ensure that there are no collisions between the machine and the treatment table or the patient. Beam paths are examined to ensure that the treatment couch does not adversely interfere with either beam delivery or with port filming. Any delivery or filming limitations should be identified and approved. Each field's blocks or MLC patterns are examined. DRRs should be used for comparisons with port films. Patient SSDs are checked. The relationships between field blocking, collimator settings, and planned wedge orientations are also assessed. All documentation is reviewed to ensure consistent adherence to the plan. The treatment-planning phase ends only when there is certainty that the plan can be consistently delivered accurately.

SUMMARY

The treatment-planning process pulls together the entire radiation oncology team—both clinical and technical staffs. The sciences of radiation oncology, biology, therapy, dosimetry, and physics collaborate to optimize a patient's treatment. This chapter discussed the role of physics and dosimetry in the treatment-planning process. The fundamental principles of photon-beam treatment planning and the basics of the treatment-planning process are described.

Review Questions

1. Isodose distributions are _____-dimensional representations of the spatial distribution of dose.
   a. One
   b. Two
   c. Three
   d. Four
2. Wedged-field isodose distributions are characterized by

increased radiation intensity under the _____ of the wedge.
   a. Heal (thicker portion)
   b. Toe (thinner portion)
   c. Both a and b
   d. Neither a nor b
3. Use of parallel-opposed fields only is contraindicated as beam energy _____ and patient thickness _____.
   a. Decreases, decreases
   b. Increases, increases
   c. Decreases, increases
   d. Increases, decreases
4. _____ corrections account for the dose effects produced by the presence of materials of density different than water or unit density.
   a. Homogeneity
   b. Heterogeneity
   c. Isocentric
   d. None of the above
5. In treatment planning, when dose delivery parameters are computed based on target-dose-delivery and normal-tissue-avoidance criteria, the process is termed _____ planning.
   a. Forward
   b. Inverse
   c. Reciprocal
   d. Reverse
6. IMRT is a treatment planning and delivery process that seeks to achieve treatment plan optimization by varying the _____ of treatment beams in addition to their position.
   a. Field size
   b. Intensity
   c. Area
   d. Energy
7. The CTV is a treatment-planning volume that includes gross visible and/or palpable disease and _____ disease.
   a. Microscopic
   b. Subclinical
   c. Both a and b
   d. Neither a nor b
8. Image _____ is a process by which images produced by different modalities can be combined to use the best features of each modality.
   a. Production
   b. Fusion
   c. Registration
   d. None of the above
9. The quality of DRRs can be improved by _____ the thickness of CT slices.
   a. Increasing
   b. Decreasing
   c. Rotating
   d. Multiplying

10. A plan-evaluation tool that simultaneously presents dose and volume information in a graphical form allowing objective plan assessment is the dose volume histogram.
    a. True
    b. False

Questions to Ponder

1. The use of heterogeneity corrections in dose calculations is becoming more commonplace because these calculations are more accurate. Most of our clinical outcome data, on the other hand, is based on homogeneous dose calculations. What are the challenges associated with clinical heterogeneity-correction implementation, if existing clinical-outcomes data is to be preserved?

2. It is clear that use of the newer technology that has become available in the field of radiation oncology produces superior radiation-dose distributions. It is also becoming apparent, however, that this technology comes at an increased cost in terms of resources needed per patient. How are these two apparently conflicting patient-treatment perspectives to be reconciled?

3. It is often necessary, in treatment planning, to make compromises between tumor control and normal-tissue complication probabilities. What are the factors that need to be considered when making these determinations?

REFERENCES

1. Anderson DW: *Absorption of ionizing radiation,* Baltimore, 1984, University Park Press.
2. Antolak JA, et al: Prostate target volume variations during a course of radiotherapy, *Int J Radiat Oncol Biol Phys* 42:661-672, 1998.
3. Bentel GC: *Radiation therapy planning,* ed 2, New York, 1996, McGraw-Hill.
4. Coia LR, Schultheiss TE, Hanks GE: *A practical guide to CT simulation,* Madison, Wisc, 1995, Advanced Medical Publishing.
5. Hendee WR: *Medical radiation physics,* St. Louis, 1970, Mosby.
6. International Commission on Radiation Units and Measurements (ICRU) Report 24: *Determination of absorbed dose in a patient irradiated by beams of x or gamma rays in radiotherapy procedures,* Bethesda, Md, 1976, International Commission on Radiation Units and Measurements.
7. International Commission on Radiation Units and Measurements (ICRU) Report 50: *Prescribing, recording, and reporting photon beam therapy,* Bethesda, Md, 1993, International Commission on Radiation Units and Measurements.
8. International Electrotechnical Commission (IEC) Performance Standard 976: *Medical electron accelerators—functional performance characteristics,* Geneva, 1989, International Electrotechnical Commission.
9. Khan FM: *The physics of radiation therapy,* ed 2, Baltimore, 1994, Williams & Wilkins.
10. Lawrence TS, et al: Clinical interpretation of dose-volume histograms: the basis for normal tissue preservation and tumor dose escalation. In Meyer JL, Purdy JA, editors: *3-D conformal radiotherapy,* Basel, Switzerland, 1996, Karger.
11. Mackie TR, Liu HH, McCulough EC: Model-based photon dose calculation algorithms. In Khan FM, Potish RA, editors: *Treatment planning in radiation oncology,* Baltimore, 1998, Williams & Wilkins.
12. Mohan R, et al: Three-dimensional conformal radiotherapy. In Khan FM, Potish RA, editors: *Treatment planning in radiation oncology,* Baltimore, 1998, Williams & Wilkins.
13. Perez CA, Brady LW: *Principles and practice of radiation oncology,* Philadelphia, 1998, Lippincott-Raven Publishers.
14. Starkschall G, Hogstrom KR: Dose-calculation algorithms used in 3-D radiation therapy treatment planning. In Purdy JA, Starkschall G, editors: *A practical guide to 3-D planning and conformal radiation therapy,* Madison, Wisc, 1999, Advanced Medical Publishing.
15. Ten Haken RK, Kessler ML: 3-D RTP plan evaluation. In Purdy JA, Starkschall G, editors: *A practical guide to 3D planning and conformal radiation therapy,* Madison, Wisc, 1999, Advanced Medical Publishing.
16. Varian Medical Systems: *C-Series Clinac: enhanced dynamic wedge implementation guide,* Palo Alto, Calif, 1996, Varian Medical Systems.
17. Verhey L, Bentel G: Patient immobilization. In *The modern technology of radiation oncology,* Madison, Wisc, 1999, Medical Physics Publishing.
18. Wong JW, Purdy JA: On methods of inhomogeneity corrections for photon transport, *Med Phys* 17:807-814, 1990.

Electron Beams in Radiation Therapy

Adam F. Kempa

Outline

Key Terms

Bremsstrahlung
Electron density
Gradient
Mass stopping power

Restricted mass stopping power
Scanning beams
Scattering foil

The goal of this chapter is to provide an accurate
overview of electron beam therapy at the student level.
To accomplish this goal, concepts dealing with the
physics of electrons and electron beams are dealt with in a
general manner. Often, important issues become obscured by
intricacy and detail. A more detailed treatment of electron
beam therapy may be found in the references listed at the end
of the chapter.

The art of radiation therapy treatment planning may be
described as making use of the unique physical properties of
various sources of radiation to optimize and individualize a
patient's treatment. Electron beams are a good example of
this concept. Selection of the energy of an electron beam
allows the choice of depth of treatment and the dose to tissues deep to the treatment volume. Basic rules of thumb may
be used to understand how the energy of an electron beam is
defined and to provide a basis for the selection of an electron
beam energy for treatment.

REVIEW OF THE PHYSICS OF ELECTRON BEAMS

Interactions of Electron Beams with Matter

Before a meaningful discussion of electron beam dosimetry
can take place, the physical differences between electron
beams and photon beams must be considered. A photon has
no charge or mass. An electron has a negative charge and a
mass approximately 2000 times smaller than that of a proton.

Electron beams' interactions with matter differ from those
of photon beams largely because of these two characteristics.
Because the electron has mass, the probability of an interaction
between the electron and an atom is greater than that of a

photon, which has no mass. Similarly, the probability of a negatively charged electron interacting with an atom's coulomb forces is greater than that of a photon with no charge.

Collisional and Radiation Interactions

Electron beams interact with matter by a combination of collisional processes and radiation processes.[5] The energy loss of these two processes is expressed in terms of mass stopping powers. The **mass stopping power** *(S/p)* is the rate of energy loss per unit length *(S)*, divided by the density of the medium *(p)*.[5] The total mass stopping power is the sum of all energy losses. This includes both losses caused by collisions of electrons with atomic electrons *(S/p)col* and radiation losses or **bremsstrahlung** production *(S/p)rad*. Bremsstrahlung (German for "braking radiation") is caused by electron decelerations when passing through the field of atomic nuclei. The expression for the total mass stopping power *(S/p)tot* is as follows[5]:

$$(S/p)_{tot} = (S/p)_{col} + (S/p)_{rad}$$

The contribution of each of these processes is affected by the energy of the electron beam and the atomic (Z) number of the irradiated material.[7]

A refinement of the total mass stopping power is the restricted mass collisional stopping power. The **restricted mass collisional stopping power** better describes the absorbed dose by accounting for energy transferred by delta rays. Delta rays are electrons scattered with enough energy to cause further ionization and excitations in other atoms.[2] All of the energy loss resulting from the interactions of the delta rays may not be deposited locally. Energy transfer by collisions of delta rays is restricted by specification of an energy below which energy losses are counted as part of the restricted collisional mass stopping power.[15] Energy losses considered as part of the restricted collisional mass stopping power relate to local absorption of dose.[15] Above this specified energy the energy losses are not counted as part of the restricted collisional mass stopping power.[15] By this mechanism a more accurate representation of absorbed dose is obtained. In the AAMP Task Group 21 the stopping power ratios were determined for monoenergetic electron beams. A further refinement of restricted mass collisional stopping powers has been incorporated in the AAMP Task Group 51 protocol.[1] The Task Group 51 protocol uses stopping power ratios for "realistic electron beams." These values reflect a spectrum of electron beam energies leading to a more precise representation of dose.

In collisional losses the predominate interaction may be described as an incident electron interacting with the electron of an atom. Low Z number materials have a greater **electron density** (number of electrons per unit mass) than high Z number materials.[15] As one would expect, collisional interactions are the predominant process by which electrons lose energy in low Z number materials. Radiation or bremsstrahlung losses occur when an incident electron interacts with the coulomb forces of the nucleus of an atom.[15] The probability of the occurrence of energy loss resulting from the radiation process increases with increasing energy or increasing Z number of the absorbing material.[7]

Energy Dependence of Electron Interactions

"For water, energy loss by collision is approximately 2 MeV/cm in the energy range of 1 to 100 MeV."[15] Radiation losses vary from 0.01 to 0.4 MeV/cm in the 1 to 20 MeV energy range.[15] A crude comparison of these values demonstrates that collisional interactions occur several times more often than radiation interactions in low Z number materials. In clinical radiation therapy in the energy range from 1 to 20 MeV, the predominant mechanism by which an electron beam loses energy is by collisional interactions in tissues because of the low Z number of tissue.[7]

Electron Beam Energy Spectrum Dependence on Depth

An electron beam emerges from the accelerator guide of the linear accelerator at a point called the "accelerator window." Before the electron beam moves through the accelerator window the energy spectrum is very narrow.[5] The electron beam then moves through various components of the linear accelerator, the accelerator window, scattering foils, ionization monitor chambers, and the air between the patient and treatment machine to the patient surface. The spectrum of the beam at the patient surface is decreased and broadened in energy because of interactions with the accelerator components.[5] As the electron beam passes into the patient, it undergoes a decrease in energy and broadening of the energy spectrum.[7] The energy spectrum of the electron beam in the patient depends on the depth in the patient and the energy spectrum at the surface of the patient.[5]

Production of Clinically Useful Electron Beams

Electron beams are most commonly produced by linear accelerators in current practice. There are several modifications of the linear accelerator required for electron beam production. The first is to remove the "target" and flattening filter used to produce x-rays from the path of the electron beam. The second is to decrease the "electron gun" current to lower the dose rate of the electron beam to clinically acceptable ranges. The reason for the reduction in the current becomes apparent when one considers the amount of current used in x-ray mode compared with that used in electron mode. "In normal electron therapy mode operation, the beam current through the electron window is on the order of 1/1000 of the beam current at the x-ray target for x-ray therapy mode."[6] Without a reduction of the current at the electron gun window, unwieldy dose rates in the thousands of centigrays per second could result.[6] A narrow electron beam commonly referred to as a "pencil beam" is produced by the linear accelerator. This pencil beam of electrons may be widened for clinical use by two methods: the use of a scattering foil or the use of a scanning electron beam.

Scattering Foils

The most common method of producing a beam wide enough for clinical use is to use a scattering foil.[6] A scattering foil is a thin sheet of a material that has a high Z number placed in the path of the pencil beam of electrons. A second scattering foil may be added to create a "dual scattering foil" arrangement. The first scattering foil is used to widen the beam; the second is used to improve the flatness of the beam.[6] Often the x-ray field flattening filter and scattering foil are mounted on a carousel arrangement (Fig. 23-1). This allows for a simple switch from photon to electron mode of operation.

Scanning Beams

Scanning electron beams are the second way that a beam wide enough for clinical purposes may be produced. The narrow pencil beam of electrons is scanned by magnetic fields across the treatment area. This constantly moving pencil beam distributes the dose evenly throughout the field. **Scanning beams** are especially useful above 25 MeV, when the thickness of the required scattering foils would result in difficulties with their mechanical size and also would cause problems with electron contamination.[6]

Advantages and Disadvantages of Scattering Foils Versus Scanning Beams

A drawback of the use of scattering foils is the production of bremsstrahlung contamination by the electron beam's inter-action with the **scattering foil.** An advantage of the use of scattering foils is that they are relatively simple and reliable when compared with the scanning beam method. An advantage of the scanning beam method is that there is none of the bremsstrahlung contamination caused by the interaction of the electron beam and the scattering foil. However, x-ray contamination from the collimators, ionization chambers, and the intervening air is still present.[6] A disadvantage of the scanning beam method is the maintenance of complex electronic systems. Failures of the scanning beam mechanism could allow the entire dose to be delivered in one small area of the patient with disastrous results.[15]

CHARACTERISTICS OF THERAPEUTIC ELECTRON BEAMS

Dosage Gradients of Clinically Useful Electron Beams

Electron beam therapy offers the ability to treat superficially located lesions with almost no dose to the deep underlying tissues. This is illustrated by Fig. 23-2, *A*. The darkened high-dose area is followed by a narrow lighter low-dose area and a white area indicating negligible dose. The implication for treatment planning is that organs and structures deep to the darkened area will receive minimal dose. This results from rapid fall-off of percent depth dose with increasing depth and is characteristic of electron beams below 15 MeV.[13]

Fig. 23-2, *B*, numerically demonstrates this rapid fall-off

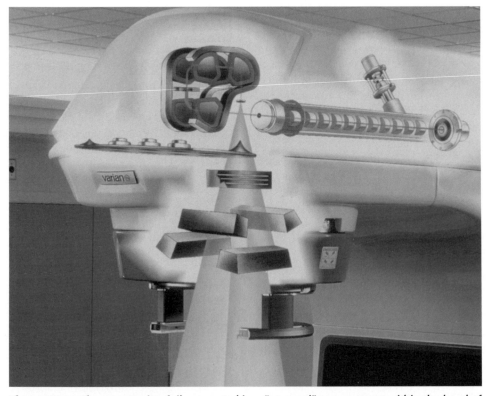

Figure 23-1. Three scattering foils mounted in a "carousel" arrangement within the head of a modern linear accelerator. *(Courtesy Varian Medical Systems.)*

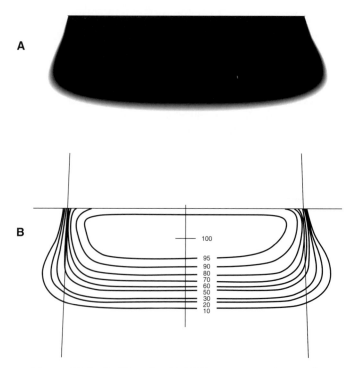

Figure 23-2. A, Film of a 12-MeV 14 × 8 cm electron beam used for obtaining isodose curves. **B,** Isodensity curves from the 12-MeV electron beam. *(From Khan F: The physics of radiation therapy, Baltimore, 1984, Williams & Wilkins.)*

of dose with depth. The rate of change of a value (dose) with a change in position is termed a **gradient.** Although the relative distances between the surface to 80% and from 80% to 10% isodose curves are approximately equal, the rates of change of isodose values are not. In the first half of the distance there is a 20% change, compared with a 70% change in isodose values in the second half of the distance. This advantageous dosage gradient may be manipulated by varying the energy of the electron beam. This may be demonstrated by a comparison of percent depth dose data in the following example (Table 23-1). The 80% isodose value is commonly used to describe the treatment depth of an electron beam. As the nominal energy of the electron beam is increased, the depth of the 80% isodose value increases from 3.5 cm at 10.6 MeV to 4.9 cm at 15 MeV. At the nominal energy of 30 MeV the rapid fall-off of dose with increasing depth is greatly diminished. The 80% isodose value is at a depth of 9 cm, and, at approximately 15 cm, 10% of the dose remains. "The clinically advantageous shape cut-off to the percentage depth dose achieved with low-energy electron beams of 10 to 15 MeV is lost at very high energies, and that consequently there is no real clinical advantage in using electron beams of energies higher than about 20 MeV."[13] Restated simply, high-energy electron beams begin to approximate the depth dose characteristics of low-energy photon beams with the disadvantage of having no "true" skin-sparing effect.

Shape of the Plot of Percent Depth Dose Versus Depth

The characteristic shape of the plot of dose versus depth for an electron beam is demonstrated in Fig. 23-3. The dose at the surface begins at approximately 85% of maximum and builds up to 100% in the first few centimeters below the surface. Beyond the 80% to 90% depth dose in Fig. 23-3, the fall-off dose with increasing depth is rapid. The curve does not reach 0 but "flattens out" at a value of a few percent. The dose in this end region is composed of bremsstrahlung-produced x-ray contamination from the interaction of the electron beam with scattering foils, ionization chambers, collimators, and the air between the patient and the treatment unit.[5] Although this dose is clinically insignificant in most cases, caution is warranted when large areas are treated, as in total body electron treatments for mycosis fungoides (cutaneous T-cell lymphoma).[7] An interesting use of this x-ray contamination has been to obtain port film radiographs of electron beam treatments.[3]

Shape of Electron Beam Isodose Curves

Electron beam isodose curves have a characteristic shape, which is described as a lateral bulge or ballooning of the isodose curves. "As the beam penetrates a medium, the beam expands rapidly below the surface due to scattering."[15] This is evident in Fig. 23-2, *B,* where the 10%, 20%, 30%, and 50% isodose curves balloon or bulge beyond the edge of the field. The lateral scattering or ballooning of electron beam decreases with increasing electron beam energy.[7]

TREATMENT PLANNING OF ELECTRON BEAM THERAPY

Electron Beam Rules of Thumb

Treatment planning using electron beams may be explained using several relationships or rules of thumb that provide estimates of several aspects of electron beams. The resulting information gained by application of the rules of thumb clarifies the use of a particular electron beam for a specific treatment application.

The first of these relationships is used to determine the energy of an electron beam. As an electron beam passes through matter, it decreases both in intensity and in energy with increasing depth. For this reason the measurement of an electron beam's energy depends on the depth of the electron

Table 23-1	Comparison of percent depth dose data for varying electron beam energies		
Nominal Beam Energy (MeV)	Percent Depth Dose/Depth (cm)		
10.6	100%/1.9	80%/3.5	10%/5.2
15	100%/2.9	80%/4.9	10%/7.1
30	100%/3.7	80%/8.7	10%/14.6

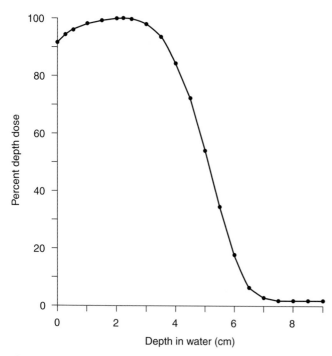

Figure 23-3. Central axis depth dose distribution measured in water. Incident energy, 13 MeV; 8 × 10 cm cone; effective source-skin distance (SSD) is 68 cm. *(From Khan F: The physics of radiation therapy, Baltimore, 1984, Williams & Wilkins.)*

beam in the phantom or patient. Although there are several methods of determining the energy of an electron beam, one method is widely used because of its practicality in the clinical setting. Simply stated, the depth of the 50% dose in centimeters (R_{50}) is multiplied by a constant (C_4). The resulting product is the mean energy of the electron (E_o) beam stated in MeV at the phantom surface[10] as follows:

$$E_o = C_4R_{50}$$

The value of the constant C_4 has varied slightly from 2.33 MeV in American Association of Physicists in Medicine (AAPM) Task Group 21 to 2.4 MeV in Task Group 25.[10] There is little difference between the final value determined by the use of either number for the constant C_4. For this reason, it is recommended that physicists select one of the two values along with other parameters and use it consistently in the calibration protocol.[10]

The second of these relationships deals with the reduction of the energy of an electron beam as it moves through matter. The energy of an electron beam at a given depth in water may be approximated based on the following relationship. The rate at which an electron beam loses energy is approximately 2 MeV/cm in water.[2] For example, an electron beam with an energy of 10 MeV incident on the phantom surface will have an energy of 6 MeV at a depth of 2 cm in water.

The third relationship deals with the practical range (E_r) in

centimeters of an electron beam in tissue. The practical range of an electron beam is determined by dividing the energy of the electron beam in MeV by 2 as follows:

$$E_r = MeV/2$$

Past the practical range within the patient, dosage drops off quickly with depth to a value of several percent. The dosage does not reach zero because of the bremsstrahlung radiation produced by the interaction of the beam with collimators, the intervening air, and the patient.

The practical range is a helpful guide in treatment planning. This simple relationship demonstrates clearly that a lesion at a depth of 4 cm is beyond the range of a 7-MeV electron beam. In a similar manner this relationship can be used in the selection of the energy of an electron beam so that critical structures receive a minimal dose.

The fourth relationship is directly related to the choice of an electron beam energy for a specific treatment depth. The depth of the 80% isodose value is often specified as treatment depth. Treatment depth may be determined by dividing the energy of the electron beam in MeV by 3 as follows:

$$80\% \text{ isodose} = MeV/3$$

In a similar manner, the depth of the 90% isodose curve may be found by dividing the energy of the electron beam in MeV by 4 as follows:

$$90\% \text{ isodose} = MeV/4$$

Use of these simple relationships gives insight into a particular treatment. For example, a patient treated with a 10-MeV electron beam will have the following: an 80% isodose at a depth of 3.3 cm, a 90% isodose line as a depth of 2.5 cm, and a range within the patient of approximately 5 cm. Structures deeper than 5 cm deep receive a minimal dose.

The relationships for the depth of the 80% and 90% isodose lines and the dose to deep structures are for homogeneous treatment volumes of tissue-equivalent material. If the treatment area overlies an air cavity such as a lung, the choice of the isodose line for treatment must take into account the increased transmission through the lung tissue. Selection of the isodose line for treatment may vary from the 70% to the 80% isodose line in an attempt to minimize the dose to the lung.[9]

Electron Beam Characteristics at the Surface

Megavoltage electron beams in the 6- to 20-MeV energy range have varying degrees of dose reduction at the skin surface. Variables that affect the surface dose include the scattering system, atomic number of the absorber, beam energy, field size, and beam collimation. Of these variables, only the last three may be manipulated for treatment-planning purposes.

The actual absorbed dose at the surface of a water equivalent medium usually is about 0.85 of the maximum in the absence of contamination of the beam.[5] Difficulties in measuring the dose at the phantom's surface have caused AAPM Task Group 25 to specify the surface dose as the dose at 0.5 cm on the central axis of the electron beam.[10] Surface dose values for electron beams in the 6- to 20-MeV range vary from 80% to 100%. In megavoltage photon beams, increased energy of the treatment beam results in a decrease in surface dose. With electron beams the reverse is true. As the energy of the electron beam increases, the surface dose and percent depth dose also increase.[8]

There is little effect of field size on both surface dose and percent depth dose of electron beams, provided the fields are of sufficient size.[5] The rule is that the electron beam's diameter (field size) in centimeters should not be less than the practical range. This rule is extended to include field sizes that are less than the practical range in either dimension.[15] For example, a 10-MeV electron beam's percent depth dose characteristics will not vary significantly as long as the diameter (field size) is 5 cm or greater ($R_p = 10$ MeV/2 = 5). "The field size dependence of the depth dose curves increases as the energy of the electron beam increases."[16] The surface dose depends on the field size in a similar manner. In general, "the smaller the diameter the larger the surface dose."[16] Increased dose produced by increasing field size continues until the diameter of the electron beam equals the practical range of the electron beam. Additional increases in field size where the diameter of the field is greater than the practical range of the electrons will not result in a significant change in dose.[17]

Electron Beam Characteristics in the Build-up Region

The region from the surface to the depth of maximum dose is at risk for being underdosed in many clinical situations. This is most true for lower-energy electron beams (less than 12 MeV). A bolus may be used to increase the dose to the surface, much as in megavoltage beams. However, the use of bolus materials in electron beam therapy is somewhat more complicated than in photon beams. It is possible to decrease the dose in an electron beam setup by use of a bolus. For this reason, "A partial bolus should never be used with electrons."[14] The dose under a small (1 × 1 cm) bolus placed in the middle of a small treatment field may decrease the surface dose by 10% to 15%.[14] Another problem, sometimes called an "edge effect," results from the use of a large bolus with an edge perpendicular to the surface, across a portion of a treatment field. Areas of increased dose and decreased dose of 20% to 30% may be produced.[4] Near the border between bolused and unbolused portions of the field, areas under the bolus have decreased dose and the unbolused areas have increased dose. In an attempt to reduce the areas of increased and decreased dose, the edge of the partial bolus may be beveled so that it forms a 45% angle with the surface. Although this eliminates the area of decreased dose near the surface, the area of increased dose remains.[14]

The use of bolus materials in electron beam therapy is not limited to increasing the dose to the surface. Hogstrom[4] iden-

tifies two other uses for bolus material in electron beam therapy: as a tissue compensator for irregular surfaces or air cavities and to shape isodose distributions to better conform to the treatment volume or decrease the dose to critical structures at depth. "A simple rule of thumb for bolus—that utilization of bolus to make the patient anatomy present itself as a water phantom results in a more uniform dose distribution."[4]

Energy Dependence of the Width of the 80% Isodose Curve

With increasing electron beam energy, the ballooning of the isodose lines decreases. "At approximately 15 MeV, the phenomenon of lateral constriction of the higher isodose values, such as at the 80% line, occurs."[15] To cover an area at depth with the 80% isodose line, a larger area must be treated on the skin surface. "A good standard is to leave a margin of at least 1 cm between the lateral edge of the target volume and the projected edge of the collimator."[4] As always, this should be based on a careful evaluation of measured data specific to the treatment machine, beam energy, and treatment cone used. It should also be noted that there is a similar constriction of the 90% isodose line for electron beams in this energy range.

Distance Correction Factors for Electron Beam Treatments

Anatomic restrictions most often require the use of electron beams at an extended source-skin distance (SSD).[10] In the AAPM Task Group 25 report, extended SSD is defined as treatments that are not more than 15 cm beyond standard SSD. This constraint will apply to the following discussion of extended SSD treatments.[10] "The use of an extended treatment distance has only minimal effect on the central-axis depth dose and the off-axis ratios."[10] For this reason it is suggested that the use of standard depth-dose curves will give an approximation that is within a millimeter at extended distances.[10] However, factors such as the output of an electron beam and the beam penumbra change dramatically with a change in treatment distance.[10]

Clinical electron beams are created by scanning a narrow pencil-width beam across the treatment area or by use of a scattering foil. In either case there is no simple point source of the electron beam from which changes in distance may be calculated. This may be resolved in two different ways: by determining an "effective point source" or by determining the position of the "virtual source." Two methods of correction of the output of electron beams relate to these methods.

Effective Point Source Method

The effective point source is defined "such that the dose varies in accordance with the inverse square law with distance from this source."[8] This method allows for use of an inverse square correction factor with the following factors[10]:

D'_{max} = The dose to D_{max} at extended distance
D_{max} = The dose to D_{max} at nominal or normal distance

SSD = Nominal or normal SSD
SSD′ = Extended SSD
SSD$_{eff}$ = Effective SSD
d$_{max}$ = Depth of maximum dose on central axis
g = Difference between the extended SSD and the nominal SSD (SSD′–SSD)
The formula is as follows:

$$D'_{max} = \frac{D_{max}\,(SSD_{eff} + d_{max})^2}{(SSD_{eff} + g + d_{max})^2}$$

Conditions such as large air gaps, small treatment field sizes, or low-energy beams may require additional modification of this formula or a new calibration measurement specific for the individual set of treatment conditions.

Virtual Source Method

One method of finding the position of a virtual point source is by "back-projection" of the 50% width of the beam profiles from several distances.[8] The point at which these back-projections intersect is termed the virtual source position.[8] The parameters for the virtual SSD output correction factor are identical to those of the effective point source method, with the following exceptions:

SSD$_{vir}$ is virtual SSD for calibration
f$_{air}$ is air gap correction factor

$$D'_{max} = (D_{max})\frac{(SSD_{vir} + d_{max})^2}{(f_{air})(SSD_{vir} + g + d_{max})^2}$$

In the virtual SSD method the variation in the inverse square law for small field sizes, low beam energy, and large air gaps is corrected by the factor fair. The factor (fair) depends on the energy, field size and extent of the air gap.[8]

IRREGULAR FIELDS AND ELECTRON BEAMS

Shielding Dependence on Electron Beam Energy

Various methods have been used to shape electron beams for clinical purposes. These include lead strips, cutouts, or masks placed directly on the patient's skin or at the end of the treatment cone or collimator. Low melting point shields that insert into the end of the treatment cone (Fig. 23-4) have also been used. The thickness of the shielding material required increases with increasing beam energy and field size. In the measurement of the transmission of shielding material, two approaches are used to address the effect of field size on the thickness of material needed. The first approach is to measure the transmission with large field sizes; this will provide a shield thickness that is appropriate to any smaller fields used.[10] A second method relates to the use of internal shields where the thickness of the shielding device is limited by the internal space available within the patient. In the case of internal shielding devices a calibration measurement under actual conditions specific to the individual patient's treatment is recommended.[10]

A rule of thumb may be used to approximate the thickness of shielding material needed in external beam treatments. "The thickness of lead in millimeters required for shielding is approximately given by the energy in MeV divided by two"[10] as follows:

MeV/2 = Shield thickness in millimeters of lead

Khan[9] suggests that an additional millimeter of lead be added to the amount indicated by the rule of thumb method to provide an "extra safety margin." Use of lead or alloys for shielding may result in an increase in dose if the thickness of the shielding material is not sufficient to reduce the dose to less than 5% of the total dose.[7] The thickness of Lipowitz alloy (Cerrobend) required may be obtained by multiplying the thickness in lead indicated by the rule of thumb by 1.2.[10]

Internal Shielding

In some cases it is appropriate to place shielding devices within the oral cavity or under the eyelids. The objective is to shield the electron beam as it exits from the volume of tissue to be treated before it reaches normal tissue. A danger in the use of internal shielding devices is that the dose to the tissues directly in front of the shield may be increased by 30% to 70% because of the electron backscatter from the shield.[7] This problem may be minimized by placing a low Z number material between the shield and the tissue. Caution should be used in the selection of the thickness of low Z number material, which should be greater than the range of the backscattered electrons. Dental acrylic is commonly used to surround the lead shield, separating it from the oral cavity and reducing electron backscatter.[7] In the case of internal eye shields, there may not be sufficient space to allow adequate thickness of both lead and low atomic Z number material to absorb the electron backscatter produced by the lead shield.[7] Lead shields thick enough to reduce dosage to "acceptable levels" may be coated "with a thin film of wax or dental acrylic (to absorb very low energy electrons)."[7]

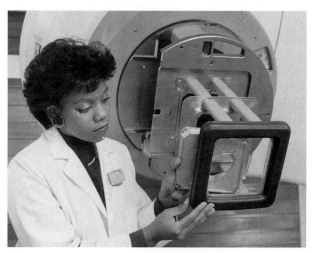

Figure 23-4. Inserting a custom shielding device into a treatment cone. *(Courtesy Varian Medical Systems.)*

Effects of Irregularly Shaped Electron Fields on Dose

An in-depth discussion of the calculation of irregular electron fields is beyond the scope of this chapter. However, situations that result in changes of dose will be identified. "Field shaping affects the output factor as well as depth dose distribution in a complex manner."[7] Variables encountered in field shaping that affect dose include the field size, the thickness of shielding material, the amount of blocking, and the treatment distance.[7] The dose rate or output factor of a clinical electron beam has a greater dependence on field size than that of a clinical photon beam.[12] The dose at any point in the patient is composed of primary and scattered radiation. The greater dependence on field size of clinical electron beams than that of photon beams results from the amount of scattered radiation that contributes to the total dose. In photon beams, approximately 10% to 30% of the dose results from scattered radiation. In electron beams, almost all the absorbed dose results from electrons that have been scattered.[12] Lateral equilibrium of these scattered electrons is an important feature in electron beam dosimetry. Lateral equilibrium is reached when the number of electrons entering an area equals the number of electrons leaving the area. This condition is met when the diameter of the field size exceeds that of the practical range of the electron beam.[12] When the diameter of the electron beam field is less than the practical range, there is a decrease in dose. The smaller the diameter of the electron beam, the greater the change in the dose because of the lack of electronic equilibrium. For this reason, changes in dose associated with irregularly shaped electron fields may be anticipated if the dimensions of any portion of the treatment field are less than the practical range (MeV/2) of the electron beam.[17] Field shaping or blocking causes changes in the output of an electron beam. The size of the change in output depends on the percentage of the area of the total treatment field that is shielded or blocked. The higher the percentage of the field that is blocked, the greater the change in output. If greater than 25% of the treatment area is blocked, measurement of the output factor for that specific treatment is recommended.[7] The effect of the electron beam energy on the output factor increases with increasing electron beam energy when blocking is used.[14] For example, at extended treatment distances (110 cm SSD), field blocking causes a large change in the output of an electron beam, which may also require measurement of the output. Olch states that "for SSD at 110 cm, almost any blockage severely changes the output factor."[14]

The use of irregularly shaped electron beams should be approached with caution. Although it has been suggested that the output factor, depth dose, and isodose distribution should be measured for any irregularly shaped electron field, this is not practical.[7] A more reasonable approach is to investigate cases of irregularly shaped electron fields in which the field edges are not greater than the practical range.[4] Computerized treatment planning of irregularly shaped electron fields by pencil-beam algorithms may resolve the uncertainties in their use. It has been demonstrated that by using treatment-planning computers with computed tomography (CT) scans, both irregular fields at nonstandard air gaps and dosage behind inhomogeneities may be calculated that are in agreement with measured data.[4] However, Hogstrom[4] indicates that careful evaluation of treatment-planning computer programs used to calculate irregularly shaped electron fields is necessary. It should be noted that the treatment-planning computer represents only half of the tools required.[17] CT images of the treatment area with the patient in treatment position can be used to obtain calculation data that are not otherwise readily available.

Tissue Heterogeneities and Their Effects on Electron Beams

"The sensitivity of high-energy electron dose distribution to the presence of tissue heterogeneities makes it essential to consider these effects in treatment planning and selection of technique."[10] The change in the dose distribution "depends on the shape, size, electron density (number of electrons/cm^3) and the effective atomic number of the heterogeneity."[11] The methods of calculating dose distributions are beyond the scope of this chapter; however, changes in the dose distributions as the result of tissue heterogeneity are described.

Small heterogeneities cause local disturbances in the dose distribution.[7] Difficulties in determining the dose distribution around small heterogeneities result from enhanced scattering effects.[11] The dose to tissues behind small bones is decreased, as might be expected, because of the shielding effect of the bone. The dose to tissues lateral to the bone is increased because of lateral scattering of the electron beam.[11] The effect of a small air cavity surrounded by tissues is somewhat different. As might be expected, the dose to tissues beyond the air cavity is increased as a result of decreased scattering of the electrons as they pass through the air cavity. Similarly, the dose to tissues lateral to the air cavity is not increased, as in the case of a bone surrounded by tissue. This results from the decreased scattering of the electrons when passing through the air cavity. The dose to tissues beyond the air cavity is also increased because of additional electron scattering from surrounding tissues.[11] Changes in dose range from a 20% underdose behind bone to a 15% to 35% overdose behind air cavities.[11]

The situation for large tissue heterogeneities of uniform density differs from that of small heterogeneities.[11] The major factor responsible for changes in the dose distribution of large tissue heterogeneities of uniform density is absorption.[11] The determination of actual dose distribution resulting from a large heterogeneity depends on the complex interrelationships of several factors. However, the effect of large heterogeneities may be discussed in a general sense.[5]

At the boundary where the electron beam leaves the bone and enters tissue, there is a small increase in dose because of increased scattering of the electrons interacting in the bone.[11] Tissues beyond the boundary of large high-density heterogeneities such as bone receive a lower dose.[5] This results in the dose distribution being moved toward the surface.[5,11] Tissues beyond low density heterogeneities, such as lung, receive a greater dose because of the reduced absorption of the lung tissue. "This results in the dose distribution being moved toward greater depth.[11] In the lung, the range of the electrons is increased by a factor of 3, with an associated increase in dose to the lung and the tissue beyond the lung."[15] An additional concern with large heterogeneities involves areas of increased and decreased dose, or "hot and cold spots," which may appear at the lateral edges of the heterogeneity.[5]

Gaps in Electron Beam Therapy

The use of combinations of two or more electron beams or electron beams and photon beams should be undertaken with great care. As previously stated, electron beam isodose curves have a characteristic shape (Fig. 23-2, *B*), which is described as a lateral bulge or ballooning of the isodose curves. Because of this characteristic shape, electron fields with adjacent treatment areas that abut each other on the surface will result in an overlap at depth.[7] Separating the treatment fields or placing a "gap" on the patient or phantom's surface results in an underdose or cold spot on the surface.[14] This is demonstrated in Fig. 23-5, which shows isodose distributions for adjacent electron fields. Note that the lowest dose to surface and superficial tissues results from the largest gap (1.5 cm). Similarly, the highest dose at depth results from the smallest gap on the surface (0.5 cm). "In a clinical situation, the decision as to whether the fields should be abutted or separated should be based upon the uniformity of the combined dose distribution across the target volume."[9] To decrease the amount that the dose will vary to a particular anatomic location the abutment line may be moved two or three times during the patient's treatment course.[4] Treatments delivered in this fashion ensure that no one anatomical area will receive all of the increased or decreased dose.

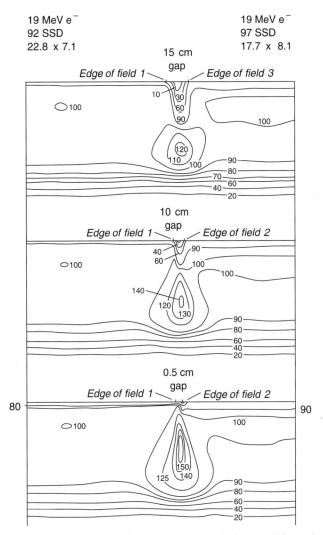

Figure 23-5. Isodose distributions for adjoining fields with the same electron beam energy with different gap widths between fields. *(From Tapley N, Almond PR, editors: Clinical applications of the electron beam, New York, 1976, Wiley.)*

APPLIED TECHNOLOGY

Clinical Applications of Electron Beams in Radiation Therapy

Correen Fraser B.S., R.T.(T)
Valerie Marable B.S., R.T.(T), CMD
Adam F. Kempa M.Ed., R.T.(T)

In the next section, three cases are presented representing the clinical application of electron beams in radiation therapy. Various principles of treatment planning covered in the preceding portion of this chapter are demonstrated. The clinical cases are followed by a summary of the cases, which is meant to underscore the treatment-planning principles outlined in each case.

Case I

Presented by Correen Fraser B.S.,R.T. (T)

A 62-year-old woman with stage $T_2N_2M_0$ intraductal carcinoma of the left breast has had a left modified radical mastectomy and axillary lymph node dissection. The patient's past medical history is significant for hypertension, diabetes, asthma, and bronchitis. Family history is negative for malignancy.

Because the incidence of residual tumor after surgery is high for intraductal carcinoma, radiation therapy is used to treat the unresected microscopic involvement. After a mastectomy, the average thickness of the chest wall is 1.5 to 2.0 cm. The major characteristics of electron beam therapy are the rapid dose fall-off, superficial dose distribution, and a skin dose of 80% to 100%, depending on the electron beam energy. With many critical structures such as lung, heart, and spinal cord underlying the chest wall, these beam characteristics make electron beam therapy an option for

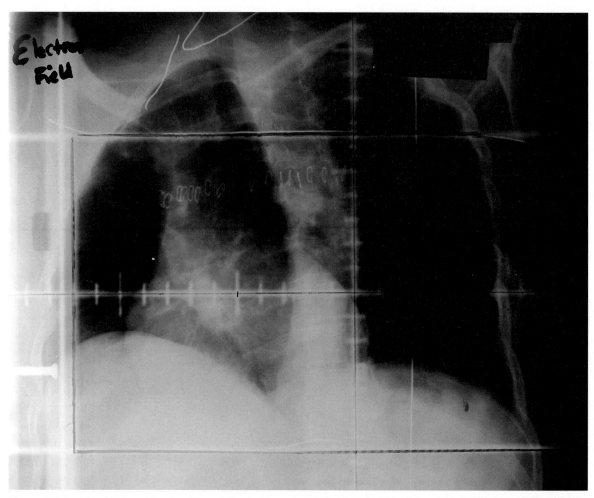

Figure 23-6. Simulator verification film of the treatment volume for chest wall irradiation. The metal clips designate the mastectomy scar and the site of possible residual disease.

chest wall irradiation. Radiation therapy machines can produce a wide range of electron beam energies. The machine used for this particular treatment is a Scanditronix MM22-Microtron, which uses a dual scattering foil system to produce electron beam energies from 3 to 20 MeV. There are many considerations when determining which electron energy to use. For chest wall electron irradiation these may include the thickness of the chest wall, the surface skin dose needed, the use of tissue-equivalent material (bolus), and underlying critical structures. A 13-MeV electron beam is prescribed for a field 24 cm wide and 13 cm long (Fig. 23-6). A 1.0-cm thick bolus material is used to increase the surface skin dose. A dose of 5000 cGy will be delivered to the chest wall in 25 fractions, 200 cGy a day, to the 90% isodose line, which lies at a depth of 4.5 cm. The resulting dose to the skin surface is about 5222 cGy. A reduced area of the chest wall will be given an additional 1000 cGy in 5 fractions, 200 cGy a day, to the 90% line with a 1.0 cm bolus.

The patient is setup and immobilized in a lateral oblique position with the left arm raised above the head (Fig. 23-7). Immobilization is achieved with the use of an alpha cradle. This position is accurately reproducible, allows the chest wall to be perpendicular to the central axis of the beam, and reduces the air gaps across the field. The central axis and borders of

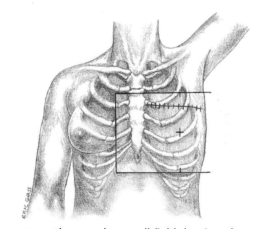

Figure 23-7. Electron chest wall field that is to be treated.

the electron field are located and marked in the simulator. Verification films and photographs are also taken at this time. In the treatment room a 100-cm SSD is set to the skin or to the top of the bolus material. The penumbra of the electron beam increases with an increase in distance between the patient skin surface and the electron cone. To avoid this problem, normal tissue and critical structures are spared by the use of an electron cone with a Cerrobend (lead alloy) block placed close to the patient skin surface. The electron cone and Cerrobend block define the field to be treated.

Case II

Presented by Valerie Marable B.S., R.T.(T), CMD

A 50-year-old black woman had a mass in her left breast found on self-examination and confirmed by mammogram and biopsy. A modified radical mastectomy was performed with an axillary dissection. Postoperative workup and all 17 axillary lymph nodes removed were both negative for disease. She was diagnosed with a $T_1N_0M_0$ adenocarcinoma of the left breast. The patient was given tamoxifen and did well for approximately 1 year postoperatively.

After 16 months the patient noted some tenderness in the left chest wall, but presumed it resulted from arthritic changes. Because of progression of symptoms and the development of a sternal mass, a biopsy was performed 2 years after initial treatment. Histologic examination confirmed locally recurrent breast cancer with metastatic disease in the sternum. She was referred to a radiation oncologist for consultation.

Examination revealed bilateral supraclavicular lymphadenopathy, which was believed to be malignant. Swelling in her upper medial left chest wall was consistent with internal mammary recurrence. CT scans were obtained to determine the dimensions of any residual masses as well as to evaluate the possibility of subclinical disease, which would affect the approach for treatment. Planning was begun for a palliative course of radiation therapy. It was decided to use a combination of photons and electrons to treat all of the disease sites with an adequate and homogeneous

dose while minimizing the dose to the lung. The dual-energy, dual-modality Siemens MD 6/15 unit was selected. This machine generates 6- and 15-MV photons and produces 5- to 14-MeV electrons with a single scattering foil. Electron and photon fields were treated on the same unit, which ensured accurate border matches. All ports were shaped with custom blocks.

Initially, 4000 cGy (200 cGy/fraction) was delivered by anteroposterior/posteroanterior (AP/PA) fields with 15-MV photons used to treat the mediastinum, left internal mammary, and bilateral supraclavicular areas (Fig. 23-8, A). A 1.5-cm bolus was placed anteriorly to ensure adequate build-up because of superficial extension of disease. The disease in the inferolateral left thorax was limited to the chest wall only. To spare underlying lung tissue a 12-MeV electron field with a 0.5 cm bolus was delivered in an oblique direction and adjoined the photon fields at the medial and superior borders. The divergence from the PA port was calculated geometrically. Because of the difficulty in matching the exit point of the PA photon field with the entrance edge of the left anterior oblique (LAO) electron port (Fig. 23-8, B) and the variance of the field size across the port, appropriate gaps were maintained between the AP and LAO ports at selected intervals. A final 1000 cGy was delivered to the sites of bulky disease using 10-MeV electrons with a 0.5 cm bolus to a total dose of 5000 cGy.

Case III

Presented by Valerie Marable B.S., R.T.(T), CMD

A 52-year-old black man had a 1-month history of sore throat, hoarse voice, and hemoptysis. He was treated unsuccessfully with antibiotics. Triple endoscopy revealed prominent exophytic lesions involving the left false cord, extending to the epiglottis, and encroaching on the entire border of the left ventricular fold. CT scans were also obtained. He was diagnosed with a $T_3N_0M_0$ squamous cell carcinoma of the larynx.

The patient adamantly refused surgical treatment, but he agreed to a definitive course of radiation therapy. He was simulated supine with his

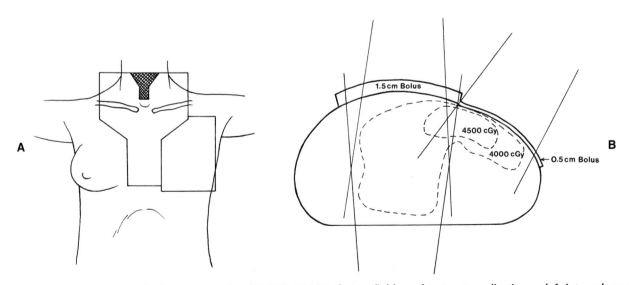

Figure 23-8. A, Anteroposterior/posteroanterior (AP/PA) 15-MV photon field used to treat mediastinum, left internal mammary, and bilateral supraclavicular areas and the oblique 12-MeV electron beam used. **B,** Cross-sectional view showing orientation of the AP/PA photon fields, oblique electron field, and bolus materials.

arms in a reproducible position, and triangulation setup marks were tattooed. Measurements were taken from stable landmarks for each tattoo as well as the chin-to-suprasternal notch distance for proper head angulation. Isodistance photographs were taken for the construction of three-dimensional compensators to maximize the homogeneity of dose with the initial larger photon ports. All fields were shaped with custom Cerrobend blocks.

A hyperfractionated approach was used with a 100 cGy/fraction delivered twice per day and a 6- to 8-hour interval between fractions. Bilateral cobalt-60 ports (Fig. 23-9, A) were treated via a Theratron 780 so as to provide a homogeneous dose to the entire target volume, which included the primary tumor plus lymphatics. At 3960 cGy the photon ports were modified (Fig. 23-9, B) to exclude the dose-limiting spinal cord. Spinal cord tolerance is generally accepted as 4500 to 5000 cGy. This amount will vary with certain circumstances, such as the patient's overall condition, the length of the spinal cord irradiated, the dose per fraction, the number of fractions per day, and the use of chemotherapy. This patient was hyperfractionated and was tentatively scheduled to receive chemotherapy at the end of the radiation course. With this in mind, his spinal cord dose for the initial photon field was kept just below 4000 cGy.

The posterior neck nodes were matched to the off-cord photon fields and treatment continued twice per day at the same dose using 7-MeV electrons up to 5500 cGy. The dose was normalized to a depth of 1.6 cm, which was the maximum build-up for the energy. This energy was selected so as to provide an adequate dose to the nodes while delivering a minimal percentage to the spinal cord. A single-foil Siemens Mevatron XX was used. The primary site was central and anterior to the spinal cord (Fig. 23-9, C). It was boosted with bilateral cobalt-60 fields, which were also given at 100 cGy/fraction twice a day to a total dose of 6600 cGy delivered in 6 weeks.

SUMMARY OF THE CLINICAL CASES

Case I details the use of an electron beam to treat a patient's chest wall after mastectomy. The goal of this treatment is to deliver a sufficient dose to the chest wall while preserving the lungs and pericardium, which are located just a few centimeters below the skin surface. A low-energy electron beam that will spare the lungs and pericardium will also deliver a low dose to the superficial tissues and skin surface. The bolus in this treatment situation may be used to shape the dosage distribution to that of the patient as well as to increase the surface dose.[5]

Case II again deals with a postmastectomy breast cancer patient. The treatment goals are slightly different from those of the first case. The patient in case II has a parasternal mass and metastatic disease in the sternum. Treatment of these areas requires a homogeneous dose to the parasternal mass as well as the sternum. A megavoltage photon beam using parallel opposed fields was chosen to deliver this homogeneous dose. A single direct electron beam with a rapid decrease in dose with increasing depth would not deliver a homogeneous dose to both parasternal mass and sternum. Additional inhomogeneities could result from the scattering of electrons by the sternum near the parasternal mass. An adjacent area of the patient's chest wall was also involved. The chest wall was well suited to a single direct electron field, which allowed a dose to be delivered to the superficial tissues while preserving the lung directly beneath it. Abutting photon and electron fields are used to deliver a homogeneous dose to the anterior surface. The anterior megavoltage photon field is opposed by a posterior photon field. Other interesting

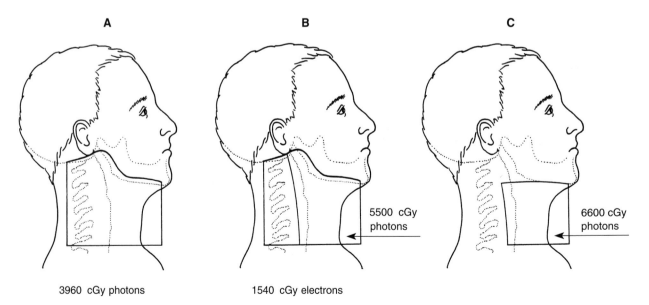

Figure 23-9. A, Treatment port used to deliver 3960 cGy with cobalt-60 photons. **B,** Modified treatment ports. Anterior port treated to 5500 cGy with cobalt-60 photons; posterior port treated to 1540 cGy with 12-MeV electrons. **C,** Primary site boosted to 6600 cGy with cobalt-60 photons.

features of this treatment include the use of bolus in both megavoltage electron and photon fields.

In case III, the goal of treatment was to deliver 5500 cGy to the lymph nodes of the patient's neck and 6600 cGy to the primary tumor. The parallel opposed cobalt-60 photons were used to provide a homogenous dose to the lymph nodes of the neck. If continued for the entire treatment course this would exceed the limit of spinal cord tolerance. A combination of electron and photon beams were used to overcome this problem. Cobalt-60 photons were used for the entire treatment course and electron beams were used at the end of the treatment course to treat the lymph nodes in the neck. This combination of cobalt-60 photons and electrons accomplished the goal of delivering 5500 cGy to the lymph nodes in the neck while limiting the dose to the spinal cord. In addition, the use of the cobalt-60 photons for the majority of the treatment course limited the dose to the patient's skin because of the skin-sparing effect of the megavoltage photon beam. To achieve the goal of delivering 6600 cGy to the primary tumor, the treatment field was reduced in size as treatment progressed.

Review Questions

1. What is the predominate mode of electron beam interaction or scattering in the 1- to 20-MeV energy range used in radiation therapy?
2. List one advantage of the use of scattering foils in electron beam therapy.
3. A patient is to be treated with a 16-MeV electron beam. Calculate the depth of the 80% and 90% isodose lines.
4. A patient has a tumor at a depth of 4 cm. What energy of electron beam should be used so that the 80% isodose line encompasses the tumor?
5. What is the range in tissue of the electron beam used in question number four?
6. List two treatment-planning considerations in the use of bolus in an electron beam used for radiation treatments.
7. Using the value of 2.4 for the constant C_4, determine the mean energy of an electron beam at the surface, whose 50% isodose value is at a depth of 5 cm.
8. A patient is to be treated with a 7-MeV electron beam. How thick (in centimeters) should a lead shield be to reduce the dose to less than 5% of the useful beam?
9. Two electron beams adjoin or abut each other on the patient's skin surface. How does this affect the dose to the patient at depth below the point where the fields abut?
10. A 12-MeV electron beam is used to deliver a dose to a 4- × 4-cm field size. What should be considered for this particular treatment?
11. A patient is to be treated with a 15-MeV electron beam to a treatment volume that measures 5 cm in width and length at depth. Discuss the selection of field size for treatment.

Questions to Ponder

1. Compare and contrast of the use of 1- to 20-MeV electron beams with that of photon beams in radiation therapy.
2. Discuss the situations in which a special calibration of an electron beam may be required.
3. Describe two specific clinical situations in which electron beam therapy is useful.
4. Compare and contrast the relationship between electron beam energy and the depth of maximum dose with that of photon beams.

REFERENCES

1. Almond PR, Biggs PJ, Coursey BM et al: AAPM's TG-51 protocol for clinical reference dosimetry of high-energy photon and electron beams. American Association of Physicists in Medicine (AAPM), *Med Phys* 26:1847-1870, 1999.
2. Cunningham R, Johns HE: *The physics of radiobiology*, ed 4, Springfield, Ill, 1983, Charles C Thomas.
3. Grimm DF, et al: Electron beam port films, *Med Dosim* 14:31-33, 1989.
4. Hogstrom KR: Treatment planning in electron beam therapy. In Vaeth JB, Meyer JL, editors: *Frontiers of radiation therapy and oncology,* vol 25, *The role of high energy electrons in the treatment of cancer,* New York, 1991, Karger.
5. ICRU Radiation Dosimetry: *Electrons with initial energies between 1 and 50 MeV, report No. 21,* Washington DC, 1972, International Commission on Radiation Units and Measurements.
6. Karzmark CJ, Nunan CS, Tanabe E: *Medical electron accelerators,* New York, 1993, McGraw-Hill.
7. Khan FM: *The physics of radiation therapy,* Baltimore, 1984, Williams & Wilkins.
8. Khan FM: Basic physics of electron beam therapy. In Vaeth JB, Meyer JL, editors: *Frontiers of radiation therapy and oncology,* vol 25, *The role of high energy electrons in the treatment of cancer,* New York, 1991, Karger.
9. Khan FM: *The physics of radiation therapy,* ed 2, Baltimore, 1997, Williams & Wilkins.
10. Khan FM, Doppke KP, Hogstrom KR et al: Clinical electron-beam dosimetry. Report of AAPM Radiation Therapy Committee Task Group No. 25. American Association of Physicists in Medicine (AAPM), *Med Phys* 18:73-109, 1991.
11. Klevenhagen SC: *Physics of electron beam therapy, medical physics handbooks,* Bristol, Great Britain, 1985, Adam Hilger.
12. McPharland BJ: *Med Dosim* 14:17, 1989.
13. Mould RF: *Radiotherapy treatment planning,* Bristol, Great Britain, 1981, Adam Hilger.
14. Olch A, et al: External beam electron therapy: pitfalls in treatment planning and deliverance. In Vaeth JB, Meyer JL, editors: *Frontiers of radiation therapy and oncology,* vol 25, *The role of high energy electrons in the treatment of cancer,* New York, 1991, Karger.
15. Perez CA, Brady LW: *Principles and practice of radiation oncology,* ed 3, Philadelphia, 1997, Lippincott.
16. Rustgi SN, Working KR: Dosimetry of small field electron beams, *Med Dosim* 17:107-108, 1992.
17. Tapley N duV: *Clinical applications for the electron beam,* New York, 1976, Wiley.

24

Electronic Charting and Image Management

Annette M. Coleman, Cara Zeidman

Outline

Key Terms

"**W***here is the chart?"*

This simple question may be the most often uttered phrase in a medical facility. As the primary tool in the health care provider's repertoire, access to the patient record is an absolute necessity when assessing patient status, planning, or delivering treatment. The chart is required by every member of the team, often by several members at once. It contains records from a variety of sources, in forms of every shape, size, and format. It provides critical information on an individual and data for assessing patterns of care in a population. In its traditional paper form its integrity can be challenged by loose or missing documents or poor handwriting; delays in access can leave details less fresh in the mind of the individual entering a report. Enter computerization, long accepted as essential to transactions of business, law, and everyday communication; computerization is integral to the operation of much of modern health care's equipment. However, it is only recently that headway is being made into the world of medical record keeping. What challenges must be addressed that have made this seemingly obvious development so slowly accepted?

The **medical records** consolidate, organize, and document an individual's health care experience. These data take the form of a sequentially recorded narrative describing the patient's medical history, medications, any test findings, treatment plans, and communication between the provider and outside consultants and between the provider and the patient. The term *medical records* reflects the plural nature of these critical documents because they are independently created and maintained by each practice or institution providing care to the individual.

Well-documented medical records demonstrate clear reasoning for a course of treatment and show attention to patient response. Caregivers follow professional guidelines to ensure that medical record keeping maintains high standards of quality and accuracy. Clinical workflow within a practice or institution steers medical record maintenance toward a standardized format. This supports the caregiver's ability to locate and read pertinent information. Entries must be made as soon after a patient encounter as possible to ensure accuracy and completion. Errors or poor documentation are potential sources of harm; therefore each caregiver is responsible for the character of the record. When corrections are required, they must be dated, initialed, and entered legibly, without masking the original error.[11]

WHY ELECTRONIC?

Traditionally, the patient record was safe in the hands of the family physician, possibly the caregiver from birth to death. Modern health care enables many caregivers to follow a patient, each having a specific focus and thus a unique perspective of the patient's overall condition (Fig. 24-1). Optimal patient care requires up to date communication of examinations and findings between multiple caregivers.

Despite the increasing complexity and goals of interconnected health care delivery, medical records continue to be primarily created and stored independent of one another by each practice or institution providing care to the individual. As a better alternative, computer software can provide shared access to all charted information. Data from electronic medical records (EMRs) are more easily accessed and sorted. Reports can be generated for individual patients, providing a comprehensive and more accurately interpreted view of their overall condition.

Converting to an **electronic medical record (EMR)** is a monumental goal. As diagnosis and treatment options become more complex, as the population becomes more mobile and assertive in its pursuit of idealized care, and as specialized care becomes more accessible, continuity and access to comprehensive "birth to death" paper records become less and less attainable. Although modern medical practice embraces the contribution of computer technology to diagnosis and treatment, applying this same technology to the medical record presents a unique set of legal, technical, and psychologic challenges. Although advantages are easily identified, conversion and acceptance requires current technology to ensure security; manage content; and provide comprehensive, accurate access to information. Legal standards governing the use of medical records have evolved over the history of medical care. Conversion to an EMR requires that it meet existing expectations while delivering on the promise

to improve health care. Data must be accessible yet protected from loss and unauthorized access to make providers and patients confident that no current benefits will be lost during the conversion.

The accessibility of electronic records aids caregivers; however, it poses risks to patient privacy and safety. Security issues must be addressed by the sources of this information, namely, those who provide the care. The data must be secure from unauthorized access and from those who might modify or destroy it. The patient must have confidence that both the security and integrity of this data is not compromised.

Public Health

In addition to the advantages to individuals, the emergence of the computerized patient record provides the framework to compile and analyze data from large populations to aid the epidemiologist's goals for improving overall public health. The National Cancer Policy Board has reported that **computer-based patient record (CPR)** systems form the backbone of improving cancer care outcomes. CPR systems provide patient data when and where it is needed, regardless of the source. They provide access to clinical and administrative data; support physician ordering and data entry; support and coordinate clinical communication between multiple organizations; and are capable of providing clinical decision support including clinical guidelines, drug interactions, and alerts for abnormal test results.[8] Population-based data reporting is much more readily accomplished with computerized systems than through retrospective medical chart review.

The history of public health is the history of how people have tried to understand the causes of disease and what can be done to reduce disease and improve health. The Department of Health and Human Services (HHS) is the principal agency that the United States federal government uses to protect the health of all Americans and provide essential human services, especially for those who are least able to help themselves. Three of the most readily recognizable public health service organizations include the following:

National Institutes of Health (NIH)—the NIH is the world's premier medical research organization, supporting some 35,000 research projects nationwide involving diseases like cancer, Alzheimer's, diabetes, arthritis, heart ailments, and acquired immunodeficiency syndrome (AIDS).

Food and Drug Administration (FDA)—the FDA ensures the safety of foods and cosmetics and the safety and efficacy of pharmaceuticals, biologic products, and medical devices (products that represent 25 cents out of every dollar in U.S. consumer spending).

Centers for Disease Control and Prevention (CDC)—working with states and other partners, the CDC provides a system of health surveillance to monitor and prevent disease outbreaks (including bioterrorism), implement disease-prevention strategies, and maintain national health statistics.[9]

Only a limited amount of funding can be applied to address health issues. When trends can be established, deci-

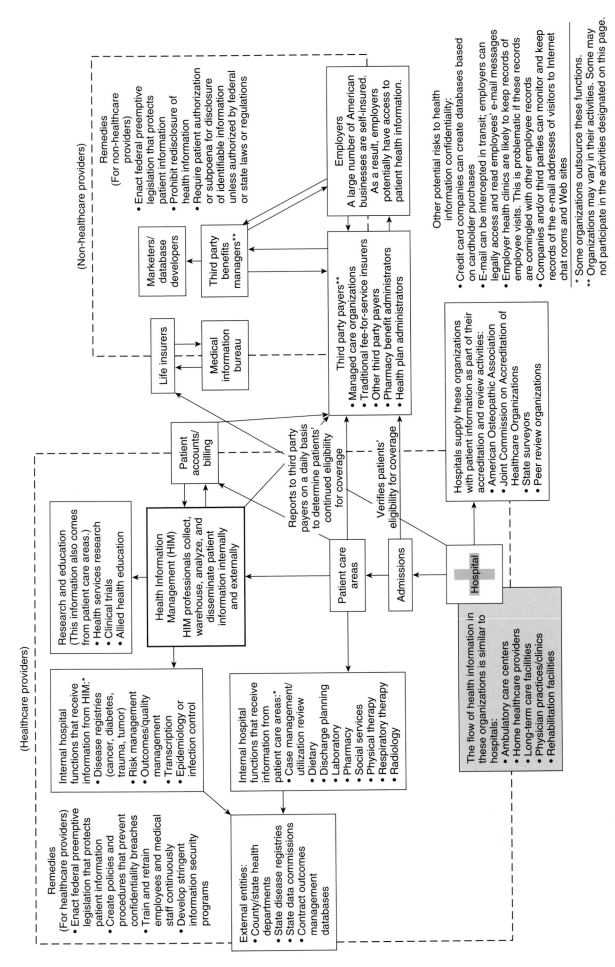

Figure 24-1. Flow of patient health information inside and outside the health care industry from the AHIMA situation analysis and position statement "Confidentiality of Medical Records." (Reprinted with permission from *J Am Health Inf Manage Assoc, Copyright 2002 by the American Health Information Management Association. All rights reserved. No part of this figure may be reproduced, reprinted, stored in a retrieval system, or transmitted, in any form or by any means, electronic photocopying, recording, or otherwise, without prior written permission of the association.*)

sions can be made regarding the allocation of that funding. These trends are determined as each patient's medical history and treatment is measured and patterns of care and outcomes are evaluated among the general population. This information must be gathered not only within a single department but also across all similar treatment centers to see trends that currently exist and paths to quality improvement. Designed to ensure quality care for the patient whose history and treatment is described, the medical record is also a source of data for measuring and evaluating patterns of care and outcomes among the general population. This data gathering is termed **abstracting.** In oncology centers this is done on an ongoing basis with a cancer registry system.

Cancer Registry

A cancer registry is an information system designed for the collection, management, and analysis of data on persons with the diagnosis of a malignant or neoplastic disease (cancer).[4] Federal law requires that diagnosis and treatment information be collected and maintained for the lifetime of any cancer patient. Lifetime follow-up is an important aspect of the cancer registry. In addition to providing accurate survival information, patient follow-up serves as a reminder to physicians and patients to schedule regular clinical examinations. Cancer registries are valuable research tools for those interested in the etiology, diagnosis, and treatment of cancer. Fundamental research of cancer epidemiology is initiated using the accumulated data. Multiple agencies use collected data to make public health decisions aimed at maximizing the effectiveness of limited public health funds, such as the placement of screening programs. An electronic repository of this information allows for a more efficient method of evaluating the data.

> Cancer registries can be classified into three general types:
> *Health care institution registry:* also known as hospital-based. These registries focus on all patients that are diagnosed and/or treated for cancer within a specific cancer center. These do not distinguish where the patient is from, the institution must follow everyone who passes through its doors. This tracking is required by law to be passed up to a state or central registry.
> *Central registries:* These are the compilations of all the health care institution registries that are then broken down by specific geographical areas. The generated data shows larger scale trends than the individual cancer center.
> *Special purpose registries:* A registry to maintain data regarding a particular type of cancer, such as brain tumors, can be established if initial data at either the institutional or central level points toward potential trends.

Standards of Care

Practitioners commonly base clinical decision making on their knowledge and experience, patient preference, and clinical circumstances. Evidence-based decision making combines this information with scientific evidence. This combination is the optimal method for defining the clinical care of individual patients.[3]

Standards of care derive from compiling the customs and behavior of the members of the profession. These are then developed into documents that reflect a consensus of how the profession is to be practiced. These documents define the acceptable scale for judging individual transgressions. This standard cannot be fixed but must adapt to incorporate newly determined therapies. Difficulties with compiling this information include data retrieval, record legibility, and lack of a standard vocabulary. Data retrieval is hampered by the physical characteristics of a paper chart. Because it is very portable, the physical chart it is often difficult to find. It may be in a physician's hands, at the treatment machine, in storage, or simply misplaced. In addition, it can only be accessed by one individual at a time. At times, a problem as basic as the legibility of a record makes it difficult to retrieve accurate information. One of the greatest obstacles to merging information is the lack of a commonly accepted vocabulary. Variances can be found not only between sites but even within an organization. This makes it difficult to merge information and compare records. Yet this merging is critical to decrease variances in practice patterns and improve outcomes across geographic and practice boundaries.

THE RADIATION ONCOLOGY MEDICAL RECORD

A patient's medical history does not begin with his or her radiation treatment. More often, patients present to the radiation oncology facility through a primary care physician or some emergency care route. As such, their primary medical record resides elsewhere. Even within a radiation oncology department, the patient's chart is used by many clinical and administrative staff members. These may include physicians, radiation therapists, physicists, medical dosimetrists, nurses, tumor registrars, and administrative staff. Each team member gathers patient information critical to her or his role so that she or he can provide efficient and effective patient care. The compilation of each team member's contribution to part of the treatment information comprises an independent radiation oncology record documenting the rationale, plan, delivery, and follow-up care given the patient in this specialty clinic (Fig. 24-2). Accessibility of the EMR to all members of the care team when and where they need it is one of its primary benefits. Design must be inclusive of the varied charting needs of each phase of and each professional contributing to care.

Consultation and Assessment

In the radiation oncology department, the radiation oncologist completes a summary of the initial patient examination. Physical findings include all signs, symptoms, and patient history information pertinent to the cancer diagnosis. Comorbidities that might affect tolerance to any proposed cancer treatment must be included in the record and in the subsequent recommendation for treatment. Dimensions of all palpable masses and size and number of nodes are recorded and diagrams made indicating the extent of disease and the

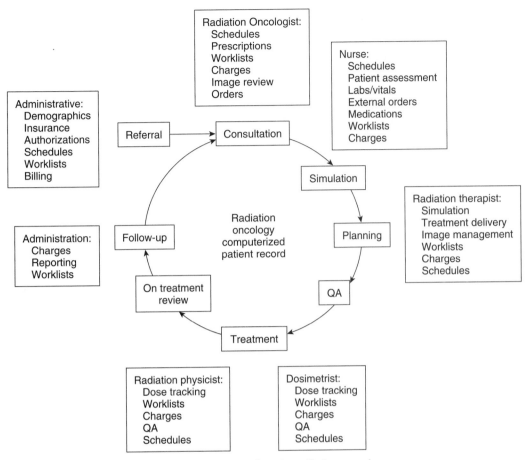

Figure 24-2. Patient flow in radiation oncology.

radiation oncologist's assessment of the patient's disease stage.

The medical record concentrates on the subjective and objective reports and findings regarding the patient under care. Initial presentation and plan for assessment and treatment is described in the **history and physical (H&P).** Expected content and a standard format for the H&P may be referred to as a **SOAP note: S**ubjective findings as reported by the patient; **O**bjective or observations of the clinician, including vital signs and physical examination; **A**ssessment of the disease or condition; and **P**lan for further examination and/or treatment.

Through conversation with the patient, a clinician records a **history of the present illness.** The **chief complaint** or reason for the visit is recorded. The **review of systems** includes the patient's description of the signs and symptoms leading to his or her presenting to the doctor, including their subjective report of overall feelings of wellness.

The physical examination adds objective observations to the medical record. Patient weight and **vital signs** including blood pressure, pulse, and respiration may be gathered along with a chief complaint at the patient's initial encounter with a nurse or other clinical specialist. The physical examination

will generally be completed and documented by the radiation oncologist, and physician extenders such as the physician assistant (PA) may be responsible in some institutions.

During the initial encounter, the patient provides a past medical history including any illnesses, injuries, surgeries, or allergies. Current medications and dose schedules are documented. Social history factors that may affect overall health expectations and concerns are discussed and recorded as they relate to the illness under care. Activities including alcohol consumption, addictions, or exposure to hazardous materials through work or home may be included in the record. Even cultural patterns such as types of food consumed or participation in traditional activities may affect overall health. Family history of major illnesses or conditions are reviewed and assessed against risk factors for the patient.

Augmenting physical examination, the patient status is further assessed, followed by a plan for treatment. Tests may be ordered to confirm diagnosis, evaluate extent of illness, or response to treatment. Clinical observations include the results of laboratory and imaging examinations. Results are reported to the ordering physician and included in the patient's record. Pathologic assessment of disease is accomplished through surgical methods and is recorded through surgical and pathology reports. Paper methods of incorporating external information limit their accessibility to the single record and are a source of potential error as information is manually transcribed from one record to another.

Additional assessments are undertaken based on the decision to treat the patient in the radiation oncology department. Specialists, including nutritionists and social workers, may conduct and document baseline interviews at the initiation of treatment, often continuing with supportive assessment and interventions throughout the course of treatment. Conclusions, interventions, and patient response to treatment are included in the medical record. Consistency of assessment is managed through developing forms that are the result of published research or may be designed by the institution or individual professional. Materials and methods used for patient self-care education must also be identified.

Dietitians assess the oncology patient's unique nutritional demands. These may stem from treatment side effects or the disease process itself. Nutrition status must be determined at the start of treatment and monitored throughout treatment. The patient's record will indicate nutritional guidelines the patient received to mitigate side effects of their treatment. Social or familial relationships affecting the patient's ability to follow direction must be documented.

Assessment continues throughout the course of treatment. Oncology patients are closely observed for physical and emotional responses. Many factors that affect a patient's well-being are included in the medical record, along with the prescribed treatment delivery. Biologic, social, and psychologic factors play a role in the patient's response to treatment and to overall quality of life. The observations and treatment guidance of several support clinicians are included in the medical record.

Pain assessment is among the most subjective quality factors to be measured and is one that changes over time. Several standardized methods for measuring pain have been developed and are in use. Physical responses to treatment, including acute reactions and interventions must be included in the record. Laboratory studies may be ordered routinely or in response to symptoms.

The radiation therapist uses the patient record to implement physician orders and to monitor and reinforce the directions of other members of the care team. Because of daily patient contact, the radiation therapist is a key contributor to daily patient assessment and carries the responsibility of ensuring that the radiation oncologist is consulted as needed. Behavioral changes of either organic or social origin may affect care and are often most readily noted by the radiation therapist. With continuous access to the EMR, the radiation therapist is able to better use it capabilities to better document and communicate with the other members of the care team.

As treatment proceeds, the medical record documents patient response. Medications, procedures, and lifestyle changes are ordered and tracked. Physical and clinical examinations are repeated and results monitored. Summary data may be collated or graphed to aid interpretation of repeated tests.

Communications, both verbal and written, between referring physicians regarding progress are included in the record. Narrative observations dictated by the physician may be transcribed into written documentation in the form of reports or letters to outside physicians or to the patients themselves. Ultimately, the EMR must provide flexible options for entering patient information.

Treatment Plan and Record

Treatment intent, whether curative or palliative, is identified before treatment planning. The proposed treatment is explained to the patient with expected results including acute and long-term reactions to irradiation of the planned area. Written consent is obtained from the patient and secured in the chart before initiating planning or treatment procedures.

The radiation oncologist determines and documents the target volume for treatment planning and the radiation prescription. Target volumes include area of known and presumed tumor with a margin included for setup variation. Radiation prescriptions include total dose to be received, the size, and pattern of fractionation. Doses to critical structures in or near the target volume must be identified and limited. Radiation therapists, dosimetrists, and physicists use these orders to generate treatment plans. Treatment plans must be approved by the radiation oncologist before treatment delivery.

The radiation treatment record presents the parameters required for the accurate reproduction of the plan and the historical record of treatment delivered. Refer to Chapter 8 for details about the treatment record.

On Treatment Review

Radiation patients meet with their oncologist during their course of treatment. This commonly takes place a minimum of once weekly throughout the course of therapy, although some treatment regimens or patients encountering problems may require more frequent monitoring. Acute response to treatment is observed and documented in the chart. Clinical tests including blood counts are routinely performed and results collected in the radiation oncology record. The oncologist records the cumulative dose along with any treatment reactions experienced by the patient. Treatment verification image record review is documented (refer to Chapter 8). Clinical decisions based on observations are documented in the medical record and include proceeding with or modifying the planned course of therapy. Modifications may range from treatment breaks to allow abatement of side effects to redefining the prescription or the entire treatment plan.

Completion and Follow-up

On completion of treatment, the patient is seen and a completion note is generated by the radiation oncologist. Completion notes summarize the treatment delivery and should be consistent with the initial plan. Any deviations from the plan must be clearly explained and supported by the treatment and completion notes. Records should also summarize any problems encountered. A follow-up plan is arranged with the patient.

Early follow-up records describe remaining and resolving acute treatment reactions and treatments administered for those reactions. Extended follow-up continues indefinitely on an annual basis to monitor late reactions and provide early intervention for negative outcomes. Imaging and laboratory tests may continue to be ordered and the results included in the patient's radiation record as needed.

In-patient Records

In addition to the medical record of the radiation department, in-patients and some residents of long-term health care facilities require an additional medical record requiring notation. The radiation therapists may document completion of daily treatment visits, and the radiation oncologist will provide weekly treatment notes. If the radiation oncologist is the admitting physician, documentation responsibilities extend to providing the admission and discharge records. Those admitted for brachytherapy procedures also require submission of operative notes.

THE PATIENT RECORD

Detailed patient identification information is a necessary component of the patient record and may be considered an adjacent record to the clinical record. Patient identifiers, or demographics, uniquely associate the medical record to an individual and facilitates both clinical and nonclinical activities. For example, birth date may be an identifier relative to other patients with the same name, and it may also be useful to provide reminder notifications of screening test recommendations. Multiple physician contacts must be included in the patient record to ensure that communication is maintained with all associated with a patient's care. In addition, this information is valuable to the practice as a tool for monitoring referral patterns for the physician or practice.

Personal information such as race or religion may affect individual care or provide important information in the public health domain. Primary language or other factors affecting communication may be noted. Emergency contacts are included to ensure multiple routes of communication and provide decision makers with a contact in the event a patient is not capable of communicating for herself or himself. Billing information including insurance or Medicare coverage also has a place in the complete patient record.

COMPUTERIZATION OF PATIENT RECORDS

Medical Informatics—Electronic Medical Records

Until recently, medical records have depended on paper and written documentation. Accessible to one caregiver at a time, charts bind collections of reports from diverse sources. Handwritten, clinical notations are entered in a diary-like chronologic order. Transcribed reports from internal and external sources are sorted and included in more or less chronologic order. Copies of any outbound documents are maintained. An individual's medical history is dispersed among several records, with unique independent records generated by each health care group visited. These characteristics present challenges to individual patient care and to analysis of patterns of care and outcomes across the population. For example, a series of test results in a single chart may require manual transcription of values to a graph to visualize rates of change over time or, as in abstracting for cancer registry, details from many, many charts are required to accurately describe patterns of presentation, treatment, and outcomes.

A wide range of computing needs from word processing to the complex algorithms used to calculate treatment plans or manage images are required to produce and maintain the radiation oncology EMR. Biomedical computing brings together computing, biology, and medicine, supporting activities such as image analysis and treatment planning. Medical informatics encompasses these elements in an evolving discipline involving the storage, retrieval, and optimal use of biomedical data, information, and knowledge for problem solving and decision-making.[2] Medical information in radiation oncology is generated on a variety of platforms and through a wide range of applications (Fig. 24-3). File format and system interfacing standards are necessary to merge information from diverse sources into a specialized patient record. In addition, medical specialties have evolved unique charting requirements; thus one tool will not be universally applicable. Computerizing the medical record may also extend its scope by making decision support tools accessible. As the knowledge base for cancer management grows, accessibility to information becomes increasingly critical to the decision-making process of defining an individual course of treatment. Links to research groups and literature sources provide access to empirical evidence published in an increasing range of journals and other forums. As recommendations are applied to an individual treatment plan, specific risks and response norms may be flagged for attention should the patient's response be inconsistent with expectations.

Medical information systems (MIS) provide database support for clinical and administrative activities. Well-designed electronic record systems facilitate process; in addition to maintaining patient records, care standards or protocols can be defined with flags to alert caregivers of required activities, ensuring that department expectations are met. Operational efficiency is further conducive of a safe and pleasant treatment environment for patients.

Data Entry

Computing with words is inspired by the remarkable human capability to perform a wide variety of physical and mental tasks without any measurements and any computations.[17] Medical records serve a number of purposes, yet are

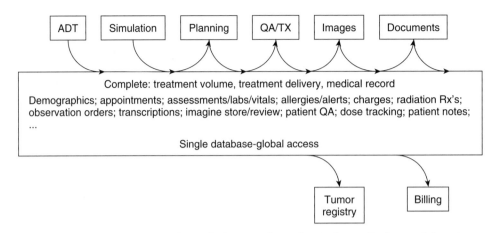

Figure 24-3. Data sources for radiation oncology electronic medical record (EMR).

primarily without computational requirements. They provide a forum for supporting treatment, create legal documents, and justify third party reimbursement. An electronic chart can guide documentation to meet external standards, expedite data entry, and create a readily queried record. Many forms are required to document each type of patient contact and may vary greatly from one facility to another. Flexibility in EMR configuration is highly desirable to meet these complex needs. Given that the EMR can play such a wide range of roles it is not surprising that some data items require a specific value, whereas others are open to free interpretation. Data can be entered in a number of ways. These include, but are not limited to, free text, drop lists, single entry, radio button selections, check boxes, and templates.

Items that can be entered in without any restriction are titled free text. One example of this is the SOAP notes that were described earlier in this chapter. The benefit of free text is that users are very comfortable with expressing their ideas without feeling forced to change either their thought process or wording. The limitation is the time required for entry and the wide range of words that can be used to describe the same clinical situation. If data is to be extracted, this variety will make it more difficult to determine trends across patients. A common example of this is as simple as the term used to describe a course of radiation therapy delivered to a patient in his or her past medical treatment.

Prior therapy

Past Rx therapy

Past RxTx

It is difficult for an abstractor or a computer program to recognize that each of these items describes the same concept. In addition, if data is to be culled out, it cannot be done without searching for each distinct item. Multiple searches are then required so that all relevant words and phrases are understood by the system. Textual reports of patient encounters are a vast source of on-line clinical information, but information in textual form is not useful for automated clinical applications, and, although electronically available, the information remains locked up within the text. Text is difficult to access because it is extremely diverse and the meanings of words vary depending on the context. Many on-line patient records are recorded in natural-language text. To be fully retrievable, however, clinical information must be structured or coded.[7]

A question having a distinct list of answers may be addressed with a selection list. The list may be in the form of radio buttons, check boxes, and drop down or full window selection menus. A user may select any item on the list but often cannot independently create items to add to the list. Lists may be published by national or international standards organizations or customized based on internal practices. An example of a standard list is the International Classification of Diseases, Clinical Modification (ICD-9-CM). These values are an agreed-on classification list that can be used to document diagnosis information. This item easily fits into an EMR because it is a standard that is used throughout the world. Shorter lists may be managed with drop down menus. Selection lists improve consistency in data entry and support reporting on cumulative data.

A compromise between complete structure and free text are templated notes (Fig. 24-4). Templated notes use selection lists to display codified phrases and generate narratives. Templates may be created for specific assessments used for a given disease, a given clinical center, or a given provider. They provide structure for the provider to ensure that all minimum assessments are done but also allow the provider to introduce his or her unique language into the charting.

Interoperability (Connectivity) and Communication Standards

The EMR manages both textual and image data. Data must be merged from a variety of providers and sources to create a comprehensive history of a particular course of care. A multitude of software applications and systems platforms exist to provide support for the many specialized activities of health care. At the same time, much of the resulting documentation must be shared with other caregivers. The demand for sharing data is the result of the desire to improve care through shared knowledge and increasing efficiency. Informed decision making is best

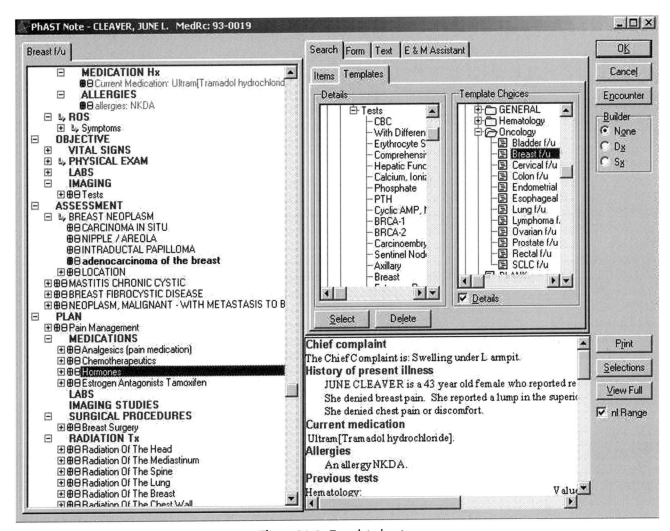

Figure 24-4. Templated note.

supported by presenting all the information available regarding a patient's problem into one database accessible to all clinicians when and where they need it. With the abundant methods of generating and storing this information, the ability to pass it electronically from one system into another grows.

Proprietary communication protocols are developed and owned by commercial entities. These are developed to meet customer needs and may become or provide a basis for industry standards. In the absence of national or international standards, proprietary protocols and interfaces can provide much needed tools for sharing information across diverse data sources. Duplication of effort occurs as various organizations produce their own solutions for common problems, a process that is wasteful in time and resources and does little to solve the overriding intercommunication problem of universal access. Standardization is sought by national and international organizations such as the **American National Standards Institute (ANSI)** or the **International Standards Organization (ISO).** These organizations accredit various specialty organizations that produce standards for industry specific requirements.

Standards organizations or committees include wide representation from the industry for which interoperability standards are being designed. As such, agreement can be a long process and results will have latitude. Standards are published in the public domain and commercial providers use them to create multisystem interface formats. Latitude exists, however, in the interpretation of standards and in what constitutes compliance. Vendor solutions generally are accompanied by compliance statements, which describe, in detail, how their system adheres to the published standard.

Two standards routinely applied in radiation therapy are Health Level 7 **(HL7)** and Digital Imaging and Communications in Medicine **(DICOM).** These standards have been further validated by the recommendation of the National Commission on Vital and Health Statistics as uniform data standards for patient medical record information (PMRI).[10]

HL7

HL7 is an ANSI accredited organization developing standards for exchanging clinical and administrative data. Specifically, HL7 defines standards for "the exchange, management and integration of data that supports clinical patient care and the management, delivery and evaluation of healthcare services."[1]

HL7 interfaces allow sharing of information available used across the entire health care facility such as admission, discharge, and transfer (ADT) data including demographics; financial information for billing; scheduling information; clinical documents such as transcriptions, orders, laboratory results, and medications; and other data. By employing HL7 interfaces, clinical and administrative information may be entered only once yet employed in any specialty department's record. This avoids wasted time and reduces error produced by multiple entries of data. Updates and corrections may be propagated through the same interface, allowing a single point of entry to disseminate corrections throughout the organization.

The Clinical Context Object Workgroup (CCOW) is another HL7 standard promoted to increase efficiency. CCOW intends to automate multiple application log-ins and synchronizes patient record selection through a single point.[1] Users of multiple applications that compliment the work process, but for which an exchange of information is inappropriate, are assisted when working on a single patient's records even though the information is managed by multiple databases.

DICOM

DICOM standards are produced by a joint committee of the National Electrical Manufacturers Association (NEMA) and the American College of Radiology (ACR) and that is affiliated with several international agencies.[5] This committee was formed to provide communication standards for sharing image information regardless of manufacturer and has included radiation therapy treatment information. This facilitates the use of picture archival and communications systems (PACS) and allows the wide distribution of diagnostic images. DICOM3 refers to the third part of the base standards and describes each type of information that is included. These information types are called information object definitions (IODs). IODs may describe image or textual information. Several IODs expressly describe radiation therapy information:

- Radiation therapy (RT) image: conventional and virtual simulation images, digitally reconstructed radiographs (DRRs) or portal images
- RT dose: dose distributions, isodose lines, dose-volume histograms (DVHs)
- RT structure set: contours drawn on images, that is, computed tomography (CT)
- RT plan: text information describing treatment plans including prescriptions and fractionation, beam definitions, and so forth
- RT beams and RT brachy: treatment session reports for external beam or brachytherapy, may be used as part of a verification and record system (V&R)
- RT treatment summary: cumulative summary information, may be used after treatment to send information to a hospital EMR[6]

DICOM IODs enable radiation therapy manufacturers to concentrate on a single internationally accepted format for interoperability between their system and others in the industry. Compliance statements should be available to describe the manufacturer's conformity with the published standard.

SECURITY AND PRIVACY

Although the ability to transfer large amounts of electronic data from one system to another holds great promise for streamlining health care and supporting clinical decision making, this same flow of information has the power to harm individuals. Transferred data must be accurately assigned to patients and data access and entry restricted to qualified individuals. Passwords are currently the most common method of restricting access to an EMR. In the future, security may include biometric technology such as fingerprint or retinal scanning.

Computerizing patient records has the potential to make private information accessible, which could be used to make unfair employment, insurance coverage, or other decisions. To facilitate the proper exchange of information while restricting access to necessary personnel, Congress passed the Health Insurance Portability and Accountability Act of 1996 **(HIPAA)**. HIPAA guidelines and regulations require security precautions to not only restrict access but to keep records of who is accessing information. To this end, regulations are being developed under the provisions of this act to standardize information sets for health care reimbursement and to restrict access to the minimum needed to provide care.[15,16] By providing standards for communicating information necessary to achieve health care reimbursement, providers are assisted in the complex process of obtaining payment for their services without endangering their patient's right to privacy.[16] In general, access to information that is identifiable to an individual is restricted except to those caregivers to whom the patient has given consent. Full disclosure is extended when the purpose of disclosure is to provide treatment decision making. Certain exceptions are included in the regulations for public health needs, certain law enforcement activities, general oversight of care (i.e., quality assurance procedures), and some research activities.[12,15]

INFORMATION SYSTEMS

The technical infrastructure that supports an EMR requires significant expertise to create and maintain. Medical or hospital **information systems** (MIS or HIS) departments may employ several specialists in areas ranging from hardware to network to application support for managing the array of requirements from running the system to ensuring that it is employed efficiently by clinicians and staff. Patient records are managed using "mission critical" software supporting the provision of quality care. Patient care and safety and legal requirements necessitate that access be secure, stable, and dependable. File servers must have backup systems in place for database protection. Backup systems might include servers with multiple hard drives recording duplicate information should one fail. Tape backups record copies of files on a regular basis, usually daily. File restoration must be periodically tested, and full backup tapes should be rotated to off-site storage so potential catastrophe, fire, flood, and so forth will not result in permanent loss of entire patient records. The complexity and criticality of these functions typically requires special expertise in information systems (IS) to provide adequate support. Larger systems in hospitals or large medical groups may necessitate developing a team to maintain systems.

Computer Network

The most common platform for the EMR is the client/server configuration. The database and program executables reside on a central computer, the **file server,** and are accessed from distributed terminals or computers, known as clients. Such systems run on networks. A **network** is a system of independent, interconnected computers or terminals communicating with one another over a shared medium, consisting of hardware and communication protocols. The most common

network protocol is the Ethernet protocol. Ethernets require special hardware, including cards within the computers and particular cables. Ethernets also use specific communication protocols to transfer information (Fig. 24-5).

A local area network **(LAN)** is geographically confined to an area in which a common communication service may be used. For larger geographic areas or when multiple LANs are to be connected, a wide area network **(WAN)** may be employed. WANs use a variety of communication services currently including telephone dial-up, T-1 or T-3 lines, or even the Internet to communicate over long or short distances.

Wireless options are currently being introduced, which promise to make computers more mobile within a facility and critical information even more accessible to approved caregivers when and where they need it. Alternatively, web-based EMRs use the Internet to gain controlled access to servers maintained by application service providers **(ASP).** Applications and data are stored off-site and maintained by the vendor. Users access servers through secure and private Internet connections, reducing information system maintenance and making charts accessible wherever an Internet connection exists.

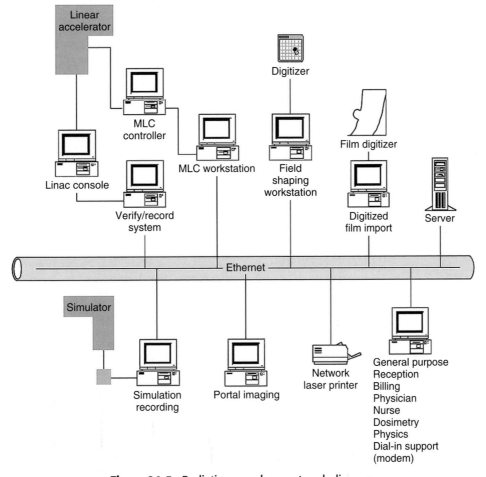

Figure 24-5. Radiation oncology network diagram.

PROCESS CONSIDERATIONS

Clinical and business decision making in the clinic depends on accessible and accurate data to produce good outcomes at reasonable costs. The analysis process generates a thorough understanding of existing processes along with performance measurements that can be referenced when measuring response to the improvement plan. Problems are defined; goals and plans for achieving those goals are formulated. Organizations may benefit from including both internal and external resources when examining workflow and identifying information needs. Internal expertise provides intimate understanding of clinic needs and dynamics, and objectivity and specialized analysis skills are gained by contracting external assistance. Systems analysts are members of the IS team and may be included in the selection and implementation process of introducing an EMR. The systems analyst is generally an external resource skilled at evaluating patterns of information use and providing objective insight. The systems analyst coordinates resources and often remains with the organization throughout the entire change process to manage purchases, installations, and workspace layouts; to produce new policies and procedures; and to measure results.[13] The EMR itself is only a tool to facilitate the process of patient care, without a detailed understanding of this process the transition will be fraught with obstacles and challenges.[14] Systems analysts perform the complex task of analyzing activities in an organization to precisely determine what must be accomplished and how it must be accomplished.

Electronic charts require more than purchasing and installing a computer program. In addition to the initial purchase, staff training and software support must be considered. There are many programs available, which perform different activities within a given department. Some program types that are commonly used in a radiation therapy department are V&R systems, radiation treatment planning systems (RTP), image management systems, scheduling systems, and billing systems. Before deciding which software package to purchase, the specific needs of the department must be analyzed to make the best decision. A radiation therapist is especially interested in a V&R system that is accurate, easy to use, and fast. A physicist is interested in a program that integrates treatment planning and imaging data. Radiation oncologists want an overall picture that does not require more than one screen to view (Fig. 24-6). The same information may be required in different forms by different members of the organization, for example, the physician or nurse may review a summary of treatment dose delivered while the therapist or physicist may have more frequent need to view the details of the treatment plan (Fig. 24-7). Finding the software package or packages that will best facilitate each team member's performance of his or her role is the goal of this

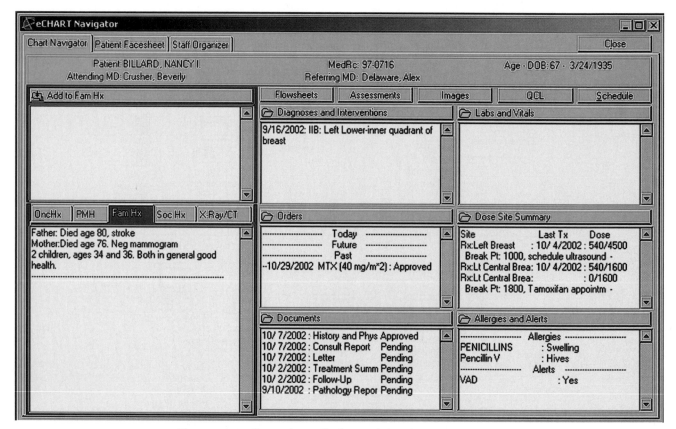

Figure 24-6. Electronic medical record (EMR) summary view.

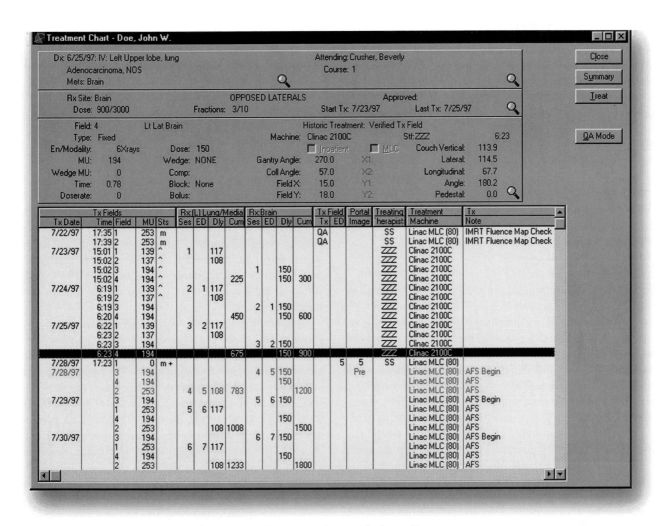

Figure 24-7. Treatment chart with dose site summary.

very important evaluation phase. Multiple software programs may be required to achieve this end.

Implementation

Once a purchase is made, the software must be configured or modified to meet the specific needs of the facility. Many people can perform this modification, including the software provider, a clinical staff member, or a systems analyst. Configuration items may include identifying staff resources and assigning security rights, describing and characterizing equipment, and building custom lists or forms for data entry. Although some configuration is completed at the time of system implementation, it must typically continue to happen as the department evolves. This may include changes as simple as adding or deleting staff members or as complex as incorporating a whole new method of treatment delivery. If multiple programs have been selected, configuration may include interfacing systems to exchange information. These interfaces are vitally important. A single point of entry ensures updates across the board and eliminates redundant data entry, a major benefit of using an EMR.

Educating the staff is the next step after configuration. This is arguably the most important step. No matter how complete the documentation of a software package is, if it is not used the benefits will be lost. Staff development is typically included with the purchase of complex systems and may be delivered through a variety of methods. Manuals can pass along a preset catalog of information but do not answer each person's individual questions and are not always accessible. Help menus often explain specific information about software functionality but are not always sensitive to the nuances of the information sought by the user. Lecture and discussion allows for the give and take of questions but requires dedicated time to effectively absorb the information. A hands-on approach does not always provide the time needed to process given information and is limited by what each user experiences. Initially, direct instruction, including lecture and hands-on experience with a knowledgeable instructor, is an effective way to support a practitioner's first use of the clinical database. Follow-up may be supported by written materials such as manuals or computerized help menus.

With time, the most common method becomes "I've seen." I've seen is similar to the child's game of "whisper down the lane." One person may learn from a primary source. He or she then shares this information with a co-worker. This co-worker shares it with the next and so on. Although this method is positive, in that the information and processes are shared, the degeneration or telescoping of the information over time must be considered. Optimal learning occurs through combining all of these methods of learning. It must be remembered that ongoing education is needed to optimally use an electronic system. Software updates and enhancements not withstanding, staff turnover and department changes such as treatment standards and staff will affect how any chart is used.

SUMMARY

Medical records consolidate, organize, and document an individual's health care experience. Whereas computers are not new to diagnosis and treatment in health care, use of computerized databases for medical record keeping is only in the early stages of acceptance. Computer software has the potential of better collecting and organizing data for the benefit of the individual, assessing standards of care, and assessing outcomes in a population. EMRs can provide simultaneous access to charted information to multiple caregivers, ensuring that information is available when and where it is needed. By providing links to research data and other decision-making tools, the electronic environment is ideal for ensuring individual patient care plans are made with as much current information possible.

Patients in the radiation oncology department are cared for by a team of professionals, each with unique contributions and expectations of the medical record. Electronic records must be capable of collecting data and describing all phases of the care process, from consultation to follow-up care. The radiation oncology department has a unique range of specialized clinical data sources. In addition to laboratory and other diagnostic reports, treatment planning, verification, and recording of treatment and imaging information must be included in the EMR.

External sources of information and outbound communication requirements are addressed using multisystem interface formats. Such interfaces are produced to reduce redundant data entry and reduce errors. Many options exist for designing interface systems including custom interfaces and standard formats. Proprietary interfaces are designed and owned by commercial entities. Nonproprietary standards are designed by professional organizations (HL7, DICOM) and are part of the public domain; these public standards are highly desirable yet can be the hardest to integrate and make available for use.

With all its potential benefits, conversion to an EMR is not a simple decision or action. Software selection must balance privacy, security, and accessibility; although information must be available to authorized individuals, it must be pro-

tected from loss or unsanctioned viewing. Software operation is dependent on the system it is installed on. Most commonly installed on networked, client/server systems, they must be sufficiently robust to have minimal downtime. A radiation oncology department may depend on other departments to ensure network stability and apply disaster recovery programs to safeguard loss of data. The EMR should incorporate process flow and the unique charting needs for a given patient population and various caregivers. To be useful in the complex medical environment it must be flexible and configurable yet provide codified data that can be easily sorted and reported on. To achieve this, the facility engages in self-examination of its processes, sometimes in collaboration with a systems analyst. Software is customized to meet department protocols and terminology before implementation. Planning for the introduction of the EMR, including sufficient staff development, is vital to the success of the transition process.

Streamlining the flow of medical information between systems and among caregivers holds great promise for improving health care. Full access to the patient's medical history is invaluable to diagnosis and treatment of illnesses, and streamlining administrative processes provides more consistent reimbursement and better use of resources. Data from many patients can be more readily compiled, providing more accurate profiles of illness and response to treatment choices. Universal introduction and acceptance, however, is a complex undertaking that places new demands on computer systems management and security and clinical practice procedures. As technical limitations are addressed, the key to successful introduction of these systems will be practitioners' ability to successfully reengineer department processes, making them safer, more secure, and more efficient.

Review Questions

1. EMRs provide what benefits over paper-based records?
   I.   Easier to use
   II. One central record
   III. Facilitate retrospective data analysis
   a. I and II
   b. I and III
   c. II and III
   d. I, II, and III
2. EMRs expedite the process of extracting data from individual patient records for evaluation of patterns of care and outcomes. This is called
   a. Analysis
   b. Compiling
   c. Interfacing
   d. Abstracting

3. The key to a well-used EMR is
   I. Software that is easy to use, easy to access, and reliable
   II. Staff development at the time of installation
   III. Staff development on an ongoing basis
   a. I and II
   b. I and III
   c. II and III
   d. I, II, and III

4. Radiation Center XYZ backs up their data every night. Each week they should carefully put this backup tape
   a. In a shipment to an off-site storage location
   b. In the back of the director's desk
   c. In a fireproof box under the treatment machine
   d. Back in the machine that runs the backup

5. HIPAA regulations provide requirements for
   a. Computerization of patient records
   b. Tracking of all individuals accessing patient information
   c. Government regulation of treatment methods
   d. Password access to patient records

6. Nonproprietary data communication standards in medicine include
   I. HL7
   II. PACS
   III. DICOM
   a. I and II
   b. I and III
   c. II and III
   d. I, II, and III

7. Standardization of file formats between software systems is easy to do because
   a. It is as simple as copying and pasting data
   b. There are a limited number of software applications and network platforms
   c. Standards organizations or committees include representation from the industry for which interoperability standards are being designed
   d. Proprietary communication protocols are developed and owned by commercial entities

8. Data gathering and interpretation is not facilitated by the use of
   a. Templates
   b. Radio button selections
   c. Free text
   d. Drop lists

9. The statement "My throat is so sore I can't eat" is an example of a(n)
   a. Subjective finding
   b. Objective finding
   c. Assessment
   d. Plan

10. Standards of care
    a. Are a fixed compilation of the customs and behaviors of a professional group
    b. Are dynamic
    c. Are an assumed activity that any person would demonstrate in a given situation
    d. Are the result of improved treatment outcomes

REFERENCES

1. *About HL7,* Ann Arbor, Mich, available at www.HL7.org (accessed May 2002).
2. Adams, RD, Wright DL: Medical informatics, virtual reality and radiation therapy, *Radiat Ther* 10(1):73-76, Spring 2001.
3. Bender D, Cormack J: *Evidence-based decision making—a clinician's guide,* presentation June 18, 2001, available at www-hsc.usc.edu/~cormack/ (accessed April 2002).
4. Cancer Registry Field: *What is a cancer registry,* available at www.NCRA-USA.org (accessed April 2002).
5. *Digital Imaging and Communications in Medicine (DICOM) part 1 information objects definitions,* Rosslyn, Va, 2001, National Electrical Manufacturers Association, available at http://medical.nema.org (accessed May 2002).
6. *Digital Imaging and Communications in Medicine (DICOM) part 3 information objects definitions,* Rosslyn, Va, 2001, National Electrical Manufacturers Association, available at http://medical.nema.org (accessed May 2002).
7. Friedman C, Hripcsak G: Natural language processing and its future in medicine, *Acad Med* 74:890-895, 1999.
8. Hewitt M, Simone JV, editors: *Enhancing data systems to improve the quality of cancer care,* report of the National Cancer Policy Board, 2000.
9. HHS: *What we do,* US Department of Health and Human Services, available at www.hhs.gov (accessed May 2002).
10. Lumpkin J: Recommendation letter of National Committee on Vital and Health Statistics to Secretary of US Department of Health and Human Services, February 27, 2002, available at www.HL7.org (accessed May 2002).
11. Midwest Medical Insurance Company Risk Management Committee: Medical record documentation: is yours a help or a hindrance in a lawsuit? *RMS Bull J Ramsey Med Soc* 91(6), Nov/Dec 1997.
12. Norris TG: Quality assurance in radiation therapy, *Radiat Ther* 9(2):161-184, 2000.
13. Silver GA, Silver ML: *Computers and information processing,* 1993, HarperCollins.
14. Smith D, Mancini-Newell L: A physician's perspective: deploying the EMR, *J Health Care Inf Manage* 16(2), Spring 2002.
15. US Department of Health and Human Services: HHS fact sheet: protecting the privacy of patients health information: summary of the final regulation, Washington, DC, Dec 20, 2000.
16. US Department of Health and Human Services: HHS fact sheet: administrative simplification under HIPAA: national standards for transactions, security and privacy, Washington, DC, Jan 22, 2002.
17. Zadeh LA: From computing with numbers to computing with words. From manipulation of measurements to manipulation of perceptions, *Ann N Y Acad Sci* 929:221-252, 2001.

PRACTICAL

APPLICATIONS

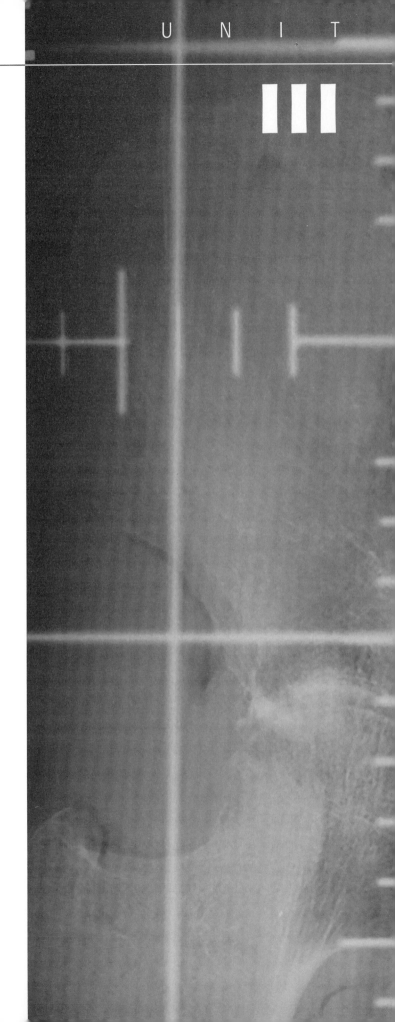

Bone, Cartilage, and Soft Tissue Sarcomas

Cheryl K. Sanders, Lisa Bartenhagen

Outline

Key Terms

CONNECTIVE TISSUE TUMORS

The skeletal system is comprised of bones or **osseous** and cartilaginous tissues; these tissues give the body its shape, form, and ability to move. Bones and cartilage possess the exceptional ability to support and protect softer tissues in the body. Bones also serve as a reservoir for fats, minerals, and other substances vital to blood cell production. The extraskeletal connective tissues include all those soft tissues that provide connection, support, and locomotion. Although bone tumors refer to malignancies involving the bone, they frequently may also include tumors of a collective group of tissues such as cartilage, joints, and blood vessels surrounding the bone. Bone marrow, responsible for blood cell production, is not spared from the attack of malignant cells. Soft tissue tumors are limited to those sarcomas arising in the extraskeletal structural connective tissues and are found throughout the human body.

BONE AND CARTILAGE TUMORS

The two types of bone tumors examined in this chapter are primary and metastatic. Malignant primary bone tumors do not constitute a major health hazard compared with other neoplastic disorders. In 2003 an estimated 2900 new cases of primary bone cancer were reported, with approximately 1400 deaths resulting from this disease.[3] In contrast, the number of metastatic bone cancers arising in various skeletal areas from other primary disease sites was far greater than the number of primary bone tumors.[2]

Primary bone tumors create a diagnostic challenge for pathologists, radiation and medical oncologists, radiologists, and orthopedic surgeons. This challenge occurs because these tumors have a vast array of presentations and biologic behaviors. This chapter presents the difficulty in diagnosing and treating these tumors. Also, because this disease often affects children, its devastating effect on the patient and family is clear.

The bone tumors covered in this chapter include osteogenic sarcoma (osteosarcoma), chondrosarcoma, fibrosarcoma, malignant histiocytoma, malignant giant cell tumors, multiple myeloma, and metastatic bone disease. Fibrosarcomas and malignant histiocytomas have been reclassified to be included in a group of tumors known as malignant fibrous histiocytoma (MFH). These tumors, along with Ewing's sarcoma, are unique among connective tissue cancers in that they affect both bone and soft tissue. For bone tumors discussed in this chapter, the former distinctions for fibrosarcomas and malignant histiocytomas (MFH) are addressed as separate histologic entities.[18]

Epidemiology

The incidence of bone cancer is highest during adolescence, with 3 instances per 100,000 people. Bone tumors account for 3.2% of malignancies in children younger than 15 years. The incidence falls to 0.2 per 100,000 for people between the ages of 30 and 35, then slowly rises until its rate for those age 60 equals that for adolescents.[52]

Multiple myeloma, a nonosseous malignant tumor arising in the marrow, should be considered a primary bone tumor. Included in this classification, multiple myeloma becomes extremely significant, accounting for approximately 35% to 43% of such tumors. Multiple myeloma is usually seen in middle-aged and older adults, peaking in the fifth and seventh decades. However, in this age bracket, multiple myeloma must be differentiated clinically and radiographically from metastatic carcinoma.[52]

Osteosarcoma, the most common osseous malignant bone tumor, is generally a tumor of adolescents and occasionally young adults, accounting for about 20% of all bone tumors. Dahlin reported that it made up 28% of such tumors in his series.[43] The next most common type of bone tumor (approximately 12% of the category) is known as chondrosarcoma (Table 25-1). Although they may be primary tumors, chondrosarcomas can also occur as secondary malignancies developing in preexisting benign lesions.[52]

Fibrosarcoma (a rare form of bone malignancy that also occurs in soft tissue), now included in MFH classifications, accounts for less than 4% of primary malignant bone tumors. In contrast, MFH is occasionally associated with bone infarctions or previous bone irradiation. These primary bone sarcomas are rare and more commonly appear as **soft tissue sarcomas (STS)**.[34,52]

Giant cell tumors of the bone generally arise in the metaphysis or epiphysis of long bones in young adults. These tumors most often arise around the knee and account for approximately 0.5% of bone tumors. The majority of these tumors are extremely aggressive benign tumors, with a small percentage (about 7%) being malignant lesions. Malignant giant cell tumors are most commonly seen in the context of previous radiation treatment portals for benign giant cell tumors. Approximately 10% of irradiated benign giant cell tumors ultimately transform into a malignancy.[52]

Metastatic bone disease accounts for approximately 60% to 65% of malignant bone lesions. Often, patients have a bone lesion resulting from the primary site located elsewhere in the body. Common primary sites are the prostate, breast, lung, kidney, and thyroid; a small percentage of bone lesions are from unknown origin. Metastatic carcinoma occurs most frequently in the spine and pelvis and becomes less frequent as the anatomic site becomes farther from the trunk. Metastatic bone lesions distal to the elbow or knee are extremely rare. They occur more often in the foot than in the hand. The primary tumor associated with these distal metastases is lung carcinoma.[52]

Ewing's sarcoma accounts for approximately 7% of bone tumors and affects a wide age range. This disease can affect anyone from the age of 5 months to 60 years, peaking in children from 11 to 17 years of age. Approximately 90% of patients are diagnosed before the age of 30, with the tumor rarely appearing in children younger than 3. Ewing's sarcoma is rarely seen among African-American and Chinese people.[2,49,52]

After osteosarcoma, Ewing's sarcoma is the most common primary malignant bone tumor in children and adolescents. This disease accounts for about 3% of childhood cancers; approximately 200 instances occur per year in the United States. This disease appears to be more predominant in males than females and affects taller people more frequently than shorter individuals.[43,52]

Etiology

Areas of prolonged growth or overstimulated metabolism appear to have a direct link with the site of the neoplasm.

Table 25-1	Frequency of primary malignant bone tumors as a function of histologic type	
Histologic Type	**Malignant Tumor**	**Frequency (%)**
Hematopoietic	Myeloma (solitary and multiple)	47
	Lymphoma (primary)	8
Osteogenic	Osteosarcoma (all types)	21
Chondrogenic	Chondrosarcoma (all types)	12
Unknown origin	Ewing's sarcoma	6
	Giant cell tumor	1
	Malignant fibrous histiocytoma (MFH)	1
Notochordal	Chordoma	4
Vascular	Hemangioendothelioma	1
Langerhans cell	Eosinophilic granuloma	1

Modified from Cox JD: *Moss' radiation oncology*, ed 7, St. Louis, 1994, Mosby.

This is seen in adult tissues affected by metabolic stimulation from long-standing **Paget's disease** (a condition characterized by excessive and abnormal bone resorption and formation), **hyperparathyroidism** (a condition caused by an abnormal parathyroid gland, resulting in a loss of calcium from the bones), chronic **osteomyelitis** (an infection of the bone or bone marrow), old bone infarcts, and fracture callous.[52] Cells that are proliferating or rapidly dividing (as occurs during the repair of bone tissue) tend to be more prone to a malignant transformation.

Another etiologic factor linked to the formation of osteogenic sarcomas, chondrosarcomas, and fibrosarcomas is radiation. Also, bone-seeking radioisotopes from occupational (old radium dial painters) and medicinal uses need to be considered as a possible factor in diagnosing these tumors. Based on laboratory observations, another suggestion is that the role of infectious agents in bone cancers (particularly osteogenic sarcomas) has been indicated.[52]

The cause of Ewing's sarcoma is unknown, but some studies have suggested a cytogenetic abnormality in the tumor. This concept could explain the higher-than-expected frequency of an osteosarcoma developing in an irradiated field in patients. Research is ongoing with the hope of a better understanding of this disease process and therefore more success in its treatment.[43]

Prognostic Indicators

The prognosis for a patient with primary bone cancer appears to be related to several factors. These include the location of the tumor, histologic grade of the tumor, presence or absence of disseminated disease, and age and gender of the patient. Overall for this diverse disease cluster, most studies conclude that tumor response to preoperative chemotherapy, as measured histologically from a resected specimen, is the most critical and powerful predictor of survival.

The prognosis for patients who have osteogenic sarcoma depends solely on the histologic grade of the malignancy and the presence or absence of metastases at the time of presentation.[14] A study done by the Mayo Clinic cited five unfavorable prognostic factors and four favorable factors.[43] The unfavorable factors are (1) treatment before 1969, (2) a duration of symptoms less than 6 months, (3) male gender, (4) a lesion in proximal extremity, and (5) younger than 10 years. The favorable factors are (1) extremity lesions respond better than axial primaries because of accessibility; (2) a longer duration of symptoms, possibly indicating a more indolent disease; (3) a smaller tumor size; and (4) a longer time interval between the presentation and appearance of the first metastatic lesion.

The prognostic indicators for patients with chondrosarcoma include the histologic grade, size of the tumor, cell type, and location. In addition, the stage of the disease, patient's age, degree of local aggressiveness, and presence or absence of pain at the time of presentation all play a part in determining how well the patient functions with the disease.[43]

The prognostic indicators for fibrosarcomas include the histologic grade, the location in the bone (medullary or periosteal), and whether the lesions arise de novo (anew) or are secondary to a preexisting bony condition.[43]

MFH of the bone carries a poorer prognosis than MFH of soft tissue. The disease is extremely aggressive and overall entails a poor prognosis for any patient with the disease.[43]

Patients diagnosed with multiple myeloma with additional signs of advanced renal disease have a poorer prognosis than those diagnosed before the disease affects the kidneys. According to a study done by the Southwest Oncology Group (SWOG), the median survival time was 26 months for patients younger than 55 years, and 20 months for patients older than 65. Other indicators may shorten the survival or remission duration of these patients. These indicators include severe anemia, hypercalcemia, and high tumor cell volume. Based on the prognostic indicators, patients diagnosed early in the disease process are much more likely to have a longer survival or remission duration.[43]

Prognostic indicators in patients who have Ewing's bone sarcoma include the location of the tumor, the amount of extension by the time the patient is diagnosed, and whether the patient is male. Pelvic tumors carry a poorer prognosis because of the greater incidence of extraosseous extension.[43]

The most important prognostic factor with Ewing's bone sarcoma is the extent of the disease at the time of the diagnosis. Several variables are directly or indirectly related to this factor, making difficult the determination of the independent significance of any factor. Patients who have a grossly metastatic disease at the time of the diagnosis usually experience a poor outcome. Early studies have shown that patients with bone or bone marrow involvement did not do as well as patients with limited pulmonary involvement. However, progress is being made in the treatment of patients who have metastatic disease. Another prognostic factor is the extension in the soft tissue component of the primary tumor, producing a less favorable prognosis than that in patients with limited or no soft tissue involvement. In addition, because it involves the bone (greater or less than 8 cm), the size of the primary may influence the likelihood of a successful outcome. High serum levels of lactic dehydrogenase appear to be associated with a poor outcome, possibly because they reflect the tumor burden or activity of the tumor. A high leukocyte count may also be associated with an increased risk of tumor recurrence.[52]

Another important factor with Ewing's bone sarcoma is the site of the involvement, which is relevant to the success of therapy. The involvement of the pelvis or sacrum is associated with a worse prognosis than that of the proximal extremities (i.e., humerus and femur) or central sites such as the ribs and vertebrae. These sites are less favorable than the involvement of a distal extremity site, which makes treatment much easier. The local recurrence rate in the primary site is 15% for children with extremity lesions, 47% for children with rib primaries, and 69% for children with pelvic tumors.[52,55]

Anatomy and Lymphatics

Bone tumors have their embryologic origin in the mesoderm, primitive mesenchyme, and/or the ectoderm cells, which give rise to the common connective tissues (Fig. 25-1). The high incidence rate of bone tumors in children supports the assumption that these neoplasms arise in areas of rapid growth. The most common site of a primary bone sarcoma is near the growth plate (Fig. 25-2). A typical long bone, as illustrated in Fig. 25-2, consists of the **diaphysis** (the main shaft of the bone), two **epiphyses** (the knoblike portions at either end of the bone), **articular cartilage** (a thin layer of hyaline cartilage covering the joint surface of the epiphyses), and the **periosteum** (the hard dense covering of the bone). The growth plate is the area in long bones where rapid cell proliferation and remodeling activity takes place.[35] This is known as the **epiphyseal line.** Because they possess large growth plates, the distal femur and proximal tibia are the two most common locations for bone tumors.[52]

Osteosarcomas are most commonly found in the distal femur or proximal tibia. The third most common site is the proximal humerus. Lesions appear in other areas, such as the proximal femur, distal tibia, and fibula, with rare occurrences in the vertebrae, ilium, facial bones, and mandible. In one study of patients 24 years or older, 41% of the lesions were found in flat bones associated with Paget's disease.[43]

Chondrosarcomas usually occur in areas such as the shoulder girdle, proximal femur, and proximal humerus. Like osteosarcomas, chondrosarcomas are rarely found in the distal extremities. However, chondrosarcomas most commonly involve the femur, with some types involving the femoral shaft arising from preexisting benign conditions.[43]

Fibrosarcomas (MFH) and giant cell tumors of the bone often arise in long, tubular bones. These bones usually include the femur and tibia.[43]

Ewing's sarcoma can be present in virtually any bone but is most frequently seen in the lower half of the body. It can occur in any part of the bone but is most commonly seen in the diaphysis. Metaphyseal involvement occurs less often, and epiphyseal involvement is rare.[43] For treatment purposes the entire medullary cavity (the cavity of the bone that contains fats or yellow marrow) of the affected bones should be considered. Generally, extension occurs through the bony cortex into the soft tissue, giving rise to a large, soft tissue component. In axial lesions the soft tissue mass is often larger than the intraosseous component.[14]

Lung metastases are the most frequent result of hematogenous spread of Ewing's sarcoma. These metastases are frequently present at the time of the diagnosis, or the lung becomes the site of initial relapse. Lymph node involvement appears uncommon, although some studies suggest more

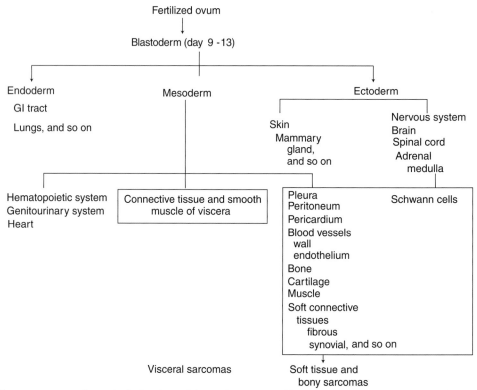

Figure 25-1. Embryonic derivation of the soft tissue and bony sarcomas. Cells of origin determine designations as particular types of soft-tissue sarcomas. *(From Rosenberg SA, Suit HA, Baker LH: Sarcomas of soft tissues. In DeVita VT, Hellman S, Rosenberg SA, editors: Cancer: principles and practice of oncology, vol 2, ed 2, Philadelphia, 1982, JB Lippincott.)*

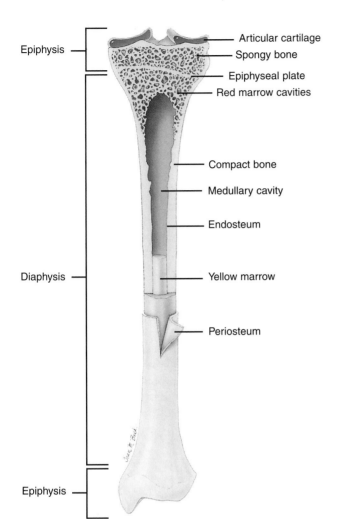

Epiphysis

Diaphysis

Epiphysis

Articular cartilage
Spongy bone
Epiphyseal plate
Red marrow cavities

Compact bone

Medullary cavity

Endosteum

Yellow marrow

Periosteum

Figure 25-2. A longitudinal section of long bone showing diaphysis, epiphyses, and articular cartilage. *(From Thibodeau GA, Patton KT: Anatomy and physiology, ed 15, St. Louis, 1996, Mosby.)*

frequent involvement may be evident with routine node sampling done during diagnosis and staging of processes. For the present, however, the true incidence of nodal involvement remains an unanswered question.[14]

Multiple myeloma can occur in any bone with **lytic** (areas of bone destruction) bone lesions demonstrated on diagnostic radiographs. However, the vertebral pedicles are rarely involved in patients who have multiple myeloma, compared with patients suffering from metastatic carcinoma.[43]

Metastatic bone disease most often involves the vertebral bodies, pelvic bones, and ribs. However, with widespread metastases, lesions are sometimes found in the humerus, femur, scapula, sternum, skull, clavicle, or ribs. Although the distal extremities are often spared from metastatic disease, lesions in the foot are more common than lesions in the hand and usually result from a primary lung carcinoma.[14]

Lymphatic spread of most bone tumors is not of great con-

cern unless the tumor arises in the trunk of the body. There the lymph vessels and nodes are more prominent and a greater chance exists of the tumor invading the lymph system. If this occurs, the microscopic tumor cells can be carried to other parts of the body through the lymphatic system.

Clinical Presentation

The most common presenting factor with bone tumors is pain in the affected area. Some swelling and locally engorged veins in instances of neglect may accompany this. Patients with osteosarcoma usually complain of nonspecific pain and swelling in the involved area that begins insidiously and progresses over a few months. Weight loss and symptoms related to anemia are also late complaints. Pathologic fractures are not commonly seen in patients with osteosarcoma.[43] Chondrosarcomas, fibrosarcomas (MFH), and giant cell tumors of the bone have symptoms similar to those of osteosarcomas, and the duration of the symptoms may be somewhat longer. Pain usually correlates with the degree of histologic aggressiveness of the disease, and rapid worsening of symptoms may indicate the histologic grade or cell type. Pathologic fractures are common in fibrosarcomas (MFH). Also seen are neurologic abnormalities in vertebral lesions, a decreased range of motion of the involved extremity, and muscular atrophy.[43]

Patients with Ewing's sarcoma also complain of pain and swelling in the affected area. The symptoms are frequently present for several months before a diagnosis is made. Patients with axial lesions especially have a prolonged duration of symptoms. In about 60% of patients a palpable mass is evident, demonstrating the propensity for this tumor to break through the cortex and involve surrounding tissue. Other symptoms include a fever, weight loss, and generalized fatigue. Occasionally, the presence of lung metastases may cause symptoms that encourage the patient to seek medical treatment early.[14,52]

Detection and Diagnosis

Patients generally have pain that tends not to be activity related and may be worse at night. A complete history of the patient is important to determine the exact duration of the symptoms. Also, an indication of a previous carcinoma may suggest a metastatic cause of a new bone lesion. It is important to bear in mind that sarcoma may develop in a previously irradiated area. A long history (usually lasting years) of symptoms from a long bone lesion may indicate a benign condition, whereas symptoms that rapidly progress over weeks or a few months usually signify a higher likelihood of a malignant process.[21,52]

Primary bone tumors are rare. This low incidence is a contributing factor in making early detection extremely difficult. The incidental finding of a bone lesion on a diagnostic radiograph is unusual. Usually, only persistent pain in a bone initiates a physician's investigation. Because pain is present early in the course of malignant lesions and they usually progress rapidly, incidental discoveries of these lesions are rare, making an early diagnosis difficult.[52]

The most important tool for a diagnosis and prognosis of a bone tumor is the radiograph. A variety of parameters are associated in accurately diagnosing a bone lesion. Some of these parameters are the permeative pattern, the sunburst periosteal reaction, the onionskin periosteal reaction, and whether the lesion is osteolytic or **osteoblastic** (pertaining to bone-forming cells). All of these indicate a bone lesion's level of advancement, its aggressiveness, and its rate of growth. Fig. 25-3 illustrates several lytic lesions of the humerus caused by metastatic renal cell carcinoma. (Fig. 25-4 shows the presence of a Ewing's sarcoma of the upper humerus.)

Computed tomography (CT) has been extremely helpful in establishing the extent of the tumor in the bone and determining the presence or absence of soft tissue masses. However, magnetic resonance imaging (MRI) has replaced CT in many instances (Fig. 25-5). MRI is used particularly in instances of highly malignant bone tumors because of the accurate detail it exhibits concerning the relationship of

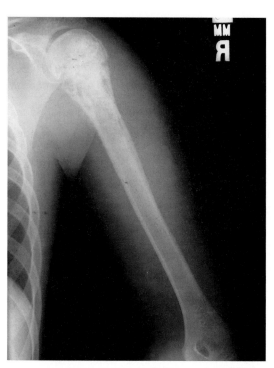

Figure 25-4. Ewing's sarcoma of the upper right humerus. Note the diffuse permeative destruction of the bone, with periosteal reaction involving the proximal portion of the humerus.

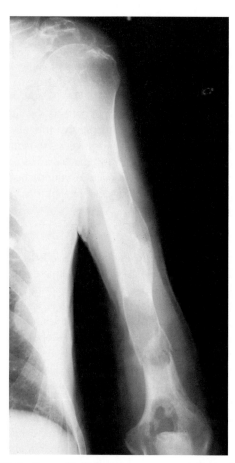

Figure 25-3. Several lytic lesions are present throughout the humerus of this patient with metastatic renal cell carcinoma. Note the destruction of the periosteum along the mid- and lower portion of the shaft.

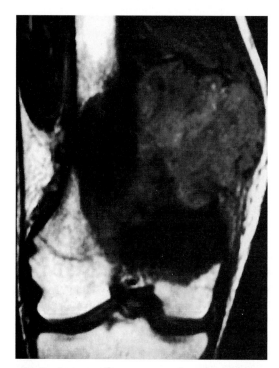

Figure 25-5. A magnetic resonance imaging (MRI) scan of an osteogenic sarcoma of the distal femur showing the intermedullary and soft tissue extent of the tumor. *(From Stark DD, Bradley WG Jr: Magnetic resonance imaging, ed 2, St. Louis, 1991, Mosby.)*

normal tissues and neurovascular structures with the tumor tissue. This is essential in planning a surgical biopsy and treatment. MRI demonstrates with high sensitivity the reactive zone of the tumor in the bone and differentiates any marrow edema adjacent to tumor tissue.

Bone scans using technetium-99m have played an important role in bone tumor evaluation. Fig. 25-6 demonstrates the diagnostic importance of a bone scan in a patient with metastatic prostate cancer. These scans are extremely sensitive and can detect tumor foci in bone that are not yet visualized on diagnostic radiographs. Therefore the extent of the tumor in the bone and the presence of skip metastases can be demonstrated accurately. Bone scans can also identify distant bony metastases even though they are extremely uncommon in primary bone tumors. For multiple myeloma, however, bone scan results are frequently negative and may underestimate the extent of the disease.[43]

The diagnosis of Ewing's bone sarcoma requires many diagnostic and some surgical procedures. The most important of these is the surgical biopsy. This procedure should be sufficient to confirm a pathologic diagnosis. The biopsy site and approach must be discussed with the surgeon and radiation oncologist before the procedure is performed. If the biopsy incision is poorly placed, the delivery of optimal irradiation therapy may be technically impossible. Many patients have a considerable associated soft tissue mass; they can undergo a soft tissue biopsy rather than a biopsy of intraosseous tissue. A soft tissue biopsy is much easier and avoids further weakening of the bone, the integrity of which is already compromised by the tumor. This is especially true in patients who have lesions in weight-bearing bones, which have increased potential for pathologic fracture.

A radiographic assessment of the primary lesion is necessary to demonstrate an expanding destructive lesion in the diaphysis. The classical appearance of Ewing's sarcoma on radiographs shows a periosteal reaction in the form of periosteal elevation with extension through the cortex, giving an onionskin appearance. CT and MRI are extremely beneficial in assessing the disease extent.[52] Because of the propensity for Ewing's sarcoma to metastasize to the lungs, a CT scan of the lungs and a radiograph of the chest are also necessary.

Pathology and Staging

Pathologic grading of primary bone tumors is intimately associated with current anatomic staging systems. Grade is determined to be either low (G1) or high (G2) grade and is nearly synonymous with early (I and II) or late (IIB and III) stage. No universally accepted staging system exists for primary bone sarcomas. The Enneking staging system classifies tumors according to the grade (G), local extent of the disease (T), determined to be either intracompartmental (T1) or extracompartmental (T2), and presence or absence of distant metastases (M). Box 25-1 shows a system that may be used in the future.[37]

In the following sections, specific treatment techniques

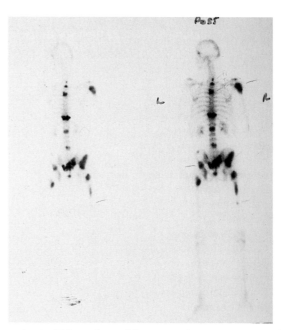

Figure 25-6. This patient with metastatic prostate cancer has diffuse disease in the right shoulder, vertebral column, and pelvic area. Bone scans with the use of technetium-99 play an important role in detecting the presence of metastatic disease. Both the anterior and posterior projections demonstrate several areas of increased uptake *(dark areas)* of the technetium-99.

are discussed regarding osteogenic sarcoma, chondrosarcoma, fibrosarcoma (MFH), giant cell tumors, multiple myeloma, Ewing's sarcoma, and metastatic bone disease. In addition, more detailed information is provided for each of these tumors. Emphasis is on the role of radiation therapy as it relates to treatment, although for some primary bone lesions, radiation therapy plays a minor role (if any) in the treatment plan.

Routes of Spread

The tendency for almost all sarcomas is to metastasize to the lungs, particularly the peripheral lung fields. Rarely, osteosarcomas metastasize to other sites. Enneking stresses the importance of skip metastasis in osteosarcomas.[43] A skip metastasis is a second, smaller focus of osteosarcoma in the same bone or a second bone lesion on the opposing side of a joint space. This phenomenon is attributed to the extensive spread by the lesion into the marrow cavity of the bone. Along with metastasis to the lung, low-grade chondrosarcomas have a tendency to recur locally.

Treatment Techniques

Osteogenic sarcoma. Osteogenic sarcoma is a relatively rare tumor but is the most frequently encountered malignant primary bone tumor. The hallmark of this disease is osteoid,

Box 25-1	Enneking Staging System for Bone Sarcomas

GRADE

Low Grade (G1)
    Parosteal osteosarcoma
    Endosteal osteosarcoma
    Secondary chondrosarcoma
    Fibrosarcoma, low-grade
    Atypical malignant fibrous histiocytoma
    Giant cell tumor
    Adamantinoma
High grade (G2)
    Classic osteosarcoma
    Radiation-induced sarcoma
    Paget's sarcoma
    Primary chondrosarcoma
    Fibrosarcoma, high-grade
    Giant cell sarcoma

LOCAL EXTENT

Intracompartmental (T1)
    Intraosseous
    Parosseous
    Intrafascial
Extracompartmental (T2)
    Soft tissue extension
    Extrafascial or deep fascial extension

DISTANT METASTASES

MO: no distant metastases
M1: distant metastases present

STAGE GROUPING

Stage	G	T	M
1A	G1	T1	M0
1B	G1	T2	M0
IIA	G2	T1	M0
IIB	G2	T2	M0
III	G1 or G2	T1 or T2	M1

Modified from Moss WT: *Radiation oncology,* ed 6, St. Louis, 1989, Mosby.

or immature, bone produced by a malignant, proliferating spindle cell stroma. This disease is the most common bone tumor encountered in the first three decades of life, with the peak incidence rate occurring in girls 13½ years old and boys 14½ years old. The peak incidence rate corresponds with growth spurts. Tall people and those affected with Paget's disease are at higher risk.[52]

The most common metastasis from osteogenic sarcoma occurs in the lung. This seems to occur in about 80% of patients within 1 to 2 years after the initial diagnosis. However, with the introduction of more aggressive surgical techniques and newer chemotherapeutic agents, researchers hope to extend the disease-free status of patients. In addition, with the aggressive resection of pulmonary nodules, these patients are potentially curable.[14,52]

The most important prognostic indicator in patients diagnosed with osteogenic sarcoma is the presence or absence of metastases at the time of the diagnosis. Other factors requiring consideration are the duration of the symptoms, size of the tumor, gender of the patient, and site of the lesion. If the duration of the symptoms has been more than 6 months, this may indicate a more indolent disease, which may respond well to aggressive surgical and chemotherapeutic treatment. Reason dictates that the smaller the tumor, the more easily it can be surgically removed and the less chance it has to metastasize. The disease appears more often in males and in those younger than 10 years at the time of the diagnosis. These patients do not seem to do as well as others. Also,

lesions that occur in the extremities (usually the lower extremity) rather than in the axial primaries are more favorable. This has to do with the easy accessibility for surgical removal of the tumor to obtain localized control. Fig. 25-7 demonstrates the classic sunburst pattern seen radiographically, which is caused by the outward extension of bony spicules.

The treatment of osteogenic sarcoma requires a multidisciplinary approach. The mainstay of treatment goals for this disease is the attainment of local control. Because this tumor is relatively chemosensitive and radioresistant, the management of the primary tumor is the surgical removal of all gross and microscopic tumors. When possible, this is achieved most easily by amputation with a wide margin of normal tissue taken at the time of the surgery. The tumor's recurrence in the stump is usually attributed to skip lesions of the tumor in the affected bone separated from the primary tumor by several centimeters of normal bone. Historically, disarticulations were used to prevent this. Because of the introduction of adjuvant chemotherapy and improved CT and MRI scanning, the removal of entire bones is not necessary unless doing so is dictated by the location and extent of the tumor.[52]

Subamputative and **limb-sparing surgery** (LSS) have been used in patients who have osteogenic sarcoma to reduce the functional and psychologic morbidity of amputation. In this procedure the bone involved with the tumor is removed and replaced by an artificial prosthesis or bone graft. This procedure can only be performed if the vascular and neuro-

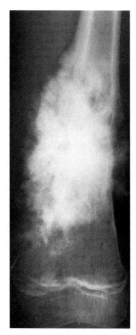

Figure 25-7. Osteogenic sarcoma of the distal femur demonstrates a classic sunburst pattern caused by the outward growth of bony spicules. *(From Eisenberg RL, Dennis CA: Comprehensive radiographic pathology, ed 2, St. Louis, 1995, Mosby.)*

logic integrity of the limb is not compromised. In many instances, preoperative chemotherapy is used to reduce the size of the tumor to make LSS possible. However, the disease-free survival rate of patients with LSS is much the same as that with patients who have undergone an amputation. Subamputative and LSS are limited to patients with tumors of the lower extremity and those who have completed most of their growth. For patients with lesions of the humerus, any preservation of function in the hand can significantly improve long-term functional results.[52]

Before 1972, chemotherapy for osteogenic sarcoma was ineffective. In 1972, however, doxorubicin (Adriamycin) or high doses of methotrexate followed by leucovorin were shown to produce objective tumor regression in 42% of patients. Since then, these two agents have been the basis for adjuvant chemotherapy. The early studies showed the importance of treatment with full-dose doxorubicin. Cisplatin has also proved to be an active agent in treating this type of tumor.[39,52]

Radiation therapy is not a treatment of choice for patients with osteogenic sarcomas. These tumors are radioresistant, and doses required for a clinical response often result in severe tissue damage and subsequent amputation. However, radiation has been used in patients for whom surgery is not feasible, but a cure with this approach is unusual. Radiation has been used to control or prevent pulmonary metastases but is of limited value in this setting. Palliative radiation therapy can be beneficial for pain control or the temporary control of metastases.[52]

Chondrosarcoma. Chondrosarcomas are malignant mesenchymal neoplasms that produce cartilage but no osteoid. The lesions are graded from 1 to 3, with 3 being the most **anaplastic** (exhibiting a loss of cell differentiation). Grading is an important prognostic indicator in this disease. The number of mitoses and the degree of cellularity are important in determining the grade of these tumors.[43]

A histologic analysis of these tumors may indicate an invasion of the adjacent joint and infiltration beyond the x-ray margin of the tumor in the marrow cavity. Areas of **necrosis** (dead tissue), cyst formation, and hemorrhage may also be present. The average tumor can range from 2 to 32 cm, with soft tissue extension possible.[43]

Low-grade chondrosarcomas do not tend to metastasize but do tend to recur locally. When this happens the tumor continues to grow and eventually evolves into a high-grade tumor. These tumors most often readily metastasize to the lungs, giving the patient a poorer prognosis and making tumor control more difficult.[14]

The prognosis of patients with chondrosarcomas depends on two factors. One factor is the histologic grade of the tumor. Low-grade chondrosarcomas are locally invasive and do not metastasize, making this tumor easier to control. High-grade tumors, in contrast, have a high frequency of metastasis, particularly to the lungs. The other prognostic indicator is the tumor's location. If the tumor is located peripherally, it is easily accessible for surgical intervention; but if it appears in the pelvis or sacral area, surgery may not be possible. Fig. 25-8 shows a large chondrosarcoma of the distal femur.

The treatment of choice for this disease is the surgical removal of the entire tumor mass, with adequate bone and

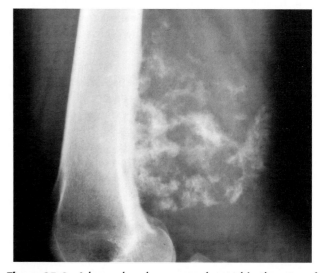

Figure 25-8. A large chondrosarcoma located in the area of the distal femur. Note the prominent dense calcification of the lesion. *(From Eisenberg RL, Dennis CA: Comprehensive radiographic pathology, ed 2, St. Louis, 1995, Mosby.)*

soft tissue margins. Radiation therapy does not usually play a role in treating these patients because of the radioresistant qualities of this type of tumor. However, in patients with an inoperable disease, radiation therapy doses of 4000 to 7000 cGy have been used with some response. To date, chemotherapeutic agents do not appear to have any substantial effect on this disease. Radioactive sulfur has been used in the past in patients who have an inoperable disease, but it has been abandoned because of its ineffectiveness and toxicity.[14,52]

Fibrosarcomas. Fibrosarcomas, frequently now classified with MFH, are locally aggressive lesions with a metastatic potential related to histologic grade. High-grade lesions behave much like classic osteogenic sarcomas, whereas low-grade lesions appear less aggressive. These lesions are found mostly in the distal femur, followed in frequency by the proximal tibia and proximal humerus. The pelvis can be involved more often than in osteogenic sarcomas, and tumors of the jaw are not uncommon.[14,43]

Prognostic indicators for fibrosarcomas include the histologic grade, the location in the bone, and whether the lesion arises de novo or secondary to a preexisting bony condition. The overall outlook for these patients is poor because of the tendency toward higher grade histology.[43]

Treatment for fibrosarcomas involving bone consists of an aggressive surgical procedure using wide or radical excision. Because these tumors have a high incidence rate of recurrence, even with aggressive surgery, postoperative radiation is now recommended. Fibrosarcomas are not highly radiosensitive, but irradiation is recommended for inoperable tumors, postoperative residual disease, and palliation. Doses of 6600 to 7000 cGy using a shrinking-field technique are recommended if radiation therapy is prescribed to control a skeletal fibrosarcoma.[43]

Malignant fibrous histiocytoma (MFH). MFH arises from **histiocytes** (a type of macrophage or phagocytic cell found in loose connective tissue) and may arise in bone or soft tissue of any part of the body. This is an extremely aggressive tumor, and, like other STSs, it metastasizes hematogenously (via the circulatory system) to the lungs. MFH of the bone requires radical surgical resection, amputation, or disarticulation. Trials are underway that include radical or limited surgical procedures combined with preoperative or postoperative chemotherapy. Responses and occasional cures have been reported in patients receiving definitive radiation therapy with and without chemotherapy. Radiation therapy has also been reported as having a beneficial palliative response in some of the affected patients.[43]

Giant cell tumors. Giant cell tumors of the bone are malignant tumors made up of a stroma of spindle or ovoid cells, in addition to numerous multinucleated giant cells dispersed throughout the tumor tissue.[14] This tumor usually causes pain, swelling, and tenderness at the lesion site. The most common site for these tumors is in and around the knee. Approximately half the lesions occur at the distal femur, and half occur at the proximal tibia. Additional common sites for

this tumor are the proximal humerus, proximal femur, sacrum, and other pelvic areas.

Giant cell tumors of the bone usually occur predominantly in the third and fourth decades of life, with some occurrences during the second decade of life. However, this condition is extremely rare for children younger than 10 years. These tumors tend to recur locally. Metastases rarely occur, but, when they do, the most affected area is the lung.

The histology of giant cell tumors is generally low grade, with areas of focally malignant cells present in the examined specimen. These lesions are treated locally because of their low propensity to metastasize. Occasionally, however, even these low-grade tumors have metastasized, with a histologic diagnosis made by a biopsy of pulmonary nodules. These nodules sometimes occur as isolated, solitary nodules with a benign giant cell tumor. A fully malignant, grade III, giant cell tumor is rarely encountered. Only about 10% of these tumors are fully malignant at the time of the initial diagnosis. However, about 20% of giant cell tumors become malignant after they have recurred locally. In addition, giant cell tumors have been reported to become fully malignant after the application of radiation therapy to obtain local control. It is unclear whether this transformation is a result of the natural history of this tumor or radiation therapy is truly an oncogenic agent. However, the occurrence of fully malignant giant cell tumors with metastatic capabilities may be an indication that radiation therapy causes malignant transformation or just is not adequate therapy to eradicate this tumor. The latter is probably closer to what can be expected because this tumor is a spindle cell sarcoma known to be radiosensitive.[14]

The prognosis of a patient who has a giant cell tumor of the bone depends primarily on the location and histology of the tumor. Tumors located in the extremity and those of low-grade histology are easily accessible for surgical intervention and have a low propensity to metastasize. Those located in the pelvic region are harder to excise; therefore local control is difficult.

The treatment of choice for giant cell tumors of the bone is surgical removal of the tumor. Benign giant cell tumors can be treated in several different ways, including curettage and bone grafting with or without cauterization, filling of the cavity with cement, application of liquid nitrogen after curettage, or surgical excision if functional results permit. Malignant giant cell tumors require a more radical surgical procedure, followed by the use of adjuvant chemotherapy. Radiation therapy is reserved for control of inoperable tumors or for palliation of symptomatic areas in patients with advanced malignant disease.[43]

Multiple myeloma. A multiple myeloma is a malignant plasma cell tumor that has several different forms. The forms constitute a spectrum from small, localized lesions to a diffuse, disseminated disease. The most frequent presentation of this disease is a disseminated disease with the involvement of multiple skeletal sites. Common complaints of patients with multiple myeloma include bone pain, bleeding, infections,

time may experience more acute side effects. The use of these two modalities together or in succession is not uncommon. The type and severity of the side effects depend on many factors, such as the type of disease, chemotherapeutic agents, and anatomic site of the radiation therapy portal. Aggressive systemic treatment (chemotherapy) may cause acute problems, including fever, neutropenia, mucositis, nausea, vomiting, and diarrhea. In addition to erythema in the irradiation field, these acute side effects are often enhanced by irradiation, depending on the location and size of the radiation fields. If metastatic bone disease is treated, patients may experience some nausea, vomiting, and diarrhea if the treatment portal includes any of the stomach or bowel. This is avoided when possible by limited fields or beam shaping to block these tissues.

Knowing when to withhold treatment (until a physician can be consulted) because of factors such as skin breakdown or a low blood count (white blood cell [WBC] count $<2000/mm^3$ or platelets $<50,000/mm^3$) is critical to effective patient care. In the treatment of patients with metastatic cancer to the bone, care must also be taken to observe and evaluate the patient's condition for further metastatic spread of the disease. Questioning the patient and family members and observing the patient is an important part of the therapist's role in the day to day treatment delivery.

Subacute and late changes of edema, fibrosis, contractures, and growth arrest can often be avoided or minimized through the use of an optimal technique. If radiation is used in children, the treatment portal may include the growth plates for the treatment of long bones causing growth deficits. Patients treated with doses of 6000 to 6500 cGy have been known to develop osteosarcoma in bones previously treated for Ewing's bone sarcoma. Another complication is the development of leukemia in these patients who have been treated with megavoltage techniques and chemotherapy. Acute and late cardiac damage has been noted in patients who have received doxorubicin; this is a major consideration for planning a patient's course of treatment (limiting radiation doses to the heart). In addition, sterility, endocrine dysfunctions, and an increased risk of hemorrhagic cystitis are concerns of physicians planning a course of treatment for patients receiving pelvic irradiation combined with cyclophosphamide.[14]

Patients undergoing treatment for Ewing's bone sarcoma are clearly at great risk for developing second primaries, leukemias, cardiac damage, and many other problems. Therefore continued follow-up for an indefinite time is necessary to intervene before the complication becomes uncontrollable. Despite the best efforts of all involved health care professionals and caregivers, many of these patients ultimately die a premature death as a result of the disease or a complication resulting from treatment. At the time of the diagnosis, all of the complications (acute and long term) must be considered before a course of treatment is planned and initiated. Modifications may be necessary for obtaining

the best technique while trying to prevent some of the complications. In general, the side effects experienced by patients with primary bone cancer are fairly well tolerated. Because the amputation of a limb is sometimes necessary to control the disease, the use of prosthetic devices allows patients to lead a somewhat normal life. If, however, patients survive into adulthood, they are at a high risk for developing a second malignancy. This makes follow-up care and close monitoring of these patients extremely important.

SOFT TISSUE SARCOMAS

A STS† is a tumor occurring in the extraskeletal connective tissue. These tissues include all those that provide connection, support, and locomotion. They are grouped together because they share similarities in appearance pathologically, as well as in clinical presentation and behaviors. Although in many respects they resemble bone tumors and are frequently associated with primary bone cancer, they may also occur in any anatomic structure containing connective tissue such as blood vessel walls and viscera.

The derivation of this complex and fascinating group of sarcomas is primarily from mesodermal structures and connective tissue cells. However, some of the soft tissues in this category arise from ectodermal structures and some from the epithelium. The muscles in the adult human are about 40% of the total body weight. The somatic soft tissues are about 50% of the total body weight. These structures are found throughout the entire body. Therefore an STS can arise anywhere in the body. The most common site at first presentation involves the extremities. Of the 1957 patients with an STS admitted to Memorial Sloan Kettering Cancer Center between 1982 and 1992, half (52%) had primaries in the upper or lower extremities. The incidence rate of the lower extremity primaries was 37%, with most primaries located in the proximal thigh and 15% in the upper limbs. Other primary sites included the retroperitoneum, trunk, viscera, and head and neck[11] (Table 25-2).

This section of the chapter presents fundamental information critical to understanding the nature of this disease, including its etiology, tissue derivation, histology, staging, grading, and patterns of spread. Factors affecting treatment decision making and options in radiation therapy treatment planning and modalities are addressed.

Epidemiology

STS is rare. Rates of incidence range from 0.57% to 0.7% of all cancers. The incidence in the United States may now be in excess of 5700 new cases per year.[33,51] The American Cancer Society's estimate for 2003 was 8,300 new cases, with 3,900 deaths resulting from the disease.[3]

STS is more common in children than adults, accounting for 6.5% of all tumors in pediatric age-groups; they are the

---

†Soft tissue sarcomas are a class of malignant tumors arising primarily but not exclusively from mesenchymal connective tissues.

Table 25-2	Incidence of soft tissue sarcoma by site
Site	**Percentage**
Lower extremity	37
Retroperitoneal/intraabdominal	14
Trunk	9
Upper extremity	15
Genitourinary	2
Visceral	13
Head and neck	5
Thoracic	5
Other	4.6

Data from Conlon KC, Brennen MF: Sarcomas. In Murphy GP, Lawrence WL Jr, Lenhard RE Jr, editors: *The American Cancer Society textbook of clinical oncology,* ed 2, Atlanta, 1995, The American Cancer Society.

fifth highest ranked cause of death for children younger than 15 years.[53] A slight predilection in incidence exists for males compared with females (45% to 46%).[3,11] The literature does not indicate significant incidence by geographical location or distribution.

The most common subtypes of STS are liposarcomas (STS arising from fat), 23%; leiomyosarcomas (STS arising from smooth muscle), 18%; MFH (deep STS showing partial fibroblastic and histiocytic differentiation with variable storiform pattern, myxoid areas, and giant cells), 18%; fibrosarcomas (STS derived from collagen-producing fibroblasts), 9%; synovial and a group of unclassified sarcomas, 8%. Extraosseous Ewing's sarcomas were originally described by Ewing as permeative destructive tumors of the bone that infiltrated adjacent muscles and spread along fascial planes. Because it is of endothelial origin, it is also a STS histologic classification characterized by round cellular composition rather than spindle-shaped cells.[22] However, because of differences in the STS histopathologic classification of criteria, precise estimates of incidence by type is difficult.[11] In the current altered identification methods and evolving classification criteria, tumors previously known as fibrosarcomas, or spindle cell sarcomas, have come to be classified as MFH. Therefore the apparent increase in MFH is an artificial one resulting from reclassification of other types of STS.

As new technologies emerge, further classification of histogenesis is possible. Electron microscopy, immunohistochemical staining for proteins unique to mesenchymal neoplasms, flow cytometry, and molecular biologic techniques are promising adjuncts in decreasing pathologic disagreements for the determination of histogenesis and tumor grade.[17]

Etiology

The etiology of STS is not known. A variety of genetic and environmental factors have been implicated. Historically, intensive radiation for benign conditions such as tuberculosis and thyroid disease gave rise to sarcomas. More recently, STS appears as a second primary resulting from high-dose irradiation for other cancers after a 5- to 15-year interval. Patients with von Recklinghausen's disease (neurofibromatosis) have small, discrete, pigmented skin lesions (café au lait spots and/or pigmented nevi) that develop into multiple neurofibromas along the course of peripheral nerves and may undergo malignant transformation. This disease is a familial disorder with a predisposition for malignant peripheral nerve tumors or malignant schwannomas (nonencapsulated tumors resulting from a disorderly proliferation of Schwann cells that includes portions of nerve fibers and typically undergoes a transformation to malignant schwannomas). Longstanding lymphedema is occasionally followed by a lymphangiosarcoma, especially after a radical mastectomy.[11,28,48] Wijnmaalen et al.[60] concluded that the future incidence of angiosarcomas in previously irradiated breasts may increase because the number of patients with long-term follow-up after conservation surgery and radiation therapy is growing rapidly.

Certain ground troops of the Vietnam War who had increased exposure to defoliant chemicals such as Agent Orange may have a higher incidence rate of STS than other soldiers serving in the war at that time.[29] Occupational exposure to vinyl chloride has been reported in association with hepatic angiosarcoma.[13] Other causes, including trauma, have also been implicated as an etiologic factor giving rise to these tumors.

Prognostic Indicators

Probably the most important prognostic factor in STS diagnosis is histologic grade, followed by site, size, resectability, presence or absence of metastasis, local invasion of a **pseudocaspsule,*** regional lymph node involvement, and local recurrence. After an accurate histologic type is determined, grading of the tumor is essential for predicting metastasis and the general outcome. In a study of 163 patients treated at the National Cancer Institute published in 1984, Costa et al.[12] graded the most common types of STS. The study indicated that the amount of necrosis present was the best predictor at that time to recurrence and overall survival.

In general, younger patients (younger than 53 years) with small, low-grade primaries (less than 5 cm) in distal extremity sites who undergo a wide resection with an intact pseudocapsule and no regional lymph node involvement or distant metastasis will probably fare better in local control and overall survival.[23,36,38,60,62,63] The use of generally favorable (small size, superficial site, and low grade) versus unfavorable (large size, deep-seated site, and high histologic grade) signs in predicting prognosis has been replaced with more precise incorporation of those factors into current staging systems (Table 25-3).

*Pseudocapsules are STS tumors surrounded by compressed normal tissue, reactive inflammation, and fibrosis that give the gross anatomic appearance of a capsule.

Table 25-3	Correlation of prognostic signs and stage	
Stage	Favorable Signs*	Unfavorable Signs†
0	3	0
I	2	1
II	3	2
III	0	3
IV	0	Evidence of mets

Modified from Holleb AI, Fink DJ, Murphy GP editors: *American Cancer Society textbook of clinical oncology,* ed 1, Atlanta, 1991, The American Cancer Society.
*Favorable signs include (1) small size, (2) superficial site, and (3) low histologic grade.
†Unfavorable signs include (1) large size, (2) deep site, and (3) high histologic grade.

Pertinent Anatomy and Natural History of Disease

Embryologically, as the blastoderm gives rise to the endodermal, mesodermal, and ectodermal layers, the basic tissue derivations for anatomic structures and their corresponding malignancies are established. The embryonic ancestry of STS begins in the primitive mesoderm. The loosely formed network of cells in the mesoderm, the primitive mesenchyme, and/or the ectoderm give rise to the most common connective tissues, such as the pleura, peritoneum, pericardium, walls and endothelium of blood vessels, bone, cartilage, muscles, and soft connective tissue. Visceral connective tissue, similar muscle organs, and smooth muscle organs (e.g., the kidney, ureters, uterus, gonads, heart, and a variety of hematopoietic tissues) all derive from the remainder of the primitive mesoderm.

Malignant tumors are usually categorized as carcinomas or sarcomas based on whether they derive from epithelial or connective tissue. Because epithelium is a morphologic and not an embryologic term, the classification of many tumors is not precise. The endothelial lining of blood vessels, lymphatics, and the mesothelial lining of body cavities in visceral organs are epithelial in type but arise from the mesoderm germ layer of the embryo. Other deviations in derivation include Kaposi's sarcoma, which is believed to arise from endothelial cells and occurs as pigmented skin lesions. Neurofibrosarcomas have their origin in the Schwann cells of the neural tube of the primitive ectoderm. They occur as tumors of the neural sheath surrounding the peripheral nerves. Sometimes they are referred to as neurogenic sarcomas, schwannomas, or malignant neurilemmomas, and they are often associated with von Recklinghausen's disease (neurofibromatosis).[11] Structural support is required for endothelial organs, so sarcomas may arise in these connective tissues that provide the organ's form and therefore its ability to function. These connective tissue cells of origin for the corresponding malignancies determine the resulting designations as particular types of STS (Fig. 25-1).

The local growth pattern of STS follows the lines of least resistance in the longitudinal axis of the **primary site compartment**—the natural anatomic boundaries surrounding the STS primary, composed of a common fascia plane(s) of muscles, bone, joint, skin, subcutaneous tissues, and major neurovascular structures.[51]

As undisturbed tumor size progresses, it pushes other structures away and forms a pseudocapsule that is made of compressed normal and fibrotic tissue. Trunk and head and neck primaries tend to invade adjacent muscle groups. Compartment boundaries of bone and fascia for these sites may act as a partial barrier to extension. Intermediate- and high-grade lesions typically undergo hematogenous metastasis, primarily to the lungs. Retroperitoneal primaries also have a high potential for lung metastasis but also spread to the liver and other abdominal structures. Lymph nodes are rarely involved. However, when lymph nodes are involved it is considered an unfavorable prognostic indicator.

Clinical Presentation

Usually STS is a painless mass that grows over several weeks or months. One study reports a median time of 4 months from the time of the initial appearance of the mass until the consultation of a physician for an investigation and diagnostic workup.[36] Because surrounding anatomy is easily compressed, readily observed and troublesome symptoms are usually absent. The size and location are such that, unless the mass interferes with the normal functioning of vital organs, tumors often become large before the initial investigative workup, especially when they arise in the buttocks and thighs. Night pain may occur with larger lesions. Fixation to other structures and the presence of warmth or distended vascularity are also regarded as ominous indications. Systemic effects and symptoms are rare with extremity STS. Tumors causing paraneoplastic syndromes with weight loss, a fever, and general malaise are generally large and retroperitoneal but may also arise in the trunk or head and neck.[51]

Detection and Diagnosis

After the discovery of the soft tissue mass, comprehensive diagnostic and staging procedures provide criteria that form the treatment-planning decision-making process. If the presence of a mass is apparent with inspection and palpation, suspicion demanding an accurate diagnosis should motivate the workup.

Imaging modalities include plain film radiography with soft tissue techniques and the use of contrast media studies to demonstrate subtle calcifications and the gross size, shape, and location of the primary tumor and occult or metastatic lesions, especially in the retroperitoneum.[40] CT of the chest is useful for demonstrating additional lesions not visualized radiographically, especially for intermediate- and high-grade lesions.[36]

CT and MRI are essential in the localization of tumors and the relationships to blood supply, nerves, tendons, musculature, supporting fascia, and bone. MRI is considered superior to CT in differentiating normal versus abnormal tissue and in determining the anatomic extent of the tumor. However, even with enhancement agents, differentiation between malignant and benign tissue and an infection is frequently difficult. A complete history and physical examination often provides supporting information to include or rule out further suspicion of benign versus infectious possibilities in the list of probabilities.

In limited instances, arteriography may be useful in demonstrating the vasculature of the tumor. Radionuclide scans may also provide additional documentation of data accumulated with MRI. Diagnostic sonography may be useful in the initial stages to discern cystic versus solid structures. In addition, positron emission tomography (PET) and MRI spectroscopy may provide other information regarding the metabolism and grade of a primary.

After the localization of the tumor, a biopsy to obtain viable tumor tissue is essential. This may be accomplished before the completion of the localization of all anatomic structures, but unless a team carefully manages the biopsy, future treatment options may be compromised.[15] Because of the presence of the pseudocapsule, an incisional biopsy is generally considered the preferred procedure. An excisional biopsy may be appropriate for extremely small lesions (less than 3 cm).[11,15,32,51] Control of bleeding during the procedure is necessary because hematomas provide a mechanism of spread. The longitudinal placement of the incision with avoidance of planes near neurovascular structures allows for later en bloc removal during definitive surgery with a predicted decrease in surgical contamination.

Pathology and Staging

Sarcomas are classified histologically and named according to the tissues in which they arise. Because histologic grade is accepted as the most critical predictor of outcomes, the importance of an accurate determination must not be underestimated.

Grading systems lack uniformity in criteria definition. Overall, however, they include the following: degree of differentiation, cellularity, amount of stroma, necrosis, vascularity, and number of mitoses. The two most commonly used classifications in staging systems are the **Musculoskeletal Tumor Society (MTS)** surgical staging system and the **American Joint Committee on Cancer (AJCC)** classifications (the classification and anatomic staging systems used for STS).

Both systems combine the anatomic stage with grade categories. The AJCC system identifies GX as grade cannot be assessed, G1 as well differentiated, G2 as moderately differentiated, G3 as poorly differentiated, and G4 as undifferentiated. Therefore anatomic stage is nearly synonymous with grade (Box 25-2). With the MTS system, G1 and G2 are simply identified as low grade or high grade.[19,24]

In the AJCC system, size as less than or more than 5 cm defines a tumor (T). A lower case a or b is added to the T, indicating a superficial or deep-seated tumor, respectively. In the MTS systems, (T) is defined by its confinement to one compartment (T1) or more than one compartment (T2). The presence of nodal involvement is equated with the presence of distant metastases.

With both systems, higher grades and an increasing anatomic extent of the disease readily correlate to an advanced stage. In all but a few specific histopathologic tumors (e.g., synovial sarcomas and rhabdomyosarcomas), lymph node involvement is rare. However, when it is present, it is considered equivalent to metastasis and becomes more important than grade in determining the stage.[51]

Routes of Spread

Posner and Brennan's evaluation of 1091 patients with STS[11] found that 22% of STS patients who had metastasis were also likely to have large (greater than 5 cm), high-grade tumors. Retroperitoneal and visceral primaries metastasized more readily than extremity lesions. Histopathologically, leiomyosarcomas spread more frequently; fibrosarcomas (MFH) are less likely to have metastases at the time of the diagnosis.

STSs initially invade aggressively along local, anatomically defined planes composed of neurovascular structures, fascia, and muscle bundles. Lymphatic extension is not common. Hematologic pathways are the primary routes of spread; the lung is the most common site of recurrence, followed much less frequently by the bones, liver, and skin (Fig. 25-15). For retroperitoneal tumors the lung is still the predominant metastatic site, but extension to the liver and other abdominal sites is also likely for recurrence. Most distant metastatic recurrences are likely to be reported within 2 years of the diagnosis and surgery.[32] Primary fibrosarcomas (MFH) originating within the brain parenchyma or its meningeal covering have a propensity for distant meningeal and distant bone metastases.[25]

Treatment Techniques

Multimodality treatments. A variety of imaging procedures has resulted in the improved demonstration of tumor localization and metastatic extension. This improvement, in addition to radical wide-margin surgical techniques, sophisticated radiation therapy treatments, and effective antineoplastic agents, has helped the general management of STS to progress to a multidisciplinary team approach, a multimodality treatment plan that may use a variety of surgical and radiation therapy techniques with or without multiagent chemotherapy. The overall treatment plan is influenced in large part by the size, site, histology classification and subtypes, stage, and grade of the primary tumor at presentation and the natural history of STS, its patterns of spread, and recurrence locally and systemically.

Surgery. In addition to providing tissue for a biopsy, aggressive surgery regardless of site or histology is a proven effective treatment whether used alone or with radiation therapy and/or chemotherapy. Despite the appearance of being encapsulated, a pseudocapsule that nearly always is assumed

Box 25-2   **AJCC Staging for Soft Tissue Sarcoma**

DEFINITION OF TNM

Primary tumor (T)*

TX   Primary tumor cannot be assessed

T0   No evidence of primary tumor

T1   Tumor 5 cm or less in greatest dimension

    T1a   Superficial tumor

    T1b   Deep tumor

T2   Tumor more than 5 cm in greatest dimension

    T2a   Superficial tumor

    T2b   Deep tumor

REGIONAL LYMPH NODES (N)

NX   Regional lymph nodes cannot be assessed

N0   No regional lymph node metastasis

N1   Regional lymph node metastasis

DISTANT METASTASIS (M)

MX   Distant metastasis cannot be assessed

M0   No distant metastasis

M1   Distant metastasis

HISTOPATHOLOGIC GRADE

GX   Grade cannot be assessed

G1   Well differentiated

G2   Moderately differentiated

G3   Poorly differentiated

G4   Undifferentiated

From Greene FL, et al.: *AJCC cancer staging manual,* ed 6, 2002, Springer-Verlag.

*Superficial tumor is located exclusively above the superficial fascia without invasion of the fascia; deep tumor is located either exclusively beneath the superficial fascia, superficial to the fascia with invasion of or through the fascia, or superficial and beneath the fascia. Retroperitoneal, mediastinal, and pelvic sarcomas are classified as deep tumors.

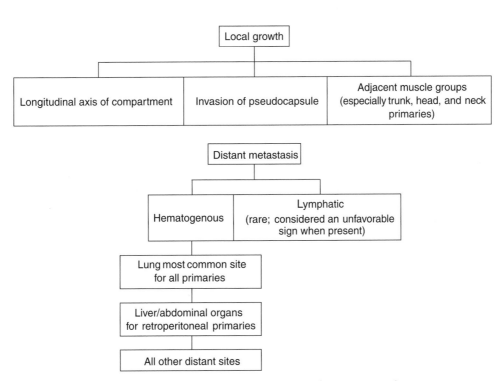

Figure 25-15. Patterns of soft tissue sarcoma (STS) spread. STS metastatic patterns progress from local invasion to the early hematogenous extension to the lung, liver, abdominal organs, and all other distant sites. Lymphatic spread is rare.

to contain invasive foci of tumor cells surrounds an STS. Therefore **shelling** out these tumors (removing the contents of the capsule) surgically is inadequate. For high-grade tumors, wide or radical margins of normal tissue are required. Wide and radical margins are defined for limb-sparing and amputation techniques for extremities. **Radical resections** include all structures in every involved compartment, whereas **wide resections** include the tumor, its pseudocapsule, and normal tissue in the compartment. If adjuvant radiation therapy is a consideration for extremity STS, a lateral incision is best for more effective lymphatic drainage and a longitudinal incision (along the long axis of the limb) is best.[20,51] When used with radiation therapy, LSS reduces the loss of function and improves local contral.[18,29,54] When radiation therapy is included in the treatment plan, factors related to operative and postoperative care to minimize wound healing complications are important. Achievement of hemostasis, avoidance of closure under tension, and use of skin flaps to eliminate dead spaces are helpful.[27] For STS tumors occurring in sites other than extremities, the disease management is particularly challenging. These sites often have fewer fascial planes to contain them and often encroach on major vasculature and adjacent organs. Despite this, for STS tumors in the head and neck, trunk, and abdomen and retroperitoneum, a properly executed surgical resection is still the most important treatment modality. Moreover, frequently these sites may not be amenable to curative doses of radiation because of the necessity of including critical dose-limiting structures, for example, brain, spinal cord, urinary bladder, kidney, and small bowel, in the tumor bed.

Radiation therapy. Based on the careful evaluation of individual patients, radiation therapy may be delivered in a variety of ways. Except for a few extremely small superficial tumors or when surgery is not medically recommended, radiation therapy is combined with surgery and, in some cases, with chemotherapy. A variety of techniques may be employed and radiation can be administered either preoperatively or postoperatively.

Preoperative radiation for STS in extremities has proven to be especially effective in improvement of local control when patients present with gross disease and/or have had previous biopsy.[6,7,15,32,45,51,53]

Generally accepted advantages include the following:
1. A smaller treatment volume will likely be possible because neither surgical manipulation nor disruption has taken place. The treatment volume will be planned from images demonstrating the extent of the tumor.
2. Because of tumor regression, less aggressive surgery may be possible.
3. The likelihood of surgical contamination caused by the release of viable tumor cells into the tumor bed or blood is reduced.
4. No delay in starting treatment is required.
5. The biologic effect of radiation is better in terms of tumoricidal activity because hypoxia associated with postoperative scarring is absent.

Disadvantages include the following:

1. Difficulties with postirradiation surgical wound healing may be more likely.
2. The precise extent and description of the tumor resulting from resection and direct observation are not available.[11,15,51]

Techniques include external beam therapy (including photon, electron, proton, and neutron beams), brachytherapy, intraoperative electron beam treatment, or some combination of these. These modalities may be delivered preoperatively and postoperatively to boost preoperative doses.

Postoperative external photon beam radiation continues to be effective for situations in which preoperative treatment is not feasible. With external beam therapy a shrinking-field technique is generally used. For extremities the initial field should include the entire compartment and/or wide margins up to 10 cm. The second volume treated is coned down to the tumor bed itself with narrower margins (±5 cm). The final volume is the primary tumor volume plus a 2- to 3-cm margin. The scar should receive the full dose by inclusion tangentially or boosted with bolus or electrons. No regional lymph nodes, except for rhabdomyosarcomas, synovial sarcomas, and epithelioid sarcomas, are included with radiation therapy techniques. Total circumferential radiation of extremities must be avoided by leaving at least a 1- to 3-cm strip of skin and soft tissue to avoid future excessive fibrosis and edema[15,32] (Fig. 25-16).

STSs in the paravertebral and head and neck tissues frequently are not amenable to complete surgical resection. In addition they often involve unfavorable geometry that may not be overcome with photon beams alone. When used in combination with megavoltage photon beams, proton beams have been effective. The physical characteristics of protons of having a finite range of penetration depths in tissue because of its Bragg peak effect and small penumbra allow manipulation of dose whereby doses to target volumes are high and the adjacent normal tissues are well within safe limits.[4,27,31]

Radiobiologically, fast neutrons should theoretically be effective in the treatment of these sarcomas. However, Bamberg et al.[4] reviewed the outcomes of a number of centers using this modality and determined that there currently is no evidence that neutron therapy is an improvement over conventional external beam treatment.

Brachytherapy is generally accomplished with catheters placed in the tumor bed at the time of resection. Iridium-192 (Ir-192) is loaded into the catheters after the fifth postoperative day to avoid wound healing problems.[9,50,61] Brachytherapy using Ir-192 is also a useful alternative for selected patients who have a recurrent extremity STS.[42] The use of high dose rate intraoperative radiation therapy (HDR-IORT) using Ir-192 has produced early encouraging results for retroperitoneal STS when combined with complete surgical resection and external photon beam radiation therapy.[1] HDR-IORT has been employed in the treatment of rhabdomyosarcoma in selected organ sites of infants and young children. Because time is critical for observation of long-term effects of radiation, this modality has been limited to

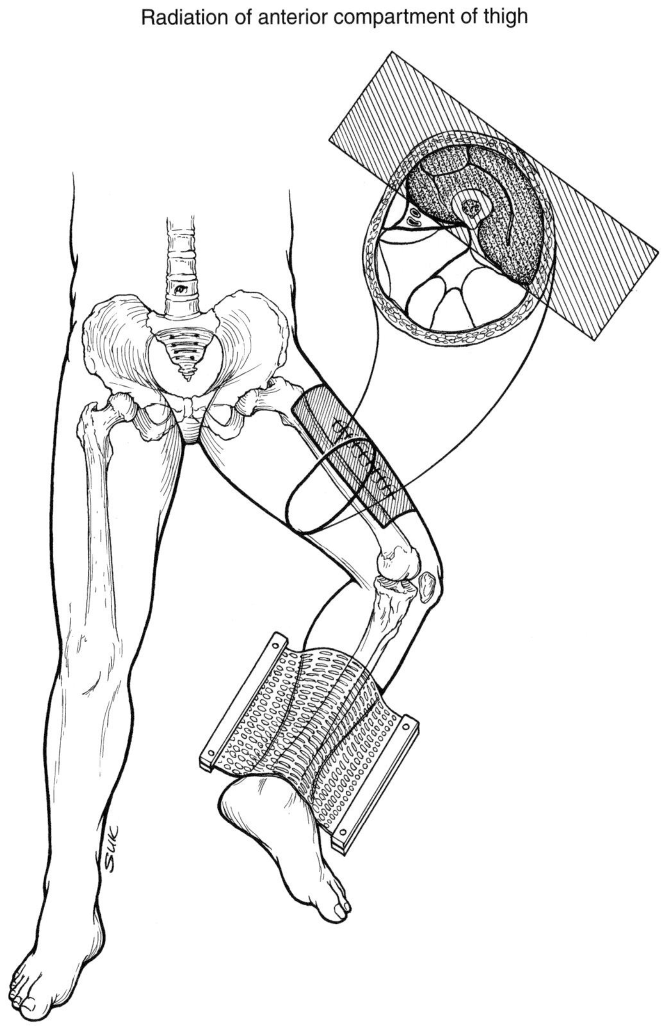

Radiation of anterior compartment of thigh

Figure 25-16. Appropriate treatment position demonstrating access to the tumor compartment.

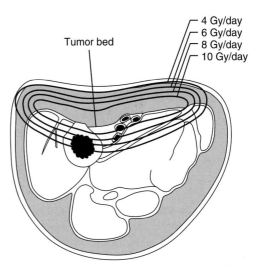

Figure 25-17. Cross section of an implant in the thigh showing the location of afterloading catheters in relation to the anterior compartment. *(From Nori D, Hilaris BS: Recent results in cancer research, vol 138, Berlin, Heidelberg, 1995, Springer-Verlag.)*

selected patients in narrowly defined clinical trials.[38] Superior results in limb salvage, functional preservation, and local control has been achieved with sealed-end temporary implants initiated 4 to 5 days following surgery involving extremity STS[41] (Fig. 25-17). Iodine-125 (I-125) is another radioactive source used in brachytherapy applications; it usually is used in limited ways and in selected patients with retroperitoneal and head and neck STS.[23,26,30] The inclusion of brachytherapy in the radiation therapy treatment plan is generally perceived as a mechanism to increase the total dose to the tumor and tumor bed when added to postoperative external beam radiation dose while maintaining safe levels of dose to surrounding normal structures. The planned brachytherapy dose depends on the way that it fits in the comprehensive treatment plan and the site involved.

Intraoperative electron beam radiation is another adjunctive modality for selected patients. This technique affords the delivery of a high dose to areas at risk with the advantage of sparing normal adjacent tissues. Doses are usually between 1000 and 2000 cGy, with a range of electron beam energies from 9 to 15 MeV.[56,57] A study evaluating IORT using both electrons and 100-kV x-ray photon beam for a variety of STS sites and histologic types reported encouraging results with recommendation for additional randomized phase III trials.[16]

Another factor in radiation therapy delivery that can be manipulated is that of altered fractionation schemes. Although used with some encouragement for Ewing's sarcoma of extremity bones, hyperfractionation (twice daily treatment), nonconventional fractionation schemes for connective tissue sarcomas continue to be recommended for further investigation and evaluation.[5,8]

Overall, STS requires high doses of radiation to achieve local control and long-term survival. A preoperative dose is usually limited to 5000 cGy with 180- to 200-cGy daily fractions. Postoperative shrinking fields are usually used to deliver a total dose of 6500 cGy with field reductions at 4500 to 5000 cGy and 5500 to 6000 cGy. With the use of a boost the total dose may exceed 7500 cGy. It is generally accepted that three-dimensional planning and external beam intensity modulation radiation therapy (IMRT) capabilities have improved the options for increased dose delivery to target volumes. These capabilities have had a positive influence in achieving currently improved long-term survival with limited morbidity. When combined with adequate surgery, modern radiation therapy techniques, and chemotherapy, the results for local and long-term control are further enhanced.

Chemotherapy. The use of chemotherapy has demonstrated some substantial advances, but optimal regimens do not appear to be established. A variety of drug programs have been investigated in which some patients have enjoyed relatively long periods of remission. The agents most often used in varying protocols include a combination of doxorubicin and dacarbazine: **CYVADIC** (cyclophosphamide [Cytoxan], vincristine, doxorubicin [Adriamycin], and dacarbazine), **ADCZ** (doxorubicin, dacarbazine, cisplatin, and vincristine), **IM** (ifosfamide methotrexate), **MAID** (methotrexate, doxorubicin, ifosfamide, and dacarbazine), and VAC (vincristine, dactinomycin, and cyclophosphamide). A study of 130 children with Ewing's sarcoma of soft tissues indicated that these sarcomas responded similar to rhabdomyosarcomas when given multimodality treatment. All of the patients received chemotherapy regimens with and without the addition of doxorubicin (DOX). Most of them also received radiation therapy. Survival at 10 years was most likely for patients with primaries in the head and neck, extremities, and trunk and for those who underwent grossly complete tumor removal before initiation of chemotherapy. No benefit was apparent from the addition of DOX to VAC chemotherapy to those patients with gross residual disease.[16] Controlled studies will continue to investigate sophisticated advances in combined modalities and their sequencing to improve the overall survival and quality of life in patients with STS.[15,17,51]

Role of Radiation Therapist

The technical competence of the radiation therapist is assumed. Although an understanding of the academic, scientific, and intellectual aspects of connective tissue sarcomas should not be minimized, the obligation to apply that information with meaningful caregiving skills is the therapist's opportunity to provide comprehensive attention to the patient. The predilection for bone and STS to occur in younger populations in anatomic sites where disfigurement is often a threat may require educational and communication techniques unique to children, teenagers, young adults, and middle-aged patients. Bony metastases may occur in elderly patients, who also require specific communication skills. The therapist's relationship with the patient is based on trust, professionalism, and knowledge of the disease. Because everyone involved in the care of the patient must fully understand the importance of daily treatments and the nature and severity of expected side effects, an assessment of the patient's physical, emotional, and coping status is essential in daily interactions with patients and their families. In this section, several roles of the radiation therapist are discussed, including the following: education, communication, assessment, and management of accessory medical equipment.

Education. Wilkinson[61] reported that 25% to 35% of clients indicate dissatisfaction with the information received about their treatment and nursing care. This report corroborated others in the literature that information about health care procedures reduces anxiety, pain, distressing side effects, and length of hospital stay.

Taenzer and Fisher's study[56] indicated that providing patient education is one of the skills that radiation therapists use most often. The educator role of the radiation therapist extends beyond dispensing information. It is an ongoing, integral part of the treatment process that includes the patient, family, and other health care team professionals. Just as traditional teachers use goals, objectives, and testing mechanisms in the educational process, therapists need to establish goals and objectives that are patient directed and then verify (test) patients for comprehension and understanding. Implementing these goals and objectives is a part of a formal or informal patient care plan custom designed to meet the needs of each patient. Teaching tools include the use of appropriate print materials written in terms easily understood by the patient and family, videos, slide-tapes, and support groups sharing information. In a study by Rainey,[47] two groups of patients undergoing their first course of radiation therapy were tested regarding the information they received. One group participated in a 12-minute slide-tape presentation that explained the way the department personnel, equipment, and related technical procedures worked together to produce a treatment plan and deliver a prescribed dose of radiation. The other group of 30 patients received a brochure to read. The data collected in the study showed those patients in the slide-tape group displayed increased understanding, lower anxiety levels, and better coping skills than the group receiving the brochure only. However, at the end of the course of treatment, both groups demonstrated equal levels of knowledge regarding their treatment. According to the data from the study, radiation therapy patients desire knowledge about their treatment, and continued intervention initiated by the therapist can have a positive effect on the patient's well being.

Just as it is important for some patients to be offered a lot of information about their treatment, others may not benefit from it. Radiation therapists are responsible for making professional evaluations and judgments concerning what and how much education is appropriate for each patient and family.

Education is not limited to patients and their families. Professional education provided by therapists is often necessary for other members of the health care team to share accurate information about radiation therapy treatment delivery and side effects, and interaction with other health professionals aids in providing optimal care for patients.

Communication. Disfigurement, loss of limbs, decreased motor functions, or a threat of any of these leads to heightened emotional responses typically described by cancer patients as feelings of denial, frustration, anger, depression, fear, grief, bereavement, rejection, and loss of control. Although Taenzer and Fisher[56] indicated that therapists reported offering emotional support and referrals to other professionals as nontechnical skills used frequently, they also indicated that these skills were among the most difficult to acquire and use effectively. Weintraub[59] described several responses from patients and families specific to radiation therapy treatment. These responses included a fear of treatment, a loss of control over health and destiny, treatment-related side effects, and financial implications of treatment.

Listening, attending, following, reflecting, touching, and questioning skills provide the basis for effective communication with the patient. Openness and assertiveness offers the patient a comfortable invitation to talk. Patients list talking to others as a therapeutic activity used in coping strategies for dealing with their cancers.[48] This is generally not different for patients with a bone or STS diagnosis and can be accomplished by the therapist on a daily basis, as well as by appropriate referrals to support groups or other health professionals as needed.

Assessment. Appraising and evaluating the patient's condition before, during, and after daily treatment is important for good cancer management of bone and STS tumors. In the treatment of patients with bone metastases, care must be taken to observe and evaluate the condition for further spread of the disease. Patient assessment and interventions obviously include the patient's pathophysiologic and emotional status. The cancericidal doses administered to achieve local control require a regular assessment of the skin's integrity. Monitoring of the anticipated erythema and dry and/or moist desquamation may necessitate a decision to withhold treatment until the radiation oncologist verifies confirmation to proceed. Many bone and STS patients are immunocompromised because of concomitant chemotherapy. Close observation for symptoms of infection and regular notation of blood values with appropriate interventions described by institutional policy is the therapist's responsibility. An evaluation of the patient's nutritional status and performance rating may also indicate the need for an intervention referral. Recognition of and responding to medical emergencies such as allergic reactions, adverse drug interactions, medical disorders, and cardiac arrest are included in the radiation therapist's purview of professional responsibilities, capabilities, and obligations.

As patients find emotional mechanisms to cope with the distress of an STS diagnosis, the radiation therapist should have the ability to recognize and support helpful responses. Identifying destructive responses is also important. Fawzy and Fawzy[23] describe reactions to behavioral, cognitive, and affective states that may be adaptive or maladaptive. These reactions are categorized as active-behavioral, active-cognitive, or avoidance methods. Radiation therapists must be comfortable with supporting healthy coping mechanisms and developing strategies to help patients alter destructive behaviors with appropriate referrals to other professionals when needed.

Monitoring medical equipment. Patients treated for connective tissue cancers may range from the very old (those with metastatic bone disease) to the extremely young (those with Ewing's sarcoma). The needs of these patients and the accessory medical equipment may include intravenous fluids, oxygen, urinary catheter, chest tubes, or shunts. In the case of pediatric and adolescent patients with these primaries, they may be recovering from radical surgery such as

amputation and/or undergoing adjuvant chemotherapy demanding appropriate observation, evaluation, and interventions. Patients treated under sedation may require additional intense monitoring and observation, for example, pulse oximeter. Attention to placement of these devices during the setup and positioning of the treatment equipment and monitoring of the patient during treatment are important for patient safety and accurate radiation dose delivery.

The radiation therapist's broad-based patient care responsibilities include the knowledge and understanding of connective tissue sarcomas as malignant processes and treatment delivery competency. The therapist is the patient's advocate in coordination of referrals for all aspects of conditions relevant to the patient's disease status and treatment.

Case Studies

Case I

A 36-year-old woman with a 1-year history of symptoms initially experienced a cracking sensation along the anterior left horizontal ramus of the mandible after opening her mouth widely. When pain developed with the cracking, she sought medical attention. The physician advised her to wait 2 weeks to see if the pain resolved. After 1 month, she returned to the physician because of increased pain. Radiographs demonstrated a suspicious lytic lesion. The patient agreed to a biopsy, which revealed an osteogenic sarcoma of the mandible.

Through consultations with the medical oncologist, surgical oncologist, and radiation oncologist, a plan of action was established. The plan called for the patient to receive two cycles of chemotherapy initially, followed by a surgical resection, two more cycles of chemotherapy, radiation therapy to the mandibular bed, a bone graft implantation, and two more cycles of chemotherapy.

The patient received her first two cycles of chemotherapy, which included doxorubicin, platinum, high-dose methotrexate, and leucovorin. She tolerated the chemotherapy fairly well, except for some morbidity from the platinum. She was then scheduled for the surgical resection, with the placement of an appliance to retain the shape of her face. She tolerated this procedure and adapted to the prosthesis quite well. After an adequate recuperation period the patient received another cycle of chemotherapy, followed by radiation therapy. She received a dose of 5000 cGy over a 5-week period.

The physician advised the patient to return for routine follow-up visits because of the aggressive nature of her disease. She followed his advice diligently, keeping her appointments as scheduled. This patient continues to be disease free 3 years after treatment.

Case II

A 52-year-old woman with a 2-year history of left calf pain and a 1-week history of dyspnea sought medical attention because the shortness of breath she experienced made work difficult. On examination the physician observed labored breathing by the patient and a mass in the left calf. The physician ordered a chest and left lower leg radiographs. The chest x-ray films revealed multiple bilateral pulmonary metastases with consolidation in the right lower lung base. The left lower leg radiographs indicated a soft tissue mass that was suspicious for a malignant process.

Biopsy results revealed a well-differentiated fibrosarcoma (MFH) of the left calf, and pulmonary washings were positive for metastatic sarcoma.

An additional metastatic workup included a CT scan of the chest, abdomen, and pelvis; an MRI scan of the lower leg; and a bone scan. The CT scan of the chest revealed extensive bilateral pulmonary metastases with a localized right pleural effusion. The bone scan showed a vague increased uptake in the left lower leg over the proximal fibular shaft, compatible with a periosteal reaction from a sarcoma. The MRI of the left lower leg revealed a 10 × 15 cm lesion deep in the posterior aspect of the left lower leg. The tumor abutted the proximal tibia and midtibia, with no evidence of cortical destruction. The patient's disease was staged as follows: T2 N0 M1 (lung).

Given all the options, the patient decided against surgery because of the morbidity involved; removal of the tumor would result in a large surgical deficit. She had an extensive vacation planned to visit family that she had not seen in several years, and it was important for her not to have difficulty walking.

The patient was immediately started on six cycles of chemotherapy using the following drugs: mesno, doxorubicin, isophosphamide, and MAID. She tolerated the chemotherapy well, complaining of fatigue, alopecia, nausea, and vomiting (controlled with antiemetics). Her hematologic status remained stable throughout the six cycles of drugs. After the completion of chemotherapy a repeat MRI scan of the lower leg and a chest x-ray film were obtained with the following results: The MRI scan demonstrated a significant reduction in the size of the tumor. The chest x-ray film revealed an excellent response with almost complete resolution of the bilateral pulmonary metastases and a complete resolution of the right localized pleural effusion.

Because the patient continued to complain of pain in the left lower leg, she was referred to the radiation oncology department for a consultation. The radiation oncologist considered all the options, including surgical intervention. Because surgery required the removal of the gastrocnemius muscle (lower calf muscle), causing a functionally impaired foot drop, the radiation oncologist decided to administer radiation therapy for the palliation of pain. High doses of radiation are needed to adequately control this disease. Therefore the radiation oncologist planned to deliver 5000 cGy in 20 fractions at 250 cGy per fraction, which is a slightly accelerated fractionation because the patient had a planned vacation. If after 5000 cGy was reached her chest x-ray film demonstrated the disease to be in remission, an additional 1250 cGy would be delivered to a reduced field. The patient tolerated her treatments well with minimal side effects. The patient had less pain and was encouraged to take her vacation and return for a follow-up.

After returning from her vacation (which was about 2 months after the completion of her treatments) the patient returned for a check-up. Her only complaint was swelling of the left ankle and limping after prolonged walking. The radiation oncologist ordered a chest x-ray film, which demonstrated the growth of the pulmonary nodules and some right pleuritic pain. She was sent home and told to call if she had any further problems before her follow-up in 1 month.

Within 3 weeks time, the patient developed some expressive aphasia and was brought into the hospital for a metastatic workup. A CT scan of the brain revealed a large, solitary lesion in the left frontoparietal region. The patient was started on a high-dose regimen of steroids and palliative radiation therapy to her whole brain. After 3 days of treatment the patient's physician discontinued the treatments. The patient subsequently succumbed to central nervous system disease 2 days later, just 5 months after her initial diagnosis.

Case III

A 15-year-old girl experienced an injury playing field hockey. She had a bruise and some soreness of the right pelvic area. After a few weeks the bruise and soreness persisted, so her parents started taking her to their family chiropractor. This went on for approximately 4 months with no relief. The girl's parents then made an appointment for her to see a physician. After a physical examination the physician noted a large right pelvic mass obscuring the right iliac crest. This prompted an immediate investigation. An ultrasound of the pelvis was obtained, revealing a solid right pelvic mass. Radiographs of the pelvis were then ordered and demonstrated an onionskin appearance of the bone of the right iliac crest with extensive soft tissue involvement, indicating a possible Ewing's sarcoma. Arrangements were then made to obtain a biopsy of the area for confirmation of the diagnosis. This was carried out a few days later, and the diagnosis of Ewing's sarcoma was confirmed.

Within the next few weeks, several consultations were scheduled with surgical oncologists, medical oncologists, and radiation oncologists. A metastatic workup was performed during this time. The patient and her parents decided to initiate chemotherapy using vincristine, doxorubicin, and cyclophosphamide (Cytoxan) in hopes of reducing the size of the tumor, which measured 10 × 15 cm. If chemotherapy resulted in regression of the tumor, surgical intervention would be considered.

The patient was started on her first course of chemotherapy, and after 2 months a dramatic regression in the soft tissue disease was noted. The tumor measured 3 × 2 cm, making surgery feasible. She was asymptomatic, except for alopecia from the chemotherapy, and had no complaints of limping or difficulty walking. She was then referred back to the surgical oncologist.

Because of the location of the tumor, surgical intervention was possible but not without risks. If the patient chose surgery, she would have a large scar around her waist and probably significant functional deficit of the right leg. The use of surgery would, however, increase the chance of local control and decrease the chance of a second malignancy caused by radiation therapy. With that information in mind, the patient and family were sent for a radiation oncology consult so they could make a decision on her extended management.

The radiation oncologist explained the immediate and long-term effects of radiation therapy. These included a possible second malignancy, intestinal obstruction, fatigue, diarrhea, and cramping. Considering all the information provided by the surgical and radiation oncologists, the patient opted for radiation therapy.

The plan was to deliver 4500 cGy through opposed anteroposterior/posteroanterior (AP/PA) portals with a 4-cm margin. After 4500 cGy was reached the area would receive a boost to 5580 cGy through opposed oblique portals to spare the anterior bowel. The patient tolerated the treatments fairly well, except for some hematologic depletion as a result of radiation therapy and chemotherapy being given at the same time. These depletions required unscheduled hospital admissions and transfusions.

Approximately 2 months after the completion of the treatment, she had a follow-up visit. No complaints were noted from the radiation therapy directly, but fatigue lingered partly because of the chemotherapy and radiation therapy. The decision was made for the patient to continue with her scheduled course of chemotherapy, with careful monitoring of her blood values.

Approximately 6 months after the initial diagnosis the patient was admitted for her final round of chemotherapy and was doing well. She tolerated her chemotherapy treatments without much morbidity and was discharged home. She was still disease free 1 year later.

Case IV

A 73-year-old woman presented to her primary care physician with an achy sensation and mass in her left forearm that had been getting progressively larger for the previous 3 to 4 months. She was advised to initiate diagnostic procedures to rule out or confirm malignancy.

The initial workup included an MRI scan, which revealed a significant tumor-like mass in the left proximal forearm. Chest radiographs were normal as were blood and chemistry values. The patient was referred to an orthopedic oncologist and a CT-guided biopsy of the mass was performed.

The result of the biopsy showed a myxoid MFH. Following consultation with the oncology team physician, the patient was referred to radiation oncology for preoperative radiation.

The radiation therapy treatment plan was to include initial preoperative radiation in hope that there would be significant tumor shrinkage allowing definitive resection with possible additional intraoperative radiation boost, Ir-192 brachytherapy implant, or postoperative external beam irradiation as deemed appropriate at the time of resection. The following treatment technique was then implemented:

Region treated: left forearm
Modality: 6-MeV photons
Technique: Left Anterior Oblique/Right Posterior Oblique (LAO/RPO) to 4600 cGy, then reduce field
Field size: 18 × 11 cm with custom blocking
Dose/fraction: 200 cGy
Number of fractions: 26
Total dose: 5200 cGy
Elapsed days: 36

The patient tolerated the treatments well with mild to moderate erythematous skin reaction. Minimal shrinkage of the tumor was detectable by examination at the completion of treatment. This was confirmed by an MRI scan. There was no compromise of neurologic or vascular status.

The patient was allowed 4 weeks to recuperate. Resection of the tumor was then performed. The margins were clear and an intraoperative boost to the initial tumor bed was also performed. The treatment parameters for the intraoperative treatment included the following:

Region treated: left forearm
Modality: 6-MeV electrons
Field size: 10-cm round IORT cone
Dose: 1000 cGy in one fraction
Normalization: prescribed to 85% isodose line
Bolus: 1-cm wet gauze placed in surgical incision
Linac setting: 1075 MU

The patient tolerated the surgery and radiation well. Surgical oncology continues to follow the patient who is disease-free after 1 year with only minimal skin changes to the treated area of the forearm.

Review Questions

1. The incidence rate of bone cancer is highest during which of the following?
   a. Infancy
   b. Adulthood
   c. Adolescence
   d. Equal for all ages

2. A nonosseous malignant tumor of the marrow is which of the following?
   a. Fibrosarcoma
   b. Chondrosarcoma
   c. Osteosarcoma
   d. Multiple myeloma

3. Bone lesions resulting from primary sites elsewhere in the body are which of the following?
   a. Osteosarcoma
   b. Multiple myeloma
   c. Metastatic disease
   d. Chondrosarcoma

4. The most common site of a primary bone sarcoma is which of the following?
   a. Epiphyseal
   b. Metaphyseal
   c. Diaphyseal
   d. None of the above

5. Neoplasms, including those in connective tissues, seen in adult tissues are affected by metabolic stimulation from which of the following?
   a. Long-standing Paget's disease
   b. Long-standing fracture
   c. Long-standing sarcoma
   d. Long-standing metastasis

6. Prognostic indicators for patients with primary bone cancer include all *except* which of the following?
   a. Age
   b. Gender
   c. Location
   d. Weight

7. The most common site of metastasis from primary bone cancer is which of the following?
   a. Brain
   b. Bowel
   c. Lung
   d. Distal extremities

8. Malignant plasma cell tumors are known as which of the following?
   a. Multiple myeloma
   b. Giant cell tumors
   c. Fibrosarcoma
   d. Melanoma

9. Which of the following may be used in treating metastatic bone disease resulting from primary prostate or breast cancer?
   a. Technetium-99
   b. Iodine-131
   c. Strontium-89
   d. Iodine-125

10. The most common prognostic factor in Ewing's sarcoma is which of the following?
    a. Gender
    b. Age
    c. Extent of the disease at the time of the diagnosis
    d. Height

11. The epidemiology of STS includes which of the following parameters?
    a. The estimated incidence in the United States is 10,000 new cases per year
    b. The incidence is more common in children than adults
    c. A slight predilection exists for incidence in females compared with males
    d. The incidence in the Pacific Northwest is significantly higher than other areas of the United States

12. Although the exact cause of STS is unknown, which of the following factors have been implicated?
    a. Prior irradiation for benign diseases
    b. Appearance as a second primary 5 to 15 years after high-dose radiation therapy for other cancers
    c. The predisposition of von Recklinghausen's disease for certain STSs
    d. Prior exposure to defoliant chemicals
    e. All of the above

13. Factors or clinical signs that are incorporated in the staging systems and considered appropriate as general prognostic indicators for STS include which of the following?
    I.   Histology
    II. Size
    III. Site
    a. I and II
    b. I and III
    c. II and III
    d. I, II, and III

14. Regional lymph nodes are generally not included in the treatment portals for STS. Which of the following are exceptions for this statement?
    I.   Rhabdomyosarcoma
    II. Synovial sarcoma
    III. Epithelioid sarcomas
    a. I and II
    b. I and III
    c. II and III
    d. I, II, and III

15. The rationale for leaving a 1- to 3-cm strip of skin and soft tissue rather than total circumferential irradiation of an extremity being treated for STS includes

a. Decreases excessive erythema
b. Promotes healing of the incision scar
c. Avoids future excessive fibrosis and edema
d. Increases future mobility for the treated limb

16. Advantages of preoperative radiation therapy for STS include
    a. Decreased difficulty with postirradiation surgical wound healing
    b. Availability of the precise extent and description of the tumor
    c. Possibility of a larger treatment volume
    d. Less aggressive surgery possible because of tumor regression

17. Intraoperative electron beam radiation usually involves energies ranging from 9 to 15 MeV with doses to which of the following range?
    a. 1000 to 2000 cGy
    b. 1500 to 2500 cGy
    c. 2000 to 2500 cGy
    d. 2500 to 3000 cGy

18. Generally, a postoperative radiation shrinking-field technique plans the first field reduction at which of the following dose?
    a. 3000 to 3500 cGy
    b. 3500 to 4000 cGy
    c. 4000 to 4500 cGy
    d. 4500 to 5000 cGy

19. With the use of a shrinking-field technique and a boost, the total dose for STS may exceed which of the following?
    a. 6000 cGy
    b. 6500 cGy
    c. 7000 cGy
    d. 7500 cGy

20. STS metastasis occurs primarily by which of the following?
    I.   Local invasion along adjacent, anatomically defined planes
    II. Hematologic pathways to the lung and other sites
    III. Extension to regional lymph nodes
    a. I and II
    b. I and III
    c. II and III
    d. I, II, and III

Questions to Ponder

1. Explain why patients with Ewing's sarcoma of the pelvis carry a poorer prognosis than patients with the same tumor of an extremity.

2. Define skip metastases and explain how radiation therapy can be used to treat these lesions.

3. Describe the shrinking-field technique and how it is used to control skeletal lesions.

4. Explain the difficulty in diagnosing primary bone tumors and the challenge that physicians face in doing so.

5. Define limb-sparing surgery, and describe its use in treating primary bone and STS tumors.

6. Consider the relationships between the surgical procedures used and radiation therapy planning for a patient who has an extremity STS. Describe, for example, the rationale for postoperative radiation therapy after a wide resection.

7. For extremity bone and STS, incomplete total circumferential radiation with an external photon beam is recommended to avoid future excessive fibrosis and edema. What is the biologic rationale for implementing this technique?

8. Despite the evidence that lymphatic involvement of STS is rare, the radiation therapy technique selected for rhabdomyosarcomas, synovial sarcomas, and epithelioid sarcomas frequently includes the regional lymph nodes. Explain the rationale for this exception.

9. A shrinking-field external beam is generally used for the treatment of an STS with radiation therapy. Discuss the biologic rationale for this technique. Why are the recommended dose ranges effective? Why is a boost with bolus or electrons to the scar frequently required?

10. The most common primary sites for STSs are the extremities (65%). The remaining sites are anywhere in the extraskeletal anatomy. Use the embryologic and morphologic ancestry of STS to explain the reason that this is true.

REFERENCES

1. Alektiar KM et al: High-dose rate intraoperative radiation therapy (HDR-IORT) for retroperitoneal sarcomas, *Int J Radiat Oncol Biol Phys* 47:157-1163, 2000.
2. American Cancer Society: *Cancer response system, malignant bone tumors,* #406057, Atlanta, 1996, The American Cancer Society.
3. American Cancer Society: *Cancer facts and figures,* Atlanta, 2003, The American Cancer Society.
4. Bamberg M, Schmidberger H, Hoffman W: *Radiotherapy in the treatment of inoperable and advanced soft tissue sarcomas in adults: recent results in cancer research,* vol 138, Berlin-Heidelberg, 1995, Springer-Verlag.
5. Barbieri E et al: Nonconventional fractionation in radiotherapy of the musculoskeletal sarcomas, *Tumori* 84:167-170, 1998.
6. Barkely H et al: Treatment of soft tissue sarcoma by pre-operative irradiation and conservative surgical resection, *Int J Radiat Oncol Biol Phys* 14:693-699, 1988.
7. Basso-Ricci S et al: An extravisceral soft tissue sarcoma: effectiveness of radiation treatment and problems of radiotherapy and radiosurgical treatment, *Panminerva Med* 34(2):69-76, 1992.
8. Bolek TW et al: Local control and functional results after twice-daily radiotherapy for Ewing's sarcoma of the extremities, *Int J Radiat Oncol Biol Phys* 35:687-602, 1996.
9. Brennan MF et al: The role of multi-modality therapy in soft tissue sarcoma, *Ann Surg* 214:3328-336, 1991.
10. Chukhlovin A: Enhanced ex vivo apoptosis of peripheral granulocytes is a sufficient factor of neutropenia following myeloablative chemotherapy, *Leukemia Res* 24:507-509, 2000.
11. Conlon KC, Brennan MF: Soft tissue sarcomas. In Murphy GP, Lawrence WL Jr, Lenhard RE Jr, editors: *The American Cancer Society textbook of clinical oncology,* ed 2, Atlanta, 1995, The American Cancer Society.
12. Costa J et al: The grading of soft tissue sarcomas: results of a clinico-histiopathologic correlation in a series of 163 cases, *Cancer* 53:530-541, 1984.
13. Dannaher CI, Taniburro CH, Yam LT: Occupational carcinogenesis: the Louisville experience with vinyl chloride-associated hepatic angiosarcoma, *Am J Med* 70:279-287, 1981.
14. DeVita VT Jr, Hellman S, Rosenberg SA: *Cancer: principles and practice of oncology,* Philadelphia, 1993, JB Lippincott.
15. Doosenbury KE, Thompson RC, Levitt SH: Extremity soft tissue sarcoma in adults. In Levitt SH, Khan FM, Potish RA, editors: *Levitt and Tapley's technological basis of radiation therapy: practical clinical applications,* ed 2, Malvern, Pa, 1992, Lea & Febiger.
16. Dubois JB et al: Intra-operative radiotherapy in soft tissue sarcomas, *Radiother Oncol* 34:160-163, 1995.
17. Eilber FR, Eckhardt J, Morton DI: Advances in the treatment of sarcomas of the extremity: current status of limb salvage, *Cancer Suppl* 54(11):2695-2701, 1984.
18. Eilber FR et al: Progress in the recognition and treatment of soft tissue sarcoma, *Cancer* 65:660-666, 1990.
19. Enneking WF: *Staging of musculoskeletal neoplasms: current concepts of disease and treatment of bone and soft tissue tumors,* Heidelberg, Germany, 1984, Springer-Verlag.
20. Enneking WF: A system for staging musculoskeletal neoplasms, *Clin Orthop* 204:9-24, 1986.
21. Evans RG: The bone. In Cox JD, editor: *Moss' radiation oncology: rationale, technique, results,* ed 7, St. Louis, 1994, Mosby.
22. Ewing J: Diffuse endothelioma of bone, *Proc N Y Pathol Soc* 21:17-24, 1921.
23. Fawzy FFI, Fawzy NW: Intervention for cancer patients, *Gen Hosp Psychiatry* 16:1511-191, 1994.
24. Fleming ID et al: *AJCC cancer staging handbook,* ed 5, Philadelphia, 1998, Lippincott-Raven.
25. Gaspar LE et al: Primary cerebral fibrosarcomas: clinicopathologic study and review of the literature, *Cancer* 72:3277-3281, 1993.
26. Glutin PH et al: Brachytherapy of recurrent tumors of the skull base and spine with I-125 sources, *Neurosurgery* 20:938-945, 1987.
27. Hug EB et al: *Combined surgery and radiotherapy for conservative management of soft tissue sarcomas: recent results in cancer research,* vol 38, Berlin-Heidelberg, 1995, Springer-Verlag.
28. Jameel-Ahmed M et al: Soft tissue sarcomas in Kuwait: a review of 114 patients, *Clin Radiol* 38:27-29, 1987.
29. Kang H et al: Soft tissue sarcoma and military service in Vietnam: case-control study, *J Natl Cancer Inst* 79:693-699, 1987.
30. Karakkousis CP et al: Feasibility of limb salvage and survival in soft tissue and survival in soft tissue sarcomas, *Cancer* 57:484-491, 1986.
31. Koehler AM, Preston WM: Protons in radiation therapy: comparative dose distribution of protons, photons and electrons, *Radiology* 104:1911, 1972.
32. Kumar PP, Good RR: Interstitial I-125 implantation in the treatment of retroperitoneal soft tissue sarcoma report of a case, *Acta Radiol Oncol* 15:37-39, 1986.
33. Lawrence W et al: Adult soft tissue sarcomas' pattern of care: survey of the American College of Surgeons, *Ann Surg* 205:349-359, 1987.
34. Maine Medical Center, Nursing Service: *Strontium 89,* Portland, Me, 1994, The Maine Medical Center.
35. Marieb E: *Human anatomy and physiology,* Redwood City, California, 1989, Benjamin-Cummings.
36. McGinn CJ, Lawrence TS: soft tissue sarcomas (excluding retroperitoneum). In Perez CA, Brady LW, editors: *Principles and practice of radiation oncology,* ed 3, Philadelphia, 1998, Lippincott.
37. Moss WT: *Radiation oncology,* ed 6, St. Louis, 1989, Mosby.
38. Nag S, Grecula J, Ruyman FB: Aggressive chemotherapy, organ preserving surgery and high dose rate remote brachytherapy in the treatment of rhabdomyosarcoma in infants and young children, *Cancer* 71:2769-2776, 1993.
39. Niederhuber JE: *Current therapy in oncology,* St. Louis, 1993, Mosby.

40. Nitti D et al: Management of primary sarcomas of the retroperitoneum, *Eur J Surg Oncol* 19:355-360, 1993.

41. Nori D, Hilaris BS: *Role of brachytherapy in the treatment of soft tissue sarcomas of the extremities-techniques and results: recent results in cancer research,* vol 138, Berlin-Heidelberg, 1995, Springer-Verlag.

42. Nori D et al: Role of brachytherapy in recurrent extremity sarcoma in patients treated with prior surgery and irradiation, *Int J Radiat Oncol Bio Phys* 209:1229-1233, 1991.

43. Perez CA: *Principles and practice of radiation oncology,* Philadelphia, ed 2, 1992, JB Lippincott.

44. Poglod R, Kraj M, Maj S: Effect of recombinant human granulocyte colony stimulating factor on granulocytopenia induced by cytotoxic chemotherapy in patients with multiple myeloma, *Materia Medica Polona* 27(3):83-89,1995.

45. Pritchard JD: Malignant tumors in bone: In Murphy GP, Lawrence WL Jr, Lenhard RE Jr, editors: *The American Cancer Society textbook of clinical oncology,* ed 2, Atlanta, 1995, The American Cancer Society.

46. Raina V et al: Whole blood harvested after granulocyte-colony stimulating factor (Neupogen) mobilization, and reinfused unprocessed after high-dose melphalan treatment, accelerates hematopoietic recovery in patients with multiple myeloma, *Cancer* 77:1073-1078, 1996.

47. Rainey L: Effects of preparatory patient education for radiation oncology patients, *Cancer* 56:1056-1061, 1985.

48. Raleigh E: Sources of hope in chronic illness, *Oncol Nurs Forum* 19:443-446, 1992.

49. Raney RB et al: Ewing's sarcoma of soft tissues in childhood: a report from the Intergroup Rhabdomyosarcoma Study, 1972 to 1991, *J Clin Oncol* 15:573-582, 1997.

50. Rosenberg SA, Suit HD, Baker LH: Sarcomas of soft tissues. In De Vita VT, Hellman S, Rosenberg SA, editors: *Cancer: principles and practices of oncology,* Philadelphia, 1993, JB Lippincott.

51. Rosier RN, Constine LS III: Soft tissue sarcoma. In Rubin PO, McDonald S, Qazi R, editors: *Clinical oncology: a multi-disciplinary approach for physicians and students,* ed 7, Philadelphia, 1993, WB Saunders.

52. Rubin P: *Clinical oncology,* Philadelphia, 1993, WB Saunders.

53. Shiu MH et al: Brachytherapy and function-saving resection of soft tissue sarcoma arising in the limb, *Int J Radiat Oncol Biol Phys* 21:1488-1492, 1991.

54. Silverberg E, Boring C, Squires T: Cancer statistics, *Cancer* 40:7-24, 1990.

55. Simon MA, Enneking WF: The management of soft tissue sarcomas of the extremities, *J Bone Joint Surg* 58(3);317-327, 1976.

56. Taenzer P, Fisher P: Psychosocial issues in radiation therapy, *Can J Med Radiat Technol* 20(2):81, 1989.

57. Tepper JE, Suit HD: The role of radiation therapy in the treatment of sarcoma of soft tissue, *Cancer Invest* 3:587-592, 1985.

58. Wallace SR et al: Abnormalities of bone marrow mesenchymal cells in multiple myeloma patients, *Cancer* 91:1219-1230, 2001.

59. Weintraub FN: Coping with cancer treatment: family response to radiation therapy. In Dow KH, Hilderly LJ, editors: *Nursing care in radiation oncology,* Philadelphia, 1992, WB Saunders.

60. Wijnmaalen A et al: Angiosarcoma of the breast following lumpectomy, axillary node dissection and radiotherapy for primary breast cancer: three case reports and a review of the literature, *Int J Radiat Oncol Biol Phys* 26:135-139, 1993.

61. Wilkinson S: Confusions and challenges, *Nurs Times* 88(35):25, 1992.

62. Willett CG et al: Intra-operative electron beam radiation for primary locally advanced rectal and rectosigmoid carcinoma, *J Clin Oncol* 9:843-849, 1991.

63. Willett CG et al: Intra-operative electron beam radiation therapy for retroperitoneal soft tissue sarcoma, *Cancer* 68:278-283, 1991.

BIBLIOGRAPHY

Rubinstein Z, Morag B: The role of radiology in the diagnosis and treatment of osteosarcoma. In Katznelson A, Nerubay J, editors: *Osteosarcoma: new trend in diagnosis and treatment,* New York, 1982, Alan R Liss.

Sapherson DA et al: Atypical progression of multiple myeloma with extensive extramedullary disease, *J Clin Pathol* 47:269-271, 1994.

Sim FH, Ivans JC, Pritchard DJ: Surgical treatment of osteogenic sarcoma at the Mayo Clinic, *Cancer Treat Rep* 62:205, 1978.

Thomas PRM et al: The management of Ewing's sarcoma: role of radiotherapy in local control, *Cancer Treat Rep* 68:703, 1984.

Trigg ME, Glaubiger D, Nesbit ME: The frequency of isolated CNS involvement in Ewing's sarcoma, *Cancer* 49:2404, 1982.

Urtasum RC, McConnachie PR: Disappearance of osteosarcoma after irradiation: immunological observations, *J Can Assoc Radiol* 27:80, 1975.

Watts HG: Introduction to resection of musculoskeletal sarcomas, *Clin Orthop* 153:31, 1980.

Weichselbaum RR, Cassady JR: Radiation therapy in osteosarcoma. In Jaffe N, editor: *Solid tumors in childhood,* Boca Raton, Fla, 1983, CRC Press.

Wist E et al: Primary retroperitoneal sarcoma: a review of 36 cases, *Acta Radio Oncol* 24:305-310, 1985.

Zelefsky MF et al: Limb salvage in soft tissue sarcoma involving neurovascular structures using combined surgical resection and brachytherapy, *Int J Radiat Oncol Biol Phys* 19:913-918, 1990.

Zornig C et al: Retroperitoneal sarcoma in a series of 51 adults, *Eur J Surg Oncol* 18:475-480, 1992.

Zornig C et al: Soft tissue sarcoma of the extremities and trunk in the adult: report of 124 cases, *Langenbecks Arch Chir* 377:28-33, 1992.

Zucker JM et al: Intensive systemic chemotherapy in localized Ewing's sarcoma in childhood, *Cancer* 52:415, 1983.

26

Lymphoreticular System

Sally Green

Outline

Key Terms

Akimbo
Ann Arbor staging system
Autologous bone marrow stem
    cell transplants
B symptoms
Contiguous
Extended-field irradiation
Involved-field radiation
Mantle field

Oophoropexy
Paraaortic field
Peyer's patches
Pruritus
Reed-Sternberg cell
Staging laparotomy
Total-nodal irradiation
Waldeyer's ring

L ymphomas are the predominant cancers of the lymphoreticular system. The two main categories of lymphomas are Hodgkin's lymphoma (also called Hodgkin's disease [HD]) and non-Hodgkin's lymphoma (NHL). Thomas Hodgkin, an English pathologist, identified lymphoma in 1832 as a clinical entity distinct from inflammation. By the end of the nineteenth century, Hodgkin's disease was distinguished from other lymphomas and leukemias.

HODGKIN'S LYMPHOMA

Hodgkin's lymphoma is treated as a separate category of lymphomas because of the presence of the **Reed-Sternberg cell** in the lymph nodes of Hodgkin's patients, and because Hodgkin's spreads in a predictable, systematic or contiguous pattern through the lymph system. The Reed-Sternberg cell is a giant connective tissue cell containing one or two large nuclei. The presence of this cell determines whether the diagnosis is Hodgkin's or NHL.

Epidemiology

In the United States approximately 7400 new cases of Hodgkin's disease were reported in 2003, with 1400 deaths.[1] Hodgkin's lymphoma accounts for only 6% of the newly diagnosed cancers per year. Approximately 1000 more cases occurred in men than in women, indicating a slight male predominance. Worldwide, Hodgkin's is more frequent in developed countries than in undeveloped countries. To date, no explanation exists to account for this phenomenon.

Hodgkin's lymphoma occurs in young people, most commonly those between the ages of 11 and 30, with the median age of 26 years at the time of the diagnosis. Another peak of incidence takes place between 75 and 80 years of age. Hodgkin's lymphoma is rare in children younger than 10 years.

Etiology

The causes of Hodgkin's lymphoma remain a mystery to researchers, who have not yet found conclusive evidence linking Hodgkin's to environmental or occupational exposure or to genetic predisposition. Although clusters of patients with Hodgkin's lymphoma are present in some communities, data have been insufficient to determine whether the origin of the disease is viral or contagious. However, components of the Epstein-Barr virus genome are in the cellular deoxyribonucleic acid (DNA) of the Reed-Sternberg cells involved in this disease. A link between a prior infection with the Epstein-Barr virus and Hodgkin's disease has been investigated. (The Epstein-Barr virus is found in the cell cultures of Burkitt's lymphoma and is also associated with infectious mononucleosis). Most cases in the United States are not Epstein-Barr virus related.[13] Another risk factor for Hodgkin's is defective T-cell functioning.

Prognostic Indicators

The histology of Hodgkin's has the least effect on the prognosis of a particular patient, whereas the stage of the disease has the greatest effect. In other words, the later the stage, the worse the prognosis. In the later stages, more bulky disease is present, and the risk of a relapse after treatment is greater with increased bulky disease.

More males than females are diagnosed with Hodgkin's lymphoma, and the prognosis is also slightly worse for males. Gender may also influence the choice of treatment, based on a consideration of toxicities to the reproductive system. Fertility may be preserved in most men through the use of radiation therapy but not with alkylating agents (chemotherapy). In women the ovaries cannot be completely protected during radiation therapy, and some women experience menopause after radiation therapy. Youth is a favorable prognostic factor, with younger patients (those in their teens to twenties) doing better than older patients, who cannot tolerate the aggressive treatment. Hodgkin's lymphoma is likewise difficult to manage in children because of the need to limit radiation therapy fields because of the effect on the growth process, especially in the skeletal system. The extent of the disease, the presence of B symptoms, the number of sites of involvement, the presence of the disease in the lower abdomen, splenic involvement, and an elevation of serum markers (such as erythrocyte sedimentation rate) are all factors influencing the natural history of the disease.

Anatomy and Lymphatics

A review of the lymphatic system is important for understanding the nature of Hodgkin's lymphoma and NHLs. The lymph system originates in the lymphatic capillaries. The capillaries merge to form the lymphatic vessels, which in turn lead to the collecting ducts that unite with the veins in the thorax (see Chapter 18).

The kidney-bean-shaped lymph nodes are less than 2 cm in length and enclosed by a capsule of white fibrous connective tissue. The lymph nodes occur in chains or clusters along the lymphatic vessels. The primary function of the lymph nodes is the production of lymphocytes and the filtration of foreign particles and cellular debris from the lymph before it is returned to the circulatory system. The major lymph nodes (Fig. 26-1) are as follows:
1. Waldeyer's ring and cervical, preauricular, and occipital lymph nodes
2. Supraclavicular and infraclavicular lymph nodes
3. Axillary lymph nodes
4. Thorax (includes hilar and mediastinal nodes)
5. Abdominal cavity (includes paraaortic nodes)
6. Pelvic cavity (includes iliac nodes)
7. Inguinal and femoral lymph nodes

After leaving the nodes, the lymph vessels merge to form the larger lymphatic trunks. The trunks drain lymph from large regions of the body and are named for the regions they serve, including the following: lumbar trunk, intestinal trunk, intercostal and bronchomediastinal trunks, subclavian trunk, and jugular trunk. The lymphatic trunks join one of two collecting ducts: the thoracic or right lymph duct. Then the lymph reenters the venous system just before the blood returns to the right atrium of the heart. The thymus and spleen are lymphatic organs whose functions are closely related to the lymph nodes. The thymus contains large numbers of lymphocytes (called thymocytes), most of which remain inactive. However, some develop into T lymphocytes, which play a part in the immune process.

The spleen is the largest lymphatic organ. It resembles a large lymph node in its structure, but its cavities are filled with blood instead of lymph. The spleen filters the blood similar to the way that lymph nodes filter lymphatic fluid, but through the action of its phagocytes, it destroys damaged red blood cells and the remains of ruptured cells carried in the blood. The splenic lymphocytes help in the body's defense against infection.

Clinical Presentation

Hodgkin's lymphoma usually appears as a painless mass that the patient discovers. The most common sites of presentation are in the neck and supraclavicular regions. Mediastinal masses are usually detected on a radiograph of the chest. Most patients have the disease above the diaphragm.

Approximately one third of the patients also experience the following systemic symptoms: unexplained fevers (over 38° C, or 100.4° F), drenching night sweats, and weight loss of 10% of their body weight in 6 months. These are referred to as **B symptoms.** Generalized **pruritus** (severe itching) and/or alcohol-induced pain in the disease-involved tissues may also be included as B symptoms but are present only in some instances.

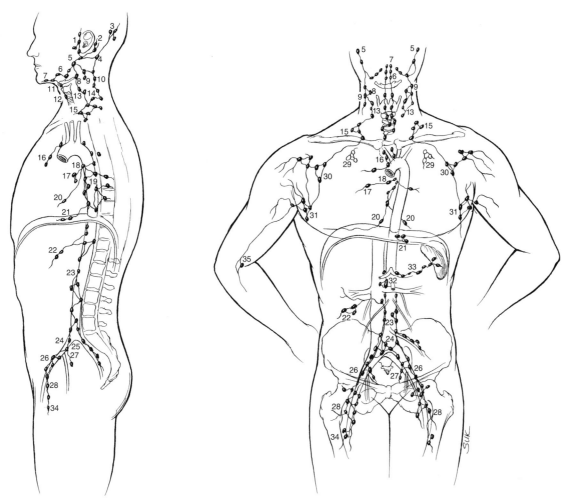

Figure 26-1. Major lymph node regions of the abdomen and pelvis. *1,* Preauricular; *2,* mastoid; *3,* occipital; *4,* upper cervical; *5,* parotid; *6,* submaxillary; *7,* submental; *8,* jugulodigastric; *9,* upper deep cervical; *10,* spinal accessory chain; *11,* infrahyoid; *12,* pretracheal; *13,* jugulo-omohyoid; *14,* lower deep cervical; *15,* supraclavicular; *16,* mediastinal; *17,* interlobar; *18,* intertracheal; *19,* posterior mediastinal; *20,* lateral pericardial; *21,* diaphragmatic; *22,* mesenteric; *23,* paraaortic; *24,* common iliac; *25,* lateral sacral; *26,* external iliac; *27,* hypogastric; *28,* inguinal; *29,* interpectoral; *30,* axillary apex; *31,* axillary; *32,* cisterna chyli; *33,* splenic; *34,* femoral; *35,* epitrochlear.

Sometimes Hodgkin's lymphoma is discovered during pregnancy, but pregnancy per se has no effect on the natural history. Pregnancy is merely coincidental because of the age-group of the patients. Patients testing positive for the human immunodeficiency virus (HIV) are not at a greater risk than the general population for developing Hodgkin's disease. However, if an HIV-infected patient contracts Hodgkin's disease, the disease appears at a more advanced stage. Treatment for these patients is a challenge because of their poor tolerance for chemotherapy and the occurrence of opportunistic infections.

Detection and Diagnosis

Enlarged lymph nodes in the neck, clavicular, or axilla regions are usually the first indication of Hodgkin's lym-

phoma. As mentioned previously, a mediastinal mass is usually discovered on a routine chest radiograph. Occasionally, these patients experience a cough, shortness of breath, or chest discomfort. The enlarged node may be the only symptom a patient experiences. However, about one third of the patients have B symptoms.[4] B symptoms include presence of fever greater than 38° C not caused by other diseases, night sweats, and weight loss greater than 10% of the body weight in 6 months. An enlarged spleen or abdomen, bony tenderness, and pleural effusion indicate a later stage of Hodgkin's disease. Enlarged groin nodes can be an early symptom, although Hodgkin's rarely originates in the groin.

The diagnostic workup includes a complete history and physical examination. Standard laboratory studies should include a complete blood and platelet count, liver and renal function tests, and blood chemistry and thyroid function tests. Occasionally, patients display anemia, leukopenia, lymphopenia, or thrombocytosis, which may be indicative of bone marrow involvement. A serum alkaline phosphatase level is a nonspecific marker of tumor activity, hepatic bone marrow disease, or bone disease.

Radiographic studies should include a chest x-ray examination, computed tomography (CT) scan, or magnetic resonance imaging scan (MRI) of the thorax for disease detection and treatment planning. A bipedal lymphangiogram is a good assessment method for detecting retroperitoneal lymph node involvement because this test is more sensitive than the CT scan in localizing these nodes. In recent years the positron emission tomography (PET) scan has been used to effectively image the thoracic and abdominal lymph nodes. A gallium scan or bone scan is optional but helpful in evaluating the mediastinum and residual disease after treatment.

A bone marrow biopsy should be restricted to patients with B symptoms or subdiaphragmatic disease. There is only a 5% chance of bone marrow involvement in patients who have Hodgkin's disease.

In the past, when radiation therapy was the only curative treatment, a **staging laparotomy** was a standard diagnostic procedure to determine the extent of the disease. If the disease extended beyond the lymph nodes to the spleen, liver, or bone marrow, the patient would not be a candidate for radiation therapy alone (total-nodal irradiation) but instead would have received chemotherapy. The laparotomy included a detailed inspection of the abdomen, a splenectomy, selected lymph node biopsies, and liver and bone marrow biopsies. It is a major surgical procedure that requires skill, time, and effort on the part of the surgeon.[6] Today the laparotomy is seldom used for several reasons. First, the use of combined modality, radiation and chemotherapy for early-stage disease has made the laparotomy unnecessary. Second, improved radiographic imaging techniques such as CT, MRI, and PET scans produce similar results to the laparotomy. Some researchers consider MRI superior to CT because it is able to detect bone marrow involvement and lymphadenopathy.[11]

The spleen is usually involved when the high paraaortic nodes are involved. It is also at risk with lymphocyte depletion or mixed cellularity histologies. The liver biopsy should be done when splenic involvement occurs, but the liver is rarely involved if the spleen is not. A peritoneoscopy with multiple liver biopsies is a viable alternative to the laparotomy.

Pathology

As mentioned previously, Hodgkin's disease is identified pathologically by the presence of the Reed-Sternberg cell. The current system used for histologic classification is the World Health Organization (WHO) modification of the Revised European-American Lymphoma (REAL) classification.[10] It divides Hodgkin's into two categories and three subcategories:

1. Nodular lymphocyte predominant Hodgkin's lymphoma (NLPHL)
2. Lymphocyte-rich classical Hodgkin's lymphoma (CHL)

Nodular sclerosing Hodgkin's lymphoma (NSHL)
Mixed cellularity Hodgkin's lymphoma (MCHL)
Lymphocyte depletion Hodgkin's lymphoma (LDHL)

CHL patients generally lack bulky disease, mediastinal disease, and B symptoms. There is a male predominance and an older median age.

NLPHL is distinguished from CHL because it is of B-cell origin, and it is the most favorable of the categories. The median age for NLPHL is in the mid-30s and there is a 3:1 male predominance. Generally the cervical or inguinal lymph nodes are involved but not the mediastinal. Eighty percent of these patients have stage I or II disease. Fewer than 10% of these patients experience any of the symptoms, and there is a 90% survival at 10 years posttreatment.[10]

CHL is characterized by the presence of typical, diagnostic Reed-Sternberg cells with a background of either nodular sclerosing, mixed cellularity, or lymphocyte depleted cells.

NSHL is the most common subtype in developed countries accounting for 60% to 80% of all cases.[10] NSHL is the type that occurs most frequently in adolescents and young adults. The mediastinum and supradiaphragmatic sites are most often involved in NSHL, and about one third of the patients experience B symptoms.

MCHL accounts for 15% to 30% of all Hodgkin's lymphomas. It can occur at any age and lacks the early adult peak of NSHL. Abdominal lymph nodes and splenic involvement are more common in MCHL.

LDHL is the least common subtype (less than 1%) in the United States. It occurs in older patients and HIV-infected patients. It usually presents with advanced disease such as spleen, liver, and bone marrow involvement and B symptoms. As a result, LPHL carries the worst prognosis of the four subtypes.

Staging

The **Ann Arbor staging system** has been the accepted method of classification for Hodgkin's disease since 1971 (Box 26-1).

These stages can be subdivided into A or B groups. An A indicates the lack of general symptoms. For example, stage IIA may indicate that two or more node regions are involved in the thorax and that the patient has not experienced any symptoms, such as fever, night sweats, and weight loss. The presence of these symptoms is indicated by a B next to the stage number (e.g., stage IB). However, the presence of B symptoms usually indicates a worse prognosis.

Routes of Spread

Hodgkin's disease has a predictable pattern of spread, and 90% of the patients have **contiguous** spread. In other words, the cancer has begun spreading to the adjacent node or region. The rapidity of the growth and spread of the disease, however, are not predictable.

Spread to the viscera occurs after spread to the adjacent lymph nodes. Obviously, visceral spread indicates a higher stage and worse prognosis.

Box 26-1	AJCC Staging Classification for Lymphoid Neoplasms

Ann Arbor Stage

Stage I: Involvement of a single lymph node region (I) or localized involvement of a single extralymphatic organ or site in the absence of any lymph node involvement (IE) (rare in Hodgkin lymphoma).

Stage II: Involvement of two or more lymph node regions on the same side of the diaphragm (II), or localized involvement of a single extralymphatic organ or site in association with regional lymph node involvement with or without involvement of other lymph node regions on the same side of the diaphragm (IIE). The number of regions involved may be indicated by a subscript, for example II_3.

Stage III: Involvement of lymph node regions on both sides of the diaphragm (III), which also may be accompanied by extralymphatic extension in association with adjacent lymph node involvement (IIIE) or by involvement of the spleen (III_S) or both (III_{ES}).

Stage IV: Diffuse or disseminated involvement of one or more extralymphatic organs, with or without associated lymph node involvement; or isolated extralymphatic organ involvement in the absence of adjacent regional lymph node involvement, but in conjunction with disease in distant site(s). Any involvement of the liver or bone marrow, or nodular involvement of the lung(s). The location of Stage IV disease is identified further by designating the specific site.

Greene FL, et al.: *AJCC cancer staging of manual,* ed 6, New York, 2002, Springer-Veriag.

The spleen becomes involved in late stages, and the likelihood of disseminated disease increases with splenic involvement. The liver and/or bone marrow are at increased risk with splenic involvement. Hodgkin's disease can also spread to the lungs and skeletal system in the late stages. It rarely involves the organ systems of the upper aerodigestive tract, central nervous system (CNS), skin, gastrointestinal (GI) tract, Waldeyer's ring, or Peyer's patches.

Treatment Techniques

Stages I and II. Radiation therapy has been the primary method of treatment for stage I and II Hodgkin's disease since the 1960s. Surgery is used only for a biopsy to determine the pathology and stage the disease or debulk large tumors. Chemotherapeutic agents historically have been used in advanced cases, usually in combination with radiation therapy. Currently, however, studies have demonstrated that combination radiation therapy and chemotherapy can effectively treat early-stage disease.[5,12,16]

Until the mid to late 1990s **total-nodal irradiation** was the standard treatment for stage I and II disease. In this method, the contiguous lymphatic chains are radiated with a cancerocidal dose. The patients are treated with anterior and posterior fields to the supradiaphragmatic lymph nodes **(mantle field)** (Fig. 26-2) and to the subdiaphragmatic lymph nodes. The subdiaphragmatic field always includes the paraaortic nodes and the spleen or the splenic pedicle, but the extent and location of the disease determines whether the pelvic, retroperitoneal, and inguinal nodes are also treated. When only the mantle field and the **paraaortic fields** are treated (without the pelvic, retroperitoneal, and inguinal nodes) it is referred to as **extended-field irradiation.** The mantle and paraaortic fields are most commonly treated sequentially, with a break in treatment occurring between fields to enable the patient to recover from the side effects of treatment. These fields require meticulous treatment planning, simulation, and frequent verification films.

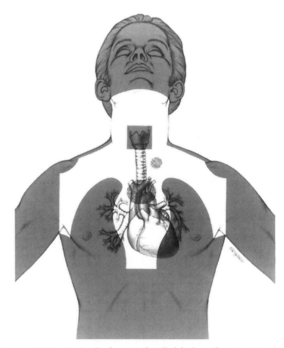

Figure 26-2. A typical mantle field for the treatment of Hodgkin's disease. Note the blocking of healthy lung tissue and humeral heads. An anterior larynx block and posterior cervical spine block are optional, depending on the location of the affected nodes. The treatment is with parallel opposed anterior and posterior fields. (From Cox JD: *Moss' radiation oncology,* ed 7, St. Louis, 1994, Mosby.)

A dose of 3500 to 4400 cGy delivered by 6- to 10-MV photons is considered the optimal dose to the mantle and paraaortic fields, with a minimum dose of 3000 to 3600 cGy. Typical fractionation was 750 to 1000 cGy per week, delivering 150 to 200 cGy per day, depending on the patient's tolerance. The rationale for this technique is to treat the clinically uninvolved nodes prophylacticly.[16]

Current studies, however, have shown that patients with

pathologic stage I and II Hodgkin's with favorable characteristics who receive mantle field radiation alone have very similar relapse-free and overall survival rates as patients who received both mantle and paraaortic irradiation.[15]

Lower doses of radiation have likewise proved effective. Many recent investigations have demonstrated that doses of 3000 cGy to 4000 cGy provide a good survival rate.[8]

Previously, chemotherapy was most commonly used in unfavorable stages I and II (A or B) and stages III and IV. It was generally reserved for patients with a worse prognosis because of the toxicity of the drugs used, especially nitrogen mustard that induced leukemia as a late-term side effect. Several regimens that are less toxic have been developed more recently and, as a result, are used in combination with limited field radiation for early-stage disease as well as for later stage disease. The ABVD regimen of doxorubicin (Adriamycin), bleomycin, vincristine, and dacarbazine has proven to be as effective and less toxic than the MOPP (mechlorethamine, vincristine [Oncovin], prednisone, and procarbazine) regimen. Other regimens currently in use include the following: VBM (vinblastine [Velban], bleomycin, and methotrexate), BEA-COPP (bleomycin, etoposide, doxorubicin [Adriamycin], cyclophosphamide, vincristine, procarbazine, and prednisone) and CVPP (cyclophosphamide, vinblastine, procarbazine, and prednisone) and the Stanford V (nitrogen mustard, doxorubicin [Adriamycin], vincristine [Oncovin], bleomycin, etoposide [VP-16], and prednisone).[7]

Using radiation therapy alone with either the total-nodal or extended-field technique reduces the acute and late drug-related toxicities and avoids drug resistance, so that chemotherapy may be used as a salvage treatment in case of recurrence. Radiation, however, is not without its own toxicities. Total-nodal and extended-field radiation increase the risk of second solid malignancies of the lung, GI tract, and breast. Therefore researchers have developed treatment regimens that combine the less toxic chemotherapy (generally ABVD) and radiation to the involved field only with a lower dose of 3000 cGy to uninvolved sites and 3600 to 4000 cGy to involved sites.[8] **Involved-field irradiation** is the treatment of the involved lymph node region only (Fig. 26-3).

Chemotherapy is used to reduce the bulky disease, either before radiation or as the entire treatment in later stages. Sometimes a split course of chemotherapy and radiation is prescribed, with alternating of the treatments. Radiation doses for combined modality treatments vary between 2500 and 4000 cGy. MOPP and ABVD regimens can be delivered alternately to prevent cells from developing a resistance to a particular drug, in the case of recurrence.

Treatment field design, and techniques: mantle field. A mantle field is illustrated in Fig. 26-2. It includes all major lymph node regions above the diaphragm: submandibular, occipital, cervical, supraclavicular, infraclavicular, axillary, hilar, and mediastinal. Anteriorly, the superior border is at the inferior portion of the mandible, and the inferior border is at the level of the insertion of the diaphragm (usually around T10).

Posteriorly, the superior border includes the occipital nodes, and the inferior border is the same as it is anteriorly (approximately T10). Laterally, the axillary nodes are included. Precise blocking is extremely important in this field. As much healthy lung as possible should be spared by blocking the lungs anteriorly and posteriorly; however, adequate margins need to be designed around sites of involvement. Some lung will be radiated because the mediastinal and hilar nodes must be included in this field. Humeral head blocks are also important to prevent future bone destruction, and a larynx block should be included anteriorly unless bulky disease is adjacent to the larynx. Posteriorly, a cord block may be needed, depending on the total dose. A posterior cord block may be used from the outset of treatment or added at 4000 cGy, unless it is contraindicated by the location of the primary tumor.

The cardiac silhouette is irradiated to a dose of 1500 cGy, but then a block shielding the apex of the heart should be added. After 3000 to 3500 cGy a subcarinal block (5 cm inferior to the carina) should also be added to shield more of the pericardium and heart.

If the pulmonary hilar nodes are involved and the patient is treated with radiation alone, partial transmission blocks should be used to deliver a low dose of 1500 to 1650 cGy to the lungs. This is considered an adequate dose for the treatment of occult, microscopic disease.

A large mediastinal mass necessitates modifications of the typical mantle field. In such instances, as the tumor decreases in size, wider lung blocks are added to protect as much lung tissue as possible. With such a mass, treatment is given more slowly: 150 cGy per day to 1500 cGy, followed by a 7- to 14-day break to allow for tumor regression and a redesign of the blocks.

Structures included in the **Waldeyer's ring** are seldom involved in patients with Hodgkin's disease. However, in these rare cases the preauricular nodes must be treated. A small Waldeyer's ring field is also treated when cervical nodes (which are superior to the thyroid notch) are involved. Parallel opposed lateral photon fields, or unilateral 6- or 9-MeV electrons, are used to treat the Waldeyer's ring. The

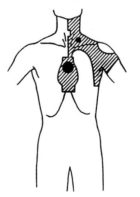
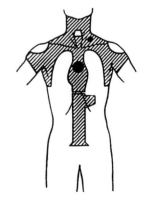
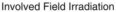

Involved Field Irradiation   Subtotal Lymphoid Irradiation

Figure 26-3. Involved-field irradiation includes areas of lymph node involvement only.

advantage of the electron field is that it spares the contralateral parotid gland. A typical dose to the preauricular nodes is 3600 cGy. Care must be taken to abut the borders of this field with the superior border of the mantle field and to ensure that the teeth are outside of the Waldeyer's ring field.

The mantle treatment may be delivered as an isocentric setup if the size of the patient allows such an isocentric configuration. The treatment distance on some mantle fields must be extended to accommodate an increase in the field dimensions. Many of the older linear accelerators have limitations on the field dimensions that are set by the manufacturer. For example, if the maximum field size that may be set at 100 cm is 40 × 40 cm and the actual treatment field must be 44 × 44 cm, the treatment distance must be extended to 110 cm source-skin distance (SSD). The method to determine the new treatment distance SSD is a simple direct proportion based on the geometrical principle of similar triangles: 44/40 × 100 = 110 (new extended SSD). Of course, the time or monitor units must increase to compensate for the decreased intensity of the beam from extending the distance.

With treatment at extended distances (particularly with older couches), alternating the position of the patient between anterior and posterior fields is occasionally necessary. For example, the patient is supine for the anterior field and prone for the posterior field. The newer couches, accommodate the extended distances better, and the patients may be treated isocentrically without turning over during treatment. However, problems with posterior gapping of the borders between the mantle and paraaortic fields can arise when the patient remains supine. For the treatment of the mantle field the patient lies supine (for anterior) with the arms **akimbo** (elbows bent) and hands on the hips (Fig. 26-4) or with hands placed above the head. The chin must be extended as much as possible to prevent exposure to the mouth, particularly from the exit dose of the posterior field. Treatment in the prone position for the posterior field forces the chin superiorly and eliminates the exit dose to the oral cavity. Body molds are helpful in reducing body movement and increasing the patient's comfort.

Inhomogeneous dose distribution. Because of the large field size, treatment at an extended distance, irregular-shaped blocks, and slanting body contours, an inhomogeneous dose distribution occurs in mantle treatments. Because the SSD and depth to the cervical, supraclavicular, axillary, and mediastinal lymph nodes vary so dramatically, so do the doses to these regions. Irregular field calculations must be done to accommodate for the irregularities in dose distribution. These dose discrepancies can be handled in numerous ways. Compensators are one method for reducing the dose variance between the various anatomic points. The use of compensators to reduce dose variation is desirable because of the positive biologic effect of reduction in variation of the daily and total doses between points.

Another way to reduce the total dose gradient between the various points of interest is the shrinking-field technique. This technique requires additional blocking as each anatomic site reaches the desired or total prescribed dose. The daily dose to each site remains the same, but the additional blocking alters the total doses. If a site must continue beyond the prescribed total dose, the additional treatments may be added to that site. This method has a slightly different biologic effect on the tissues as a result of the varying daily doses.

Subdiaphragmatic fields. The most common treatment of the subdiaphragmatic fields is the treatment of the paraaortic nodes and the spleen or splenic pedicle when no evidence of subdiaphragmatic disease is present. The inferior border of the mantle field determines the superior border, with a gap between to avoid overdosing of the spinal cord. The inferior border is typically L4 or L5 or below the bifurcation of the aorta (Fig. 26-5).

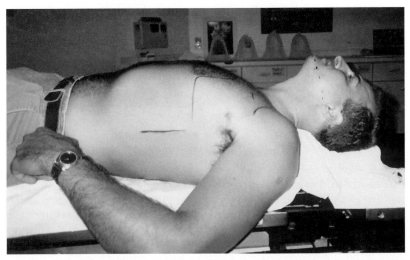

Figure 26-4. Typical patient positioning for a mantle field. Note the position of the arms (akimbo), the chin position, and the leveling marks on the patient's side.

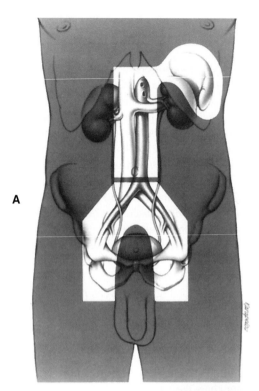
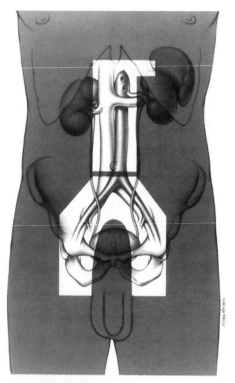
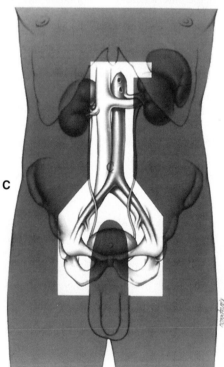

Figure 26-5. Several treatment alternatives for subdiaphragmatic field arrangements. **A,** The paraaortic field must include the spleen if the spleen is still intact. The pelvic irradiation is done only if subdiaphragmatic disease is present and can be administered separately from the paraaortic fields to improve patient tolerance. **B,** Paraaortic treatment including the lymph nodes of the splenic pedicle after a splenectomy. **C,** Field arrangement when the paraaortic and pelvic fields are treated simultaneously. This is the classic inverted Y technique. *(From Cox JD: Moss' radiation oncology, ed 7, St. Louis, 1994, Mosby.)*

The classic total-nodal irradiation technique includes an inverted Y field. Included in the inverted Y field are the retroperitoneal, common iliac, and inguinal lymph nodes. The full inverted Y is seldom treated as a prophylactic measure, but it is treated for subdiaphragmatic disease. Sometimes it is also used for stage IB or IIB disease. If the pelvis is not included in the treatment fields, the radiation method is referred to as subtotal lymphoid irradiation.

Blocking in the subdiaphragmatic fields is also extremely important because of the presence of the liver, kidneys, and bone-marrow-containing pelvic bones and reproductive organs. A low dose to the liver is delivered with partial transmission blocks of 50% to deliver 2000 to 2200 cGy if (1) the spleen is involved, (2) radiation alone is used as a primary treatment, or (3) the liver is involved.

A lymphangiogram is a valuable tool in delineating the precise location of the lymph nodes to enable the most precise blocking. The ovaries overlie the iliac lymph nodes; therefore an **oophoropexy** can be performed to reduce the risk of infertility. During this procedure the ovaries are clipped behind the uterus. A midline block of 10 half-value layer (HVL) may then be placed to shield the gonads. In male patients, no special blocking is used to protect the testes unless the inguinal and femoral nodes are irradiated. In such instances, the dose to the testes may be as high as 10%. This dose can be reduced to 0.75% to 3% with the use of a 10-HVL midline block. The inguinal and femoral nodes are treated only if disease appears in these nodes or adjacent to them.

Gapping methods. When extremely large fields are treated above and below the diaphragm, an appropriate separation, or gap, must be left between the fields on the skin surface to account for the normal divergence of the edges of the beams. Further discussion of gapping methods and calculations appears in Chapters 8 and 21.

The involved-field radiation includes only the affected lymph node region such as the supraclavicular, ipsilateral cervical or the inguinal nodes. Adjuvant chemotherapy is always used before irradiation of involved fields. See Fig. 26-3 for an example of involved-field radiation.

Stage III and IV. Advanced stages of Hodgkin's disease (stages IIIA, IIIB, and IV) are usually treated with chemotherapy with or without radiation therapy. Chemotherapy is also used for patients who relapse after radiation therapy; this is referred to as "salvage therapy." The original chemotherapy employed was the MOPP regimen; however, recent studies have proven the ABVD regimen to be as effective, and there is no risk of leukemia, as there is with the MOPP regimen. Other drug combinations currently in clinical trials are a MOP-BAP (mechlorethamine, Oncovin, prednisone, bleomycin, Adriamycin, and procarbazine) hybrid or an ABVD with MOPP/ABV.[14]

The debate continues on the role of adjuvant radiation therapy for advanced-stage Hodgkin's lymphoma. Patients receiving chemotherapy tend to relapse at the original site of the disease. When involved-field radiation therapy is used following chemotherapy, there is a lowered risk of local relapse.[15] To further the argument for radiation therapy, 20% of stage III and IV patients fail to enter a complete remission after their initial chemotherapy. Clinical trial outcomes indicate that late-stage patients receiving consolidative irradiation after chemotherapy obtained an 82% to 85% disease-free survival rate.[15] Unfortunately, patients treated with radiation after chemotherapy experienced more deaths from causes other than Hodgkin's than those who received additional chemotherapy. It is therefore generally recommended that only stage III patients with NSHL and bulky nodal involvement receive adjuvant radiation therapy.[15]

Autologous bone marrow stem cell transplants and peripheral blood stem-cell transplants have been used when Hodgkin's disease becomes resistant to standard treatment with chemotherapy and radiation. Experience has proven that it is best to perform the autologous stem-cell transplant soon after the first treatments fail. However, if the patient remains in remission for a long period after the first treatment, a second course of either radiation or chemotherapy is recommended.[1] In preparation for the bone marrow transplant, low-dose total body irradiation (TBI) may be used to deplete the bone marrow function of the patient.

Radiation may also be used for palliation to prolong survival and provide symptomatic relief. It may be used to alleviate pain, to decrease the tumor mass to eliminate obstructions, and to improve the overall quality of life.

Because the initial doses of radiation range from 2500 cGy to 4000 cGy, additional treatment with radiation to affected sites is entirely possible. Twice a day treatment may be necessary for a rapidly growing, chemotherapy-resistant tumor.[15]

Pediatric treatments. Children and adolescents may be treated with chemotherapy alone or in combination with involved-field radiation therapy. High-dose, extended-field radiation therapy is seldom used in childhood cases because of the long-term effects on the growth process, cardiac toxicities, and the occurrence of second malignancies (particularly lung, breast, and GI tract). Likewise, systemic therapy alone has undesirable side effects: myelosuppression, gonadal injury, and secondary acute myelogenous leukemia (AML). Researchers have achieved excellent treatment outcomes and reduced treatment side effects with combined modality treatments that use lower does and smaller volumes of radiation therapy and fewer cycles of less toxic chemotherapy. Involved-field radiation may be reduced to as low as 15 to 25 cGy, and the chemotherapy regimens of MOPP/ABVD have proved to be highly effective.[12]

Side effects. Acute side effects of radiation treatment are dependent on the size of the fields treated. The following is a list of side effects for the mantle and paraaortic fields:

- Fatigue
- Occipital hair loss (may be permanent, depending on the dose)
- Skin erythema
- Sore throat (esophagitis)
- Altered taste (especially with preauricular nodes)

- Transient dysphagia from radiation-induced esophagitis
- Dry cough
- Nausea
- Occasional vomiting
- Diarrhea (rare)

Most of the side effects are managed by good nursing care, which may include an antiemetic, the application of nongreasy skin creams, protection from sunlight, additional rest, an altered diet (soft, bland foods and no alcohol), throat lozenges, and diarrhea medication. Because the course of treatment is relatively short for each phase of treatment, patients with Hodgkin's disease usually manage their side effects well.

Late-stage complications depend on the treatment technique, total dose, and irradiated volumes. Most of the complications result from the mantle field treatment. They include the following:

- Mild radiation pneumonitis (depending on the volume of the lung treated) 6 to 12 weeks after the end of treatment
- Hypothyroidism in one third of the patients
- Herpes zoster
- Transient xerostomia, which requires careful, permanent dental care
- Increased dental caries
- Radiation carditis, which occurs in fewer than 5% of the patients
- Lhermitte's syndrome, which is a transient complication consisting of numbness, tingling, or electric sensations (caused by head flexion)

Patients are at increased risk for lung, breast, and GI cancers after mantle treatment. In addition, breast cancer in previously irradiated Hodgkin's patients tends to be a more aggressive than in normal populations.[9] Treatment-related second malignancies and cardiac complications are the main causes of death other than Hodgkin's disease itself in long-term survivors.[15]

Xerospermia can result in men after pelvic irradiation if no precautions are taken. With precautions the sperm count diminishes during treatment but returns to normal levels afterward. The MOPP, but not the ABVD, regimen causes sterility in men.

In women older than 30 years, even with oophoropexy and well-planned pelvic irradiation precautions, the scattered dose may be sufficient to decrease ovarian functions and cause menopausal symptoms. Younger women do not experience these menopausal symptoms. Chemotherapy also affects women similarly. Combined chemotherapy and radiation therapy, however, may affect menstrual function and fertility in younger women.

Psychosocial problems that patients with Hodgkin's disease commonly experience include depression (associated with the low energy levels during treatment), marital difficulties, and a decrease in sexual interest. Patients who have recovered from Hodgkin's disease sometimes are denied coverage by insurance providers because of an increased risk of later disease.

Results of Treatment

Stages IA and IIA. Most studies indicate that patients with stage IA disease have a cure rate of approximately 90% with radiation therapy as the only form of treatment.[14] Eighty percent of stage IIA patients achieve a cure with radiation therapy alone. Stage IA and IIA patients with favorable prognostic factors (sedimentation rate of less than 40 to 50, patient age of 40 to 50 or younger, lymphocyte predominant or nodular sclerosing histology, and no bulky adenopathy) have an 80% relapse-free survival rate at 5 to 10 years with mantle field, paraaortic, and splenic radiation therapy and no laparotomy.[14] To date, the treatment of early stage, favorable disease with ABVD chemotherapy and involved-field or extended-field radiation has proved to be equivalent in overall survival and failure-free survival rates. However, statistics on 15-year survival are not yet available on this group of patients.[14]

Stages IB and IIB. It is recommended that patients with B symptoms receive combination chemotherapy with or without additional radiation therapy, because 25% of these patients relapse after radiation.[14] Patients in this category have a similar survival rates to patients in stages IA and II A. The 10-year relapse-free rate is 78% to 88%. However, the subgroup that experiences fevers and weight loss has a 10-year-survival relapse-free rate of 48% to 57%, regardless of the type of therapy.[14]

Stages I and II, with bulky mediastinal involvement. Patients in this group have no difference in survival rates as stages IA and IIA, but their relapse rates are as high as 50%. These patients are at special risk for developing complications related to treatment. Usually, chemotherapy is used first to reduce the mediastinal disease and to allow for more narrow lung radiation therapy fields.

Subdiaphragmatic stages I and II. Approximately 10% of patients with Hodgkin's disease have this type of disease. Current practice recommends that patients with subdiaphragmatic presentation should receive chemotherapy and involved-field radiation.[14] This treatment avoids the extended pelvic and abdominal field irradiation of the inverted Y and splenic field techniques, which have serious side effects to the bone marrow. Such treatment also eliminates the need for a laparotomy.

Stage IIIA. A summary of 11 studies that used combined chemotherapy and radiation showed a 10-year survival rate of about 80% to 90% for patients. With radiation alone the 10-year survival rate declined to 68% to 80%.[15]

Stages IIIB and IV. The 10-year survival rate is 43% to 51% with the use of systemic MOPP or ABVD. Radiation may be added to treat bulky disease, and doing so increases the 5-year disease-free survival rate to as much at 82%.[15]

Treatment for relapse must be individualized. Generally, patients who received radiation alone are candidates for chemotherapy. Some researchers recommend the delivery of low-dose radiation (1500 to 2500 cGy) to the previously treated areas after chemotherapy and 3500 to 4400 cGy to the previously untreated areas.

Pediatric treatment outcomes. Long-term, disease-free survival for early-stage pediatric patients treated with combined chemotherapy and radiation therapy ranges from 85% to 96% of the cases. Children and adolescents with advanced stage, who have received combined modality treatments, achieved from 77% to 93% disease-free survival. Treatment results for pediatric Hodgkin's patients receiving chemotherapy alone range from 60% to 100% for all stages.[12]

Role of Radiation Therapist

For patients who have Hodgkin's disease the radiation therapist plays a vital role not only in delivering the radiation but also in assisting with side-effect management education and offering psychologic support during treatment.

Of course, the first priority of the therapist is the accurate delivery of the prescribed radiation dose. Positioning the patient consistently is vital for the accuracy of the treatments. Leveling marks on the side of patients assist in ensuring that the patient is lying consistently flat. The use of horizontal marks on the shoulders (in alignment with the central axis) as a positioning guide for the arms is also helpful. For treatment of the paraaortic field the gap measurement must be measured precisely and daily to prevent an overdose or underdose.

Accuracy in block placement can mean the difference in shielding disease or in delivering an unnecessary dose to healthy tissue. Custom blocks should always be fabricated because of the complex blocking necessary to shield the lungs and heart. Fig. 26-6 demonstrates the use of shielding in a minimantle field. The use of multileaf collimators simplifies the need for custom blocking; however, because of the complex block arrangements and the limits of the multileaf collimators, additional custom blocks may be necessary. Verification films should be taken at least weekly to ensure accuracy.

Because of the addition of cord blocks, cardiac blocks, and shrinking fields, the maintenance of accurate records is critical. Clear and precise notes should be written in the charts, indicating all blocking changes. Verification films should be taken before changes in blocking, especially before the addition of the cord block.

The blood counts require rigorous monitoring because the radiation and/or chemotherapy effects on the bone-marrow. Again, the therapist should pay close attention to the counts and ensure that they are taken as prescribed.

Communication is the second priority of a good therapist. The patient must be informed about daily procedures and any additional occurrences, such as portal images or new blocking. As the treatment progresses, the therapist plays an important role in the management of side effects. Frequently, the therapist is told first of these side effects. According to institution policies, the therapist may advise the patient regarding the way to handle the side effects or refer the patient to a nurse, dietitian, or physician. Communication with the family (and other professionals involved with the patient's care) about the side effects is also important.

Because of the daily contact with the patient, the therapist is in the position of evaluating the patient's physical and emotional needs. Many times, referral to another agency or individual (such as a social worker, support group, or chaplain) is appropriate.

Case Study

J.K., a 28-year-old white woman, had been in good health up to 6 weeks before her initial consultation. At that time, she noticed swelling in her lower neck. A biopsy revealed NSHL. Her weight had remained stable, she had no energy loss, and she did not exhibit any B symptoms. At the time of the biopsy a chest radiograph also revealed mediastinal adenopathy, classifying J.K.'s disease as stage IIA (more than one involved area on the same side of the diaphragm).

The patient had a tonsillectomy at age 4. Seven years before her diagnosis, J.K. had a benign lymph node removed from the high cervical area. She smoked lightly in high school and had an occasional glass of wine.

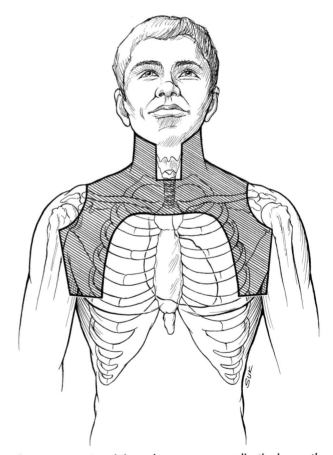

Figure 26-6. A minimantle, or supramediastinal mantle field, for disease limited to the cervical, supraclavicular, or axilla regions. Note the use of blocks to shield the lungs. Treatment is delivered anteriorly and posteriorly with parallel opposed portals.

She had no family history of cancer, although her maternal grandmother had a bilateral mastectomy for reasons unknown to the patient.

In addition to the biopsy and chest radiograph, a liver function test and CT scan were performed. The outcomes were negative for any abdominal involvement. Therefore the conclusion was made that a bone marrow biopsy was unnecessary. During physical examination the physician did not find any organomegaly, masses, inguinal adenopathy, or epitrochlear lymphadenopathy. J.K. was also presented to a tumor board. The tumor board recommended a lymphangiogram to serve as an additional diagnostic procedure and assist in the treatment planning. The consensus of the tumor board was that radiation alone would be the optimal treatment for this patient.

J.K. was treated with parallel-opposed mantle fields to 4140 cGy in 25 fractions (180 cGy per day) over 35 elapsed days with 6-MV photons. The mantle field measured 33 × 29.5 cm anteriorly and 31 × 29.5 cm posteriorly, both at 105 cm SSD. She was treated in the supine position for the anterior field and the prone position for the posterior field.

After a month break from the completion of the mantle fields, she received radiation therapy to the paraaortic lymph nodes and spleen anteroposteriorly/posteroanteriorly (AP/PA) to 3960 cGy in 22 fractions over 29 elapsed days. This field measured 25 × 17 cm and was treated at 105 SSD in a spade field configuration. The superior border was T10, and the inferior border was between S1 and S2.

During the mantle field treatment, J.K. experienced severe nausea and vomiting, beginning after the third fraction. Prochlorperazine (Compazine) was given, without much relief, followed by metoclopramide (Reglan) after a dose of 1620 cGy (9 fractions) was delivered. Metoclopramide brought some minor relief, but on the fifteenth treatment, intramuscular injections of pyridoxine (HexaBetaline) were given and resulted in dramatic improvement. During this time, J.K. lost 10 pounds and experienced headaches, a sore throat, and a dry mouth. She also had difficulty swallowing. She was instructed to drink tepid liquids, and she was given throat lozenges and Tylenol no. 3. By the end of the mantle treatment course, she had regained two of the pounds that she had lost.

J.K. tolerated her paraaortic treatments better. When she returned 1 month after the completion of the mantle field, she was feeling better, was eating well, and had good energy levels. At 3060 cGy, she experienced some nausea and vomiting, which were relieved by metoclopramide. Her total weight loss during the last half of treatment was only 3¾ pounds.

About 1 month after the completion of her treatments, J.K. experienced a herpes outbreak on her right chest wall, which cleared in about a week. She experienced no other late or chronic side effects.

Three years posttreatment, J.K. gave birth to a second child. Five years after the completion of her treatment, a suspicious nodule appeared in her neck and was removed. The biopsy revealed that it was benign. She remains free of any evidence of disease 8 years after the diagnosis.

NON-HODGKIN'S LYMPHOMA

NHL may arise anywhere that the lymph travels. It may occur in the lymph nodes, a group of lymph nodes, an organ such as the stomach or lung, or any combination of these. NHLs differ from Hodgkin's disease in several ways, including the following:

1. They occur primarily in older persons. The median age is 65.

2. They can originate in the lymph nodes or in extranodal tissue.
3. They are more likely to spread randomly, rather than in an orderly pattern.
4. NHLs encompass a wide variety of diseases, which the experts continue to attempt to classify into appropriate categories.

Epidemiology

The incidence of lymphomas has increased 65% since the 1970s. The most recent projections from the American Cancer Society estimate new cases in the United States in 2003 and deaths from NHL in 2003.[1] The male/female ratio is similar to that of Hodgkin's disease in that there is a slight male predominance. In the United States, white males have a higher incidence than African Americans, Japanese Americans, Chinese Americans, Hispanics, and Native Americans. Worldwide, the incidence of NHL varies greatly from country to country. For example, Burkitt's lymphoma is common in Africa and Papua New Guinea but rare in other countries, although patients with acquired immunodeficiency syndrome (AIDS) tend to get this form of lymphoma. Lymphomas are the third most common childhood malignancy, accounting for 10% of all childhood cancers. Two thirds of these childhood lymphomas are NHL.[5]

The median age is 65, but lymphoma incidence actually peaks in the 80 to 84 age-group. The incidence has tripled for patients older than 65.[5] Researchers have yet to explain this increase in incidence.

Etiology

Researchers have discovered that lymphomas are genetic alterations of the B or T lymphocyte cells.[5] The exact causes of NHL, however, are largely unknown. However, researchers have identified many risk factors such as exposure to particular infectious agents and reduced immune function. Burkitt's lymphoma is caused by the Epstein-Barr virus. Serologic (blood) studies have shown an association between human T-cell leukemia/lymphoma virus (HTLV-1) and T-cell leukemia/lymphoma. AIDS patients have a 165% increased risk of developing NHL in the first 3.5 years after their AIDS diagnosis.[5] Other immunosuppressed patients, such as those having heart and kidney transplants, are also at increased risk.

People exposed to ionizing radiation are at a greater risk of developing lymphomas. There is an increased incidence of lymphomas in atomic bomb survivors who were exposed to 100 cGy or more. Patients who received radiation therapy for ankylosing spondylitis (a chronic inflammatory disease affecting the spine, which was formerly treated with radiation) are at risk for contracting lymphomas. Hodgkin's patients treated with chemotherapy are at a 20-fold risk of developing NHL, and patients receiving chemotherapy in general are at a greater risk of developing NHL. There is also an increased incidence in patients who take phenytoin to control seizures, in agricultural workers exposed to herbicides, and in industrial workers exposed to solvents and vinyl chloride. Recent studies have identified higher incidences in women with high dietary intake of *trans* unsaturated fats[1] and in people who participate in recreational drug use.[5]

Aside from the histology of the disease, age is an important prognostic factor. The younger the patient, the better the prognosis, in part because older patients have less tolerance to the treatment. Older patients also tend to have more advanced disease at the time of diagnosis. Unfortunately, 50% of NHL patients are older than 60 years.

Clinical Presentation

The signs and symptoms of NHL are similar to those of Hodgkin's lymphoma: enlarged lymph nodes, fever, night sweats, fatigue, itching, and weight loss. Unlike Hodgkin's, however, NHL may arise in a wide variety of sites, most commonly in the lymph nodes, GI tract, and Waldeyer's ring. Lymphomas of the CNS commonly occur in AIDS patients.

Clinically, lymphomas can appear as enlarged nodes or are discovered when the patient has symptoms related to the site and extent of tumor involvement. For example, shortness of breath or a cough is symptomatic of lung involvement. Abdominal pain or a change in bowel habits may indicate pelvic disease. Symptoms of brain involvement are headaches, vision problems, and seizures. Disease outside the lymph system is more common in intermediate- and high-grade lymphomas. Generally, when the lymphoma occurs outside the nodes, such as in the GI tract or CNS, the course of disease is worse. Waldeyer's ring is the least worrisome of all of the extranodal sites.

Systemic symptoms (as seen in Hodgkin's disease patients) are rare, occurring in only 10% to 15% of the patients at the time of presentation, and no conclusive evidence exists as to whether the presence of symptoms plays a part in the overall prognosis. Distinguishing the importance of the histology from that of the stage of disease is difficult.

Detection and Diagnosis

The diagnostic workup defines the extent of the disease and assists in the decision on the treatment course. The history and physical examination are, of course, the standard first steps, as are the cytologic evaluations. Included in the blood tests are a complete blood count, an HIV test, a blood chemistry, a urinalysis, serum lactate dehydrogenase (LDH), liver function tests, and serum alkaline phosphatase. A bone marrow biopsy is necessary because bone marrow involvement is common in many lymphomas; however, an MRI may be just as sensitive, if not more sensitive than a biopsy and can also identify CNS involvement.[5] A chest radiograph; a CT of the abdomen, pelvis, neck and chest; and a bone scan are also part of the first line of diagnostic tests. PET scans have been increasingly used for staging as well.

Further diagnostic tests may include a gallium whole-body scan and upper GI or small bowel series. A CT scan of the brain may be recommended if previous tests or symptoms indicate possible disease at these sites. A lymphangiogram of the pelvis and abdomen are done if the CT scan shows abnormal results.

Pathology

There are two types of lymphoid tissue: primary (central) lymph tissue and peripheral (secondary). The primary lymphoid tissue harbors the lymphoid precursor cells, both B and T cells. The peripheral tissue is where the antigen-specific reactions occur. The primary lymphoid tissues are the bone marrow and the thymus. The bone marrow produces the precursor B cells (which make antibodies) and precursor T cells (which are responsible for the regulation of the immune system). Most lymphomas in the United States are of B-cell origin. The immature T-cell precursors must migrate to the thymus in the anterior mediastinum to undergo maturation.

Peripheral lymphoid tissues are the lymph node, the spleen, and mucosa-associated lymphoid tissue found in the epithelium of the nasopharynx and oropharynx (Waldeyer's ring), the GI tract, the distal ileum **(Peyer's patches),** the colon, and rectum. Lymphomas arising out of these mucosa-associated tissues are referred to as mucosa-associated lymphoid tissue (MALT) lymphomas.

Features that best predict the prognosis of lymphomas are size, shape, and pattern of the cells. Small and round or angulated cells are called cleaved cells. Other lymphomas may be composed of large cells or combinations of small and large cells. Intermediate-sized lymphocytes with rapidly dividing cells are characteristic of aggressive, high-grade lymphomas.

In the normal lymph nodes are microscopic clusters or follicles of specialized lymphocytes. In lymphomas, some lymphocytes arrange themselves in a similar pattern called a follicular, or nodular, pattern. These lymphomas and small cell lymphomas tend to be low grade and follow a slower or indolent course with an average survival time for patients of 6 to 12 years.

The more aggressive lymphomas (intermediate and high grade) lose their normal appearance by the diffuse involvement of tumor cells that are usually moderate or large sized.

Lymphomas can be histopathologically classified as follicular (or nodular) and diffuse, with 40% appearing as follicular and 60% as diffuse. The follicular lymphomas are of B-cell origin and tend to run an indolent course with prolonged survival. Although many patients have advanced disease, the median survival for patients with follicular types is 5 to 7 years. Follicular lymphomas usually appear below the diaphragm, and the involvement of the mesenteric lymph nodes is common. Children seldom get follicular lymphomas, and these lymphomas do not commonly involve Waldeyer's ring.

Diffuse lymphomas can be of B or T cell origin and run a more aggressive course. Ironically, they usually appear with more localized disease, but they spread quickly to other nodes and extranodal sites. There is also an increase in bone marrow and Waldeyer's ring involvement. The lymphatics are the most common site of recurrence with either type.

Grading. Lymphoma classification systems have continually evolved since the 1950s. The current system commonly used is the Revised European-American Classification of Lymphoid Neoplasms (REAL) that has been combined with the World Health Organization (WHO) classification of hematologic malignancies (Table 26-1). The REAL classification system combines morphology, immunophenotype, genetic features, and clinical features to define disease entities and is a major advancement over the former systems.

Staging

Categorizing lymphomas into staging systems is as complex as grading them. As research continues, particularly with HIV patients, additional light is shed onto this disease

---

Table 26-1	Updated European-American classification of lymphoid neoplasms/World Health Organization classification of lymphoid neoplasms (REAL/WHO classification)*

B-CELL NEOPLASMS

Precursor B-cell neoplasms
Precursor B-lymphoblastic leukemia/lymphoma (B-ALL/LBL)
Mature (peripheral) B-cell neoplasms
  B-cell chronic lymphocytic leukemia/small lymphocytic lymphoma
  B-cell prolymphocytic leukemia
  Lymphoplasmacytic lymphoma
  Splenic marginal zone B-cell lymphoma (±villous lymphocytes)
  Hairy-cell leukemia
  Plasma cell myeloma/plasmacytoma
Extranodal marginal zone B-cell lymphoma of MALT type
Mantle-cell lymphoma
Follicular lymphoma
Nodal marginal zone B-cell lymphoma (±monocytoid B cells)
Diffuse large B-cell lymphoma
Burkitt lymphoma

T- AND NK-CELL NEOPLASMS

Precursor T-cell neoplasm
  Precursor T-lymphoblastic lymphoma/leukemia (T-ALL/LBL)
Mature (peripheral) T-cell neoplasms
  T-cell prolymphocytic leukemia
  T-cell granular lymphocytic leukemia
  Aggressive NK-cell leukemia
  Adult T-cell lymphoma/leukemia (HTLVI+)
  Extranodal NK/T-cell lymphoma, nasal type
  Enteropathy-type T-cell lymphoma
  Hepatosplenic $\gamma\delta$ T-cell lymphoma
  Subcutaneous panniculitis-like T-cell lymphoma
  Mycosis fungoides/Sézary syndrome
  Anaplastic large-cell lymphoma, primary cutaneous type
  Peripheral T-cell lymphoma, unspecified
  Angioimmunoblastic T-cell lymphoma
  Anaplastic large-cell lymphoma, primary systemic type

HODGKIN'S DISEASE

Lymphocytic predominance, nodular ± diffuse areas
Classical Hodgkin's disease
  Nodular sclerosis
  Mixed cellularity
  Lymphocyte depletion
  Lymphocyte-rich classical Hodgkin's disease

From Harris NL, et al: Lymphoma classification—from controversy to consensus: the R.E.A.L. and WHO classification of lymphoid neoplasms, *Ann Oncol* 11(suppl 1):3-10, 2000.
MALT, Mucosa-associated lymphoid tissue; *NK,* natural killer.
*More common entities are in italics.

process. Although the Ann Arbor system is most commonly used for the staging of NHLs, it is not completely satisfactory. In contrast to Hodgkin's disease, many patients with NHL have advanced disease. The Ann Arbor system also fails to account for bulky disease, which plays a significant role in lymphomas because many patients have advanced disease but experience relatively long survival. Although the diaphragm plays an important role in the staging of Hodgkin's disease, it is insignificant in the progression of lymphomas. Therefore a major factor in the Ann Arbor system is inconsequential in NHLs.

Treatment Techniques

NHLs include a wide variety of clinical diseases, and the treatment choices depend largely on the specific subtype, the extent of the disease, patient's age, and general health. Choices of treatment fall into five categories[5]:

1. No initial therapy (for indolent, low-grade disease)
2. Chemotherapy
3. Radiation therapy
4. New biologic therapies
5. Stem-cell transplants

Surgery is used only for diagnostic purposes, because it is ineffective in controlling the progression of the disease. The most common practice is to administer chemotherapy with or without radiation for most patients. The stage and grade, more than the particular treatment regimen, determines the ultimate outcome of treatment.[16]

Localized disease involving only one site or two immediately adjacent sites, with tumors less than 10 cm in diameter and no systemic symptoms, has a high likelihood of cure. This may be true for all subtypes, but most studies have been conducted on diffuse, histologically aggressive lymphomas.

Chemotherapy is administered to treat occult disease and reduce the risk of distant failure. Generally it is given as the sole treatment, depending on the particular lymphoma, or before radiation therapy. The chemotherapy dose can be reduced by half when radiation therapy follows immediately. Likewise, the radiation dose can be reduced when treatment is combined with chemotherapy. Multiagent chemotherapy has proven more effective than single agent because the multiagent regimens prevent cellular sensitization to any one drug.[5] Formerly, the most common treatment for stage I and nonbulky stage II diffuse, aggressive NHL was the CHOP regimen (cyclophosphamide, hydroxydaunorubicin [doxorubicin] vincristine [Oncovin], and prednisone), given in three or four cycles and followed by radiation therapy to the involved site and adjacent lymph nodes.

Since CHOP was introduced in the 1970s, there has been no apparent change in mortality from lymphomas in the United States.[2] Therefore new regimens have been developed, including the following[5,7]:

1. CVP (cyclophosphamide, vincristine, prednisone)
2. m-BACOD (methotrexate, bleomycin, doxorubicin, cyclophosphamide, vincristine, dexamethasone)
3. FND (fludarabine, mitoxantrone, and dexamethasone)
4. ProMACE/CytaBOM (prednisone, doxorubicin, cyclophosphamide, etoposide, cytarabine, bleomycin, vincristine, methotrexate, leucovorin)
5. PACEBOM (prednisolone, doxorubicin [Adriamycin], cyclophosphamide, etoposide, bleomycin, vincristine, methotrexate)

Cure is rare for patients with disseminated, low-grade NHL. However, patients who are asymptomatic at the time of the diagnosis can be monitored closely without therapy until symptoms occur, and a substantial portion of these patients have spontaneous remissions. If the symptoms can be improved or the patient is unwilling to proceed without therapy, treatment usually includes radiation therapy, single-agent chemotherapy, or a combination chemotherapy regimen with or without radiation therapy. Complete remissions can be achieved in most patients, and the remissions tend to last for extended periods. Interferon-*a* has been used successfully in combination with CHOP. Patients receiving this treatment have a longer remission time and a higher rate of survival than those treated with CHOP alone. Monoclonal antibodies, such as Rituximab have proven to be effective in the treatment of relapsed B-cell NHLs.[17]

Autologous bone marrow and stem cell transplants have proven to be very effective (50% 5-year survival) for treating either stage III and IV NHLs or for treating recurring disease.[4,5]

Current data indicate that 60% to 80% of adults with diffuse, aggressive NHL in stage II to IV can achieve complete remissions. Long-term, disease-free survival can be achieved in 30% to 50% of these patients. Larger doses of chemotherapy are given to patients who have histologically aggressive disease.[16]

Patients infected with HIV are particularly prone to NHLs. These lymphomas usually have a B cell origin, are often associated with the Epstein-Barr viral genome in the tumor, and frequently occur in unusual extranodal sites such as the brain. Unfortunately, because of their already suppressed immune system, these patients do not tolerate treatment well. If no opportunistic infection occurs, the patients can tolerate some therapy and often respond well to treatment. The choice of chemotherapeutic agents for this population remains controversial.

Radiation therapy. The role of radiation therapy in the treatment of lymphomas varies substantially from that in the treatment of Hodgkin's disease. Although NHLs are sensitive to radiation, only a small portion of patients obtain a cure if treated with local or regional radiation alone. This is because there is a high probability of disease spread to other lymphatic or organ sites. Therefore most lymphomas are treated with both radiation to the involved site and chemotherapy for systemic treatment.

Because lymphomas are radiosensitive, they regress quickly; however, radiation does not always alter the natural history of these diseases. In the study of treatment regimens, true survival and disease-free relapse must be distinguished.

Typically, radiation is given to the site of involvement, with coverage to the draining nodal groups on the same side of the diaphragm. Although total-nodal radiation can be used for stages I and II, it is not a common practice in the United States. The reason for this is that, although longer disease-free survival accompanies total-nodal radiation, there is no change in overall survival rates.

Radiation therapy is a standard management for stage I and II low-grade lymphomas, especially for patients younger than 40 years. Doses of 35 to 45 Gy are recommended for local control. Intermediate-grade lymphomas are generally treated with a CHOP regimen followed by 30 to 35 Gy of radiation therapy.[16]

Radiation therapy alone is used to treat stage I and II follicular lymphomas and the low-grade B cell lymphoma of MALT. Follicular and mantle cell lymphomas can be curatively treated with 30 to 36 Gy with a boost to 36 to 40 Gy to the involved or regional field. The recurrence rate after 10 years is only 10%. MALT lymphomas may be treated with either surgery alone or local or regional radiation therapy of 30 Gy.[5]

Investigation of new treatments for late-stage lymphomas include the use of interferon-*a* (an antitumor agent) alone, in combination with chemotherapy, or as an adjuvant to chemotherapy; monoclonal antibodies; and high-dose chemotherapy with fractionated total-body radiation followed by bone marrow transplantation.

If a patient relapses, the same chemotherapy is often used. However, two additional agents have proved effective in the treatment of relapses: fludarabine and 2-chlorodeoxyadenosine (2-Cd-A). High-dose rate chemotherapy, radiation, and bone marrow transplantation are also used for the treatment of relapse in stages I and II. Radiation alone may also be used to reduce bulky disease and/or to relieve pain.

The 5-year survival rate is 90% for patients in stages I and II and 80% for those in stages III and IV. The average survival time for patients with low-grade lymphomas is 6 to 12 years.

Intermediate-grade lymphomas can be divided into favorable and unfavorable tumors. Favorable tumors are those less than 4 to 10 cm in diameter in which the LDH level is normal and no B symptoms are present. For patients with favorable stage I and II disease, treatment options include the following[7]:

1. Chemotherapy alone (CHOP)
2. Chemotherapy and radiation therapy
3. Primary radiation alone to the site, particularly if the patient is unable to tolerate the chemotherapy

The 5-year survival rate for patients with stage I intermediate-grade lymphomas is 80% to 90% and 70% to 80% for patients in stage II.[7]

Unfavorable lymphomas in stages I, II, III, and IV are treated with combination chemotherapy. Regimens include CHOP, mBACOD (methotrexate, bleomycin, doxorubicin, cyclophosphamide, vincristine, and dexamethasone), ProMACE/CytaBOM, and MACOP-B (methotrexate, adri-amycin, cyclophosphamide, vincristine, and prednisone). The survival rate is significantly lower for these patients than it is in the earlier stages. A 5-year survival rate of 40% to 50% is the norm for these patients.[7]

High-grade and lymphoblastic lymphomas usually receive multiagent chemotherapy with prophylactic CNS radiation. Stage IV patients have extensive disease, usually with bone marrow involvement, and/or CNS involvement along with a high LDH level. Generally, these patients have done poorly with conventional therapy and may benefit from intensive chemotherapy and radiation, followed by bone marrow transplantation.

The 5-year survival rate is 80% for patients with limited disease and 20% for patients with extensive disease involving the bone marrow or CNS.

AIDS-associated lymphomas are usually intermediate- and high-grade lymphomas and are highly aggressive. Of course, the condition of the patient dictates the treatment.

If given total-nodal irradiation at high doses, patients with stage III nodular lymphomas achieve a 33% remission rate after 10 years. However, with diffuse lymphomas, only 10% of the patients survive 10 years after total-nodal radiation. Chemotherapy (either a single alkylating agent or a combination of agents) is usually used for this stage.

Unless the disease originates in the mediastinum, mediastinal spread is rare. The mantle technique is commonly used in instances of mediastinal involvement. A minimantle or supramediastinal mantle is appropriate if no mediastinal disease or upper abdominal disease is present. Anteriorly, the inferior border for a minimantle field should be at the level of the inferior portion of the head of the clavicles; posteriorly, it should be at the inferior surface of the shaft of the clavicles (Fig. 26-6).

Preauricular nodes are frequently involved in the diffuse lymphomas and are at high risk in patients with cervical adenopathy. In such instances, these nodes should be treated with a prophylactic dose of 3600 cGy, administered in right and left lateral ports over 4 weeks.

Subdiaphragmatic treatment.   Mesenteric lymph node involvement is common with lymphomas occurring inferior to the diaphragm. In such instances, the whole abdomen is treated with the following four-field techniques[16] (Fig. 26-7).

1. An AP/PA field extending from the dome of the diaphragm to the iliac crest (unless the tumor is at the level of the iliac crest, and then the field continues to the floor of the pelvis) is treated initially. The lateral portions of the ileum should be blocked to protect the iliac bone marrow, and the right lobe of the liver and the kidneys should also be protected. Over 2 to 3 weeks, 1500 cGy should be delivered at a rate of 150 cGy per day.
2. After the AP/PA course of treatment, the upper abdomen is treated from lateral fields, based on the initial isocentric setup. If abdominal disease is massive, the pelvic portion may continue with an AP/PA configuration. The posterior margin of these fields should be anterior to the kidneys but should include the paraaortic nodes. Anteriorly, the field should

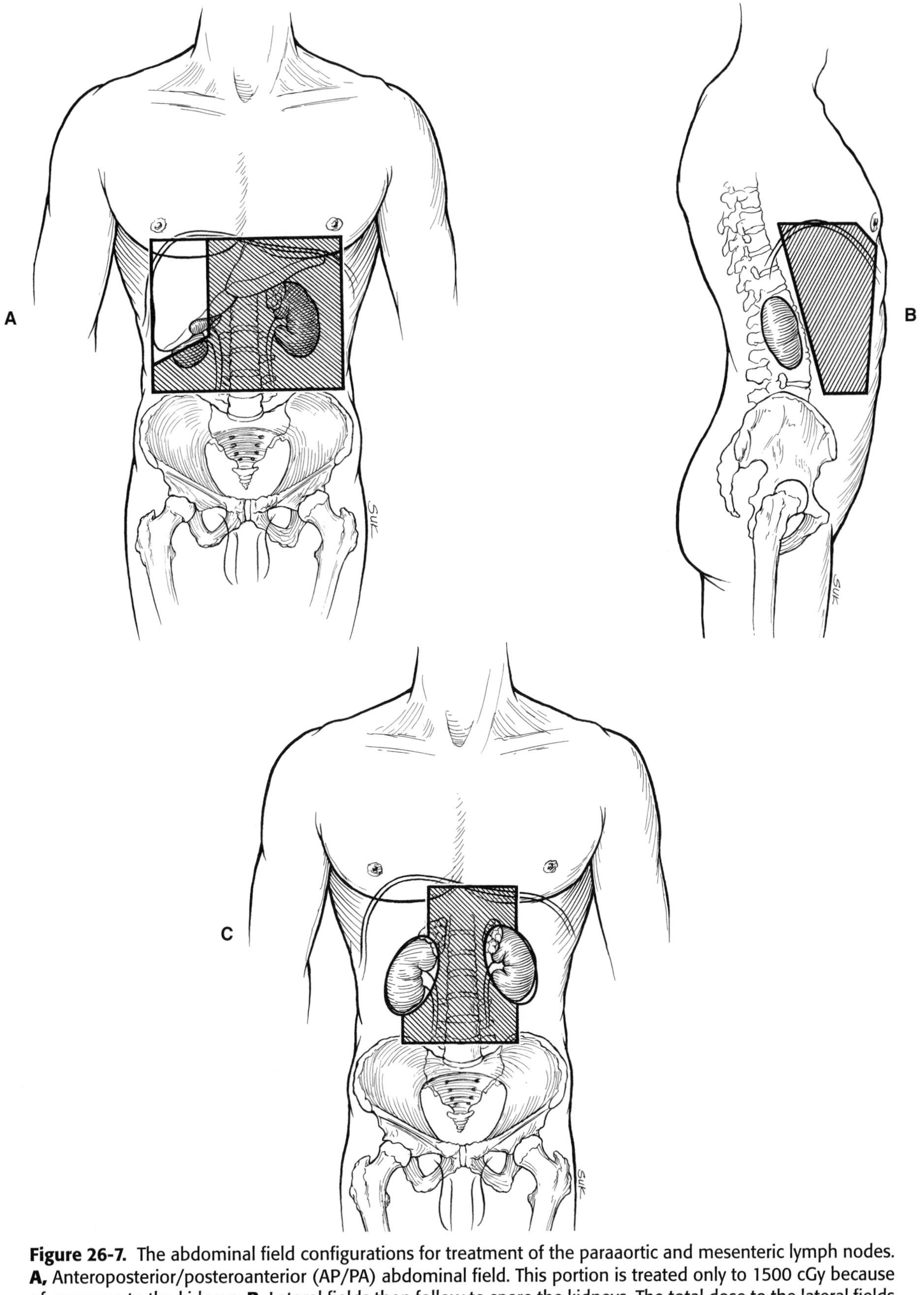

Figure 26-7. The abdominal field configurations for treatment of the paraaortic and mesenteric lymph nodes. **A,** Anteroposterior/posteroanterior (AP/PA) abdominal field. This portion is treated only to 1500 cGy because of exposure to the kidneys. **B,** Lateral fields then follow to spare the kidneys. The total dose to the lateral fields should be 1500 cGy. **C,** AP/PA paraaortic fields with five half-value layer (HVL) kidney blocks. The total dose to all three fields is 4500 cGy.

include the anterior abdominal wall. Another 1500 cGy over a 2-week period should be given, bringing the total dose to 3000 cGy over 4 to 5 weeks. If the disease is on the posterior abdominal wall, the kidneys cannot be shielded. If the kidneys lie in the same plane as the paraaortic nodes, the lateral fields should be omitted.

3. Finally, a wide AP/PA paraaortic field (10 to 12 cm) is treated with kidney blocks, delivering 1500 cGy in another 2-week period. The lateral margins of such a field should extend from the lateral margins of one kidney to the lateral margins of the other, with five HVL kidney blocks.

The total dose delivered to the whole abdomen is 4500 cGy in 6 to 7 weeks. Pelvic irradiation may continue on an AP/PA basis throughout this period of abdominal irradiation if blood counts permit. Midline blocks should be no higher than the symphysis pubis.

When total-body irradiation is used for palliation in advanced cases of nodular lymphocytic lymphoma or nodular mixed lymphoma, 150 cGy to the midplane should be delivered over 5 weeks. Two or three fractions should be delivered weekly for a total of 30 cGy per week. The major complications of such treatment are thrombocytopenia or leukopenia. The platelet counts must be closely watched, with counts taken before each treatment.

Central nervous system and gastric lymphomas. NHL is about 60 times more common in AIDS patients than in the general population.[3] These patients typically have high-grade and large-cell immunoblastic-type lymphomas and Burkitt's lymphoma. These lymphomas commonly occur in the CNS, with two thirds appearing with cerebral disease. Extranodal sites are also common in these lymphoma-AIDS patients.

Surgery is necessary for a diagnosis, but an excision is not necessarily therapeutic. Radiation therapy improves the median survival time but only to 15 months. A typical radiation field is a whole-brain field with extension to the upper cervical spinal cord and occasionally the orbit if it is at risk. Doses above 5000 cGy may lead to longer survival rates. Chemotherapy can be effective if the patient's immune system is not already severely depressed.[16]

Lymphomas of the GI tract are the most common of the extranodal lymphomas. They are most commonly diffuse, large-cell lymphomas. They appear with gastric symptoms, and a diagnosis is obtained via an endoscopic biopsy. The regimens recommended for such cancers are surgery and chemotherapy, a biopsy, chemotherapy and radiation therapy, or a biopsy and radiation therapy. One third of the patients have unresectable disease at the time of surgery. Surgery delays chemotherapy administration and causes morbidity from the functional loss of the stomach. A 10% mortality rate accompanies this surgery.[16]

Bone marrow transplants have been conducted increasingly with lymphoma patients. Allogenic or autologous transplants can be done. Frequently, these transplants are performed if the therapy for relapse or primary disease has failed. Typically, bone marrow transplants are done for aggressive cell types.

Side effects. The side effects of radiation therapy treatment for lymphomas depend on the areas treated. For example, if a patient receives radiation in a mantle or the Waldeyer's ring field, the side effects will be a dry mouth, difficulty swallowing, a loss of appetite, mucositis, mouth sores, a candidal infection, altered taste, redness of the skin, a sore throat, possible hair loss, transient dysphagia from esophagitis, and a dry cough.

Management of these side effects therefore includes eating small, frequent meals and avoiding extremely hot or cold fluids and/or alcohol. Good skin care includes the use of aloe vera or an approved topical application if the skin begins to redden. The patient must be cautioned, however, not to have the skin care product on at the time of treatment because of increased skin irritation. For this reason, many centers do not recommend any skin creams until after the radiation therapy. Corn starch, however, is allowed and works effectively at relieving skin irritations.

Abdominal treatment is sure to cause nausea and vomiting. Antiemetics such as prochlorperazine (Compazine) and trimethobenzamide (Tigan) should be taken 30 minutes before the treatment to control the vomiting or nausea. The use of tetrahydrocannabinol (THC) or marijuana (Marinol) is sometimes prescribed to control the nausea and improve the appetite for these patients. Fatigue is also common in this group of individuals, and plenty of rest should be encouraged. Patients who work full time should be strongly encouraged to limit their work hours during treatments. Also, help at home in dealing with family stress (e.g., child care and meal preparation) should be investigated.

If the pelvis is treated, diarrhea may occur, depending on the dose. In such instances a low-fiber diet should be recommended, and diarrhea medications may be indicated.

Vomiting and low blood counts are the primary side effects of total-body irradiation. Chronic effects of NHL treatments are caused more by the chemotherapeutic drugs than by the radiation therapy. Alkylating agents used in the treatment of NHL and Hodgkin's disease can cause sterility and the risk of a second cancer (usually leukemia). No risk is involved if the patient is treated by radiation alone to limited fields.

Results of Treatment

Patients with stage I and II follicular lymphomas have excellent survival rates with radiation therapy alone. The patients have an 80% to 100 % 5-year survival rate, assuming that no abdominal disease is present.

Patients with localized stage I and II large-cell lymphomas typically receive adjuvant chemotherapy after the site of involvement is treated. Some groups use chemotherapy without adjuvant radiation as the primary treatment with good results, but these groups generally experience increased morbidity.

Patients with high-stage, indolent, nonaggressive lymphomas have several options. These options include no treatment, combination chemotherapy, combination chemotherapy and radiation therapy, low-dose TBI total lymph node irradiation, and chemotherapy with TBI and bone marrow transplantation.

In stage III nodular lymphoma patients, a 5- to 10-year survival rate exists, with conservative management of patients who do not have symptoms and are feeling well. The treatment for these patients tends to be a small-field, low-dose radiation therapy for symptom relief. Patients who receive intensive chemotherapy have good responses but high rates of relapse.

Patients with nodular mixed lymphomas receive good results (possibly cures) with the C-MOPP (cyclophosphamide, Oncovin, procarbazine, prednisone) regimen.

Total lymphoid radiation for stage III has resulted in a 30% freedom-from-relapse rate at 10 years; results are the same for whole-body radiation. Similar results occur for stage IV, but total-nodal radiation is not considered appropriate for these patients.

For stage III and IV diffuse histology, chemotherapy is the mainstay, with the C-MOPP or BACOP regimens being used. Of the patients in this group, 40% achieve long-term freedom from relapse.

Role of Radiation Therapist

The radiation therapist's role in treating the lymphoma patient is similar to that for the Hodgkin's disease patient. Accuracy is the primary concern. If abutting fields are present, the therapist should be careful to match fields or measure gaps with extreme accuracy.

The therapist must be aware of the importance of blocking the critical structures in the fields (i.e., spine, liver, and kidney). Keeping precise records is vital, and clear notes should be written to indicate blocking changes. Portal images should be taken before the onset of blocking changes, particularly in regard to the liver and kidney blocks because these structures have extremely low tolerances to radiation. (The liver's maximum tolerance is 3000 cGy, and the kidney's maximum tolerance is only about 2300 cGy.) Therefore precision in block placement is paramount.

Blood counts should be taken regularly for these patients. Monitoring these counts and ensuring that the blood is drawn often become the duty of the therapist.

Because they tend to be older than the Hodgkin's disease patients, NHL patients may have worse overall health and may rely on the therapist for additional. As with all patients, communications and instructions must be clear. Communication is critical, not only with the patients but also with their families, especially as side effects require management.

SUMMARY

New forms of NHL are being identified as a result of advances in immunologic molecular diagnosis and the use of special techniques. Enteropathy-associated (small intestine disorder) T-cell lymphomas and mantle-cell–derived lymphomas are two such diseases.

Further investigation has shown NLPHL to be a B-cell proliferation that may progress to a high-grade B-cell NHL. Also, many cases of LDHL have been reclassified as T-cell NHL. The relationship between Hodgkin's disease and non-Hodgkin's large-cell anaplastic lymphoma has likewise become increasingly blurred. Therefore current research continues to shed new light on these disease processes, which increasingly are appearing more interrelated.

Treatment advances are also being continually developed. The hope is that the prognosis will improve for patients in all the categories of lymphomas.

Case Study

M.T. is a 30-year-old woman with intermediate-grade, large-cell NHL. In September she developed chest pain, which worsened until December, when she had a chest x-ray examination. A 10.5-cm mediastinal mass was discovered on the radiograph. A biopsy then revealed the intermediate-grade, large-cell lymphoma. At the time of the workup, M.T. experienced superior vena cava syndrome. Chemotherapy began shortly. ProMACE/CytaBOM was delivered in six cycles, the last of which ended in April of the following year. The patient tolerated the chemotherapy well. Chest radiographs and CT scans showed the near total resolution of the mediastinal mass, and no evidence of tumor involvement existed outside the chest.

M.T. has no family history of carcinoma. She works as an accountant and does not use cigarettes or alcohol. She has not experienced any of the following: headaches, dizzy spells, nausea, vomiting, shortness of breath, coughing, diarrhea, constipation, and abdominal pain. Her appetite and energy level are good. In addition, she does not exhibit cervical, supraclavicular, axillary, or inguinal adenopathy.

Because of the size of the initial mass, limited radiation therapy was given to the involved field only. Over 31 days, 3960 cGy of 6-MV photons were delivered in 22 fractions to the involved field. M.T. experienced fatigue at 1080 cGy, which was unusual for such a limited field of treatment and after only six fractions. However, the fatigue resolved within the week, and the patient felt much better by the twelfth fraction. She experienced an unrelated bladder infection, which was cleared up with trimethoprim/sulfamethoxazole (actrim DS).

After the completion of the radiation, she was seen in follow-up in August of the same year. To date, she has not experienced any further side effects nor any chronic effects. M.T. has been disease free since this time.

Review Questions

1. Which lymph nodes are typically treated in a mantle irradiation field?
   a. hilar
   b. paraaortic
   c. inguinal
   d. Waldeyer's ring

2. Which of the following is not a B symptom?
   a. fever above 38° C
   b. night sweats
   c. itching
   d. weight loss
3. Which subtype of Hodgkin's disease offers the most favorable prognosis?
   a. Lymphocytic predominance
   b. Nodular sclerosis
   c. Mixed cellularity
   d. Lymphocytic depletion
4. When treating a posterior mantle field, the superior field border should be high enough to include which lymph node group?
   a. Paraaortic
   b. Hilar
   c. Occipital
   d. Axillary
5. Which of the following may be seen as an *acute* complication of treatment?
   a. Radiation pneumonitis
   b. Lhermittes syndrome
   c. Fatigue
   d. All of the above
6. NHL differs from HD in which of the following ways?
   I. Occur in older persons
   II. Can originate in extralymphatic tissues
   III. Less likely to spread randomly
   a. I and II
   b. I and III
   c. II and III
   d. I, II, and III
7. Subdiaphragmatic field arrangements used in the inverted Y commonly include:
   a. Paraaortic nodes
   b. Inguinal nodes
   c. Both a and b
   d. Neither a nor b
8. Chemotherapy treatment regimens have had an increasing role in lymphoma management?
   a. True
   b. False
9. Which of the following radiographic studies are commonly used in the diagnostic workup of lymphoma
   I. Thoracic CT scan
   II. PET scan
   III. MRI
   a. I and II
   b. I and III
   c. II and III
   d. I, II, and III
10. AIDS associated lymphomas are usually intermediate- and high-grade disease and are highly aggressive
    a. True
    b. False

Questions to Ponder

1. Compare and contrast the differences between Hodgkin's disease and NHL, including the causes, clinical presentation, routes of spread, prognosis, and treatment modalities.
2. Why is the Ann Arbor staging system appropriate for Hodgkin's disease but difficult to apply to NHLs?
3. Which is the greater prognostic factor, the stage or the histologic subtype in Hodgkin's disease? How does this differ in NHLs?
4. For the treatment of a subdiaphragmatic lymphoma with a four-field abdomen technique, which structures need to be blocked or protected?
5. Compare and contrast involved-field radiation with total-nodal radiation and explain when each method is used.
6. What considerations must the therapist keep in mind daily when setting up a Hodgkin's disease patient for a mantle field and for a paraaortic field?

REFERENCES

1. American Cancer Society: available at http://www3.cancer.org (accessed April 2003).
2. Armitage JO: Treatment of non-Hodgkin's lymphomas, *N Engl J Med* 328:1023-1029, 1993.
3. Beral V, et al: AIDS-associated non-Hodgkin's lymphoma, *Lancet* 337:805-809, 1991.
4. Bolwell B: Autologous bone marrow transplantation for Hodgkin's disease and non-Hodgkin's lymphoma, *Semin Oncol* 21(suppl 7):86-96, 1994.
5. DeVita VT, Hellman S, Rosenberg SA, editors: *Cancer: principles and practice of oncology,* ed 6, Philadelphia 2001, Lippincott, Williams & Wilkins.
6. Dietrich PY, et al: Second primary cancers in patients continuously disease-free from Hodgkin's disease: a protective role for the spleen? *Blood* 84:1209-1215, 1994.
7. Dollinger M, Rosenbaum EH, and Cable G: *Everyone's guide to cancer therapy,* ed 1, Kansas City, MO, 1991, Andrews and McMeel.
8. Duhmke E, et al: Low dose radiation is sufficient for the noninvolved extended-field treatment in favorable early-stage Hodgkin's disease: long term results of a randomized trial of radiotherapy alone, *J Clin Oncol* 19:2905-2914, 2001.
9. Gaffney DK, et al: Breast Cancer after mantle irradiation for Hodgkin's disease: correlation of clinical, pathologic and molecular features including loss of heterozygosity at BRCAI and BRCA2, *Int J Radiat Oncol Biol Phys* 49:539-546, 2001.
10. Harris NL, et al: A revised European American Classification of Lymphoid Neoplasms. A proposal from the International Lymphoma Study Group, *Blood* 84:1361-1392, 1994.
11. Hoane BR, et al: Comparison of initial lymphoma staging using computed tomography (CT) and magnetic resonance (MR) imaging, *Am J Hematol* 47:100-105, 1994.
12. Hudson MM, Donaldson SS: Treatment of pediatric Hodgkin's lymphoma, *Semin Hematol* 36:313-323, 1999.
13. Jarrett R, Mackenzie J: Epstein Barr virus and other candidate viruses in the pathogenesis of Hodgkin's disease, *Semin Hematol* 36:260-269, 1999.
14. National Cancer Institute: Hodgkin's disease, available at http://www.oncolink.org/types/article.cfm?c=10&s=35&ss=280&id=9037 (accessed 4/19/2003).
15. Ng AK, Mauch PM: Radiation therapy in Hodgkin's lymphoma, *Semin Hematol* 36:290-302, 1999.

16. Perez CA, Brady LW: *Principles and practice of radiation oncology,* ed 3, 1998, Lippincott, Philadelphia, pp 1963-2012.

17. Wood, AM: Rituximab: an innovative therapy for non-Hodgkin's lymphoma, *Am J Health Syst Pharm* 58:215-229, 2001, available at http:www.ncbi.nlm.nih.gov (accessed September 1, 2001).

BIBLIOGRAPHY

Advanti R, Horning S: Treatment of early stage HD, *Semin Hematol* 36:270-281, 1999.

Armitage JO, et al: Salvage therapy for patients with lymphoma, *Semin Oncol* 21(suppl 7):82-85, 1994.

Bonadonna G: Modern treatment of malignant lymphomas: a multidisciplinary approach, *Ann Oncol* 5(suppl 2):5-16, 1994.

Dasher B, Wiggers N, Vann AM: *Portal design in radiation therapy,* ed 1, Atlanta, 1994, RL Bryan.

Dreger P, et al: Stem-cell transplantation for chronic lymphocytic leukemia: the 1999 perspective, *Ann Oncol* 11(suppl 1):49, 2000.

Fisher RI: Diffuse large-cell lymphoma, *Ann Oncol* 11(suppl 1)29-33, 2000.

Ghielmini SF, et al: The effect of Rituximab on patients with follicular and mantle-cell lymphoma, *Ann Oncol* 11(suppl 1):123, 2000.

Gladstein E, Kaplan HS: *Determination of tumor extent and tumor localization of Hodgkin's disease and non-Hodgkin's lymphomas: technical basis of radiation therapy practical clinical consideration,* Philadelphia, 1984, Lea & Febiger.

Gonzalez C, Mederios J: Non-Hodgkin's lymphomas and the Working Formulation, part 2, *Contemp Oncol* 43-55, 1993.

Harris NL, et al: Lymphoma classification—from controversy to consensus: the R.E.A.L. and WHO classification of lymphoid neoplasms, *Ann Oncol* 11(suppl 1):3-10, 2000.

Holleb AI, Fink D, Murphy GP: *American Cancer Society textbook of clinical oncology,* ed 1, Atlanta, 1991, American Cancer Society.

Horning SJ: Follicular lymphoma: have we made any progress? *Ann Oncol* 11(suppl 1):23-27, 2000.

Horning SJ, et al: The Stanford experience with combined procarbazine, Alkeran and vinblastine (PAVe) and radiotherapy for locally extensive and advanced stage Hodgkin's disease, *Ann Oncol* 3:747-754, 1992.

Kaminski MS, et al: Radioimmunotherapy of B-cell lymphoma with (^{131}I) AntiB (Anti CD-20) antibody, *N Engl J Med* 329:459, 1993.

Khan KM: *The physics of radiation therapy,* ed 1, Baltimore, 1984, Williams & Wilkins.

Kuniyoshi M, et al: Prevalence of hepatitis B or C virus infection in patients with non-Hodgkin's lymphoma, *J Gastroenterol Hepatol* 2:215-219, 2001.

Linch DC, et al: A randomised British national lymphoma investigation trial of CHOP vs. a weekly multi-agent regimen (PACEBOM) in patients with histologically aggressive non-Hodgkin's lymphoma, *Ann Oncol* 11(suppl 1):87-90, 2000.

Loeffler M, et al: Meta-analysis of chemotherapy versus combined modality treatment trials in Hodgkin's disease, *J Clin Oncol* 16:818-829, 1998.

Maartenese E, et al: Different age limits for elderly patients with indolent and aggressive non-Hodgkin lymphoma and the role of relative survival with increasing age, *Cancer* 89:2667-2676, 2000.

Mao Y, Hu J: Non-Hodgkin's lymphoma and occupational exposure to chemicals in Canada, *Ann Oncol* 11(suppl 1):69, 2000.

Mikhaell NG, et al: 18-FDG-PET for the assessment of residual masses on CT following treatment of lymphomas, *Ann Oncol* 11(suppl 1):147, 2000.

Noordijk EM, et al: Combination of radiotherapy and chemotherapy is advisable in all patients with clinical stage I & II Hodgkin's disease—six year results of the EORTC-GPMC controlled clinical trials H7-VF, H-7-F & H7-U, *Int J Radiat Oncol Biol Phys Suppl* 39:173, 1997 (abstr).

Ozsahin M: Early stage Hodgkin's disease: to mantle or not to mantle? *J Clin Oncol* 19:3298, 2001.

Sonneveld P, et al: Full-dose chemotherapy for non-Hodgkin's lymphoma in the elderly, *Semin Hematol* 31(suppl 3):9-12, 1994.

Wirth A, et al: Long term results of mantle field irradiation alone in 261 patients with clinical stage I & II supradiaphragmatic Hodgkin disease, *Int J Rad Oncol Biol Physics Suppl* 39(2), 1997.

Leukemia

Susan B. Belinsky, Mary Ann McKenney

Outline

Key Terms

Auer rods
Diplopia
Ecchymoses
Epistaxis
Leukoencephalopathy
Menorrhagia
Nadir

Papilledema
Petechiae
Pluripotent
Progenitors
Pruritus
Purpura
Stomatitis

Leukemia is a heterogeneous group of neoplastic diseases of the hemopoietic system affecting approximately 30,600 cases per year.[1] It is broadly divided into acute and chronic types, based on the disease's natural history. Acute leukemia progresses quickly and is characterized by proliferation of undifferentiated cells in the bone marrow, whereas chronic leukemia is distinguished by a slower progression of disease and the uncontrolled expansion of mature cells. Acute and chronic leukemias are further subdivided into myelogenous leukemias (those arising directly or indirectly from hemopoietic stem cells) and lymphocytic leukemias (those arising from other cells populating the bone marrow). Therefore consideration of three factors (natural history of the disease, degree of cellular maturation, and dominant cell line) results in the four main subtypes of leukemia (Table 27-1): acute lymphocytic leukemia (ALL), chronic lymphocytic leukemia (CLL), acute myelogenous leukemia (AML, which is sometimes referred to as acute nonlymphocytic leukemia [ANLL]), and chronic myelogenous leukemia (CML).

HISTORICAL PERSPECTIVE

The first documented description of a case of leukemia appears to be that of Alfred Velpeau, a French surgeon, who

Table 27-1	The four main subtypes of leukemia	
Natural History of the Disease	**Lymphocytic**	**Myelogenous**
Acute	ALL	AML
Chronic	CLL	CML

ALL, Acute lymphocytic leukemia; *AML*, acute myelogenous leukemia; *CLL*, chronic lymphocytic leukemia; *CML*, chronic myelogenous leukemia.

in 1827 recorded his observations. Dameshek and Gunz[2] described the case:

His patient, a 63-year-old florist and seller of lemonade, who had abandoned himself to the abuse of spirituous liquor and of women without, however, becoming syphilitic, fell ill in 1825 with a swelling of the abdomen, fever, and weakness. He died soon after admission to the hospital and was at autopsy found to have an enormous liver and spleen, the latter weighing ten pounds. The blood was thick, like gruel . . . resembling in consistency and color the yeast of red wine.

In 1844 Alfred Donné reported his microscopic observations of leukemia cells in his treatise "Cours de Microscopie." His studies included the examination of a postmortem sample of blood from a woman who had suffered from a large abdominal tumor and diarrhea as well as samples collected in vivo from other patients. Donné is credited with the first known observation of leukemic cells and the establishment of the disease as a hematologic condition.[4]

In 1845, Rudolf Virchow, a German physician, referred to the blood taken from a patient with splenic enlargement and massive accumulations of white blood cells as *weisses blut* (white blood). In 1847, Virchow first used the term leukemia. A decade later, Virchow described two types of leukemia: splenic and lymphatic. The advent of staining techniques in microscopy in the late nineteenth century permitted the morphologic subdivision of the myelogenous and lymphocytic leukemias.[14]

Because of the unique nature of each of the four subtypes of leukemia, they are discussed separately in this chapter.

PERTINENT ANATOMY

Leukemia develops during the formation of the constituent elements of the blood and lymphocytes. The hemopoietic process through which mature erythrocytes, neutrophils, eosinophils, basophils, monocytes, and platelets are formed and the lymphopoietic process through which lymphocytes are formed begin at the most primitive level with the pluripotent stem cells. These cells have a self-renewing capability and generate differentiating cells of multiple lineages. The cells of the **pluripotent** stem cell pool differentiate into either myeloid or lymphoid stem cells (Fig. 27-1). The myeloid stem cell pool provides the **progenitors** for the six types of blood cells, whereas the lymphoid pool provides the progenitors for the classes of lymphocytes. In the normal course of differentiation and maturation, these cells eventually become fully mature, functional blood cells and lymphocytes. During leukemic development the production of the hemopoietic or lymphopoietic progenitors is uncontrolled and greatly accelerated, resulting in incomplete or defective cellular maturation. Acute leukemia involves the rapid proliferation of primitive, undifferentiated stem cells, whereas cellular differentiation is largely preserved in chronic leukemia.

The symptoms of leukemia result from the leukemic cells' interference with normal processes. The leukemic cells accumulate in the bone marrow, impairing the body's normal production of adequate supplies of red blood cells (RBCs), white blood cells (WBCs), and platelets. The decrease in the number of these necessary blood components in the circulating blood results in anemia; thrombocytopenia; neutropenia; and the related symptoms of fatigue, pallor, bleeding, and infection.

With the acute leukemia subtypes the accumulating leukemic cells are immature or have undergone a defect in maturation. ALL is characterized by the invasion of the bone marrow by leukemic lymphoblasts. AML results from the proliferation of defective or incompletely matured cells derived from the pluripotent hemopoietic stem cell pool.

In chronic leukemia the maturation of the cells is preserved, but unregulated proliferation results in the accumulation of leukemic cells in the bone marrow. CLL is a disorder of morphologically mature, but immunologically less mature, lymphocytes. An increased proliferation of these short- and long-life lymphocytes and the prolonged survival of the long-life lymphocytes results in an enormous accumulation of these cells in the marrow, blood, lymph nodes, liver, and spleen. This causes an enlargement of the involved organs and a decrease in bone marrow function. CML involves the replacement of marrow cells with mature myeloid cells that are insensitive to the normal proliferation control mechanisms.

ACUTE LYMPHOCYTIC LEUKEMIA

Epidemiology

The acute subtypes account for approximately 50% of all instances of leukemia in the United States.[1] ALL is the most common of the pediatric malignancies, and approximately 80% of children with acute leukemia have the ALL subtype. There are approximately 3600 new cases a year with an age-adjusted incidence of 1.4 per 100,000.[1,9]

ALL is primarily a disease of children, with its incidence peaking between the ages of 2 and 10 years. It is relatively uncommon in persons over the age of 14.[5] The incidence of ALL is higher among males than females. The disease is

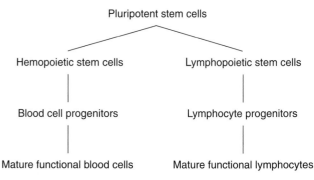

Figure 27-1. Hemopoiesis and lymphopoiesis.

more common among whites than blacks and has a higher incidence among Jews than non-Jews.

Etiology

The causes of acute leukemia are unknown. Physical and chemical agents have been associated with increased instances of leukemia. The markedly higher incidence of acute leukemia among survivors of the atomic bomb explosions in Japan has suggested that ionizing radiation may play a role in leukemogenesis. Japanese atomic bomb survivors had a 10- to 15-fold increase in the incidence of acute leukemia, with a greater increase in the incidence of ALL than AML. Benzene derivatives and other hydrocarbons and alkylating agents such as cyclophosphamide have been associated with an increased risk of acute leukemia.

Heredity appears to play a role in the development of acute leukemia. If one identical twin is diagnosed with acute leukemia, the risk of the other twin developing the disease within 6 months is approximately 20%. Down syndrome is associated with a 10- to 30-fold increased risk of acute leukemia.

Naturally occurring retroviruses and the human T-cell lymphotropic virus have been implicated as causative agents in instances of adult ALL but not childhood ALL.

Prognostic Indicators

More than 75% of patients with ALL can be expected to experience a complete remission, although the duration of the remission and subsequent potential for cure appear to be related to a number of factors, including clinical variables such as age and white blood count (WBC) at the time of the diagnosis.[10] ALL in children younger than 2 and older than 10 years carries a poor prognosis. The prognosis is the worst for an infant younger than age 1 year.[5] In adult ALL, advancing age is an adverse prognostic sign, with patients older than 50 years faring worse than younger patients. An initial leukocyte count of less than 10,000/mm³ is more favorable than a count of 20,000 to 49,000/mm³. A WBC greater than 50,000/mm³ is the least favorable.[11]

Other features with prognostic value include central nervous system (CNS) leukemia at the time of the diagnosis; a mediastinal mass; massive organomegaly and/or adenopathy; and biologic qualities of the leukemic cells such as the immunophenotype, cytogenetics, and deoxyribonucleic acid (DNA) content. Poor performance status, impaired organ function, and low serum albumin levels are unfavorable prognostic indicators.

Clinical Presentation

The symptoms of ALL at the time of presentation stem from the suppression of the normal blood components that causes anemia, thrombocytopenia, neutropenia, and associated symptoms. A nonspecific flulike malaise is common, with fatigue and pallor resulting from the anemia. Thrombocytopenia is manifested by oozing gums, **epistaxis** (nose bleeds), **petechiae** (tiny red spots on the skin caused by the escape of

small amounts of blood), **ecchymoses** (discoloration of the skin caused by the escape of blood into tissues), **menorrhagia** (excessive menstrual bleeding), and excessive bleeding after dental procedures. Neutropenia causes an increased susceptibility to respiratory, dental, sinus, perirectal, and urinary tract infections. Other common symptoms at the time of presentation are liver, splenic, and testicular enlargement. The disease at times may mimic rheumatoid arthritis with joint swelling, bone pain, and tenderness, often causing a child to limp or refuse to walk. Unlike AML, the symptoms of ALL rarely occur more than 6 weeks before the diagnosis. Vomiting, headaches, **papilledema** (swelling of the optic disc), neck stiffness, and cranial nerve palsy are indicative of CNS involvement.

Detection and Diagnosis

A blood cell count is one indicator for detecting ALL. Thrombocytopenia and anemia occur in most patients (two-thirds) at the time of the diagnosis. Leukocyte counts vary from low to high. An abnormal increase in white cells indicates a poor prognosis.

Immunophenotyping includes a morphologic evaluation, special stains, electron microscopic examination, and surface marker studies. It can establish a diagnosis in 90% of the patients.[11]

A bone marrow aspiration biopsy is necessary to make a definitive diagnosis. The amount of leukemic blast cells is the determinant for a definitive diagnosis. A biopsy revealing greater than 25% leukoblasts is positive for leukemia.

Other abnormalities may be present at the time of the diagnosis. These include hyperuricemia and several metabolic abnormalities, hyperkalemia, hypomagnesemia, hypocalcemia, and hypercalcemia. Of the patients identified with having ALL, 30% have low serum levels of immunoglobulins at the time of the initial diagnosis.

Leukemic infiltrates of the liver, periosteum, and bone may be present. A mediastinal mass may be present in some high-risk patients. This can be demonstrated on a chest radiograph.

Extramedullary leukemia is important in regard to relapse. The two most common sites for extramedullary leukemia are the CNS and testes (sanctuary sites, because they are "hidden" from most chemotherapy agents). A diagnosis of these two sites is obtained through a cytologic examination and a wedge biopsy, respectively.

Pathology

ALL is characterized by an unregulated proliferation of lymphoblasts. The disease cells limit the production of other healthy cells by overcrowding and inhibiting cell growth and differentiation.

Staging and Classification

The two major means to classify ALL are based on the morphologic appearance and immunologic surface markings.

The morphologic classification used is the French-American-British (FAB) system. This classification divides lymphoblastic leukemias into three levels (L1, L2, and L3). These divisions of ALL are based on the cell size, nuclear shape, number, prominence of nuclei, and amount and appearance of cytoplasm. These levels are as follows[11]:

L1—a small cell with a high nucleus; a regular cytoplasm ratio; or a clefted cell and small, inconspicuous nucleoli

L2—larger blast cells with irregular nuclear membranes, one or more prominent nucleoli, and a relative abundance of cytoplasm

L3—large lymphoblasts with round to oval prominent nucleoli and basophilic cytoplasm

Most pediatric ALLs are L1. L3 carries a poor prognosis and is associated with B-cell ALL.

Immunologic classification identifies the surface-marking characteristic of blast cells. Approximately 15% to 20% of patients with ALL are categorized by T-cell markers. About 80% to 85% of the patients are classified by B-cell with 20% to 25% accounting for pre-B-cell lineage type. Ninety percent of these cases are identified by the common ALL antigen positive (CALLA⁺). This cell type reacts to an antibody made from a surface antigen generally found in ALL cells.[11]

Treatment Techniques

Treatment techniques used for ALL are radiation therapy, chemotherapy, and bone marrow transplantation. These three modalities are used alone or in combination with each other. The use of these drugs and regimens may vary among institutions. Protocols are also frequently updated and changed as new information is discovered.

If radiation therapy is administered, four different techniques may be used for treating ALL. All the treatment techniques and devices discussed in this chapter are those used at Tufts-New England Medical Center's Radiation Oncology Department and Dana Farber/Brigham and Women's Hospital Cancer Center, Departments of Radiation Oncology. Most radiation oncology facilities use similar types of treatment techniques; however, Dana Farber/Brigham and Women's Hospital Cancer Center uses two 4-MV linear accelerators simultaneously to treat leukemic patients.

The New England Medical Center's Radiation Oncology Department experience. The patient may receive total body radiation with the dose totaling 1200 cGy. For 3 consecutive days, 200 cGy is given two times a day (bid). This dose is used to immunosuppress the patient in combination with a bone marrow transplant.

The dose rate set on the treatment unit is 10 cGy per minute, prescribed at midplane at the central region, the umbilicus. This low dose rate is necessary to spare late-responding tissues. These tissues include all visceral organs. The most common example is the lung.

A helmet field may be used to encompass the meninges. The helmet dose is 1800 cGy, delivered 200 cGy each day for 9 consecutive days.

The CNS technique is a combination of a helmet and spine field. This technique is used to treat positive cells in the cerebral spinal fluid. The helmet field is treated to a total dose of 2400 cGy. The dose is delivered 150 cGy each day for 16 days. This is combined with a field to encompass the entire spine. The spine receives a total of 1500 cGy, with 150 cGy each day for 10 days.

The final treatment technique for ALL is a testis field. This field receives 400 cGy for a single fraction and is commonly used with total body irradiation treatment.

Field design and critical structures. With total body irradiation the field size used is 40 × 40 cm. This is the largest jaw size that can be set on the treatment unit. The gantry is then placed in the lateral position. The patient sits in the diamond-shaped box with the knees toward the chest, the arms by the side, and the forearms on the side of the knees (Fig. 27-2). The arms are placed in this position to act as compensators for the lungs. This position is necessary to place the entire person in the beam. The diamond-shaped box is about 5 feet from the gantry, so that the light field covers the exact outer rim of the box, ensuring total coverage of the patient. The patient's eyes and face should be looking straight ahead.

Half of the treatment is given in this manner. Then the box, which is on wheels, is rotated 180 degrees. The second half of the treatment is given to the patient's other side. The patient is treated from the right and left lateral positions. After the completion of one lateral treatment field, the box is rotated manually 180 degrees and the other lateral is treated.

Thermoluminescent dosimeters (TLDs) are placed between the patients ankles, knees, and thighs once during a treatment to check midline doses. To even the dose over the uneven surfaces of the body, lead compensators are placed on a Lucite tray in the beam. The compensators are positioned over the thinnest body parts, such as the head and neck area, and the foot and ankle areas.

The field design for a helmet field is derived from specific anatomic landmarks; the field size should cover the meninges and C2, with fall-off around the head (Fig. 27-3). The patient lies supine on a plastic head cup for stability and comfort. The lenses of the eyes should be blocked with an adjustable block.

The spinal cord is a critical structure for the treatment of the head to the level of C2. (The helmet field is used as described previously.) With spinal cord involvement, there should be a recorded dose for this particular site.

For the treatment of the CNS, the patient is placed in the prone position. Numerous head holders, such as the Smithers or Osborne holders (Fig. 27-4), comfortably stabilize the head. The patient's chin should be tucked slightly to avoid a crease in the neck (Fig. 27-5). This is a critical match area and should be flat with no skin folds.

The field arrangement is in two volumes. The first field arrangement is the cranial volume, which includes two lateral parallel opposed ports with the helmet field design arrangement. The second volume is the spinal field, which contains

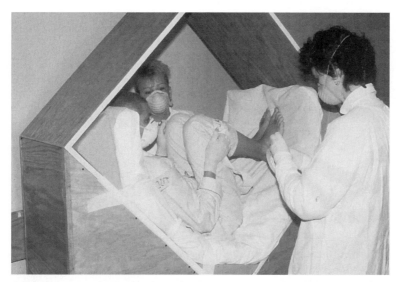

Figure 27-2. New England Medical Center's custom-made immobilization device for total body irradiation.

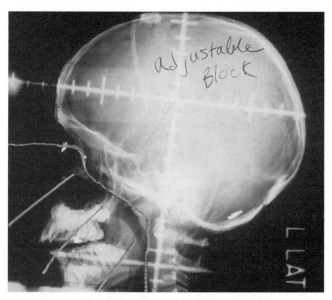

Figure 27-3. Simulation film for a helmet field that covers the meninges encompassing C2.

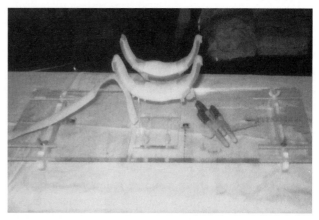

Figure 27-4. A Smither's headholder for total central nervous system treatments.

the entire spine. To encompass the entire spine, the field may have to be treated in two parts. A gap calculation must be done for the two fields. The match is at the level of the spine. In addition to the gap calculation just mentioned, another is done for the match of the spine and helmet field. The gap calculations are done to ensure coverage of the entire CNS with no cold spots (see Chapter 8).

The field size of these beam arrangements depends on the contour of the patient. The field must include the entire spine and the whole brain, including C2.

Another technique used to ensure that all the meninges

are being treated is the feathering technique. With this technique the junctions are shifted by changing the lengths of all fields. This is done daily with three different match lines. The marks are differentiated by three colored marks drawn on the patient's skin. These marks correspond to the same colored pens used to record information in the treatment chart.

The only border that must remain stable is the posterior border of the spine. A block is positioned at the posterior border of the spine for stability. As the length of the fields shift, the border with the blocked area remains stable.

The critical structures included in a CNS field are the lenses of the eyes, which are blocked with a moveable clinical block. The spinal cord is another critical structure, which receives a 1500 cGy dose.

Testis radiation for the treatment of ALL is usually in

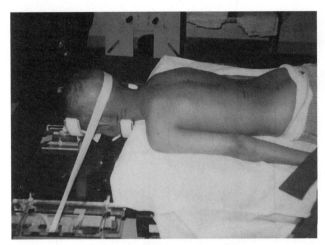

Figure 27-5. A patient immobilized through the use of the Smither's headholder. *(Courtesy Tufts-New England Medical Center's Radiation Oncology Department.)*

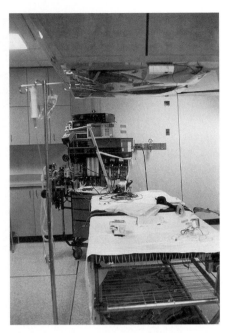

Figure 27-6. A dedicated TBI unit that has been in place since the early 1980s. It consists of two opposed 4-MV stationary linear accelerators, one mounted in the ceiling and the other in a pit under the floor.

combination with total body irradiation. The field design is a simple setup. The patient lies supine in a lithotomy position, and a field is set up to encompass the entire organ. The testis field is treated with electrons.

The Brigham and Women's Hospital/Dana Farber Cancer Institute's Radiation Oncology Department experience. There is a one of a kind dedicated TBI unit that has been in place since 1983. It consists of two opposed 4-MV stationary linear accelerators, one mounted in the ceiling and the other in a pit under the floor (Fig. 27-6). Patients lie supine on a canvas-covered frame large enough to accommodate the tallest person. The field size at a distance of 205 cm is 75 × 200 cm. Both radiation beams run at the same time. The treatment room is equipped with positive pressure and high-efficiency particulate air (HEPA) filtered air and thoroughly cleaned daily for use by immunosuppressed patients.

The patient has a chest simulation and customized 85% transmission lung shields are cut and placed anterior to posterior to lower the dose to the lungs to within 5% of the prescribed dose to decrease the incidence of interstitial pneumonitis. A portal imager verifies lung shield placement.

Fractions range from 150 to 200 cGy per treatment given bid 5 to 6 hours apart to a total dose of 1200 to 1400 cGy. The dose rate is 10 cGy/min. The dose is calculated to the midline of the patient at the umbilicus, and the average treatment time for a child and an adult is 15 and 20 minutes, respectively. The fractionated irradiation and low dose rate give time for the repair process to take place yet allow destruction of leukemic cells.

For those children in whom anesthesia is indicated a portable anesthesia machine is set up with television (TV) cameras focused on the monitors and the child (Fig. 27-7). A team of anesthesiologists delivers propofol (Diprivan), a very quick-acting anesthetic. It can be delivered easily through a

central line and the children recover rapidly and become fully awake posttreatment. They may have clear liquids for an hour or two before they must begin fasting again for their afternoon treatment.

In some situations a C2 whole brain boost may be treated prophylactically. The daily dose to the brain is in the range of 150 to 200 cGy to a total dose of 750 to 1000 cGy in addition to the TBI. Also, if indicated, an electron boost of 1000 cGy to the testes may be given.

The dose to the C2 whole brain is delivered by lateral opposed fields. The patient is supine and simulated in a head cup with a thermoplastic mask. The field covers the meninges and C2 fall-off around the head. Custom shielding blocks the face and lenses of the eyes.

The chemotherapy treatment techniques used in treating ALL are divided into four groups: induction, consolidation, prophylaxis of overt CNS disease, and maintenance therapy.[5] Induction therapy typically involves the use of prednisone or dexamethasone, vincristine, and L-asparaginase. These chemotherapeutic agents are given immediately after the diagnosis to eradicate all detectable leukemia. Consolidation therapy uses high-dose intravenous methotrexate, etoposide (VP-16), and L-asparaginase begins after remission has been achieved. Maintenance therapy involves the use of intravenous mercaptopurine (6-MP) and systemic methotrexate. The chemotherapeutic agent shown to be most effective in preventing overt CNS disease in several clinical trials is methotrexate. This drug is given either systemically or intrathecally. The

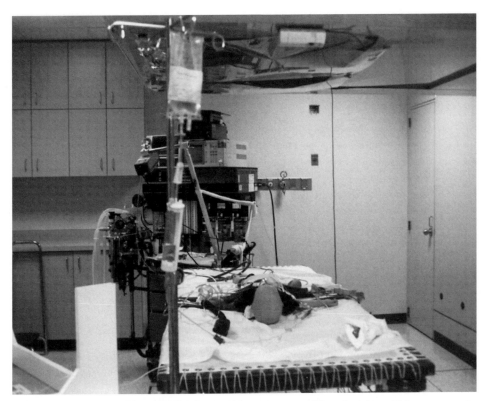

Figure 27-7. A portable anesthesia machine set up with television (TV) cameras to monitor a pediatric case, a child in whom anesthesia is indicated.

duration of chemotherapeutic treatment has been shortened from a range of 3 to 5 years to 1 ½ to 2 ½ years.[5]

Another treatment technique used for ALL is bone marrow transplantation. Bone marrow transplantation, which was considered an experimental procedure until about 20 years ago, is the treatment of choice for several diseases, including ALL, AML, and CML. The procedure involves the harvesting of healthy marrow from a suitable donor. The marrow is then infused into a patient whose diseased marrow has been destroyed or ablated by chemotherapy or TBI. The transplanted marrow finds its way into bone marrow cavities and begins supplying the patient with normal, healthy hemopoietic cells.

The most desirable donors are identical twins because they are generally identical to the patient for all transplantation antigens. Allogeneic transplants, available to 20% to 30% of patients, use human leukocyte antigen (HLA) histocompatible siblings as donors. In recent years, bone marrow registries have been developed to locate and use nonrelated histocompatible donors. Some success has been achieved with the use of marrow from donors in whom only a partial match of transplantation antigens is present.

For potential bone marrow donors, risks are small and primarily related to anesthesia. The aspiration of bone marrow is a technically simple transplant procedure done in the operating room under sterile conditions and anesthesia.

Multiple aspirations are drawn from the donor's anterior and posterior iliac crests. A small amount of heparin is used to prevent clotting.

The marrow recipient is treated before the transplant with a large dose of cyclophosphamide and TBI or with chemotherapy alone (busulfan and cyclophosphamide). These measures reduce the leukemic cell load and impair the host's ability to reject the donor marrow. After an intravenous injection the donor marrow cells migrate to the recipient's marrow cavities and begin to produce normal cells in the blood within 2 to 4 weeks.

Autologous bone marrow transplants involve the reinfusion of a patient's own marrow that has been harvested and cryopreserved while the patient was in remission. Leukemic cells are removed from the collected marrow through the use of monoclonal antibodies directed against cell-surface antigens that are expressed on leukemic blasts but not on normal stem cells.

Factors that lead to failure in bone marrow transplants are recurrent leukemia (primarily in autologous donors) and graft versus host disease, which occurs in about 50% of patients. This condition may exist only as a slight skin rash, or it may progress to a life-threatening syndrome involving the skin, liver, and/or gastrointestinal tract.[12]

Side effects. Patients receiving TBI experience numerous side effects. The gastrointestinal side effects include nausea, vomiting, diarrhea, anorexia, and malaise. Mucosa of the mouth, pharynx, bladder, and rectum may be affected.

Normal secretions are inhibited and their functions are impaired. The integumentary side effects include skin reactions, itching, tingling, bruising, and dry and inelastic skin that cracks easily. Alopecia can occur, as well as blanching or erythema of the skin and mucous membrane. A respiratory-related side effect is interstitial pneumonitis. These side effects are acute and subside in time.

Chronic side effects include permanent sterility and cataracts of the eyes (easily reversed with surgery). Hepatic fibrosis and radionecrosis of the genital tissue, muscle, and kidney are also chronic side effects.

The side effects for helmet and CNS radiation are skin reactions and hair loss for the integumentary system. The hemopoietic reactions are a decrease in blood counts and **leukoencephalopathy** (demyelinating brain lesions). Nausea and vomiting are the gastrointestinal side effects. The effect on the CNS is somnolence syndrome, characterized by drowsiness and malaise that is self-limiting. Serious injury to the tissue or blood vessels in the brain can lead to lethargy, seizures, spasticity, paresis, difficulty with movements, and Lhermitte's sign.

Lhermitte's sign may develop if the spine receives radiation treatment. This syndrome is characterized by a sensation of an electric shock in the arms, legs, or neck when the patient flexes the neck. These are the acute symptoms of helmet and CNS radiation.

The chronic side effects include neuropsychologic deficits, intellectual deficits, and cataract formation. Growth retardation and hypothalamic-pituitary dysfunction are a result of irradiation to the brain and CNS. Hypothalamic-pituitary dysfunction is an abnormality in the hormonal secretions that include growth hormones, thyroid hormones, adrenal hormones, and sex-related hormones. Myelopathy is another side effect causing irreversible injury to the spinal cord. Secondary tumors are also seen as a late effect. These tumors can be benign or malignant.

Chemotherapy has many side effects. The results from the cytotoxicity for each drug are different. The effects of vincristine are anorexia, constipation, and a metallic taste in the mouth. Neurologic effects include jaw pain, **diplopia** (double vision), vocal cord paresis, impotence, general motor weakness, and loss of deep tendon reflexes. The effects on the skin are alopecia and dermatitis.

Prednisone and dexamethasone are hormones, the effects of which are an exaggeration of normal physiologic action, suppression of immune function, hypertension, hyperglycemia, increased appetite, muscle weakness, diabetes, and fluid retention. Gastric irritation, osteoporosis, cataracts, menstrual irregularity, and a modification of tissue reactions leading to infection or slow tissue healing are other side effects of prednisone and dexamethasone.

L-Asparaginase causes gastrointestinal reactions such as anorexia, nausea, and vomiting. Neurologic reactions such as lethargy, progressive malaise, headaches, and confusion often result from this drug. Immunologic reactions can be seen secondary to a decreased number of lymphoblasts. The blood chemistry as a result of this agent has the following abnormalities: hypoalbuminemia, hyperglycemia, or altered blood-clotting factors. Elevated blood urea levels or pancreatic enzymes are also seen. Fever and chills are common side effects of this drug.

Etoposide (VP-16) causes bone marrow depression and gastrointestinal problems such as nausea and vomiting, **stomatitis,** and diarrhea. Cardiovascular effects include hypotension and anaphylaxis. The integumentary side effect is alopecia. Hepatotoxicity, parotitis, and radiation recall are considered major side effects.

Most side effects for 6-MP are gastrointestinal including nausea, vomiting, diarrhea, and anorexia. Myelosuppression is commonly seen with the administration of this agent. Hyperpigmentation of the skin is also seen, and hepatotoxicity is considered a major side effect.

Patients treated with methotrexate develop a rapid onset of bone marrow depression, with **nadir** (the lowest point) occurring in 10 to 14 days. Side effects include nausea, vomiting, stomatitis, pharyngitis, diarrhea, and renal dysfunction. Alopecia and a rash with associated erythema and **pruritus** (itching) are integumentary effects. Brown pigmentation of the skin and photosensitivity are other effects. Infertility and congenital malformation may result from this drug.

Case Study

A 12-year-old boy with recurrent ALL is considered for TBI before a bone marrow transplant. At age 3, he exhibited easy bruisability, fatigue, and coughing. Blood work performed at that time revealed a high white blood cell count, anemia, and thrombocytopenia. A bone marrow aspiration that extracted marrow from the patient's anterior iliac crest was done. A diagnosis of ALL was made at that time. After the diagnosis a chest x-ray examination was done to check for mediastinal involvement, thymic enlargement, and pleural effusion. No changes were seen.

His first course of treatment was chemotherapy. He received a chemotherapeutic regiment of prednisone, vincristine, and L-asparaginase and was placed in remission.

Approximately 14 months later, the patient exhibited testicular swelling. He received modified chemotherapy and radiation to his testes and remained in remission.

About 10 months later, the patient developed a nonproductive cough and a low-grade fever. These symptoms were treated with antibiotics, and they resolved. Approximately 3 months later, he showed increased fatigue and a nonproductive cough. A complete blood count (CBC) at this time was significant for a white count of 400,000/mm³ with 19% blasts. He had an immature T-cell, FAB classification of L2. A chest radiograph taken at that time revealed a mediastinal mass. He also exhibited hepatosplenomegaly.

The patient was scheduled to receive a regimen of vincristine, prednisone, and L-asparaginase. His family was tested, and his brother had an HLA match. The patient was enrolled in an in-house protocol for bone marrow transplantation: high-dose cyclophosphamide (Cytoxan) and TBI, followed by a bone marrow transplant.

ACUTE MYELOGENOUS LEUKEMIA

Epidemiology

The incidence rate of AML is approximately 10,500 cases per year.[1] AML typically occurs in patients over 40 years of age with a median age of 65 years at time of diagnosis.[7] In contrast to ALL (the predominant pediatric leukemia), approximately 90% of adults with acute leukemia have the myelogenous subtype. The incidence of AML is slightly higher among white males, with the gender difference being more obvious in older patients.[3]

Etiology

Risk factors for AML are similar to those for ALL. Exposure to ionizing radiation appears to increase a person's risk for developing the disease. An increased incidence of AML has occurred in military personnel at Nevada bomb test sites and patients treated with radiation for ankylosing spondylitis, menorrhagia, and thymic enlargement. Patients receiving thorium dioxide (Thorotrast) for radiologic examinations showed an increased risk of AML. Fanconi's anemia and Bloom syndrome (genetic disorders with a chromosome breakage tendency) and exposure to benzene and alkylating agents have also been associated with AML risk.[11]

Prognostic Indicators

Unfavorable prognostic variables of AML are similar to those of ALL. Unfavorable signs include an age older than 50 years, myelodysplastic syndrome, a poor performance status, impaired organ function, and low serum albumin. Children with AML have a poorer prognosis than those with ALL. As with ALL, a WBC of less than 20,000/mm^3 is more favorable than a WBC of 20,000 to 49,000/mm^3. A WBC of greater than 50,000/mm^3 is the least favorable. For AML the age, tumor burden at the time of diagnosis, and drug sensitivity of the leukemic cells are more important than cell morphology in predicting survival.

Clinical Presentation

The onset of AML may be abrupt, although most patients experience a 1- to 6-month prodromal period, during which symptoms are present. As with ALL, symptoms at the time of presentation include nonspecific flulike symptoms. Fatigue, pallor, and dyspnea on exertion are secondary to anemia. Petechiae, **purpura** (hemorrhage under the skin), epistaxis, gingival bleeding, and gastrointestinal or urinary tract bleeding may result from reduced platelet production. Neutropenia may result in a susceptibility to local infections, such as skin abscesses, or systemic infections with accompanying fever, chills, and site-specific symptoms. The sensation of an enlarged spleen may be present.

Detection and Diagnosis

Specific tests for detecting AML include CBCs, differential leukocyte and platelet counts, and blood smears. Abnormal blood counts lead to the detection of AML. Thrombocytopenia, anemia, and an increased leukocyte count should be suspect in patients with these conditions. Another form of detection is that of chromosomal abnormalities, which occur in 30% to 50% of patients with AML.[11]

The circulation of **Auer rods** (structures present in the cytoplasm of myeloblasts, myelocytes, and monoblasts) in the leukemic cells is central to the diagnostic finding of AML. A definitive diagnosis is made via a bone marrow aspiration and biopsy. In AML the bone marrow is hypercellular. The diagnosis is made based on the percentage of blast cells. If more than 30% blast cells are present, acute leukemia is the diagnosis. A staining procedure is the final step to determine a differential diagnosis of AML. In summary, a diagnosis of AML is based on the circulation of Auer rods in leukemic cells, an increase in leukemic blast cells, and a decrease in normal precursors.

Immunophenotyping that includes a morphologic evaluation, special stains, electron microscopic examination, and surface marker studies can establish a diagnosis in 90% of AML patients.[11] Morphologic evaluations are based on monoclonal antibodies reacting with a surface antigen that is expressed on the membrane of the leukemic cell.

Pathology

AML results from the unregulated proliferation of early precursor cells that have lost the ability to differentiate in response to hormonal signals and cellular interactions. This proliferation or clonal disease involves the hemopoietic stem cells or pluripotent cells. The result is a gradual accumulation of undifferentiated cells in marrow or other organs.

These undifferentiated cells have a decreased proportion of blast cells in the S or M phase of the cell cycle compared with normal bone marrow blast cells. Because of this decrease of blast cells in these specific phases, the cells do not reach maturity or are defective at maturity.

Staging and Classification

For a morphologic evaluation the FAB system is used. AML is categorized in different maturation states, from M0 (undifferentiated) to M7 (megakaryocytic). They are as follows[3]:

M0—minimal evidence of maturation exists.

M1—the cells tend to have fine azurophil granules and may have few Auer rods. Minimal evidence exists of differentiation along the rest of the granulocytic or monocytic lineages.

M2—the number of blast cells is greater than 30%, and the less than 20% of monocytic precursors have abundant cytoplasm and moderate to marked granularity.

M3—the acute promyelocytic leukemia (APL) predominant cell is heavily granulated with azurophil granulation. Many cells have bundle of Auer rods whose nucleus is often bilobed or kidney shaped.

M4—the myeloid precursors or other granulocytic precursors are between 20% and 80% of the nonerythroid nucleated cells. The monocytic cells comprise 20% or more of the nonerythroid nucleated cells.

M5—the proportion of granulocyte precursors is less than 20%.
M6—fewer than 30% of the cells are of myeloid or monocytic lineage, and more than 50% are megaloblastic erythroid precursors.
M7—this state is often associated with extensive marrow fibrosis that has an increase in reticulin or collagen.

Other classifying techniques include cytochemical, immunologic, and chromosomal studies.

Treatment Techniques

The treatment techniques for AML are radiation therapy, chemotherapy, and bone marrow transplantation. These three techniques are used in a combined fashion.

Radiation therapy is administered to the whole body (TBI). It is given bid for 3 days, with a total dose of 1200 cGy. (See the ALL treatment technique section on pp. 616-620 for further details.)

The chemotherapy treatment techniques for treating AML are divided into two groups: remission induction and postinduction consolidation/maintenance. The drugs used in remission induction therapy are cytosine arabinoside combined with an anthracycline antibiotic such as daunorubicin, doxorubicin, or idarubicin.[7] Cytosine arabinoside (Cytarabine) is used for consolidation/maintenance therapy. Cytosine arabinoside mimics the natural building blocks of ribonucleic acid (RNA) and DNA to prevent the cell from growing. The other chemicals used in the regiment, the anthracycline antibiotics, impede cell survival by interacting directly with the nuclear DNA.

Bone marrow transplantation is the final treatment technique used in treating AML. (See p. 619 for a description of the bone marrow transplantation procedure.)

Field design and critical structures. The field design and critical structures are described in the section on ALL on p. 616.

Side effects. Bone marrow depression, which occurs in 4 to 7 days, and immunologic suppression are the hemopoietic side effects of cytosine arabinoside. Nausea, vomiting, esophagitis, stomatitis, diarrhea, and ulceration are common gastrointestinal problems. Renal effects include urinary retention and thrombophlebitis. Rashes and alopecia are skin reactions. In the reproduction system, mutagenic and teratogenic problems arise.

Bone marrow depression also occurs after the use of the anthracycline antibiotics. With these drugs, common gastrointestinal problems are abdominal pain and stomatitis. Myocardial toxicity is the dose-limiting factor for daunorubicin. The integumentary effects are alopecia, hyperpigmentation of the nail beds, and sun sensitivity. Reproductive side effects are teratogenic or mutagenic. The urine turns red after one or two administrations.

Case Study

A 41–year-old mother of two was considered for total body irradiation followed by bone marrow transplantation. She initially complained of heavy menstrual periods and progressive fatigue. She noted dyspnea on exertion, petechiae, and some gingival bleeding.

About 2 months later, a blood test was performed and the patient was found to have pancytopenia with a WBC of 900/mm³, the hematocrit at 17%, and platelet count was 80,000/mm³. A bone marrow aspiration and biopsy showed myeloblasts, and the diagnosis of AML was made.

The patient received induction chemotherapy with cytosine arabinoside and daunorubicin. This treatment was complicated by neutropenia, a fever, and a rash that she developed over her body.

She had her first postremission consolidation therapy 1 month later, with cytosine arabinoside combined with hydrocortisone. She tolerated this treatment well. Her maintenance therapy consisted of 6-thioguanine, vincristine, and prednisone. This treatment caused diarrhea, anorexia, and dermatitis.

The patient now awaits her TBI and bone marrow transplant. Her brother is a 5.6 HLA match. She is being prepared for a bone marrow transplant and is having a second cycle of consolidation therapy.

CHRONIC LYMPHOCYTIC LEUKEMIA

Epidemiology

CLL affects approximately 7300 cases per year and accounts for approximately 30% of the leukemia cases in the United States. CLL is nearly twice as common as the chronic myelogenous subtype. The incidence of CLL increases with age, with 71 as the average age of onset. The disease is rare in persons younger than 40 years. CLL affects approximately 5.2 persons per 100,000 between 35 and 59 years of age and 30.4 persons per 100,000 between 80 and 84 years.[9] The disease affects twice as many males as females and is less common among Japanese and other Asian populations.[3] CLL occurs with equal frequency among black and white people.

Etiology

Heredity appears to play a role in the development of CLL. First-degree relatives of persons with CLL have a two- to seven fold increase in risk, and the familial clustering of CLL is the most notable of all the leukemias. Immunologic factors such as immunodeficiency syndromes and viruses have been associated with CLL. Several small studies have attempted to determine a suspected link between CLL and chemicals (primarily carbon tetrachloride and carbon disulfide) used in the rubber industry. CLL is the only leukemia for which an association with radiation exposure has not been established. In addition, retroviruses have not been linked with this disease.[3]

Prognostic Indicators

Prognostic factors for CLL include the stage at the time of diagnosis, age, doubling time of the peripheral blood lymphocyte count, and pattern of bone marrow involvement. The T-cell variety of CLL tends to run a more aggressive clinical course and results in shorter survival times.[11]

Clinical Presentation

This subtype is characterized with minimal changes in their blood count.[8] CLL most often occurs as incidental findings on blood tests taken during routine medical visits, with lymphocyte counts often equal to or higher than 10,000/mm³. Patients are frequently asymptomatic, with abnormalities found only on peripheral blood smears and a bone marrow biopsy. Complaints include fatigue, fever, night sweats, and weight loss. Lymphadenopathy may be present in CLL, and the spleen is almost always enlarged. Complaints of uncomfortable neck masses are common at later stages.

Detection and Diagnosis

Blood tests are used to detect CLL. Patients always exhibit lymphocytosis. Other manifestations of the disease are anemia and thrombocytopenia. Laboratory tests that determine monoclonal surface immunoglobulin and B-cell markers are important to the diagnosis. Phenotyping of leukemic lymphocytes reveals a B-cell origin in 95% of CLL cases.[11]

Other factors leading to the detection and diagnosis of CLL include the enlargement of lymph nodes and the spleen. Of patients with CLL, 50% have chromosomal abnormalities.

Pathology

The origin of CLL may be in the bone marrow lymphoid tissue.[11] A pathologic examination of CLL reveals an increased proliferation of leukemic cells in the bone marrow, blood, lymph nodes, and spleen, with resulting organ enlargement and decreased bone marrow function.[3]

Staging and Classification

One classification system for CLL is the Rai's staging system.[8] With this system the three major prognostic groups used to categorize patients are as follows:

Stage 0—low risk
Stages I and II—intermediate risk
Stages III and IV—high risk

These stages are based on the presence of adenopathy, splenomegaly, anemia, and thrombocytopenia.[6] Most patients are in the intermediate-risk category, followed by an equal percentage for the other prognostic groups.

The Binet staging system categorizes patients into three stages based on the involvement of five specific anatomic sites: the cervical nodes, axillary nodes, inguinal nodes, spleen, and liver. These stages are as follows[11]:

Stage A—no cytopenia and involvement of up to two sites
Stage B—involvement of three or more sites
Stage C—anemia, thrombocytopenia, or both

Cytochemistry is used to classify CLL according to two subtypes: B-cell CLL and T-cell CLL.[3]

Treatment Techniques

The optimal treatment for CLL is unknown. It is believed that some patients with an early stage of the disease will not

benefit from treatment. Chemotherapy is administered for progressive anemia and thrombocytopenia. The drugs used primarily are chlorambucil, an alkylating agent, and prednisone. Chlorambucil prevents the separation of the strands of DNA, which is necessary for cell replication.[11]

Other treatment techniques are radiation therapy and surgery. Palliative radiation therapy is used for localized masses of lymphoid tissue and/or an enlarged spleen. The treatment is given in an anteroposterior/posteroanterior (AP/PA) fashion to a dose of 500 cGy, delivering 100 cGy per day for 5 days.

The surgery used for treating CLL is the splenectomy. An enlarged spleen causes cytopenia, which is the result of accelerated removal or excessive pooling of platelets or RBCs. A splenectomy is used in a situation in which markedly enlarged spleen produces cytopenia.

Field design and critical structures. The field design for treating a spleen is clinical. The field must encompass the entire spleen with a 1-cm margin around the organ. Field setups are done through palpation or a fluoroscopy. Simulation is necessary to localize the spleen field and to ensure that the kidney is safely out of the field. Iodinated contrast is used for this intravenous pyelogram procedure.

Side effects. Cloramabucil causes bone marrow depression. Gastrointestinal side effects include anorexia, nausea, and vomiting. Dermatitis and urticaria are other side effects. Reproductive side effects include mutagenesis, teratogenesis, and sterility.

Prednisone causes gastrointestinal peptic ulcers and pancreatitis. Metabolic responses include centripetal obesity, hyperlipidemia, hyperosmolar nonketotic coma, and immunosuppression. The neurologic side effect is pseudotumor cerebri. Glaucoma and cataracts may also appear. Hypertension, skin striae, amenorrhea, and impaired wound healing are also side effects

Case Study

Mrs. W. is a 68-year-old woman who was diagnosed with CLL 2 years ago. She was treated at a neighborhood health center for a thyroid condition. During a routine blood test, her differential count showed a lymphocytosis of 67% (WBC was 10,800/mm³). Her hematocrit had dropped from an average of 36% to 32.2%. Therefore she was referred for further evaluation.

The patient's initial history revealed night sweats and a fever. She had chronic sinus congestion and hearing loss. She denied having a cough, shortness of breath, or chest pain, but she did note slight fatigue. Her spleen was enlarged.

Her physical examination showed clear lungs, no hepatomegaly, and no arthritis. Her blood work showed a hemoglobin of 11.6 g/100 ml, a hematocrit of 35.1%, a mean corpuscular volume (MCV) of 90.1 mm³, and unremarkable red blood cell (RBC) morphology. Her WBC was 11,700/mm³. These results indicate that the hemoglobin and hematocrit at the lower limits of normal. The lymphocytosis was consistent with CLL stage O. Peripheral blood lymphocyte markers were obtained, revealing 63% B cells. This is also consistent with CLL stage O.

About 10 months after diagnosis, Mrs. W. developed neuropathy with pain and numbness of her feet. A neurologist examined her and no pathologic changes were identified. A few months later, she developed leg ulcers. At this point, she was started on a treatment of prednisone. Her pain improved, and her ankle ulcers healed.

Mrs. W. is presently asymptomatic, and her prognosis is excellent.

CHRONIC MYELOGENOUS LEUKEMIA

Epidemiology

CML accounts for approximately 15% of all leukemias.[6] The incidence of this disease, which is rare in childhood and uncommon before the age of 20, peaks among persons in their mid-40s. A slight predominance of cases exists among males.

Etiology

The cause of CML is unknown. Radiation and benzene exposure have been linked with the development of the disease, but no other environmental or genetic factors have been clearly implicated as causes. The identification of the Philadelphia chromosome by Nowell and Hungerford in 1960 and its presence in 95% of CML patients has led to much interest regarding its possible etiologic role in this disorder.

Prognostic Indicators

The prognosis for patients with CML is affected by numerous factors, including the spleen size, platelet count, hematocrit, gender, and percentage of blood myeloblasts. The disease typically transforms into an acute leukemia after a chronic phase of about 4 to 6 years, when the patient enters a blast crisis. A patient in the active phase of the disease has a median survival time of approximately 2 years.[6]

Clinical Presentation

The natural history of CML is divided into three stages: chronic, accelerated, and acute phase, or blast crisis. The early phase of the disease is usually insidious; clinical symptoms are generally mild and nonspecific. Malaise, fatigue, heat intolerance, sweating, and easy bruising are common complaints. Symptoms related to splenic enlargement include vague discomfort in the left upper quadrant (LUQ), early satiety, weight loss, and peripheral leg edema. Within 3 to 4 years, most patients undergo a transformation to a blast crisis. At this stage, all the organs of the body are invaded by leukemic blast cells, and the circulating blood count can reach several hundreds of thousands per cubic millimeter. During the blast crisis, symptoms include fever, bone pain, and more pronounced weight loss.

The active-disease phase of CML, as defined by the Chronic Leukemia Myeloma Task Force, is characterized by weight loss greater than 10% of the body weight in less than 6 months, fever, extreme fatigue, anemia, thrombocytopenia, organ involvement (other than lymph nodes, spleen, bone marrow, and liver), and progressive or painful enlargement of the spleen.

Detection and Diagnosis

The detection and diagnosis of CML is difficult. This disease is insidious and generally not detected, except incidentally. Specific indicators lead to a diagnosis. These abnormal indicators include mild to moderate anemia and leukocytosis. Myeloblasts, promyelocytes, and nucleated red cells, which indicate CML, are present in the blood. Bone marrow specimens reveal increased granulocytic and often megakaryocytic hyperplasia. Another indicator of CML is a low or absent leukocyte alkaline phosphatase (LAP) score. The most important diagnostic factor for detecting CML is the presence of the Philadelphia chromosome.

Pathology

CML pathogenesis is a result of abnormal hemopoietic stem cells that give rise to progeny that have the Philadelphia chromosome.[11] Because of the abnormal stem cell pool, an increased proliferation of granulocytic and megakaryocytic cells exists. Erythropoiesis is impaired.[13]

Staging and Classification

The three distinct stages of CML are the chronic (or stable) phase, accelerated phase, and acute phase (or blast crisis). (For a further description of stages, see the clinical presentation section.)

Treatment Techniques

The three treatment techniques for treating CML are radiation therapy, chemotherapy, and bone marrow transplantation. Radiation therapy is delivered to the spleen and total body. The treatment technique for the spleen is the same as that for CLL. (See the treatment techniques section for CLL on p. 623.) The treatment technique for TBI is the same as that for ALL.

In chemotherapy the drugs used are alpha-interferon, busulfan, and hydroxyurea. Alpha-interferon is an immunotherapeutic drug. Busulfan is an alkylating agent given orally. It causes a gradual reduction of the leukocyte count toward normal, an increase in the RBC count, and a decrease in the spleen size. Hydroxyurea blocks DNA synthesis by inhibiting a ribonucleotide reductase.

The final treatment technique for CML is bone marrow transplantation. (See the treatment technique section for ALL on p. 616.) Allogeneic bone marrow transplantation is the only curative treatment for CML. The success rate for patients is lower when they are in the accelerated phase, especially if they have developed a blast transformation.

Field design and critical structures. The spleen field design is explained in the CLL section on p. 623. The TBI field design is explained in the ALL section on p. 616.

Side effects. Alpha-interferon side effects include flulike symptoms: fever, chills, malaise, muscle aches, anorexia, and weigh loss. The side effects of busulfan include pancytopenia and delayed bone marrow depression. Gastrointestinal side effects are diarrhea, nausea, and vomiting. Interstitial pulmonary fibrosis is a pulmonary side effect. In the integumentary system, alopecia, hyperpigmentation, and muscle wasting occur. In the reproductive system, testicular atrophy and gynecomastia occur in males. Amenorrhea and sterility are other reproductive side effects. Cataract formation also occurs.

Hydroxyurea affects the hemopoietic system, with bone marrow depression, rapid leukopenia, and erythrocytic abnormalities. The gastrointestinal side effects are anorexia and diarrhea. Facial erythema and maculopapular rash are integumentary reactions. The reproductive side effect is teratogenic.

Case Study

A 17-year-old girl with CML complained of a 1-month history of fatigue, easy bruising, and the passing of large blood clots during a menstrual period. Blood work was performed and revealed a WBC of 78,000/mm^3. A blood smear showed numerous myeloid forms consistent with CML. Her hematocrit was 35%, and her platelet count was 204,000/mm^3.

A bone marrow biopsy and aspiration were performed and found to be consistent with CML. Her LAP score was 36. Cytogenetics showed a translocation of the chromosomes 9 and 22. This is consistent with a Philadelphia chromosome.

The patient was first given alpha-interferon. She tolerated this well, aside from some mild flulike symptoms and diarrhea. About 3 months later, the patient received 500 cGy to her spleen. This was followed by TBI and a bone marrow transplant 1 week later.

ROLE OF RADIATION THERAPIST

Because of the systemic nature of the disease, chemotherapy is the front-line treatment for leukemia. Radiation therapy plays a relatively small, although significant, role in the management of this group of diseases. Therapists who work in health care facilities in which bone marrow transplants are not performed or in which specialized pediatric oncology services are not provided may see few leukemia patients. Issues relating to scheduling treatments and communicating with and providing support and reassurance for children and their parents must be taken into consideration in departments that routinely treat leukemia patients. Therapists should work closely with the child life specialist assigned to pediatric oncology patients to gain a better understanding of the patients' and their families' status.

In treating children who have leukemia, therapists must be prepared to communicate with and provide support for the patients and their parents. The radiation oncology experience may evoke fear; the equipment is large and imposing, and the child has most likely undergone numerous painful medical

procedures. Sufficient time should be allowed for an explanation of the procedures and the provision of necessary support. Creative methods of eliciting the cooperation of a young child (e.g., stuffed animals and rewards for holding still) and extreme patience may be necessary if anesthesia for daily treatment must be avoided. Exposure of the anatomic areas to be treated may cause emotional concern for a young patient and must be considered and respected by the treatment team. Therapists must be aware of the concerns of the patient's parents, who often have had to subject their child to painful medical procedures and are themselves coping with issues of denial, acceptance, and possible loss.

Last-minute changes and delays in scheduling often accompany the treatment of leukemia patients. Radiation therapists should be aware of these modifications and realize that the flexibility of daily treatment schedules is frequently necessary. Children who require anesthesia for their daily treatments not only need extra time and equipment for treatment but also require careful coordination of radiation oncology, anesthesia, and nursing schedules. The radiation oncologist may need to set up treatment fields daily for leukemia patients treated for an enlarged liver or spleen. The radiation oncologist palpates the organ and modifies the field as needed. Patients treated for the control of blood counts may need to have blood drawn and blood count results reported before each treatment. Extra time may be required for positioning and precise matching of multiple fields for CNS treatment.

TBI in preparation for bone marrow transplantation requires special attention and consideration by the radiation therapist. As much as $1\frac{1}{2}$ hours need to be set aside in the treatment schedule for each of these procedures. If bid treatment is prescribed, major interruptions in the daily treatment schedule can occur, requiring the rescheduling of other patients' appointments. Because the bone marrow transplant patient's immune system is compromised, the treatment room and machine must be scrubbed with disinfectant before the patient's arrival. The treatment team must use reverse isolation techniques (i.e., gown, gloves, and mask). Extra time and patience is required to ensure that the patient is in a position that can be maintained for the actual treatment. Because an extended source-skin distance (SSD) is required to achieve the necessary field size, the actual treatment (beam on) time required to deliver the prescribed dose is often as long as 45 minutes. The patient may experience nausea during treatment. The treatment must then be interrupted, and the patient must be allowed to move and walk around until the nausea subsides. At that time the patient can be repositioned, and the treatment can be resumed.

Present Outcomes

The most exciting outcomes that have taken place in the last 50 years are in the area of pediatric leukemia. The most common form of pediatric leukemia is ALL. Because of the advancement of multidisciplinary therapeutic interventions, children's survival has gone from 4% in 1962 to 5-year survival rates of 75% to 80%.[11]

Over the years treatment advances for AML have improved the remission rates substantially.[11] Adults with AML in the induction phase of therapy go into complete remission roughly 60% to 70% of the time.[11] Of this cohort, there is a survival rate of 3 years or more and a possible cure rate in 15% of this population.[11] It is important to note that the younger the individual is when diagnosed will ultimately result in a better remission rate than when the diagnosis is made in the older adult.[11,]

Because there is no definitive therapy for cure for CLL, the 5-year survival rate is 60%.[11] This survival rate is determined by the stage of the disease at presentation. Leukemia is not treated in the early stages of CLL. This subtype of leukemia occurs predominately in the senior population. The disease progresses slowly. Oncologists treat CLL in a conservative manner. Typically no treatment is given in the early stages.[11]

In general, CML has no treatment cure. The survival rates depend on what phase the individual has developed. In the accelerated phase, survival is approximately 1 year or less, and in the more severe phase, after blast transformation, individuals live only a few months.[11] There are longer survival rates for those individuals who are undergoing lymphocytic transformation.[11]

Review Questions

1. Which of the following concerning CLL is not true?
   a. It is a disease of children
   b. It resembles CML but with a malignant lymphoid cell line
   c. It can be confused with lymphoma
   d. Therapy is usually reserved until the patient is symptomatic
2. Which of the following is a specific characteristic of CML?
   a. A disease of children
   b. Philadelphia chromosome
   c. Requirement of prophylactic central nervous system radiation
   d. Presentation with an enlarged spleen
3. Which of the following is not a common symptom associated with acute leukemia at the time of presentation?
   a. Fatigue
   b. Easy bleeding and bruisability
   c. Nausea and vomiting
   d. Fever
4. Which of the following leukemias has not been associated with previous radiation exposure?
   a. CML
   b. CLL
   c. AML
   d. ALL

5. Anatomic sites that are potential sanctuaries for leukemic cells are the
   I. Testes
   II. Spleen
   III. Central nervous system
   a. I and II only
   b. I and III only
   c. II and III only
   d. I, II, and III
6. Which of the following is NOT one of the main subtypes of leukemia?
   a. ALL
   b. AML
   c. CCL
   d. CLL
7. The primary treatment modality for leukemia is
   a. Surgery
   b. Immunotherapy
   c. Ionizing radiation
   d. Chemotherapy
8. The most documented etiologic factor for leukemia in humans is
   a. Surgery
   b. Immunotherapy
   c. Ionizing radiation
   d. Chemotherapy
9. Which type of leukemia essentially has no cure?
   a. ALL
   b. AML
   c. CLL
   d. CML
10. Splenomegaly indicates:
    a. An enlargement of the liver
    b. An enlargement of the spleen
    c. An increase in the circulating platelets
    d. A better than average prognosis for ALL and CLL

Questions to Ponder

1. Discuss the main factors that differentiate the four subtypes of leukemia.
2. Describe the various treatment techniques used for the four main subtypes of leukemia.
3. Describe the systems used to classify the leukemias.
4. Differentiate between detection and diagnosis in reference to the specific subtypes of leukemia.
5. Describe the different types of bone marrow transplantation techniques.

REFERENCES
1. American Cancer Society: *Cancer facts and figures,* Atlanta, 2003, American Cancer Society.
2. Dameshek W, Gunz F: *Leukemia,* ed 2, New York, 1964, Grune & Stratton.

3. DeVita V, Hellman S, Rosenberg S: *Cancer principles and practice of oncology,* Philadelphia, 1993, JB Lippincott.
4. Freireich EJ, Lemak NA: Milestones in leukemia research and therapy, Baltimore, 1991, John Hopkins University Press.
5. Halperin EC, et al: *Pediatric radiation oncology,* Philadelphia, 1999, Lippincott Williams & Wilkins.
6. JAMA: *Leukemia research,* available at http:jama.ama-assn.org (accessed April 11, 2003).
7. The Leukemia and Lymphoma Society: *Acute myelogenous leukemia,* available at http://www.leukemia-lymphoma.org (accessed April 11, 2003).
8. The Leukemia and Lymphoma Society. *Chronic lymphocytic leukemia,* available at http://www.leukemia-lymphoma.org (accessed April 11, 2003).
9. National Cancer Institute: *Surveillance, epidemiology, and end results,* available at http://seer.cancer.gov (accessed April 11, 2003).
10. St. Jude's Children's Hospital: Leukemia in children-21st century treatment, 2002, available at http://www.stjude.org (accessed May 13, 2002).
11. Scigliano E, et al: The leukemias. In Rubin P, editor: *Clinical oncology: a multidisciplinary approach for physicians and students,* ed 8, Philadelphia, 2001, WB Saunders.
12. Thomas ED: Bone marrow transplantation, *CA J Clin* 37:291-296, 1987.
13. University of Pennsylvania: Oncolink, available at http://www.oncolink.com (accessed May 14, 2002).
14. Wiernik PH, et al: *Neoplastic diseases of the blood,* New York, 1991, Churchill Livingstone.

BIBLIOGRAPHY

American Cancer Society: *Clinical oncology,* Atlanta, 2000, American Cancer Society.
Brager BL, Yasko J: *Care of the client receiving chemotherapy,* Reston, Va, 1984, Reston Publishing.
Henderson ES, Han T: Current therapy of acute and chronic leukemia in adults, *CA J Clin* 36:322-350, 1986.
Tarbel N, Mauch P, Chin L: Total body irradiation. In *JCRT handbook,* Boston, 1994, Joint Center for Radiation Therapy.
Washington CM, Leaver DT, editors: *Principles and practice of radiation therapy: introduction to radiation therapy,* St. Louis, 1996, Mosby.

Endocrine System

Tammy Newell, Robert D. Adams

Outline

Key Terms

The endocrine system is composed of multiple glandular organs responsible for complex metabolic regulatory functions. The principal organs of this system include the following glands: pituitary (which resides in the sella turcica at the base of the brain), thyroid, and adrenal. Also included are the parathyroid glands and specialized cells in the pancreas called the islets of Langerhans, which are referred to as the endocrine portions of the pancreas. Each of these organs (or specialized portions of them) produces hormones under complex feedback-control mechanisms that affect various functions to meet ongoing metabolic needs and stresses of the organism. The master regulatory gland of this system is the pituitary. This gland produces many hormones under the influence of the hypothalamus, which directly affects the function of other endocrine organs. This sophisticated mechanism of stimulation and inhibition of endocrine organ function is critical for maintaining metabolic homeostasis (stability) and providing the organism with the ability to respond to various stresses.

Many disorders of the endocrine organs can result in disruption of this complex surveillance and response system. These disorders may be related to benign, congenital, degenerative, traumatic, autoimmune, or infectious processes that may affect the function of one or many organs in the endocrine system. The result can range from minor to potentially life-threatening dysfunction. Probably the most widely recognized endocrine dysfunction is insufficient insulin production by the islet cells of the pancreas, or diabetes mellitus. Although this is a complex multisystem disease, the abnormality in glucose metabolism caused by insulin deficiency can be disastrous. This situation is remedied through the supply of insulin via an injection to reestablish homeostasis of glucose metabolism.

The function of the endocrine system may also be affected

by neoplastic change in the various glands. Although true primary malignancies of these organs are rare, they are important to consider because of the wide-ranging effects they can have on the organism as a whole. Metabolic function altered by neoplastic change in various endocrine organs can produce clinical syndromes that are often well recognized. These syndromes can lead the clinician to perform various diagnostic studies to confirm the suspicions related to an endocrine gland tumor. This chapter discusses neoplastic lesions of the thyroid, pituitary, and adrenal gland. Pancreatic tumors, which can display endocrine and exocrine function, are discussed in Chapter 32.

THYROID CANCER

Epidemiology

Although thyroid cancers are the most common of the endocrine malignancies (accounting for approximately 90% of all new cases and 63% of deaths), they represent only 1.3% of all cancers. Women have a higher incidence rate than men, with approximately a 2.3:1.0 ratio. Young adult females have a fivefold risk compared with males.[12]

Etiology

Unlike other endocrine glands for which the incidence of malignancy is rare, thyroid cancer has several recognized etiologic factors.

External radiation to the thyroid gland, particularly before puberty, is the only well-documented etiologic factor. Approximately 25% of the patients who receive between 2 cGy and several hundred cGy of external radiation to the thyroid gland develop thyroid carcinoma. These carcinomas are usually a low-grade papillary subtype.[12]

Many studies have been conducted on the inhabitants of Nagasaki and Hiroshima after the explosion of the atomic bomb in 1945. Out of 20,000 heavily and lightly exposed individuals examined every year since 1959, approximately 0.2% have developed thyroid cancer. Again, most of these cancers have been papillary.[12]

After the radioactive fallout from a nuclear test in the Marshall Islands, the inhabitants have annually been studied systematically and compared with a nonexposed population. According to the results in 1974, 34 of 229 exposed persons developed thyroid lesions. Three of the total number of patients developed cancers. Those irradiated before the age of 20 showed the highest incidence rate of thyroid nodularity.[12]

The Chernobyl incident of 1986 has produced conflicting studies on the increase of thyroid cancer, probably because of the extremely short interval between radiation exposure and tumor occurrence. One study conducted 4½ years after the Chernobyl reactor accident showed no significant difference in thyroid nodularity among persons residing in highly contaminated and control villages.[16] However, another study's data confirm that the neoplasms increasingly diagnosed between 1986 and 1991 among children of the Republic of Belarus were thyroid carcinomas.[8] In the Cancer Registry of Belarus, 101 instances of thyroid cancer in children younger than 15 years had been noted between 1986 and 1991, in contrast to only 9 cases between 1976 and 1985.[8]

External radiation for benign disease, especially in young patients, was a widespread practice in the United States in the 1930s, 1940s, and 1950s. X-rays or radium was used to treat benign conditions such as acne, tonsillitis, hemangiomas, and thymic enlargement. Young patients who received radiation for malignant conditions, such as mantle irradiation for Hodgkin's disease, demonstrated an increased risk of developing thyroid cancer.[12,15]

The latent (time) period between exposure and incidence of abnormalities varies with age. The average **latent period** in infants is 11 years, and in adolescents it is 15 to 30 years. Whether adults develop cancer at a higher rate after exposure is questionable.[12]

Prolonged stimulation of the thyroid gland with a thyroid-stimulating hormone (TSH) in laboratory animals has produced thyroid cancer. However, no human population studies have been done that support this hypothesis.[20]

Some other, less well-defined, factors include the following[3]:

- Long-standing, nontoxic colloid goiter in relation to papillary and anaplastic carcinoma
- The relationship of follicular adenomas as premalignant lesions to follicular carcinomas
- The role of genetics for medullary carcinoma*

Prognostic Indicators

Age, gender, histologic subtype, and capsular invasion are prognostic. Lesions confined to the gland have an overall better prognosis than those demonstrating capsular invasion. Patients with well-differentiated thyroid carcinoma (papillary and follicular) have a better prognosis than those with undifferentiated carcinoma (anaplastic).

Anatomy

The thyroid gland, consisting of a right and left lobe, lies over the deep structures of the neck; is close to the larynx, trachea, parathyroid glands, and esophagus; and is anterior and medial to the carotid artery, jugular vein, and vagus nerve.[12] (See Fig. 28-1 for the anatomy of the thyroid gland and its anatomic relationships to surrounding structures.)

The lateral lobes are approximately 5 cm in length and extend to the level of the midthyroid cartilage superiorly and the sixth tracheal ring inferiorly. These lobes are connected in the midline by the **isthmus** at the level of the second to fourth tracheal rings. The thyroid gland weighs approximately 25 g.[12]

Lymphatic capillaries are arranged throughout the gland and drain to many nodal sites. These sites include the internal jugular chain, Delphian node (anterior cervical node), pretracheal nodes, and the paratracheal nodes in the lower neck.[12] Superior

---

*A large proportion of cases are familial, occurring as part of two complex endocrine syndromes: multiple endocrine neoplasia (MEN) IIa and IIb.

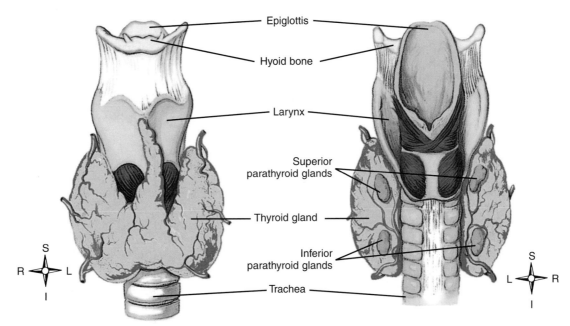

Figure 28-1. Anatomy of the thyroid gland. *(From Thibodeau GA, Patton KT, editors: Anatomy and physiology, St. Louis, 1999, Mosby.)*

mediastinal lymphatics can be considered the lowest part of the cervical lymphatic system. If it is involved, this represents significant regional spread of disease.[12]

Physiology

The thyroid gland produces several hormones, including thyroxine (T4) and triiodothyronine (T3), which are responsible for metabolic regulation. Thyroidal function is regulated by pituitary and hypothalamic hormones, which respond to complex systemic negative feedback mechanisms based on metabolic needs. The TSH produced in the pituitary gland causes direct stimulation of thyroid cells to produce and release hormones that are critical for carbohydrate and protein metabolism.

The production of these hormones relies on the thyroid gland's ability to remove iodine from the blood. Without sufficient amounts of iodine, several clinical disorders can be observed from the resultant deficiency in thyroid-hormone production. Functional disorders of the thyroid gland are characterized by hyperactivity (**hyperthyroidism**) or underactivity (**hypothyroidism**).

Disorders from hypothyroidism can include the following[25]:
- **Cretinism**—this disorder appears in infants shortly after birth. Symptoms include stunted growth, abnormal bone formation, retarded mental development, a low body temperature, and sluggishness.
- **Myxedema**—this disorder occurs if hypothyroidism develops after growth. Symptoms include a low metabolic rate, mental slowness, weight gain, and swollen tissues caused by excess body fluid.

Disorders from hyperthyroidism can include the following[25]:
- **Graves' disease**—this disorder is characterized by an elevated metabolic rate, abnormal weight loss, excessive perspiration, muscular weakness, emotional instability, and exophthalmos.
- **Goiter**—this disorder is a physical sign of an enlarged thyroid gland. Overstimulation by TSH causes an enlargement of thyroid cells. If this is associated with increased hormone production, it is referred to as toxic goiter.

In addition, a specialized subgroup of cells exists in the thyroid known as C-cells. These produce calcitonin, which is a hormone involved in calcium metabolism.

Clinical Presentation

Most patients with thyroid cancer have a palpable neck mass, which is often detected during a routine physical examination. Almost 25% of young people with differentiated thyroid carcinoma present because of a palpable cervical lymph node metastasis as a result of occult primary thyroid cancer.[12] These occult, differentiated thyroid cancers can go undetected for years because of their indolent nature. A biopsy should be performed on persistent, enlarged lymph nodes found in children, teenagers, and young adults, with a clinical differential of Hodgkin's disease, benign inflammatory disease, or papillary carcinoma of the thyroid gland.[12]

Lesions in the thyroid gland should arouse suspicion if they exhibit extreme hardness, appear fixed to deep structures or skin, and are associated with recurrent laryngeal nerve paralysis (hoarseness).

Anaplastic carcinomas are usually large, hard, and fixed; grow rapidly; and occur in older patients. Patients can appear with symptoms related to compression and/or invasion of the esophagus, airway, or recurrent laryngeal nerves. Symptoms include pain, dysphagia, dyspnea, stridor, and hoarseness.[12]

Most patients with medullary carcinoma initially have an asymptomatic painless mass.[12] They may appear with systemic symptoms of diarrhea related to vasoactive substances (calcitonin) produced by the tumor. This usually represents an advanced stage of the disease. (See Table 28-1 for clinical symptoms and signs of patients with thyroid carcinoma.)

Detection and Diagnosis

Clinical presentation cannot determine a diagnosis of carcinoma. For confirmation of the diagnostic suspicion of cancer, a biopsy (most important), specialized imaging studies, and laboratory testing are necessary.

Laboratory testing includes an analysis of the thyroglobulin and calcitonin levels. Thyroglobulin levels cannot distinguish between a benign tumor and differentiated thyroid cancer.[12,22] Postoperatively, however, elevated levels indicate residual, recurrent, or metastatic differentiated thyroid cancer and can be correlated with iodine-131 (I-131) imaging for the detection of thyroid cancer. As such, thyroglobulin levels may be useful for monitoring patients who have an established diagnosis of thyroid cancer. Calcitonin levels that are elevated preoperatively indicate C-cell hyperplasia and/or medullary thyroid cancer.[9,12] Postoperative elevated levels indicate residual, recurrent, or metastatic medullary thyroid carcinoma.

Imaging studies include radionuclide imaging, ultrasonography, computed tomography (CT), and magnetic resonance imaging (MRI). Each examination can provide useful information for the diagnosis of thyroid cancer.

Radionuclide thyroid imaging is commonly used to evaluate the function and anatomic location of a palpable thyroid nodule through the localization of hot or cold spots in the gland. By this means the detection of occult cancers in high-risk patients can be accomplished. This imaging technique

Table 28-1	Clinical symptoms and signs in 106 patients with thyroid carcinoma		
Symptoms and Signs	Patients (66) with Papillary Carcinoma (%)	Patients (33) with Follicular Carcinoma (%)	Patients (7) with Anaplastic Carcinoma (%)
Hoarseness	9	15	55
Dysphagia	11	12	28
Pain and pressure	8	6	28
Dyspnea	3	6	43
Increasing size	56	75	85
Solitary nodule	60	65	14
Multinodular	33	20	70
Found in routine examination	27	30	0

Modified from Ureles AL, et al: Cancer of the endocrine glands. In Rubin P, editor: *Clinical oncology: a multidisciplinary approach for physicians and students,* Philadelphia, 1993, WB Saunders.

can detect a primary lesion in patients with suspected regional and distant thyroid cancer metastases. In addition, radionuclide imaging can detect local-regional or distant metastases in patients with known thyroid cancer. Patients previously treated for thyroid cancer are typically monitored with repeat scans.

The four radiopharmaceuticals most commonly used for radionuclide imaging of the thyroid are I-131, I-125, I-123, and technecuium-99m (Tc-99m). A thyroid nodule can image in three ways: (1) **cold thyroid nodule** (no radionuclide uptake), (2) **warm thyroid nodule** (slightly higher concentration than the rest of the thyroid gland), and (3) **hot thyroid nodule** (radionuclide uptake much higher than the rest of the thyroid gland).[12] (See Fig. 28-2 for normal thyroid imaging

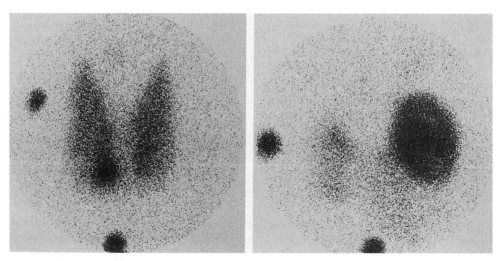

Figure 28-2. Normal thyroid imaging. *(From Bernier DR, et al: Nuclear medicine technology and techniques, St. Louis, 1994, Mosby.)*

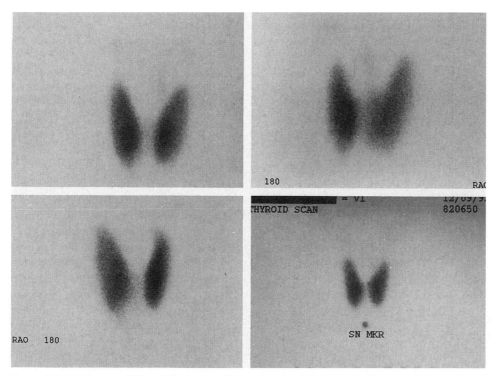

Figure 28-3. Abnormal thyroid imaging. *(From Bernier DR, et al: Nuclear medicine technology and techniques, St. Louis, 1994, Mosby.)*

and Fig. 28-3 for abnormal thyroid uptake.) Most cold nodules are thyroid adenomas or colloid cysts, with only 15% to 25% representing thyroid cancers. If multiple cold nodules appear, the incidence of the malignancy drops to 5%.[12]

The incidence rate of cancer with warm or hot nodules is low and usually represents a functioning adenoma or areas of normal tissue in an otherwise diseased gland. Some metastatic, well-differentiated follicular carcinomas accumulate radioiodine. Most metastatic, differentiated thyroid tumors do not accumulate radioiodine until all normal thyroid tissue has been ablated. This happens because normal-functioning thyroid tissue preferentially accumulates iodinated radiopharmaceuticals relative to the tumor.

Ultrasonography can determine whether a nodule is solid or cystic. This technique is used as a complementary test to radionuclide imaging. A nodule found to be solid through ultrasonography has a 30% probability of being a cancer.[12,21]

A CT scan cannot differentiate between a benign or malignant lesion. However, it can show the local and regional extent of advanced or recurrent cancer.[12] CT can also help a radiation oncologist in treatment planning if the use of external beam radiation is anticipated.

MRI can be useful in depicting lesion margins, lesion extent, tissue heterogenicity, cystic or hemorrhagic regions, cervical lymphadenopathy, invasion of adjacent structures, and additional nonpalpable thyroid nodules.[12,14,17]

A needle biopsy in some circumstances can obviate surgery by differentiating malignant from nonmalignant lesions. Two types of needle biopsies are needle aspiration cytology (performed with a small-gauge needle) and core needle biopsy (performed with a large-cutting biopsy needle of the Silverman type).

Both biopsies have a false-negative rate of up to 10%. A needle biopsy is indeterminate for follicular carcinoma because it cannot be diagnosed by cytologic or histologic criteria. However, a needle biopsy may play a role in the management of anaplastic thyroid malignancies and lymphomas because the diagnosis is more obvious.[12]

Pathology

Malignant thyroid neoplasms are divided into four categories: (1) papillary and mixed papillary-follicular, (2) follicular, (3) medullary, and (4) anaplastic. Rare tumors that account for less than 5% of thyroid malignancies include the following[12]:

- Lymphoma and plasmacytoma
- Squamous cell and mucin-producing carcinoma
- Teratoma and mixed tumors
- Sarcoma, carcinosarcoma, and hemangioendothelioma
- Metastatic carcinoma to the thyroid
- Thyroid cancer at unusual sites, including the median aberrant thyroid gland, lateral aberrant thyroid gland, and struma ovarii

Differentiated thyroid cancers include papillary, mixed papillary-follicular, and follicular carcinomas. These tumors arise from the thyroid follicle cell and can usually be treated with I-131 and thyroid hormone suppression.[12]

Papillary and mixed papillary-follicular cancers are the most common types of thyroid cancer, representing 33% to 73% of all malignant thyroid lesions. As previously mentioned, papillary carcinoma is the type most frequently seen in irradiated individuals. These tumors are slow growing, are nonaggressive, and have an excellent prognosis. This type of cancer is two to four times more common in females than males. The peak for occurrence is in the third to fifth decade of life, although the cancer can occur at any age. In children younger than 15 years, papillary carcinoma accounts for 80% of thyroid cancers.[12]

Follicular carcinoma accounts for 14% to 33% of all thyroid cancers. These tumors have the greatest propensity to concentrate I-131. They are two to three times more common in women than men, with the average age for a diagnosis from 50 to 58 years. They rarely occur in children. Follicular carcinoma has a worse overall prognosis than papillary carcinoma.[12,31]

Medullary thyroid cancer represents 5% to 10% of all thyroid cancers. About 80% of medullary thyroid cancers appear spontaneously, with 20% occurring as part of familial multiple endocrine neoplasia (MEN) syndromes (IIa, IIb, or III). No gender differentiation is seen between spontaneous and familial forms. With regard to age, however, spontaneous forms occur from the fifth decade on, whereas familial forms have been seen in patients younger than 10 and as old as 80 years. Medullary carcinoma has a worse prognosis than papillary, mixed papillary-follicular, and possibly follicular cancers, although it has a better prognosis than anaplastic carcinoma.[12]

Anaplastic carcinoma carries the worst overall prognosis. It is more aggressive than the previously mentioned types, and a patient's life expectancy is usually short after the diagnosis is established. Anaplastic carcinoma represents 10% of all malignant thyroid lesions. The age of occurrence is from 40 to 90 years, with the incidence in women outnumbering that in men by four to one.[12]

Staging

The American Joint Committee on Cancer has staged thyroid cancers according to the histologic type and age of the patient (Box 28-1).

Routes of Spread

Each pathologic classification has its own route of spread, which ranges from slow growing to extremely aggressive.

Papillary and mixed papillary-follicular carcinomas metastasize to regional lymph nodes through lymphatic channels. At the time of operation, 50% to 70% of these carcinomas have cervical lymph node metastases, although the presence of metastases in regional lymph nodes does not significantly worsen the prognosis. Bloodborne metastases can occur.

Follicular cancers have a tendency to invade vascular channels and metastasize hematogenously to distant sites,

including the bone, lung, liver, and brain. Lymph node metastases are uncommon.

Medullary thyroid cancer can vary from indolent to rapidly fatal growth patterns. Medullary carcinoma spreads regionally before displaying distant metastases, with up to 50% of patients having regional metastases at the time of the diagnosis. Metastases occur hematogenously and through lymphatic routes involving mainly the cervical nodes, lung, liver, and bone.

Anaplastic carcinoma displays local invasion of structures such as the trachea. Skin invasion is also seen, giving rise to dermal lymphatic metastases on the chest and abdominal walls. Regional neck nodes are often involved, although sometimes the primary tumor is so extensive that the regional node status is difficult to assess.[12]

Treatment Techniques

Surgery. Papillary carcinoma and mixed papillary-follicular carcinomas are rarely invasive and seldom require the resection of the muscles of the neck, internal jugular vein, esophagus, or trachea. Radical neck dissections are warranted only if nodes are grossly involved with metastatic disease. Because papillary and mixed papillary-follicular carcinomas are usually indolent diseases, prophylactic or elective neck dissections are no longer performed. During radical neck dissections, special care is taken to spare the recurrent laryngeal, vagus, spinal accessory, and phrenic nerves. Care is also taken to preserve the parathyroid glands.[29]

For small, lateralized lesions that do not show extrathyroidal involvement nor lymph node metastasis, lobectomy including removal of the isthmus is required. Surgery for mixed papillary-follicular carcinoma is the same as that for papillary carcinoma, unless vascular invasion or bloodborne metastases are present, in which case the lesion is treated as follicular cancer.

For encapsulated follicular carcinoma confined in the thyroid, a lobectomy including the isthmus can often successfully control the disease. In early stages in which the spread to cervical lymph nodes is rare, prophylactic neck dissection is not needed. If a second lesion is present in the contralateral lobe, a total or near-total thyroidectomy is performed, usually with good results.[29] If follicular carcinoma is extrathyroidal or metastatic disease is present, a bilateral total thyroidectomy is mandatory.

For medullary carcinoma that is sporadic and intrathyroidal, a lobectomy plus isthmus removal is required. If the lesion has extended beyond the thyroid to involve lymphatics and/or soft tissue, a radical en bloc resection is required. Because regional lymph nodes occur in 50% of the patients, an elective neck dissection may be advisable.[29] In the familial form, in which the cancer is generally bilateral, a total thyroidectomy is warranted.

For undifferentiated (anaplastic) carcinoma, surgery is

Box 28-1	American Joint Committee on Cancer and the International Union Against Cancer Tumor-Node-Metastasis Classification for Carcinoma of the Thyroid Gland

PRIMARY TUMOR (T)

TX   Primary tumor cannot be assessed

T0   No evidence of primary tumor

T1   Tumor 2 cm or less in greater dimension limited to the thyroid

T2   Tumor more than 2 cm but not more than 4 cm in greatest dimension limited to the thyroid

T3   Tumor more than 4 cm in greatest dimension limited to the thyroid or any tumor with minimal extrathyroid extension (e.g., extension to sternothyroid muscle or perithyroid soft tissues)

T4a   Tumor or any size extending beyond the thyroid capsule to invade subcutaneous soft tissues, larynx, trachea, esophagus, or recurrent laryngeal nerve

T4b   Tumor invades prevertebral fascia or encases carotid artery or mediastinal vessels

All anaplastic carcinomas are considered T4 tumors.

T4a   Intrathyroidal anaplastic carcinoma – surgically resectable

T4b   Extrathyroidal anaplastic carcinoma – surgically unresectable

REGIONAL LYMPH NODES (N)

Regional lymph nodes are the central compartment, lateral cervical, and upper mediastinal lymph nodes.

NX   Regional lymph nodes cannot be assessed

N0   No regional lymph node metastasis

N1   Regional lymph node metastasis

N1a   Metastasis to level VI (pretracheal, paratracheal, and prelaryngeal/Delphian lymph nodes)

N1b   Metastasis to unilateral, bilateral, or contralateral cervical or superior mediastinal lymph nodes

DISTANT METASTASIS (M)

MX   Distant metastasis cannot be assessed

M0   No distant metastasis

M1   Distant metastasis

STAGE GROUPING

Separate stage groupings are recommended for papillary or follicular, medullary, and anaplastic (undifferentiated) carcinoma.

PAPILLARY OR FOLLICULAR

Under 45 years

I	Any T	Any N	M0
II	Any T	Any N	M1

PAPILLARY OR FOLLICULAR

45 years and older

I	T1	N0	M0
II	T2	N0	M0
III	T3	N0	M0
	T1	N1a	M0
	T2	N1a	M0
	T3	N1a	M0
IVA	T4a	N0	M0
	T4a	N1a	M0
	T1	N1b	M0
	T2	N1b	M0
	T3	N1b	M0
	T4a	N1b	M0
IVB	T4b	Any N	M0
IVC	Any T	Any N	M1

MEDULLARY CARCINOMA

I	T1	N0	M0
II	T2	N0	M0
	T3	N0	M0
III	T1	N1a	M0
	T2	N1a	M0
	T3	N1a	M0
IVA	T4a	N0	M0
	T4a	N1a	M0
	T1	N1b	M0
	T2	N1b	M0
	T3	N1b	M0
	T4a	N1b	M0
IVB	T4b	Any N	M0
IVC	Any T	Any N	M1

ANAPLASTIC CARCINOMA

IVA	T4a	Any N	M0
IVB	T4b	Any N	M0
IVC	Any T	Any N	M1

effective on only a few occasions. Surgery is often necessary to alleviate a central airway obstruction resulting from extrinsic compression of the larynx and upper trachea caused by this aggressive malignancy. A tracheotomy is usually required to preserve a patient's airway. Radical surgical attempts are not always justified or technically possible because growth into soft tissue and deeper structures of the neck is often present.[12]

For malignancies that metastasize to the thyroid (an extremely rare situation), the treatment varies with primary sites, including the larynx, esophagus, lung, kidney, rectum, and skin. A biopsy is usually needed to differentiate a metastasis from a primary thyroid cancer.

Side effects of surgery can include tumor hemorrhage, damage to parathyroid gland resulting in temporary or permanent hypoparathyroidism, and temporary or permanent vocal cord paralysis.

Radioactive iodine. Radioactive iodine is used to treat papillary, mixed papillary-follicular, and follicular cancers. Indications for radioactive iodine include the following:

- Inoperable primary tumor
- Thyroid capsular invasion
- Thyroid ablation after a partial or subtotal thyroidectomy
- Postoperative residual disease in the neck and recurrent disease
- Cervical or mediastinal nodal metastasis
- Distant metastasis

The routine use of I-131 after surgery in small, lateralized, well-differentiated cancers is debatable; thyroid suppression therapy alone may be adequate. Because normal thyroid tissue has a greater propensity than differentiated thyroid cancer to absorb iodine, the consensus seems to be that all normal tissue should be ablated to allow residual or metastatic disease to accumulate I-131. An ablation dose administered after a thyroidectomy may vary from 50 to 100 mCi. If a tracer dose of radioiodine reveals persistent thyroid activity after this procedure, a second ablation dose is needed. (See Box 28-2 for guidelines for patients receiving I-131.)

After all normal thyroid tissue is ablated, I-131 (for differentiated thyroid cancers) can be used to treat local and regional disease and distant metastasis. Some of the side effects are listed in Box 28-3.

Thyroid hormonal therapy. Thyroid hormone suppression therapy is routinely given for differentiated thyroid cancers, although its effectiveness remains unproved. Differentiated thyroid carcinoma grows under the stimulation of TSH. Thus through the lowering of TSH levels, tumor activity should be decreased.[12]

External beam radiation. Responsiveness to external beam radiation varies according to histologic type. Among differentiated thyroid cancers, papillary and mixed papillary-follicular carcinomas are more radiosensitive than follicular carcinomas. Medullary thyroid cancer is less radiosensitive than papillary carcinoma. In general, anaplastic carcinomas are not very responsive.

External beam radiation can be used alone or in conjunction with I-131 and surgery. Following are several indications for its use:

- Inoperable lesion
- Patient physically unfit for surgery
- Incomplete surgical removal of thyroid carcinoma
- Superior vena cava syndrome
- Skeletal metastases in which minimal accumulation of I-131 occurred
- Residual disease involving the trachea, larynx, or esophagus

In differentiated thyroid cancer for the curative treatment of inoperable localized disease or in patients with gross residual disease, tumor doses should be 6500 cGy in 7 weeks (180 to 200 cGy daily). The radiation field should include the entire thyroid gland, neck, and superior mediastinum. The dose to the spinal cord and other organs at risk should be considered, with a cord block added around 4500 cGy. For metastatic bone involvement, doses of 3500 to 4500 cGy in 3 to 5 weeks are recommended.[12]

Several field arrangements can be used to deliver an adequate dose to the neck and mediastinum. Through anteroposterior/posteroanterior (AP/PA) portals, 4500 cGy can be given at the midplane to the neck and mediastinum. An additional dose (for a total tumor dose of 6500 cGy) can be delivered through anterior obliques or opposed oblique portals.

For the simulation of a thyroid cancer patient, the head should be extended to avoid exposure to the mouth, with the use of an immobilization device for reproducibility. So that adequate tumor coverage is ensured, the tumor volume should be wired out, and a CT scan of the treated area should be obtained for treatment planning. Dose distribution must be considered through this area, especially the cord dose.

For medullary carcinoma that has not extended below the clavicles, radiation therapy can be considered. The recommended dose is 5500 to 6500 cGy in 6 to 7 weeks. The treatment fields should encompass the primary lesion, bilateral cervical node chains, and superior mediastinum. For residual disease after a surgical resection, a dose of 5000 to 6000 cGy in 5 to 5½ weeks is recommended.

For bone metastasis, radiation therapy is warranted and often effective.

Anaplastic carcinoma is the least radiosensitive of all the thyroid cancers. Tumor control is seldom accomplished, even after a dose of 6000 cGy to the primary lesion, neck, and superior mediastinum.[12]

Case Study

A 34-year-old woman underwent a right hemithyroidectomy about 10 to 12 years ago for benign disease. A needle aspiration biopsy 2 years ago also showed benign disease, after exhibiting a cold nodule on a thyroid scan. Other than this asymptomatic nodule, the patient had no other symptoms. Because of its persistence, this left-sided nodule was excised. Pathology showed follicular carcinoma with capsular invasion. No obvious vascular invasion was present. The patient was advised to have a complete

Box 28-2	**Guidelines for Patients Receiving Iodine-131 (I-131)**

PLANNING

Order I-131 at least 48 hours in advance. Schedule patient for hospital admission.

ROOM PREPARATION

Must cover the following with plastic bags: telephone receiver, telephone, food table, basin faucet handles, nurse call set. Disposable plastic-lined paper next to bed, commode, and shower. Two radiation waste containers in room for laundry and foods/paper. A safety shield must be placed at the head of bed.

PATIENT PREPARATION

Instruct to wear footies when ambulating. Instruct to keep outside door closed and bathroom door open at all times. Obtain vital signs and blood and urine samples before I-131 administration.

ADMINISTRATION

Patient must wear hospital gown with a "chuck" around neck and in lap. Personnel administering I-131 should wear gown, gloves, and mask. Vial containing I-131 should be vented in nuclear medicine hood to allow any volatile I-131 to escape just before administration if possible. During administration, the patient should sit on the side of the bed in front of the I-131, which is in a lead vial on a covered table. Open vial with T-bar, insert drinking straw, put small amount of water in vial (along straw so it does not splash). Patient takes I-131 through straw with additional water placed in lead vial to remove as much I-131 as possible. Swish and swallow several cups of water to rinse I-131 from oral cavity. Do not remove straw from vial; bend it over and carefully place lead cap on.

INITIAL SURVEY

Within 15 minutes, measure the radiation exposure rate at 1 m from the midline of the patient's abdomen in both anteroposterior (AP) and lateral directions. Calculate the average. Patient may be released when same readings show less than 30 mCi of I-131 or less than 5 mr/hour at 1 m, which is usually about 24 to 48 hours after 100 mCi was given but is variable. An inventory or survey form with initial activity and exposure rate, nursing instructions, and decontamination form should be posted on the room door. Do not collect urine unless lead container is available and there is a specific reason.

SAFETY

At <30 mCi I-131, patient can be discharged (or exposure rate of 5 mr/hour at 1 m).

Visiting is discouraged; limit to 0.5 hr/day per visitor, no children younger than 18 years or pregnant women. Visitors should wear gown, gloves, and mask and sit in designated chair across room. If they come close to patient, they should sit behind lead shield. Patients should wear hospital gowns, not personal clothing (I-131 in sweat, breath) and should leave bed only to go to bathroom or designated chair. They should drink copious amounts of water to speed release of unused radioactivity, shower frequently, flush toilet several times after each use. Males should urinate seated. There should be no personal items except those to be disposed of at discharge. After discharge, patients should practice good personal hygiene for 1 to 2 days. Do not hold children closely for 2 to 3 days.

Modified from Grigsby PW and Luk K: Thyroid. In Perez, CA, Brady LW, editors: *Principles and practice of radiation oncology,* Philadelphia, 1998, Lippincott-Raven.

Box 28-3	**Side Effects of I-131**

- Inflammation of salivary glands
- Nausea
- Vomiting
- Fatigue
- Bone marrow suppression (only after repeated administrations)

lobectomy of the left thyroid gland or an I-131 ablation of the remaining thyroid gland. The patient elected surgical ablation.

Histopathologically, the resected lobe showed focal areas of residual follicular carcinoma with areas of infiltration into the stroma. A careful examination with the patient under anesthesia revealed no evidence of lymph node involvement. A thyroid scan after surgery showed no uptake in the neck. The patient was made hypothyroid for several weeks and then underwent an I-125 scan that showed residual uptake in the left neck, probably corresponding to the previous bed of the left thyroid lobe. No uptake was present on the right side, and there was no cervical lymph node involvement. No other activity was seen on the body scan. The patient was referred for I-131 thyroid treatment of the residual tumor in the left neck.

The acute risks of nausea and potential long-term risks of solid and hematologic cancer induction was discussed with the patient. The precautions to be taken by the patient and her family, with specific regard to exposure to the children, were carefully outlined. The advised procedures were based on the National Council on Radiation Protection (NCRP) recommendations for people ingesting radioactive material for therapeutic purposes.

With her consent, the patient was given 30 mCi of I-131 via a capsule. The dose was relatively low because the patient effectively had a total thyroidectomy and was young. After observation for 1 hour without any nausea or vomiting and with the exposure rate being measured and recorded, the patient was discharged. A 6-month repeat thyroid scan showed no residual uptake in the left neck.

PITUITARY TUMORS

Pituitary tumors are less aggressive than many central nervous system tumors, although pituitary neoplasms still pose problems as a result of local growth causing compressive and destructive effects and endocrine abnormalities caused by pituitary hormone dysfunction. The pituitary is composed of an anterior, posterior, and intermediate lobe. Tumors of the posterior and intermediate portion are virtually unknown. This section addresses tumors arising from the anterior pituitary gland, or adenohypophysis.

Epidemiology and Etiology

Pituitary tumors are most always benign, with malignancies accounting for fewer than 1% of all pituitary tumors.[2] These neoplasms represent 10% of all intracranial tumors, although small, asymptomatic adenomas appear in approximately 25% of all pituitary glands examined at autopsy. With the increasing quality of diagnostic studies, these pituitary neoplasms are now estimated to account for 30% of all intracranial tumors.[23]

Pituitary adenomas can be classified as functioning or nonfunctioning, as related to the hormones they produce. Hormone production often serves as a diagnostic and treatment-response marker. Pituitary adenomas categorized as functioning are as follows:

- **Prolactin (PRL)**-secreting tumors are the most common, representing 65% of all functioning pituitary adenomas. These neoplasms grow large and show little tendency toward local invasion.[23,28]
- **Growth hormone (GH)**-secreting tumors represent 15% of all pituitary adenomas and are more likely to be locally invasive.[28]
- **TSH**-secreting tumors represent fewer than 1% of all pituitary adenomas.
- **Adrenocorticotrophic hormone (ACTH)**-secreting tumors are more likely to be invasive compared with the other functioning adenomas.[23]

Chromophobe adenomas, which are nonfunctioning, are usually larger than functioning tumors and tend to exhibit invasive characteristics.[18] Patients usually have visual symptoms caused by the compression of the optic chiasm or a headache, rather than syndromes associated with the hyper-

Table 28-2	Clinical effects of excess secretion of pituitary hormones
Hormones	**Clinical Effects**
ACTH	Cushing's disease
GH	Giantism, acromegaly
Prolactin	Females: infertility
	Males: impotence, decreased libido
TSH	Hyperthyroidism

ACTH, Adrenocorticotrophic hormone; *GH,* growth hormone; *TSH,* thyroid-stimulating hormone.

secretion of pituitary hormones. These syndromes are listed in Table 28-2.

Pituitary tumors can occur at any age, from infancy to old age, although they are rarely found before puberty and are most commonly diagnosed in middle-aged and older patients.[28] No significant difference exists in the prevalence of adenomas among men and women.

Because of the rarity of malignant pituitary tumors, little knowledge of the etiology exists. Hardy et al.[11] have found an association between PRL-secreting tumors in women and the use of oral contraceptives. However, no clear etiologic link has been determined.

Prognostic Indicators

The prognosis depends on the type of adenoma and a combination of other factors, including the following: (1) the extent of the abnormalities (through mass effect or hormonal alterations), (2) the success of the treatment in normalizing endocrine activity and/or relieving pressure effects, (3) the morbidity caused by the treatment, and (4) the effectiveness of the treatments in preventing a recurrence.

Anatomy

The pituitary gland is 1.3 cm in diameter and located at the base of the brain. Attached to the hypothalamus by a stalk-like structure (the **infundibulum**), the pituitary gland lies in the sella turcica of the sphenoid bone. The gland is divided structurally and functionally into an anterior lobe **(adenohypophysis),** a posterior lobe **(neurohypophysis),** and an intermediate lobe. The blood supply to the adenohypophysis is from several superior hypophyseal arteries, and the blood supply to the neurohypophysis is from the inferior hypophyseal arteries.[25] The pituitary gland is close to critical structures of the central nervous system, such as the optic chiasm (superiorly) and the cavernous sinuses and their contents (laterally). (See Fig. 28-4 for the anatomic relationships.) Related to topographic anatomy, the pituitary gland is positioned behind the temporomandibular joint (TMJ) and midplane behind the nasal bone (i.e., between the eyes).

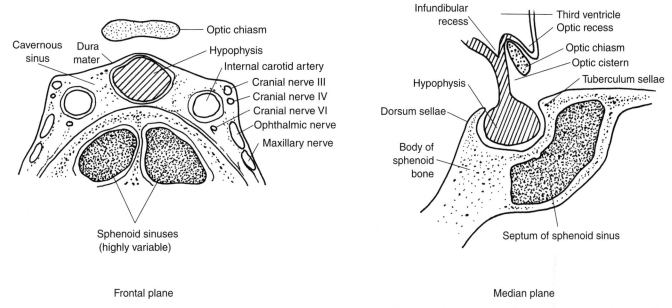

Figure 28-4. Frontal and median planes of the pituitary fossa region. *(Redrawn with permission from Perez CA, Brady LW, editors: Principles and practice of radiation oncology, Philadelphia, 1992, JB Lippincott.)*

Physiology

Derived from the endoderm, the adenohypophysis forms the glandular part of the pituitary. The glandular cells (acidophils and basophils) are responsible for the secretion of seven hormones.

Acidophils secrete the following:

- **GH**—controls body growth
- **PRL**—initiates milk production

Basophils secrete the following:

- **TSH**—controls the thyroid gland
- **Follicle-stimulating hormone (FSH)**—stimulates egg and sperm production
- **Luteinizing hormone (LH)**—stimulates other sexual and reproductive activity
- **Melanocyte-stimulating hormone (MSH)**—relates to skin pigmentation
- **ACTH**—influences the action of the adrenal cortex

The release of these hormones is stimulated or inhibited by the chemical secretions from the hypothalamus, which are called regulatory, or releasing, factors. The posterior lobe or neurohypophysis secretes oxytocin (which causes smooth muscle contractions) and antidiuretic hormone (ADH) or vasopressin, which regulates free water resorption in the kidneys.[25]

Clinical Presentation

Hormonal effects. Functioning pituitary tumors retain hormone-producing capabilities, although they are unresponsive to regulatory mechanisms and produce hormones regardless of metabolic needs.[23] Hypersecretion of pituitary hormones results in varied clinical presentations, depending on the type of secreting tumor. PRL-secreting tumors pro-duce clinical symptoms such as amenorrhea and galactorrhea, which are detected easier in premenopausal versus postmenopausal women. The hypersecretion of GH produces clinical symptoms such as weight gain; thickening of the bones and soft tissues of the hands, feet and cheeks; and overgrowth of the jaw and tongue. Patients are hypertensive and commonly complain of headaches and lassitude. This clinical syndrome is referred to as acromegaly, if hypersecretion occurs after puberty, and giantism, if it happens before puberty.[27] (See Table 28-2 for more hypersecreting syndromes.)

In some instances, local compressive effects of the tumor in the pituitary itself may cause deficient production of hormones normally synthesized in the gland. Hormones that have target organs (such as ACTH [adrenals], TSH [thyroid], and FSH [ovaries and testes]) can cause an array of abnormalities that result from a loss of pituitary hormonal action.[7] These clinical manifestations are listed in Table 28-3.

Pressure effects. The most common manifestation of an expanding pituitary lesion is headache, which occurs in 20% of all patients.[7,23] Local pressure on the lining of the sphenoid sinus and traction on the diaphragma sellae produce these headaches.

Visual acuity and field defects are other clinical manifestations and signify extension beyond the sella. Suprasellar extension of these tumors causes pressure effects on the inferior aspect of the optic chiasm, resulting in visual symptomatology, which is usually progressive. The presentation may be altered visual acuity, but more commonly, visual field defects are observed. The most common field defect is **bitemporal hemianopsia** (loss of peripheral vision

Table 28-3	**Clinical manifestations of pituitary hormones**	
Hormone	**Target Tissue**	**Clinical Effects**
ACTH	Adrenal cortex	Postural hypotension; impaired tolerance of stress (trauma, surgery); can lead to shock
Prolactin	Gonads	Gonadal atrophy; loss of FSH reproductive function; LH decreased gonadal hormones
TSH	Thyroid	Hypothyroidism (fatigue, slow or slurred speech, bradycardia, decreased reflexes, cold intolerance)
GH	Bones, muscles, organs	Decreased bone growth; lethargy; hypoglycemia

Modified from Donehower MG: Endocrine cancers. In Baird SB, McCorkle R, Grant M, editors: *Cancer nursing: a comprehensive textbook,* Philadelphia, 1991, WB Saunders.
ACTH, Adrenocorticotrophic hormone; *FSH,* follicle-stimulating hormone; *LH,* luteinizing hormone; *TSH,* thyroid-stimulating hormone; *GH,* growth hormone.

bilaterally). If pressure effects on the optic chiasm persist for significant periods, the result can be permanent visual field defects or blindness. In rare instances, these tumors can extend laterally into the cavernous sinuses (Fig. 28-4) and cause characteristic cranial nerve deficits.

Detection and Diagnosis

Patients with functional tumors have characteristic endocrine abnormalities that are associated with the hypersecretion of hormones. The clinical syndromes from Table 28-2 prompt medical attention. Laboratory testing, which can directly measure hormone levels, can confirm pituitary hormone dysfunction and strongly suggest the diagnosis. The expanding growth of nonfunctioning tumors into the suprasellar area causes pressure symptoms such as headache, visual disturbances, and impairment of various cranial nerves.[28] These symptoms often bring the patient to medical attention and prompt diagnostic studies.

The principal imaging study for the pituitary gland is CT or MRI. MRI is superior to CT in delineating the extent of the tumor process relative to normal critical structures such as the optic chiasm, vascular structures, cranial nerves, and cavernous sinuses just lateral to the pituitary gland (Fig. 28-4). MRI provides detailed anatomic information in transverse, sagittal, and coronal projections. This information is invaluable to the neurosurgeon and radiation oncologist in determining a therapeutic approach.

Pathology

Pituitary tumors are sinusoidal, papillary, or diffuse.[18] Although pituitary tumors appear encapsulated, no true capsule exists. Neoplasms are formed of tightly packed cells that remain separate from normal tissue without a membrane.

Neoplasms are classified according to size. **Microadenomas** are less than 1.0 cm, and **macroadenomas** are greater than 1.0 cm.[18,28] This classification is important because predictions of the prognosis can be made from the tumor size. Larger adenomas are surgically more difficult to remove with complete resections, and recurrence is more common in this group.

Pituitary tumors can also be classified according to their growth patterns (by expansion or invasion) and are separated into intrahypophyseal, intrasellar, diffuse, and invasive adenomas. **Intrahypophyseal tumors** stay in the pituitary gland, whereas **intrasellar lesions** grow within the confines of the sella. **Diffuse adenomas** usually fill the entire sella and can erode its wall. **Invasive neoplasms** have a more rapid growth rate and tend to erode outside the sella to invade neighboring tissues such as the posterior pituitary gland, sphenoid bone, and cavernous sinus. These neoplasms may even penetrate into the brain and third ventricle. Invasive adenomas are classified as malignant adenomas when metastases are present. Malignant adenomas metastasize via cerebrospinal fluid (CSF) or vascular pathways. This is extremely rare.

Staging

Because most tumors are benign, no true staging exists. However, pituitary tumors have been classified into four grades according to the extent of expansion or erosion of the sella. This system also types tumors into four categories based on suprasellar extension (Box 28-4).

Treatment Techniques

The primary goal of treatment is to normalize pituitary hormonal function or relieve local compressive and/or destructive effects of the tumor. In some instances, both factors must be ameliorated. This can be accomplished surgically, therapeutically with radiation, medically, or with a combination of these modalities. An obvious secondary goal is to prevent recurrence.

Surgery. Surgery plays a significant role in the management of pituitary tumors. Before 1970, craniotomies were performed with an associated operative mortality rate of 2% to 25%. Currently, the less invasive transsphenoidal approach is widely used, decreasing the mortality rate to 0.9%. Complications of this surgery are CSF leakage, infection (meningitis), and visual pathway defects, with a combined morbidity rate of about 14%.[28] (See Fig. 28-5 for a depiction of the transsphenoidal approach.) In summary, the two main

Box 28-4	Hardy and Vezina's Pituitary Tumor Classification

Grade I—sella of normal size, but with asymmetry
Grade II—enlarged sella, but with an intact floor
Grade III—localized erosion or destruction of the sella floor
Grade IV—diffusely eroded floor
Type A—tumor bulges into the chiasmatic cistern
Type B—tumor reaches the floor of the third ventricle
Type C—more voluminous tumor, with extension into the third ventricle up to the foramen of Monro
Type D—extension into temporal or frontal fossa

Courtesy of Jules Hardy, MD, and Jean L. Vézina, MD.

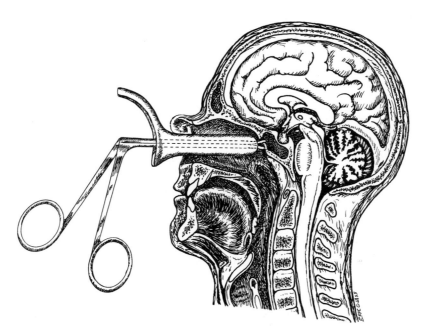

Figure 28-5. Anatomic root for a transsphenoidal hypophysectomy.

surgical approaches are the transfrontal approach (transfrontal craniotomy) and the transsphenoidal approach, which allows direct access to the pituitary gland without disturbance of the central nervous system structures.

Transsphenoidal surgery is reported to permanently control 70% to 90% of small adenomas. Results with larger adenomas are less satisfactory, although the debulking of large tumors decompresses vital structures.[23] Transsphenoidal surgery results in the improvement of visual field defects in 80% of patients. Only 4% of patients experience worsening of visual field defects with transphenoidal surgery. Results are the same with a craniotomy, with a higher percentage of visual impairment related to the surgical procedure.[26,28]

Characteristic hormonal abnormalities show favorable responses after surgery. If surgical intervention of functioning adenomas is successful, the response in terms of the normalization of hormone levels is almost immediate. Symptomatic relief is seen in 94% of patients with acromegaly, although the recurrence rate after 10 years is 8% to 10%. Results are generally satisfactory for patients with Cushing's syndrome (ACTH-producing adenomas). Although results vary, remission occurs in 80% to 86% of patients, with a recurrence rate over 10 years of 8% to 10%.[28] Similar, excellent results are achieved with PRL-secreting adenomas.

Radiation therapy. Surgery is often only one part of the overall management for a pituitary adenoma. Although the role of postoperative radiation therapy is controversial, it has been shown in various series to reduce recurrence rates compared with surgery alone. Radiation therapy alone has also been used to control pituitary tumors in patients who refused surgery or those who were medically unfit.

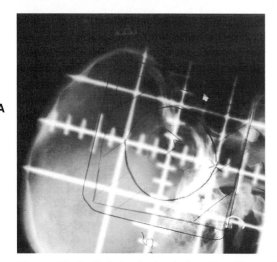

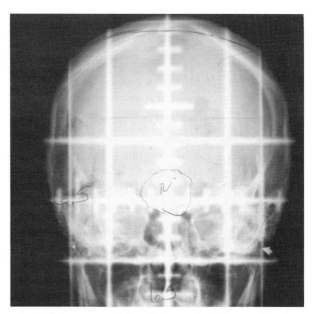

Figure 28-6. A, Lateral simulation film illustrating the portal used for external irradiation of pituitary adenoma. **B,** Anteroposterior (AP) simulation film.

Postoperative radiation therapy is used as an adjunctive modality in the following circumstances:

- An incompletely resected invasive tumor
- Tumors demonstrating suprasellar extension with an associated visual field defect
- Large tumors in which the risk of attempted removal is relatively high
- Persistent hormonal elevation after surgery

Radiation therapy techniques. With any treatment technique a precise target volume must be defined through the use of MRI, CT, surgical, and clinical findings. The treatment volume should be slightly larger than the target volume, allowing for day-to-day variations in the treatment setup. The head must be immobilized to ensure reproducibility and accuracy. The patient's chin is usually tucked to avoid radiation exposure to the eyes. Lead markers on the outer canthus of each eye during simulation documents the eye position with respect to the radiation beam. The use of three tattoos (two lateral and one midline) aids in repositioning. Verification portals should be taken routinely to document the field location. (See Figs. 28-6 and 28-7 for examples of simulation and portal film.)

With the advent of high-energy megavoltage linear accelerators (i.e., 10 to 18 MeV) and multiple-field treatment approaches, the dose-volume distribution to the pituitary gland has been greatly enhanced. This results in a more precise dose delivered to the tumor volume, a reduction in the dose to normal central nervous system structures, increased tumor-control probability, and decreased treatment-related morbidity.

The optimization of dose-volume distribution is illustrated in various treatment plans shown in Figs. 28-8, 28-9,

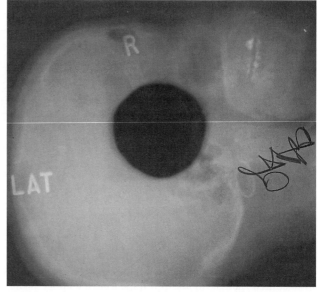

Figure 28-7. Lateral verification film (portal image) on a therapy machine.

and 28-10. These treatment plans show an obvious advantage of high-energy photons and multifield or rotational arrangements to accomplish the goal of optimizing the dose to the target tissue while minimizing the dose to nontarget, normal tissue. This is of paramount importance in the pituitary gland because of the critical normal tissue surrounding it. (See Fig. 28-11 for a treatment portal of a superimposed lateral and vertex.)

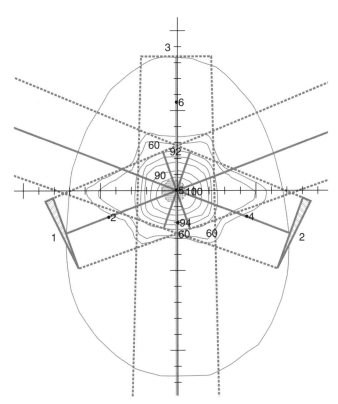

Figure 28-8. Isodose curves for a 2-cm-diameter tumor volume, with the use of a 15-MV linear accelerator and three portal arrangement: an open vertex and two 110-degree posterior oblique, 30-degree wedge fields.

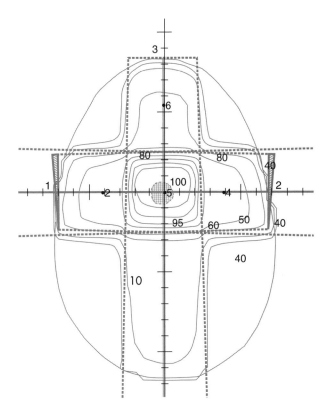

Figure 28-9. Isodose curves for a 2-cm-diameter tumor volume, with the use of a 15-MV linear accelerator and three portal arrangement: open vertex and two lateral 15-degree wedge fields.

Other strategies not widely available are used to treat pituitary adenomas. These strategies include proton beam therapy and stereotactic radiosurgery (see Chapter 7).

Proton beam therapy. Because of the proton beam's physical characteristics (i.e., a Bragg peak with a rapid dose fall off at depth), the dose can be precisely delivered within millimeters of a defined target directly related to the beam's energy. This is a particularly attractive feature for treatment near critical structures such as the optic chiasm and the temporal lobe, areas in which an excessive radiation dose can produce devastating clinical consequences.

Stereotactic radiosurgery. Stereotactic radiosurgery uses a high-energy photon beam with multiple ports of entry convergent on the target tissue. This is typically done as a single, large fraction of treatment with the patient immobilized in a stereotactic head frame. After being rigidly positioned, the patient undergoes a planning CT scan to define the tumor volume and determine the multiports of entry. With the patient immobilized the entire time, this procedure takes several hours and requires several images on the treatment unit to ensure accuracy.

This technique may not be an optimal approach to this particular disease because pituitary neoplasms are benign and high single-fraction treatment can produce significant normal-tissue morbidity if an uncertainty exists regarding the target volume treated. With improved technology, stereotactic radiation may eventually be delivered as fractionated treatment, making it more desirable in this circumstance.

Results of Treatment

The treatment of pituitary adenomas shows results that are favorable. Surgery for microadenomas is generally curative. Series with radiation therapy alone have demonstrated excellent disease-free survival rates of up to 85% at 5 and 10 years. A direct comparison between the results of different treatment approaches is difficult to make because of the various criteria used to select the optimal treatment, as previously described. However, surgery and radiation therapy alone or in combination clearly produce excellent results.

Case Study

A 32-year-old woman came to the emergency room with a history of headaches. During examination the patient demonstrated features of acromegaly. She had a 2-year history of progressively enlarging hands and feet and pain in the joints of the upper extremities. She noted that her shoe size had increased from an 8 to a 10 over this period. She complained of amenorrhea for approximately the past year but denied any visual symptoms.

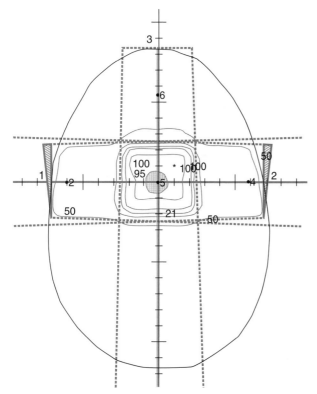

Figure 28-10. Isodose curves for a 2-cm-diameter tumor volume, with the use of a 4-MV linear accelerator and three portal arrangement: open vertex and two lateral 30-degree wedge fields.

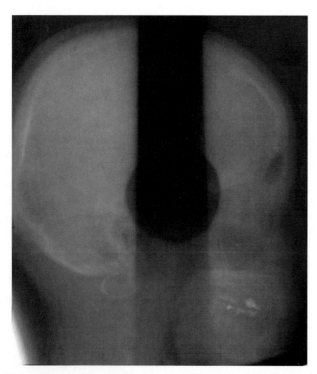

Figure 28-11. A vertex therapy machine portal that is used to deliver a portion of dose without irradiation of the temporal lobes.

As part of the initial workup, a brain MRI scan showed findings consistent with a pituitary macroadenoma measuring about 1.5 cm in diameter and extending into the suprasellar cistern anterior to the optic chiasm. A slight elevation of the optic chiasm was present. The cavernous sinuses appeared free of tumor extension. The floor of the sella was eroded, and the tumor appeared to extend partially into the sphenoid sinus. The GH was 150 ng/ml (normal range, 1 to 10 ng/ml), and a transsphenoidal hypophysectomy was advised.

After surgery the patient had a remarkable reduction in the GH level and a reversal of some of the clinical findings of acromegaly. However, with the persistent elevation of GH and radiographic (erosion of sella) and surgical findings (involving the sphenoid sinus), the patient was at an extremely high risk for recurrence of her adenoma. A course of radiation therapy directed at the pituitary fossa, sphenoid sinus, and cavernous sinus region was recommended to improve the probability of local control and normalization of the GH level.

In a supine, immobilized position the patient was treated via a three-field technique through the use of 6-cm-diameter circular fields with 10-MV photons. Right and left lateral opposed fields in combination with a superior vertex field angled 15 degrees off the horizontal were used. CT and MRI scans were performed through the treatment volume to aid in the treatment planning. This three-field arrangement was treated at 180 cGy per fraction. Equal weighting was provided from each field for 25 treatment fractions to accomplish 4500 cGy to the pituitary fossa, which included the sphenoid sinus.

The patient tolerated the therapy well but still complained of headaches and fatigue at the completion of the therapy. About 3 months after the external beam radiation therapy, the patient continued to show regression of her acral changes. This regression was characterized by thinning facial characteristics, smaller hands, and smaller feet. An MRI scan at that time showed no evidence of a tumor. During subsequent follow-up visits the patient continued to do well, with decreasing GH levels. Approximately 2 years after the therapy the patient's GH level was 3.0 ng/ml.

ADRENAL CORTEX TUMORS

Neoplasms of the adrenal glands are rare, with malignant tumors accounting for only 0.04% of all cancers.[4] Tumors arising in the adrenal glands are classified according to the portion of the gland from which they arise. This includes tumors arising from the **cortex** (outer portion of the gland) and those from the **medulla** (inner portion of the gland). The cortex and the medulla, which make up the adrenal gland (Fig. 28-12), have distinct histologic features and physiologic functions. In general, the cortex manufactures steroid hormones that are critical in metabolic regulation, and the medulla produces epinephrine (adrenalin) under the regulation of the autonomic nervous system.

Epidemiology and Etiology

Adrenocortical tumors are extremely rare, with only 150 to 300 instances in the United states per year (of which, approximately 10% are malignant).[30] Men and women are affected equally, although hyperfunctioning malignancies are more common in women. Tumors arise more commonly in the left

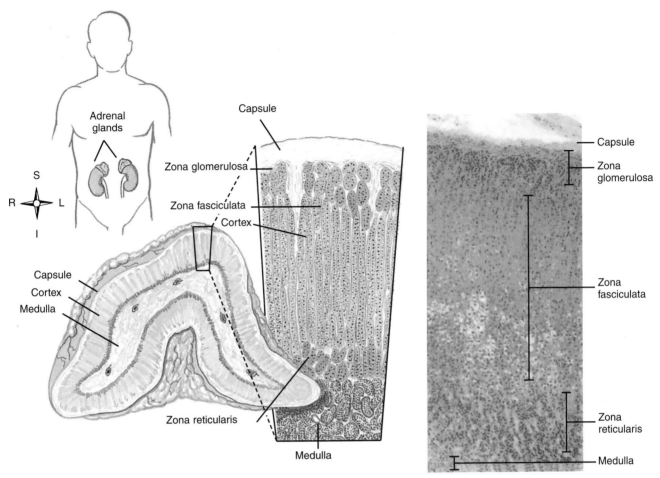

Figure 28-12. Anatomy of the adrenal gland. *(From Thibodeau GA, Patton TK, editors: Anatomy and physiology, St. Louis, 1999, Mosby.)*

gland than the right. Although the median age is 50 years, the ages in two series ranged from 1 to 80 years.[4,6]

Adrenal adenomas are benign neoplasms that can be found in 2% of all adults, according to an autopsy series.[25] These adenomas are rarely associated with serious medical illness. However, in some circumstances these can cause hypersecretion of normally produced steroid hormones, giving rise to various clinical syndromes. Many adrenal masses represent metastatic disease typically from lung cancer.

Prognostic Indicators

The stage of the disease at the time of diagnosis closely parallels survival rates. Most patients have advanced disease at the time of presentation. Only 30% of patients have a tumor confined to the adrenal gland.[4]

The ability of the surgeon to achieve curative resection is another prognostic factor because surgery is the only modality that has demonstrated a significant effect on survival rates. All patients should have close postoperative surveillance for the detection of abdominal and distant metastases while they are still resectable.

A young age at the time of diagnosis is a favorable prognostic factor.

Anatomy

The adrenal glands are paired organs located on the superior pole of the kidneys. These glands have a yellow cortex and dark brown medulla. They derive their blood supply from the adrenal branches of the inferior phrenic artery, aorta, and renal artery.[4] The lymphatic drainage is to the paraaortic nodes. The normal adrenal gland weighs approximately 20 g.

Physiology

The adrenal cortex produces steroid hormones, including glucocorticoids, mineralocorticoids, and sex hormones, which are responsible for metabolic regulation. These hormones include cortisol, aldosterone, estrogen, and androgen. The cells of the adrenal cortex that manufacture these hormones are regulated by the ongoing stresses and needs of an individual's metabolism. The normal functioning adrenal cortex can respond instantaneously to meet metabolic demands and maintain homeostasis.

Clinical Presentation

Because of the location of adrenal cortex tumors in the abdomen and the inaccessibility for physical examination, many patients develop symptoms of pain from advanced cancer. Alternatively, clinical manifestations of symptoms related to excess hormone production may prompt medical attention. Well-described syndromes are associated with the excessive production of hormones from the adrenal cortex. These are listed in Table 28-4.

In a series of 47 patients with adrenocortical carcinoma reported by Cohn et al.[5] symptoms relating to a nonfunctioning tumor included an abdominal mass in 77% of the patients, weight loss in 46%, fever in 15%, and distant metastases in 15%. Many patients have more than one symptom at the time of diagnosis. In the same series, symptoms relating to functional tumors included Cushing's syndrome in 26% of the patients, mixed Cushing's syndrome and virilization in 24%, virilization in 15%, and feminization in 9%.

Detection and Diagnosis

Patients may exhibit functioning or nonfunctioning tumors. With functioning tumors the clinical syndromes from Table 28-4 often lead to the diagnosis and can be easily confirmed with laboratory testing. In nonfunctioning tumors, pain is the presenting symptom and is often associated with locally advanced disease.

The principal imaging study for the adrenal gland is CT or MRI. These scans often suggest the diagnosis of an adrenal neoplasm and demonstrate the local and regional extent of the disease. (See Fig. 28-13 for an abdominal CT scan of a suspected adrenal neoplasm.) A definite tissue diagnosis requires a needle biopsy under CT guidance.

Table 28-4	Clinical manifestations of adrenocortical hormone excess	
Hormone	**Syndrome**	**Clinical Manifestations**
Aldosterone	Conn's syndrome (aldosteronism)	Hypernatremia, hypokalemia, hypertension, neuromuscular weakness and paresthesias, electrocardiographic and renal function abnormalities
Cortisol (ACTH)	Cushing's syndrome	Acid-base imbalance, hypertension, obesity, osteoporosis, hyperglycemia, psychoses, excessive bruising, renal calculi
Sex hormones (testosterone, estrogen, and progesterone)	Virilization (in women)	Male pattern baldness, hirsutism, deepening voice, breast atrophy, decreased libido, oligomenorrhea
	Feminization (in men)	Gynecomastia, breast tenderness, testicular atrophy, decreased libido

From Donehower MG: Endocrine cancers. In Baird SB, McCorkle R, Grant M, editors: *Cancer nursing: a comprehensive textbook,* Philadelphia, 1991, WB Saunders.
ACTH, Adrenocorticotrophic hormone.

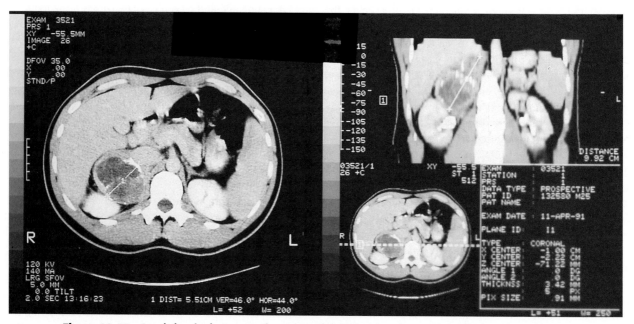

Figure 28-13. An abdominal computed tomography (CT) scan of a suspected adrenal neoplasm.

Pathology

Adrenocortical tumors are usually large, single, rounded masses of yellow-orange adrenocortical tissue. Because they are usually large at the time of diagnosis, they have considerable hemorrhage, necrosis, and calcification.[4]

In a series of 38 patients conducted by Karakousis et al.[13] tumors were graded according to the cells' resemblance to normal adrenal cortical cells. Well-differentiated (grade I) tumors were distinguished from adenomas by the presence of capsular and vascular invasion and abnormal mitoses. The survival rate for grade I and II tumors is significantly greater than that for grade III tumors.

Staging

No true staging system exists because so few cases are reported. However, an example of a conventional staging system for adrenocortical carcinoma is presented in Box 28-5. This system stages according to the size of the tumor and the extent to which it has advanced locally or distantly.

Routes of Spread

Adrenocortical carcinomas can grow locally into surrounding tissues. However, these carcinomas may also spread to regional paraaortic nodes, lung, liver, and brain.[1,4]

Local invasion or distant metastases are often present at the time of diagnosis. Tumors on the right side involve the kidney, liver, and vena cava (often by direct extension of the tumor). Tumors on the left side often involve the kidney, pancreas, and diaphragm.

Treatment Techniques

Surgery is the treatment of choice. A complete resection is not always feasible because of invasion to adjacent vital structures such as the spleen, kidney, and parts of the pancreas. Although the resection of adrenal carcinomas is not always for cure, debulking results in decreased pain. Radiation therapy has a limited role, but it may be used as an adjunct to surgery to improve local control and for the palliative treatment of metastatic disease.

The use of systemic treatment in the management of adrenocortical cancer has been disappointing. Most reported series have evaluated patients with locally advanced or metastatic disease. Mitotane is an adrenolytic drug that has demonstrated limited but favorable responses. About a 40% response rate is observed in patients with advanced disease. Some studies have suggested that patients who receive mitotane as adjuvant treatment after surgical resection (i.e., without obvious evidence of metastatic disease) may realize significantly improved disease-free survival.[24] Whether this confers a true overall survival benefit or a delay in the development of metastatic disease is not clear.

Because of the rarity of this malignancy, cytotoxic chemotherapy has not been widely studied. However, some evidence suggests that agents having activity alone or in combination against adrenocortical carcinoma include doxorubicin

(Adriamycin), cisplatin, etoposide (VP-16), cyclophosphamide (Cytoxan), and 5-fluorouracil (5-FU). The role of these agents in an adjuvant setting is far from clear.[10]

ADRENAL MEDULLA TUMORS

Epidemiology and Etiology

Approximately 400 medullary tumors are diagnosed in the United States per year. These are called pheochromocytomas, and only 10% of these have cytologic features that are malignant.[30] The peak incidence of this tumor is in the fifth decade of life, but it can be seen at any age. These tumors may be bilateral in various familial syndromes and can be associated with MEN syndromes. In addition, this type of tumor has been observed in patients with von Recklinghausen's disease (type I neurofibromatosis).

Anatomy

The anatomy of adrenal medulla tumors is discussed in the section on adrenal cortex tumors.

Clinical Presentation

A well-recognized clinical syndrome is associated with pheochromocytomas. The symptoms include hypertension, severe headache, nervousness, palpitations, excessive

---

Box 28-5 Staging System for Adrenocortical Carcinoma

T = Extent of the primary tumor
  1 = <5 cm and confined to the adrenal gland
  2 = >5 cm but <10 cm or adherence to the kidney
  3 = >10 cm or invasion of surrounding structures including the renal vein
M = Presence and type of metastases
  0 = no demonstrable metastases
  1 = regional lymphatics
  2 = distant metastases, (e.g., liver, lung, bone)
R = Tissue remaining after resection
  0 = tumor completely excised
  1 = tumor entered at operation
  2 = tumor tissue remaining after resection
D = Degree of histologic differentiation
  1 = differentiated, no capsular or vascular invasion
  2 = moderately undifferentiated, capsular or vascular invasion
  3 = anaplastic, capsular and vascular invasion
Stage 1 = 3 or fewer; (e.g., T1 M0 R0 D1)
Stage 2 = 4 and 5; (e.g., T2 M0 R1 D2)
Stage 3 = 6 and 7; (e.g., T3 M1 R1 D2)
Stage 4 = 8 or more; (e.g., T3 M2 R2 D3)

Modified from Bradley EL: Primary and adjunctive therapy in carcinoma of the adrenal cortex, *Surg Gynecol Obstet* 141:507, 1995.

perspiration, angina, blurred vision, and abdominal and chest pain. These are mediated by the excessive production of epinephrine associated with these tumors. Symptoms vary little among benign and malignant tumors and are often sporadic.[4]

Detection and Diagnosis

These tumors are suspected based on the clinical presentation. CT or MRI scans are used to assess the extent of disease. Laboratory testing, which measures urinary or plasma catecholamines (vanillylmandelic acid [VMA] and precursors of epinephrine), can help confirm the diagnosis. A needle biopsy can establish a tissue diagnosis but may not be necessary if the clinical, radiographic, and laboratory findings support the diagnosis.

Pathology and Staging

Adrenal medulla tumors are well-delineated, circumscribed tumors ranging from dark red, through gelatinous pink, to gray-brown or gray. The tumor size varies from 1 cm to 30 cm, with areas of hemorrhage and necrosis.[19]

Routes of Spread

The metastatic pattern of malignant pheochromocytomas is similar to that of adrenocortical carcinoma.

Treatment Techniques

Surgery is the treatment of choice for these tumors. Malignant tumors may grow extensively into surrounding structures, making a complete resection impossible. Persistent elevation of blood pressure indicates residual tumor or metastatic disease.[19]

The surgical resection of benign pheochromocytomas results in a normal life expectancy, and patients with malignant pheochromocytomas can be maintained for many years. Patients with extraadrenal malignancy have a poorer prognosis.

Results of Treatment

Adrenocortical carcinoma. The outcome for patients treated with this disease is poor. The 5-year survival rates for all stages range between 25% and 40%. The stage at diagnosis and ability to resect the disease has a significant effect on its outcome. Because most patients (65% to 75%) have advanced-stage disease, the ability to accomplish a curative resection is minimized and survival rates decrease.[5]

Adrenal medulla-pheochromocytoma. Because the majority of these tumors are benign and the surgical resection is often complete, results of treatment are excellent. Most patients live a normal life span.

Case Study

A 26-year-old man was in a normal state of health until approximately 2 months before presentation, at which time he experienced right flank pain and sought medical attention. His past medical history was unremarkable, except that 7 years before, he had sustained a blunt, right-sided chest wall and flank injury. A physical examination demonstrated no evidence of cushingoid changes, hyperaldosteronism, or virilism (signs of a functioning tumor). His blood pressure was normal, and he denied having flushing, sweats, palpitations, and diarrhea.

As part of the initial workup, an intravenous pyelogram (IVP) showed partially calcified mass above the right kidney that was pushing the kidney inferiorly and posteriorly. A CT scan was performed and showed a 10-cm mass that appeared to be involving the right adrenal gland with obvious extrinsic compression of the right kidney. No direct invasion of the inferior vena cava was evident. Obvious hypodense regions and calcified areas were present in this tumor mass. Neither adenopathy nor liver abnormalities were obvious. For a determination of the vascular supply of the tumor before surgery, an arteriogram was performed. It showed a single vessel with a trifurcate artery coming off the aorta serving this tumor mass. The venous phase of the arteriogram showed no gross invasion of the vena cava. Preoperative urinary VMAs and metanephrines (laboratory testing done to rule out pheochromocytoma) values were normal. A preoperative chest x-ray examination was unremarkable.

At the time of surgery, a rock-hard mass was encountered in the upper quadrant above the kidney overlying the entire right renal vein and inferior vena cava. This mass appeared to be involved with peritumoral inflammation and fibrosis. This was an extremely arduous resection secondary to the fibrous adherence to the local structures. A clear cleavage plane was established between the kidney and mass. However, dense adherence was encountered over the inferior vena cava, requiring a resection of a portion of the cava to remove the mass. A lymph node overlying the right renal vein was encountered and surgically resected. At the completion of the procedure, induration that spread in a sheetlike manner was behind the cava. The consensus was that additional resection was not possible.

The patient had an uneventful surgical recovery. Histologically, this proved to be a high-grade adrenocortical carcinoma. Because of concern for a residual tumor overlying the vena cava and in the retroperitoneal space behind the cava, the patient was sent for a radiation oncology consultation. The radiation oncologist felt that, because there was gross residual disease, the patient was indeed at risk for local regional recurrence and that postoperative external beam treatment was indicated to secure the optimal probability of local control.

The patient was treated in the supine position with combined proton beam and megavoltage (10-MV photon) radiation therapy. The patient received a total dose of 6000 cGy. The photon portion of the treatment included the delivery of 3280 cGy via a parallel-opposed AP/PA pair of Cerrobend-shaped fields, weighted with a ratio of 1:1. Subsequently, 720 cGy in four fractions were given via a parallel-opposed lateral wedge pair of MLC-shaped fields, weighted with a ratio of 2R:1L. The patient then received 2000 cGy from proton beam therapy. The characteristic properties of the proton beam allow a maximum target dose while limiting radiation exposure to surrounding structures. A high-resolution, contrast-enhanced CT scan with the patient in the treatment position was performed to delineate the primary target volume and neighboring critical dose-limiting structures. The dose to the spinal cord was 4600 cGy; the cauda equina received 4500 cGy, 30% of the right kidney received less than 4000 cGy, and the left kidney received less than 5 Gy.

Other than mild fatigue and mild intermittent nausea, the patient tolerated the treatment well. The patient was sent to a medical oncologist to discuss an adjuvant chemotherapy program. The patient received four cycles of adjuvant chemotherapy with cisplatin and doxorubicin over a 4-month period. Other than minimal weight loss and fatigue, the patient tolerated this treatment well.

Approximately 30 months have passed since the completion of the postoperative external beam radiation therapy. Since that time the patient has undergone a complete radiographic staging with a CT scan of the thorax, abdomen, and pelvis. There is no evidence of recurrence.

ROLE OF RADIATION THERAPIST

Education of the patient and family members during radiation therapy is aimed at helping the patient understand the goals and importance of treatment and the potential side effects. Symptoms experienced during treatment are often difficult to endure and affect the patient's ability to consent to the completion of treatments. However, with the support of family and health care professionals and with information for controlling side effects, the patient can successfully complete a course of therapy. Open communication between the patient and supporting staff members (nursing, dietary, and social services) is of utmost importance in abating and controlling symptoms during and after a course of treatment.

The following are some potential side effects patients can experience while receiving radiation to glands of the endocrine system:

1. Fatigue is a common side effect of most patients receiving radiation therapy. Daily treatments and biologic effects of the disease and radiation can cause fatigue. Poor nutrition, depression, and family and financial worries are all contributing factors. Scheduling appointments around rest or meal times can aid in combating fatigue. The therapist should discuss the daily activity level with the patient to assess potential problems, and family members should be encouraged to assist in daily activities (e.g., meal preparation) to allow for rest time.
   Appointments with the social services department can reduce financial worries and aid in emotional support. The therapist should encourage patients and family members to discuss their concerns and fears with each other.

2. Skin reactions can be painful and irritating to the patient. The therapist should advise the patient to avoid harsh creams, soaps, and lotions in the irradiated area. Hot water and sun exposure to the treated area should also be avoided. After a reaction starts the therapist should communicate with the physician, and depending on the degree of desquamation (dry or moist), a treatment break may be warranted.
   For patients who may have a tracheostomy a plastic cannula should replace a metal one, allowing it to stay in place during treatments. This will aid in preventing the enhancement of a skin reaction at the tracheostomy site.
   Loose-fitting clothes, especially cotton, should be worn to prevent rubbing and further irritation.

3. Hair loss **(alopecia)** can occur in the irradiated field as a result of the radiosensitivity of hair follicles. High-dose radiation may cause alopecia or delayed hair regrowth. The therapist should try to give the patient and family an appraisal for the potential and degree of hair loss and a time frame for its approximate occurrence. The therapist should inform patients to use mild shampoo and avoid excessive hair washing, which only dries and irritates the skin. In addition, the therapist should inform the patient and family that the new hair may have a different quality, texture, and color. If hair loss becomes significant, the use of a wig or turban may be indicated. Therapists should inform patients of national programs (e.g., "Look . . . Feel Better") that promote positive feelings and attitudes.

4. Dysphagia (difficulty swallowing) is often present in thyroid patients before the start of treatments as a result of the disease process. Early in the treatment, the patient may describe the feeling of "a lump in the throat." The therapist should encourage the patient to eat frequent meals consisting of high-protein and caloric foods. Eggnog, frappes, Ensure, Sustecal, and shakes supply high-protein and caloric intake and are soothing and easy to swallow.
   The patient should be advised to avoid commercial mouthwash, hot food and drinks, smoking, spicy food, and alcoholic beverages. If available, a dietary consultation should be scheduled within 1 week of the start of treatments.

Visual changes resulting from the disease can also cause a patient to be depressed. Simple pleasures such as reading or watching television can no longer be enjoyed. Unfortunately, little can be done to alter these effects caused by damage to the optic nerve; even treatment may not reverse the damage already inflicted on the nerve. However, audiotapes of best-selling books are available and may offer some enjoyment to the patient. The therapist can also encourage a family member to take time out to read the daily paper or a novel to the patient. The therapist should try to encourage family participation so that the patient does not feel left out.

Endocrine neoplasms can cause an array of previously discussed hormonal upsets, which can result in changes in emotions, appearance, and abilities. An altered body image can lower a patient's self-esteem. Patients with hair loss, hormonal syndromes, or acromegalic features may have misconceived notions of the way others perceive them. The therapist should be alert to these changes, allowing patients to express their feelings, promoting support from family members, and offering support to the family. Illness not only affects the patient but also the family because aggression and anger is often directed toward the family members.

The therapist should offer outside counseling (e.g., "I Can Cope") that is aimed at supporting families and patients through difficult times. Seeing other patients in similar circumstances lets patients know that they are not alone, their feelings are normal, and help is available.

Before the initiation of radiation therapy, the therapist should discuss the treatment process with the patient and family. The therapist should inform them that holding still is of the utmost importance for the delivery of proper treatment. In addition, the therapist should assure them that, although alone in the room, the patient is being carefully monitored. The therapist should take them into the room, explain positioning procedures, show them the monitors and intercom, and clearly explain that the machine will stop and someone will come in if help is needed. The therapist must give them a sense of control. The more they understand, the less anxiety they will feel, making the overall treatment process more tolerable.

Before educating patients and their families, therapists should educate themselves. Therapists should read the consultation, know the basics, and be prepared to address any specific questions or concerns a patient may wish to discuss. The patient must feel comfortable and confident in the therapist, allowing for open communication and trust throughout the duration of the treatment. A lack of trust can inhibit communication and cause undue stress for the patient and family.

Therapists must present themselves in a professional manner. After all, patients are entrusting themselves to the therapist, with little understanding and with much apprehension for what is before them.

Review Questions

1. _____ cancers are the most common of the endocrine malignancies.
   a. Thyroid
   b. Pituitary
   c. Adrenal gland
   d. Parathyroid
2. Radioactive iodine-131 is used in the treatment of which tumors?
   a. Thyroid
   b. Pituitary
   c. Adrenal gland
   d. Parathyroid
3. Of all functioning pituitary adenomas, prolactin-secreting tumors affect the _____ as a target organ.
   a. Thyroid
   b. Pancreas
   c. Breast
   d. Uterus
4. X-rays or radium was used in the past to treat which of the following benign conditions?
   a. Acne
   b. Rashes
   c. Tonsillitis
   d. All of the above
5. Which of the following is an indication for the use of radioactive iodine?
   a. Inoperable primary tumor
   b. Thyroid capsular invasion
   c. Distant metastasis
   d. All the above
6. What are the pituitary tumors that stay within the pituitary?
   a. Intrasellar
   b. Diffuse
   c. Intrahypophyseal
   d. Invasive
7. Which of the following would not be considered an endocrine-type tumor?
   a. Breast
   b. Thyroid
   c. Adrenal gland
   d. Pituitary
8. Which of the following is not a hormone secreted by the pituitary gland?
   a. ZH
   b. TSH
   c. FSH
   d. ACTH
9. Proton beams are sometimes used in the treatment of _____ tumors.
   a. Breast
   b. Thyroid
   c. Adrenal gland
   d. Pituitary
10. Which of the following does not belong?
    a. Medulla
    b. Cortex
    c. Follicular
    d. Mineralocorticoids, glucocorticoids

Questions to Ponder

1. Discuss the diagnostic tests for a patient suspected of having a low-grade, early-stage malignancy.
2. Discuss the role of I-131 in the management of a patient with papillary or follicular cancer. Why is this iodine-based pharmaceutical useful in thyroid cancer?
3. Discuss the clinical syndromes that can be associated with adrenocortical carcinoma and the factors mediating these symptoms.
4. Explain which imaging studies should be suggested for a patient suspected of having an adrenal neoplasm.
5. Describe the critical structures in proximity to the pituitary gland and the effect of the tumor mass and pressure on these structures. Discuss the presenting symptoms related to the tumor mass and pressure on these structures.
6. Explain for a pituitary adenoma the criteria for postoperative radiation therapy management and the various radiation treatment techniques.
7. As a radiation therapist, discuss the way you would help a patient deal with the physical and emotional changes brought about by an endocrine malignancy. List some of the resources available to patients and their families.

REFERENCES

1. Alkire KT: Cancer of the pancreas, hepatobiliary and endocrine system. In Baird SB, et al, editors: *A cancer source book for nurses,* Atlanta, 1991, American Society Professional Education Publication.

2. Arafah B, Brodkey J, Pearson O: Acromegaly. In Santen R, Manni A, editors: *Diagnosis and management of endocrine related tumors,* Boston, 1984, Martinus Nijhoff.

3. Block MA, et al: Clinical characteristics distinguishing heredity from sporadic medullary thyroid carcinoma, *Arch Surg* 115:142, 1980.

4. Brennan MF: Cancer of the endocrine system. In DeVita VT Jr, Hellman S, Rosenberg SA, editors: *Cancer principles and practice of oncology,* ed 6, Philadelphia, 2001, JB Lippincott.

5. Cohn K, Gottesman L, Brennan M: Adrenocortical carcinoma. Presented at the seventh annual meeting of the American Association of Endocrine Surgeons, Rochester, Minnesota, April 14-15, 1986.

6. DeAtkine AB, Dunnick NR: The adrenal glands, *Semin Oncol* 118:131-139, 1991.

7. Donehower MG: Endocrine cancers. In Baird SB, McCorkle R, Grant M, editors: *Cancer nursing: a comprehensive textbook,* Philadelphia, 1991, WB Saunders.

8. Furmanchuk AW, et al: Pathomorphological findings in thyroid cancers of children from the Republic of Belarus: a study of 86 cases occurring between 1986 (Ôpost-Chernobyl') and 1991, *Histopathology* 21:401-408, 1992.

9. Graze K, et al: Natural history of familial medullary carcinoma: effects of program for early diagnosis, *N Engl J Med* 299:980, 1985.

10. Hajjar RA, Hickey RC, Samaan NA: Adrenal cortical carcinoma: a study of 32 patients, *Cancer* 35:549, 1975.

11. Hardy J, Beauregard H, Robert F: Prolactin secreting pituitary adenoma: transsphenoidal microsurgical treatment. In Robyn C, Garter M, editors: *Progress in prolactin physiology and pathology,* Amsterdam, 1978, Elsevier/North Holland Biomedical Press.

12. Hay I: Thyroid cancer. In Tepper J, Gunderson S, editors: *Clinical radiation oncology,* Philadelphia, 2000, Churchhill Livingston.

13. Karakousis CP, Rao U, Moore R: Adenocarcinomas: histologic grading and survival, *J Surg Oncol* 29:105-111, 1985.

14. Kroop SA, et al: Evaluation of thyroid masses by MR imaging. Presented at the Radiological Society of North America 71st scientific assembly annual meeting, Chicago, November 17-22, 1985.

15. Mazzaferri EL, et al: Papillary thyroid carcinoma: the impact of therapy in 576 patients, *Medicine* 56:171, 1977.

16. Mettler FA, et al: Thyroid nodules in the population living around Chernobyl, *JAMA* 268:616-619, 1992.

17. Mountz JM, Glazer GM, Sissom JC: Evaluation of thyroid disease using MR imaging and scintigraphy. Presented at the Radiological Society of North American 71st scientific assembly annual meeting, Chicago, November, 1985.

18. Murali R: Tumors of the nervous system. In Nealon TF Jr, editor: *Management of the patient with cancer,* Philadelphia, 1986, WB Saunders.

19. Newsome HH Jr, Kay S, Lawrence W Jr: The adrenal gland. In Nealon TF, editor: *Management of the patient with cancer,* ed 3, Philadelphia, 1986, WB Saunders.

20. Sambade MC, et al: High relative frequency of thyroid papillary carcinoma in northern Portugal, *Cancer* 51:1754, 1983.

21. Scheilbe W, Leopold GR, Woo VL: High resolution real-time ultrasonography of thyroid nodules, *Radiology* 13:413, 1979.

22. Schneider AB, et al: Plasma thyroglobulin in detecting thyroid carcinoma after childhood head and neck irradiation, *Ann Intern Med* 86:29, 1977.

23. Schreiber NW: Endocrine malignancies. In Groenwald SL, editor: *Cancer nursing principle and practice,* Boston, 1987, Jones & Bartlett.

24. Schteingart DE, et al: Treatment of adrenal carcinoma, *Arch Surg* 117:1142-1146, 1982.

25. Thibodeau G, Patton K: *Anatomy and physiology,* ed 4, New York, 1999, Mosby.

26. Trautmann JC, Law ER Jr: Visual status after transsphenoidal surgery at the Mayo Clinic, 1971-1982, *Am J Ophthalmol* 96:200-208, 1983.

27. Varia MA: Pituitary tumors. In Tepper J, Gunderson S, editors: *Clinical radiation oncology,* Philadelphia, 2000, Churchill Livingston.

28. Varia MA: Central nervous tumors: pituitary tumors. In Tepper J, Gunderson S, editors: *Clinical radiation oncology,* Philadelphia, 2000, Churchhill Livingston.

29. Wang Chi-an: Thyroid cancer. In Wang CC, editor: *Clinical radiation oncology: indications, techniques and results,* Littleton, Mass, 1988, PBG Publishing.

30. Wittes RE: *Manual of oncologic therapeutics 1989/1990,* Philadelphia, 1989, JB Lippincott.

31. Wool MS: Management of papillary and follicular cancer. In Greenfield LD, editor: *Thyroid cancer,* Boca Raton, Fla, 1978, CRC Press.

BIBLIOGRAPHY

Cady B, et al: The effect of thyroid hormone administration upon survival in patients with differentiated thyroid carcinoma, *Surgery* 6:978-983, 1983.

Denny JD, Marty R, Van Herle AJ: Serum thyroglobulin: a sensitive indicator of metastatic well differentiated thyroid carcinoma. Society of Nuclear Medicine western regional meeting II, Las Vegas, 1977.

Hardy J, Vezina JL: Transsphenoidal neurosurgery of intracranial neoplasm. In Thompson RA, Green JR, editors: *Advances in neurology,* vol 15, New York 1976, Raven Press.

Van Herle AJ: Pathophysiology of thyroid cancer. In Greenfield LD, editor: *Thyroid cancer,* Boca Raton, Fla, 1976, CRC Press.

29

Respiratory

Donna Stinson, Paul E. Wallner

Outline

Key Terms

This chapter discusses lung cancer as it relates to the practice of radiation therapists. The focus is on bronchogenic carcinoma, although mesothelioma is discussed in a limited fashion. Technically, **bronchogenic carcinomas** are primary tumors of the lung that arise in the bronchi. Frequently, however, the term is used to refer to lung cancers collectively, including those that arise in pulmonary alveoli or pleural surfaces. Etiology and epidemiology related to age, gender, causes, occupational exposure, and prognosis are highlighted. The section on the anatomy of the respiratory system describes the organs of the system, physiology, blood supply, and lymphatics. The signs and symptoms of lung cancer are discussed through clinical presentations of local, regional, and metastatic disease. Also discussed are methods of detection and diagnosis. Various types of radiographic imaging techniques including emerging technologies such as positron emission tomography (PET) scans, laboratory studies, and relevant findings are identified. The details of pathology and staging, including histologic cell types, location, and prognosis, are discussed. Direct, lymphatic, and hematogenic routes of spread are also described. Surgical and chemotherapeutic treatment techniques are discussed, with radiation therapy covered in detail. The section on field design and critical structures elaborates on the methods used for the definitive treatment of lung cancer and includes examples of the following: parallel-opposed fields, boost fields, multiple-field combinations, intensity modulated radiation therapy (IMRT), frequently treated critical structures, off-axis points, customized beams, and doses. The impact of altered fractionation and protraction is discussed. Side effects; clinical presentations; the therapist's role in patient education, communication, and assessment; and the use of accessory medical equipment are described.

CANCER OF THE RESPIRATORY SYSTEM

Epidemiology and Etiology

Cancers of the bronchial tree, lung, and pleural surfaces represent the most common invasive malignancies in the United States. According to the American Cancer Society, approximately 170,000 new cases are diagnosed and approximately 157,000 deaths are caused by the disease each year.[22] Considered as a group, these malignancies represent 13% of all new cancers in the United States and 28% of all cancer deaths.[9]

Age and gender. Over the past five decades, there has generally been an absolute increase in new cancers with some leveling of the increase, especially in white males, over the past decade. In 1950, the male/female ratio was approximately 6:1; however, an increase in female incidence has now produced a ratio of almost 1:1.[6] In 1987, lung cancer surpassed breast cancer as the leading cause of cancer-related deaths in women.[7]

Causes. The most common cause of lung cancer is significant tobacco exposure, which is generally defined as more than one pack of cigarettes per day. Although tobacco product manufacturers have consistently denied absolute proof of the link, epidemiologic data strongly suggest an unequivocal causal relationship. Also, an apparent dose-response consistency is related to a higher incidence of lung cancers with (1) an increased duration of smoking, (2) an increased use of unfiltered cigarettes, and (3) an increased number of cigarettes consumed.[52] The use of chewing tobacco, cigars, and pipes is generally associated with a higher incidence of malignancies in the upper aerodigestive tract rather than the lung.

Occupational exposure. Additional causative factors include fumes from coal tar, nickel, chromium, and arsenic and exposure to various radioactive materials. Especially dangerous are agents with alpha emissions in their various daughter products, such as uranium and radon. The Environmental Protection Agency estimates that radon is the second leading cause of lung cancer in the United States and has recommended guidelines for various levels of radon exposure.

Radon may be present in various levels in soil. Also, depending on the type of home construction, ventilation, insulation, and size, radon may be found in high quantities inside parts of a home.

Pollution and genetic factors may be synergistic in their causative effect, adding to the risk above and beyond the various exposures indicated. However, these relationships are somewhat more difficult to prove.

Prognosis. Although numerous factors effect prognosis, the most significant variables include the following: (1) stage—extent of the disease (Box 29-1), (2) clinical performance status—measured by scales such as the **Karnofsky Performance Scale**[27] (Box 29-2), and (3) weight loss[1]—especially greater than 5% of the total body weight over 3 months. Multiple studies have clearly demonstrated the independent nature of each of these variables in determining the prognosis.[14,17,18] This effect is so marked that prospective clinical trials for definitive disease management frequently exclude patients who are in an advanced clinical stage (although the disease is apparently limited to the chest), patients with a Karnofsky Performance score of less than 70 or patients with weight loss greater than 5%. Individuals with advanced intrathoracic disease, extrathoracic extension, a Karnofsky score below 70, or weight loss greater than 5% rarely survive more than 2 years.

Malignant **mesothelioma** of the pleural surfaces has been increasing at a greater rate than other types of lung cancers, presumably related to the long latent period existing between carcinogenic exposure and development of the disease. Approximately 8 million individuals have been exposed to significant levels of asbestos (the primary etiologic agent), and estimates suggest that by the year 2030, perhaps 300,000 new cases per year may be evident. Because asbestos exposure had previously occurred in primarily male-dominated industries, the incidence of mesothelioma is seen overwhelmingly in men. Nonoccupational asbestosis and asbestos-related mesothelioma may occur in women.[34]

Asbestos fibers inhaled in industries such as mining, asbestos-material manufacturing and insulation, railroads, shipyards, pipe insulation, and gas mask producers are primarily associated with the production of mesotheliomas. Many types of asbestos particles exist, all of which have potential risks, but the longer and thinner strands produce more chemical reactivity and greater carcinogenesis.

Because metastatic disease to the lung represents a common occurrence for other primary tumor sites, the definitive establishment of the lung disease as primary or secondary is appropriate in most instances. This determination usually has significant implications for subsequent decisions regarding additional evaluation, management, and prognosis.

Anatomy

Organs of the system. The respiratory system consists of the nose, pharynx, larynx, trachea, and both lungs. Air is conducted from the nose; through the pharynx, larynx, and trachea; and into the lungs. Because cancers of the upper respiratory system (nose, pharynx, and larynx) are discussed in Chapter 30, only the anatomy of the trachea and lungs are included in this section.

The lower respiratory system consists of the trachea and lungs. The trachea is the major airway in the thoracic cavity. The wall is composed of rings of cartilage, smooth muscle, and connective tissue. Epithelial cells line the trachea. The trachea begins at the inferior border of the larynx and ends at the level of the fifth thoracic vertebra (T5), where it bifurcates.[50] This bifurcation is called the **carina,** the area in which the trachea divides into two branches. Anatomically and radiographically, the carina corresponds to the level of the fourth and fifth thoracic vertebra (T4 and T5). At the bifurcation the trachea divides into the right and left primary

Box 29-1 — AJCC Staging System for Lung Cancer

TX Primary tumor cannot be assessed, or tumor proven by presence of malignant cells in sputum or bronchial washings but not visualized by imaging or bronchoscopy

T0 No evidence of primary tumor

Tis Carcinoma in situ

T1 Tumor 3 cm or less in greatest dimension, surrounded by lung or visceral pleura, without bronchoscopic evidence of invasion more proximal than the lobar bronchus

T2 Tumor with any of the following features of size or extent:

More than 3 cm in greatest dimension
- Involves main bronchus, 2 cm or more distal to the carina
- Invades the visceral pleura
- Associated with atelectasis or obstructive pneumonitis that extends to the hilar region but does not involve the entire lung

T3 Tumor of any size that directly invades any of the following: chest wall (including superior sulcus tumors), diaphragm, mediastinal pleura, parietal pericardium; or tumor in the main bronchus less than 2 cm distal to the carina but without involvement of the carina; or associated atelectasis or obstructive pneumonitis of the entire lung

T4 Tumor of any size that invades any of the following: mediastinum, heart, great vessels, trachea, esophagus, vertebral body, carina; or separate tumor nodules in the same lobe, or tumor with a malignant pleural effusion

Regional lymph nodes (N)

NX Regional lymph nodes cannot be assessed

N0 No regional lymph node metastasis

N1 Metastasis in ipsilateral peribronchial and/or ipsilateral hilar lymph nodes, and intrapulmonary nodes including involvement by direct extension of the primary tumor

N2 Metastasis in ipsilateral mediastinal and/or subcarinal lymph node(s)

N3 Metastasis in contralateral mediastinal, contralateral hilar, ipsilateral or contralateral scalene, or supraclavicular lymph node(s)

Distant metastasis (M)

MX Presence of distant metastasis cannot be assessed

M0 No distant metastasis

M1 Distant metastasis present

Stage grouping

Occult carcinoma	TX	N0	M0
0	Tis	N0	M0
IA	T1	N0	M0
IB	T2	N0	M0
IIA	T1	N1	M0
IIB	T2	N1	M0
	T3	N0	MO
IIIA	T1	N2	M0
	T2	N2	M0
	T3	N1	M0
	T3	N2	M0
IIIB	Any T	N3	M0
	T4	Any N	M0
IV	Any T	Any N	M1

With permission from American Joint Committee on Cancer (AJCC), Chicago, Illinois: AJCC Cancer Staging Manual, ed 6, New York, 2002, Springer-Verlag.

---

bronchi. These bronchi begin a branching process that is similar to the structure of a tree (the bronchial tree). The primary bronchi are also called the right and left mainstem bronchi. The primary bronchi form branches of decreasing size until finally reaching the microscopic level where gases are exchanged. First, the mainstem bronchi form branches called the secondary bronchi. These lobar bronchi continue to divide into smaller, tertiary bronchi. Also called the segmental bronchi, these tertiary bronchi divide into smaller branches known as bronchioles. Bronchioles are microscopic structures that further divide into alveolar ducts. Many capillaries supply the alveolar ducts. Gases diffuse across the alveolar-capillary membranes. Oxygen and carbon dioxide exchanges take place at this microscopic level.[50]

The **hilum** of the lung is the area in which the blood, lymphatic vessels, and nerves enter and exit each lung. The **mediastinum** refers to the anatomy between the lungs including the heart, thymus, great vessels, and other structures that help position the lungs on either side of the midline.[3]

Physiology

Ventilation is the term for oxygen and carbon dioxide exchange to the external environment (i.e., breathing). The physiology of the respiratory system begins as air is inhaled into the body. Air moves inferiorly along the trachea and enters the lungs at the mainstem bronchi. The bronchi divide into many branches. As the branching increases, the cartilage decreases and the amount of smooth muscle in the structures increases.

A respiratory unit is composed of the bronchioli, alveolar ducts, atria, and alveoli. Gas exchange takes place from these units into the lung capillaries and is called external respiration. Oxygenated blood moves from these capillaries and major vessels in the lungs to the heart, where it is pumped throughout the body. Oxygenated blood is carried in the arteries and

Box 29-2	Karnofsky Performance Scale

100	Normal; no complaints; no evidence of disease
90	Ability to carry on normal activity; minor signs or symptoms of disease
80	Normal activity with effort; some signs or symptoms of disease
70	Self-care; inability to carry on normal activity or do active work
60	Requirement of occasional assistance, but ability to care for most personal needs
50	Requirement of considerable assistance and frequent medical care
40	Disability; requirement of special care and assistance
30	Severe disability; hospitalization indicated, although death not imminent
20	Extreme sickness; hospitalization necessary; active support treatment necessary
10	Moribund; rapid progression of fatal processes
0	Dead

Modified from Macleod CM, editor: *Evaluation of chemotherapeutic agents,* New York, 1949, Columbia University Press.

then exchanged in cells throughout the body for deoxygenated blood. From the capillaries, further exchanges take place through the interstitial fluid to the cells. This is known as internal respiration, a process in which oxygen and carbon dioxide exchanges take place at the cellular level as a result of changes in pressure. Thus carbon dioxide is removed from the cells, returned through the venous system to the capillaries in the lungs, and finally exhaled through the respiratory units in the following order: (1) alveoli, (2) alveolar ducts, and (3) bronchioli to the external environment.[50]

Blood supply and lymphatics. The lymphatic system is important in lung cancer because it is one of the principal routes of regional spread. Lymph nodes and channels permeate the respiratory system. At many points the lymphatics anastomose (connect) with pulmonary arteries and veins. Lymphatics of the lungs are classified in several ways. They are grouped anatomically according to the tumor, node, metastases (TNM) staging system into mediastinal and intrapulmonic nodes[3] (Box 29-3).

Flow between the mediastinal nodes is complicated and difficult to predict. As an example, mediastinal nodes connect directly with the subcarinal, pretracheal, and diaphragmatic channels.[16] Lymphatic flow is influenced by lung pressures, the diaphragm, movements of the chest wall, and motions of other local organs and vessels.[24]

Mediastinal nodes are subdivided into those in the superior mediastinum and inferior mediastinum, and further classified by number and location. The superior mediastinal nodes include (1) highest mediastinal, (2) upper paratracheal,

(3) pretracheal and retrotracheal, and (4) lower paratracheal (including azygos nodes). Inferior mediastinal nodes include (1) subcarinal, (2) paraesophageal (below the carina), and (3) pulmonary ligament.[3]

The other major groups of lymph nodes include (1) aortic, (2) subaortic A-P window, (3) paraaortic (ascending aortic or phrenic), (4) hilar, (5) intralobar, (6) lobar, (7) segmental, and (8) subsegmental.[3]

The blood supply of the respiratory system is similar to that of the lymphatics. Many of the vessels have similar names. For example, the vessels that supply the trachea are called the tracheal veins and arteries.

The location of the lungs in relation to the circulatory system is important. In fact, the two systems are linked. The lymph channels that drain the heart flow into the mediastinal nodes at the level of the carina.[24] At the carina the lymphatic drainage of the lungs meets with the cardiac flow of the lymph. From this region of the bifurcation of the trachea, access to the circulatory system occurs as the flow enters the thoracic duct and aorta.

In addition, the lymph nodes have arterial and venous blood supplies. Cancer cells trapped in the lymph nodes form emboli that can leave the node through its own blood vessels.[24]

When bronchogenic carcinoma of the lung is treated with radiation, the fields generally include the tumor and draining blood and lymph vessels. A simple field design, such as a mediastinum, includes all the lymphatics and blood vessels that flow in the area of the carina. Structures such as the hilum of each lung, aorta, thoracic duct, esophagus, vertebral bodies, and others are included in fields of this nature. The lungs, mechanics of respiration, blood, and lymphatic supplies are considered in planning a course of radiation therapy for patients with lung cancer.

Clinical Presentation

The signs and symptoms of lung cancer are often insidious and especially difficult to differentiate from the symptoms of

Box 29-3	Respiratory System Lymphatics

Mediastinal nodes
1. Superior mediastinal
2. Tracheal
3. Aortic
4. Carinal and subcarinal
5. Pulmonary ligaments

Intrapulmonic (hilar, bronchopulmonic) nodes
1. Mainstem bronchus
2. Interlobar
3. Lobar

chronic obstructive pulmonary disease that often occur. Presenting features are associated with (1) local disease in the bronchopulmonary tissues, (2) regional extension to the lymph nodes, chest wall and/or neurologic structures, and (3) distant dissemination.[8]

Local disease. Symptoms related to local disease extent are generally among the earliest complaints, with evidence of a cough in approximately 75% of patients. This cough may be severe and unremitting in 40% of the patients. Hemoptysis (blood associated with the cough) may be present in up to 60% of patients and may be the first sign of disease in up to 5% of patients. Approximately 15% of patients complain of a recent onset of dyspnea (shortness of breath), and a similar percentage exhibit chest pain.

Regional disease. Regional extension of disease (usually to the central mediastinal, paratracheal, parahilar, and subcarinal lymph nodes) may produce pain, coughing, dyspnea, and occasionally an abscess formation secondary to an obstructive pneumonia. Disease extension into the mediastinum may be manifested as dysphagia (difficulty swallowing) because of esophageal compression. Compression of the superior vena cava, especially in lesions of the right lobe extending into the mediastinum, may produce a **superior vena cava syndrome** associated with increasing dyspnea; facial, neck, and arm edema; orthopnea (an inability to lie flat); and cyanosis (a blue tinge to the lips). Hoarseness may occur as a result of compression or invasion of the recurrent laryngeal nerve, especially on the left side, where the nerve takes a somewhat longer course. Dyspnea may occur secondary to phrenic nerve involvement, producing diaphragmatic paralysis.

Less common are apex tumors of the lung. Apical tumors may be Pancoast tumors, but certain criteria other than anatomic location must be met. A patient with a true **Pancoast tumor** has a tumor in the superior sulcus and a clinical presentation that includes (1) pain around the shoulder and down the arm, (2) atrophy of the hand muscles, (3) Horner's syndrome, and (4) bone erosion of the ribs and sometimes the vertebrae.[28,36] Pancoast tumors involve the cervical sympathetic nerves that cause Horner's syndrome. Classically, **Horner's syndrome** includes an ipsilateral (same-side) miosis (contracted pupil), ptosis (drooping eyelid), enophthalmos (recession of the eyeball into the orbit), and an ipsilateral loss of facial sweating. Arm and shoulder pain is caused by brachial plexus involvement, and these tumors may extend upward into the neck. Erosion of the first and second ribs may cause arm pain. Not all apical tumors are Pancoast tumors.

Metastatic disease. Distant metastasis is generally associated with anorexia (loss of appetite), weight loss, and fatigue. Approximately 2% of patients with lung cancer may demonstrate **paraneoplastic syndromes** that are thought to represent distant manifestations of the effect of chemicals or hormones produced by these tumors.[25] Typically, symptoms of paraneoplastic syndromes may affect nerves, muscles, and

endocrine glands. These symptoms may be improved but rarely controlled for significant periods in the absence of primary tumor control. A frequently seen phenomenon associated with lung cancer is hypertrophic pulmonary osteoarthropathy, which is manifested by clubbing of the distal phalanges of the fingers (Fig. 29-1). Although this finding is most frequently associated with benign, long-standing chronic obstructive pulmonary disease, it may be seen as a presenting sign of lung cancer.

Individuals at high risk for the development of lung cancer because of habits such as tobacco consumption, occupational exposures, and/or significant exposure to passive smoke are often encouraged to consider routine chest x-ray screenings. A number of trials have been attempted with the use of annual chest x-ray screenings alone or with the addition of annual sputum cytologies. Most of these attempts to diagnose disease at an earlier stage have not been associated with significant improvement in long-term survival rates and have been largely abandoned, except in some industrial settings.

Detection and Diagnosis

Radiographic imaging. Conventional chest x-ray examinations using posteroanterior (PA) and lateral projections remain the principal method of lung cancer detection, although estimates show that approximately 75% of the natural history of the disease has occurred at the time of first radiographic appearance.[41] Conventional computed tomography (CT) scans may be suggestive of malignant disease, but the diagnosis is frequently not definitive, although some improvement may be obtained with a contrast-enhanced study, demonstrating variations in blood flow. Low-dose spiral CT may be effective in detecting tumors as small as 6 to 10 mm. Studies are under way to evaluate the use of this modality for screening of high-risk populations. One study completed in the United States, demonstrated findings positive for tumor in 2.7% of screened individuals versus 0.7%

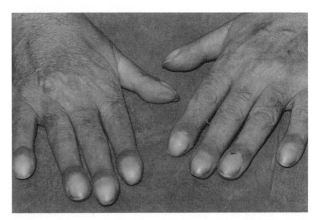

Figure 29-1. Hypertrophic pulmonary osteoarthropathy (clubbing).

detected by conventional chest radiograph. Unfortunately, the high rate of false-positivity presents a significant drawback to this approach, both in cost and morbidity.[46]

Fig. 29-2 shows a radiograph of an abnormal anterior chest, whereas the CT scan demonstrates that the tumor has already invaded the chest wall.

At the initial presentation the most frequent findings include a solitary soft tissue lesion, mediastinal widening secondary to lymphatic extension, parabronchial or parahilar lymphadenopathy, and pleural effusion (Fig. 29-3). Obstructive pneumonias may occur with endobronchial extension sufficient to produce bronchial obstruction. Solitary lesions are frequently irregular in contour and marginal distinctness. These lesions, if connected to a bronchus, may eventually break down to produce a thick-walled abscess with an air-fluid level. Long-standing obstructive pneumonias may also lead to abscess formation.

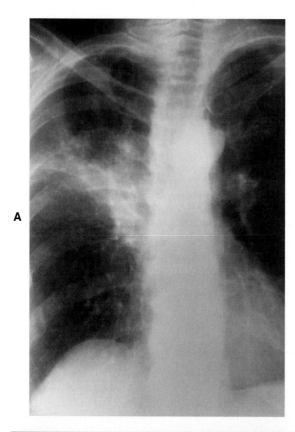

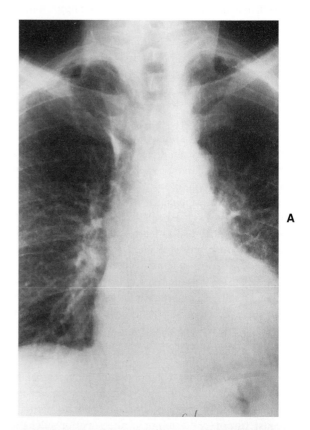

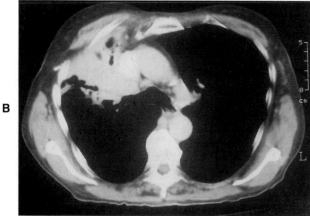

Figure 29-2. A, A posteroanterior (PA) chest radiograph showing a right upper lobe tumor. **B,** A computed tomography (CT) scan demonstrates the involvement of the chest wall.

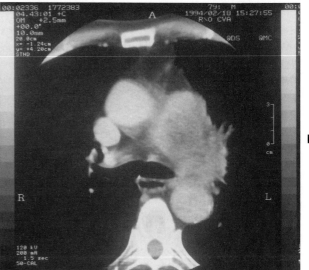

Figure 29-3. A, A posteroanterior (PA) chest radiograph showing midline disease. **B,** A computed tomography (CT) scan demonstrates the involvement of the mediastinum.

Chest radiographs that are suspicious for lung cancer must lead to other diagnostic interventions. Because a histologic (or cytologic) diagnosis is essential for appropriate management decisions, the next steps in evaluation frequently include CT of the chest to evaluate the following: (1) the primary finding itself, (2) the possibility of other pulmonary lesions, (3) the involvement of mediastinal and paramediastinal structures, and (4) pleural or extrapleural thoracic involvement. Fig. 29-4 demonstrates a right upper lobe tumor that has invaded the midline structures, whereas the CT scan shows mediastinal extension.

CT examinations are often crucial in selecting sites for a biopsy. CT examinations should involve the upper abdomen for an evaluation of the liver and adrenal glands, which are frequent sites of metastatic spread. CT scans have become an invaluable aid in the preoperative determination of resectability.

Patients in whom lesions are too peripheral for bronchoscopy or for whom bronchoscopy has failed to demonstrate endobronchial disease may be candidates for a CT-directed percutaneous fine needle aspiration (PFNA). This procedure is highly effective and associated with a small risk of pneumothorax. PFNA is frequently carried out on an outpatient basis with postprocedure time for monitoring of the respiratory status and blood pressure.

Magnetic resonance imaging (MRI) studies have been helpful in evaluation of mediastinal and paravertebral disease and PET scans have become a frequently used tool for determining if peripheral nodular lesions are benign or malignant. Incidentally detected pulmonary nodules in asymptomatic patients may be categorized on the basis PET positivity as probably malignant (Fig. 29-5). 18F-2-Deoxy-D-glucose (FDG) PET is accurate in more than 90% of patients with lesions as small as 10 mm. Additional uses for PET scanning include staging, especially for evaluation of normal-sized nodes; determining extent of primary tumor and small adrenal metastases; evaluating recurrent lung cancer (postoperative/radiation fibrosis vs. active tumor), and evaluating therapeutic response and prognostic potential.[37]

Except for bone scans, radioisotope studies have been supplanted primarily by CT scans of various organs, with much greater sensitivity and selectivity resulting.

Laboratory studies. Pulmonary function studies are beneficial primarily for determining a patient's ability to withstand various types of treatment, especially because many of these patients have preexisting compromised pulmonary function from their chronic pulmonary disease.

Sputum cytology may be positive in up to 75% of patients with lung cancer. These cytologies are of limited use, however, because of the difficulty in determining the precise sites of disease based on expectorated sputum and because specific tissue subtyping may be difficult.[15]

Bone marrow biopsies are of limited value except in individuals who have small-cell, undifferentiated carcinoma of the lung in which up to a 40% incidence of bone marrow involvement exists.

A histologic evaluation is generally sought and usually obtained through interventional routes that include surgery.

Hematologic and serum chemical evaluations of the blood are important and should include a complete blood count (CBC), serum calcium, alkaline phosphatase, lactic dehydrogenase (LDH), and serum glutamic oxaloacetic transaminase (SGOT). Serum calcium elevation is indicative of osseous disease. Alkaline phosphatase, LDH, and SGOT may be indicative of liver or bone involvement.

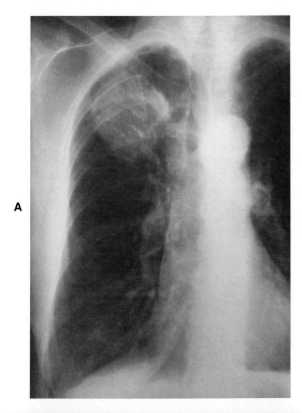

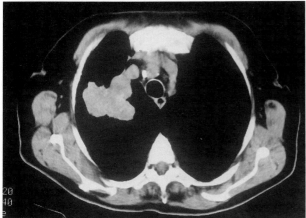

Figure 29-4. A, A posteroanterior (PA) chest radiograph showing a right upper lobe tumor. **B,** A computed tomography (CT) scan demonstrates the involvement of midline structures.

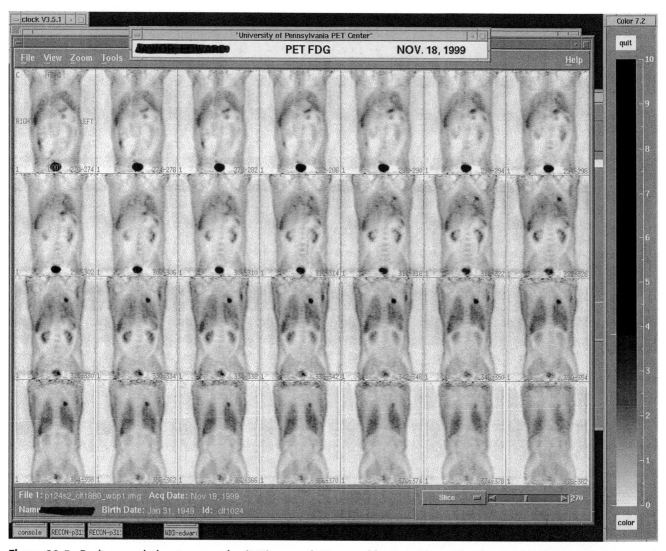

Figure 29-5. Positron emission tomography (PET) scan of 53-year old man with previously resected right lower lobe (RLL) lesion with radiographic changes in the RLL and left upper lobe (LUL). PET suggests that only the LUL is tumor.

Surgery. Tumor histology is most frequently obtained through a fiberoptic bronchoscopy because up to 75% of lesions may be visible in this fashion. The **bronchoscope,** which is a curved flexible tube, is used to examine the bronchial tree, to obtain a specimen for biopsy, or in some cases to remove a foreign body. Endobronchial brushing and endobronchial biopsy or a transbronchial biopsy provides a true-positive diagnosis in more than 90% of patients with visible lesions. The patency of bronchi and sites of bleeding can also be established.[40]

A pleural biopsy is used most frequently for pleural-based diseases such as mesothelioma. Thoracentesis (removal of fluid from the chest) or a pleural biopsy may be invaluable in the presence of pleural effusion because malignant effusion adversely affects the prognosis.

CT-directed percutaneous needle biopsy can confirm malignancy in 90% to 95% of lesions greater than 2 cm and in approximately 60% of smaller lesions.[37]

Video-assisted thoracoscopy is used routinely in diagnosis and management of small pulmonary nodules. The procedure involves the insertion of a tube into the chest and visualization of intrathoracic contents on a television monitor. Video-assisted thoracoscopy may be especially beneficial with pleural-based disease or if no dominant masses are demonstrated. The procedure may also assist in staging.[37]

A **mediastinoscopy,** which also uses a small flexible tube, is frequently used for the evaluation of the superior mediastinal extent of disease. If surgical intervention is anticipated, a formal, open mediastinotomy may also be used.

Advanced disease. CT scanning of the brain is used primarily for small-cell, undifferentiated carcinomas and adenocarcinomas of the lung. Both of these have a high risk for central nervous system metastasis.

The use of formal thoracotomy for diagnosing and staging

has generally been abandoned because of the availability of less-invasive interventional studies.

Pathology

Histologic cell types. The World Health Organization (WHO) has established a histologic classification of lung cancer that includes 12 primary tumor types with additional subtypes (Box 29-4). Although little question exists whether these categories are distinct pathologically, they are somewhat cumbersome from a clinical perspective, and more frequently the nomenclature of small cell lung cancer (SCLC) and non small cell lung cancer (NSCLC) are used. This breakdown is appropriate because of the distinct clinical differences between the small cell anaplastic carcinoma and the group of non small cell lesions, including adenocarcinoma, large cell carcinoma, and epidermoid (squamous cell) carcinoma, which act in a similar fashion clinically. Mesothelioma of the lung remains a distinct, although less frequent, category.[23,34]

Location. Squamous cell (epidermoid) carcinoma is usually associated with tobacco consumption, occurs most frequently in men, and is often located centrally in proximal bronchi. This lesion represented the most common form of primary pulmonary malignancy until the recent rise in the incidence of adenocarcinomas, which now account for approximately 40% of lung cancers in North America.[45] Adenocarcinomas are less frequently associated with tobacco consumption, occur most often in women, and are frequently more peripheral in location, arising in bronchioles or alveoli. Small cell carcinomas and large cell carcinomas each represent approximately 20% of the remaining lesions,

with small cell lesions tending to occur more centrally and large cell lesions appearing more peripherally. SCLC is prone to early spread, and fewer than 10% of these patients have diagnoses of limited stage disease.

Prognosis. Because of its predisposition for early metastasis, SCLC's prognosis is poor with only 10% to 15% of patients surviving 3 years. NSCLC has a better prognosis with 15% to 20% of patients surviving 5 or more years. Survival is significantly better in early-stage disease when surgery is undertaken for curative intent, with 5-year survivals approaching 60% or higher for clinical stages IA and IB.[12,35,48]

Staging

The use of clinical and pathologic staging represents an attempt to compare similar cases with regard to the effectiveness of treatment and the prognosis. Before the 1970s, conventional chest x-ray examinations, radioisotope scanning, and serum chemistry analyses were routinely used as the basis for clinical staging. Subsequent evidence has indicated the unreliability of these procedures for accurate evaluation of disease extent.

The advent of CT in the 1970s enhanced the ability to determine resectability before formal thoracotomy by enabling greater definition of the mediastinum, lymph nodes, and chest-wall invasion. In many instances the presence of these factors was felt to be a contraindication to curative resection, and during the 1970s and 1980s the frequency of surgical intervention in lung cancer declined.

Improvements in local control and systemic chemotherapy have increased the interest in surgical intervention, even

---

Box 29-4	**World Health Organization Histologic Classification of Lung Cancer[51]**

I. Epidermoid carcinoma
II. Small cell anaplastic carcinoma
  1. Fusiform cell type
  2. Polygonal cell type
  3. Lymphocyte-like (oat cell) type
III. Adenocarcinoma
  1. Bronchogenic
    a. Acinar, with or without mucin formation
    b. Papillary
  2. Bronchoalveolar
IV. Large cell carcinoma
  1. Solid tumors with mucin-like content
  2. Solid tumors without mucin-like content
  3. Giant cell carcinoma
  4. Clear cell carcinoma
V. Combined epidermoid and adenocarcinoma
VI. Carcinoid tumors

VII. Bronchial gland tumors
  1. Cylindromas
  2. Mucoepidermoid tumors
  3. Others
VIII. Papillary tumors of the surface epithelium
  1. Epidermoid
  2. Epidermoid with goblet cells
  3. Others
IX. Mixed tumors and carcinomas
  1. Mixed tumors
  2. Carcinosarcoma of the embryonal type (blastoma)
  3. Other carcinosarcomas
X. Sarcomas
XI. Unclassified
XII. Mesotheliomas
  1. Localized
  2. Diffuse

Modified from World Health Organization: *International histologic classification of tumors,* no. 1-20, Geneva, 1978, World Health Organization.

in the presence of mediastinal lymph node involvement. This intervention has necessitated a greater use of pathologic staging. A frequently used system is the TNM system proposed by Mountain and Carr and accepted by the American Joint Committee on Cancer[3] (see Box 29-1).

Routes of Spread

Direct.   As tumor cells continue to reproduce, the size of the mass increases. The mass itself may grow into surrounding structures. This is called local extension.[38] Tumors of the lungs are most likely to extend to the ribs, heart, esophagus, and vertebral column.[11] They may grow silently for long periods. Patients may seek medical attention for pain related to local extension.

Tumors that are not encapsulated have an ability to invade and attach themselves to local structures such as the chest wall, diaphragm, pleura, and pericardium. When tumors are continuous with local structures, they are called fixed, an ominous prognostic sign. In lung cancer, direct invasion constitutes a T3 tumor (i.e., a minimum of stage III).[3]

Direct extension can occur through the visceral pleura into the pleural cavity. A malignant pleural effusion may occur as fluid in the pleural cavity accumulates. Another possible route of local extension is through the hila. A tumor at or near the midline may grow directly into the hilum of the opposite lung.

Lymphatic.   Cancer cells break from the tumor mass and enter the lymphatics through two known routes. First, the cells can be trapped in the nodes as the lymphatic fluid is filtered. The cells continue to colonize in the nodes and eventually pass from one node to the next. This lymphatic spread is also called regional extension.[38] Second, cancer cells may grow through the lymph node and gain access to the circulatory system through blood vessels supplying the node.

The lymphatics that drain the lungs are the mediastinals and intrapulmonic channels (see Box 29-2). The lymphatics of the other organs in the thoracic cavity play an important role in the spread of lung cancer. The diaphragm, esophagus, pleural cavity, and heart are all in intimate relationship to the lungs.

The drainage of the diaphragm runs through the muscle to the aorta, inferior vena cava, and esophagus. Periesophageal lymphatics connect to the cardiac lymphatics because the heart lymph flows in the direction of the periesophageal nodes. From there the flow is toward the thoracic duct. Some of the nodes of the diaphragm drain toward the stomach and pancreas.[24] Drainage continues to the right lymphatic duct.

The pleural surfaces are rich in lymphatic channels. These superficial channels drain into the hilum and connect to the veins and arteries at the bronchioles. Also, the intercostal nodes (between the ribs) have many anastomoses. Drainage flows from the nodes between the ribs to the parasternal, paravertebral, and internal mammary nodes[2] and then to the thoracic duct.

Lymphatics that drain the heart meet at the bifurcation of the trachea. Lymphatics from the left coronary and pulmonary arteries also connect to the cardiac nodes.[16] Thus channels from the heart and lungs meet in the area of the carina.

Hematogenous.   The circulatory system plays a major role in the distant spread of disease.[38] At the bifurcation of the trachea the lymphatic drainage from the lungs, diaphragm, esophagus, pleural cavity, heart, stomach, and pancreas converges.[24] The drainage then has access to the entire body through the circulatory system at the thoracic duct and aorta.

The thoracic duct drains the left side of the body. The lymph moves medially and superiorly from the lungs into the thoracic duct. After moving through the thoracic duct, the lymph enters the circulatory system at the left subclavian vein (Fig. 29-6). From the right side of the body the lymph

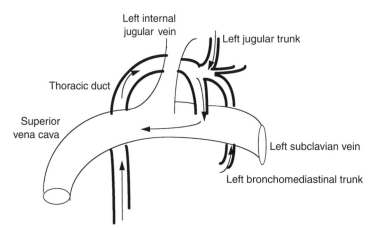

Figure 29-6. The role of the thoracic duct in lymphatic drainage of the left chest. The lymph moves superiorly through the thoracic duct (left lymphatic duct) and joins the venous portion of the circulatory system at the level of the left subclavian vein.

moves superiorly and medially into the right lymphatic duct. From the right lymphatic duct the lymph flows into the right subclavian vein[50] (Fig. 29-7).

Tumors also gain access to the circulatory system through blood vessels feeding the local lymphatic structures. In addition, spread occurs when malignant cells pass into blood vessels that supply the tumor.[24] Therefore lung cancer has access to the circulatory system from a variety of directions.

Common sites for metastasis. After gaining access to the circulatory system, tumors of the lung set up colonies in virtually any site. These metastases, or secondary growths, occur most commonly in the cervical lymph nodes, liver, brain, bones, adrenal glands, kidneys, and contralateral lung.[3]

Contralateral spread from hilum to hilum occurs as cells break away from the tumor and move to the area of the carina. Pressure changes as a result of respiration or gravity may transport the cell into the other hilum and then eventually into a resting place in the other lung. A "new" tumor may then begin to grow.

Treatment Techniques

The primary purpose of clinical and pathologic staging of lung cancer is to guide decision making regarding treatment goals. In the absence of demonstrable extrathoracic extension and despite poor long-term survival probability, patients should be considered as candidates for definitive or curative therapy. Individuals with extrathoracic metastasis, severe chronic obstructive pulmonary disease, or other limiting underlying medical problems may be candidates for palliative therapy or supportive care alone. After these decisions are made, despite the fact that lung cancer has been evaluated in clinical trials for decades, an extraordinary degree of controversy exists regarding appropriate management.

All conventional modalities (i.e., surgery, radiation, and chemotherapy) alone or in combination have been studied extensively. Newer modalities such as immunotherapy and radiolabeled monoclonal antibodies are also being investigated. Even in circumstances in which combined modalities appear to be advantageous, uncertainty remains concerning the most appropriate tactics of sequencing and dose modifications.

Surgery. Patients who are able to tolerate surgery and have intrathoracic disease of a limited nature, without pleural effusion or evidence of mediastinal extension, should be considered for definitive surgical intervention. Even with CT scanning and careful attention to the mediastinum and paramediastinal tissues, only approximately 20% of all patients with lung cancer may be considered candidates for surgery. Of those lung cancers, up to 90% may be resectable. Patients with complete resections (i.e., no evidence of a tumor at the resection margin and no evidence of regional lymphatic extension) have a 60% to 70% five-year survival rate for clinical stage IA disease; a 50% to 60% five-year survival rate for clinical stage IB disease; and a 50% to 60% five-year survival rate for clinical stage IIA disease. Increasing stage, based on tumor extent or lymph node involvement, significantly reduces 5-year survival and decreases the potential for total excision.[19,48,49]

Although limited wedge resections using video-assisted thoracoscopy have been associated with good results for limited-stage disease, if feasible, a lobectomy with regional lymph node sampling is the preferred procedure. Lesions that are central and involve a mainstem bronchus may require a total pneumonectomy. In this situation, careful attention must be given to preoperative and postoperative pulmonary function. If surgery is to be considered as primary therapy, there has been significant interest in the addition of radiation

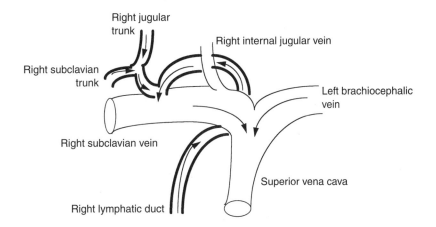

Figure 29-7. The role of the right lymphatic duct in the drainage of the right chest. The lymph moves superiorly via the right lymphatic duct and enters the venous phase of the circulatory system at the level of the right subclavian vein.

in a preoperative or postoperative setting. Although preoperative radiation had been used frequently, especially for apical tumors, most studies have failed to demonstrate a significant improvement in survival or increased resectability.[5,12,35]

Surgery may be used occasionally for palliative purposes, but indications in this regard are relatively limited.

Chemotherapy. Although many bronchogenic cancers will respond to single-agent chemotherapy, these responses are rarely complete and are typically short-lived. Numerous trials have demonstrated improvements in response using combined multiple-agent drug programs over single-agent regimens, but issues related to increasing intensity and diversity of drug therapy remain unproved. The most effective single-agent drug remains cisplatin with newer agents such as paclitaxel, docetaxel, vinorelbine, gemcitabine, and irinotecan,[5] all demonstrating moderate (20% to 50%) response as single agents, and improvement in response including 5-year survival, when used in combination with cisplatin or carboplatin. Phase III trials comparing combined-modality chemotherapy and radiation have demonstrated improvements in survival from 13% at 2 years, and 6% at 5 years, up to 26% at 2 years, and 17% at 5 years for appropriate combinations.

SCLC may respond dramatically to chemotherapy if combinations such as cisplatin and etoposide (VP-16) are used in combination with radiation for intrathoracic disease and alone for extensive disease.[12,35]

Radiation. There is little evidence to suggest that postoperative radiation improves local control and/or survival in the absence of local residual disease or mediastinal-paramediastinal lymphadenopathy. A number of studies have suggested an improvement in 3- and 5-year survival with postoperative radiation if lymph nodes are positive and there is residual local disease. In addition, studies have demonstrated a reduction in local-regional failure.[13,21]

The evidence of improvement in local-regional control and survival with the addition of systemic chemotherapy to external radiation now suggests that this combination of modalities represents the standard of care for patients with local residual disease postoperatively or for unresectable disease patients in whom radiation fields can encompass known disease and who are not candidates for surgical intervention. The precise timing of chemotherapy and radiation, for example, sequential or concurrent, remains controversial, the precise definition of radiation fields and time-dose relationship also is unproved.

The Cancer and Acute Leukemia Group B (CALGB) have studied hyperfractionation techniques of 120 cGy bid to a total of 6960 cGy, which did not demonstrate improvement of results above and beyond those of conventional radiation. Studies of hyperfractionated accelerated radiation (360 cGy at 150 cGy three times daily for 12 days to a total of 5400 cGy) demonstrated a slight improvement in local regional control, but similar studies carried out by the Radiation Therapy Oncology Group, with concurrent chemotherapy, failed to demonstrate improvement and did produce significant toxicity.

Current standard therapy would generally include concurrent, sequential, or alternating chemotherapy and radiation, using radiation tumor doses between 4500 to 5400 cGy at 180 to 200 cGy per fraction, one fraction per day and five fractions per week.[10,12,20]

Recent literature has suggested that increasing doses and reduced morbidity are possible using three-dimensional planning with CT simulators and conformal radiation, or IMRT.[11,35,44] Although dose escalation has been achievable without a concomitant increase in morbidity, improvements in local control and/or survival have not as yet been demonstrated.

Advanced disease. Palliative radiation is effective and commonly used for control of osseous and brain metastases. Skeletal pain can be relieved for extended periods in up to 90% of patients treated. If architectural bone disruption occurs, as in the case of vertebral body compression or pathologic fracture, the probability of pain relief is reduced. Generally, doses between 3000 to 4000 cGy in 200 to 300 cGy daily dose fractions are sufficient for pain relief and bone healing. In those instances in which a pathologic fracture has occurred or evidence exists of impending fracture based on the loss of bone calcium (based on empirical observations rather than specific measurement), consideration should be given to internal fixation before radiation. If internal fixation is carried out, palliative radiation can begin within several days if the surgical incision can be avoided. If the incision is within the treatment field, initiation of radiation should be delayed for 7 to 10 days, providing for satisfactory wound healing. Many patients treated for palliation of osseous metastases will have received previous systemic chemotherapy, and careful attention must be paid to the stability of blood counts.

Patients developing brain metastases may present with seizures, headaches, focal or motor sensory deficits, gait disturbance, visual or speech changes, changes in memory, or personality alteration. Patients with seizure activity should receive antiseizure medication such as phenytoin (Dilantin) and moderate to high-dose corticosteroids such as dexamethasone or prednisone. In the absence of seizure activity, there has been no demonstrated benefit to antiseizure therapy. Patients in whom significant intracranial edema is demonstrated on CT or MRI studies may note a rapid relief of symptoms with immediate initiation of high-dose corticosteroids, but these agents generally provide only short-term symptomatic relief. Radiation doses of 3000 to 4000 cGy in 10 to 15 fractions produce symptomatic relief in 35% to 75% of treated individuals. Patients in generally good clinical condition with apparent solitary intracranial metastases may benefit from surgical excision followed by radiation.

Signs and symptoms related to partial or complete obstruction of the superior vena cava may be evident in up to 5% of all lung cancer patients and may be secondary to extrinsic pressure on the vena cava or direct tumor extension into the vessel. Superior vena cava syndrome is considered an oncologic emergency requiring immediate initiation of palliative external beam radiation therapy, frequently in combination with high-dose corticosteroid therapy. Usual radiation techniques include three to four fractions of 300 to 400 cGy, followed by a reduction of the daily dose to 180 to 250 cGy. Depending on the patient's general clinical status, extent of disease, and intent of therapy, the total dose is usually 4500 to 5000 cGy. Approximately 85% of patients treated for vena cava obstruction will experience some relief of symptoms within 2 to 3 weeks, but long-term survival is rare.

For control of hemoptysis, radiation doses of 3000 to 4000 cGy in 2 to 3 weeks using a small field are generally sufficient if the site of bleeding can be well localized. Hemoptysis secondary to a small endobronchial lesions or obstruction may be improved or relieved entirely using endoscopic laser fulguration in conjunction with external radiation, conventional low-dose rate brachytherapy, or high-dose rate after-loading brachytherapy.

Field Design and Critical Structures

Parallel-opposed fields. The simplest fields used in the treatment of lung cancer are anterior and posterior parallel-opposed mediastinal fields, which typically include the primary tumor volume and adjacent mediastinum (Fig. 29-8). Typically, AP/PA (anteroposterior/posteroanterior) field arrangements are designed to include the primary tumor volume (defined by radiographic techniques) with a 2.0- to 2.5-cm margin of apparently normal tissue. If induction chemotherapy is used, the definition of tumor volume should be that obtained before initiation of chemotherapy. If a primary tumor is located in an upper lobe, or involves the mainstem bronchus, ipsilateral supraclavicular lymph nodes may be included. Ipsilateral hilar and superior mediastinal lymph nodes should be included with a 2.0-cm margin along with subcarinal lymph nodes to at least 5.0 cm below the carina. If the primary lesion involves the lower lobe or inferior mediastinum, the field should extend to the bottom of T10 or to the diaphragm. Although contralateral hilar lymph nodes had been routinely included in AP/PA fields in the past, they are generally excluded at present, unless disease involves the contralateral mediastinum, subcarinal, or contralateral hilar region.

When possible, normal tissues should be shielded to provide only the appropriate margins as noted previously. Ideally, this shielding is accomplished with customized blocking, such as alloys, Cerrobend, or multileaf collimation (MLC) (Fig. 29-9).

Boosts fields. Boost fields are used to deliver a high

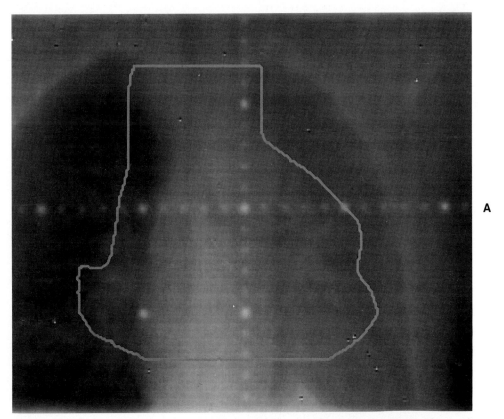

A

Figure 29-8. A, Field shape for a tumor in the hilum and mediastinum includes the mediastinum, carina, bilateral hila, tumor mass, and adjacent routes of extension.

continued

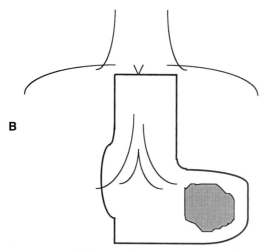

Figure 29-8, cont'd. B, Field shape for a tumor in the hilum and mediastinum includes the mediastinum, carina, bilateral hila, tumor mass, and adjacent routes of extension.

dose to a small volume. With boost fields the radiation dose is generally delivered to the gross tumor volume only, excluding regional lymph nodes. Boost fields may be administered using AP/PA, or multiple-field combinations, using custom blocking, MLC, wedge filters, or other types of tissue compensation (Fig. 29-10). Care must be taken to calculate doses to adjacent critical structures, such as the spinal cord, to ensure safe doses to those tissues.

Multiple-field combinations. Generally, the definitive treatment of lung cancer requires multiple-field combinations with alterations in weighting, shaping, and tissue compensation to enable delivery of tumoricidal doses to primary and lymph node tissue and safe doses to critical normal tissues. Because patients with bronchogenic cancers typically have compromised pulmonary function before initiation of radiation, the use of progressively reduced field sizes becomes even more essential.

Accurate positioning of the patient is essential, and lasers should be used when possible. A sagittal laser and lasers aligned with marks on the sides of the patient increase the accuracy of the setup. Of critical importance is the arm

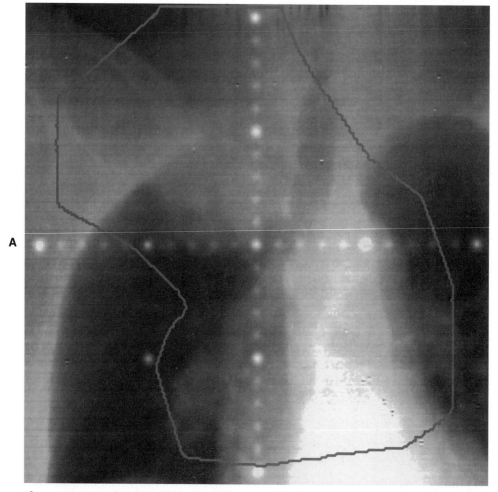

Figure 29-9. A, Shrinking fields. Parallel-opposed fields for right upper lobe (RUL) tumor.

continued

position with off-cord boosts because the probability of the patient rolling to one side or the other increases if the arms are raised above the patient's head. In addition, the spinal cord can receive doses above tolerance if lasers are not aligned properly. Geographical misses can occur if the patient is not aligned accurately for every treatment. This goal of reproducibility is improved with the use of lasers for alignment.[47]

Critical structures. Three critical structures are frequently of concern in fields used to treat lung cancer: the spinal cord, heart, and normal lung.[38] Conceivably, the dose tolerances of these organs can be exceeded. Therefore doses to these structures must be carefully documented during planning and throughout the treatment course. Fields are designed so that organ tolerance is not exceeded. Advance planning before organ tolerance is reached is critically important so that the optimal dose distributions can be achieved.[11]

The first critical structure considered is the spinal cord.

Doses of radiation required to control lung cancer exceed the spinal cord tolerance of 4500 to 5500 cGy[43] (Table 29-1). Although higher spinal cord tolerance doses are discussed in the literature,[33,43] radiation oncologists generally take a conservative approach to the spinal cord dose by prescribing treatments that do not exceed the 4500 cGy limit.[25] Standard practice for radiation therapists is to require a written order for all cord doses greater than 4500 cGy. In charting daily treatments, radiation therapists should monitor a spinal cord dose column to ensure that tolerance is not exceeded. Frequently, the cord receives a daily dose that is higher than the prescribed dose to the tumor. The quality of a patient's life will be diminished and even death may result if these standards are not followed.

If cord tolerance is exceeded, neurologic signals that normally move along the spinal cord will be blocked. Demyelination of the oligodendrocytes that conduct nerve impulses is responsible for some of the neurologic complications. In addition, damages in the form of fibrosis and

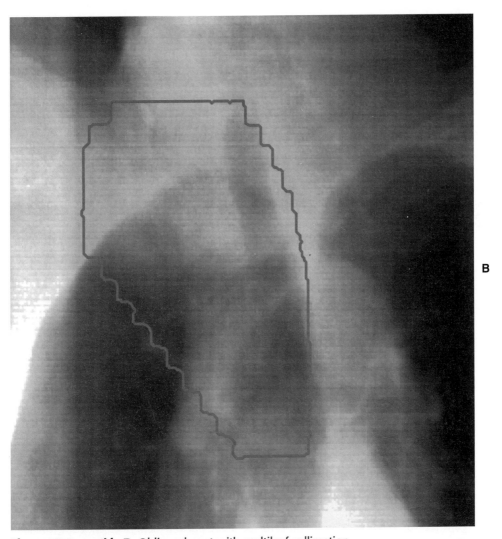

B

Figure 29-9, cont'd. B, Oblique boost with multileaf collimation.

occlusion of capillaries and arterioles result in a reduced blood supply to the neurons and oligodendrocytes in the region treated. Because nervous system tissue has severely limited or no regenerative abilities, damage is irreparable.[42] Clinical manifestations of cord damage such as myelitis (inflammation of the spinal cord) can occur. Depending on the level of the cord affected, quadriplegia or paraplegia may follow. Necrosis and infarction of the cord can occur. When transection of the cord occurs, Brown-Séquard's syndrome results, with paralysis and loss of sensations such as pain and temperature.[38]

During the planning process the depth of the spinal cord must be determined. If available, CT images are useful; the depth of the cord in the patient is determined from the images of the individual vertebral bodies in the field to be treated. In simulation, **orthogonal radiographs**[47] are taken to determine the cord depth. Generally, anterior and lateral films of the thorax (orthogonal radiographs) are taken at right angles. The physical depth of the cord in the patient is measured from the image through the use of a demagnification calculation.

The depth of the spinal cord is important for two reasons. First, tumoricidal doses exceed the tolerance of the spinal

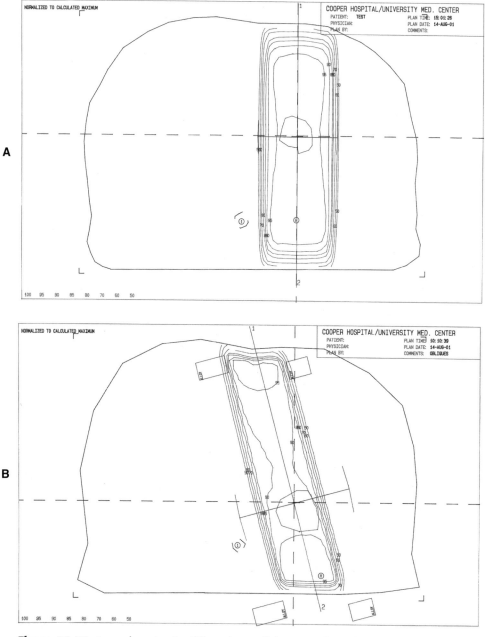

Figure 29-10. Lung boosts. **A,** Off-cord, parallel-opposed fields. **B,** Off-cord, parallel-opposed oblique fields.

continued

cord. Second, because the depth of the spinal cord varies along the vertebral column, the dose calculated to one point in the spinal cord is not the same for the remainder of the cord. For example, the depth of the cord in the lower cervical area may be 5 cm, whereas the depth in the lower thorax may be 8 cm. If the tumor is close to the midplane (approximately 10 cm), overdoses to both areas of the spinal cord can occur (Fig. 29-11). Even if cord tolerance is considered in the prescription, the dose the patient receives to the cord must be monitored closely because the dose along the length of the field varies as the depth of the cord changes.

Avoiding the spinal cord with boost fields can be challenging, particularly considering the normal curvature of the vertebral column. With oblique and lateral fields, collimator rotations may be used to follow the curvature of the spinal column. The angle of rotation is calculated through the use of a geometrical slope formula. Blocking the cord may be useful, but the transmission of radiation through the block or MLC should be considered. Spinal cord tolerance can be exceeded with beam transmission through the shielding and with scatter radiation that occurs in the patient (under the shadow of the shielding projected on the skin).

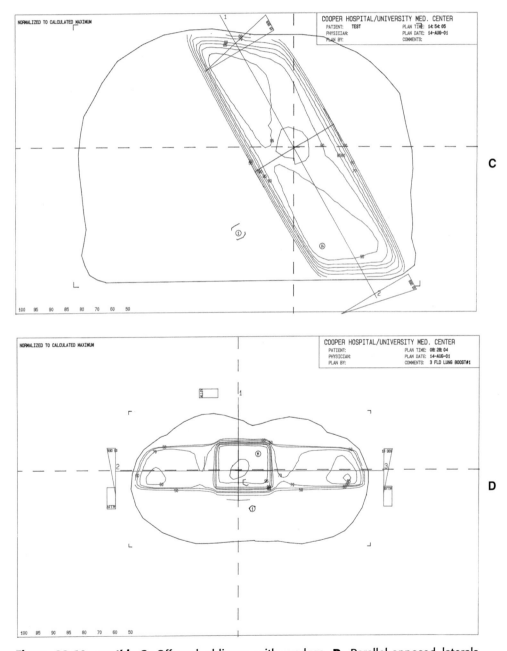

Figure 29-10, cont'd. C, Off-cord obliques with wedges. **D,** Parallel-opposed laterals. (Note the amount of uninvolved lung.)

continued

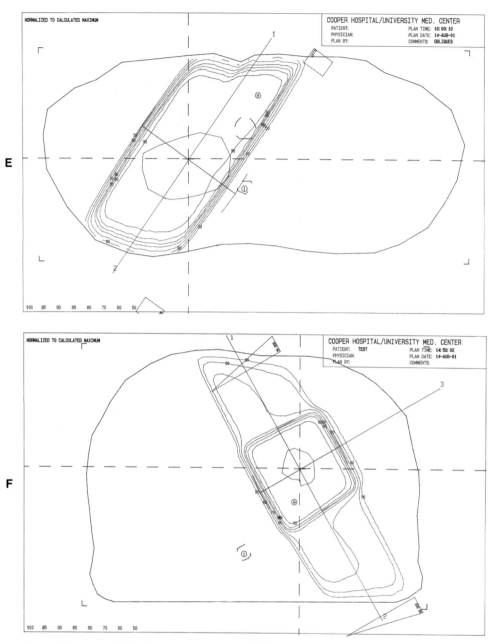

Figure 29-10, cont'd. E, An open anterior field weighted 0.7 and two posterior obliques with equal weighting. **F,** Two off-cord obliques with wedges and an open field. (Note the position of the spinal cord in relation to the open field.)

continued

When the spinal column is not midplane the image of the anterior field is different from that of the posterior field. This is caused by divergence. The effect of divergence can be seen through a comparison of the disc spaces on the anterior and posterior images. When fields are exactly parallel-opposed the images may not be identical.[4]

Magnification-measuring devices are used during simulation. Devices such as beaded trays are used so that comparisons can be made between the images and actual patient anatomy. Magnification-measuring devices are used for com-

paring objects of a predetermined size with objects of an undetermined size.[47] For example, fiducial trays containing the beads are placed above the patient in the head of the simulator. The spacing of the beads is such that the image projects a 2 cm (sometimes 1-cm) space between the beads at the axis of the machine. Through the use of a 100 cm isocentric unit the space between the beads is 2 cm at 100 cm. If the image is produced at a 140 cm source-film distance (SFD), a direct relationship exists between the space between the beads on the film and the space at the axis. With the use of a

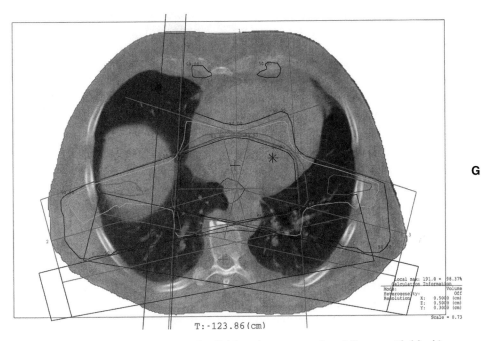

G

Figure 29-10, cont'd. G, Open anterior field and two posterior obliques with blocking.

Table 29-1	Organ tolerances[44]	
Organ	**TD 5/5 (cGy)**	**TD 50/5 (cGy)**
Spinal cord	5000	6000
Normal lung	2000	3000
Heart	4300	5000
Esophagus	5000	5500
Bone marrow	2500	3500
Skin	5500	7000
Liver	3500	4000
Bone	6500	7000

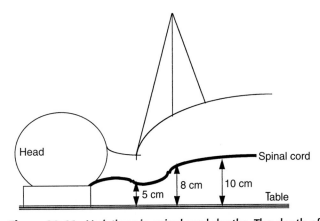

Figure 29-11. Variations in spinal cord depths. The depth of the cervical spinal cord is closer to the posterior surface than that of the thoracic cord.

ratio, the space is calculated to 2.8 cm. Other devices such as rulers, rings, or coins accomplish the same goal; a known dimension is used to find an unknown dimension.

In the planning of treatments for patients with lung cancer, magnification-measuring devices are particularly useful in finding the spinal cord depth. The cord depth can be determined from the lateral orthogonal film. The amount of the simulation table on the film causes a distortion because of the width of the table and the distance the beam travels. Tables can be marked with a radiopaque wire in the center to reduce distortion.[4] Alternatively, the therapist can palpate the spinous processes and carefully tape on the patient's back a piece of solder wire that will relate the vertebral column to the skin surface. During simulation in the supine position the wire will be in contact with the table, thereby indicating the table on the radiographic image.

The second critical structure in the treatment of lung cancer is the heart. When 60% or more of the heart is treated with 4500 to 5500 cGy, pericarditis (inflammation of the pericardium) and pancarditis (inflammation of all parts of the heart) may result[43] (Table 29-1). Long-term complications can follow because of damage of the interstitial components of cardiac tissue, and the resulting fibrosis may damage the valves.[38]

In the planning of fields for lung tumors near the heart, the volume of the heart treated should be considered. In particular, when parallel-opposed beams are weighted anteriorly to reduce the spinal cord dose, the dose to the heart should also be measured so that tolerance is not exceeded The use of chemotherapy should be monitored closely. Drugs such as doxorubicin (Adriamycin) have cardiac toxicity that has a synergistic effect when the drug is used in combination with radiation.[38]

The third critical structure to be considered in the treatment of lung cancer is the normal lung. The major complication that occurs is radiation pneumonitis, followed by fibrosis. Pneumonitis occurs from 1 to 3 months after radiation. Fibrosis occurs from 2 to 4 months after treatment.[38] Pneumonitis is the clinical manifestation of vascular, epithelial, and interstitial injuries. Patients exhibit dyspnea, fevers, night sweats, and/or cyanosis.[11] The chronic phase consists of severe dyspnea and coughing, clubbing of the fingers, and an abscess that can be followed by infection and sepsis.

The volume of lung treated and the total dose must be considered to avoid complications related to the lung. The dose tolerance to the lung generally ranges from 2000 to 3000 cGy[43] (Table 29-1). Large volumes of lung are projected to have at least a 50% complication rate at 3000 cGy (TD 50/5, or 50% of the patients in 5 years). Fraction sizes range from 180 to 200 cGy. Care is taken throughout the planning process to minimize the amount of noncancerous lung in the fields. Customized beams such as reduced and boost fields, shielding blocks, and off-cord arrangements are used to limit the beam transmission through unaffected lung. The nature of lung tissue itself is notable. Lung density is less than the density of other tissue because of the presence of air (oxygen and carbon dioxide) in the organs. Therefore the dose to the tumor and lung tissue is increased by 15% to 20%.[26,38] Heterogeneity corrections can be used to compensate for this phenomenon.[31]

Other structures included in fields designed to treat lung cancers are important but not critical. The esophagus, bone marrow, skin, and sometimes the liver with right lower lobe lung tumors have dose tolerances identified in Table 29-1. Generally, however, tolerance of these organs is not exceeded.

Off-axis points.   Typically, doses are calculated to the center of a field. With lung tumors, however, knowledge about the structures not in the center is important. For the calculation of doses to off-axis points, two measurements are needed: (1) the source-skin distance (SSD) to each point and (2) the corresponding patient thickness at each point. Depending on the institution, the physical measurement of the size of the patient may be referred to as the patient thickness, separation, interfield distance (IFD), or diameter. The physical measurement of a patient's size is determined through the use of calipers. SSDs are determined by reading and recording the distance that the optical distance indicator shows. Doses to the various points vary according to the inverse square law and attenuation.

Distances vary with patient size and anatomic variations. In Fig. 29-12, the SSD to the center is 90 cm, and the distance at the supraclavicular point is 93 cm. The patient measures 20 cm at the center and 14 cm at the supraclavicular point. Each anatomic point at which doses are needed will be measured. The SSDs and the corresponding patient diameters must be recorded. These distances and diameters work with each other. When the 90-cm SSD and 20 cm separation are accurate, the patient must measure 22 cm at the mediastinum if the 89 cm SSD to that point is correct (100 − 11 = 89) (Table 29-2). A patient with a left upper lobe tumor will have off-axis points to include the tumor, supraclavicular nodes, and mediastinum.

Customized beams.   Optimal patient care frequently requires combinations of several types of field designs. For example, multiple fields with boosts, collimator rotations, and weighting may be needed to deliver the best dose distribution. Mixed beams of photons and electrons may be used to meet specific clinical challenges, such as a mass extending through the chest wall. Also, dual-energy accelerators have the capacity to customize the beam to an effective energy level that is not possible with a single-energy conventional accelerator. Beam arrangements are selected to cover the tumor and simultaneously limit the dose to the normal tissue.

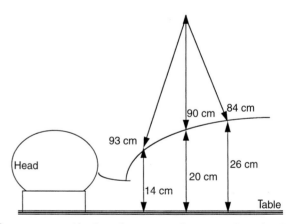

Figure 29-12. Sloping chest. Superior, central, and inferior borders have different distances and corresponding patient measurements.

Table 29-2	Comparison of points and distances		
Point	**SSD (cm)**	**Diameter (cm)**	**Midplane Depth**
Center	90	20	10
Mediastinum	89	22	11
Supraclavicular	93	14	7
Mass	91	18	9

SSD, Source-skin distance.

Specific anatomic features, such as a **kyphosis** (excessive curvature of the spine), need special attention. With curvatures of the spine the collimator can be rotated to follow the vertebral column. Another approach is the use of a customized shield (alloy) to tailor the field to meet the individual patient's anatomy without rotating the collimator.

There is increasing evidence that the use of IMRT may enable delivery of higher doses to irregularly shaped tumor volumes with sparing of normal tissue structures. Extensive studies in this regard have been carried out for tumor sites such as the prostate, but the normal movement of the lung and mediastinal structures during respiration presents added challenges in this regard. IMRT techniques have not as yet been adopted for routine use.

If oblique fields are needed to boost the lung tumor and at the same time avoid treating the spinal cord, the varying depths of the spinal cord often present challenges. With the use of a collimator "twist," one section of the spine is included, whereas another section may be excluded in the fields. The use of shielding may solve this dilemma. However, if collimator rotations are used, care must be given to changing the rotation for the parallel-opposed field. With the clinical application of the concept of mirror images,[4] an anterior field with a 175 degree rotation off the 180 degrees requires a 5 degree twist in the opposite direction for the posterior field. The posterior collimator position therefore is 355 degrees so that the volume treated in these fields is truly parallel-opposed.

Compensators are used to adjust dose distributions for anatomic features such as a barrel-shaped chest. Either a customized device is made or a standard wedge, C-wedge (compensating wedge),[26] is used to improve the dose distribution. Compensators attenuate the beam. They are useful for correcting surface irregularities. Also, spinal cord dose variations resulting from spinal column curvature can be adjusted with the use of a compensator. A compensator is useful if the inferior thorax measures significantly more than the superior thorax.[30] Examples include C-wedges, conventional compensators (i.e., lead, brass, aluminum, plastic, or Lucite), and computerized custom compensators. Bolus can be used to reduce surface irregularities, but the loss of a skin-sparing effect usually precludes its use in clinical practice.[30]

Wedges can be used to help shape dose distributions. In particular, wedges are useful for the delivery of boost doses with laterally located tumors. Multiple-field arrangements that include a three- or four-field wedge and open field combinations are examples of the use of the wedges' beam-shaping characteristics (Fig. 29-13, *E* and *F*).

Doses. Total doses vary depending on the intent of therapy and precise tissue. Patients treated with a curative intent typically require higher doses and more complex field arrangements. Patients treated with palliative intent generally have the option of lower total doses, shorter courses of therapy, and more simple field arrangements. Definitive doses to control or cure localized SCLC generally range from 4500 to 5400 cGy at 180 to 200 cGy per fraction. Doses for definitive management of NSCLC generally range from 6000 to 7500 cGy at 180 to 200 cGy daily dose fractions. When used with systemic chemotherapy, especially concomitantly, total doses may be somewhat reduced.[10]

Definitive doses to control or cure localized bronchogenic carcinomas range from 6000 to 7500 cGy[9,11,36] (Table 29-3). Initial field arrangements are generally prescribed between 4000 and 4500 cGy. Boost fields follow in various combinations until tumoricidal doses are achieved. Various fraction patterns can be used, depending on whether conventional fractionation, hyperfractionation, accelerated fractionation, or accelerated hyperfractionation is prescribed.[30,45] **Conventional fractionation** uses a 180 or 200 cGy dose given once per day. The other fraction patterns change the conventional approach by altering the fraction size, daily dose, number of treatment days, and/or total dose in an effort to improve patient tolerance and survival. Table 29-4 displays these different approaches to fractionation in a hypothetical patient.

Palliative treatment is given to relieve symptoms. For lung cancer, treatment can be given to relieve an airway obstruction. In these situations the total tumor dose ranges from 4000 to 5000 cGy,[38] depending on the patient's response.

For a patient with superior vena cava syndrome, initial doses are high for the first one to three treatments and range from 350 to 400 cGy.[9] Because of the large volume and high doses, the daily dose must be reduced after the initial treatments. Initial prescribed doses are generally 350 to 1200 cGy, followed by 200 cGy fractions to a total dose of 4500 to 5000 cGy.

Brachytherapy can be used in the treatment of lung cancer. High-dose-rate (HDR) remote afterloading is used in the treatment of bronchial disease.[29] For example, during a course of external beam radiation a supplemental dose of radiation can be given with HDR, using 500 cGy for two to four treatments. In the event of recurrent disease, HDR may also be useful, particularly if spinal cord tolerance has been reached or the airway is compromised.

Side Effects

Classification. During courses of radiation therapy, patients may experience side effects classified as acute or chronic. The short-term reactions that occur during treatment and subside after the course is completed are known as acute side effects. Chronic side effects are long-term effects of radiation treatments.

Clinical presentation. With lung cancer, common acute side effects are dermatitis, erythema, and esophagitis. Routine departmental skin care is recommended. Dysphagia associated with inflammation of the esophagus occurs at approximately 3000 cGy. Esophagitis can be relieved by medication or diet. Oral medications include liquid antacids

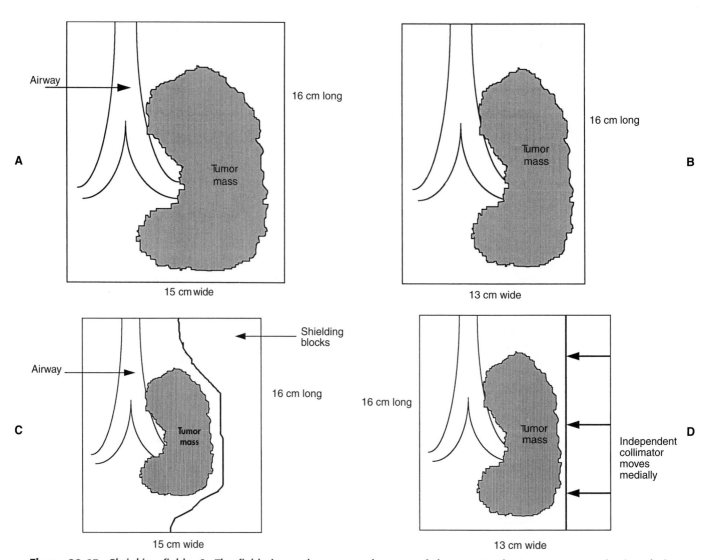

Figure 29-13. Shrinking fields. **A,** The field size and tumor at the start of therapy. **B,** The tumor mass reduction during therapy and the field width reduction. **C,** Shielding added to block uninvolved lung with smaller tumor mass. Shrinking fields. **D,** Width reduction to accommodate a smaller tumor size through the use of an independent collimator (beam off-sets).

Table 29-3	External beam treatment doses	
Treatment Approach		**Total Dose (cGy)**
Primary radiation		6000-7500
Surgery + radiation (postoperative)		5000-6500
Chemotherapy + radiation		3000-5000
Palliation and/or recurrence		4000-5000
Preoperative (superior sulcus)		3000-4500

Modified from Cox JD, editor: *Moss' radiation oncology: rationale, technique, results,* ed 7, St. Louis, 1994, Mosby; DeVita V, Hellman S, Rosenburg S: *Principles and practice of oncology,* ed 4, Philadelphia, 1993, JB Lippincott; and Pancoast HK: Superior pulmonary sulcus tumor, *JAMA* 99:17.

and mucosal anesthetics such as lidocaine hydrochloride.[38] Nutritional suggestions include foods that are soft, moist, and nonspicy and liquids at room temperature or slightly chilled. Patients may also experience coughing, dry throat, and excessive mucous secretions.

A chronic side effect caused by irritation of the trachea and bronchi is a dry, nonproductive cough. Other chronic effects include fibrosis of the lung and subcutaneous fibrosis of the skin.

Complications are different from side effects because they are usually a result of doses that exceed organ tolerance. Complications are serious and, in the case of pneumonitis, may be life threatening. If spinal cord tolerance is exceeded, myelopathy may occur. With serious neurologic complications the resulting infections can lead to death.

Table 29-4	**Fraction patterns and total doses for primary radiation**			
Type of Fractionation	**Fraction Size**	**Daily Dose**	**Treatment Days**	**Total Dose (cGy)**
Conventional fractionation	180-200	180-200	30-34	6000-6120
Hyperfractionation	120	240	30	7200
Accelerated fractionation	160	320	19	6080
Accelerated hyperfractionation	160	320	23	7360

Role of Radiation Therapist

Education.   Opportunities exist for the radiation therapist to evaluate the patient daily for needs related to education, communication, and assessment. Frequently, patients need education regarding testing procedures such as x-ray examinations and blood tests. The information should include the reason that the tests are needed, the location and time to report, and special requirements such as fasting and other preparations. Procedures that seem uncomplicated to medical professionals may be overwhelming to patients and family members. Radiation therapists should take time to explain carefully and at the appropriate level the how, why, and when details of a particular study. Patient education is important from the time of consultation and continues to the last day of treatment. Education continues when patients return for follow-up visits. Patients have a right to this education as defined in the "Patient's Bill of Rights" supported by the American Hospital Association. At any point, a patient can refuse care (i.e., refuse further treatment). When possible the therapist must try to ensure patient understanding. Sometimes questions can be one-sided; the patient is not given the opportunity to indicate an understanding of the information received. The therapist should use a questioning style permitting the patient to reflect an answer that indicates an understanding of the explanation. Because patient compliance is important to achieve the goal of therapy, whether definitive or palliative, education is critical.

Communication.   Communication with patients and family members is essential. Details related to daily treatments, appointment times, and the length of treatment require initial education followed by frequent reinforcement. Communication is almost continuous throughout the day. As related to the patient, the scheduling of daily treatments and other planning times throughout the course of therapy requires reinforcement. Also of concern to patients is the management of the other commitments in their lives. Radiation therapists need to be sensitive and responsive to the demands placed on the patient by competing forces. For example, the scheduling of a simulation appointment for off-cord boosts and subsequent patient notification should be done in advance. In this way the patient is given the opportunity to determine the best way to keep this appointment. If a problem arises, enough time should exist for the therapist and patient to collaborate in a positive manner on the way to work through the patient's special needs and concerns.

Assessment.   Assessment is the process of evaluating a patient's condition. With lung cancer therapy, as with other types of treatment, the condition of a patient's skin should be assessed before daily treatment is given. Ongoing monitoring of dermatitis and erythema and appropriate skin care is necessary to prevent skin breakdown. If the skin is blistered, cracked or open, and oozing, treatment should be withheld until a physician's medical opinion is obtained.

A nutritional evaluation of the ability to swallow solid foods, liquids, and medications should be done to determine whether dietary counseling or medical intervention is required. Adequate fluid intake is particularly important to prevent dehydration because patients may reduce or stop their fluid intake as a result of the discomfort associated with esophagitis.

The status of blood counts should be reviewed. White blood cell counts of 2000/mm^3 or less and platelets of 50,000/mm^3 or less should not be treated without a written order. Patients receiving chemotherapy must be monitored closely.

Changes in a patient's condition can be observed during therapy. As described previously, lung cancer metastasizes to the central nervous system and skeletal system. Clinically, evidence of brain metastasis may be observed with personality changes, headaches, and visual disturbances. With spinal metastases, patients may complain of severe neck and/or back pain and they may describe bowel and/or bladder dysfunctions such as incontinence. In addition, patients may experience leg and/or motor weakness that the therapist may observe as an unsteady gait or limp. Symptoms related to pleural or pericardial effusion include dyspnea, increased respiratory effort, chest pain, a change in a cough, or a fever.[23] Such observations must be reported to the radiation oncologist for medical evaluation.

Medical problems unrelated to lung cancer and radiation therapy occur. If a patient has symptoms or describes a problem with which a therapist is unfamiliar, the therapist should refer the patient to the radiation oncologist. For cardiac or respiratory arrest, therapists should respond appropriately. Knowledge of living wills is important. In particular, if a patient having a cardiac arrest has a do not resuscitate (DNR) or similar order, that request should be honored.

Accessory medical equipment. Accessory medical equipment used with lung cancer may include oxygen tanks, respirators, and intravenous (IV) bottles. This equipment must be maneuvered cautiously to avoid collision hazards. Oxygen tanks must be maneuvered close to the treatment tables, and the catheter must be kept free from table and gantry motions. IV bottles should remain above a patient's head to allow the fluid to move with gravity and prevent backflow or clotting. Because fluid moves from areas of high pressure to low pressure, the IV fluid flows from the bottle above the head (high pressure) into the vein (low pressure). When the bottle is placed at a level below the head, the pressure gradient changes and blood flows into the IV tubing because the pressure in the vein is greater than the bottle pressure. With chest tubes, the bottle must remain below the patient. The pressure in the chest cavity is greater than the pressure in the bottle. Because of this pressure difference, the fluid flows from higher pressure (chest) to lower pressure (bottle). When the table is raised, the bottle should not be placed on the table because the pressure gradient change forces the fluid from the bottle into the chest. Caution must be observed to ensure that the attached lines are long enough to reach to adjacent stretchers and/or poles.

Patients with superior vena cava syndrome are transported to the treatment units on stretchers with respirators, oxygen tanks, IV lines, and cardiac and other monitoring equipment. A team approach is needed to safely move the patient and accessory equipment to and from the treatment table.

Case Studies

Case I

A 61-year-old woman had increasingly severe right-arm pain and hypersensitivity for approximately 2 years. She complained of sharp pains that radiated down the arm to the hand. She also described numbness in the fingers and episodes of arm weakness. She had a long smoking history of approximately 40 years. During the past 3 years, she smoked approximately two packs per day.

A chest radiograph demonstrated an ill-defined density in the apex of the right lung. A CT scan demonstrated a right apical mass with destruction of the second rib posteriorly and extension into the muscular tissues of the posterior thoracic wall. An MRI scan demonstrated right paraspinal disease at T1, T2, and T3. A percutaneous, CT-directed needle biopsy was done, and histologic evaluation revealed a mixed adenocarcinoma and squamous cell carcinoma consistent with bronchogenic carcinoma.

The patient consulted a surgeon, who felt the lesion was resectable and advised that she receive preoperative radiation therapy. A second surgical opinion was more doubtful about the resectability of the tumor, even after radiation therapy, and recommended that the patient be treated with definitive radiation therapy only.

A course of anticipated preoperative radiation therapy began with anterior and posterior parallel-opposed-shaped portals measuring 18.5 × 15 cm on the 4-MV linear accelerator (Figs. 29-14 and 29-15). A conventional fraction pattern of 180 cGy each day was used. Shrinking fields were used, and at 3780 cGy the field size was reduced to 13.5 × 9 cm through the use of an isocentric technique. Treatment to the right upper medi-

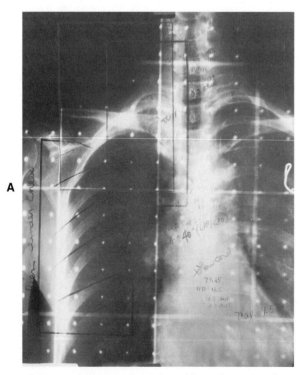
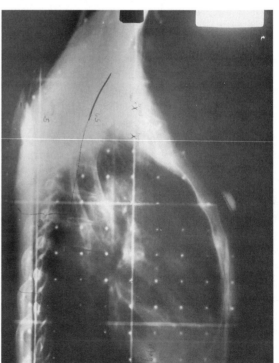

Figure 29-14. Anterior **(A)** and lateral **(B)** simulation films with planning information for blocks, measurements, and boost fields.

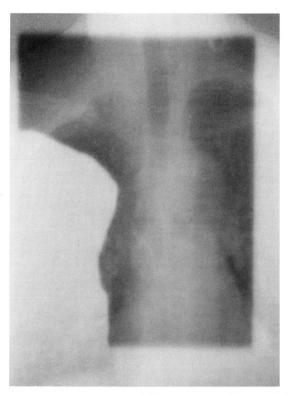

Figure 29-15. Anterior portal film for 18.5 × 15 cm fields treated to 3780 cGy.

astinum, apex of the right lung, and supraclavicular region continued to a dose of 5544 cGy (Fig. 29-16).

A repeat MRI scan failed to reveal significant tumor resolution in the paravertebral region. Therefore surgical intervention was not recommended. The radiation volumes were reduced again, and radiation to the tumor was boosted through the use of 13.5 × 6 cm oblique fields to 7358 cGy (Fig. 29-17).

The patient tolerated the course of radiation therapy satisfactorily, with increasing weight and stable blood counts. During the initial portion of therapy, she complained of minimal dysphagia and later of mild pruritus of the skin secondary to a dry skin reaction. She also noted complete resolution of the shoulder and arm pain, with cessation of the need for analgesics and improved strength in the right arm.

Case II

A 52-year-old man had a routine chest x-ray examination that revealed a right hilar mass. A CT scan of the chest revealed a 3-cm mass in the posterior aspect of the right upper lobe and a soft tissue mass surrounding the right mainstem bronchus with narrowing (see Fig. 29-3). Significant adenopathy was present in the middle mediastinum, the anterior mediastinum anterior to the aortic arch, the aortic pulmonary window, the subcarinal region, and the right hilum. A bronchoscopy demonstrated diffuse submucosal tumor involvement of the right mainstem bronchus with associated narrowing. Bronchial brushings were positive for poorly differentiated large cell carcinoma. Because of complaints of headaches, a CT scan was done that was negative for metastasis.

A

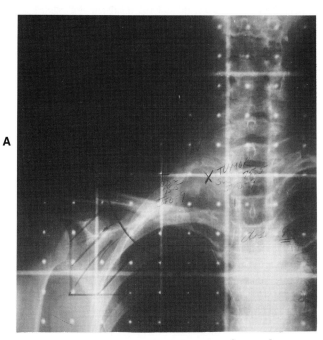

B

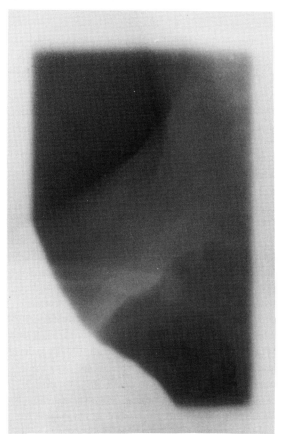

Figure 29-16. Simulation **(A)** and portal **(B)** films for 13.5 × 9 cm right upper lobe fields treated to 5544 cGy.

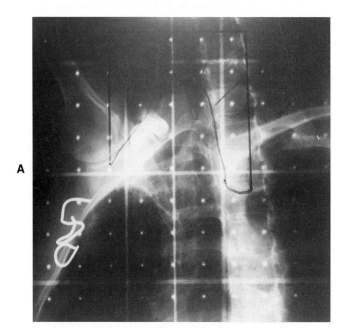
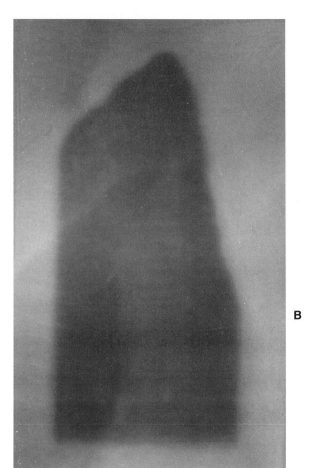

Figure 29-17. Simulation **(A)** and portal **(B)** films for 13.5 × 6 cm oblique boost fields treated to 7358 cGy.

He described shortness of breath and wheezing when lying flat, and his best position was on his left side. He had a 7-lb weight loss over the past few months. His medical history was significant for hypertension and congestive heart failure as a result of a cardiomyopathy of unknown etiology diagnosed 11 years ago. His last episode of heart failure was 1 year ago. He had a significant smoking history of one to two packs per day for 25 years, but he quit 10 years ago. He was staged T1 N3 M0, with poorly differentiated large cell carcinoma. His tumor was surgically unresectable.

The plan was to start chemotherapy for three cycles and follow with radiation therapy.[32,39] He began radiation therapy on the week after the last cycle of chemotherapy. The long-term risks because of his cardiomyopathy were explained. These risks included heart damage possibly leading to myocardial infarction, pericardial effusion, and arrhythmia. The total dose planned was 6000 cGy through the use of conventional fractionation, with two dose evaluation points at 3600 and 5000 cGy to the carina. The initial fields were parallel-opposed, 19.5 × 15.5 cm with alloys, and 4 MV. An 80 cm SSD was used (Fig. 29-18). At 3600 cGy to the carina the fields were changed to a three-field isocentric technique consisting of two obliques with wedges, shielding blocks, and an open field (right posterior oblique, left anterior oblique, and right anterior oblique) (Figs. 29-19 and 29-20). After eight treatments in this manner, the fields were changed again at 5040 cGy. The tumor was boosted to a total dose of 5940 cGy through the use of 11 × 6.5 cm parallel-opposed field (AP/PA)

(Figs. 29-21 and 29-22). The treatment was given in 33 fractions over 46 days. The patient had a significant loss of appetite and esophagitis, which were treated with oral megestrol (Megace) and viscous lidocaine (Xylocaine), respectively. A local skin reaction occurred in the treated field, and the patient was given routine skin care instructions.

Review Questions

Essay

1. Describe three criteria related to an individual's tobacco exposure that appear to increase the risk of developing lung cancer.
2. What are three variables that appear to affect significantly the prognosis of patients with lung cancer?
3. Name the two groups of lymphatics that are primarily responsible for the regional spread of bronchogenic carcinoma.
4. With conventional fractionation, what is the commonly accepted definitive dose range for localized bronchogenic carcinomas?

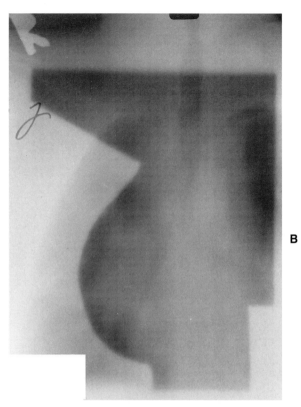

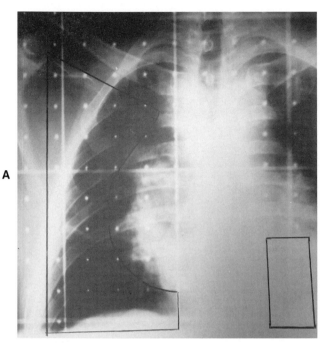

Figure 29-18. Anterior simulation **(A)** and portal **(B)** films for 19.5 × 15.5 cm fields treated to 3600 cGy.

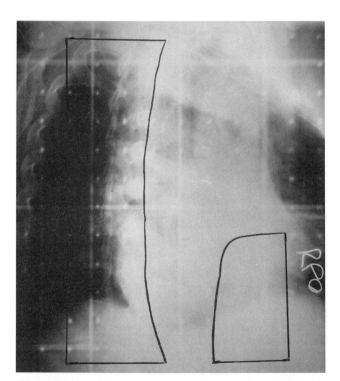

Figure 29-19. Oblique simulation film of a three-field technique treated to 5040 cGy.

5. List at least three common acute side effects a patient may experience during the course of treatment.

Multiple Choice

6. Microscopically, diffusion of oxygen and carbon dioxide takes place at which of the following
   a. Bifurcation of the trachea
   b. Right and left primary bronchi
   c. Bronchiolar ducts
   d. Alveolar-capillary membranes
7. Symptoms associated with local disease include which of the following?
   I. Hemoptysis
   II. Dyspnea
   III. Orthopnea
   a. I only
   b. II only
   c. I and II only
   d. I, II, and III
8. Symptoms associated with regional disease include which of the following?
   I. Dysphagia
   II. Superior vena cava syndrome
   III. Orthopnea

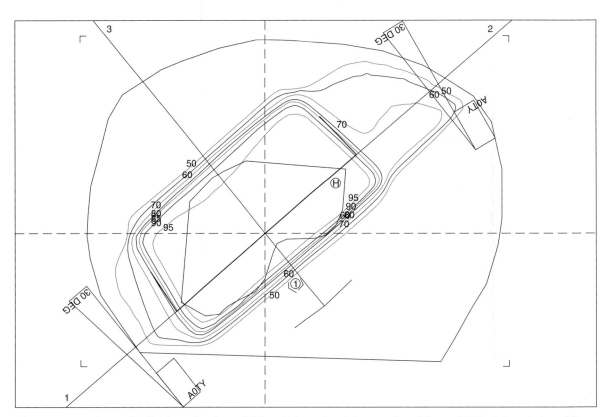

Figure 29-20. Dose distribution of a three-field technique for right anterior oblique (RPO), left anterior oblique (LAO) and right anterior oblique (RAO) fields.

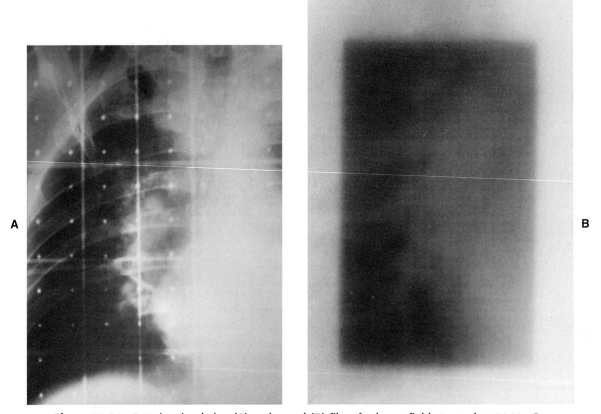

Figure 29-21. Anterior simulation **(A)** and portal **(B)** films for boost fields treated to 5940 cGy.

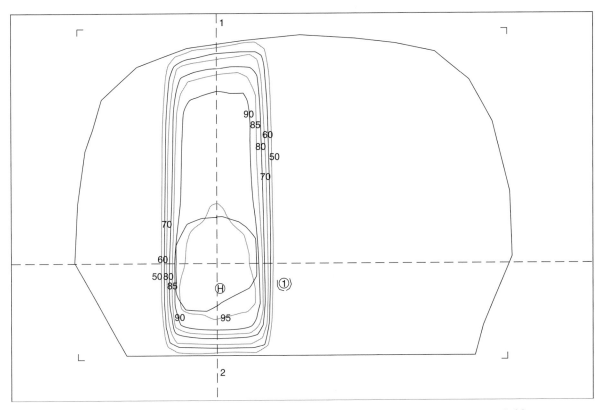

Figure 29-22. Dose distribution of parallel-opposed boost fields for 11 × 6.5 cm fields.

a. I only
b. II only
c. I and II only
d. I, II, and III

9. In what part of the lung are primary squamous cell carcinomas usually found?
   a. Superiorly
   b. Centrally
   c. Laterally
   d. Peripherally

10. Critical structures frequently located in the treatment fields for lung cancer include which of the following?
    a. Normal lung and trachea
    b. Esophagus and trachea
    c. Spinal cord and heart
    d. Heart and esophagus

Questions to Ponder

1. Discuss reasons that the incidence of lung cancer is rising.
2. Compare and contrast the various issues related to radiosensitivity and radiocurability of lung cancer.
3. What are common signs and symptoms of bronchogenic carcinomas? What are uncommon signs and symptoms?
4. Discuss the nonrespiratory signs and symptoms of lung cancer (i.e., neurologic findings).
5. Analyze the anatomic considerations in treatment field design.

REFERENCES

1. Bauer M, et al: Prognostic factors in cancer of the lung. In Cox JD, editor: *Syllabus: a categorical course in radiation therapy: lung cancer,* Oak Brook, Ill, 1985, Radiological Society of North America.
2. Baum GL, Wolinski E: *Textbook of pulmonary diseases,* ed 5, New York, 1994, Little, Brown and Co.
3. Beahrs OH, et al: *AJCC Manual for staging of cancer,* ed 5, Philadelphia, 1997, JB Lippincott.
4. Bentel GC, Nelson CE, Noell KT: *Treatment planning and dose calculation in radiation oncology,* ed 4, New York, 1989, Pergamon Press.
5. Choy H, MacCrae RL Irinotecan in combined modality therapy for locally advanced non-small cell lung cancer, *Oncology* 15:31-36, 2001.
6. Chung CK, et al: Evaluation of adjuvant postoperative radiotherapy for lung cancer, *Int J Radiat Oncol Biol Phys* 8:1877-1880, 1982.
7. Clark R, Idh DC: Small-cell lung cancer treatment progress and prospects, *Oncology* 12:647-658, 1998.
8. Cohen MH: Signs and symptoms of bronchogenic carcinoma. In Straus MJ, editor: *Lung cancer clinical diagnosis and treatment,* New York, 1977, Grune & Stratton.
9. Cox JD and Ang KK editors: *Radiation oncology: rationale, technique, results,* ed 8, St. Louis, 2003, Mosby.
10. Curran WJ Jr: Combined modality therapy for limited stage small cell lung cancer, *Semin Oncol* 28:1422, 2001.
11. DeVita V, Hellman S, Rosenberg S, editors: *Principles and practice of oncology,* ed 6, Philadelphia, 2001, JB Lippincott.

12. Dillman RO, et al: A randomized trial of induction chemotherapy plus high dose radiation vs. radiation alone in stage III non-small cell lung cancer, *N Engl J Med* 323:940-945, 1999.

13. Eisert DR, Cox JD, Komaki R: Irradiation for bronchial carcinoma: reasons for failure. I. Analysis as a function of dose-time-fractionations, *Cancer* 37:2655-2670, 1976.

14. Emami B, et al: Phase I/II study of treatment of locally advanced (T3/T4) non-oat cell lung cancer with high dose radiotherapy (rapid fractionation): radiation therapy oncology group study, *Int J Radiat Oncol Biol Phys* 15:1021-1025, 1988.

15. Erozan YS, Frost JK: Cytopathological diagnosis of lung cancer, *Semin Oncol* 1:191-198, 1974.

16. Fishman AP: *Pulmonary diseases and disorders,* ed 2, New York, 1988, McGraw-Hill.

17. Fletcher GH, editor: *Textbook of radiotherapy,* ed 3, Philadelphia, 1980, Lea & Febiger.

18. Gazdar AF: Pathology's impact on lung cancer management, *Contemp Oncol* 3(11):22-31, 1993.

19. Ginsberg RJ: Multi-modality treatment of resectable non-small lung cancer, *Clin Lung Cancer* 1(3):194-200, 2000.

20. Gordon GS, Vokes EEL: Chemoradiation for locally advanced unresectable non-small carcinoma of the lung, *Oncology* 13:1075-1084, 1999.

21. Green N, et al: Postresection irradiation for primary lung cancer, *Radiology* 116:405-407, 1975.

22. Greenlee RT, Hill-Harmon MB, Thun M: Cancer statistics 2001, *CA Cancer J Clin* 51:1, 2001.

23. Groenwald SL, et al: *Manifestations of cancer and cancer treatment,* Boston, 1992, Jones & Bartlett.

24. Haagensen CD, et al: *The lymphatics in cancer,* Philadelphia, 1972, WB Saunders.

25. Hall TC, editor: Paraneoplastic syndromes, *Ann N Y Acad Sci* 230:367-377, 1974.

26. Kahn FM: *The physics of radiation therapy,* ed 2, Baltimore, 1994, Williams & Wilkins.

27. Karnofsky DA, Burchenal JH: The clinical evaluation of chemotherapeutic agents in cancer. In Macleod CM, editor: *Evaluation of chemotherapeutic agents,* New York, 1949, Columbia University Press.

28. Komaki R: Preoperative radiation therapy for superior sulcus lesions, *Chest Surg Clin North Am* 1:13-35, 1991.

29. Komaki R, Garden AS, Cundiff JH: Endobronchial radiotherapy. In Roth HA, Cox JD, Hong WK, editors: *Advances in diagnosis and therapy of lung cancer,* Cambridge, Mass, 1993, Blackwell.

30. Levitt SH, Kahn FM, Potish RA: *Levitt and Tapley's technological basis of radiation therapy practical clinical applications,* ed 2, Philadelphia, 1992, Lea & Febiger.

31. Mah K, van Dyk J: On the impact of tissue inhomogeneity corrections in clinical thoracic radiation therapy, *Int J Radiat Oncol Biol Phys* 21:1257-1267, 1991.

32. Mantravadi RVP, et al: Unresectable non-oat cell carcinoma of the lung: definitive radiation therapy, *Radiology* 172:851-855, 1989.

33. Marcus RB, Million RR: The incidence of myelitis after irradiation of the cervical spinal cord, *Int J Radiat Oncol Biol Phys* 19:3-8, 1990.

34. Mew D, Pass H: Malignant mesotheliomas: a clinical challenge, *Contemp Oncol* 3(12):50-67, 1993.

35. Murray N: Small-cell lung cancer at the millennium: radiotherapy innovations improve survival while new chemotherapy treatments remain unproven, *Clin Lung Cancer* 1(3):181-190, 2000.

36. Pancoast HK: Superior pulmonary sulcus tumor, *JAMA* 99:17, 1932.

37. Patz EF Jr, Erasmus J: Positron emission tomography imaging in lung cancer, *Clin Lung Cancer* 1:42-48, 1999.

38. Perez CA, Brady LW, editors: *Principles and practice of radiation oncology,* ed 3, Philadelphia, 1998, JB Lippincott.

39. Rapp E, et al: Chemotherapy can prolong survival in patients with advanced non-small-cell lung cancer: report of a Canadian multicenter randomized trial, *J Clin Oncol* 6:633-641, 1988.

40. Richardson RH, et al: The use of fiberoptic bronchoscopy and brush biopsy in the diagnosis of suspected pulmonary malignancy, *Am Rev Respir Dis* 109:63-66, 1974.

41. Rigler LG: The earliest roentgenographic signs of carcinoma of the lung, *JAMA* 195:655, 1966.

42. Rubin P, editor: *Radiation biology and radiation pathology syllabus,* Reston, Va, 1975, American College of Radiology.

43. Rubin P, Casarett GW: *Clinical radiation pathology,* Philadelphia, 1968, WB Saunders.

44. Rubin P editor, Williams J asst. editor: *Clinical oncology a multidisciplinary approach for physicians and students,* ed 8, Philadelphia, 2001, WB Saunders.

45. Seydel HG, et al: Hyperfractionation in the radiation therapy of unresectable non-oat cell carcinoma of the lung: preliminary report of a RTOG pilot study, *Int J Radiat Oncol Biol Phys* 11:1841-1847, 1985.

46. Siegfried JM: Lung cancer screening in high risk populations, *Clin Lung Cancer* 1(2):100-106, 1999.

47. Stanton R, Stinson D: *Applied physics for radiation oncology,* Madison, Wisc, 1996, Medical Physics Publishing.

48. Strauss GM: Potential treatment options for early stage non-small cell lung cancer patients, clinical decision-making in non-small cell lung cancer, *Cancer* 48:6-9, 1998.

49. Tazelaar HD: Screening, pathologic classification, prognostic factors and staging: clinical decision-making in non-small lung cancer, *Cancer* 48:3-6, 1998.

50. Tortora GJ, Grabowski SR: *Principles of anatomy and physiology,* ed 9, New York, 2001, HarperCollins College Publishers.

51. World Health Organization: *International histologic classification of tumors,* no. 1-20, Geneva, 1978, World Health Organization.

52. Wynder EL, Hoffmann D: *Tobacco and tobacco smoke: studies in experimental carcinogenesis,* New York, 1967, Academic Press.

BIBLIOGRAPHY

American Cancer Society: *Cancer facts and figures 2001,* Atlanta, 2001, American Cancer Society.

Nakhashi H, et al: Results of surgical treatment of patients with T3 non-small cell lung cancer, *Ann Thorac Surg* 46:178-181, 1988.

Schultheiss TE: Spinal cord radiation "tolerance": doctrine versus data, *Int J Radiat Oncol Biol Phys* 19:219-221, 1990.

Valley JF, Mirimanoff RO: Comparison of treatment techniques for lung cancer, *Radiother Oncol* 28:168-173, 1993.

Head and Neck Cancer

Ronnie Lozano

Outline

Key Terms

PERSPECTIVE

The management of head and neck malignancies requires a multidisciplinary team approach, with an understanding that this disease can produce significant morbidity and survival cannot be measured only in terms of mortality.[3] Reducing the deformity, maintaining the reduction, and restoring the function are essential to the management of head and neck cancer. The cure of cancer, with preservation of structure, function, and esthetics, has become more evident with advances in modern radiation oncology, based on technologic gains in radiation physics and insights into radiation biology and pathophysiology.[14] From a structural standpoint, mutilation is no longer an acceptable condition of cure because of its psychosocial stresses. Treatment that causes the permanent loss of vision, smell, taste, or hearing should be evaluated concerning its effect on quality of life and survival. Maintaining food paths and airways is vital, but the treatment decision should also preserve the patient's ability to interact as a human. The loss of the ability to speak results in significant changes in the patient's lifestyle, it can significantly alter the patient's quality of life. With early detection techniques, head and neck cancers involving the larynx and other upper aerodigestive sites treated by radiation therapy allow for preservation of voice and swallowing. With the continued improvements in imaging using computed tomography (CT) and magnetic resonance imaging (MRI) and the increasing accuracy of three-dimensional (3D) conformal treatment (including intensity-modulated radiation therapy [IMRT]) tumors involving the head and neck area can be eliminated with preservation of vision and minimal neurologic impairment.[14]

The effective management of patients with head and neck

cancer involves the close cooperation of the radiation oncologists, medical oncologists, dentists, maxillofacial prosthodontists, nutritionists, head and neck surgeons, neurosurgeons, plastic surgeons, oral surgeons, pathologists, oncology nurses, radiologists, social workers, radiation therapists, speech therapists, pain service, and neurology service without forgetting the patient's involvement. The patient may decide to select a treatment approach that offers a slightly lower probability of survival in return for a better functional or cosmetic result if the treatment is successful.[14] This is an important reason to bring the patient into the decision-making process regarding treatment. Despite many major advances, the treatment of locoregional recurrence remains a major challenge as indicated by low success rates for salvage therapy. Most patients with locoregional recurrence develop progressive disease resulting in a high degree of suffering.[10]

NATURAL HISTORY OF THE DISEASE

Head and neck cancer has been marked in American history by public accounts and newspaper articles describing the extensive suffering and death of Ulysses S. Grant in the late 1800s. This event significantly added to the public fears of cancers and the useless treatments of that era. Today, only one third of affected patients present at an early disease stage. An estimated two thirds of patients present with locally advanced disease, either at the primary site or in the cervical lymph nodes, stages III and IV.[9] The lungs are the most common site of distant metastasis. Other sites of distant metastasis include the mediastinal lymph nodes, liver, brain, and bones. The incidence of distant metastasis is greatest with tumors of the nasopharynx and hypopharynx. A direct correlation appears to exist between the bulk of cervical nodal disease and the development of distant metastasis. Atypical metastatic spread may occur in patients who have had a radical neck dissection or previous radiation therapy. These patients are at high risk of developing atypical metastasis to the neck and to subcutaneous and cutaneous sites. Tumors may also spread along the nerves. Direct nerve invasion may occur from tumors in the affected area. Nerve routes are an important consideration in treatment planning. High-grade parotid tumors are known to involve the facial nerve and to cause paralysis.[10] The *standard* treatment for these patients is either surgery with preoperative or, more commonly, postoperative radiation therapy or is primary radiation therapy followed by surgery. A combination of chemotherapy and radiation therapy is used in patients with inoperable or unresectable (stage III and IV) disease in an attempt to increase cure rates over radiation therapy alone. The advantage of the treatment combinations is the preservation of cosmesis and function that result compared with radical surgeries such as the laryngopharyngectomy.[9]

Epidemiology

Head and neck cancers account for approximately 5% of the overall incidence of cancer in the United States and 2% of all cancer deaths.[10] The American Cancer Society estimated approximately 39,400 new cases in 2003 and approximately 11,200 deaths yearly in the country. Tumors of the upper aerodigestive tract occur mostly in men from the age of 50 continuing through their 60s; however, recent evidence suggests that these tumors are becoming more common in young people younger than 40.[5] The incidence rate of tongue and oral cavity cancers in females is on the rise, notably because more women are smoking. Approximately half of all squamous cell carcinomas of the upper aerodigestive tract occur in the oral cavity. Cancers of the nasopharynx and hypopharynx are extremely common in Southeast Asia, Hong Kong, and southern China. A decreased incidence of nasopharyngeal carcinoma (NPC) in successive generations of Chinese born in America suggests an etiologic role for environmental factors.[9] Tumors of the oral cavity and base of tongue are more common in India, which also indicates a strong environmental and cultural influence in the prevalence of this type of disease. In the Indian subcontinent, oral SCC may account for 50% of all cancers. The high incidence is owed to the chewing of *pan,* a mixture of betel leaf, lime, catechu, and areca nut.[5,14] The alkaloids released when the nut is chewed provoke excessive and abnormal synthesis of collagen by cultured fibroblasts causing submucous fibrosis. Environmental and genetic predisposition results in nasopharynx cancer being the most common tumor in the Kwantung province of southern China. Recurrences usually occur within the first 2 years and rarely after 4 years, establishing a 5-year follow-up for most sites. Generally, for most sites, 5-year survival for stage I is 75% to 90%; for stage II, survival is 40% to 70%; for stage III, survival is 20% to 50%; and for stage IV, 10% to 30%. For all stages, the 5-year survival rate for oral cavity and pharynx is 55% in whites and 34% in blacks. Most 5-year survivors will be alive at 10 years. In whites, the 5-year survival rate improved from 43% in the period 1960 to 1963 to 55% in the period 1974 to 1976. Little change has occurred from then until the most recent surveillance period of 1986 to 1993. The adjusted years of life lost decreased from 23.1 in 1970 to 19.9 in 1985. Evidence suggests that improved locoregional control decreases dissemination and metastases reflecting an improved overall survival.[14]

Etiology and Predisposing Factors

The large number of disease processes that can affect the head and neck region can have a multitude of histologic appearances. This is a reflection of the many specialized tissues present and at risk for specific diseases. This chapter refers to those tumors of an epithelial character arising from the mucosal lining of the aerodigestive tract. The most common sites of the aerodigestive tract affected are the oral cavity, pharynx, paranasal sinuses, larynx, thyroid gland, and salivary glands. Risk factors for head and neck cancer include tobacco and alcohol use, ultraviolet (UV) light exposure, viral infection, and environmental exposures.

Smoking. Tobacco was first introduced to western civilization by the Spanish explorers of America in the early sixteenth century. At first, it was simply smoked in pipes, but, as it became more popular, it was also chewed and snuffed. Cigarettes were first made in Spain in the midseventeenth century, and in the twentieth century they became the most popular form of the tobacco habit. The incidence of head and neck cancers correlates most closely with the use of tobacco. Head and neck tumors occur six times more often among cigarette smokers than nonsmokers. The mortality from laryngeal cancer appears to rise with increased cigarette consumption. For the heaviest smokers, death from laryngeal cancer is 20 times more likely than for nonsmokers.[12] Pipe and cigar smoking results in extensive intraoral **keratosis.** Unfiltered cigarettes cause lip carcinoma, especially when habitually held in the same place.[5] The use of unfiltered cigarettes or dark, air-cured tobacco is associated with further increases in risk.[12] Cigar smoking is often misperceived as posing a lesser health risk than cigarette smoking based on the decreased incidence of cancers associated with smoking (larynx, lung cancer). The incidence of cancer is actually higher at other sites where pooling of saliva and associated carcinogens tend to occur (i.e., the oropharynx, esophagus).[12] Although production and consumption of pipe tobacco has decreased over the recent years, there has been an increase in cigars and cigarillos.[15]

Alcohol. Alcohol consumption alone is a risk factor for the development of pharyngeal and laryngeal tumors.[12] Pure ethanol has never been shown to be carcinogenic to oral tissues, but three etiologic factors have been identified:

1. Liver damage and secondary nutritional deficiencies (i.e., B complex vitamins that increase the susceptibility of oral mucosal to environmental carcinogens).
2. Alcohol may directly damage mucosa and make it more permeable.
3. Impurities present in alcoholic beverages may be associated with the disease process.[5]

Smoking, tobacco, and alcohol. This combination has been regarded as the most important risk factor for this disease. Alcohol seems to have a synergistic effect on the carcinogenic potential of tobacco. This combination facilitates the pathogenic effects of the thousands of substances of the combustion mainstream of a cigarette. These include tars (the basis for the tobacco taste) or aromatic hydrocarbons that contain the most potent carcinogens. Evidence suggests that ethanol suppresses the efficiency of deoxyribonucleic acid (DNA) repair after exposure to nitrosamine compounds.[10] Nitrosamines (N'nitrosonornicotine) has been identified as the most potent noncombustible product in snuff and chewing tobacco that possess carcinogenic activity.[15]

Other forms of tobacco. There is a higher frequency of premalignant and malignant oral lesions in young Americans because of the increasing use of smokeless tobacco.[14] Smokeless tobacco users frequently develop premalignant lesions, such as oral **leukoplakia** (thick, white patches on the mucous membrane that are slightly raised), at the site where the tobacco quid rests against the mucosa. Over time, these lesions may progress to invasive carcinomas.[12] Tobacco may clearly induce a benign clinical condition involving the oral mucosa in the form of a red or white lesion that progresses to a malignant tumor.[15] Other carcinogens are found in smaller quantities in addition to the nitrosamines mentioned previously (hydrocarbons and polonium). The nitrosamine levels far exceed those permitted in food preservatives by the Food and Drug Administration. Nicotine levels are high and serve as a potent factor in habituation, addiction, and hypertension. The most common conditions found with the use of smokeless tobacco are gingival recession, hyperkeratosis, and staining. The risk of oral epithelial dysplasia or carcinoma increases with long-term use.[15]

UV light. Exposure to UV is a risk factor for the development of lip cancer. At least 33% of lip cancer patients have outdoor occupations.

Occupational exposures. Occupations associated with greater risk include nickel refining (laryngeal cancer), furniture and woodworking (cancers of the nasal cavity and paranasal sinuses), and steel and textile workers (oral cancer).[10]

Radiation exposure. Exposure, particularly in childhood, is implicated in the development of thyroid cancer and salivary gland tumors.[14]

Viruses. Increasing evidence suggests a role for viruses in the development of head and neck cancer. Nasopharyngeal cancer has been linked to the Epstein Barr virus (one of 8 herpes viruses that infect human tissue) and viral DNA has been identified in nasopharyngeal tissue.[10] Epstein-Barr virus has been associated with NPC in all races.[14] Herpes simplex virus-1 (HSV-1) is the well-known cause of primary herpetic stomatitis and of recurrent herpes labialis (cold sores). The virus remains latent in the trigeminal or other sensory ganglion for an entire lifetime. Reactivation occurs to produce recurrent lesions or to be shed asymptomatically in the saliva. The virus has the ability to transform cells to a malignant phenotype under certain conditions. In an experimental situation, the infected cells can become immortal in cell culture and will invade and metastasize if they are injected into an experimental animal. Experiments with hamsters show that if tissue is exposed to low doses of the tobacco carcinogen benzo(a)pyrene and to HSV-1 simultaneously, tumors can be produced.[15] This may have implications for smokers with HSV-1; they may have an increased incidence of oral cancer. Human papillomavirus (HPV) has also been linked to head and neck carcinogenesis.[10] HPV has been found in oral papillomas, in leukoplakia lesions, and in oral carcinomas. Laryngeal papillomatosis and carcinoma of the larynx have been linked with HPV.[14] Evidence is based on animal models; conclusive proof of higher risk linked to viruses requires further research.

Syphilis. Syphilis was implicated in tongue carcinoma in the preantibiotic era. Past reports of patients with oral cancer have indicated positive histories for syphilis; however, little evidence currently supports as association between syphilis and oral cancer.[14,15]

Diet. Dietary factors include nutritional deficiency (vitamin A and E), especially in alcoholics, most prevalent in females.[14] The Plummer-Vinson syndrome (esophageal web, iron deficiency anemia, dysphasia from glossitis) is associated with a high incidence of postcricoid and tongue carcinoma, most prevalent in Europe. Epidemiologic data suggest that fruits, vegetables, and carotenoids may have a preventive role.[10] Evidence suggests that mucosal atrophy, as a result of nutritional deficiencies, leads to an increase in mitotic activity and diminished repair capacity of cells, creating an increased susceptibility to cancer.[5]

Marijuana. Chronic abuse of marijuana has been linked to head and neck cancer, but the degree of risk is unknown.[10,12]

Dentures and poor oral hygiene. Although lacking studies with conclusive evidence, some carcinomas develop in areas covered by or adjacent to a prosthetic appliance. Although the risk is low, chronic denture irritation in addition to other unidentified factors may possibly promote neoplastic activity (Figs. 30-1 and 30-2). The same principle may apply to patients who have poor oral hygiene or jagged teeth or filings that may act as irritants. Denture material per se has not been shown to be carcinogenic.[15]

Genetics. Genetic predisposition to head and neck cancer has been suggested by its sporadic occurrence in young adults and in nonusers of tobacco and alcohol.[10] Studies of human cancer of certain specific types have shown that some families have an increased incidence of cancer, implying a genetic influence. Examples include retinoblastoma in childhood or breast and colon cancers. No such evidence has been presented for oral cancer.[15] Increased susceptibility to environmental carcinogens has been attributed to genetic anomalies. An association with the Bloom syndrome and the Li-Fraumeni syndrome has been implicated in head and neck cancers.[15] It is estimated that squamous cell carcinoma of the

head and neck requires the accumulation of 8 to 11 mutations, and 4 to 7 genetic mutations may be sufficient for the development of salivary gland malignancies.[14]

Prognostic Indicators

In general, the morbidity of treatments increases and the prognosis decreases as the affected area progresses backward from the lips to the hypopharynx, excluding the larynx. Lesions that cross the midline, exhibit **endophytic** growth (invasion of the lamina propria and submucosa), have cranial nerve involvement, have fixed nodes or a fixed lesion in the anatomic compartments, are poorly differentiated, and are nonsquamous cell cancers represent advanced growth and have an unfavorable prognosis.

Anatomy and Physiology

The organs of the head and neck region serve dual purposes in that respiratory and digestive activities take place. For a better appreciation of this complex system, a brief anatomic review is necessary.

The staging and classification of head and neck tumors are based on subsite involvement, which concerns nearly 50% of the patients. Understanding the physiologic relationships of adjacent structures in the head and neck region is of paramount importance. The opening of the nasal cavities into the nasopharynx (Fig. 30-3) provides a natural pathway for tumor spread. During the act of swallowing, the soft palate elevates and prevents food from entering the nasopharynx. Tumors in this location do not allow this activity to occur. An enlargement of the pharyngeal tonsil can obstruct the upper air passage and allow breathing only through the mouth, resulting in the passing of unfiltered, cool, dry air to the lungs. Collectively, the tonsils are bands of lymphoid tissue that provide protection against airway infections and form a barrier between the respiratory tubes (nasopharynx) and

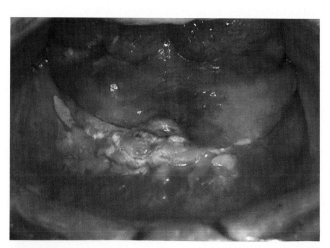

Figure 30-1. Carcinoma developed under a lower denture in anterior alveolar mucosa after a 15-year history of leukoplakia. *(From Silverman S: Oral cancer, ed 4, Hamilton, Ontario, 1998, BC Decker.)*

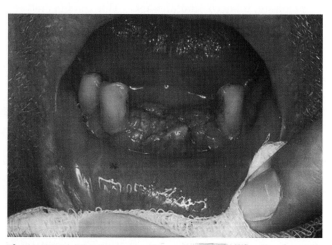

Figure 30-2. Verrucous carcinoma developed under the saddle of a lower partial denture. *(From Silverman S: Oral cancer, ed 4, Hamilton, Ontario, 1998, BC Decker.)*

digestive tubes (oropharynx and hypopharynx). In addition, knowing the location of a cervical vertebral body provides boundary locations of the soft tissue aspects of the head and neck region. The first cervical vertebra (C1) lies at the inferior margin of the nasopharynx, whereas the second and third cervical vertebrae (C2 and C3) are at the level of the oropharynx. The epiglottis is in line with C3, whereas the true vocal cords lie along the fourth cervical vertebra (C4) (Fig. 30-3).

Any tumor of the salivary glands can involve lymphatics, major cranial nerves, and arterial neck blood flow (Fig. 30-4, *A* and *B*). Tumors in this area can cause facial paralysis, nerve pain, and interruption of the neck muscles' blood supply (Figs. 30-5 and 30-6).

As mentioned, tumors can damage the cranial nerves, which control the major senses. The involvement of the cranial nerves leads to signs and symptoms that can point to a

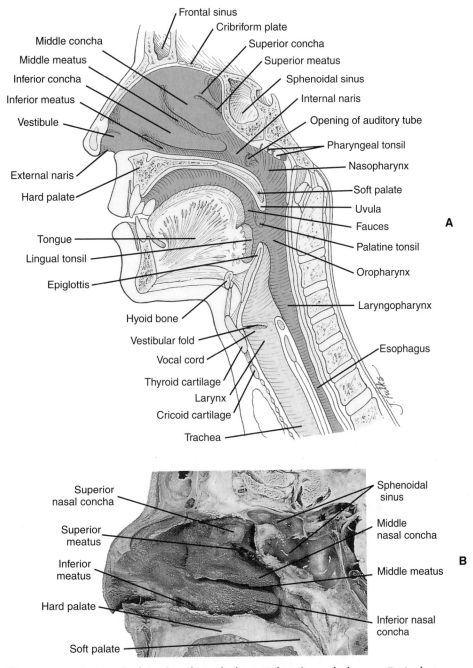

Figure 30-3. A, A sagittal section through the nasal cavity and pharynx. **B,** A photograph of a sagittal section of the nasal cavity. *(From Seeley RR, Stephens TD, Tate P, editors: Essentials of anatomy and physiology, ed 3, St. Louis, 1996, Mosby.)*

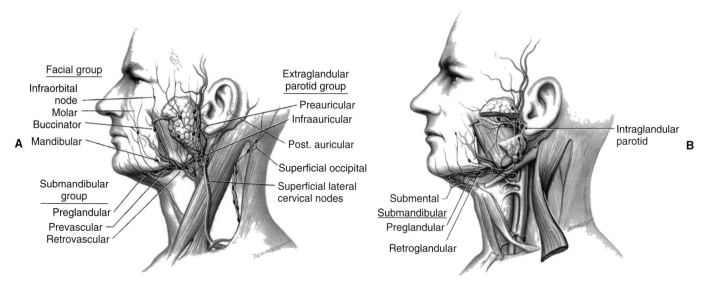

Figure 30-4. **A,** Extraglandular parotid, facial, and superficial submandibular nodes. **B,** The deep submandibular and parotid lymph nodes. *(From Haagensen CD: The lymphatics in cancer, Philadelphia, 1972, WB Saunders.)*

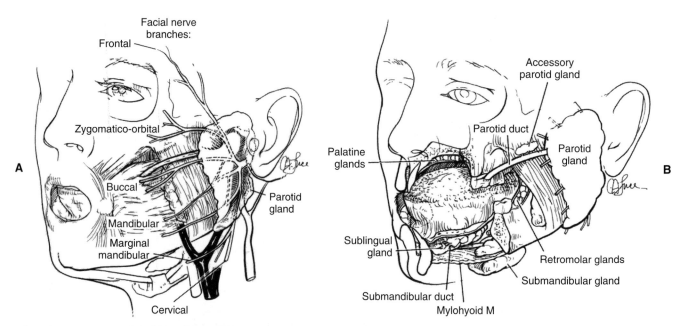

Figure 30-5. Anatomic relationships of the major salivary glands. **A,** Facial nerves. **B,** Portion of mandible removed to show minor salivary glands in the palate. *(From McCarthy JG: Plastic surgery: vol 5, tumors of the head and neck and skin, Philadelphia, 1990, WB Saunders.)*

possible location of a tumor. Table 30-1 lists the 12 cranial nerves and their associated functions.

Lymphatics. The lymphatics of the head and neck and their involvement exhibit a direct correlation to the prognosis. Nearly one third of the body's lymph nodes are located in the head and neck area. The neck may be divided into levels or classifications that group cervical lymph nodes into six levels[14] (Fig. 30-7, *A* and *B*). Fig. 30-7, *A*, depicts the major chains of the head and neck. Some nodes have two names.

For example, the jugulodigastric node is called the subdigastric node, the node of Rouvière is also called the lateral retropharyngeal node, the spinal accessory chain is also called the posterior cervical lymph node, and the mastoid node is also called the retroauricular node.

Because a metastatic cervical lymph node is clinically present in many of the tumors found in the head and neck area, an assessment of node involvement dictates the size of the radiation portal and the treatment plan. For example, in

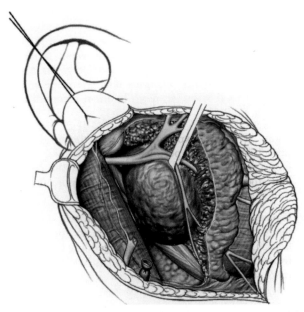

Figure 30-6. Deep lobe parotid tumor. Lesion exposed by retraction of facial nerve. *(From Silver CE, Rubin JS: Atlas of head and neck surgery, ed 2, New York, 1999, Churchill, Livingstone.)*

Table 30-1	Cranial nerves and their functions	
Name (number)	**Function**
Lung	Liver, adrenal glands, bone, and brain
Breast	Lungs, bone, and brain
Stomach	Liver
Anus	Liver and lungs
Bladder	Lungs, bone, and liver
Prostate	Bone, liver, and lungs
Uterine cervix	Lungs, bone, and liver

Figs. 30-8 and 30-9 the **jugulodigastric** group (the group of neck nodes below the mastoid tip) receives nearly all the lymph from the head area and is usually treated, whereas the Rouvière node is included as the minimum target volume for nasopharyngeal cancer. This node is inaccessible to the surgeon, and, because of its proximity to the carotid artery, it can be a problem if not treated.

The port size of the irradiated fields in the head and neck area are large because of the risk of nodal spread. As shown in Fig. 30-9 the inferior cervical nodes are clinically positive for tumor in 6% to 23% of the cases for nasopharyngeal cancer. For this reason the supraclavicular area requires treatment,

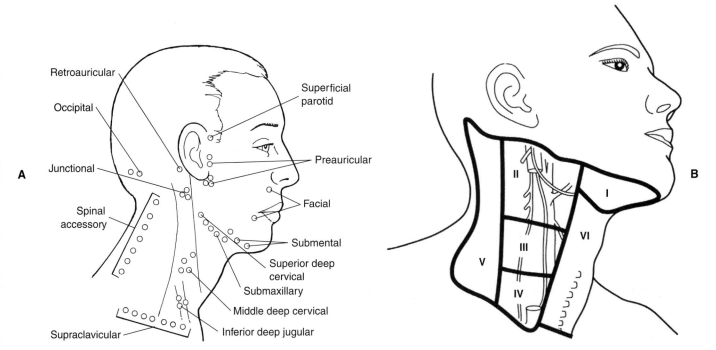

Figure 30-7. A, Lateral view of the head and neck. **B,** Nodal grouping by regions as generally used by the head and neck surgical oncologist. *(A from Moss WT, Cox JD: Radiation oncology: rationale, technique, results, St. Louis, 1987, Mosby; B from Rubin P: Clinical oncology: a multidisciplinary approach for physicians and students, ed 8, Philadelphia, 2001, WB Saunders.)*

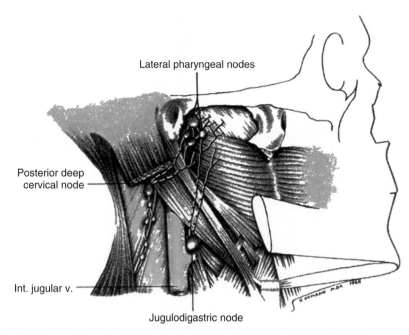

Figure 30-8. Major lymphatic drainage of the nasopharynx. *(From Leibel S: Textbook of radiation, Philadelphia, 1998, WB Saunders.)*

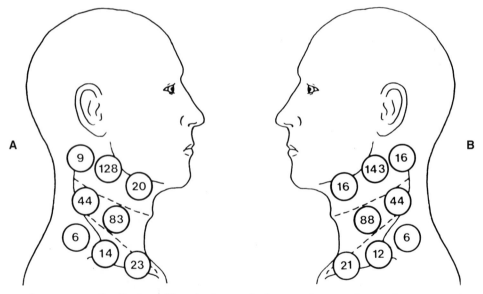

Figure 30-9. Distribution of lymphadenopathy in 204 of 271 patients who presented with enlarged nodes. **A,** Right cervical region. **B,** Left cervical region. *(From Cox JD: Moss' radiation oncology: rationale, technique, results, ed 7, St. Louis, 1994, Mosby.)*

which an anterior port can accomplish. Generally, hematogenous spread below the neck is rare, except in NPC or in cancer of the parotid gland. More than 75% of all head and neck cancers recur locally or regionally above the clavicle.

NPC with known bilateral cervical node involvement has shown a 25% chance of bloodborne distant spread first to the bone and then to the lung. In addition, for non-NPC disease there is a higher risk of the development of a second primary

than distant spread. The normal lymphatic drainage by site is listed in Box 30-1.

Clinical Presentation

Most head and neck cancers are infiltrative lesions found in the epithelial lining. They can be raised or indurated (hard and firm). These growths are sometimes classified as endophytic tumors, which are more aggressive and harder to con-

---

Box 30-1 — **Lymphatic Drainage by Site**

ORAL CAVITY

1. Lips into the submandibular, preauricular, and facial nodes
2. Buccal mucosa into the submaxillary and submental nodes
3. Gingiva into the submaxillary and jugulodigastric nodes
4. Retromolar trigone into the submaxillary and jugulodigastric nodes
5. Hard palate into the submaxillary and upper jugular nodes
6. Floor of mouth into the submaxillary and jugular (middle and upper) nodes
7. Anterior two thirds of the tongue into the submaxillary and upper jugular nodes

OROPHARYNX

1. Base of the tongue into the jugulodigastric, low cervical, and retropharyngeal nodes
2. Tonsillar fossa into the jugulodigastric and submaxillary nodes
3. Soft palate into the jugulodigastric, submaxillary, and spinal accessory nodes
4. Pharyngeal walls into the retropharyngeal nodes, pharyngeal nodes, and jugulodigastric nodes

NASOPHARYNX

1. Retropharyngeal nodes into the superior jugular and posterior cervical nodes

SINUSES

1. Retropharyngeal and superior cervical nodes

LARYNX

1. Glottis—extremely rare nodal involvement
2. Subglottis into the peritracheal and low cervical nodes
3. Supraglottis into the peritracheal, cervical submental, and submaxillary nodes

---

Box 30-2 — **Common Symptoms by Site**

Oral cavity—swelling or an ulcer that fails to heal
Oropharynx—painful swallowing and referred otalgia
Nasopharynx—bloody discharge and difficulty hearing
Larynx—hoarseness and stridor
Hypopharynx—dysphagia and painful neck node
Nose and sinuses—obstruction, discharge, facial pain, diplopia, and local swelling

---

Box 30-3 — **Common Clinical Presentations by Site**

1. A high cervical neck mass often represents metastases from the nasopharynx.
2. Positive subdigastric nodes are often the site of metastases from the oral cavity, oropharynx, or hypopharynx.
3. Positive submandibular triangle nodes arise from the oral cavity.
4. Midcervical neck masses are associated with tumors of the hypopharynx, base of tongue, and larynx.
5. Preauricular nodes frequently arise from tumors found in the salivary glands.

---

trol locally. **Exophytic** tumors are noninvasive neoplasms characterized by raised, elevated borders. Specific signs and symptoms correlate with anatomic sites. Box 30-2 provides a list of the common symptoms by site. A cervical lymph node mass can be present clinically in cancers from any of these sites. In an adult, any enlarged cervical node that persists for 1 week or more should be regarded as suspicious and should be evaluated for a malignancy.

Detection and Diagnosis

Careful examination and inspection of the head and neck via indirect laryngoscopy, palpation, and fiberoptic endoscopy are of paramount importance. A systemic, step-by-step examination of all the anatomic compartments for any suspicious growths or nodes is needed. Nodes that are hard, greater than 1 cm, nontender, nonmobile, and raised probably contain metastatic disease. The number of nodes should also be assessed. The location of neck masses can often suggest the site of the primary tumor. Box 30-3 lists common clinical presentations relative to the origin of the head and neck primary cancers.

Biopsies are performed on all suspicious lesions to determine a precursor benign condition or to evaluate the predominate malignant growth pattern (grading). A fine-needle aspiration biopsy (FNAB) is performed for most neck masses.

Radiographic studies performed routinely include CT, MRI, and x-ray examinations of the skull, sinuses, and soft tissue. For symptomatic patients, barium swallow is recommended, along with a radiograph of the chest and bone scans to rule out metastases. Positron emission tomography (PET) may be useful in locating occult tumor in situations of an unknown primary and in ascertaining tumor recurrence after treatment.

Anti–Epstein-Barr virus antibody titers (immunoglobulin G and immunoglobulin A) are fairly specific for NPC and may aid in the diagnosis of cervical node cancer with unknown primary.

Pathology

More than 80% of head and neck cancers arise from the surface epithelium of the mucosal linings of the upper digestive tract. These cancers are mostly squamous cell carcinomas. Adenocarcinomas are found to a lesser extent in the salivary glands. Squamous cell carcinomas seen in the head and neck region include lymphoepithelioma, spindle cell carcinoma, verrucous carcinoma, and undifferentiated carcinoma. Lymphoepithelioma occurs in places of abundant lymphoid tissue (i.e., the nasopharynx, tonsil, and base of the tongue). Patients with this histologic type have a better cure rate with radiation therapy than patients with squamous cell carcinoma.[6]

Spindle cell carcinoma has a nonneoplastic background and responds to radiation therapy in much the same manner as squamous cell carcinoma. Verrucous carcinoma is most often found in the gingiva and buccal mucosa. This type of carcinoma has an indolent pattern of growth and is associated with chewing tobacco or snuff. Verrucous carcinomas tend to be exophytic, have distinct margins, and look like warts. They are often hyperkeratotic, treated according to their appearance alone, and watched for further growth.

Undifferentiated lymphomas are similar histopathologically to undifferentiated carcinomas and should be treated as carcinomas if doubt exists after microscopic evaluation. Box 30-4 lists some cancer cell types found in the head and neck region. Tumor grading is classified as G-1 (well differentiated), G-2 (moderately well differentiated), or G-3 (poorly differentiated). A variety of nonepithelial malignancies, melanomas, soft tissue sarcomas, and plasmacytomas can also occur in the head and neck region.

Staging

The staging system for head and neck cancers is based mostly on clinical diagnostic information that determines the size, extent, and presence of nodes positive for tumor. The surgical-pathologic classification is crucial for determining the need or type of adjuvant therapy.

In 2002, the American Joint Committee on Cancer (AJCC), in collaboration with the Union Internationale Contre le Cancer, updated the tumor, node, metastasis (TNM) staging system for cancers of the head and neck. Box 30-5 contains a version of the AJCC/TNM classification system by site, nodal status, and the stage groupings.[10] The T system used varies with each anatomic site. Cancers found in the lip, oral cavity, oropharynx, salivary gland, or thyroid gland are size oriented. Designations are as follows:

T1 <2 cm
T2 >2 cm or = 4 cm
T3 >4 cm
T4 >4 cm, with invasion of adjacent structures

The nasopharynx, hypopharynx, larynx, and maxillary antrum are classified according to the involvement of the anatomic subsite by the depth of extension. The N classifications are uniform for all sites, except for the thyroid. The sizes and locations of nodes determine the N designation.

Stage groupings can exhibit a wide spectrum of diseases. Stage IV disease is always distant metastasis. However, in the head and neck region, MO as N2 or N3 with any T disease (which is usually curable) is possible. The TNM classification alone is not adequate for choosing the best method of treatment. The staging workup should include evaluating the primary lesion size, examining the depth of invasion into surrounding anatomic subsites, and mapping and measuring the cervical or at-risk nodal stations. Careful attention is given to the mobility of the nodes. Fixed nodes result in a poor prognosis. Contrast-enhanced CT and MRI scans can define the size and shape of the tumor better than a clinical evaluation. 3D multiplanar imaging has made staging much more precise and accurate for deeply invading disease or in the assessment of inaccessible neck nodes.

Routes of Spread

Physiologically, the head and neck region has distinct anatomic compartments. As a malignant lesion starts to grow, it exhibits a somewhat unique tendency of direct invasion. Figs. 30-10 and 30-11 depict open-mouth views that demonstrate a tumor's expected location of infiltration and thus determine the size of the target volume during irradiation. Fig. 30-12 is a lateral view of the anatomic subdivision of the head that shows the underlying or adjacent structures. (See also Fig. 30-3 for anatomic locations.) Box 30-6 lists areas of the head and neck region and the expected direct spread of a tumor in each area.

PRINCIPLES OF TREATMENT

General Principles

Radiation and surgery are the major curative modalities. The eradication of the disease, maintenance of physiologic function, and preservation of social cosmesis determine the best

---

Box 30-4	Head and Neck Cancer Cell Types

SQUAMOUS CELL CARCINOMA

Lymphoepithelioma
Spindle cell carcinoma
Verrucous carcinoma
Undifferentiated carcinoma
Transitional cell carcinoma
Keratinized carcinoma
Nonkeratinized carcinoma

ADENOCARCINOMA

Malignant mixed carcinoma
Adenocystic carcinoma
Mucoepidermoid carcinoma
Acinic cell carcinoma

Box 30-5	AJCC Staging System for Head and Neck Cancer

PRIMARY TUMOR (T)

(General—for all sites)

TX   No available information on primary tumor

T_0 No evidence of primary tumor

TIS   Carcinoma in situ

ORAL CAVITY AND OROPHARYNX

T_1 Greatest diameter of primary tumor < or = 2 cm

T_2 >2 cm or = 4 cm

T_3 > 4 cm

T_4 Massive tumor, with deep invasion into maxilla, mandible, pterygoid muscles, deep tongue muscle, skin, and soft tissues of neck

HYPOPHARYNX

T_1 Tumor confined to region of origin

T_2 Extension into adjacent region or site, without fixation of hemilarynx

T_3 Extension into adjacent region or site, with fixation of hemilarynx

T_4 Massive tumor invading bone or soft tissues of neck

NASOPHARYNX

T_1 Tumor confined to one site or identified during biopsy only (no tumor visible)

T_2 Involvement of two sites within nasopharynx

T_3 Extension into nasal cavity or oropharynx

T_4 Invasion into skull and/or cranial nerve involvement

LARYNX

Glottic

T_1 Confinement to true vocal cords; normal mobility; includes anterior or posterior commissure

T_2 Supraglottic or subglottic extension; normal or impaired mobility

T_3 Confinement to larynx proper; cord fixation

T_4 Cartilage destruction and/or extension out of larynx

Supraglottic

T_1 Confinement to site of origin; normal mobility

T_2 Extension to glottis or adjacent supraglottic site; normal or impaired mobility

T_3 Confinement to larynx proper; cord fixation and/or extension into hypopharynx or preepiglottic space

T_4 Massive tumor; cartilage destruction and/or extension out of larynx

Subglottic

T_1 Confinement to subglottic region

T_2 Glottic extension; normal or impaired mobility

T_3 Confinement to larynx proper; cord fixation

T_4 Massive tumor; cartilage destruction and/or extension out of larynx

NODAL METASTASIS (N)

NX   Nodes cannot be assessed

N_o No clinically positive nodes

N_1 Single, clinically positive, ipsilateral node; < or = 3 cm

N_{2a} Single, clinically positive, ipsilateral node; >3 or = 6 cm

N_{2b} Multiple, clinically positive, ipsilateral nodes; all < or = 6 cm

N_{3a} Clinically positive, ipsilateral node(s); one > 6 cm

N_{3c} Contralateral, clinically positive node(s) only

DISTANT METASTASIS (M)

MX   Not assessed

M_0 No distant metastases identified

M_1 Distant metastasis present

Site specification

    PUL—pulmonary

    OSS—osseous

    BRA—brain

    LYM—lymph nodes (noncervical)

    MAR—bone marrow

    PLE—pleura

    SKI—skin

    OTH—other

STAGE GROUPING

Stage I $T_1 N_0 M_0$

Stage II $T_2 N_0 M_0$

Stage III $T_3 N_0 M_0,$ $T_1 T_2,$ or $T_3 N_1 M_0$

Stage IV $T_4 N_0$ or $N_1 M_0$

           Any T N_2 or $N_3 M_0$

From Greene, et al: *AJCC cancer staging handbook,* ed 5, Philadelphia, 2002, Springer-Verlag.

modality. The ability to cure and eradicate the disease without severe complications necessitates extremely selective treatment criteria. Radiation therapy is indicated in most head and neck cancers because the tumors located in this region are often inaccessible to the surgeon's knife. The goals of treatment, however, can only be achieved through a multidisciplinary approach involving the many specialists, but the patient often plays an important role. Emphasis is given to age and general condition, comorbidity factors (associated diseases; i.e., emphysema, cardiovascular disease), habits and lifestyle, occupation, and patient's desires. Small primary lesions with nodes negative for tumor are generally treated with one modality (surgery or radiation therapy). Small lesions with involved nodes may need both surgery and radiation therapy for control of neck disease. Large primary lesions (T3 and T4), extensive cervical node disease, or both usually need surgery and irradiation[14] (Fig. 30-13). Follow-up at regular intervals to detect early recurrence,

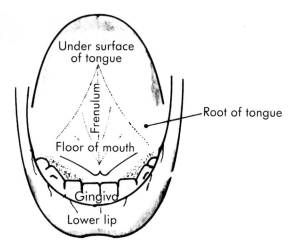

Figure 30-10. A front open-mouth view of the floor of the mouth with the tongue raised. *(From Cox JD: Moss' radiation oncology: rationale, technique, results, ed 7, St. Louis, 1994, Mosby.)*

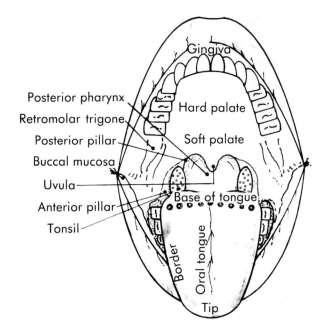

Figure 30-11. A front open-mouth view of the oral cavity. *(From Cox JD: Moss' radiation oncology: rationale, technique, results, ed 7, St. Louis, 1994, Mosby.)*

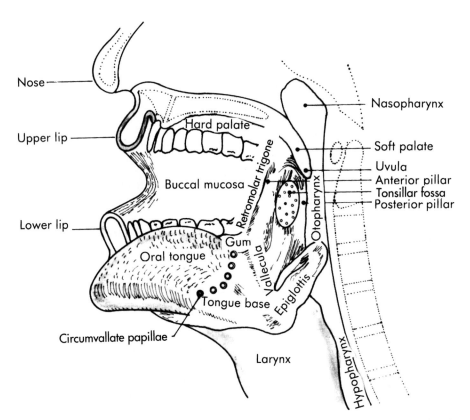

Figure 30-12. A lateral view of the oral cavity and oropharynx depicting anatomic subdivisions. *(From Cox JD: Moss' radiation oncology: rationale, technique, results, ed 7, St. Louis, 1994, Mosby.)*

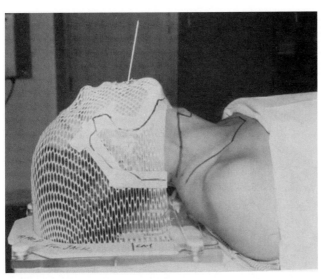

Figure 30-15. Treatment position of a patient with nasopharyngeal carcinoma. *(From Leibel S: Textbook of radiation oncology, Philadelphia, 1998, WB Saunders.)*

piece rigidly supported by and referenced to a solid base plate placed under the patient's head.[8]

The lateral photon portals of the typical head and neck treatment should encompass as much of the clinical target volume as possible without having the entrance beam (as determined by the light field on the skin) go through the shoulder. The shoulders may be displaced inferiorly as much as possible to maximize the utility of the lateral portals. Inferior displacement of the shoulders can be accomplished by the patient's pulling on two ends of a strap wrapped around a footboard.[9] In a similar fashion, a shoulder strap with Velcro adjustments can be placed around the patient's wrists and feet while the knees are bent; then the patient straighten the knees to pull the shoulders down. Patients with short necks or those unable to displace their shoulders inferiorly pose a treatment-planning problem. One solution involves the use of lateral fields that are angled inferiorly to obtain better inferior coverage. This is done by rotating the foot of the treatment table 10 to 20 degrees away from the gantry.

Accurate and reproducible treatment has always been an important aspect of high-quality radiation therapy. Its importance today has grown with increased interest in 3-D conformal therapy and dose escalation. The objective of tumor control with these new techniques involve higher doses while using tighter target margins and at the same time limiting the dose to adjacent normal tissues.

THE ORAL CAVITY

Anatomy

The oral cavity extends from the skin-vermilion junction of the lip to the posterior border of the hard palate superiorly and the circumvallate papillae inferiorly. Subdivisions within the oral cavity include the anterior two thirds of the tongue (anterior to the circumvallate papillae), lip, buccal mucosa, lower alveolar ridge, upper alveolar ridge, retromolar trigone, floor of mouth, and hard palate (Figs. 30-10, 30-11, and 30-12). Oral cavity cancers, the most common aerodigestive tract carcinomas, occur mostly (80%) in men between the ages of 55 and 65. Alcohol and tobacco have a **synergistic** (a combined effect greater than the individual effect) etiologic history.

Clinical Presentation

Patients who have oral cavity cancer often demonstrate poor oral and dental hygiene. In females, Plummer-Vinson syndrome (iron deficiency anemia) is considered an important etiologic factor. Because premalignant conditions are usually asymptomatic, the general practitioner or dentist is responsible for clinical detection. Early diagnosis is essential for a good prognosis.

As previously stated, leukoplakia and **erythroplasia** (a premalignant well-circumscribed reddish patch) represent severe dysplastic changes and should be regarded as serious pathologic problems. Most often, oral cavity cancers appear as nonhealing ulcers with little pain. Localized pain is considered a symptom of advanced disease.

Diagnostic Procedures

Inspection and palpation are important first steps. The malignant ulcer is typically raised, centrally ulcerated, with indurated edges and an infiltrated base. Biopsy is mandatory. Imaging modalities include both CT and MRI for staging of advanced tumors.

Histopathology

Squamous cell carcinoma accounts for 90% to 95% of the histopathologic types, either well or moderately well differentiated. Unusual variants of squamous cell carcinoma include verrucous carcinoma and spindle cell squamous cell carcinoma. Adenocarcinomas of the salivary gland may also be identified.

Staging

The staging system is listed in Box 30-5.

Metastatic Behavior

Cervical lymph node involvement at the time of presentation is uncommon, and oral cavity cancer demonstrates the lowest incidence (except glottic cancer) of nodal metastasis in the head and neck region. Bloodborne spread occurs in fewer than 20% of patients. Of those patients, most have cervical node involvement at the time of presentation and advanced-stage disease.

GENERAL TREATMENT TECHNIQUES

Early-stage (<1 to 1.5 cm) and premalignant lesions are candidates for surgery alone. If inadequate surgical margins and

Box 30-8	Five-Year Survival Rates for Head and Neck Cancer
Stage I—30%-95%	
Stage II—30%-85%	
Stage III—15%-70%	
Stage IV—5%-60%	

Modified from Rubin P: *Clinical oncology*, ed 8, Philadelphia, 2001, WB Saunders.

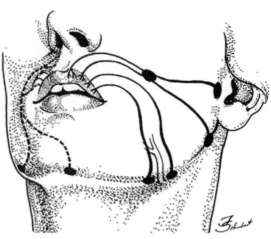

Figure 30-16. Lymphatics of the upper lip drain into buccal, parotid, upper cervical, and submandibular nodes. Lymphatics of the skin of the upper lip *(dotted line)* may cross midline to terminate in submental and submandibular nodes of the contralateral side. *(From Cox JD: Moss' radiation oncology: rationale, technique, results, ed 7, St. Louis, 1994, Mosby.)*

neck node involvement are present, combination radiation therapy and surgery is indicated. The sequence of the therapy is usually dictated by the first treatment's design. If radical surgery is planned, the radiation therapy should not be given before surgery. Elective irradiation of the lymph nodes is included if a lesion demonstrates a high rate of spread or has a history of bilateral movement (anatomically) via the lymphatics. A 5-year follow-up plan is recommended because lesions in most sites recur within 2 years and rarely after 4 years. The expected 5-year survival rates are listed in Box 30-8.

Lip

The lymphatics of the upper lip drain into the submandibular and preauricular nodal beds (Fig. 30-16). Lymphatics from the mid-lower lip and anterior floor of the mouth rain into the submental nodal group (Fig. 30-17). Lymphatics from the oral tongue drain into the anterior cervical chain; more anteriorly placed lesions drain lower in the neck than lesions placed more posteriorly (Fig. 30-18).

Lip cancer is treated with radiation in the same manner as skin cancer. Successful control is achievable by external beam therapy, interstitial implants, or both. Single, anterior source-skin distance (SSD) ports, given 100- to 200-kVp x-rays or 3- to 7-MeV electrons at the 100% isodose line is a common regimen. Protracted treatment schedules (4 to 6 weeks) with deliveries of 200 to 300 cGy per day can be given for lesions less than 2 cm. Larger, bulkier lesions require doses of 5000 to 6000 cGy. Regional (submental) lymphatics are rarely treated, whereas patients with advanced-stage or recurrent disease should have neck irradiation. Face shielding must be constructed to delineate the target volume and thus only expose 1 to 2 cm of normal tissue. A lead shield is designed and positioned in place to expose the lip lesion. The lesion may be treated with 100-KVP x-rays through a cone. To reduce dose to teeth and gums, a *stent* coated with wax or a low-atomic-number compound (tissue equivalent) can be made to fit over the teeth. A stent is a lead shield that may consist of two sheets of lead (each ⅛ in. thick) overlaid with one sheet of aluminum and is coated with wax or vinyl. The face mask shielding should also be coated with wax to reduce the electron scatter to the adjacent tissues. Exit radiation to the bone and gums must be

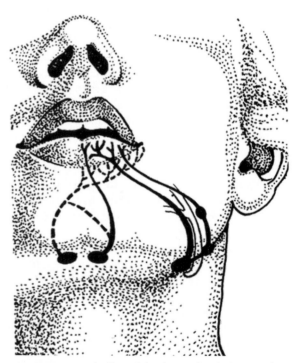

Figure 30-17. Lymphatics of the lower lip drain to submental and submandibular nodes. Sometimes disease involves facial nodes. Lymphatics of the skin of the lower lip *(dotted line)* may cross midline to end in submental or submandibular nodes on the contralateral side. *(From Cox JD: Moss' radiation oncology: rationale, technique, results, ed 7, St. Louis, 1994, Mosby.)*

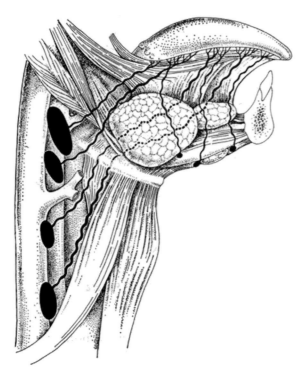

Figure 30-18. Lymphatics of the tongue, illustrating that the more anteriorly they originate in the tongue, the lower in the neck their draining nodes may lie. *(From Cox JD: Moss' radiation oncology: rationale, technique, results, ed 7, St. Louis, 1994, Mosby.)*

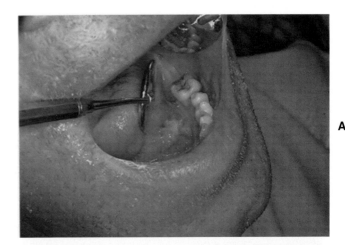

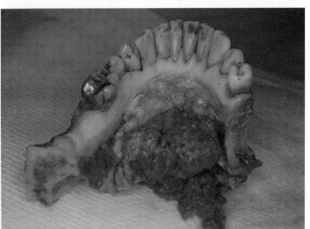

Figure 30-19. A, A deeply infiltrating squamous cell carcinoma involving the entire anterior floor of mouth and mandible. **B,** Treatment involved composite resection followed by radiation. Reconstruction was critical to function, appearance, and quality of life. *(From Silverman S: Oral cancer, ed 4, Hamilton, Ontario, 1998, BC Decker.)*

controlled at safe levels to prevent progressive, long-term physiologic changes. With megavoltage electron energies a tissue compensator is sometimes used to make the dose more uniform. The expected 5-year survival rate is 85%.

Floor of Mouth

The medical literature suggests that at some institutions most cancers of the floor of the mouth are treated with resection (Fig. 30-19). Megavoltage external beam alone gives inferior control results, even for T1 lesions.[11] However, reports of several studies show that good local control may be achieved with a combination of external irradiation interstitial implants or intraoral cone.[9]

Cancers in this area arise on the anterior surface on either side of the midline. They can spread to the bone and tongue. About 30% of these cancers have involvement of submaxillary and subdigastric nodes. Therefore opposed lateral ports are used. If the lesion is small and confined to the floor of the mouth, the tip of the tongue is elevated out of the portal with a cork or a bite block and tongue depressor (tongue blade). Bite blocks may also serve to spare the roof of the mouth from incidental irradiation. If the lesion has grown into the tongue, the tongue is flattened to reduce the superior border of the portal (Fig. 30-20, *A* and *B*). A small stainless steel pin may be inserted into the posterior border of the tumor and

serves as a marker for treatment planning (simulation) and brachytherapy.[11] The entire width of the mandibular arch is included in the port. The superior border is designed to spare the maxillary antrum. An off-cord boost via opposed laterals occurs at 4500 cGy. If the neck nodes are clinically positive for tumor, the lateral ports are enlarged to include all the upper cervical nodes, and an anterior, bilateral, supraclavicular neck field is added.

The lateral borders of the anterior supraclavicular field extend to the coracoid process. The inferior borders extend horizontally 1 to 2 cm below the suprasternal notch, and the superior borders abut via (megavoltage x-ray) the lateral borders at the thyroid notch. The supraclavicular field is taken to 5000 cGy. The bilateral neck fields receive a minimum of 5000 cGy, with boost fields added to bring the dose to 6000 to 7000 cGy. The reduced boost fields can be treated with an intraoral cone, needle implants, or small external photon

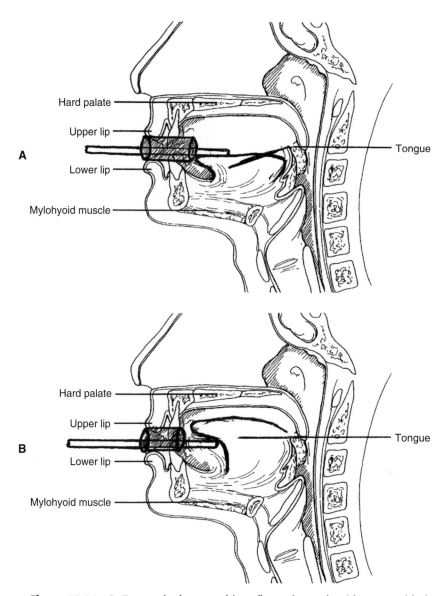

Figure 30-20. A, Tongue is depressed into floor of mouth with tongue blade and cork or bite block if tumor invasion includes the tongue. **B,** Tip of tongue is displaced from treatment field when a lesion is limited to the anterior floor of mouth. Tongue blade is positioned under the tongue.

beams. This is followed by radical neck dissection or limited nodal resection depending on the extent of disease.[1] Despite good local control, actuarial survival of these patients is poor, because of a significant number of deaths from intercurrent disease or a second primary cancer.[9]

Tongue

Both the anterior tongue and the base of the tongue are discussed in this section. The reader is advised that only the anterior two thirds is included in the oral cavity. The base of tongue is considered to be in the oropharynx. The oral tongue is the freely mobile portion of the tongue that extends anteri-

orly from the line of circumvallate papillae to the undersurface of the tongue at the junction of the floor of the mouth. It is composed of four areas: the tip, the lateral borders, the dorsum, and the undersurface (nonvillous surface of the tongue).

Small tumors arising in the anterior two thirds of the tongue also known as the oral tongue are usually resected. Radiation therapy is used in patients who are medically inoperable. Postoperative radiation therapy to the primary site and the cervical lymph nodes is used to cover margins positive for tumor, extensive primary tumor with bone or skin invasion, and multiple nodes positive for tumor. The anterior tongue drains into the submandibular lymph nodes, whereas the posterior portion of the tongue drains more to the jugulodigastric, posterior pharyngeal, and upper cervical lymph nodes.

Lesions of the tongue usually appear on the lateral borders near the middle and posterior third section. The lesions can be large and still confined to the tongue (Figs. 30-21, 30-22, and 30-23). Only a limited number of tongue cancers can be excised. Therefore external beam irradiation can achieve the best control with interstitial boost fields.

Lesions on the tip of the tongue are seen first and are commonly in an early stage, whereas lesions at the base and posterior one third of the tongue invade the floor of the mouth, the tonsils, or the muscles; are advanced; and have a higher incidence of nodal metastasis. An early-stage lesion of the tongue can be cured with a local excision or **hemiglossectomy** (surgical removal of half the tongue). For the preservation of speech and swallowing functions, external beam irradiation is the best choice for large T3 to T4 lesions. Iridium-192 implants follow the external beam. Fig. 30-24 depicts radiation ports for the base of a tongue. A depressor is sometimes inserted to push the tongue back and keep as much of the mandible out of the field as possible. The subdigastric and submaxillary nodes must always be included in the port. A three-field technique that uses isocentric lateral-opposed fields is employed, with the posterior borders encompassing the upper cervical nodes and the superior border aligned to miss the maxillary antrum matched to a lower anterior neck field.[9] External beam is delivered to a dose of 5400 cGy in 30 fractions with 180 cGy per fraction. The fields are reduced off the spinal cord at 4500 cGy. At that point the tongue and upper anterior neck are boosted with photons and posterior neck is treated with electrons for a total dose of 5400 cGy. Palpable nodes are treated with electrons, and additional 600 cGy brings the total dose to 6000 cGy. The patient then undergoes an iridium implant and a neck dissection.[9]

Buccal Mucosa

The buccal mucosa is the mucous membrane lining the inner surface of the cheeks and lips. Most lesions originate on the lateral walls; have a history of leukoplakia; and appear as a raised, exophytic growth. As it grows, the lesion invades the skin and bone. Usually, the patient notices a bump with the tip of the tongue. Pain is not associated with this lesion unless the nerves to the tongue or ear become involved. Advanced lesions bleed. Early lesions often appear as an inflammatory process, so care should be taken during a biopsy to obtain a correct diagnosis.

Stensen's duct can become obstructed. This enlarges the parotid gland, thereby necessitating surgical intervention. Small (1 cm) lesions can be excised, whereas larger lesions are treatable with combination surgery and radiation therapy,

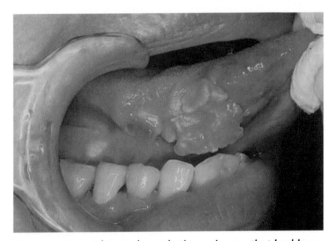

Figure 30-22. Advanced exophytic carcinoma that had been noticed for more than 6 months. *(From Silverman S: Oral cancer, ed 4, Hamilton, Ontario, 1998, BC Decker.)*

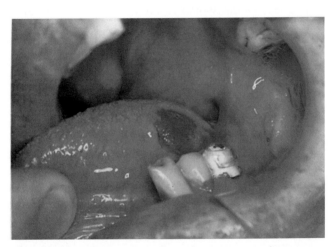

Figure 30-21. Squamous cell carcinoma presenting as erythroleukoplakia and thought to be irritation from a temporary crown. *(From Silverman S: Oral cancer, ed 4, Hamilton, Ontario, 1998, BC Decker.)*

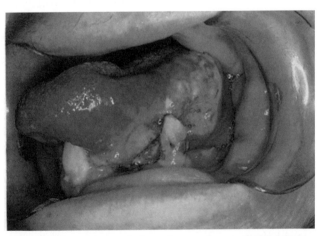

Figure 30-23. Advanced ulcerative carcinoma that had been noticed for more than 6 months. *(From Silverman S: Oral cancer, ed 4, Hamilton, Ontario, 1998, BC Decker.)*

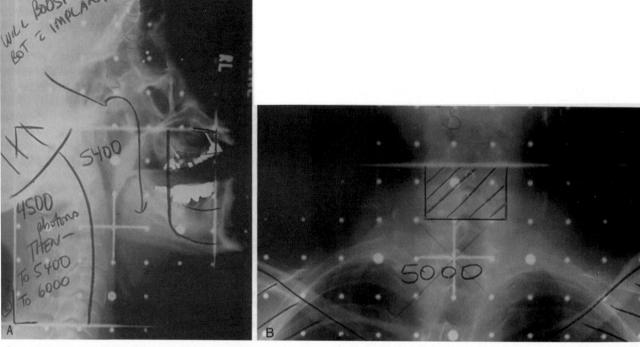

Figure 30-24. A and **B,** Simulation film, base of tongue, external beam radiation therapy. Patients are immobilized using custom designed Aquaplast masks and placement of a bite block. The superior border includes the retropharyngeal and upper jugular lymph nodes (levels I, II). The inferior border is at the hyoid bone; clinically this is just above the thyroid notch and can be palpated. The posterior border is placed at the posterior aspect of the spinal process. The anterior border is approximately 2 cm from the primary tumor. Even in the situation of a small primary, both the lateral and anterior neck are treated. The treatment field should include lymph node levels I, II, III, and V. There should be generous coverage of the retropharyngeal nodes. *(From Leibel S: Textbook of radiation oncology, Philadelphia, 1998, WB Saunders.)*

radical surgery, or radical radiation therapy alone. If radiation therapy is chosen as a treatment modality, a single-plane photon or electron beam that spares contralateral tissues can be used. The submaxillary and subdigastric nodes are at risk. If positive for tumor, these nodes require a controlling dose. Radiation therapy usually consists of 5500 to 6000 cGy in 6 weeks, followed by a boost of 2000 cGy sparing the mandible.[1] A total additional dose of up to 3000 cGy has been documented through an interstitial implant.[9] In advanced tumors, radiation therapy is followed by surgical resection of the lesion and regional lymph nodes. Fibrosis of the cheek and trismus are not infrequent complications following curative radiation therapy. T1 lesions can be treated with oral cone alone, 6000 cGy in 15 fractions or an implant to deliver 6000 cGy in 6 to 7 days. Large buccal mucosal tumors may be treated with 3D-conformal therapy, delivering 7500 cGy with sparing of normal structures using right anterior and left anterior oblique beams (Fig. 30-25). The 5-year absolute survival rate is 53% and the determined survival rate is 65% for patients treated with radiation therapy alone.[9]

Hard Palate

The hard palate is the semilunar area between the upper alveolar ridge and the mucous membrane covering the pala-

tine process of the maxillary palatine bones. It extends from the inner surface of the superior alveolar ridge to the posterior edge of the palatine bone. Hard palate carcinomas are rare and are mostly adenocarcinomas. Most malignant tumors of the hard palate are of minor salivary gland origin. Squamous cell carcinoma is rare. They tend to spread to the bone and invade the maxillary antrum. Adenoid cystic types spread hematogenously to lungs and bone and along the second branch of the fifth cranial nerve to the middle fossa. These types of tumors seldom metastasize to lymph nodes. Surgical resection is the usual treatment, with postoperative radiation therapy given as needed. Extensive disease requires radiation therapy. Cancers in this area have been noted to be the result of secondary spread from the upper gum. A history of ill-fitting dentures or trauma is common. Except for early superficial lesions, most tumors of the hard palate and upper gingival are treated with surgery. Postoperative radiation therapy is added in high-risk patients. The patient may be treated definitively with opposed-lateral fields or wedge pairs to 6500 or 7000 cGy in 6.5 to 7.5 weeks. Postoperative doses of 6200 to 6500 cGy are delivered in 6.5 to 7.0 weeks. A balloon filled with water can be used to compensate for postsurgical tissue defects.[9]

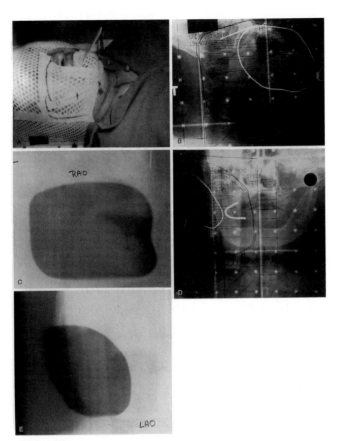

Figure 30-25. A, Patient in marks with portals marked for three-field three-dimensional (3D) plan to treat buccal mucosa. **B,** Right anterior oblique port simulation film. **C,** Right anterior oblique port film. **D,** Left anterior oblique port simulation film. **E,** Left anterior oblique port film. *(From Leibel S: Textbook of radiation oncology, Philadelphia, 1998, WB Saunders.)*

Retromolar Trigone

The retromolar trigone is the triangular space behind the last molar tooth. Carcinomas of this area are rare. Lesions can cause tongue pain, ear-canal pain, or, if the muscles become involved, trismus. Indirect extension into the anterior tonsillar pillar or the buccal mucosa occurs early. A lesion may be indistinguishable from carcinomas of the anterior tonsillar pillar; most are moderately differentiated squamous cell carcinomas. X-ray examinations are needed to detect bone invasion. Lymphatic spread occurs to the submaxillary and subdigastric nodes. Early lesions may be treated with external beam irradiation alone using mixed electrons and photons with single lateral fields or parallel opposing fields with 2:1 loading favoring the diseased side. A usual dose of 6500 to 7500 cGy in 6 to 7.5 weeks is delivered.[9] Treatment techniques may also involve anterior and lateral wedged pair fields or anterior and posterior oblique fields using wedges. Small, well-defined lesions may be boosted via an intraoral cone using an electron beam. Large lesions that involve the

base of tongue and invade bone may be treated using parallel opposed lateral fields to the primary lesion and cervical nodes. An anterior field is included to treat the lower cervical nodes and bilateral supraclavicular fossa.[1] Surgery is noted to be reserved for salvage of radiation therapy failures. Moderately advanced lesions are usually managed with resection and postoperative radiation therapy. A 5-year determinate survival rate of 83% has been reported.

THE PHARYNX

Anatomy

The pharynx is subdivided into three anatomic divisions: the oropharynx, nasopharynx, and hypopharynx (Fig. 30-26). Attention should be provided to the distinct anatomic structures that define each subdivision.

Clinical Presentation

The most common symptoms include persistent sore throat, painful swallowing, and referred otalgia. Enlargement of cervical nodes are presented. Fetor oris, dyspnea, dysphasia, hoarseness, dysarthria, and hypersalivation may indicate advanced disease.[14]

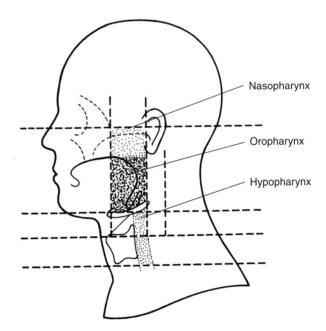

Figure 30-26. Subdivisions of the pharynx. The oral cavity (not shown) lies anterior to the oropharynx and is bounded by the vermilion border of the lips. The lines indicated on this figure can be determined with respect to the following palpable structures: zygomatic arch, external auditory canal, mastoid process, hyoid bone, thyroid cartilage, and cricoid cartilage. *(From Rubin P: Clinical oncology: a multidisciplinary approach for physicians and students, ed 8, Philadelphia, 2001, WB Saunders.)*

Diagnostic Procedures

Inspection includes indirect mirror examination (essential), palpation, biopsy (essential), and CT and MRI imaging to detect occult primaries and defining anatomic extensions three-dimensionally.

Histopathology

These tumors are predominately squamous cell carcinomas (90%). Well-differentiated squamous cell carcinomas are less common than in the oral cavity. Lymphoepithelioma may occur in the tonsil and base of tongue. Minor salivary gland carcinomas have been identified in this region. Non-Hodgkin's lymphoma is seen in approximately 5% of tonsillar malignancies.

Staging

The staging system is listed in Box 30-9.

Metastatic Behavior

Cervical lymph node involvement is common with oropharyngeal carcinoma. Base of tongue tumors may have palpable nodes on presentation. The incidence of bilateral neck disease is up to 40%. Tonsillar lesions have palpable metastatic nodes at diagnosis in 60% to 70% of cases, pharyngeal wall lesions have involved nodes in 50% to 60% of cases, and soft palate carcinoma metastasizes about 40% to 50% of cases to the jugulodigastric nodes. Bilateral nodal disease is frequent, and retropharyngeal node involvement is common. Hematogenous metastasis is associated with tonsillar and base of tongue primaries. Lung is the most common site for hematogenous metastasis.

GENERAL TREATMENT TECHNIQUES

Oropharynx

The **oropharynx** consists of the base of the tongue, the tonsils (fossa and pillars), the soft palate, and the oropharyngeal walls. The oropharynx is situated between the axis and C3 vertebral bodies. The soft tissue regions include the anterior tonsillary pillars, the soft palate, the uvula, the base of the tongue, and the lateral-posterior pharyngeal walls (Figs. 30-3 and 30-12). Tumors in this region and their treatment can have a profound effect on all of the basic aerodigestive functions. The tonsils are the most common site of disease. Clinically, a sore throat and pain during swallowing are the most common presenting symptoms. Upper spinal accessory nodes are involved bilaterally in 50% to 70% of the patients. Early T1 to T2 lesions are treatable with external beam irradiation alone. Large ports are required for T3 to T4 lesions that encompass the cervical and supraclavicular neck nodes.

Fig. 30-27 shows a typical field for treatment of early stage cancer of the soft palate. The anterior border is 2 cm from known tumor; the superior border should be 1.5 to 2.0 cm superior to the soft palate. If there is extension into the tonsillar fossa, the field should encompass the medial pterygoid muscle at its insertion into the pterygoid plate. The posterior border is at the posterior spinous processes, and the inferior border at the level of the hyoid. This is matched to a low anterior neck field, with the spinal cord blocked on the lateral portals. With more advanced-stage lesions, the field may have to include portions of the base of tongue, tonsillar fossa, tonsillar pillars, soft palate, and medial pterygoid muscle. For more advanced tumor, the pterygoid plates up to the base of skull should be covered, and, if there is extension into the nasopharynx or hypopharynx, this area too must be incorporated into the treatment field. For neck nodes clinically negative for tumor, all patients receive 5000 cGy to 5400 cGy in 5 to 6 weeks. An additional boost to therapeutic doses to the neck or neck dissection follows for patients whose neck nodes are clinically positive for tumor. The preference is neck dissection for palpable nodes.[7]

Acute mucosal reactions are common, and complications from the radiation pose a significant medical problem. The soft palate and tonsils have the best prognosis.

Hypopharynx

The hypopharynx (Figs. 30-3 and 30-12) is composed of the pyriform sinuses, postcricoid, and *lower posterior* pharyngeal walls below the base of the tongue. It is anatomically situated between the vertebral bodies C3 to C6. The cricoid cartilage represents the inferior border, and the epiglottis is the superior border.

Typically, disease of the hypopharynx is advanced. There is a high rate of nodal metastasis (70%), and the tumor is highly infiltrative. Treatment can also be debilitating. The rare T1 to T2 lesions are controllable through radiation or surgery. The pyriform sinus is the site of highest incidence of hypopharyngeal cancer. Most patients receive combined radical surgery and radiation therapy for curative purposes. Tumors of the posterior pharyngeal wall are considered unresectable. Radiation therapy consists of large fields, including the entire pharynx and upper cervical esophagus and extending superiorly to include the nasopharynx vault; superior deep, middle, and low jugular; and Rouviere's (lateral retropharyngeal) lymph nodes at the base of the skull. The large fields are treated to 4500 cGy and are then reduced off the spinal cord. The smaller fields are continued to 6500 to 7000 cGy or 7500 cGy with a twice daily (bid) regimen. Attention is brought to a required sharp edge to treat the primary and Rouviere's lymph node while shielding the spinal cord.[1]

The radiation ports for tonsillar, pharyngeal wall, and posterior cricoid are similar stage for stage. Fig. 30-28 depicts a typical field alignment for treatment of the region of the hypopharynx. Cumulative postoperative dose of 6300-7000 cGy is delivered to the primary tumor bed after a field reduction off of the spinal cord at 4500 cGy and a second field reduction to exclude low-risk regions of the neck after 5400 cGy. The dose is divided in daily fractions of 180 cGy each. Posterior neck is boosted with appositional electron fields to

PRIMARY TUMOR (T)

T_x Primary tumor cannot be assessed
T_0 No evidence of primary tumor
Tis   Carcinoma in situ

Nasopharynx

T_1 Tumor confined to the nasopharynx
T_2 Tumor extends to soft tissues
T_{2a} Tumor extends to the oropharynx and/or nasal cavity without parapharyngeal extension[1]
T_{2b} Any tumor with parapharyngeal extension[1]
T_3 Tumor involves bony structures and/or paranasal sinuses
T_4 Tumor with intracranial extension and/or involvement of cranial nerves, infratemporal fossa, hypopharynx, orbit, or masticator space

Oropharynx

T_1 Tumor 2 cm or less in greatest dimension
T_2 Tumor more than 2 cm but not more than 4 cm in greatest dimension
T_3 Tumor more than 4 cm in greatest dimension
T_{4a} Tumor invades the larynx, deep/extrinsic muscle of tongue, medial pterygoid, hard palate, or mandible
T_{4b} Tumor invades lateral pterygoid muscle, pterygoid plates, lateral nasopharynx, or skull base or encases carotid artery

Hypopharynx

T_1 Tumor limited to one subsite of hypopharynx and 2 cm or less in greatest dimension
T_2 Tumor invades more than one subsite of hypopharynx or an adjacent site, or measures more than 2 cm but not more than 4 cm in greatest diameter without fixation of hemilarynx
T_3 Tumor measures more than 4 cm in greatest dimension or with fixation of hemilarynx
T_{4a} Tumor invades thyroid/cricoid cartilage, hyoid bone, thyroid gland, esophagus or central compartment soft tissue[2]
T_{4b} Tumor invades prevertebral fascia, encases carotid artery, or involves mediastinal structures

REGIONAL LYMPH NODES (N)

Nasopharynx

N_x Regional lymph nodes cannot be assessed
N_0 No regional lymph node metastasis
N_1 Unilateral metastasis in lymph node(s), 6 cm or less in greatest dimension, above the supraclavicular fossa[3]
N_2 Bilateral metastasis in lymph node(s), 6 cm or less in greatest dimension, above the supraclavicular fossa[3]
N_3 Metastasis in a lymph node(s) >6 cm and/or to supraclavicular fossa
N_{3a} Greater than 6 cm in dimension
N_{3b} Extension to the supraclavicular fossa[3]

Oropharynx and Hypopharynx

N_x Regional lymph nodes cannot be assessed
N_0 No regional lymph node metastasis
N_1 Metastasis in a single ipsilateral lymph node, 3 cm or less in greatest dimension
N_2 Metastasis in a single ipsilateral lymph node, more than 3 cm but not more than 6 cm in greatest dimension, or in multiple ipsilateral lymph nodes, none more than 6 cm in greatest dimension, or in bilateral or contralateral lymph nodes, none more than 6 cm in greatest dimension

N_{2a} Metastasis in a single ipsilateral lymph node more than 3 cm but not more than 6 cm in greatest dimension
N_{2b} Metastasis in multiple ipsilateral lymph nodes, none more than 6 cm in greatest dimension
N_{2c} Metastasis in bilateral or contralateral lymph nodes, none more than 6 cm in greatest dimension
N_3 Metastasis in a lymph node more than 6 cm in greatest dimension

DISTANT METASTASIS (M)

M_x Distant metastasis cannot be assessed
M_0 No distant metastasis
M_1 Distant metastasis

STAGE GROUPING: NASOPHARYNX

Stage	T	N	M
0	Tis	N_0	M_0
I	T_1	N_0	M_0
IIA	T_{2a}	N_0	M_0
IIB	T_1	N_1	M_0
	T_2	N_1	M_0
	T_{2a}	N_1	M_0
	T_{2b}	N_0	M_0
	T_{2b}	N_1	M_0
III	T_1	N_2	M_0
	T_{2a}	N_2	M_0
	T_{2b}	N_2	M_0
	T_3	N_0	M_0
	T_3	N_1	M_0
	T_3	N_2	M_0
IVA	T_4	N_0	M_0
	T_4	N_1	M_0
	T_4	N_2	M_0
IVB	Any T	N_3	M_0
IVC	Any T	Any N	M_1

HISTOLOGIC GRADE (G)(OROPHARYNX, HYPOPHARYNX)

G_x Grade cannot be assessed
G_1 Well differentiated
G_2 Moderately differentiated
G_3 Poorly differentiated

STAGE GROUPING: OROPHARYNX AND HYPOPHARYNX

Stage	T	N	M
0	Tis	N_0	M_0
I	T_1	N_0	M_0
II	T_2	N_0	M_0
III	T_3	N_0	M_0
	T_1	N_1	M_0
	T_2	N_1	M_0
	T_3	N_1	M_0
IVA	T_{4a}	N_0	M_0
	T_{4a}	N_1	M_0
	T_1	N_2	M_0
	T_2	N_2	M_0
	T_3	N_2	M_0
	T_{4a}	N_2	M_0
IVB	T_{4b}	Any N	M_0
	Any T	N_3	M_0
IVC	Any T	Any N	M_1

With permission from American Joint Committee on Cancer (AJCC), Chicago, Illinois, *AJCC Cancer Staging Manual*, ed 6, New York, 2002, Springer-Velag.

Notes
1. Parapharyngeal extension denotes posterolateral infiltration of tumor beyond the pharyngobasilar fascia.
2. Central compartment soft tissue includes prelaryngeal strap muscles and subcutaneous fat.
3. Midline nodes are considered ipsilateral nodes.

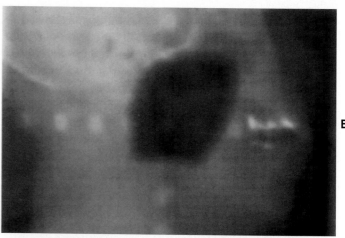

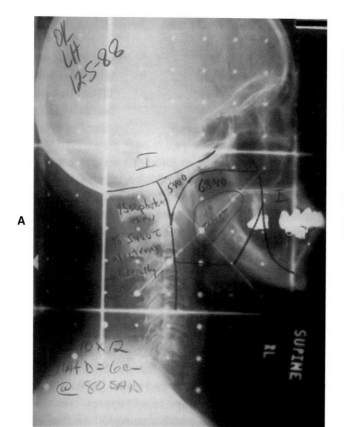

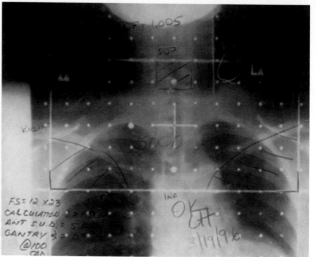

Figure 30-27. A, B, and **C,** Simulation films and port film of boost field for patient with early-stage cancer of the soft palate. *(From Leibel S: Textbook of radiation oncology, Philadelphia, 1998, WB Saunders.)*

5400 cGy if nodes are negative for tumor or 6300-7000 if nodes are positive for tumor.[9] The inferior border of the lateral port is difficult to treat because of interference of the shoulders. Care must be taken to ensure that the shoulders are pulled down toward the feet and remain that way during treatment. Note that the lateral retropharyngeal and jugular chain nodes are treated, even if they are clinically negative for tumor. Anterior **shine over** (falloff) is usually not necessary from the laterals unless the larynx is involved. Substantial soft tissue, cord damage, airway damage, or fibrosis is possible with these fields if the radiation dose to the critical organs is not carefully monitored. Full-course therapy can last 7 to 8 weeks.

Five-year survival rates greater than 70% has been reported for early lesions. However, most cases are advanced, and overall survival rarely exceeds 25%. Radical treatment measures achieve better locoregional control, but the 5-year survival outcomes are little improved compared with conservative measures. This result is related to the discovery of

hematogenous metastases despite improved locoregional control.[14] The need for improved systemic therapy has been cited.

Nasopharynx

The nasopharynx includes the *posterosuperior* pharyngeal wall and *lateral* pharyngeal wall, the eustachian tube orifice, and adenoids. The nasopharynx is a cuboidal structure lying on a line from the zygomatic arch to the **external auditory meatus (EAM),** extending inferiorly to the mastoid tip. The nasopharynx lies behind the nasal cavities and above the level of the soft palate (Fig. 30-3). The nasal cavity drains into the nasopharynx via the two posterior nares and also has on its lateral walls the two eustachian tubes, which connect to the middle ear. Disease in the nasopharynx can mimic an inflammatory process and cause considerable respiratory or auditory dysfunction.

Cranial nerve involvement occurs frequently. The ninth to the twelfth cranial nerves can be affected by enlargement of

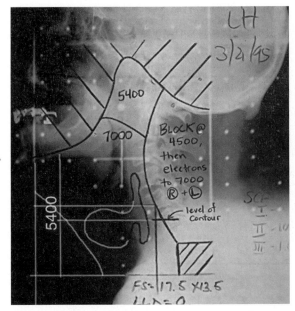

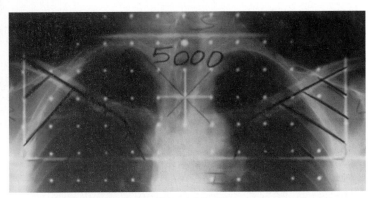

A

B

Figure 30-28. A, Typical lateral photon portals, cone-down fields, and doses for hypopharyngeal cancer. Level of contour is indicated. Horizontal white line above of contour and vertical dark line posterior to thyroid cartilage delineate the region encompassed by tissue compensators. Anterior curved white line delineates the skin surface at the anterior neck. A strip of the superior and anterior neck is blocked after 5400 cGy, as indicated by the vertical white line inside the anterior border of the treatment portal. **B,** Typical low anterior neck portal. *(From Leibel S: Textbook of radiation oncology, Philadelphia, 1998, WB Saunders.)*

the retropharyngeal nodes (Fig. 30-8), as can the external carotid artery. Because of its proximity to the base of the brain, a lesion can directly invade the third cranial nerve and most commonly involves the sixth cranial nerve. Any cranial nerve involvement signifies advanced, widespread disease. Ninety percent of these lesions are squamous cell carcinoma or its variants. NPC has a tendency toward poor differentiation and unusual growth patterns. The World Health Organization recommend the following nomenclature:

Type 1: keratinizing squamous cell carcinoma (30% of cases)

Type 2: nonkeratinizing carcinoma (50% to 70% of cases)

Type 3: lymphoepithelioma (25% of cases)

Nonkeratinizing carcinoma and lymphoepithelioma are variants of squamous cell carcinoma. Surgical intervention in the nasopharynx is extremely difficult. This disease is not associated with tobacco consumption. NPC is associated with the Epstein Barr virus and the age distribution is bimodal, with a small peak in adolescence and young adulthood and the major peak occurring between 50 and 70 years. The disease is uncommon in white populations, comprising of only 2% of all head and neck cancer in the United States.[14] There is a high incidence in southern China (57% of all head and neck cancers) and Middle Eastern countries; the high incidence in southern China may be attributed to nitrosamines in salted fish. Seventy-five percent to 85% of NPC patients have cervical nodes that are clinically positive for tumor, with about half of all cases having bilateral or contralateral disease. Radiation ports are large to encompass all the nodes

and at-risk tissue. The lateral retropharyngeal (node of Rouviere), which usually cannot be surgically removed, and jugulodigastric nodes are nearly always treated as tumor volume during any cone-down procedure.

NPC demonstrates an overall incidence of 25% of blood-borne metastasis. The nodal disease can be extensive while the primary lesion is small. Patients with bilateral cervical nodes have up to a 40% to 70% likelihood of developing a distant metastasis with bone and lung being the most common sites. NPC disease spreads to adjacent subsites quickly and demonstrates a 30% to 40% local recurrence rate. For these reasons, aggressive, large-volume curative radiation therapy is necessary.

Fig. 30-29 depicts a three-field setup. Opposing laterals with a matching anterior supraclavicular field are used to deliver a minimum of 5000 cGy to all areas. Subsequent cone-down fields boost the dose to 6500 cGy, with careful consideration of the dose to the spinal cord, optic nerve, pituitary, and brainstem. An electron boost of 7000 cGy to bulky disease or nodes positive for tumor is warranted if lymphadenopathy is present. Recurrences are treatable with small, multiple ports; arcs; or brachytherapy. Any external beam reirradiation should avoid the same surface-entrance points. Concomitant chemotherapy should be used along with radiation for stage III and IV (localized) tumors. Retreatment of local failures with a combination of external beam followed by an intracavitary brachytherapy boost is considered feasible.

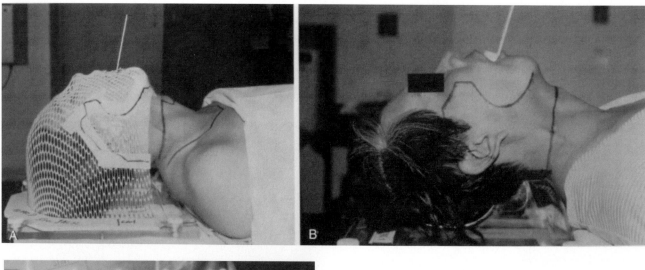

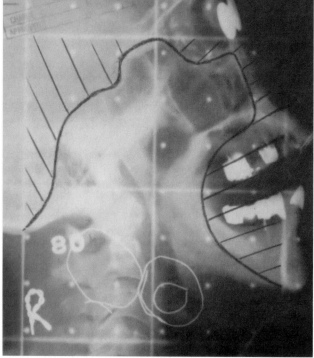

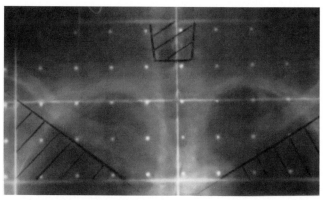

Figure 30-29. A, Treatment position of a patient with nasopharyngeal carcinoma. The neck is extended, a tongue blade with a cork attached to one end is inserted between the incisor teeth to depress the tongue. The head is immobilized. **B,** Outline of the primary treatment field on the face and neck. **C,** Initial lateral photon portal of a patient with T1N2 carcinoma of the nasopharynx. The neck nodes are outlined with metallic wires. **D,** Typical low anterior neck portal. A 2 × 2 cm block is placed at midline over the spinal cord at the junction of the lateral and anterior fields. *(From Leibel S: Textbook of radiation oncology, Philadelphia, 1998, WB Saunders.)*

This disease has an overall 45% survival rate. Survival decreases from 50% to 60% for T1 lesions to 10% to 20% for T4 lesions treated with radiation alone. Overall, lymphoepithelioma has a better prognosis that squamous cell carcinoma. Local control has improved with radiation therapy. Unlike other head and neck tumors, adjuvant chemotherapy seems to improve both local control and survival.[14]

Larynx

The larynx is contiguous with the lower portion of the pharynx above and is connected with the trachea below. It extends from the tip of the epiglottis at the level of the lower border of the C3 vertebra to the lower border of the cricoid cartilage at the level of the C6 vertebra. The larynx is subdivided into three sites (Fig. 30-30): the glottis, supraglottis, and subglot-

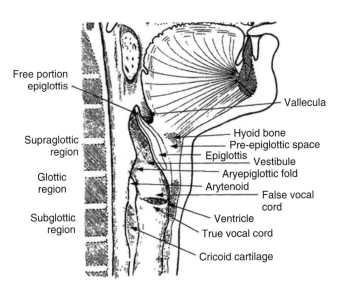

Figure 30-30. Anatomic regions and structures of the larynx. *(From Leibel S: Textbook of radiation oncology, Philadelphia, 1998, WB Saunders.)*

tis region. Glottic cancer accounts for roughly 65% of the cases, and the supraglottic region accounts for 25% to 33% of cases. The remainder of the larynx cancers appear in the subglottic area.

Cancers of the larynx are the most common cancers of the upper aerodigestive tract. The ratio of glottic to supraglottic carcinomas is about 3:1. Carcinomas of the glottis (true vocal cord) are not considered life threatening, and the choice of therapy is based on the preservation of speech and maintenance of the airway. Larynx cancer is mostly (90%) a male-dominated disease, with a peak incidence in the 50- to 60-year age-group. Laryngeal carcinomas display an extremely high association with smoking. The use of black tobacco is associated with a higher risk than the use of blond tobacco. People who employ their voices extensively in their work also appear to be at higher risk. The role of alcohol has been associated with the incidence of supraglottic cancer; the role of alcohol related to glottic cancer is not clear.

Recent studies have involved a molecular basis for laryngeal cancer. Mutation of the *p53* gene is common; it is seen in 47% of the patients who are smokers but in only 14% of nonsmokers. This mutation has been identified in 55% of the tumors among drinkers and 20% among nondrinkers.[9]

A persistent sore throat and hoarseness are classic presenting symptoms. Cervical lymph node involvement, if present, is seen in supraglottic lesions but not in glottic lesions. Carcinoma in situ (TIS) is common on the vocal cords. Glottic lesions are well to moderately differentiated, with supraglottic lesions being less differentiated and more aggressive. About 65% to 75% of glottic lesions appear on the anterior two thirds of one cord. Cord mobility is a factor in the classification of the lesions. Radiation therapy is the primary choice of treatment for nonfixed surface lesions that have not extensively infiltrated muscle, bone, or cartilage.

Glottic cancer is treated with opposing lateral fields, 5×5 cm (for T1 and early T2) to 6×6 cm. Wedges are indicated if the tissue inhomogeneities produce unacceptable hot spots in the posterior margins. Daily doses can be 200 to 220 cGy, up to a total dose of 6000 to 7000 cGy, depending on the size of the lesion and mobility of the cord. Large, fixed lesions need more aggressive therapy.

The radiation port's borders can be clinically determined before simulation. Fig. 30-31 depicts a typical lateral port.

The typical radiation field borders are as follows:

Superior—top of hyoid bone
Inferior—cricoid cartilage
Anterior—1- to 1½-cm shine over (flash)
Posterior—just anterior to the vertebral body

Large T3 to T4, transglottic lesions are treated with radiation alone. In the event of a recurrence, salvage surgery is an option. However, the voice is usually sacrificed. Radiation therapy offers the best method of voice preservation.

Supraglottic lesions are frequently large and bulky but (despite appearances) do not usually invade the inferior false cord or the ventricles. These lesions tend to spread superiorly to the epiglottis.

Lymph node metastasis is expected in 40% to 50% of the patients. Therefore the radiation ports are much larger than the glottic ports. Posteriorly, the spinal accessory chain is included in the lateral treatment fields, then boosted superficially. Superiorly, the field border extends along the mandible (Fig. 30-32). If necessary, an anterior bilateral

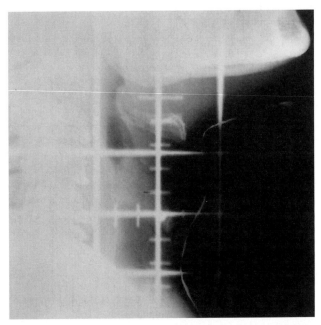

Figure 30-31. A simulation film of a lateral port, T1N0 glottic cancer. *(From Cox JD: Moss' radiation oncology: rationale, technique, results, ed 7, St. Louis, 1994, Mosby.)*

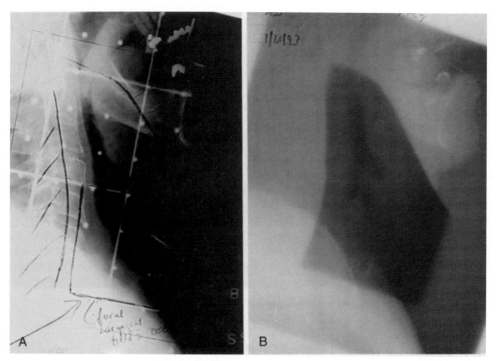

Figure 30-32. A, Simulation film of a supraglottis lateral port. **B,** Port film of a supraglottic lateral port. *(From Leibel S: Textbook of radiation oncology, Philadelphia, 1998, WB Saunders.)*

supraclavicular field is matched to the laterals. The midline block, placed below the cricoid, should only shield the trachea and cord. Because of the risk of blocking tumor, no midline block is used in some instances, thereby requiring that a safety block be placed in the lateral fields at the match line junction. Positioning and immobilizing the head is critical for this type of treatment port.

Surgery can control 80% of supraglottic T1 to T2 lesions, whereas radiation therapy offers 75% local control. Radiation therapy alone for T3 to T4 supraglottic lesions is contraindicated. Relapses are treated with surgery. The tumor dose needed to achieve control is 6600 to 7000 cGy. Electron beam boosts are needed for the cervical lymph nodes. Subglottic cancers are treated with a total laryngectomy, with postoperative radiation therapy given for any residual disease.

Survival rates are good for glottic cancer: 80% to 90% without cord fixation, 50% to 60% if fixation exists. Patients with supraglottic cancers have a 60% to 70% 5-year survival rate with nodes negative for tumor, but this rate drops to 30% to 50% if clinical nodes positive for tumor are present.[14]

Salivary Glands

The salivary glands consist of three large, paired, major glands—the parotid, submandibular, and sublingual glands—and many smaller minor glands located throughout the upper aerodigestive tract. They have major roles in digestion and tooth protection. The parotid gland is the largest of the three salivary glands, is located superficial to and partly behind the ramus of the mandible, and covers the masseter muscle. It fills the space between the ramus of the mandible and the anterior border of the sternocleidomastoid muscle. The parotid contains an extensive lymphatic capillary plexus, many aggregates of lymphocytic cells, and numerous intraglandular lymph nodes in the superficial lobe. Lymphatics drain from more laterally on the face, including parts of the eyelids, diagonally downward and posteriorly toward the parotid gland, as do the lymphatics from the frontal region of the scalp. Associated with the gland, both superficial and deep, are parotid nodes that drain down along the retromandibular vein to empty into the superficial lymphatics and nodes along the outer surface of the sternocleidomastoid muscle and into upper nodes of the deep cervical chain. Lymphatics from the parietal region of the scalp drain partly to the parotid nodes in front of the ear and partly to the retroauricular nodes in back of the ear, which, in turn, drain into upper deep cervical nodes.[13]

Tumors of the salivary gland are rare, constituting from 4% to 7% of all cancers of the head and neck region.[9,14] The parotid is the site of highest incidence of salivary glands tumors (85%). Of these tumors, nearly two thirds are benign. Tumors of the minor salivary glands account for 2% to 3% of all head and neck cancers, about 75% of these are malignant.[14] The submandibular gland is involved in about 10% of all instances. Low-dose ionizing radiation in childhood may account for some cases of malignant salivary gland tumors.

Patients with breast cancer have a higher risk, but firm evidence of this association is lacking.[9] Most major and minor salivary cancers are of unknown origin and etiologic factors are poorly understood. However, risk factors such as dental radiographs have been implicated for both benign and malignant salivary gland tumors. Exposure to hardwood dust has been linked to the development of nasal cavity and paranasal sinus minor salivary gland adenocarcinomas.[7] The incidence is about equal between genders with a slight male predominance.

Histologically, the more common cell types for malignant tumors are adenoid cystic, mucoepidermoid, and adenocarcinoma. Most patients develop an asymptomatic parotid mass lasting on average from 4 to 8 months before presentation.[7] Presenting symptoms are localized swelling and pain, facial palsy, and rapid growth. Facial nerve involvement is highly suggestive of a malignancy. Incisional biopsies are not routinely performed. A diagnosis via a lobectomy is done.

The incidence of cervical node involvement varies according to the histologic subtype. High-grade mucoepidermoid tumors display a 44% rate of metastatic behavior. The rate for this behavior is 5% in adenoid cystic tumors, 21% in malignant mixed tumors, 37% in squamous cell carcinoma, and 13% in acinic cell carcinoma. Hematogenous metastases are common and range from about 13% for acinic cell carcinoma to 41% for adenoid cystic carcinoma. Lung metastases from adenoid cystic carcinomas may lie quiescent for years after initial presentation.[14]

Although tumors in this area are mostly benign, the risk of local recurrence is high. They are treated as low-grade cancer and are optimally treated via total resection, with generous margins for sparing facial nerves. Radiation therapy is given postoperatively for residual, recurrent, or inoperable lesions. In the postoperative case, the primary resection bed is given 6000 cGy to 6300 cGy if the margins are clear; 7000 cGy to 7500 cGy are delivered if there is gross residual disease. The neck that is clinically negative for tumor is generally treated to 5000 cGy.[14] High-grade mucoepidermoid and undifferentiated cancers of the parotid often spread to ipsilateral lymph nodes but seldom involve contralateral lymph nodes. Consequently the target volume is commonly designed to fit the local invasion and lymphatic spread. Because the opposite side is seldom at risk, most cancers of the parotid can be irradiated with a wedge pair or electron to spare the brainstem, spinal cord, and opposite parotid. A strip of bolus should be placed over the scar to raise the surface dose and prevent recurrence in the scar. The patient may be positioned on the side with the lateral side of the head up, when it is necessary to irradiate the parotid and cervical lymph nodes, or supine, when irradiating a local field.[8]

Treatment is administered by one of several external beam techniques. Fields are best designed with the aid of 3D simulation and treatment planning. Treatment may be delivered using a wedge-pair technique, the ipsilateral photon and high-energy electron combination, or an opposed lateral field if the target volume extends beyond the midline. The usual wedge pair is a superior oblique and inferior oblique combination directed away from the opposite oral cavity and orbit. This involves rotating the table 90 degrees off the usual axis. An anterior and posterior oblique combination is possible if the exit beam is not through the contralateral orbit (requires maximum extension of the neck). This may involve matching the low-neck portal to the primary fields. It is important to use CT scan-based treatment planning to derive the maximum benefit from a wedge-pair technique.[1,9,11] An ipsilateral mixed-beam treatment using photons and high-energy electrons produces a homogeneous dose distribution and delivers 3000 cGy or less to the opposite salivary glands.[11] IMRT treatment, sparing dose to the parotid gland, has advanced considerably in recent years, providing better dose distributions.

Care should be taken to monitor the dose to the base of the brain and contralateral maxillary antrum with this technique. Local control with conventional fractionated radiation therapy is only about 25%. High linear energy transfer neutron radiation seems to be more effective. Studies in Britain have shown significant improvement in locoregional control using fast neutrons. However, long-term survival shows no improvement because of metastases. Modern hospital-based neutron radiation therapy facilities allow precise beam shaping and cause fewer side effects than occurred with the older, laboratory settings. In addition, improved results have been reported using **accelerated fractionation.**[14] Accelerated fractionation regimens provide similar dose levels of radiation therapy in a shorter amount of overall time. This counteracts quick cellular proliferation of aggressive tumors by giving more dose in shorter time. Care must be taken to limit heightened side effects.

Maxillary Sinus

The maxillary sinus is a pyramid-shaped cavity lined by ciliated epithelium and bound by thin bone or membranous partitions. Carcinomas arising from the ciliated epithelium or mucous glands perforate the bony walls almost from the start. The roof of the maxillary sinus is also the floor of the orbit. Tumors involving the superior portion of the sinus readily extend into the orbit (Fig. 30-33). The more posterior wall, or infratemporal surface, separates the sinus from the pterygopalatine fossa and the posterosuperior alveolar nerves. The nasal surface of the antrum is visible through the nostril, with the ostium of the sinus inferior to the middle turbinate. The alveolar process and hard palate separate the maxillary sinus from the oral cavity.[4]

Maxillary sinus disease accounts for 80% of all sinus cancers. Patients with this type of cancer have a history of long-standing sinusitis, nasal obstructions, and bloody discharge. These cancers are mostly squamous cell carcinomas and tend to invade the floor of the orbit, ethmoid sinuses, hard palate, and zygomatic arch. Displacement of the eye is common. Physical examination should include inspection and bimanual palpation of the orbit, oral and nasal cavities, and

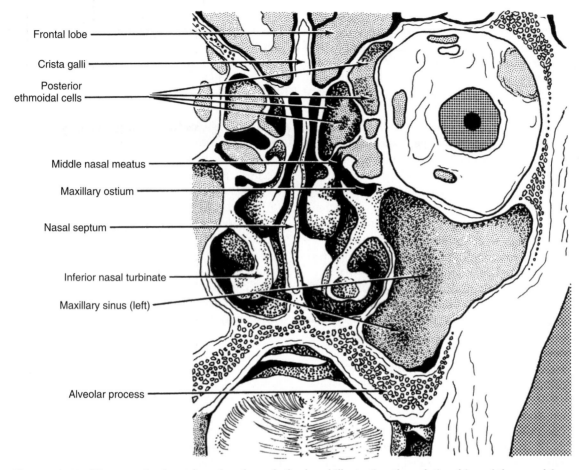

Frontal lobe

Crista galli

Posterior
ethmoidal cells

Middle nasal meatus

Maxillary ostium

Nasal septum

Inferior nasal turbinate

Maxillary sinus (left)

Alveolar process

Figure 30-33. Diagram of a frontal section through the head illustrating the relationships of the nasal fossa to the paranasal sinuses, orbit, and hard palate. *(From Cox JD: Moss' radiation oncology: rationale, technique, results, ed 7, St. Louis, 1994, Mosby.)*

nasopharynx and direct fiberoptic endoscopy. Neurologic examination should evaluate cranial nerve function, because nasal cavity and paranasal sinus tumors are frequently associated with cranial nerve palsies, especially of the trigeminal branches. Cervical lymph nodes are palpated for adenopathy. Imaging has essentially replaced surgical exploration for staging and tumor mapping in this region. The most useful studies are CT and MRI. CT defines early cortical bone erosion more clearly (Fig. 30-34), whereas MRI better delineates soft tissue and can differentiate among opacification of the sinuses resulting from fluid, inflammation, or tumor. MRI may demonstrate subtle perineural spread and involvement of the cranial nerve foramen and canals. In addition, the visualization of sagittal and coronal images using MRI advances visualization compared with CT in evaluating intracranial or leptomeningeal spread[9] (Fig. 30-35).

Cervical nodal spread is uncommon, but, if it is present, the submandibular node is the first station involved and will be treated. Surgery is the principle treatment for control of small lesions of the nasal septum or those limited to the infrastructure of the maxillary sinus. Although primary radiation

therapy for small lesions have a high cure rate, this approach has a significant chance of optic nerve injury from the high dose required to achieve good tumor control.[9]

Most cases warrant treatment with combined surgery and radiation therapy. However, massive tumors with extensive involvement of the nasopharynx, base of skull, sphenoidal sinuses, brain, or optic chiasm are considered unresectable. Some institutions have performed studies using radiosensitizing chemotherapy for unresectable squamous cell carcinoma of the nasal cavity and paranasal sinuses. Hyperfractionated regimens may allow the delivery of higher doses if radiation therapy alone is used for larger lesions.[9]

A classic technique for radiation therapy involves preoperative doses of 6000 cGy, which are delivered via an external beam, wedged-pair technique. Lateral and anterior ports are custom designed to follow the expected route of spread. If the orbit is involved, eye blocking should not be used. Care should be taken to miss the cord and contralateral lens. Angling the anterior beam a few degrees off the vertical spares brain tissue. If the nasal cavity is at risk, bolus material should be inserted to improve dose homogeneity. Angling

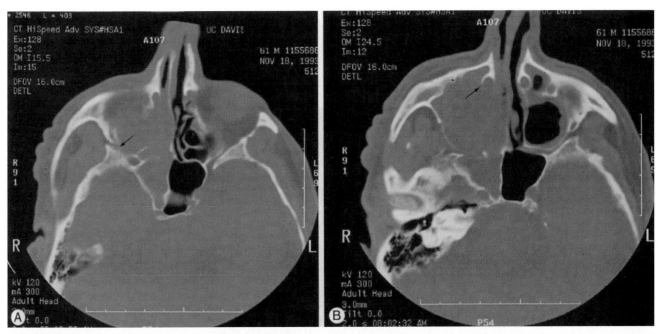

Figure 30-34. Computed tomographic images of a right maxillary antrum carcinoma eroding the medial and lateral walls of the maxillary sinus, extending into the pterygopalatine fossa *(A arrow)*. Eroding lacrimal duct *(B arrow)*. *(From Leibel S: Textbook of radiation oncology, Philadelphia, 1998, WB Saunders.)*

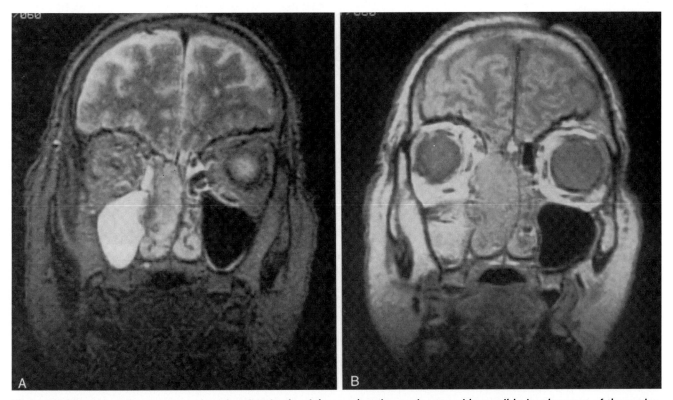

Figure 30-35. Magnetic resonance imaging (MRI) of a right nasal cavity carcinoma with possible involvement of the periorbital fat **(A)** and a coexisting fluid-filled maxillary antrum that is uninvolved by the tumor **(B).** MRI is able to distinguish sinusitis and fluid-filled sinus from tumor on a T2 signal. *(From Leibel S: Textbook of radiation oncology, Philadelphia, 1998, WB Saunders.)*

the lateral port a few degrees off the horizontal plane spares the contralateral optic nerve and lens. Extensive disease may require the use of bilateral wedged fields. Attempts to shield the lacrimal gland and to retract the upper lid superior to the beam edge should be emphasized to reduce eye injury[4] (Figs. 30-36 and 30-37). Four fields, using an anterior and two lateral wedged portal plus an intraorbital electron portal, is reported to be more commonly used that the three-field technique (without using the anterior electron portal).[9]

It is most advantageous to base the treatment volume on treatment planning CT, with MRI correlation. The complex anatomy of this region and the presence of numerous critical,

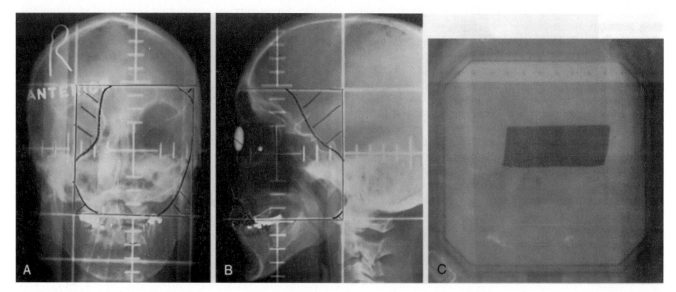

Figure 30-36. Simulation films of a patient undergoing postoperative radiation therapy for a locally advanced paranasal sinus tumor requiring left orbital exenteration. The treatment volume encompasses all the ipsilateral nasal cavity and sinuses including the frontal sinus and orbital bed, contralateral ethmoidal sinus and nasal cavity, and medial maxillary sinus. The patient was treated using a four-field technique that included left and right lateral photon portals, an anterior photon portal, and an electron portal to make up the dose to the left orbital bed, which was blocked from the lateral portals to protect the contralateral eye. **A,** Anterior photon portal including the entire orbital bed. **B,** Lateral photon portal blocking the eye (a dime is placed over the intact eyelid and a canthal marker is placed over the bony canthus). **C,** Anterior electron portal film. *(From Leibel S: Textbook of radiation oncology, Philadelphia, 1998, WB Saunders.)*

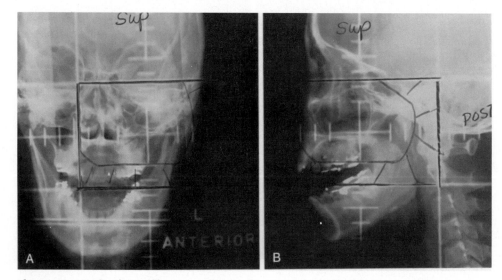

Figure 30-37. Simulation films of wedged-pair setup for a limited lesion involving the maxillary antrum only. The treatment volume includes the ipsilateral maxillary sinus and the nasal cavity. **A,** Anterior portal. **B,** Lateral portal. *(From Leibel S: Textbook of radiation oncology, Philadelphia, 1998, WB Saunders.)*

dose-limiting structures (optic nerves, chiasm, eyes, lacrimal gland, pituitary, brainstem, etc.) renders these tumors ideal candidates for a sophisticated treatment-planning system.[9] A 3D system allows careful definition and comprehensive visualization of the tumor and normal anatomy through beam's eye view. The use of nonaxial and non-coplanar fields allow greater flexibility in treatment planning so that dose distribution conforms to tumor volume in 3D space, sparing the surrounding normal tissue to a greater extent. This type of treatment planning has great potential for improving tumor control by allowing dose escalation that has not been possible with conventional two-dimensional (2D) treatment-planning systems. Compared with a conventional treatment plan, which routinely includes one half to one third of the ipsilateral eye (Figs. 30-36 and 30-37), greater sparing of the ipsilateral eye is possible without sacrificing tumor control by using a 3D conformal plan (Figs. 30-38 and 30-39). Doses volume histograms are also produced for target and the normal structures to provide graphic presentation of each structure receiving percentage dose.

The presentation of inhomogeneity corrections for air cavities and dense bone is a significant advantage of this type of conformal planning system. The extensive air cavities and sloping surfaces present in the paranasal sinuses can distort the isodose curves for electron treatment planning generated by a conventional system resulting in an overdose to critical structures. The ability to optimize and show the effects of inhomogeneity corrections addresses this issue.

The 5-year survival rate is poor because of recurrent disease and invasion of the brain and skull. An overall survival rate is typically 20% to 30%, but with combined therapy survival may approach 75% for early-stage lesions.[14]

MANAGEMENT OF SYMPTOMS AND MORBIDITY

The incidence of morbidity is related to the treatment technique employed, the size of the irradiated volume, the time/dose fractionation scheme used, the location and the extent of the disease, and the patient's age and nutritional status. The early- and late-responding tissues are affected differently by these factors. The interaction of radiation in cells is random and has no selectivity for any structure or site. This forms the basis of the great challenge in radiation therapy.

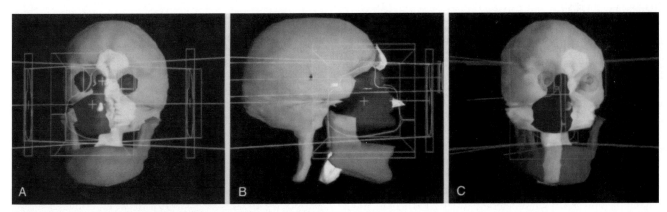

Figure 30-38. Three-dimensional beam's eye views: four-field technique using opposed lateral portals and anterior photon and electron portals. **A,** Anterior view. **B,** Lateral view. **C,** Oblique view. *(From Leibel S: Textbook of radiation oncology, Philadelphia, 1998, WB Saunders.)*

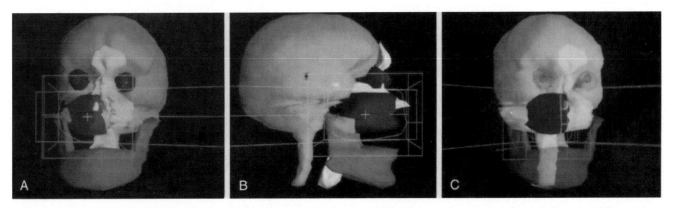

Figure 30-39. Three-dimensional beam's eye views: wedged-pair portals. **A,** Anterior view. **B,** lateral view. **C,** Oblique view. *(From Leibel S: Textbook of radiation oncology, Philadelphia, 1998, WB Saunders.)*

The amount of dose prescribed to eradicate a cancer ultimately is dependent on normal tissue tolerance. Radiosensitivity is the innate sensitivity of cells, tissues, or tumors to radiation. Both normal and cancer cells are affected by radiation. Cells vary in their expressed sensitivity to radiation. Generally, rapidly dividing cells are most sensitive (e.g., mucosa) and nondividing or slowly dividing cells generally are less radiosensitive or radioresistant (e.g., muscle cells, neurons). Exceptions include small lymphocytes and salivary gland cells, which are nondividing but are radiosensitive. The incidence of morbidity is also higher when radiation therapy and surgery are combined. The difficulties consist of delayed wound healing because of impaired blood supply and infection.[1] Specific curative doses for head and neck cancers are listed in Box 30-7. The tissue tolerance doses (TD 5/5 and TD 50/5), the radiation doses to which a normal tissues can be irradiated and continue to function, are listed in Table 30-3. The radiation therapist should know the dose limitations to the specific tissues included in the typical head and neck port. Table 30-3 provides an approximate dose-tissue response schedule for a conventional fractionation scheme. The student may also refer to the chapter on radiobiology (Chapter 4).

Periodontal Disease and Caries

Because healing is poor after treatment, extractions of carious teeth after radiation therapy is not recommended. Aggressive extractions after high doses can lead to osteoradionecrosis. The teeth should be extracted before radiation therapy if the patient has carious teeth.

Nutrition

At the time of diagnosis, many patients will have lost a significant amount of weight. Maintaining adequate nutrition is a major problem for these patients, because both the tumor and treatment side effects, such as mucositis from both chemotherapy and radiation therapy (after 2000 cGy to 3000 cGy), may contribute to this problem. Placement of a gastrostomy tube or nasogastric feeding may be required to maintain adequate nutrition.

Mucositis/Stomatitis

The epithelial cells of the mucous membrane lining the oral cavity are extremely radiosensitive. Inflammation of the oral mucous membranes with edema and tenderness can occur. A pseudomembrane may form along the mucosal surface. This membrane can slough off, leaving a friable, painful ulcerated surface. Areas that are adjacent to metallic tooth fillings within the treatment field may develop an increased reaction because of scatter radiation from the filling. Dental accessories may be available to eliminate scatter during treatment. Mouth care should involve avoiding drying agents, such as alcohol or glycerine-based products, and brushing and rinsing the oral cavity frequently. Instruct patient and family about an oral-care regimen and the need for routine follow-up with a dentist (Box 30-10).

Xerostomia

Xerostomia occurs after 1000 cGy to 2000 cGy and may be permanent after 4000 cGy, posing a significant long-term side effect. The patient then becomes at risk for dental caries and oral infections. When the salivary glands are within the treatment field, the saliva becomes scant and is thick and ropy. In some patients, pilocarpine hydrochloride (Salagen) has been useful in stimulating the production of saliva.[12] The use of saliva substitutes is required along with other oral lubricants; XeroLube or vegetable oils help decrease the sensation of mouth dryness. The use of reinforced daily fluoride application to the teeth may strengthen the tooth enamel and minimize dental caries.

Table 30-3	Approximate dose-tissue response schedule for a conventional fractionation scheme	
Response		**Dose (cGy)**
Dry mouth		2000
Erythema		2000
Brachial plexus		5500
Spinal cord		4500
Lhermitte's sign		2000-3000
Mandible, teeth and gums		5000-6000
Mucositis		3000
Ears		4000
Cataracts		500-1000
Dry eye		4000+
Optic nerve		5000
Retina		5000
Trismus		6000
Laryngitis		5000

Box 30-10	Recommended Oral-Hygiene Program

- Clean teeth and gums daily with a soft brush after meals.
- Use fluoride toothpaste or fluoride rinses daily.
- Floss daily.
- Rinse the mouth with salt and a baking-soda solution (1 qt water, 1/2 Tsp salt, 1/2 tsp baking soda).
- See a dentist regularly during treatment for a teeth and gum examination.
  To reduce the severity of any head and neck complication, the patient should be encouraged to avoid the following:
- Spicy hot foods, course or raw vegetables, dry crackers, chips, and nuts
- Smoking, chewing tobacco, and alcohol
- Sugary snacks
- Commercial mouthwash that contains alcohol because it drys the mouth
- Cold foods and drinks

Cataract Formation

One of the most radiosensitive tissues in the head and neck area is the lens of the eye, and formation of cataracts, which can be removed surgically, may develop following doses lower than 1000 cGy.[1]

Lacrimal Glands

Irradiation of the lacrimal gland may cause a dry painful eye. Severe dry-eye syndrome has been reported in 100% of patients receiving more that 5700 cGy. Obstruction to the tear duct, which is rare and usually associated with tumor involvement of the lacrimal duct, causes a constantly wet eye.[1]

Taste Changes

Treatment may affect the taste buds, which line the tongue and other parts of the oral cavity. The sensation affected (sweet, sour, salty, or bitter) varies; reports indicate that the sweet sensation is affected more than the salty sensation.[2] The incidence is dose dependent. The taste buds are radiosensitive; atrophy and degeneration is noted at 1000 cGy. Although some recovery may occur within a few months after treatment, many patients continue to report persistent taste changes for several months following irradiation. The therapist should educate the patient and family regarding temporary or permanent effects and maintenance of nutritional status. One should encourage the patient to identify and consume foods that have or retain some taste (sweet and sour foods retain some taste). Patients should be encouraged to chew foods longer to allow more contact of the food with the taste buds. The sense of taste and smell are closely linked. Because the olfactory senses are not affected, having the patient smell the food before eating it can give the sense of some taste.[2]

Skin Reactions

Most patients will experience some degree of acute skin effects. Affects vary depending on total dose, dose of daily fraction, type and energy of radiation used, the use of radiosensitizing/chemotherapy agents (methotrexate, 5-fluorouracil), the use of beam modifiers (bolus material), and individual differences among patients (complexity and nutrition). Reactions range from mild erythema or dryness to dry or moist desquamation. Adhering to principles of good wound care and maintaining a clean environment is recommended. Moisturizing lotions and gels can be applied to areas of dry desquamation, after consulting the radiation therapist, nurse, or oncologist. Hydrocortisone cream can be applied to irritated, inflamed skin but should not be used on areas of moist skin reactions because it may enhance infection.[2] Box 30-11 lists elements of a recommended skin care program.

ROLE OF THE RADIATION THERAPIST

The extent of radiation therapy side effects varies from patient to patient. During the initial consultation the radiation oncologist should inform the patient of all possible complications that can arise from the treatment or disease process; this is usually accomplished while completing an informed consent. The entire oncology team is responsible for assessing the efficiency of the treatment in terms of the health and well-being of the patient. The importance of adequate knowledge regarding treatment complications is to be emphasized to the radiation therapy student. The radiation therapist's role in patient assessment and as a gatekeeper to direct care or to avoid significant patient reactions (perhaps by interrupting treatment) depends on this knowledge.

Head and neck cancer patients need to know that the side effects encountered are site specific and dose dependent. Patients also need to understand that communicating any discomfort they are experiencing to the radiation therapists or other team members is vital to good cancer treatment management of the head and neck region. Radiation therapists should encourage patients to express any fears they have about the side effects; disease outcomes; or procedures that can alter speech, food intake, or breathing. Patients should also be informed that follow-up after treatment is an important aspect of head and neck cancer because they are at risk for a recurrence. Radiation therapists should give patients explicit instructions regarding physical changes to look for in tissue color, texture, new growths, or unexplained pain. Patients should be instructed to seek medical advice as soon as possible.

Soreness of the throat and mouth is expected to appear in the second or third week of standard fractionated external beam therapy. Minor irritations often remain for about a month after treatments end. Lidocaine (Xylocaine) viscus or dyclonine are good liquid pain relievers. Over-the-counter medication (approved by a physician) such as Ora-gel for babies and Ambusol can provide temporary relief.

Denture wearers may notice that the dentures no longer fit as a result of swelling of the gums. Loss of saliva is a common side effect of radiation to the oral cavity. Sipping cool carbonated drinks during the day may alleviate some of this.

Box 30-11	Recommended Skin-Care Program

- Wash the skin with lukewarm water, pat dry, and do not wash off marks.
- Use mild soaps (e.g., Basis, Neutrogena).
- Use water-based lotions or creams (e.g., Aquaphor, Eucerin).
- Avoid lotions with perfume and deodorants.
- Avoid direct sunlight.
- Do not use straight razors.
- Avoid tight-fitting collars and hat brims.
- Do not use aftershave lotions or perfumes.
- Apply only nonadherent, hydrophilic dressings to wounds.

Lemon drops (sugar free) help promote saliva production and taste. The radiation therapist should instruct the patient to choose foods that are easy to eat. As chewing and swallowing become more difficult, the therapist should recommend more liquid, semisolid meals moistened with sauces and gravies to make eating easier. Artificial saliva is a possible remedy; a physician should be consulted.

The cancer care team including the therapist should instruct the patient about wound care, cleaning of tracheostomies, and speech-rehabilitation options. The therapist should be mindful of any weeping surgical sites or a change in the healing process that can indicate an infection. Proper skin care during treatment is an important aspect of patient care management. To better facilitate communication with a speech-impaired patient, the therapist should provide a pad and pencil. Hand signals should be arranged with the patient in the event something goes wrong in the treatment room during beam-on conditions. The radiation therapist must understand that the head and neck cancer patient will undergo some structural and functional losses; the therapist should be ready to answer any questions or provide for the specific needs of the patient.

FUTURE DIRECTIONS

Greater results in radiation therapy my be achieved by the use of techniques such as 3D conformal therapy (including IMRT), proton-beam therapy, or intracavitary boost delivery for limited tumors. A report on proton-beam therapy for nasopharyngeal tumors has shown promising results. It suggests that the use of proton beams result in a significant increase in dose with increased sparing to normal tissue. The high cost and time-consuming planning is noted to be a disadvantage.[7] An example of the advantages of 3D conformal therapy has been cited in the section for maxillary tumors. Computer-assisted multileaf collimators with a real-time portal imaging device allow the delivery of multiple beams with minimal human interventions. This development adds to available quality assurance, which is growing in importance as treatment volumes become more specific with escalating doses. Intracavitary brachytherapy has allowed the delivery of higher doses to the tumor. Local control has been reported to be enhanced. In a recent review on nasopharyngeal brachytherapy, the results of boost brachytherapy after external irradiation were promising but should be confirmed in a large-scale randomized trial.[7] Fast neutrons have been investigated clinically; potential advantages over photons include less dependence on tumor oxygenation, less absorption of bone, and shorter overall treatment time. Results of treatment for primary or recurrent unresectable (T4) tumors of the paranasal sinus include complete regression in 86% of cases with local control to 68%. The disadvantages included adverse skin reactions, blindness, or pain development, although overall local control rates are as high as 88%. Clinical trials of neutron treatment to salivary gland tumors show great advantages as well.[7]

Review Questions

1. Multiple tumor types are included in the head and neck region. Which type of primary tumor is most common?
   a. Adenocarcinoma
   b. Squamous cell carcinoma
   c. Basal cell carcinoma
   d. Fibrosarcoma

2. The primary lymphatic drainage of the lower lip would be to
   a. Submental nodes
   b. Submaxillary nodes
   c. Subdigastric node
   d. The posterior cervical chain

3. What normal organ would be at most risk of radiation damage when treating the maxillary antrum?
   a. Brain
   b. Eye
   c. Skin
   d. Pituitary

4. The most common sign/symptom of oral cancer is
   a. Ulceration
   b. Hoarseness
   c. Odynophagia
   d. Xerostomia

5. The most commonly involved group of nodes in oropharyngeal cancer is the
   a. Submandibular nodes
   b. Retropharyngeal nodes
   c. Jugulodigastric nodes
   d. Supraclavicular nodes

6. In glottic cancer, a tumor confined to the larynx with cord fixation is staged as a
   a. T1
   b. T2
   c. T3
   d. T4

7. Palpation of the cricoid cartilage indicates the inferior border of the
   a. Oral cavity
   b. Oropharynx
   c. Larynx
   d. Hypopharynx

8. For patients with carious teeth, when is dental work recommended when anticipating oral cavity irradiation?
   a. Following treatment
   b. Preceding treatment
   c. Both a and b
   d. Neither a nor b

9. Parotid gland tumors may be treated with which of the following treatment techniques?
   a. Wedged-pair technique (superior-inferior combination)

b. Ipsilateral photon and high-energy electron combination
c. Opposed lateral field
d. All of the above

10. Tumors of the head and neck may involve the cranial nerves that control our major senses. This may lead to signs and symptoms that can point to a possible location of a tumor. The cranial nerve that may be involved in facial paralysis is the cranial nerve.
   a. XII
   b. I
   c. VIII
   d. VII

Questions to Ponder

1. Most head and neck cancers are grouped together by anatomic site. Why then is there such diverse difference in biologic and clinical behavior between the same cell type and structures that are only a few millimeters apart?

2. What is the reason for the high incidence of a second primary for patients with early-stage squamous cell disease that was cured?

3. Are there biologic markers that can be identified early and will decrease the toxicity and morbidity from treatments?

4. Will nonstandard radiation therapy fractionation schemes improve survivability at the expense of second malignancies?

5. Does chemotherapy have a role in the elective treatment of premalignant conditions seen in head and neck disease?

REFERENCES

1. Bentel GC: *Radiation therapy planning,* ed 2, New York, 1996, McGraw-Hill.
2. Bruner DW: *Manual for radiation oncology nursing practice and education,* Pittsburgh, 1998, Oncology Nursing Press.
3. Bruner DW: *Outcomes in radiation therapy: multidisciplinary management,* Boston, 2001, Jones & Bartlett.
4. Cox JD, Ang KK: *Radiation oncology: rationale, technique, results,* ed 8, St. Louis, 2003, Mosby.
5. Dimitroulis G: *Oral cancer: a synopsis of pathology and management,* Boston, 1998, Butterworth-Heinemann.
6. Fajardo LF: *Radiation pathology,* New York, 2001, Oxford.
7. Harrison LB: *Head and neck cancer: a multidisciplinary approach,* Philadelphia, 1999, Lippincott.
8. Khan F: *Treatment planning in radiation oncology,* Philadelphia, 2000, Lippincott.
9. Leibel S: *Textbook of radiation,* Philadelphia, 1998, Saunders.
10. Lenhard E, Osteen R, Gansler T: *American Cancer Society's clinical oncology,* Atlanta, 2001, American Cancer Society.
11. Levitt S: *Levitt and Tapley's: technological basis of radiation therapy: clinical applications,* ed 3, Philadelphia, 1999, Lippincott.
12. Pazdur R: *Cancer management: a multidisciplinary approach,* ed 5, New York, 2001, PRR.
13. Perez CA: *Principles and practice of radiation oncology,* ed 3, Philadelphia, 1998, Lippincott.
14. Rubin P: *Clinical oncology: a multidisciplinary approach for physicians and students,* ed 8, Philadelphia, 2001, Saunders.
15. Silverman S: *Oral cancer,* ed 4, Hamilton, Ontario, 1998, BC Decker.

BIBLIOGRAPHY

DeVita V: *Cancer: principles and practice of oncology,* Philadelphia, 2001, Lippincott.
Mills S: *Tumor of the upper aerodigestive tract and ear,* 2000, Armed Forces Institute of Pathology.
Myers E: *Cancer of the head and neck,* Philadelphia, 1996, Saunders.
Rice D: *Surgical pathology of the head and neck,* Philadelphia, 2000, Lippincott.

Central Nervous System

Robert D. Adams, Linda Langlin, Dennis Leaver

Outline

Key Terms

Blood-brain barrier (BBB)
Cerebellum
Cerebrospinal fluid (CSF)
Cerebrum
Debulking
Edema
Gamma knife
Intracranial pressure (ICP)
Karnofsky Performance Scale
  (KPS)
Necrosis
Papilledema
Positron emission tomography
  (PET)
Radiation necrosis
Radiosensitizers
Regeneration
Tentorium
Ventricles

Central nervous system (CNS) tumors include brain and spinal cord tumors. The tumors can be primary or secondary (metastatic) and benign or malignant. Some are regarded as benign because of slow growth rates and their response to therapy.[20]

In recent years, radiation therapy has played a significant role in the treatment of CNS tumors, provided a means of increased survival time, resulted in a regression of the effects of neurologic deficit, and enhanced the quality of life of many patients with brain tumors.[15]

Although CNS tumors rarely metastasize, they are often locally invasive and create significant problems. Structures that become involved with these neoplasms are not capable of **regeneration** (repair or regrowth). Tumors of the CNS, even if benign histologically, are considered malignant in part because of their inaccessible location.[19] As shown in Table 31-1, many different cell types are believed to produce CNS and spinal axis tumors. Because CNS tumors arise in different areas of the cranium and spinal axis, the belief is that different molecular and genetic mechanisms are at work during various times of life.

CANCER OF THE CNS

Epidemiology

Approximately 18,300 cases of primary brain tumors and other nervous system tumors are diagnosed annually in the United States. Brain tumors account for 1.5% of all malignancies. About 80% of CNS tumors involve the brain, whereas 20% involve the spinal cord. Primary CNS neoplasms result in 11,000 deaths annually.

The incidence rate is 5 per 100,000 people and varies according to race, gender, and age. Brain tumors are the second leading cause of death in children (behind leukemia).

Table 31-1	Classification of tumors of the central nervous system

I. Neuroepithelial tumors
    Astrocytic tumors
    Astrocytoma
    Anaplastic astrocytoma
    Glioblastoma
    Oligodendroglial tumors
    Oligodendroglioma
    Anaplastic oligodendroglioma
    Ependymal tumors
    Ependymoma
    Anaplastic ependymoma
    Mixed gliomas
    Oligoastrocytoma
    Anaplastic oligoastrocytoma
II. Choroid plexus tumors
III. Neurologic tumors
    Ganglioglioma
    Anaplastic ganglioglioma
    Neurocytoma
IV. Pineal parenchymal tumors
    Pineocytoma
    Pineoblastoma
V. Embryonal tumors
VI. Medulloepithelioma
    Ependymoblastoma
    Primitive neuroectodermal tumors (PNET)

VI. Tumors of the cranial /spinal nerves
    Schwannoma (neurilemoma)
    Neurofibroma
VII. Tumors of the meninges
    Atypical meningioma
    Anaplastic meningioma
VIII. Mesenchymal tumors, benign
IX. Mesenchymal tumors, malignant
    Hemangiopericytoma
    Chondrosarcoma
    Malignant fibrous histiocytoma
    Rhabdomyosarcoma
X. Uncertain histologies
    Hemangioblastoma
XI. Hemopoietic neoplasms
    Malignant lymphomas
    Plasmacytoma
XII. Cysts/tumorlike lesions
    Rathke cleft cyst
    Epidermoid cyst
    Dermoid cyst
XIII. Sellar tumors
    Pituitary adenoma
    Caniopharyngioma

Modified from Wara WM, Bauman GS, Sneed PK et al: Brain, brain stem and cerebellum. In Perez C, Brady L, editors: *Principles and practice of radiation oncology,* ed 3, Philadelphia, 1998, Lippincott-Raven.

Age is a dominant variable, with the incidence of CNS tumors in older patients appearing to rise. Nelson et al.[19] attributes this increase to three possible factors: (1) an increase in life expectancy, (2) the increasing availability and use of computed tomography (CT) and magnetic resonance imaging (MRI), and (3) an increased interest in geriatrics and an overall improvement in health care of the elderly. Most CNS tumors occur in persons between the ages of 50 and 80. The incidence is higher than 20 per 100,000 for older men and fewer than 2 per 100,000 for children younger than 15.[15] Most brain tumors occur in two age peaks: childhood (3 to 12 years) and later in life.[10,25]

Many different tumors types are included in the CNS category. However, gliomas comprise 50% of all primary brain tumors in adults.[17] The most common location of these tumors is the **cerebrum,** which is the largest part of the brain and consists of two hemispheres (Fig. 31-1). The functions of the cerebrum include interpretation of sensory impulses and voluntary muscular activities; it is the center for memory, learning, reasoning, judgment, intelligence, and emotions. Gliomas commonly occur in persons between the ages of 40 and 74.[18]

Approximately 45% of childhood tumors are gliomas

with most involving the **cerebellum** and to a lesser degree the brainstem (Fig. 31-1). The cerebellum is the part of the brain that plays a role in the coordination of voluntary muscular movements.

Primary brain tumors are relatively uncommon. However, cerebral metastases occur in approximately 30% of patients with cancer and are the most common brain lesions. The most common primary site of disease responsible for producing brain metastases is the lung. Most metastatic lesions occur in the cerebral hemispheres. Single metastases occur 40% to 45% of the time. Brain metastases may be the only indication of malignant disease. These metastases can occur early in the disease process or may not appear until years later.

Long-term survival for patients with CNS tumors is uncommon.[23] Factors such as the patient's age, Karnofsky Performance Status, and neurologic signs and symptoms at the time of diagnosis are important in the chances for survival.

Most spinal-axis tumors are extradural (on the outside of or unconnected to the dura mater). They are predominantly metastatic carcinomas, lymphomas, or sarcomas; they are rarely chordomas. Most primary spinal-axis tumors are intradural (within or enclosed by the dura mater).

Etiology

Little is known concerning the cause, development, and growth mechanisms of CNS tumors. Increasingly, a genetic link is thought to exist. Weingart and Brem[24] have noted recent reports implicating several growth factors, protein kinase C, and the *p53* gene with tumor growth and progression. However, absolute proof of a genetic predisposition for all CNS tumors in unavailable. According to Filippini and Artuso,[11] fewer than 1% of patients are known to have inherited disorders, although certain genetic disorders have been associated with CNS tumors.

Tuberous sclerosis (a disease involving the CNS and cutaneous sites) is associated with astrocytomas, glioblastomas, ependymomas, and ganglioneuromas. von Recklinghausen's disease is associated with meningiomas, multiple ependymomas, and optic gliomas. It is marked by the occurrence of multiple neurofibromata on the skin along the course of the nerves. von Hippel–Lindau disease is associated with hemangioblastomas and characterized by lesions involving the retina, the cerebellum, and sometimes the spinal cord. Brain tumors are also associated with polyposis coli in Turcot's syndrome.

Because gliomas are the most common type of CNS tumors, they have received the most attention in studies focusing on the identification of amplified genes. The first gene shown to be amplified was the *epidermal growth factor receptor (EGFR)* gene.[8] Cytogenic observation provided the first evidence that gene amplification may be occurring in glioblastomas. Studies have now shown that gene amplification occurs in up to 50% of glioblastomas.[3,4]

The *p53* gene on chromosome 17 encodes a nuclear phosphoprotein that may be a suppressor gene. Gliomas have been associated with mutations and deletions of chromosome 17. Studies indicate that this occurs more often in high-grade than low-grade gliomas. These mutations and deletions are also involved in tumor progression from low- to high-grade gliomas.[24]

Chromosome abnormalities have been identified in high-grade and low-grade tumors. Studies to date suggest that low-grade tumors tend to have fewer chromosome abnormalities than high-grade tumors.[18,19]

Protein kinase C has also been associated with the growth of gliomas. Activity rates of protein kinase C are increased in malignant gliomas compared with normal brain and are associated with increased proliferation rates.

Environmental factors also may play a role in the cause of CNS tumors. The association between chemical exposure and brain tumors is limited to a few occupations. People exposed to pesticides, herbicides, and fertilizers and workers in the petrochemical industries and health professions have demonstrated a higher incidence rate than normal. The only documented link associates gliomas with vinyl chloride and rubber manufacturing industries. The incidence of increased brain tumors has been the same for both genders in most countries; therefore occupational exposure is not a likely explanation for the increases.[13] Studies revealing potential links to *N*-nitroso compounds, power magnetic fields, dental amalgams, x-rays, and passive smoking have generated considerable interest.[1] None of these links have been validated, but occupational exposure to metals, paints, and some hydrocarbons may be associated with excess risks that contribute to parental exposure as an added risk for the later development of CNS tumors. Excessive numbers of tumors have resulted from postnatal exposure to high doses of irradiation for tinea capitis, which is a fungus skin disease of the scalp similar to ringworm.

Viral infections have recently been associated with the development of CNS neoplasia in animals. Immunocompromised patients who have CNS lymphomas also have a high incidence of the Epstein-Barr virus. Trauma does not seem to influence the incidence to CNS neoplasia.

Only a small incidence of CNS tumors occurring after treatment for another malignancy has been documented. Patients with acquired immunodeficiency syndrome (AIDS) and those receiving transplants have an increased risk for primary CNS lymphoma, but not for gliomas. Because these patients are immunologically compromised, whether this problem is a cause or an effect needs further investigation.

Prognostic Indicators

Several factors have been identified as prognostic indicators for CNS disorders. The three most important factors are age, the performance status, and tumor type. In numerous clinical trials involving malignant gliomas, these prognostic factors have had a greater influence on survival than the type or extent of the therapy being evaluated. Unfortunately, one of the most common adult brain tumors, glioblastoma multiforme (GBM), is one of the most lethal and, despite years of clinical research, progress has been slow and disappointing.[19]

The prognosis tends to be better in younger patients, with one exception. Children younger than of 4 present a particular problem with respect to a treatment regimen. Therapy must be modified because of the developing brain, which is more sensitive to radiation; therefore radiation treatment in children younger than 4 years must be avoided if possible.

Doses may be modified to prevent later learning difficulties. Late effects after CNS treatment in children is an area of concern. A study by Avizonis et al[2] focused on several areas of interest. Mean IQ scores after treatment indicated slightly decreased scores as whole-brain dose radiation increased. However, learning disabilities can be overcome so that the children can go on to lead productive lives. Another area monitored in the study, the regrowth of hair, appeared to be dose related, with diminished regrowth as the dose increased. The measured late effects after radiation did not seem to vary with regard to age at the time of treatment, gender, tumor type, or tumor location.

The mortality rate for both genders and for blacks and whites has increased since 1950, and that trend seems to be continuing. The mortality rate for adolescents and young adults remains unchanged or has decreased slightly over the past 30 years.

The location of the tumor is of great importance, serving as a natural prognostic indicator for survival time and neurologic deficits. In addition, **the Karnofsky Performance Scale (KPS)** measures the neurologic and functional status, allowing for measurements of the quantity and quality of neurologic defects. The KPS ranges from 0 to 100 and is measured in decades. Patients who are able to work have scores in the 80, 90, or 100 range. Patients who are unable to work but can still care for themselves have scores in the 50 to 70 range (Box 31-1). Patients who are chronically ill from the disease process have scores of 40 or below.

Tumor grade rather than size is the primary factor involved with prognosis. The tumors are normally grouped into benign or low-grade and malignant or high-grade categories. The presence or absence of necrosis in a tumor has prognostic significance. **Necrosis** is the death of a cell or cell group resulting from disease or injury. The process is caused by the action of enzymes and can also affect part of a structure or an organ.

Low-grade tumors have cellularity patterns that look similar to those found in reactive hyperplasia, whereas marked cellularity has been recognized in high-grade tumors, with necrosis seen in the most aggressive tumors. Typically, the higher the grade, the shorter the survival time.

Almost all patients experience a recurrence (with high-grade tumors) postoperatively, and 80% of all recurrences are within a 2-cm margin.[5]

Tumor type and especially the grade of the tumor have the most profound influence on the prognosis of patients with brain tumors.

Anatomy and Lymphatics

The brain is one of the most complex organs in the body (Fig. 31-1). It is composed of two cerebral hemispheres and two cerebellar hemispheres. The cranial bones, meninges, and **cerebrospinal fluid (CSF)** provide an outer covering of protection for the brain.

The **ventricles** are cavities that form a communication network with each other, the center canal of the spinal cord, and the subarachnoid space. They are filled with CSF. These cavities are the right and left lateral ventricles and the third and fourth ventricles. The lateral ventricles are located below the corpus callosum and extend from front to back. Each opens into the third ventricle. The lateral ventricles are able to communicate with the third ventricle via the interventricular foramen, which is a small oval opening. The third ventricle is connected to the fourth ventricle. The fourth ventricle lies between the cerebellum and inferior brainstem. Three small openings also allow the CSF to pass into the subarachnoid space. The openings also allow communication

Box 31-1 Karnofsky Performance Scale

PERFORMANCE CRITERIA

Able to carry on normal activity; no special care needed	100	Normal; no complaints; no evidence of disease
	90	Ability to carry on normal activity; minor signs or symptoms of disease
	80	Normal activity with effort; some signs or symptoms of disease
Unable to work; able to live at home and care for most personal needs; a varying amount of assistance needed	70	Self-care; inability to carry on normal activity or do active work
	60	Occasional care for most needs required
	50	Considerable assistance and frequent medical care required
	40	Disabled; special care and assistance required
Unable to care for self; required equivalent of institutional or hospital care; disease may be progressing rapidly	30	Severely disabled; hospitalization indicated, although death not imminent
	20	Extremely sick; hospitalization necessary; active supportive treatment necessary
	10	Moribund; fatal processes progressing rapidly
	0	Dead

PERFORMANCE SCALE (EASTERN COOPERATIVE ONCOLOGY GROUP)

Grade
0 Fully active; able to carry on all predisease activities without restriction (Karnofsky score of 90 to 100)
1 Restricted in physically strenuous activity, but ambulatory and able to carry out work of a light or sedentary nature, such as light housework or office work (Karnofsky score of 70 to 80)
3 Capable of only limited self-care; confined to bed or chair 50% or more of waking hours (Karnofsky score of 30 to 40)
4 Completely disabled; Unable to carry on any self-care; totally confined to bed or chair (Karnofsky score of 10 to 20)

Modified from Carter S et al: *Principles of cancer treatment,* New York, 1982, McGraw-Hill.

with the cord and subarachnoid space (Fig. 31-1).

The supratentorial and infratentorial regions comprise the two major intracranial compartments, the cerebral and cerebellar hemispheres. The **tentorium** (a fold of dura mater, or the outer covering of the brain) separates these compartments. It passes transversely across the posterior cranial fossa in the transverse fissure and acts as a line of separation

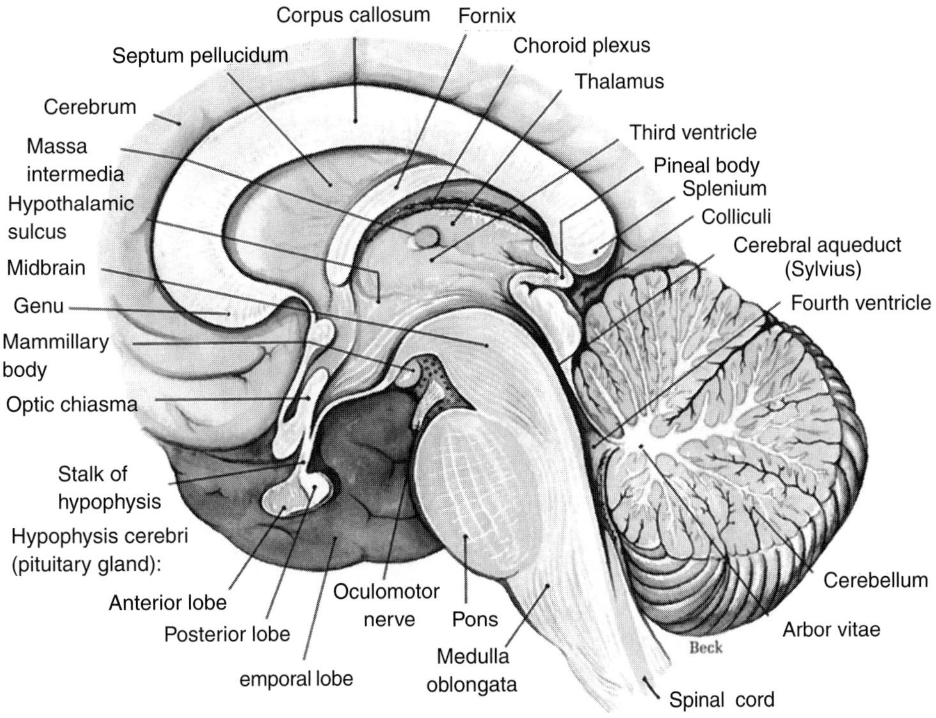

Figure 31-1. Sagittal section through the midline of the brain. *(From del Regato JA, Spjut HJ, Cox JD: Ackerman and del Regato's: cancer: diagnosis, treatment, and prognosis, ed 6, St. Louis, 1985, Mosby.)*

between the occipital lobe of the cerebrum and the upper cerebellum. The cerebral hemispheres and the sella, pineal, and upper brainstem regions are located in the supratentorial region. The infratentorial region, which leads to the upper spinal cord, houses the brainstem, pons, medulla, and cerebellum.

The CNS is composed of 40% grey matter and 60% white matter. The grey matter contains the supportive nerve cells and related processes. It forms the cortex, or outer part of the cerebrum, and surrounds the white matter. The white matter is composed of bundles of nerve fibers, axons carrying impulses away from the cell body, and dendrites carrying impulses toward the cell body. The nerve cells process and integrate nerve impulses from other neurons. The spinal cord is also composed of a grey substance that forms the inner core, which contains the nerve cells. The outer layer, or white substance, is the location of the nerve fibers. The grey matter varies at different levels of the spinal cord.

The blood supply for the brain comes from the internal carotid arteries and vertebral arteries via the circle of Willis. The blood that enters the brain contains oxygen, nutrients, and energy-rich glucose, which is the primary source of energy for the brain cells. If the blood supply to the brain is interrupted, dizziness, convulsions, or mental confusion may result.

The spinal cord is the continuation of the medulla oblon-

gata and forms the inferior portion of the brainstem. The anterior and lateral portions contain motor neurons and tracts, whereas the posterior portions contain the sensory tracts. The motor neurons are nerve cells that convey impulses from the brain to the cord. This system allows communication between the spinal cord and various parts of the brain. The cord continues down to the level of the first and second lumbar vertebrae. This is an important anatomic reference point for the radiation therapy student. Many times doses to the spinal cord must be calculated, and it is important to have an understanding of where the spinal cord ends. From the spinal cord come 31 pairs of nerves. The spinal cord is surrounded by the same material that surrounds the brain. The CSF flows between the arachnoid and pia arachnoid. Blood is supplied to the cord from the vertebral arteries and radicular branches of the cervical, intercostal, lumbar, and sacral arteries (Fig. 31-2). No lymphatic channels exist in the brain substance.

The **blood-brain barrier (BBB),** which hinders the penetration of some substances into the brain and CSF, exists between the vascular system and brain. Its purpose is to protect the brain from potentially toxic compounds. Substances that can pass through the BBB must be lipid soluble. Water-soluble substances require a carrier molecule to cross the barrier by active transport. Lipid-soluble substances include alcohol, nicotine, and heroin. Examples of water-soluble

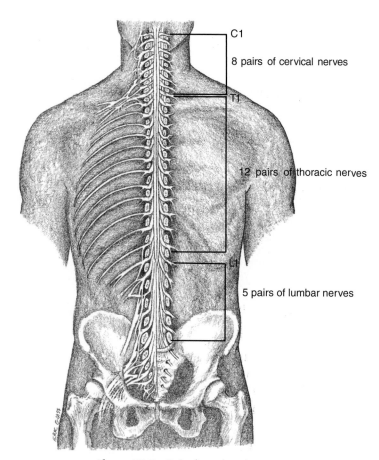

C1

8 pairs of cervical nerves

T1

12 pairs of thoracic nerves

L1

5 pairs of lumbar nerves

Figure 31-2. Spinal cord and nerves.

substances are glucose, some amino acids, and sodium. Various drugs pass the barrier with varying degrees of difficulty but never easily. Tumor cells infiltrating normal brain tissue cannot be reached by drugs that do not cross the BBB (Fig. 31-3).

The CSF is a clear, colorless fluid resembling water. The entire CNS contains 3 to 5 oz of this fluid, which is composed of proteins, glucose, urea (a compound formed in the liver and excreted by the kidney), and salts. The CSF performs several functional roles, including buoyancy to protect the brain, a link in the control of the chemical environment of the CNS, a means of exchanging nutrients and waste products with the CNS, and a channel for intracerebral transport. Blockage of CSF, because of tumor growth, may have disastrous effects on the patient. If the flow of CSF is interrupted it may contribute to increased **intracranial pressure (ICP),** which is pressure that occurs within the cranium.

Natural History of Disease and Patterns of Spread

With few exceptions, most gliomas tend to spread invasively because they do not form a natural capsule that inhibits growth. These neoplasms are unique because they do not metastasize through a lymphatic drainage system and rarely metastasize outside the CNS unlike many epithelial tumors and tumors of connective tissue origin that commonly metastasize to lymph nodes and other distant anatomic locations. The common route of spread for medulloblastomas and primitive neuroectodermal tumors (PNETs) is via CSF to points in the CNS.

Local invasion and CSF seeding provide the major patterns of spread for CNS tumors. These tumors tend to have cells that can invade normal brain. Drop metastases occur via the CSF and can form secondary tumors. The confines of the brain itself limit the spread of disease, but local recurrence is a major concern. Secondary seeding may grow along nerve roots, causing pain or cord compression. Although the lumbosacral area is the most frequent site of CSF seeding, any area along the spinal axis can become involved. Hematogenous spread is rare.

CNS tumors are characterized by their heterogeneity, which makes understanding their biology difficult.[16] With an improved understanding of the reason and way that CNS tumors develop, grow, and progress, new treatment approaches can be developed and implemented.

Clinical Presentation

As stated, the location of the tumor correlates with the presenting symptoms. Table 31-2 provides an excellent correlation between common symptoms and tumor location. The

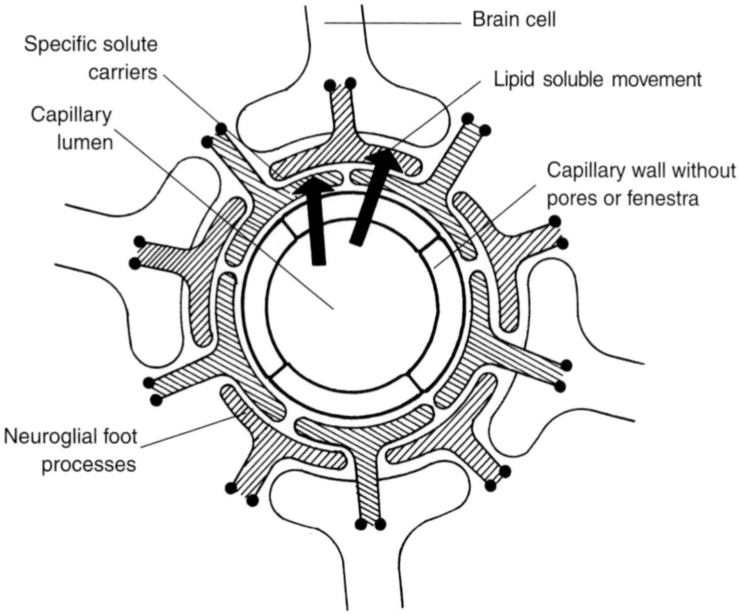

Figure 31-3. Blood-brain barrier. *(Redrawn from Maisey M, Britton KE, Gilday DL: Clinical nuclear medicine, ed 2, New York, 1992, Chapman and Hall.)*

initial symptom may be a headache, which is usually worse in the morning. This is due to the differences in the CSF drainage from the recumbent to upright positions. Seizures and difficulties with balance, gait, and ambulation are also common presenting signs. Focal signs are usually unilateral. Other neurologic symptoms can include aphasia, hemiplegia, and paresis. Ocular symptoms may result in decreased vision, oculomotor defects, proptosis, and ophthalmic defects. Other presenting signs may be expressive aphasia, sensory aphasia, mental and personality changes, short-term memory loss, hallucinations, and changes in intellectual functions. Increased ICP can result from the obstruction of CSF flow. The symptoms can result from direct invasion of the tissue by the tumor, destruction of brain tissue and bone, and increased pressure.

Patients with spinal cord tumors have pain, weakness, loss of sensation, and bowel- and bladder-control problems. Although pain may be an early symptom, additional symptoms may signal a cord compression or vascular problems. Weakness usually occurs in the distal part of the extremity first and progresses proximally. Rapid deterioration of motor and sensory functions soon follows. Immediate treatment is required for patients who have a sudden onset of symptoms so that permanent paralysis may be prevented (Table 31-3). In contrast to brain lesions, the symptoms are more frequently bilateral.

Detection and Diagnosis

The initial workup is critical to a definitive diagnosis, and a complete history and physical examination are necessary. Because some CNS tumors are genetic, associated with

exposure to chemicals, or related to infection, previous medical, family, and social histories are extremely important.

Information gathered from people other than the patient may also be beneficial in making a diagnosis. Mental changes, personality changes, and changes in behavior are not often noticed by the patient but are noticed by other individuals. Symptoms of long duration may indicate a slow-growing tumor, whereas the sudden onset of symptoms may point toward a tumor of higher grade and size.

A neurologic workup includes an evaluation in several key areas. The patient's mental status at the time of the diagnosis often reflects changes in behavior, mood, thought and speech patterns, and intelligence. Intellectual function is crucial, and the level of consciousness must be evaluated quickly. One test for intellectual function includes orientation to person, place, and time and the quickness of the responses to these questions. Further intellectual functions are determined by studying speech, memory, and logical thought processes.

Coordination skills (including walking, balance, and gait), sensations, reflexes, and motor skills are also examined. Lesions that inhibit motor function tend to affect fine motor skills first and produce a spastic paralysis. Sensory functions can be tested with a pin, temperature, and vibrations. These functions can be affected before motor skills. Reflexes may be hyperactive with intracranial tumors early but may become hypoactive in later stages.

If spinal cord tumors are suspected, the evaluation of motor, sensory, and reflex functions is also important. Sensory testing is helpful in determining the level of the lesion. Motor testing may reveal weakness.

Table 31-2

Symptoms, signs, and diagnostic characteristics of various intracranial tumors

Tumor	Common Symptoms	Common Signs	Diagnostic Characteristics*
PRIMARY			
Malignant astrocytoma	Headache, seizure, unilateral weakness, mental changes	Focal presentation related to tumor location	Enhancing CT lesion, tumor blush on angiography
Glioblastoma multiforme (GM)			Hypodense interior of enhanced CT lesion
Astrocytoma with anaplastic foci (AAF)			No hypodense interior enhanced CT lesion
Brain stem or thalamus	Nausea, vomiting, ataxia	Increased intracranial pressure (papilledema), abducens and oculomotor nerve defects	May not enhance on CT scan; biopsy may not be appropriate
Meningioma (B, M)	Localized headache, seizure	Focal presentation related to tumor location	Enhancing CT lesion associated with dura
Astrocytoma (B, M)	Headache, seizure, unilateral weakness, mental changes	Focal presentation related to tumor location	May not enhance on CT
Cerebral	Headache, seizure, unilateral weakness, mental changes	Focal presentation related to tumor location	
Cerebellar	Occipital headache	Increased intracranial pressure (papilledema), abducens and oculomotor nerve defects, coordination	
Brain stem or thalamus	Nausea, vomiting, ataxia	Increased intracranial pressure (papilledema), abducens and oculomotor nerve defects, coordination	May be seen only on MR image biopsy may not be appropriate
Optic nerve	Ocular changes	Ocular changes	Detailed CT scan
Pituitary (B, M)	Vertex headache, ocular changes	Ocular and endocrine abnormalities	Hormone analysis, resection histopathology
Medulloblastoma (M)	Morning headaches, nausea, vomiting	Coordination, increased intracranial pressure (papilledema), abducens and oculomotor nerve defects	CT scan, careful lumbar puncture recommended
Ependymoma (B, M)	Morning headaches, nausea, vomiting	Coordination, increased intracranial pressure (papilledema), abducens and oculomotor nerve defects	CT scan, careful lumbar puncture recommended
Hemangioma, arteriovenous malformation (B, M)	Migrainous headache	Focal presentation related to tumor location	Angiography, biopsy may not be appropriate
Neurilemoma, schwannoma, neurinoma (B, M)	Unilateral deafness, vertigo	Ipsilateral acoustic and facial or trigeminal nerve defects	CT scan, resection gives histopathology
Oligodendroglioma (B, M)	Insidious headache, mental changes	Focal presentation related to tumor location	Radiographic calcification
Sarcoma (M), neurofibroma (B)	Focal presentation related to tumor location	Focal presentation related to tumor location	
Pinealoma (B, M), dysgerminoma	Various (ocular, vestibular, endocrine)	Parinaud's syndrome, endocrine changes, ocular changes, increased intracranial pressure (papilledema), abducens and oculomotor nerve defects	Biopsy or resection may not be obtained, markers in CSF misinformative
Lymphoma (M), reticulum cell sarcoma, microglioma	Focal presentation related to tumor location	Focal presentation related to tumor location	Soft CT enhancement
Unspecified (B, M)	Focal presentation related to tumor location	Focal presentation related to tumor location	
OTHER			
Craniopharyngioma	Headache, mental changes, hemiplegia, seizure, vomiting (and ocular changes)	Cranial nerve defects (II-VII)	Bone erosion, mass effective for base of skull
Syringomyelia, syringobulbia	Pain, weakness	Sensory level, paresis	MR imaging, CT scan, myelogram, biopsy not appropriate
Midline granuloma syndrome, lymphoid granulomatosis	Various (ocular, vestibular, endocrine)	Various (ocular, vestibular, endocrine)	Diagnosis presumed
Arachnoiditis		Fasciculations	

Modified from Wara WM, et al: Brain, brain stem and cerebellum. In Perez C, Brady, editors: *Principles and practice of radiation oncology,* ed 3, Philadelphia, 1998, Lippincott-Raven.

*Unless noted, a biopsy is assumed.

B, Benign; *M,* malignant; *CT,* computed tomography; *MR,* Magnetic resonance, *CSF,* cerebrospinal fluid.

Table 31-3	Clinical manifestations of spinal cord tumors
Location	**Findings**
Foramen magnum	Eleventh and twelfth cranial nerve palsies; ipsilateral arm weakness early; cerebellar ataxia; neck pain
Cervical spine	Ipsilateral arm weakness with leg and opposite arm in time; wasting and fibrillation of ipsilateral neck, shoulder girdle, and arm; decreased pain and temperature sensation in upper cervical regions early; pain in cervical distribution
Thoracic spine	Weakness of abdominal muscles; sparing of arms; unilateral root pains; sensory level with ipsilateral changes early and bilateral with time
Lumbosacral spine	Root pain in groin region and sciatic distribution; weakened proximal pelvic muscles; impotence; bladder paralysis; decreased knee jerk and brisk ankle jerks
Cauda equina	Unilateral pain in back and leg, becoming bilateral when the tumor is large; bladder and bowel paralysis

Modified from Levins V, Guten P, Leibel S: Neoplasms of CNS. In DeVita VT, Hellman S, Rosenberg SA: *Cancer: principles and practice of oncology,* ed 4, Philadelphia, 1993, JB Lippincott.

Ophthalmoscopy is a test designed to check for **papilledema** (edema of the optic disc), which results from increased ICP. Visual fields may decrease and blind spots increase as the disease progresses. An increase in ICP is usually the result of the flow of CSF becoming obstructed. This can indicate an increase in the tumor mass. If CSF flow is obstructed or production of the fluid is changed, hydrocephalus may appear on CT scans. Infection, **edema** (swelling caused by the abnormal accumulation of fluid in interstitial spaces), or hemorrhage may also cause rising pressure.

Invasion, irritation, and compression of the brain by the tumor cause symptoms. Benign tumors generally cause symptoms produced by pressure, whereas malignant tumors can cause pressure and destruction of CNS tissue The initial presentation of symptoms depends on different anatomic locations. The involvement of specific regions of the brain generally produces symptoms specific to the areas controlled by those regions, thereby making tumor localization possible (Table 31-4).

Therefore patients typically have symptoms that reflect the site of involvement. For example, if a tumor occurs in the frontal portion of the brain, symptoms likely to be identified include personality changes, memory defects, gait disorders, and speech difficulties. Lesions occurring in the parietal regions of the brain can produce symptoms such as loss of vision, spatial disorientation, and seizures.

Radiographs of the skull may show several changes that have occurred as a result of an ongoing tumor process. The pineal body may be calcified and deviated, increasing pressure may show erosion of the posterior clinoid process, or calcification of certain tumors may be seen. Radiographs may show a hammered-metal appearance, which results from chronic pressure on the inner table of the skull. This condition is seen more often in radiographs of children. Erosive changes also may occur if the tumor invades the skull by eroding through the dura or outermost, toughest, and most fibrous membranes covering the brain and spinal cord.

The CT scan can distinguish the CSF, blood, edema, and tumor from normal brain tissue. The risks to the patient are minimal with CT. The use of iodine-based contrast to enhance the study increases the risk of an allergic reaction. Localization of the tumor is achievable through the use of a contrast-enhanced study. This also provides information regarding tumor extension, grade, and growth patterns. An area of higher or lower x-ray scattering power differentiates between necrosis or edema and calcification. Contrast-enhanced volume is indicative of a tumor. If used in conjunction with MRI, CT can confirm calcification or verify hemorrhage (Fig. 31-4).

MRI is useful for showing the normal anatomic structure and changes in the parenchyma. Having several advantages over CT scanning, MRI is the best noninvasive procedure. After radiation therapy or surgery, MRI provides a method of evaluating tumor response or recurrence. Iodine contrast is not necessary to perform the procedure, reducing the risk for a patient's reaction. Tumors smaller than 1 cm can be detected. With MRI, three-dimensional imaging is possible and bone artifacts are absent. MRI scans may be displayed in transverse, sagittal, and coronal sections, whereas CT is only displayed in the transverse section. Contrast-enhanced studies can be performed through the use of gadolinium, which is a non–iodine-based intravenous (IV) contrast agent. Gadolinium helps differentiate between edema and the tumor and can detect surface seeding. MRI may not be able to detect treatment-related changes from recurrent disease. CT is more cost effective, allowing for more economical use in follow-up posttreatment (Fig. 31-5).

Brain scans using technetium-99m (^{99m}Tc) provide information concerning blood flow and demonstrate vascular lesions and those altering the BBB. These studies are no longer widely in use because of the availability of better diagnostic tools.[6]

Positron emission tomography (PET) is a beneficial diagnostic tool that may be useful in determining differences between necrosis and malignancy, which are associated with areas of high metabolism. PET uses radionuclides and CT to help detect lesions. PET incorporates the localizing ability of CT scanning with the ability of the isotopic agent to concentrate in lesions and help differentiate between various types of CNS lesions, infections, and degenerative processes.[19]

A stereotactic biopsy (a procedure commonly performed during neurosurgery to guide the insertion of a needle into a specific area of the brain) allows all areas of the tumor and

| | Table 31-4 | Brain tumor localization chart | | |

Frontal	Parietal	Temporal	Occipital
SYMPTOMS			
Often asymptomatic until late	Symptomatic earlier than frontal lobes	Speech disorders (left hemisphere dominant; not only for right-handed, but for most left-handed persons)	Seizures (relatively less common, but with auras including flashing lights and unformed hallucinations)
Symptoms of increased ICP	Symptoms of increased ICP		
Bradyphrenia	Loss of vision		Loss of vision
Personality changes	Spatial disorientation	Loss of smell (superior lesion)	Tingling (early)
Libido changes	Tingling sensation	Disturbance in hearing, tinnitus, etc.	Weakness (late)
Impetuous behavior	Dressing apraxia	Speech disturbance	
Excessive jocularity	Loss of memory	Uncinate fits	
Defective memory	Seizures (focal sensory epilepsy)	Seizures with vocal phenomena in aura, including speech arrest	
Urinary incontinence	Weakness (anterior extension)	Hallucinations, dreams, déja vu	
Seizures (generalized, becoming focal)		Space-perception disturbances	
Gait disorders		Dysarthria	
Weakness		Dysnomia	
Loss of smell		Disturbance of comprehension	
Speech disorder			
Tonic spasms of fingers and toes			
SPECIFIC CEREBRAL FUNCTIONS			
		Dysarthria	Visual agnosia
Behavioral problems (anterior location)	Anosognosia	Sensory asphasia	Visual impulses
Labile personality	Autotopagnosis	Defective hearing	
Mental lethargy	Visual agnosia	Defective memory	
Defective memory	Graphesthesia (X)		
Motor aphasia	Loss of memory		
	Proprioceptive agnosia		
CRANIAL NERVE FUNCTIONS			
Anosmia (inferior lesion)	Hemianopsia	Superior quadrantanopsia (X) (could be homonymous hemianopsia with tumor extension)	Macular-sparing hemianopsia
Nerve VI palsy with increased ICP	Papilledema (with increased ICP)		Horizontal nystagmus
Papilledema with increased ICP		Central weakness of the cranial nerve VI	
Foster Kennedy's syndrome		Papilledema with increased ICP	
Proptosis			
MOTOR SYSTEM			
Contralateral weakness (late)	Weakness	Dysdiadochokinesia (early)	Late appearance of motor signs, manifested by drift or dysdiadochokinesia
Paresis (flaccid spastic)	Atrophy	Drift (secondary in later stages, involving arm more than leg)	
Disturbed gait (midline lesion)	Clumsiness		
Automatism	Dysdiadochokinesia		
Persistence of induced movement (Kral's phenomenon)	Independent movements (unrecognized by patient)		
Diagonal rigidity [arm (X); leg (-)]			
Loss of skilled movement (X)			
Urinary incontinence (superior lesion)			
SENSORY FUNCTIONS			
Rare involvement initially, unless invasion of sensory area (posterior lesion)	Dysesthesias (tingling)(X)	Initially minimal	Somatosensory disturbances earlier than motor changes as adjacent structures are involved
	Pallesthesia (loss of vibratory sense)(X)		Visual phenomena, such as persisting images, unformed hallucinations, and aura
	Loss of touch, press, and position sense (X), but pain and temperative usually unaffected		
REFLEX CHANGES			
Tonic plantar reflex	Babinski's sign	May occur contralateral to tumor	No effect in early stages
Hoffmann's sign	Hoffmann's sign		
Grasp reflex			
Babinski's sign			

Modified from Karlsson UL et al: In Perez C, Brady L, editors: *Principles and practice of radiation oncology,* ed2 Philadelphia, 1992, JB Lippincott.
ICP, Intracranial pressure; *(X),* contralateral; *(-),* ipsilateral.

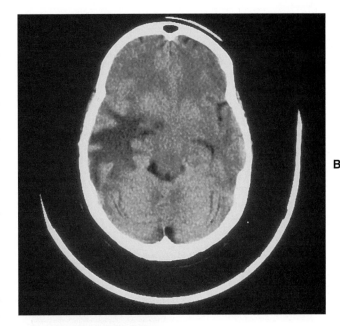

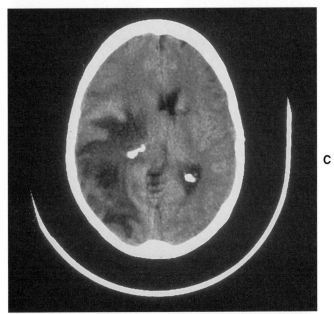

Figure 31-4. **A** and **B,** Noncontrast computed tomography (CT) scans of the head. Extensive edema can be seen through the white matter of the right temporal, parietal, and occipital lobes. A relatively well-circumscribed central area of low density appears to represent necrotic debris in the nidus (nucleus) of a tumor. This is strongly suggestive of a glioblastoma. **B** and **C,** Edema results in a midline shift approaching 1 cm to the left. **C,** Calcifications in the choroid plexus.

its borders to be studied before surgery causes changes in the appearance of the tumor. A biopsy is indicated if a lesion is deep seated, is probably malignant, and occurs in older or debilitated patients who cannot tolerate a surgical procedure. The risks of a biopsy include approximately a 30% rate of inadequate diagnosis.[19] Other risks include hemorrhage in the area of the biopsy and postoperative swelling.

Debulking procedures are performed if the tumor location is accessible and the tumor volume is large. Debulking accomplishes a reduction in tumor size and the opportunity to obtain a pathologic diagnosis. A reduction in tumor size may sometimes make it easier to treat with postoperative radiation therapy.

Cerebral angiography has value for planning surgical intervention as a means for surgeons to study the intrinsic vasculature (blood supply) of the tumor and surrounding blood vessels. However, this tool is of little value in establishing a definitive diagnosis.

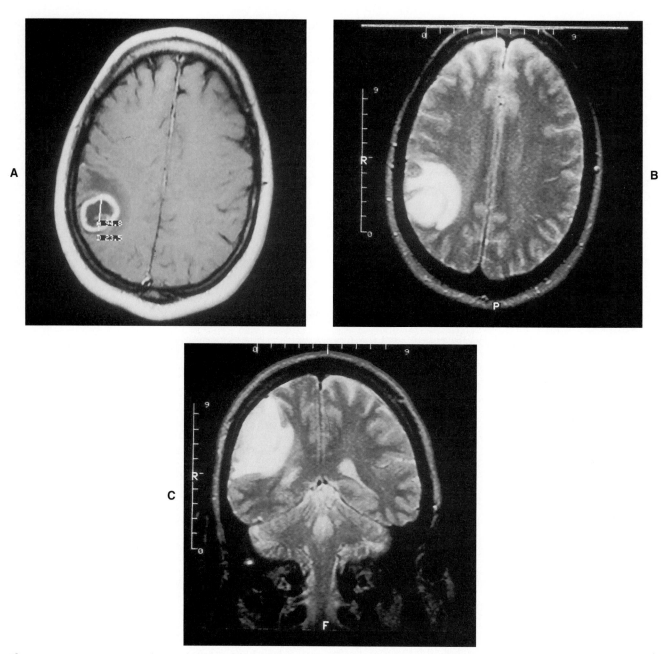

Figure 31-5. A 3-cm mass located in the right posterior parietal lobe with surrounding edema. The peripheral aspect of the lesion exhibits gadolinium enhancement. **A,** An axial magnetic resonance imaging (MRI) cut showing a lesion with a necrotic center. **B,** The mass is enhanced by gadolinium and shows surrounding edema. **C,** A coronal cut.

Because electroencephalography is imprecise and not specific for brain tumors, it is of little diagnostic value. Pneumoencephalography and ventriculography are now obsolete.

Pathology

The most important prognostic factor for CNS tumors is the histopathologic diagnosis. Benign lesions are indicative of a better prognosis, and the potential for a cure with the use of

surgery and/or radiation therapy exists. Intracranial tumors are considered locally malignant based on the limited space for expansion in the cranium. Treatment of the neuralaxis is indicated for some histopathologically malignant lesions such as medulloblastoma because of the risk of metastatic seeding.

Tumor growth is not hindered in most gliomas because CNS tumors do not form a natural capsule to contain them. Cellularity patterns differ according to the tumor grade. Low-grade tumors exhibit reactive hyperplasia with low cellularity, whereas marked cellularity is common in high-grade tumors. Necrosis is an important feature in high-grade tumors. Survival rates, with or without treatment, are clearly associated with tumor grade. Histopathology is more important than anatomic staging in determining the clinical outcome and behavior of the tumor. In other words, the cell type associated with brain tumors is more important than the size of the tumor. Tissue diagnosis should be obtained in all patients with a brain tumor. The few exceptions include patients with diffuse intrinsic brainstem gliomas and optic nerve gliomas.[19]

Staging

No universal staging system is currently in use, and problems result because of the lack of a standardized method of staging. The American Joint Committee on Cancer uses a system based on the grade, tumor, metastasis (GTM) classification. Grade (G) has prognostic significance, ranging from well differentiated to poorly differentiated (G1 to G3).

The Kernohan grading system has also been used. It is also a four-grade system, but it is difficult to use. The Kernohan system considers cellularity, anaplasia, mitotic figures, giant cells, necrosis, blood vessels, and proliferation.

Treatment Techniques

A multidisciplinary approach is necessary for the treatment of CNS tumors (Table 31-5). A biopsy is extremely important for diagnostic purposes and essential for therapeutic decision making.

Surgery. With the development of new surgical techniques, preoperative evaluation is even more important to further aid the surgeon. The tumor size and extent should be determined before surgery. The introduction of microsurgery, the ultrasonic aspirator, the laser, and perioperative ultrasound have made the surgeon's job easier. Computer-assisted stereotactic neuronavigation provides a new tool with the potential for great medical value.

When possible, surgery should be performed on tumors that are symptomatic and offer a chance for complete resection. **Debulking** is indicated with a large tumor volume and if a complete resection is not possible. Surgery can range from a debulking procedure to complete microsurgical removal. The primary goal for surgery is to remove the tumor and to obtain a histologic diagnosis. Surgery can be limited by the tumor location and extent, patient status, and risk of causing debilitating neurologic deficits. The patient's chances for survival are not enhanced by partial removal of the tumor. Tumor recurrence occurs from residual tumor that invades healthy brain tissue. Decreases in morbidity and mortality rates result from an earlier diagnosis, the use of steroid therapy, improvements in anesthetic techniques, and improved surgical methods. Surgical approaches to tumors depend on anatomic pathways, the tumor size, and the tumor location. According to Fransen and de Tribolet,[12] general opinion in the surgical world is that early and radical excision

Table 31-5	Multidisciplinary treatment decisions for various brain tumors		
Tumor Type	**Surgery**	**Radiation Therapy**	**Chemotherapy**
Astrocytoma (low grade)	Gross total resection* followed by observation	At tumor progression, postop RT 50-55 Gy	NR
	Gross total resection*	Postop RT 50-55 Gy	NR
Astrocytoma, mixed astrocytoma (high grade)	Gross total resection*	Postop RT 60-70 Gy + 50-60 Gy BT/RS	BCNU (patients <60 years)
Oligodendroglioma	Gross total resection*	Postop RT 60-70 Gy + 50-60 Gy BT/RS	NR
Anaplastic oligodendroglioma	Gross total resection*	Postop RT 60-70 Gy	PCV
Meningioma	Subtotal resection	Postop RT 50-55 Gy	NR
	Gross total resection	NR	
Malignant meningioma	Gross total resection*	Postop RT 60 Gy	
Ependymoma	Subtotal resection	Postop RT 54-59 Gy	
	Gross total resection	Postop RT 54 Gy + RS boost	
Medulloblastoma, anaplastic ependymoma	Gross total resection*	Postop RT 30-36 Gy to entire brain and spine; 20-25 Gy tumor boost	
Spinal cord tumors	Biopsy vs. resection	Postop RT 50 Gy	BCNU
CNS lymphoma	Biopsy	WBI 40-45 Gy	MTX or MAC

From Nelson D, et al: Central nervous system tumors. In Rubin P, editor: *Clinical oncology—multidisciplinary approach for physicians and students,* ed 8, Philadelphia, 2001, WB Saunders.
BCNU, Carmustine; *BT,* brachytherapy; *CNS,* central nervous system; *MAC,* multiagent chemotherapy; *MTX,* methotrexate; *NR,* not recommended; *PCV,* procarbazine, lomustine (CCNU), and vincristine; *Postop RT,* immediate postoperative radiation therapy (unless otherwise stated); *RS,* radiosurgery; *WBI,* whole brain irradiation.
*Gross total resection where possible; also includes subtotal resection or biopsy.

provide the best chance for a good outcome because of an accurate histologic diagnosis, control of a mass effect, and cytoreduction, which allow or enhance adjuvant therapy.

Surgery also plays a crucial role in the management of some spinal cord tumors. Surgery can establish a diagnosis and make possible the removal of the tumor. Because of the location of the cord, a surgical resection is difficult at best to perform and impossible in some instances. Serious neurologic deficits are always a risk.

Radiation therapy. Radiation therapy is indicated for malignant tumors that are incompletely excised, inaccessible from a surgical approach, and associated with metastatic lesions.

Several factors are considered in determining the doses for treatment. Tumor type, tumor grade, and patterns of recurrence are particularly important. The radioresponsiveness of the tumor must also be considered.[14] The total dose must be limited by normal tissue tolerance because **radiation necrosis** (tissue destruction) develops if tissue tolerance is exceeded. The risk of tumor progression must be balanced against the potential risk of necrosis when the dose is determined. In addition, consideration should be given to the side effects that may be induced. These side effects include acute reactions (or those encountered during the course of treatment), early-delayed reactions occurring from a few weeks until up to 3 months after treatment, and late-delayed reactions occurring months to years later. Threshold doses and the therapeutic ratio also must be considered.

Several approaches are available for treating tumors of the brain, depending on the type of disease, tumor location and extent, and whether the spinal axis requires treatment. Because brain malignancies can result from primary brain tumors, metastases from another site, or meningeal involvement, each type of malignancy must be handled appropriately.

The total surgical resection of a brain tumor for cure is an extremely difficult task to accomplish, partly because of the difficulty in obtaining generous enough resection margins in brain tissue. Radiation therapy usually follows surgery in an attempt to prevent tumor regrowth or recurrence. In the past, whole-brain irradiation has been used via lateral portals with a boost to the tumor bed after initial treatment. With the advent of CT and MRI, more accurate tumor localization allows smaller fields to be simulated and treated. Smaller field designs and unique configurations through the use of specialized blocking make simulation and daily reproducibility of the setup an even more important part of the treatment process.

If brain metastases are present from another primary site of involvement, whole-brain irradiation is the preferred treatment. Even with a solitary mass, occult disease is often present, although undetected. Therefore the whole brain should be treated.

Simulation provides the foundation for all radiation treatment (see Chapter 20). The simulation procedure should be carefully explained to the patient before it begins. The patient's understanding of the complexity of the procedure

and the necessity for daily reproducibility of the treatment setup should be stressed. Patients should be aware of the importance of their compliance and cooperation in relation to the outcome of the treatment. Accurate reproducibility is a must. Head rotation and tilting create the potential for difficulties in reproducibility. Immobilization is extremely important and can be achieved through the use of head-holding devices. The use of an immobilization system is beneficial for treating patients via lateral ports to a limited brain field with the patient in the supine position. The use of a thermoplastic mask greatly reduces errors in the reproducibility of the setup.

Lateral portal fields are used for treating the whole brain. The inferior margin of the field intersects the superior orbital ridge and external auditory meatus (EAM). In selecting the field size, 1 cm of flash or shine over should be seen at the anterior, posterior, and superior borders of the field. The flash reduces the chances of clipping any of the anatomy as a result of the field size being too small. The fields may be treated isocentrically or with a fixed source-skin distance (SSD). Isocentric setups are quicker to set up and carry out because the patient and table are not moved between lateral fields. This approach also reduces error rates.

For complex treatment to the craniospinal axis (the brain and spinal cord) the patient is simulated and treated most frequently in the prone position (Fig. 31-6). Lateral fields are used for treatment of the whole brain, whereas a gapped posterior field is used for treatment of the spinal cord. Care must be taken to match the beam divergence, allowing no overlap. Hot or cold spots can be avoided by feathering the gap. This can be accomplished by shifting the gap by 1 cm every 1000 cGy. Other methods of feathering the gap can be used. This approach allows a 1-cm gap between fields daily. With this technique the length of the brain and spine fields change daily. The central axis of the spine fields is shifted superiorly to accommodate the gap. The central axis of the brain field remains constant, whereas the field size changes. The treatment volume for gliomas is determined by the tumor's extent, which (as shown by CT and MRI) includes the gross tumor volume (GTV) and related tumor edema. Because tumor cells have been found in edema, this area should be included in the treatment field with a 2.5-cm margin for malignant tumors and a 1.0 to 2.0-cm margin for benign tumors.

Conventional therapy has been enhanced through the use of three-dimensional treatment planning, portal imaging, and multileaf collimators. Irregularly shaped fields can be created in seconds through the use of these collimators, eliminating the need to construct custom blocks. Three-dimensional treatment planning allows the use of multiple non-coplanar fields to a well-defined target volume. Checking the accuracy of the patient's setup before treatment is now possible through the use of portal imaging.

As a result of radiation treatments to the cranium, temporary hair loss occurs with doses ranging from 2000 to 4000 cGy. With doses of greater than 4000 cGy, hair loss may

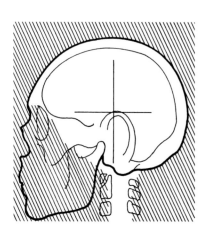
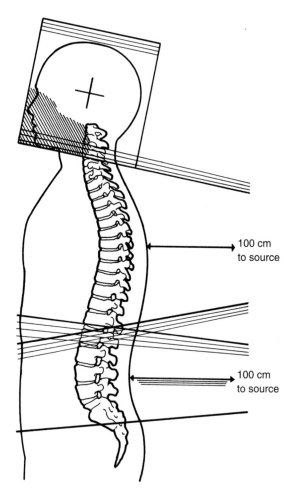

Figure 31-6. Helmet field and craniospinal field setup. *(Redrawn from Wara WM, et al: Brain, brain stem and cerebellum. In Perez C, Brady L, editors: Principles and practice of radiation oncology, ed 3, Philadelphia, 1998, Lippincott-Raven.)*

be permanent. Erythema, tanning, dry and moist desquamation, and edema are also side effects of the treatments. Early-delayed reactions include drowsiness, lethargy, a decreased mental status, and a worsening of symptoms. These reactions can occur up to 3 months after treatment, are usually temporary, and disappear without therapy. The occurrence of apparently new symptoms at this time is not necessarily indicative of treatment failure or the need for any change in therapy. Radiation necrosis (tissue death resulting from the effects of radiation) is a complication that rarely occurs from 6 months to many years after irradiation. Late reactions are usually irreversible and progressive. Radiation cataracts can be avoided by shielding or keeping the eyes out of the field.

Chemicals that enhance the lethal effects of radiation are known as **radiosensitizers.** Hypoxic cell sensitizers and halogenated pyrimidines are under investigation. Hypoxic cells are more radioresistant than well-oxygenated cells. The use of sensitizers makes the cells more susceptible to the radiation without increasing the radiation effects to the normal tissue, which is well oxygenated. Halogenated pyrimidines are used with deoxyribonucleic acid (DNA) to increase the sensitivity

of the cells to radiation and ultraviolet light.[21] Mitotically active tumor cells use these compounds more than replicating normal glial cells and vascular cells.

Interstitial implants (brachytherapy) are done with the use of radioactive seeds that are temporarily placed in tumors. Adjacent normal tissue is spared from excessively high doses because of the rapid decrease of dose outside the high-dose volume. Conceptually normal tissue can better tolerate the low-dose rate (given over a longer period as compared with external beam radiation therapy), so a higher dose can be delivered. Interstitial implants provide a less invasive treatment modality than surgery if recurrence occurs. Interstitial irradiation (IIR) may provide an alternative in the treatment of infants and children. Brachytherapy may be beneficial to patients suffering from recurrent disease, but it does not play a major role in the management of the disease.

Stereotactic radiosurgery is an important treatment option for patients with CNS tumors. The process combines stereotactic localization techniques with a sharply collimated beam to direct the dose of radiation to a specific, well-defined lesion. The patient is positioned in a halo device that is used as an immobilization device to ensure the accuracy and reproducibility of the treatment setup. The target volume should be spherical and only up to 3 cm at its maximum dimension. Accuracy approaches 1 mm. A necrosing dose of radiation can be given in a single-fraction treatment or in multiple fraction. A local dose to the tumor can be increased while sparing surrounding tissue. The process can be accomplished with the use of different sources of radiation. Heavy charged particles, a **gamma knife** using multiple cobalt-60 sources (a type of radiosurgery with a sharply defined field, considered by some to be equivalent to resecting the irradiated region), and linear-accelerator–based systems can be used with comparable results. The role of radiosurgery in the management of primary, metastatic, and recurrent disease is still under investigation.

Chemotherapy Progress has been slow in the area of chemotherapeutic drugs. Several reasons account for this. According to Chatel, Lebrun, and Freny,[7] the number of effective drugs is limited, adjuvant therapy has not changed the time to progression, adjuvant chemotherapy only slightly increases the percentage of survival at 18 and 24 months, a 20% to 25% response rate exists when drugs are given at recurrence, and multidrug therapy does not seem to be more efficient than single-agent chemotherapy. Other reasons for the difficulty in finding useful drugs include the small number of patients with CNS tumors for use in clinical trials compared with more prevalent diseases, difficulties measuring the tumor response, and the fact that one measurement of response is survival time. Effective chemotherapy for CNS tumors is furthered hindered by the BBB, which impedes the penetration of the drugs into the brain. "High concentration in cerebral tumors can nevertheless be reached because of the frequent extensive disruption of the BBB, but tumor cells infiltrating normal tissue are theoretically inaccessible to drugs that do not cross the BBB."[9]

Chemotherapeutic drugs can be administered orally, intravenously, directly into the tumor bed, and by direct carotid perfusion. Most chemotherapeutic drugs cause cytotoxic effects by disrupting DNA synthesis in rapidly dividing cells.

The designing of new drugs that allow better penetration of the BBB and can exhibit better distribution and lower toxicity has become extremely important. Limited studies suggest that the drug concentrations in the area around the tumor or in normal brain may be lower than those in the tumor itself, where the BBB is inefficient. The concentrations of drugs in the normal brain tissue decreases as the distance from the tumor increases. Therefore drug concentrations in the brain surrounding the tumor may be too low to eliminate infiltrating tumor cells. This can be a reason for therapeutic failures.[9] The nitrosourea drugs are lipid soluble, allowing them to cross the BBB. Because of this ability, these drugs can work against brain tumors.

Drugs of choice for CNS neoplasms include carmustine, procarbazine, vincristine, and Lomostine. Multiagent chemotherapy plays a major role in the treatment of recurrent gliomas (Table 31-6).

Role of Radiation Therapist

Patient education is a primary goal of the physician, radiation therapist, and oncology nurse. Although the physician and nurse initially discuss treatment procedures, side effects, skin care, nutrition, and psychosocial issues with the patient and family members, the emotional state of those persons at that time is generally not conducive to remembering and complying with all the information they are given. It becomes the responsibility of the therapist, who sees the patient daily, to reiterate and reinforce all these educational issues with the patient.

Daily contact allows the therapist to build a professional bond of trust, understanding, and communication with the patient. The therapist must be ready to step in and provide patients with emotional support, answers to their questions and concerns, and referrals to persons they may need to see (e.g., social worker, pastor, nutritionist, business office personnel, and support groups).

In addition, the therapist's daily contact also allows monitoring of the patient's mental and physical well-being. Some patients still feel overwhelmed, angry, and vulnerable and are in denial at the beginning of treatments.

A separate patient-waiting area allows patients to talk and share their thoughts with other persons who have the same concerns. This area allows discussions regarding issues the patient may not be able to discuss with family members.

Patients undergoing treatment for CNS neoplasms can expect specific side effects. Most commonly, patients complain of fatigue. Reassuring patients that this is not unusual helps them a great deal to cope with the situation. Explaining to patients that the body requires plenty of rest while it tries to heal itself from the disease and effects of daily treatment eliminates some concern. Suggesting that patients pamper themselves and take a nap when they feel tired, rather than fight the fatigue, is an option.

A proper diet is a must for the healing process and well-being of the patient. If food becomes unappealing in looks, taste, and smell, the patient will not want to eat. The patient can try eating smaller portions several times a day rather than sitting down to a large meal. Large portions are sometimes discouraging to someone with no appetite. A change in the location of eating can sometimes help, as well as having someone else cook. Nutritional supplements should be available to patients, including different kinds of supplements so patients can then purchase the brand that appeals to them most.

Frequent blood tests are not required, with the exception of patients receiving craniospinal irradiation. The white cell count and platelet counts may decrease in patients treated with craniospinal irradiation. These counts require close monitoring in the event the patient requires a break in treatment until the situation corrects itself.

Permanent hair loss for persons being treated for primary brain tumors occurs. A loan closet with wigs, turbans, and kerchiefs ranging in a wide variety of colors and styles should be available to patients. Shops specializing in these items should also be suggested. Therapists should caution patients to use a mild shampoo to prevent skin irritation. Moisturizing

Table 31-6	**Response Rates for Single-Agent and Multiagent Therapy in Brain Tumors**					

Investigators (ref. no)	Tumor Type	No. Patients	Drug(s)	Other Therapy	Response Rate (%)
SINGLE AGENT					
Yung et al[203]	Recurrent glioma	29	Carboplatin (IV)	PRT	48
Fujiwara et al[204]	Malignant glioma	6	ACNU (IA)—high dose	—	50
		6	ACNU (IA)—low dose	—	17
Eyre et al[205]	Low-grade glioma	54	CCNU	RT	54
				RT	79
Watanable et al[206]	Malignant glioma	19	MCNU (IA)	RT	43
		7	MCNU (IA)		33
Chauveinc et al[207]	Malignant glioma	10	ACNU (IA)	RT	30
	Anaplastic astrocytoma	17	ACNU (IA)	RT	65
Prados et al[208]	Recurrent glioma	41	Paclitaxel	PRT + PCT	35
Fujiwara et al[209]	Malignant glioma	20	Carboplatin (IA)	—	12.5
		22	ACNU (IA)	—	45
Forsyth et al[210]	Recurrent glioma	18	Docetaxel	—	0
Newlands et al[211]	Malignant glioma	27	Temozolomide	RT	30
	Recurrent glioma	48	Temozolomide	PRT	25
Cloughesy et al[212]	Recurrent glioma	19	Carboplatin (IA)	—	70
Phuphanich et al[213]	Recurrent glioma	25	All-trans-retinoic acid	PRT	12
Kuratsu et al[214]	Recurrent glioma	37	MX2 (IV)	—	11
Clarke et al[215]	Recurrent glioma	49	MX2 (IV)	—	43
MULTIAGENT					
Coyle et al[216]	Recurrent glioma	27	MOP	PRT ± PCT	52
Watne et al[217]	Recurrent glioma	79	PCV	—	60
Galanis et al[218]	Recurrent low grade glioma	61	PCV	± PCT	19
	Recurrent anaplastic astrocytoma			± PCT	11
	Recurrent oligodendrogliomas			± PCT	25
	Recurrent glioblastoma			± PCT	4.3
Soffietti et al[219]	Recurrent oligodendrogliomas	26	PCV	± PRT	62
Hildebrand et al[220]	Recurrent glioblastoma	26	PCD	—	12
	Recurrent anaplastic astrocyloma	11	PCD	—	55
van den Bent et al[221]	Recurrent glioma	16	Cisplatin + etoposide	RT	31
Brandes et al[222]	Recurrent glioma	51	Procarbazine + tamoxifen	PCT	30
Dazzi et al[223]	Malignant glioma	18	BCNU + cisplatin	RT	54

From Rubin P: *Clinical oncology: a multidisciplinary approach for physicians and students*, ed 8, Philadelphia, 2001, WB Saunders.
IV = intravenous; IA = intra-arterial; ACNU = nimustine; CCNU = lomustine; MCNU = ranimustine; BCNU = carmustine; MX2 = KRN8602 (novel morpholino-anthracycline); MOP = mechlorethamine + vincristine + procarbazine; PCV = carmustine + vincristine + procarbazine; PCD = dibromodule + carmustine + procarbazine; RT = radiation therapy, PRT = previous radiation therapy; PCT = previous chemotherapy.

creams can be prescribed for dry desquamation and other products for moist desquamation. Therapists can also recommend skin conditioners if erythema tanning occurs.

The patient should be cautioned against exposing to direct sunlight areas of the body being treated. The radiation from the sun in combination with the radiation from treatment enhances the adverse side effects.

Most patients begin to feel a sense of security that develops over the course of treatment from the daily contact with the therapy team. When treatment ends, patients feels a sense of loss and abandonment after weeks of daily attention being focused on them and their needs. In some facilities, patients can be called 1 week to 10 days after the completion of treatment (before the first follow-up visit) just to check on them and evaluate their physical and mental condition. This may provide the patient with a sense of ongoing care.

The therapist must also be watchful for signs of medical complications that may arise as a result of the treatment. Early intervention of potential problems can prevent unnecessary suffering later in the course of treatment. Attention to detail regarding treatment setups and parameters is a must, and providing professional, competent, efficient, and accurate treatment in a relaxed and friendly atmosphere completes the role of the therapist.

Case Study

A 31-year-old white man noted a change in vision and headaches. An initial workup included an MRI scan about 4 months later that revealed gadolinium enhancement in the region of the hypothalamus. Separate disease was noted in the corpus callosum. The pineal gland was enlarged but not enhanced.

A spinal MRI showed no evidence of spinal tumors. An additional workup included serum alpha-fetoprotein (AFP) and human chorionic gonadotropin (HCG), which were within normal limits. A lumbar puncture for cytology was performed. CSF was negative for malignant cells. The patient's history revealed that, at the age of 15, the patient was treated for failure to grow and diabetes insipidus. Diabetes insipidus sometimes occurs for years before other symptoms develop. A CT scan performed at that time revealed a questionable suggestion of abnormality in the hypothalamic region but apparently was not pursued. The patient was treated at the time with growth hormones, thyroid supplements, and vasopressin with response.

A biopsy was performed via a right frontotemporal craniotomy 5 months after the onset of symptoms. A preoperative diagnosis considering the patient's long history indicated a glioma. A postoperative diagnosis was probable hypothalamic glioma. A pathology report was positive for hypothalamic germinoma with metastasis to the corpus callosum. Several special stains of the biopsy specimen were used to confirm this diagnosis, and several pathologists reviewed the slides because the patient's history was unusual for a diagnosis of germinoma.

The patient's visual-field deficits were unchanged postoperatively. The craniotomy incision healed well.

The patient presented himself for radiation therapy consultation shortly after surgery. His history revealed panhypopituitarism manifested by hypothyroidism, high prolactin levels, adrenal insufficiency, diabetes insipidus, and abnormal testosterone levels. The family history was unremarkable. The patient's mental status was intact. A neurologic review was within normal limits. Vision testing revealed greater deficits on the right. The patient had blurred vision on the right and denied having a headache.

Because the patient had metastasis to the corpus callosum, he was a candidate for curative radiation therapy to the cranial spinal axis. Risks and benefits of the treatment were explained to the patient. Side effects during treatment can include skin irritation, hair loss, and fatigue. The white cell count and platelet counts tend to become lower in adults who are treated with craniospinal irradiation. The patient's blood counts were monitored weekly. Long-term risks included radiation damage to the brain, lens with cataract formation, and spinal cord.

Because there was no seeding to the spinal cord, the plan was to administer 2550 cGy in 17 fractions to the craniospinal axis. After this a cone-down boost of 2500 cGy was given to the gross disease, as seen on an MRI scan. The craniospinal axis was treated with 6-MV photons. The boost to the cone-down used 10-MV photons. If seeding to the spinal column had been present, those areas would also have been boosted.

The patient was simulated in the prone position with an alpha cradle to ensure reproducibility. Lateral fields to the whole brain and a posteroanterior (PA) spinal field were planned. Multileaf collimation was used to shape the portals.

The patient experienced minimal nausea after his first treatment. Prochlorperazine (Compazine) spansules given before further treatments helped relieve this problem. The patients blood counts dropped after receiving 750 cGy. Because the white count was below 1000/mm³, the patient was given time off with orders for a stat complete blood count to be done before resuming treatment. A 1-week break resolved this problem. He was cautioned not to use a toothbrush because of his decreased platelet count. He was told to sponge his teeth or gargle. The patient's visual deficits remained unchanged since the beginning of treatment.

Shifting of the fields to incorporate a gap began at 2100 cGy. A cone down began after 2500 cGy. At 3090 cGy the patient experienced less nausea but had complaints of altered taste with salty taste buds. At 3990 cGy he was doing well but had flulike symptoms. He continued to have poor visual acuity but had improved visual-field changes with a decrease in bilateral hemianopsia. The patient finished treatment at a total dose of 5070 cGy. He had only a 1-week break because of falling blood counts. The patient was suffering from severe fatigue and had complaints of indigestion and gastric reflux. He lost a total of 10 lb during treatment.

The patient was feeling well and eating better at the time of his 1-month follow-up visit. He continued to have some fatigue, which the oncologist felt would resolve itself after a little more time. The patient was able to regain some of the weight he had lost. Vision testing revealed no papilledema. The patient's vision was still poor, and he was unable to read a page in a book. Visual fields revealed marked improvement in the inferior aspect fields. Cranial nerves III to XII were intact. No motor or sensory abnormalities were present, and cerebellar findings were intact. There was epilation over his skull consistent with the treatment portal. No evidence existed of skin changes along his spine or cranium. A recent MRI scan showed no evidence of remaining germinoma.

At a follow-up 3 months later, the patient had a good appetite with his energy level improving, although he was still having problems gaining weight. An ophthalmologist examined the patient for his poor vision. Other than magnifying glasses, nothing could be done to help him. Optic nerve deficits were again noted with greater difficulty on the right than left. The patient had moderate alopecia with patchy regrowth. His blood counts had improved and were expected to continue to do so. The long-term survival prognosis for patients who have germinomas is 85% at 5 years. The patient is doing well 6 years after completion of treatment.

Review Questions

1. Karnofsky Performance Status (KPS) is
   a. A measure of the biologic grade of the tumor
   b. A measure of the neurologic and functional status of the patient
   c. Measured in cGy
   d. Measures the chance of 5-year survival
2. What is the purpose of the blood-brain barrier?
   I. To hinder the penetration of some substances into the brain and CSF
   II. To protect the brain from potentially toxic substances
   III. To protect the brain from radiation
   IV. To prevent the passage of lipid- or water-soluble substances into the brain
   a. I and III
   b. II and III
   c. I and II
   d. II and IV

3. Which of the following are important factors to consider in the initial workup for a definitive diagnosis of CNS neoplasms?
   a. Family and social histories
   b. Changes in behavior or personality
   c. Difficulties with speech, memory, or logical thought processes
   d. All of the above

4. What is the best approach to treating CNS neoplasms?
   a. Surgery and radiation
   b. Surgery and chemotherapy
   c. Radiation and chemotherapy
   d. A multidisciplinary approach

5. Surgery for CNS neoplasms can be limited by which of the following?
   a. Tumor location and extent
   b. Patient status
   c. Risk of causing neurologic deficits
   d. All of the above

6. What is the most common brain lesion?
   a. Astrocytoma
   b. Glioma
   c. Metastatic
   d. Medulloblastoma

7. Little is known concerning the _____, development, and growth mechanisms of CNS tumors.
   a. Etiology
   b. Dose response
   c. Effects of alcohol
   d. BBB

8. Which of the following does not provide protection for the brain?
   a. Cerebellum
   b. Cranial bones
   c. Meninges
   d. Cerebrospinal fluid (CSF)

9. Weakened proximal pelvic muscles, impotence, bladder paralysis, and decreased knee jerk may be signs of a spinal tumor in the _____ region.
   a Cervical
   b. Upper thoracic
   c. Lower thoracic
   d. Lumbosacral

10. Side effects from radiation treatment of primary brain tumors include
    a. Dry and moist desquamation
    b. Edema
    c. Hair loss
    d. Spinal cord damage

Questions to Ponder

1. Explain the benefits and risks involved in treating patients who have CNS neoplasms with surgery, radiation therapy, and chemotherapy.

2. What are some of the presenting signs and symptoms you would anticipate with patients who have CNS tumors?

3. What is the purpose of the feathered-gap technique for treating patients to the craniospinal axis?

4. Analyze the expected side effects from radiation therapy to the CNS?

REFERENCES

1. Ahlbom A: A review of the epidemiologic literature on magnetic fields and cancer, *Scand J Work Environ Health* 14:337-343, 1991.
2. Avizonis VN, et al: Late effects following central nervous system radiation in a pediatric population, *Neuropediatrics* 23:228-234, 1992.
3. Bigner SH, et al: Gene amplification in malignant human gliomas, *J Neuropathol Exp Neurol* 47:191-205, 1988.
4. Bigner SH, et al: Characterization of the epidermal growth factor receptor in human gliomas, cell lines, and xenografts, *Cancer Res* 50:8017-8022, 1990.
5. Black KL, Ciacci M: The limits of treatment of malignant gliomas, *West J Med* 158:65-66, 1993.
6. Bruner J: Neuropathology, cell biology, and new diagnostic methods, *Curr Opin Oncol* 5:441-449, 1993.
7. Chatel M, Lebrun C, Freny M: Chemotherapy and immunotherapy in adult malignant gliomas, *Curr Opin Oncol* 5:464-473, 1993.
8. Collins VP: Amplified genes in human gliomas, *Semin Cancer Biol* 4:27-32, 1993.
9. Donnelli MG, Zucchetti M, D'Incali M: Do anticancer agents reach the tumor target in the human brain? *Cancer Chemother Pharmacol* 30:251-260, 1992.
10. Farwell J, Dohrmann GJ, Flannery JT: Central nervous system tumors in children, *Cancer* 40:3123-3132, 1977.
11. Filippini G, Artuso A: International incidence of CNS tumors in children, *Ital J Neurol Sci* 13:395-400, 1992.
12. Fransen P, de Tribolet N: Surgery for supratentorial tumors, *Curr Opin Oncol* 5:450-457, 1993.
13. Frelich R, Huang P, Topham A: Cancer current—brain and CNS tumors Delaware 1980-1989, *Del Med J* 64:571-573, 1992.
14. Hall EJ: *Radiobiology for the radiologist*, ed 5, New York, 2000, Lippincott Williams & Wilkins.
15. Wara WM, et al: Brain, brain stem and cerebellum. In Perez C, Brady L, editors: *Principles and practice of radiation oncology*, ed 3, Philadelphia, 1998 Lippincott-Raven.
16. Laem OD, Mork SJ, DeRidder L: The transformation process. In Rosenblum ML, Wilson CB, editors: *Brain tumor biology: progress in experimental research*, Basel, 1984, Karger.
17. Louis DN, Cavenee WK: Neoplasms of the central nervous system. In Devita VT, Hellman S, Rosenberg SA, editors: *Cancer principles and practice of oncology*, ed 5, Philadelphia, 1997 Lippincott-Raven.
18. Myers MH, Gloechler Ries LA: Cancer patients survival ratio: SEER program results for 10 years of follow-up, *CA Cancer J Clin* 39:21-32, 1989.
19. Nelson D, et al: Central nervous system tumors. In Rubin P, editor: *Clinical oncology—a multidisciplinary approach for physicians and students*, ed 8, Philadelphia, 2001, WB Saunders.
20. Ranskoff J, Koslow M, Cooper P: Cancer of the CNS and pituitary. In Holleb A, Fink D, Murphy G, editors: *American Cancer Society textbook of clinical oncology*, Atlanta, 1991, American Cancer Society.
21. Salmon I, et al: DNA histogram typing in a series of 707 tumors of the central and peripheral nervous system, *Am J Surg Pathol* 17:1020-1028, 1993.
22. American Cancer Society: *Cancer facts and figures 2003*, Atlanta, 2003, American Cancer Society.
23. Vertosich F Jr, Selker RG: Long term survival after the diagnosis of malignant glioma: a series of 22 patients survive more than 4 years after diagnosis, *Surg Neurol* 38:359-363, 1992.

24. Weingart J, Brem H: Biology and therapy of glial tumors, *Curr Opin Neurol Neurosurg* 5:808-812, 1992.

25. Youmans JR: *Neurological surgery,* vol 3, Philadelphia, 1973, WB Saunders.

BIBLIOGRAPHY

del Regato JA, Spjut HJ, Cox JD: *Ackerman and del Regato's: cancer: diagnosis, treatment, and prognosis,* ed 6, St. Louis, 1985, Mosby.

Griffin C, et al: Chromosome abnormalities in low grade CNS tumors, *Cancer Genet Cytogenet* 60:67-73, 1992.

Digestive System

Leila Bussman

Outline

Key Terms

Abdominoperineal resection
Achalasia
Anterior resection
Barrett's esophagus
Chronic ulcerative colitis
Endocavitary radiation therapy
Esophagitis
Familial adenomatous polyposis
Gardner's syndrome

Hereditary nonpolyposis
  colorectal syndrome
Intraoperative radiation therapy
  (IORT)
Leukopenia
Odynophagia
Orthogonal radiographs
Peritoneal seeding
Plummer-Vinson syndrome
Tenesmus
Three-point setup
Thrombocytopenia

This chapter discusses the three major malignancies of the gastrointestinal system that are managed with radiation therapy (i.e., cancers of the rectum, esophagus, and pancreas). Colorectal cancer is the most common gastrointestinal malignancy and is associated with the best prognosis. Cancers of the esophagus and pancreas are usually diagnosed with advanced-staged disease and do not have many long-term survivors.

COLORECTAL CANCER

Epidemiology and Etiology

The incidence of colorectal cancer has been steadily declining since 1980. However, about 138,900 new cases are projected in the United States each year.[25] The disease affects men and women equally. Cancer of the colon is ranked third in incidence in comparing men and women separately. The risk of developing cancer of the large bowel increases with age. The incidence rate for persons younger than 65 years is 19.2 cases per 100,000, compared with 337 cases per 100,000 for persons older than 65.[14] Cancer of the large bowel more commonly affects the rectum or distal colon. However, an increase has occurred in right (proximal) colon lesions, especially in older women. The reason for this is unclear, but the increase may be the result of earlier detection of precancerous lesions in the distal colon. Colorectal cancer is the second leading cause of cancer death in the United States, accounting for approximately 57,000 deaths annually.[2,8,14,48,61]

The cause of colorectal cancer has largely been attributed to a diet high in animal fat and low in fiber. The excess fat in a person's diet may act as a promoter of the development of colon cancer. The intake of fiber into diets may act as an inhibitor, diluting fecal contents and increasing fecal bulk, resulting in quicker elimination, and therefore minimizing the exposure of the bowel epithelial lining to the carcinogens.[14,48,64] Some authors suggest that the type of fiber consumed determines the effectiveness of reducing or neutralizing mutagens in the diet. Cellulose and wheat bran have been considered more effective than alternate forms of fiber in reducing the mutagen formation.[8,64] A diet high in fiber is considered an effective means of preventing the development of colon cancer. However, further studies are needed to determine the effectiveness of different types of fiber sources.

Other principle factors in the development of colon cancer include the following: **chronic ulcerative colitis,** carcinomas arising in preexisting adenomatous polyps, and the hereditary cancer syndromes. These syndromes are **familial adenomatous polyposis** (FAP) and hereditary nonpolyposis colorectal syndrome (HNPCC).[14,48,52,64]

Individuals also at an increased risk for the development of colorectal cancer are those persons whose first-degree relative developed colorectal cancer or adenomatous polyps before age 60. An increased risk also exists if two or more first-degree relatives at any age developed colorectal cancer or adenomatous polyps in the absence of a hereditary syndrome.[61]

Chronic ulcerative colitis usually occurs in the rectum and sigmoid area of the bowel but may spread to the rest of the colon. This condition is characterized by extensive inflammation of the bowel wall and ulceration. A patient experiences attacks of bloody mucoid diarrhea up to 20 times a day. These attacks persist for days or weeks and then subside, only to recur.[58] The risk of developing colon cancer depends on the extent of bowel involvement, age of onset, and severity and duration of the active disease.[8,14,57] The earlier the age at onset and the longer the duration of the active disease, the higher the risk of developing cancer. Studies have shown the risk to be 3% at 15-years duration, increasing to 5% at 20 years.[8,14,57] Only 1% of patients with a diagnosis of colorectal cancer have a history of chronic ulcerative colitis.

Adenomatous polyps are growths that arise from the mucosal lining and protrude into the lumen of the bowel. They are classified as tubular or villous, based on their growth pattern and microscopic characteristics. Polyps are considered a precursor to the development of a malignancy.[8,14,52,57,64] The larger the polyp, the greater the risk of malignant transformation.[8,14,52] Villous adenomas are 8 to 10 times more likely than tubular adenomas to be malignant.[8,52,57]

Virtually all patients with the hereditary condition FAP, if left untreated, develop colon cancer.[8,14,48,57] FAP is characterized by the studding of the entire large bowel wall by thousands of polyps. Persons affected with this disease do not have polyps at birth. Progression to extensive involvement of the colon usually occurs by late adolescence. The cause of FAP is associated with a mutation on the adenomatous polyposis coli gene on chromosome 5.[46,61] FAP is treated by the complete removal of the colon and rectum. **Gardner's syndrome** is another inherited disorder similar to FAP. Patients with Gardner's syndrome have adenomatous polyposis of the large bowel and other abnormal growths, such as upper gastrointestinal polyps, periampullary tumors, lipomas, and fibromas.[8,14,57]

The frequent occurrence of colorectal cancer in families without polyposis has been termed **hereditary nonpolyposis colorectal syndrome** (HNPCC).[2,8,14] The cause of HNPCC has been attributed to mutations in repair genes located on chromosomes 2, 3, or 7. HNPCC has classically been defined as colorectal cancer that develops in three or more family members. At least two must be first-degree relatives and involve people in at least two generations with one family member being diagnosed before the age of 50.[61] Patients with this family history of colon cancer usually develop right-sided colon cancers at a much younger age than the general population. These patients are also at an increased risk for the development of a second cancer of the colon and adenocarcinomas of the breast, ovary, endometrium, and pancreas.[8,14] Individuals with this family history should undergo physical examinations regularly and consider genetic testing.

Anatomy and Lymphatics

Cancer of the large bowel is usually divided into cancer of the colon or rectum because the symptoms, diagnosis, and treatment are different based on the anatomic area involved. A major factor determining the treatment and prognosis is whether a lesion occurs in a segment of bowel that is located retroperitoneally or intraperitoneally. This is discussed further in the section on the anatomy and lymphatic drainage of these areas.

The colon is divided into eight regions: the cecum, ascending colon, descending colon, splenic flexure, hepatic flexure, transverse colon, sigmoid, and rectum. Located intraperitoneally, the cecum, transverse colon, and sigmoid have a complete mesentery and serosa and are freely mobile (Fig. 32-1).[8,30,48,51] Lesions occurring in these regions can usually be surgically removed with an adequate margin unless the tumor is adherent or invades adjacent structures.[8,28,47] Treatment failure or recurrence is most likely attributed to peritoneal seeding.

Located retroperitoneally, the ascending and descending colon and the hepatic and splenic flexures are considered immobile. They lack a true mesentery and a serosal covering on the posterior and lateral aspect. Because of the retroperitoneal location and lack of a mesentery for these regions, early spread outside the bowel wall and invasion of the adjacent soft tissues, kidney, and pancreas are common. Thus adequate surgical margins are more difficult to achieve and may result in a local recurrence.[8,30,48]

The rectum is continuous with the sigmoid and begins at the level of the third sacral vertebra. Like the sigmoid, the upper rectum is covered by the peritoneum but only on its lateral and anterior surfaces. The peritoneum is then reflected over the anterior wall of the rectum onto the seminal vesicles and bladder in males or the vagina and uterus in females, forming a cul-de-sac termed the rectovesical pouch or rectouterine pouch, respectively. The lower half to two thirds of the rectum is located retroperitoneally. Three transverse

system were based on studies showing that penetration through the bowel wall, the number of nodes positive for tumor, and tumor adherence to adjacent structures were important predictors of survival.[8,48] In the MAC system, Gunderson and Sosin created separate categories for tumors that microscopically or grossly (B2m or B2g) involved surrounding organs or structures.[8]

The TNM system incorporated these changes into the current system (Table 32-1), which is similar to the MAC system.[8,21] The revisions in the staging systems reflect that the two most important prognostic indicators of survival are the number of nodes positive for tumor and depth of penetration through the bowel wall.[8,30]

Routes of Spread

As implied in the staging system, malignancies of the large bowel usually spread via direct extension, lymphatics, and hematogenous spread. Direct extension of the tumor is typically in a radial fashion, penetrating into the bowel wall rather than longitudinally.[8]

Lymphatic spread occurs if the tumor has invaded the submucosal layer of the bowel. The initial lymphatic and venous channels of the bowel wall are found in the submucosal layer. Lymphatic spread is orderly. The initial nodes involved for rectal cancer are the perirectal nodes.[8,30] Approximately 50% of patients have nodes positive for tumor.[30]

Bloodborne spread to the liver is the most common type of distant metastasis. The mechanism of spread involves the venous drainage of the gastrointestinal system (the portal circulation). The second most common site of distant spread is the lung. This spread results from tumor embolus into the inferior vena cava (IVC).[8]

Lesions may also spread within the peritoneal cavity. The growth of a tumor through the bowel wall onto the peritoneal

Table 32-1	TNM colorectal staging systems
T1	Tumor invades submucosa
T2	Tumor invades muscularis propria
T3	Tumor invades through the muscularis propria into subserosa or into pericolic or perirectal tissues
T4	Direct extension into other organs or structures and/or perforation of visceral peritoneum
N0	Nodes negative
N1	1-3 regional nodes positive
N2	4 or more positive regional nodes
M0	No distant metastasis
M1	Distant metastasis

Modified from Fleming ID et al, editors: *AJCC manual for staging of cancer,* ed 5, Philadelphia, 1997, Lippincott-Raven.

Box 32-1	AJCC Staging Classification for Colorectal Cancer

PRIMARY TUMOR (T)

TX	Primary tumor cannot be assessed
T0	No evidence of primary tumor
Tis	Carcinoma *in situ*: intraepithelial or invasion of lamina propria
T1	Tumor invades submucosa
T2	Tumor invades muscularis propria
T3	Tumor invades through the muscularis propria into the subserosa, or into non-peritonealized pericolic or perirectal tissues
T4	Tumor directly invades other organs or structures, and/or perforates visceral peritoneum

REGIONAL LYMPH NODES (N)

NX	Regional lymph nodes cannot be assessed
N0	No regional lymph node metastasis
N1	Metastasis in 1 to 3 regional lymph nodes
N2	Metastasis in 4 or more regional lymph nodes

DISTANT METASTASIS (M)

MX	Distant metastasis cannot be assessed
M0	No distant metastasis
M1	Distant metastasis

STAGE GROUPING

Stage	T	N	M	Dukes	MAC
0	Tis	N0	M0	–	–
I	T1	N0	M0	A	A
	T2	N0	M0	A	B1
IIA	T3	N0	M0	B	B2
IIB	T4	N0	M0	B	B3
IIIA	T1-T2	N1	M0	C	C1
IIIB	T3-T4	N1	M0	C	C2/C3
IIIC	Any T	N2	M0	C	C1/C2/C3
IV	Any T	Any N	M1	–	D

HISTOLOGIC GRADE (G)

GX	Grade cannot be assessed
G1	Well differentiated
G2	Moderately differentiated
G3	Poorly differentiated
G4	Undifferentiated

With permission from American Joint Committee on Cancer (AJCC), Chicago, Illinois: *AJCC Cancer Staging Manual,* ed 6, New York, 2002, Springer-Verlag.

surface of the colon can result in tumor cells shedding into the abdominal cavity. These shedded cells then take up residence on another surface (i.e., peritoneal lining, cul-de-sac) and begin to grow. This process is called **peritoneal seeding.** The implantation of tumor cells onto a surface at the time of surgery is another mechanism of spread.[8,32]

Treatment Techniques

Surgery is considered the treatment of choice. The tumor, an adequate margin, and draining lymphatics are removed. The type of procedure depends on the location of the tumor. For colon tumors the removal of a large segment of bowel, adjacent lymph nodes, and the immediate vascular supply by procedures such as a right hemicolectomy or left hemicolectomy is common. For rectal cancer the two most common procedures are the anterior and abdominoperineal (AP) resection.

The **anterior resection** involves the removal of the tumor plus a margin (an en bloc excision) and immediately adjacent lymph nodes.[18] The bowel is then reanastomosed. Therefore a colostomy is not required. This procedure is used in the treatment of colon cancers and select rectal cancers.[7,8] Patients with disease in the upper third or middle third of the rectum (6 to 12 cm above the verge) are usually candidates for this sphincter-preserving surgery.[7,18,25,44]

An **abdominoperineal resection** is used in patients with rectal cancer in the lower third (distal 5 cm) of the rectum.[7] An anterior incision is made into the abdominal wall to construct a colostomy. Then a perineal incision is made to resect the rectum, anus, and draining lymphatics, pulling the entire en bloc specimen out through the perineal opening. Because of the narrow, bony configuration of the pelvis and closeness of adjacent structures (i.e., prostate and vagina), adequate margins laterally, anteriorly, and posteriorly are difficult.[44,48] Surgical clips placed to outline the tumor area assist the radiation oncologist in the design of treatment portals.[7,48] The final phase of the procedure involves the reconstruction or reperitonealization of the pelvic floor through the use of an absorbable mesh, omentum, or peritoneum. This is extremely important for the patient who needs postoperative radiation therapy. Reperitonealization allows the small bowel to be displaced superiorly, reducing the amount of small bowel in the treatment field and minimizing the treatment toxicity from radiation therapy.[7,18,48]

Radiation therapy. Radiation therapy is most commonly used as an adjuvant treatment postoperatively for rectal cancer. However, preoperative radiation therapy and radiation alone may also be used in selected patients.[7,28-30,48]

Postoperative adjuvant radiation therapy and concurrent chemotherapy is advocated based on the high local failure rate of surgery alone in rectal cancer patients who have nodes positive for tumor or tumor extension beyond the wall. Postoperative radiation therapy and chemotherapy is the only adjuvant treatment approach consistently shown to improve survival rates in rectal cancer patients and is preferred over other adjuvant approaches such as preoperative radiation ther-

apy. A major advantage of postoperative adjuvant treatment is that the physician has pathologic confirmation of the extent of the tumor spread through the wall to nodes or distant sites. This information is critical in determining whether adjuvant treatment is necessary.[49] Studies have shown that patients with nodes positive for tumor but with a tumor confined to the bowel wall (C1) have a 20% to 40% recurrence rate.[8,30,48] A similar local recurrence rate (20% to 35%) is found with B2 and B3 lesions, tumors that extend through the bowel wall with or without adherence and nodes for tumor. A patient with both poor prognostic factors (extension through the wall and nodes positive for tumor [C2 and C3]) has almost twice the risk for local recurrence. Various studies have reported recurrence rates in these patients of 40% to 65% in a clinical series and up to 70% in a reoperative series.[32,33]

Endocavitary radiation therapy is a sphincter-preserving procedure done for curative intent in a select group of patients with low- to middle-third rectal cancers that are confined to the bowel wall. Papillon established the following characteristics for patients eligible for this procedure: no extension of the tumor beyond the bowel wall, a maximum tumor size of 3 × 5 cm, a mobile lesion with no significant extension into the anal canal, a well- to moderately well-differentiated exophytic tumor that is accessible by the treatment proctoscope (≤10 cm from the anal verge).[27,53] Patients receive four doses of 3000 cGy each, separated by a 2-week interval. This is done on an outpatient basis through the use of a 50-kVp contact unit (4-cm source-skin distance [SSD]), with 0.5- to 1.0-mm aluminum filtration at a dose rate of 1000 cGy per minute. Treatments are delivered directly to the rectal tumor through an applicator inserted into the rectum and held in place by the radiation oncologist (Fig. 32-5). If the size of the lesion exceeds the diameter of the applicator (3 cm), overlapping fields are necessary. Treatment results have been excellent with this technique. Papillon reported only a 11% locoregional failure rate with a 5-year follow-up out of 207 patients treated.[48,53]

Radiation alone has also been used in patients who are medically inoperable or who have locally advanced rectal cancer and are deemed unresectable.[7,48] In this setting, radiation provides palliation and is rarely curative. Radiation combined with chemotherapy (5-fluorouracil [5-FU]) has proved more effective than radiation alone in relieving symptoms, decreasing tumor progression, and increasing overall survival. Preoperative radiation (≥45 Gy) has resulted in 50% to 75% of patients becoming resectable, but 35% to 45% of the patients still experience local recurrence, necessitating additional treatment.[48]

Chemotherapy. The addition of adjuvant chemotherapy combined with radiation therapy in the postoperative setting in high-risk rectal and colon cancer patients (MAC B2-C3) has demonstrated an increase in overall survival rates (Fig. 32-6).[13,31,32,49,48] The Gastrointestinal Tumor Study Group (GTSG) and Mayo Clinic/North Central Cancer Treatment Group (NCCTG) have performed many random-

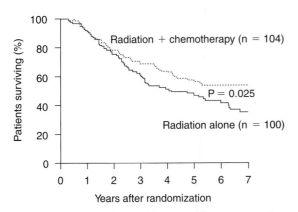

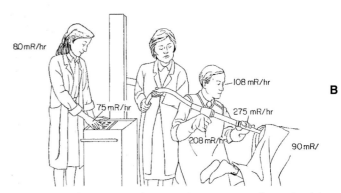

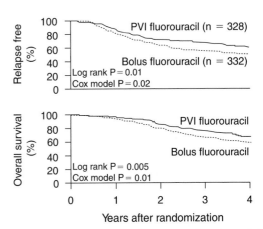

A and B

Figure 32-5. **A** and **B,** Sphincter-preserving endocavitary radiation therapy of the low rectal tumor. *(Courtesy Dr. Alan J. Stark.)*

Figure 32-6. Improved survival rates with postoperative radiation and chemotherapy versus radiation alone. *(Modified from Krook JE, et al: Effective surgical adjuvant therapy for high-risk rectal carcinoma, N Engl J Med 324:713, 1991.)*

Figure 32-7. A comparison of protracted venous infusion (PVI) fluorouracil and bolus fluorouracil. Improved relapse-free and overall survival rates occur with PVI. *(Modified from O'Connell, et al: Improving adjuvant therapy for rectal cancer by combining protracted-infusion fluorouracil with radiation therapy after curative surgery, N Engl J Med 331:502, 1994.)*

ized trials of adjuvant therapy for rectal cancer (Fig 32-7). These studies have demonstrated a decreased disease recurrence and improved survival rates with a combination of 5-FU and pelvic radiation therapy. Current studies are employing 5-FU plus leucovorin or levamisole. Six months of 5-FU plus leucovorin has proven to be as effective as 5-FU plus levamisole for 12 months for advanced-stage colon cancer.[26,37,43]

Field design and critical structures. Patients receiving postoperative adjuvant radiation therapy for rectal cancer are at a high risk for local recurrence. These patients include those with extension beyond the bowel wall, tumor adherence (MAC B2-3), or lymph nodes positive for tumor (MAC C1-3). The treatment fields are typically designed to encompass the primary tumor volume and pelvic lymph nodes, shrinking the field to treat the primary target volume to a higher dose. Anatomic boundaries of the portals depend on whether the patient underwent an anterior resection or AP resection directly relating to the areas at risk for recurrence. For patients with rectal cancer, most recurrences occur in the

posterior aspect of the pelvis, including metastasis to the internal iliac and presacral lymph nodes.[30,48] These two nodal groups are not included in a standard surgical resection for rectal cancer and need to be encompassed in radiation portals.[48] For irradiation of the pelvis the dose-limiting structure is the small bowel. Radiation treatment techniques and the field design must take into consideration the amount of small bowel in the field to minimize treatment-related toxicities. The reduction of the small-bowel dose is achieved through patient positioning and positioning devices, bladder distention, multiple-shaped fields, and dosimetric weighting.[8,30,48] The dose delivered to the large volume (tumor plus regional nodes) is 4500 cGy, with the coned-down volume (primary tumor bed) receiving 5000 cGy to 5500 cGy in 6 to 6½ weeks. Doses in excess of 5000 cGy are not achievable unless the small bowel can be excluded from the field.[7,30,48]

Usually, a four-field posteroanterior/anteroposterior (PA/AP) and opposed laterals or three-field technique (PA and opposed laterals wedged) is used, allowing a homogenous dose to the tumor bed while sparing anterior structures, including the small bowel. For patients who have undergone an anterior resection the superior extent of the field is placed 1.5 cm superior to the sacral promontory, which correlates to L5-S1 innerspace.[7,30,48] Depending on the superior extent of the lesion and clinical indications, the field may need to be placed at the L4-L5 interspace or extend superiorly to include the paraaortic lymph node chain.[30] The more superi-

orly the field extends, the more precautions are necessary to avoid small-bowel injury and complications. The width of the PA/AP fields is designed to provide adequate coverage of the iliac lymph nodes. This border is placed 2 cm lateral to the pelvic brim and inlet. The inferior border generally includes the entire obturator foramina, although this may vary depending on the location of the lesion. The recommended inferior margin is 3 to 5 cm on the gross tumor preoperatively or below the most distal extent of dissection postoperatively (Fig. 32-8).[30] A rectal tube is inserted at the time of simulation. Barium or Gastrografin contrast (30 to

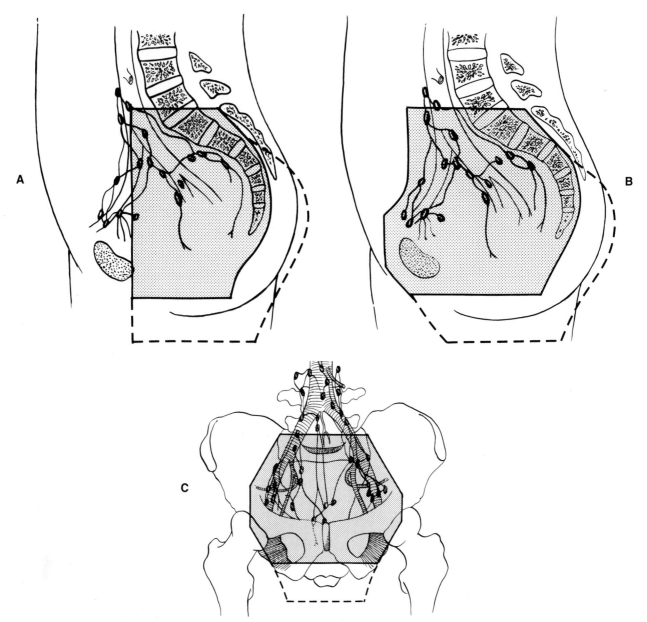

Figure 32-8. Radiation treatment fields. In all figures the dotted line indicates the field extension to be used after an abdominal-perineal resection. **A,** A standard lateral field. **B,** A lateral field to include external iliacs in patients who have involvement of structures with external iliac lymph node drainage. **C,** A standard anteroposterior/posteroanterior (AP/PA) field.

40 cubic centimeters) is injected into the rectum to facilitate the localization of critical structures and design of treatment fields. Lead shot or a BB is placed on the anal verge to reference the perineal surface on simulation films.

Lateral treatment portals and prone positioning with full bladder distention allows the small bowel to be excluded from the treatment volume. This position also assists in the localization of critical posterior structures. Anatomically, the rectum and perirectal tissues are extremely close to the sacrum and coccyx. In locally advanced disease the tumor may spread along the sacral nerve roots, resulting in tumor recurrence in the sacrum. Therefore the posterior field edge is placed 1.5 to 2.0 cm behind the anterior bony sacral margin. In advanced situations the entire sacral canal plus a 1.5-cm margin is recommended.[30,48] This margin allows day-to-day variances in the patient setup caused by movement. Anteriorly, the field border is placed at the anterior edge of the femoral heads to ensure coverage of the internal iliac nodes. The lower third of the rectum lies immediately posterior to the vaginal wall and prostate, placing these organs and their draining lymphatics at risk for involvement. If the rectal lesion has invaded anterior structures (prostate or vagina), the anterior border is placed on pubic symphysis for inclusion of the external iliac nodes (Fig. 32-8, *B*).[7,30,48] In female patients a tampon soaked with iodinated contrast is inserted into the vagina to ensure adequate coverage of the vagina in the radiation portals.

The use of a CT simulator rather than a fluoroscopic simulator allows the physician to more accurately localize and outline the pertinent anatomic structures described previously. With conventional simulation, these structures are transferred onto the simulation radiograph from measurements taken off a previous CT scan. Errors in measurements or the shift of anatomic structures because of change in patient position from the original scan may result in inadequate margins. The CT simulator software enables physicians to digitize in different colors the target volume and critical normal structures, such as the rectum, bladder, and lymph nodes on each CT slice. The intimate relationships of target versus normal tissues are available at the time of simulation and with the patient in treatment position. This assists the physician and the dosimetrist in the accurate placement of the isocenter and in the design of the fields. A digitally reconstructed radiograph (DRR) is produced which shows the radiation field outline, the treatment isocenter, and pertinent anatomic structures (Fig. 32-9). The CT images can be sent electronically directly to dosimetry for treatment planning.

The CT simulation procedure requires the radiation therapist to position the patient prone on a positioning device ensuring elbows are "in" so that they will not hit the sides of the CT gantry during the scan. It is extremely important to get the patient as straight as possible before the scan because they cannot be repositioned once the scan is complete. Contrast is typically placed in the rectum and tubes removed before scan-

ning. Unlike fluoroscopic simulation, a more dilute mixture of contrast (15-cc water and 5-cc Gastrografin) is used to prevent artifacts on the CT images. A tampon soaked with a more dilute iodinated contrast may be used in female patients. A reference isocenter or three points are placed on the patient's pelvis and marked with small BBs. The reference isocenter is used to ensure that the patient did not move during the scan. The reference isocenter is also used as the zero coordinates from which the treatment isocenter will be marked. After the reference isocenter is placed, couch parameters, scanning limits, and length of pilot or scout are recorded. A typical scan may extend from the level of the second lumbar vertebrae to below the lesser trochanters. Following the scan, the physician will determine the treatment isocenter and give the therapist the measurements to shift anterior or posterior and so forth to the appropriate location. The therapist then places marks or tattoos on the treatment isocenter or three points. Most CT simulators are not equipped with a patient marking system like a conventional simulator is. Only the treatment isocenter or three points can be marked. It is helpful if the radiation therapist uses the sagittal laser to place additional straightening lines superior and inferior to the isocenter. The patient may proceed to treatment following the completion of the treatment plan.

In patients having an AP resection the field design is similar, except the posterior and inferior borders are extended to include the entire perineal incision. The perineal region is included in the treatment volume to decrease the risk of tumor recurrence in the scar from implantation of tumor cells

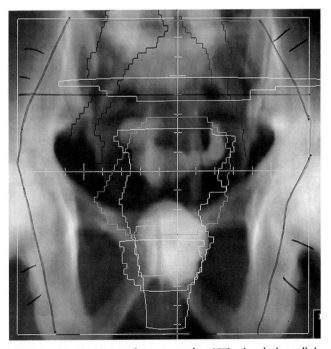

Figure 32-9. Computed tomography (CT) simulation digitally reconstructed radiograph (DRR) of standard posteroanterior (PA) field.

at the time of surgery. The entire perineal scar is outlined at the time of simulation with solder wire or lead BBs. The posterior and inferior margins are established by placing the field edge 1.5 to 2.0 cm beyond the radiopaque perineal markers. This corresponds to flashing the posterior and inferior perineal skin surfaces (see Fig. 32-8).[30,48] The perineal scar is then bolused (thickness/energy dependent) during the PA treatment. The buttocks are taped apart, and bolus is placed on the entire perineal scar to have a controlled measurable bolusing effect. Because of the tangential radiation beam, the perineal tissue and thinner upper thigh tissue may exhibit acute skin reactions, requiring interruption of the planned treatment course. In male patients the penis and scrotum are shifted superiorly under the pubic region to lessen this reaction. Alternatively, the reaction to male genitalia can be reduced by the use of a three-field technique (PA and laterals).

An extrapelvic colon cancer field design should include an initial margin of 3 to 5 cm beyond the tumor plus high-risk nodal groups and adjacent structures. If the tumor invaded or was adherent to an organ such as the ovary or stomach, the majority of the organ and its draining lymphatics should be encompassed in the treatment portal unless the organ was completely resected. Adherent structures should be included with a 3- to 5-cm margin. Usually, an anteroposterior/posteroanterior (AP/PA) technique is used. However, CT treatment planning and clip placement may determine that a multifield approach more optimally spares normal tissue. The initial large volume is treated to 4500 cGy with a shrinking-field technique used to boost the tumor bed (with a 2- to 3-cm margin) an additional 540 to 900 cGy.[30,48]

Dose-limiting structures for treating an ascending or descending colon cancer include the kidney and small bowel. Contrast studies for assessing renal function and kidney localization films should be performed before treatment or at the time of simulation to ensure the adequate sparing of at least one kidney. For example, when treating a right-sided colon lesion, 50% or more of the right kidney may be in the field; therefore the left kidney must be spared.[30,48] For limiting the dose to the small bowel the patient can be treated in the decubitus position, resulting in a shift of the bowel away from the treated area and reducing the volume of the small bowel in the field. For a right-sided colon lesion the patient is simulated by lying on the left side, outlining the field based on surgical clips and preoperative imaging studies. A special tabletop device can be used that supports the patient's upper back and buttock-thigh region to aid in stability and reproducibility of the setup. Contrast in the small bowel at the time of simulation demonstrates whether an adequate shift of the small bowel takes place to make these fields feasible.

In patients with locally advanced colorectal cancer or recurrent disease, local control is difficult to achieve. This is due to the limited surgical options because of fixation of the tumor to pelvic organs (prostate, uterus) or unresectable structures such as the presacrum or pelvic sidewall. If microscopic residual disease exists, an external beam dose of 6000 cGy or greater is necessary to provide a reasonable chance for control. This dose is even higher ($\geq$7000 cGy) if gross residual disease exists.[29,35] These doses exceed the normal tissue-tolerance dose of abdominal or pelvic structures and cannot be safely delivered with conventional external beam irradiation.[28,29]

Intraoperative radiation therapy. Intraoperative radiation therapy (IORT) is a mechanism for supplementing the external beam dose to assist in obtaining local control of the tumor while sparing dose-limiting normal structures.[24] IORT is a specialized boost technique similar to brachytherapy. As the name implies, IORT involves an operative procedure requiring general anesthesia. The radiation oncologist and surgeon must work closely with one another to determine whether IORT is appropriate and which diagnostic tests would be helpful in planning the IORT and external beam radiation treatments. A contraindication for IORT is the presence of distant metastasis. The surgeon and radiation oncologist also determine the optimal sequence of surgery and external radiation by discussing the benefits and side effects of each.[28,35]

Patients undergoing an IORT procedure receive a dose of 1000 to 2000 cGy of electrons in a single fraction directly to the tumor bed. Critical dose-limiting structures (i.e., kidney, bowel) are shielded or surgically displaced out of the radiation portal so that these normal tissues receive little or no radiation. This dose, delivered in a single fraction, is two to three times the dose if delivered at conventional fractionation of 180 to 200 cGy/fraction. For example, an IORT single dose of 1500 cGy equals 3000- to 4500-cGy fractionated external radiation. When adding the effective IORT dose to the 4500 to 5000 cGy, delivered with conventional external beam radiation, the total effective dose equals 7500 to 9500 cGy.[28,35] A dose this high cannot be safely given with standard external irradiation.

The IORT dose is calculated at the 90% isodose line, with the energy and dose delivered depending on the depth or amount of residual disease. Electron energies of 9 to 12 MeV are used after a gross total resection or minimal residual and high energies of 15 to 18 MeV are used for patients who have recurrent disease with gross residual or unresectable disease.[28,30] The target volume is encompassed in a lucite cylinder that projects from the patient and is docked to the treatment head of the linear accelerator. The beam of electrons travel through the lucite cylinder directly onto the tumor bed (Fig. 32-10).

The precise role of IORT in the treatment of large bowel cancer has not been definitively documented. Although some data suggest better local control and survival rates with this form of treatment, this improvement is possibly due to the selection of the most favorable patients for this form of treatment rather than an effect of the treatment itself. Moreover, toxicity can be significant. Further study is needed before IORT becomes a widely accepted tool in the treatment of colorectal cancer.

next most frequent type is basaloid, or cloacogenic, cancer. These tumors occur in the region of the dentate line where the epithelium is in transition. Also found in this region are adenocarcinoma (arising from the anal glands), mucoepidermoid tumors, and melanoma. Cancers occurring in the perianal region are typically squamous or basal cell carcinomas consistent with skin cancers.

The most commonly used staging system is the AJCC system. This is a clinical system in which tumors are staged according to their size and extent (Box 32-2).

Tumors of the anal canal spread most frequently by direct extension into the adjacent soft tissues. Lymphatic spread occurs relatively early, whereas hematogenous spread to the liver or lungs is less common.

Treatment Techniques

An AP resection with a wide perineal dissection is the most common surgical procedure for anal cancer. This procedure results in an overall survival rate of 50%. Combination radiation therapy and chemotherapy (5-FU and Mitomycin C) is now advocated as the preferred method of treatment. Radiation alone is advocated for patients who cannot tolerate chemoradiation.[62] Studies have shown that the multimodality (radiation and chemotherapy) approach provides good local control and colostomy-free survival.[47,60,62] Most series report

survival rates from 50% to 80% at 5 years, with a local control rate of 60% to 80%.[60]

A variety of radiation techniques exist for the treatment of anal cancer. Most use a four-field or AP/PA pelvic-field approach including a boost to the tumor bed with a perineal electron field or another multifield technique. The pelvic field extends from the lumbosacral-sacroiliac region to 3 cm distal to the lowest extent of the tumor (noted by a radiopaque marker at the time of simulation). The inferior border typically flashes the perineum, resulting in brisk erythema and moist desquamation of the perineal tissues. The lateral border may extend to include treatment of the inguinal lymph nodes on the AP field only, placing that field edge at the midlateral aspect of the femoral heads. The PA field is kept narrower because the anteriorly located inguinal nodes do not receive much contribution from the posterior field. This also avoids an excessive dose to the femoral heads, yet encompasses the tumor bed and deep pelvic nodes. Anterior electron fields centered over each inguinal region and abutting the PA lateral border are used to further supplement the dose to the inguinal lymph nodes.[62]

The dose regimen used with radiation alone is 6000 to 6500 cGy delivered to the region of the primary tumor. This dose is reduced to approximately 4500 to 5040 cGy if concomitant chemotherapy is used. With either technique, field

---

Box 32-2 — AJCC Staging System for Anal Cancer

DEFINITION OF TNM

The following is the TNM classification for the staging of cancers that arise in the anal canal only. Cancers that arise at the anal margin are staged according to the classification for cancers of the skin.

Primary Tumor (T)
TX Primary tumor cannot be assessed
T0 No evidence of primary tumor
Tis Carcinoma in situ
T1 Tumor 2 cm or less in greatest dimension
T2 Tumor more than 2 cm but not more than 5 cm in greatest dimension
T3 Tumor more than 5 cm in greatest dimension
T4 Tumor of any size invades adjacent organ(s), e.g., vagina, urethra, bladder (involvement of the sphincter muscle[s] alone is not classified as T4)

Regional Lymph Nodes (N)
NX Regional lymph nodes cannot be assessed
N0 No regional lymph node metastasis
N1 Metastasis in perirectal lymph node(s)
N2 Metastasis in unilateral internal iliac and/or inguinal lymph node(s)
N3 Metastasis in perirectal and inguinal lymph nodes and/or bilateral internal iliac and/or inguinal lymph nodes

Distant Metastasis (M)
MX Distant metastasis cannot be assessed
M0 No distant metastasis
M1 Distant metastasis

STAGE GROUPING

Stage	T	N	M
Stage 0	Tis	N0	M0
Stage I	T1	N0	M0
Stage II	T2	N0	M0
	T3	N0	M0
Stage IIIA	T1	N1	M0
	T2	N1	M0
	T3	N1	M0
	T4	N0	M0
Stage IIIB	T4	N1	M0
	Any T	N2	M0
	Any T	N3	M0
Stage IV	Any T	Any N	M1

With permission from American Joint Committee on Cancer (AJCC), Chicago, Illinois: *AJCC Cancer Staging Manual,* ed 6, New York, 2002, Springer-Verlag.

reductions are implemented after a dose of 4500 cGy to reduce small-bowel toxicity.

In conclusion, radiation therapy alone or in combination with chemotherapy is a viable treatment option, providing sphincter preservation and satisfactory cure rates in patients with anal cancer.

ESOPHAGEAL CANCER

Epidemiology and Etiology

Cancer of the esophagus accounts for 1% of all cancers in the United States, with approximately 14,000 cases annually. Men are more commonly affected than women (9900 vs. 3300, respectively), and a higher incidence is reported in blacks than in whites (13.1 vs. 3.5 per 100,000).[5,17,25] Most of these cancers are diagnosed in patients between 55 and 65 years of age. Esophageal cancer is a nearly uniformly fatal disease, with the estimated deaths in the United States numbering approximately 13,000 annually.[5,25]

Cancer of the esophagus occurs with the greatest frequency in northern China, northern Iran, and South Africa. In China, one northern county (Hebi) has an incidence rate of 139.8 persons per 100,000 occurring in persons 30 years of age or older, whereas another county in China has a rate of only 1.4 persons per 100,000. This has been attributed to environmental and nutritional factors.[17,20,58]

The most common and important etiologic factors in the development of squamous cell cancer of the esophagus in Western countries are excessive alcohol and tobacco use. Alcohol and tobacco abuse are associated with 80% to 90% of all cases diagnosed in North America and Western Europe. The combination of these two factors has a synergistic effect on the mucosal surfaces, increasing the risk of esophageal cancer and other aerodigestive malignancies. Esophageal cancer is commonly found as a second primary after a previous diagnosis of head and neck cancer.[17,20,58]

Dietary factors have also been implicated in the development of cancer of the esophagus. Diets low in fresh fruits and vegetables and high in nitrates (i.e., cured meats and fish, pickled vegetables) have been cited as risk factors for persons from Iran, China, and South Africa, respectively.

Other conditions predispose individuals to the development of esophageal cancer. They include achalasia, Plummer-Vinson syndrome, caustic injury, and Barrett's esophagus.

Achalasia is a disorder in which the lower two thirds of the esophagus has lost its normal peristaltic activity. The esophagus becomes dilated (termed megaesophagus), and the esophagogastric junction sphincter also fails to relax, prohibiting the passage of food into the stomach. Clinical symptoms include progressive dysphagia and regurgitation of ingested food. Patients with achalasia have a 5% to 20% risk of developing cancer of the esophagus.[57,58]

Plummer-Vinson syndrome (also known as Paterson-Kelly syndrome) is an iron-deficient anemia characterized by esophageal webs; atrophic glossitis; and spoon-shaped, brittle fingernails. This syndrome occurs mostly in women.

Caustic injuries and burns caused by the ingestion of lye are responsible for 1% to 4% of esophageal squamous cell cancers. Malignancies develop in the scarred, or stricture, area years after an injury.[57,58]

Barrett's esophagus is a condition in which the distal esophagus is lined with a columnar epithelium rather than a stratified squamous epithelium. This mucosal change usually occurs with gastroesophageal (GE) reflux. One theory to explain this phenomenon is that chronic chemical trauma resulting from reflux causes the mucosa to undergo metaplasia.[57,58] Adenocarcinoma of the esophagus occurs in 2.4% to 8.3% of patients who have Barrett's mucosa.[20]

Prognostic Indicators

Tumor size is an important prognostic tool. According to a series by Hussey et al., patients with tumors less than 5 cm in length had a better 2-year survival rate (19.2%) than patients with lesions larger than 9 cm (1.9%).[20] Tumors ≤5 cm in length were more often localized (40% to 60%), whereas tumors larger than 5 cm had distant metastasis 75% of the time.[20,58] Other factors indicating a poor prognosis are weight loss of 10%, a poor performance status, and patients older than 65.

Anatomy and Lymphatics

The esophagus is a thin-walled 25-cm-long tube lined with stratified squamous epithelium. The esophagus begins at the level of C6 and traverses through the thoracic cage to terminate in the abdomen at the esophageal gastric (E-G) junction (T10-T11).

For accurate classification, staging, and recording of tumors in the esophagus, the AJCC has divided the esophagus into four regions: cervical, upper thoracic, middle thoracic, and lower thoracic. Because lesions are localized by an endoscopy, reference is made to the distance of the lesion from the upper incisors (front teeth). This distance is also used in defining each region (Fig. 32-13).[21,58]

The cervical esophagus extends from the cricoid cartilage to the thoracic inlet (suprasternal notch [SSN]), corresponding to vertebral levels C6 to T2-3 and measuring about 18 cm from the upper incisors. The thoracic inlet (SSN) to the level of the tracheal bifurcation (carina)—24 cm from the incisors—defines the upper thoracic portion. The middle thoracic esophagus begins at the carina and extends proximally to the E-G junction, or 32 cm from the incisors. The lower thoracic portion includes the abdominal esophagus and is approximately 8 cm long at a level of 40 cm from the incisors.[14,21,58]

The esophagus lies directly posterior to the trachea and is anterior to the vertebral column. Located laterally and to the left of the esophagus is the aortic arch. The descending aorta is situated lateral and posterior to the esophagus (Fig. 32-13). During an endoscopy an indentation is visible where the

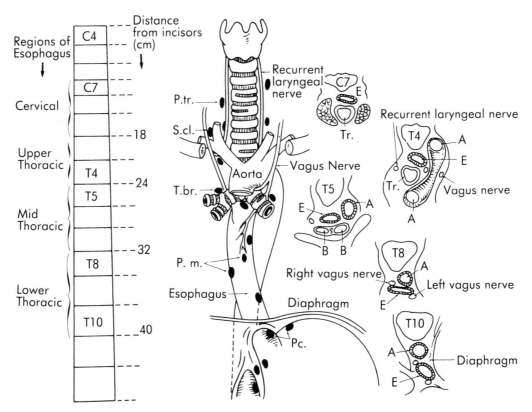

Figure 32-13. The relationship of the esophagus with surrounding anatomic structures, including divisions of the esophagus and their location from the upper central incisors. *(From Cox JD: Moss' radiation oncology: rationale, techniques, results, ed 7, St. Louis, 1994, Mosby.)*

aorta and left mainstem bronchus are in contact with the esophagus. Because of the esophagus' intimate relationship with these structures, tumors are often locally advanced, fistulas may occur, and surgery is often not feasible.[15,51,58]

Histologically, the esophagus consists of the usual layers of the bowel common to the gastrointestinal tract (i.e., the mucosa, submucosa, and muscular layers). However, the esophagus lacks a serosal layer. The outermost layer, the adventitia, consists of a thin, loose connective tissue. This is another factor contributing to the early spread of these tumors to adjacent structures.[20,51]

The esophagus has numerous small lymphatic vessels in the mucosa and submucosal layers. These vessels drain outward into larger vessels located in the muscular layers (Fig. 32-14). Lymph fluid can travel the entire length of the esophagus and drain into any adjacent draining nodal bed, placing the entire esophagus at risk for skip metastasis and nodal involvement.[19,20,51,58]

Although the entire length of the esophagus is at risk for lymphatic metastasis, each region still has primary or regional nodes that specifically drain the area. For example, the upper third (cervical area) of the esophagus drains into the internal jugular, cervical, paraesophageal, and supraclavicular lymph nodes. The upper and middle thoracic portion has drainage to the paratracheal, hilar, subcarinal, parae-sophageal, and paracardial lymph nodes. Finally, the principal draining lymphatics for the distal or lower third of the esophagus include the celiac axis, left gastric nodes, and nodes of the lesser curvature of the stomach (Fig. 32-15). Lymphatic spread is unpredictable and may occur at a significant distance from the tumor. Nodes positive for tumor outside a defined region represent distant metastasis rather than regional spread. For example, supraclavicular nodal involvement in a primary tumor located in the cervical esophagus is considered regional lymph node involvement, but this would be a distant metastasis for tumors arising in the thoracic esophagus.[15,21]

Clinical Presentation

The most common presenting symptoms are dysphagia and weight loss, which occur in 90% of patients. Patients complain of food sticking in their throat and may point to the location of this sensation. Initially, patients have difficulty with bulky foods, then with soft foods, and finally even with liquids. Patients may recall having this difficulty in swallowing for 3 to 6 months before the diagnosis. Regurgitation of undigested food and aspiration pneumonia may also occur. **Odynophagia** (painful swallowing) is reported in approximately 50% of patients. Symptoms of a locally advanced tumor include the following: hematemesis (vomiting blood),

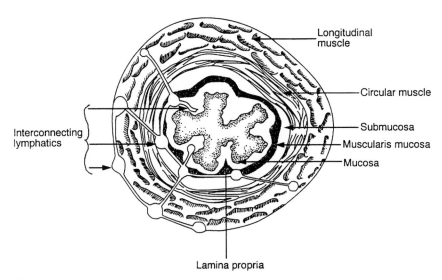

Figure 32-14. Lymphatic vessels located in the wall of the esophagus. *(From Cox JD: Moss' radiation oncology: rationale, techniques, results, ed 7, St. Louis, 1994, Mosby.)*

coughing (caused by a tracheoesophageal fistula), hemoptysis, Horner's syndrome, or hoarseness as a result of nerve involvement.[17,20,58]

Detection and Diagnosis

A thorough history and physical examination should be performed. Information should be obtained regarding weight loss and the use of alcohol and tobacco. The physical examination should include palpation of the cervical and supraclavicular lymph nodes and abdomen to assess potential spread to the nodes or liver. A chest radiograph and esophagogram are necessary for localizing the lesions causing the dysphagia. Esophagograms depict characteristic features of esophageal cancers. The reported incidence of tumors located in each third of the esophagus varies in the literature. Lesions in the upper third of the esophagus occur with the least frequency, accounting for 10% to 25% of tumors. Approximately 40% to 50% of tumors are located in the middle third of the esophagus, and 25% to 50% are located in the lower third.[17,20,58]

A CT scan of the chest and upper abdomen should be obtained. This scan may demonstrate extramucosal spread and invasion of adjacent structures such as the trachea or aorta. Spread to lymph nodes in the thorax and abdomen can be also assessed. Bloodborne metastases to the liver and adrenals may be imaged via CT, although small lesions may not be detectable.

An ultrasound of suspicious liver nodules is performed to differentiate metastasis from a cystic mass.[17,20,58] Laboratory studies include a CBC and blood chemistry group to assess the liver and kidney function.

A histologic confirmation is obtained during an esophagoscopy. A rigid or flexible endoscope can be used to examine the entire esophagus, obtaining brushings and biop-

sies of all suspicious lesions. EUS is also helpful for visualizing the tumor, its depth of invasion, and lymph node status.[1,9,21,58] A bronchoscopy should also be performed for all upper- or middle-third lesions to detect any possible communication of the tumor with the tracheobronchial tree.[17,20,58]

Pathology and Staging

The most common pathologic types of esophageal cancer are squamous cell carcinoma and adenocarcinoma. Squamous cell carcinomas are found most frequently in the thoracic esophagus. Adenocarcinoma typically occurs in the distal esophagus. Adenocarcinoma is often found with Barrett's esophagus or is believed to be an extension of a gastric cancer into the esophagus. In the United States, adenocarcinoma has been increasing in frequency. A variety of other epithelial tumors arise in the esophagus but are rare. These include adenoid cystic carcinoma, mucoepidermoid carcinoma, adenosquamous carcinoma, and undifferentiated carcinoma.[20,58]

Nonepithelial tumors also arise in the esophagus, although this is rare. Leiomyosarcoma (a tumor of the smooth muscle) is the most common nonepithelial tumor. Leiomyosarcomas yield a more favorable prognosis than squamous cell carcinomas. Malignant melanoma, lymphoma, and rhabdomyosarcoma are other nonepithelial tumors that can occur in the esophagus.[20,58]

The AJCC staging system for esophageal cancer is shown in Box 32-3.

Routes of Spread

Because the esophagus is distensible, lesions are large before causing obstructive symptoms. Spread is usually longitudinal. Occasionally, skip lesions may be present at a significant distance from the primary lesion. This is principally due to

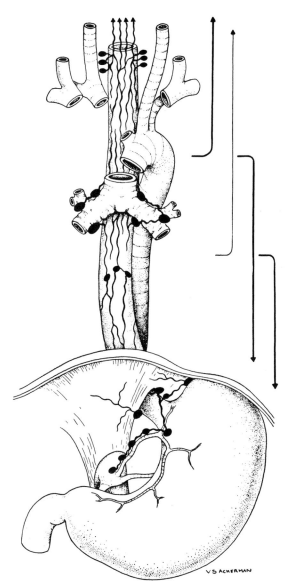

Figure 32-15. Lymphatic drainage of the esophagus. The arrows represent potential spread to cervical, mediastinal, and subdiaphragmatic lymph nodes, based on the location of the esophageal lesion. Subdiaphragmatic involvement is unusual in the upper-third tumors. *(From del Regato JA, Spjut HJ, Cox JD: Ackerman and del Regato's cancer: diagnosis, treatment, and prognosis, ed 6, St. Louis, 1985, Mosby.)*

submucosal spread of the tumor through interconnecting lymph channels. Locally advanced disease, invasion into adjacent structures, and early spread to draining lymphatics are common in esophageal cancer. Distant metastasis can occur in many different organs, with the liver and lung being the most common.

Treatment Techniques

The treatment of esophageal cancer is highly complex and technically difficult. Most patients have locally advanced or metastatic disease at the time of diagnosis and require multi-modality treatment. Treatment is usually categorized as curative or palliative and may be given with surgery or radiation for the local-regional problem. Patients who receive either modality (surgery or radiation) alone have a significant risk of local recurrence and distant metastasis. The primary goal of either treatment is to provide relief of the dysphagia and a chance for cure. The current nonsurgical standard for the treatment of esophageal cancer is combined chemotherapy and radiation therapy.[29,40]

A variety of surgical techniques exist for the resection of esophageal cancer. In many centers, surgical resection is limited to the middle and lower thirds of the esophagus. The cervical esophagus is not considered a surgically accessible site in many institutions and is often managed with radiation therapy and chemotherapy. Curative surgery usually involves a subtotal or total esophagectomy. The type of procedure chosen depends on the location of the lesion and extent of involvement. Typically, the entire esophagus is removed. The continuity of the gastrointestinal system is maintained by placing either the stomach or left colon in the thoracic cavity. The Ivor Lewis procedure consists of a laparotomy and right thoracotomy to remove the esophagus and mobilize the stomach into the thoracic cavity (Fig. 32-16). A total thoracic esophagectomy also requires multiple surgical incisions. A laparotomy is performed to mobilize the stomach, and a thoracotomy is performed to remove the esophagus. However, a third incision is made at the neck to assist in the anastomosis of the stomach to the remaining cervical esophagus (Fig. 32-17).[1,9,10,17,58,59]

Both of these procedures are technically difficult and associated with a high morbidity and mortality rate. Operative mortality rates from either procedure have ranged from 8% to 31%, although recent studies have demonstrated a decrease in these rates. Complications from surgery include anastomotic leaks (which can be life threatening), respiratory failure, pulmonary embolus, and myocardial infarctions. Strictures, difficulty in gastric emptying, and GE reflux are mechanical side effects resulting from surgery.

Even after a curative resection most patients fail distantly with bloodborne spread to the lungs, liver, or bone.

Radiation therapy. Radiation therapy alone or with chemotherapy has been routinely used for the treatment of esophageal cancer. Radiation therapy with chemotherapy is considered the current nonsurgical treatment of choice for esophageal cancer.* Recent studies demonstrated a clear advantage for radiation therapy and chemotherapy compared with radiation therapy alone.[1,9,10,30,59] Preoperative chemoradiation followed by curative surgery is also being evaluated. Preliminary results show a slight improvement in survival. Radiation and concomitant chemotherapy remain the treatment standard.[1,9,10,59]

Chemotherapy. The poor survival rates resulting from esophageal cancer are associated with the high percentage of

---

*References 1, 9, 10, 22, 30, 44, 59.

DEFINITION OF TNM

Primary Tumor (T)

TX Primary tumor cannot be assessed
T0 No evidence of primary tumor
Tis Carcinoma in situ
T1 Tumor invades lamina propria or submucosa
T2 Tumor invades muscularis propria
T3 Tumor invades adventitia
T4 Tumor invades adjacent structures

Regional Lymph Nodes (N)

NX Regional lymph nodes cannot be assessed
N0 No regional lymph node metastasis
N1 Regional lymph node metastasis

Distant Metastasis (M)

MX Distant metastasis cannot be assessed
M0 No distant metastasis
M1 Distant metastasis
    Tumors of the lower thoracic esophagus:
    M1a Metastasis in celiac lymph nodes
    M1b Other distant metastasis

Tumors of the midthoracic esophagus:
M1a Not applicable
M1b Nonregional lymph nodes and/or other distant metastasis
Tumors of the upper thoracic esophagus:
M1a Metastasis in cervical nodes
M1b Other distant metastasis

STAGE GROUPING

Stage 0	Tis	N0	M0
Stage I	T1	N0	M0
Stage IIA	T2	N0	M0
	T3	N0	M0
Stage IIB	T1	N1	M0
	T2	N1	M0
Stage III	T3	N1	M0
	T4	Any N	M0
Stage IV	Any T	Any N	M1
Stage IVA	Any T	Any N	M1a
Stage IVB	Any T	Any N	M1b

With permission from American Joint Committee on Cancer (AJCC), Chicago, Illinois: *AJCC Cancer Staging Manual,* ed 6, New York, 2002, Springer-Verlag.

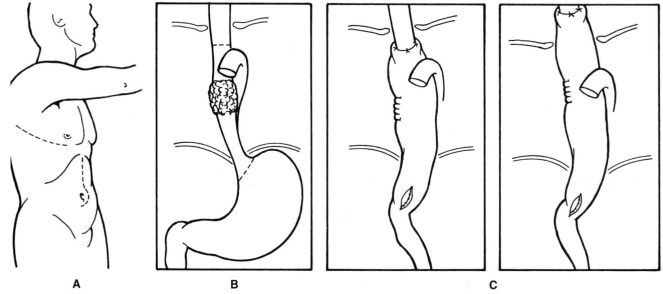

Figure 32-16. The Ivor Lewis procedure. **A,** Laparotomy and right thoracotomy. **B,** Tumor and margin of resection. **C,** Mobilization of the stomach into the chest cavity with anastomosis to the remaining esophagus (esophagogastrostomy). *(Redrawn from Ellis FH Jr: Esophagogastrectomy for carcinoma: technical considerations based on anatomic location of lesion, Surg Clin North Am 60:273, 1980.)*

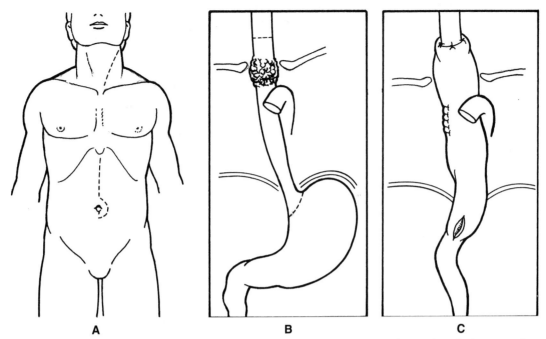

Figure 32-17. A, Laparotomy and left cervical incision. **B,** Tumor and margin of the resection. **C,** Mobilization of the stomach into the chest cavity with anastomosis to the cervical esophagus via a neck incision. *(Redrawn from Ellis FH Jr: Esophagogastrectomy for carcinoma: technical considerations based on anatomic location of lesion, Surg Clin North Am 60:275, 1980.)*

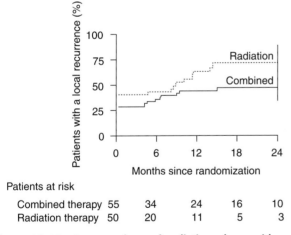

Patients at risk

Combined therapy	55	34	24	16	10
Radiation therapy	50	20	11	5	3

Figure 32-18. A comparison of radiation alone with combined radiation and chemotherapy regarding the time to a local recurrence in patients with esophageal cancer. *(From Herskovic A, et al: Combined chemotherapy and radiotherapy compared with radiotherapy alone in patients with cancer of the esophagus, N Engl J Med 326:1596, 1992.)*

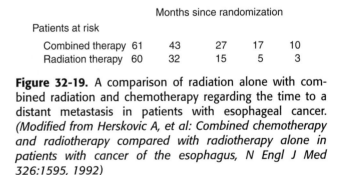

Patients at risk

Combined therapy	61	43	27	17	10
Radiation therapy	60	32	15	5	3

Figure 32-19. A comparison of radiation alone with combined radiation and chemotherapy regarding the time to a distant metastasis in patients with esophageal cancer. *(Modified from Herskovic A, et al: Combined chemotherapy and radiotherapy compared with radiotherapy alone in patients with cancer of the esophagus, N Engl J Med 326:1595, 1992)*

patients who fail locally and with distant metastases after curative treatment. The addition of combination chemotherapy has resulted in a decrease in local and distant failures and an increase in the overall survival rate compared with radiation alone (Figs. 32-18 and 32-19).[40]

Continuous infusion 5-FU and cisplatin are administered during weeks 1, 5, 8, and 11 of the radiation therapy treatments. Combined modality therapy has definite local control and survival benefits. However, the side effects from this regimen are worse.[10] New drugs and different combinations of chemotherapy and radiation are being researched. Paclitaxel is one drug being evaluated.[1,59]

Field design and critical structures. Esophageal cancer spreads longitudinally with skip lesions up to 5 cm from the primary. Regional spread to draining lymphatics is a common early presentation and must be taken into consideration in the design of the radiation field. The cervical, supraclavicular, mediastinal, and subdiaphragmatic (celiac axis) lymph node regions are at risk. The degree to which these nodal groups are at risk depends on the location of the primary tumor. Supraclavicular nodes are involved more often with a proximal lesion than a distal lesion. However, neck or abdominal nodal-disease involvement can occur with any esophageal primary site.[1,10,23,59]

Because of the potential for longitudinal spread of these cancers, radiation portals encompassing the areas at risk are typically large. For tumors of the thoracic esophagus the anatomic borders included in the treatment field extend from above the supraclavicular fossa to the esophagogastric junction. This volume is necessary for including the regional lymphatics and encompassing the primary tumor with a 5-cm margin above and below the gross disease.

Lesions of the upper third of the esophagus are treated with a field that begins at the level of the thyroid cartilage and ends at the level of the carina. In patients with tumors of the distal third of the esophagus the inferior margin must include the celiac-axis lymph nodes, which are located at the T12-L1 vertebral level. The superior extent of the treatment field should include the mediastinal nodes and may not include the supraclavicular nodes because they are at a low risk of being involved.[1,20,36,58,59]

The standard technique for treating the initial large fields is an AP/PA field, followed by shrinking fields of various arrangements. For treatment with radiation alone the prescribed dose is 65 Gy. With combined radiation and chemotherapy the total dose is 50 Gy to minimize normal tissue toxicity. Both of these doses exceed the radiation-tolerance dose of the spinal cord, which is 45 to 50 Gy. Careful dosimetry planning is necessary to avoid overdosing the spinal cord. AP/PA fields are used initially; as cord tolerance is approached, an off-cord technique is implemented. With three-dimensional (3D) conformal planning capabilities, the AP/PA fields and oblique off-cord fields are frequently treated simultaneously. The AP/PA fields are discontinued as cord tolerance is reached. A variety of off-cord field arrangements can be used, depending on the location of the tumor. The most common field arrangements are oblique radiation portals. Many institutions use a three-field approach: an anterior field and two posterior-wedged obliques, especially for lesions of the thoracic esophagus. Two anterior-wedged obliques or parallel-opposed oblique fields have also been used for lesions of the upper third of the esophagus (Fig. 32-20).[20,36,58] Another common off-cord technique in distal esophageal lesions is opposed laterals with AP/PA fields.[1,9,10,59]

For the simulation of a patient with esophageal cancer a variety of patient positions have been advocated. Some authors advise placing the patient in the prone position, using gravity to help place the esophagus at a greater distance from the spinal cord. This facilitates lower cord doses without compromising the tumor dose.[11,20] More universal is the standard supine position for patient simulation and treatment. Older patients and those who are more ill can tolerate this position easier and for a longer time than the prone position.

Other patient-positioning issues deal with the placement of the patient's arms. Because lateral treatment-field arrangements may be used, the patient's arms are often positioned above the head, with the patient clasping the elbows or wrists. This position can be difficult for the patient to hold and maintain, causing reproducibility problems later during treatment. Custom-made immobilization devices such as body casts, foaming cradles, and vacuum-bag devices greatly assist the daily reproducibility of the setup. Without a custom-made device, measurements of the elbow-to-elbow separation will assist in the consistency of the daily setup.

For the simulation of patients with their arms along their sides for isocentric fields, the elbows should be bent slightly out from the body so that a set of marks can be placed on the thoracic cage for a **three-point setup.** This is extremely important if the lateral positioning marks are on the arms and shoulders, because they are in an upper-third esophageal lesion. The arms are mobile and are not reliable for positioning and maintaining the established isocenter daily. Therefore a second set of three reference points are placed lower on the thoracic cage and are used to establish the isocenter. The upper three points are used to maintain the shoulder position. The anteroposterior SSD, or setup distance, is double-checked and maintained, especially with oblique treatment fields.

Orthogonal radiographs are taken 90 degrees apart at the time of the initial simulation. This includes an anterior film (defining the actual treatment volume) and a lateral film (establishing the isocenter or depth). Both films should be taken with barium contrast in the esophagus to delineate the esophagus and its relationship to normal structures. These radiographs, along with multiple-level contours or a CT scan with the patient in treatment position, assist the dosimetrist in planning the necessary off-cord field arrangements (Fig 32-21). After the treatment plan is complete a second simulation is often needed to film the oblique treatment fields.

CT simulation more accurately defines the location of the target volume, lymph node regions, and spinal cord interface than a conventional simulation. CT simulation also allows pertinent information to be obtained in one procedure instead of having a postsimulation treatment-planning CT scan. A second simulation to film the obliques or boost fields is not required with CT simulation. All fields can be designed from the original CT scan and treatment isocenter.

The patient will typically be positioned supine with arms above the head in an immobilization device as described previously. The device is measured to ensure that it fits inside the scanner and a photograph of patient setup is taken. Oral contrast used for CT imaging may be given to the patient

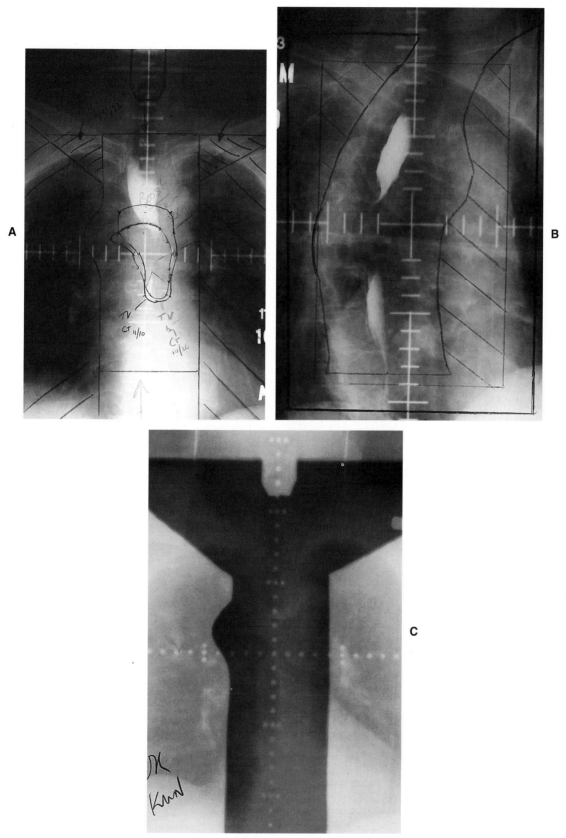

Figure 32-20. Radiation treatment fields for cancer of the esophagus. **A,** An anteroposterior/posteroanterior (AP/PA) field with barium to localize the esophageal lesion. **B,** Off-cord oblique fields. **C,** Port film of the initial anteroposterior field.

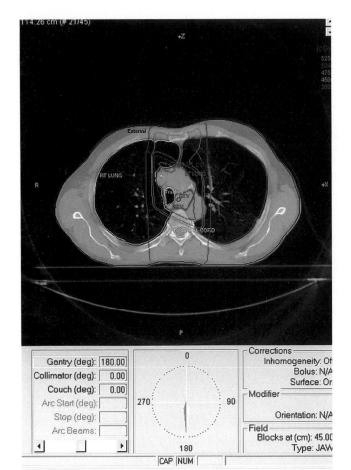

Figure 32-21. Isodose distribution resulting from anteroposterior/posteroanterior (AP/PA) and parallel-opposed obliques. AP/PA fields are discontinued as cord tolerance is reached. Note the sparing of the spinal cord with oblique fields.

30 minutes to 1 hour before the scan. A pudding-type contrast may also be given at the time of the CT simulation to visualize the esophagus. Patients with severe dysphagia may not be able to tolerate this, especially in the supine position.

The radiation therapist will ensure that the patient is straight and place reference marks on the thoracic cage and place radiopaque markers on these marks for visualization on the scan. The coordinates of these reference marks, superior and inferior scanning limits, pilot or scout length will all be recorded. A scan from above the mandible to iliac crest to include the entire esophagus and stomach may be obtained. Following the scan, the physician will digitize in different colors the target volume and critical anatomy as listed previously. The treatment isocenter will also be identified. The therapist is given the measurements to shift anterior or posterior and so forth from the reference marks to the appropriate location. The therapist then places marks or tattoos on the treatment isocenter or three points. Because the CT Sim is not equipped with field localization graticule like a conventional simulator, only the three points can be marked on the

patient's skin. Additional straightening lines drawn superiorly and inferiorly on the anterior chest using the sagittal laser are beneficial. Patient setup information, such as positioning and immobilization devices, is recorded at the time of simulation. Field size parameters and gantry and/or couch angles will be recorded once planning is complete. The patient will proceed to treatment following the completion of the treatment plan. 3D conformal treatment planning may be done to spare vital organs such as heart, lungs, and spinal cord.[59] A DRR of a treatment field with pertinent anatomy identified and a transverse CT Sim image of the treatment isocenter is seen in Fig. 32-22. A block check with contrast may be done on a conventional simulator to verify field design and patient setup before treatment.

Side effects.   After 2 weeks of radiation treatment, patients begin to experience **esophagitis.** They complain of substernal pain during swallowing and the sensation of food sticking in their esophagus. Patients may be unable to eat solid foods and require a diet of bland, soft, or pureed foods. In addition, patients should eat small, frequent meals that are high in calories and protein (Table 32-3). High-calorie liquid supplements such as Carnation Instant Breakfast and Ensure are good alternatives for a high-calorie snack during the day or at bedtime.[16,40,66]

To ease the pain of swallowing, the physician may suggest that the patient take liquid analgesics or viscous lidocaine before meals. These drugs provide local and systemic pain relief. Esophagitis can become severe by the end of the treatment and may even require the placement of a nasogastric tube.

Concomitant chemotherapy increases the sensitivity of the esophageal mucosa to radiation. Therefore more severe esophagitis and possibly ulceration may occur. The radiation tolerance of the esophagus is 65 Gy delivered with 1.8- to 2.0-Gy fractions. When concurrent chemotherapy is administered, the total radiation dose safely delivered is 50 Gy, based on the increased treatment-related toxicities associated with combined-modality treatment. Decreased blood counts, nausea, and vomiting also occur with chemotherapy. A break in a patient's treatment may be necessary if the leukocyte or platelet count becomes too low.

Radiation pneumonitis or pericarditis may occur if a large volume of lung or heart is in the radiation field. Proper field shaping, multiple fields per day, and careful dosimetry greatly reduce the likelihood of severe complications. Perforation and fistula formation can result from rapid shrinkage of a tumor that was adherent to the esophageal-tracheal wall.

Long-term side effects from irradiating the esophagus include stenosis or stricture as a result of scar formation. Dilatations of the esophagus can be performed, relieving the obstructive symptoms and restoring the patient's ability to swallow.* Transverse myelitis is a late complication that

---

*References 1, 9, 10, 20, 40, 58, 59.

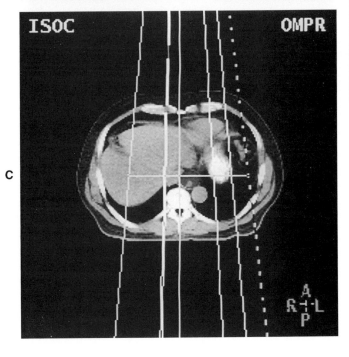

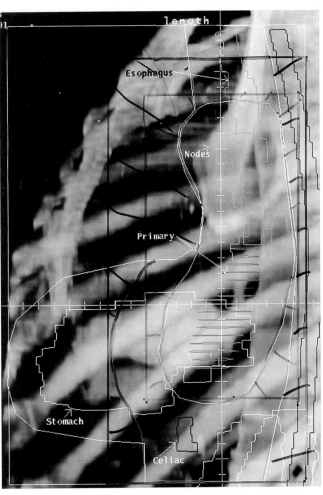

Figure 32-22. Computed tomography (CT) simulation digitally reconstructed radiographs (DRRs) of radiation treatment fields for cancer of the esophagus. **A,** Anteroposterior/posteroanterior (AP/PA) field with pertinent anatomy identified. **B,** Off-cord oblique field. **C,** CT simulation image at treatment isocenter. Note divergent beam outline.

should not occur if the radiation treatments are delivered and planned precisely and accurately.

Role of Radiation Therapist

Patients receiving radiation therapy for esophageal cancer require a lot of supportive care. They usually experience substantial weight loss as a result of the tumor's obstructive process and are nutritionally compromised. Esophagitis, as a result of the treatment, can cause more weight loss and further debilitate the health of the patient. The therapist should question patients about the way they are feeling, their appetite, and their food intake. Dietary suggestions regarding recommended foods or those to avoid should be made available to the patient. Some radiation therapy centers have

Table 32-3	Dietary guidelines for patients receiving thoracic irradiation	
Recommended Foods	**Foods to Avoid**	
Cottage cheese, yogurt, and milk shakes	Hot and spicy foods	
Puddings	Dry to coarse foods	
Casseroles	Crackers, nuts, and potato chips	
	Raw vegetables, citrus fruits, and juices	
Scrambled eggs	Alcoholic beverages	
Meats and vegetables in sauces or gravies		

printed sheets for the therapist or nurse to give to the patient. Many centers also have a dietitian to whom the patient may be referred for meal planning and dietary supplements.

Esophagitis can be emotionally and physically draining for these patients. The therapist should try to monitor the patient's emotional well-being as much as the physical aspects. The therapist should inform the patient about local cancer support groups that assist in coping with side effects of radiation treatments and disease.

Case Study

A 70-year-old man presented to his local physician complaining of episodes of sharp pain in the lower part of his midchest. His social history is significant in that he is a former smoker of 1 to 1.5 packs a day for 15 years. He continues to chew tobacco and consumes two drinks of alcohol per day. A barium swallow of the upper gastrointestinal area was obtained, demonstrating a filling defect in the lower esophageal region. An endoscopy was performed revealing a mass in the distal esophagus that was biopsied and found to be an adenocarcinoma. The patient was referred to the cancer center and was seen by one of the gastroenterologists. An EUS was performed that confirmed the mass located at 37 to 42 cm from the incisors in the area of the GE junction. The lesion was exophytic and involved 50% to 75% of the esophagus circumferentially without significant involvement of the stomach. Suspicious paraesophageal and subcarinal lymph nodes located at 28 cm from the incisors were biopsied and found to be adenocarcinoma grade 3. A CT scan of the chest and upper abdomen was obtained. The examination revealed a 3- to 3.5-cm lesion in the GE junction. The liver was negative for distant metastasis. The patient was a staged a stage III (T3, N1, M0). It was recommended that the patient undergo preoperative chemoradiation consisting of 5040 cGy in 28 fractions with concomitant 5-FU and cisplatin followed by a 4-week interval, restaging and surgery as indicated. The patient was treated with AP/PA fields including tumor and regional lymph nodes to a dose of 3060 cGy then off-cord parallel opposed obliques were used. A cone-down boost of the obliques was implemented at 4500 cGy to bring the total dose to 5040 cGy.

PANCREATIC CANCER

Epidemiology and Etiology

Cancers of the pancreas account for approximately 2% (31,000) of all cancers diagnosed annually in the United States. Pancreatic cancer is the fourth leading cause of cancer-related deaths in the United States, with approximately 30,000 deaths occurring annually. Pancreatic cancer has a high mortality rate and is considered one of the deadliest malignancies. It occurs more commonly in men than women, with incidence and mortality rates greater in African Americans than in whites. The disease rarely occurs in persons younger than 40 years with most patients in the 50- to 80-year-old age-group.[25,43,63]

No known cause exists for the development of pancreatic cancer, although a higher incidence seems to occur in smokers. Hereditary nonpolyposis colorectal cancer, familial breast cancer associated with the *BRCA2* mutation, and hereditary pancreatitis have been implicated as risk factors for the development of pancreatic cancer. Exposure to industrial chemicals such as benzidine and beta napthylamine over an extended period is related to an increased incidence of pancreatic cancer. However, definitive evidence establishing a causal relationship is lacking.[6,33,43,63]

Anatomy and Lymphatics

The pancreas is located retroperitoneally at the L1-L2 level and lies transversely in the upper abdomen. The pancreas is divided into three anatomic regions: the head, body, and tail. The head of the pancreas is located in the C-loop of the duodenum. The body lies just posterior to the stomach near the midline and is anterior to the IVC. Extending laterally to the left, the tail terminates in the splenic hilum. The pancreas is in direct contact with the duodenum, jejunum, stomach, major vessels (IVC), spleen, and kidney. Tumors of the pancreas commonly invade these structures and are therefore usually unresectable at the time of diagnosis.[6,17,33]

Numerous lymph node channels drain the pancreas and its surrounding structures. The main lymph node groups include the superior and inferior pancreaticoduodenal nodes, porta hepatis, suprapancreatic nodes, and paraaortic nodes. Tumors arising in the tail of the pancreas drain to the splenic hilar nodes (Fig. 32-23). Most patients have advanced local and/or metastatic disease at the time of diagnosis.[6,15,33]

Clinical Presentation

The four most common presenting symptoms of pancreatic cancer are abdominal pain, anorexia, weight loss, and jaundice. Tumors arising in the head of the pancreas may obstruct the biliary system, resulting in jaundice. Tumors that occur in the body or tail of the pancreas are not associated with obstruction of the biliary system and commonly involve severe pain and weight loss. Pancreatic cancers occur most frequently in the head of the pancreas.[6,36,43]

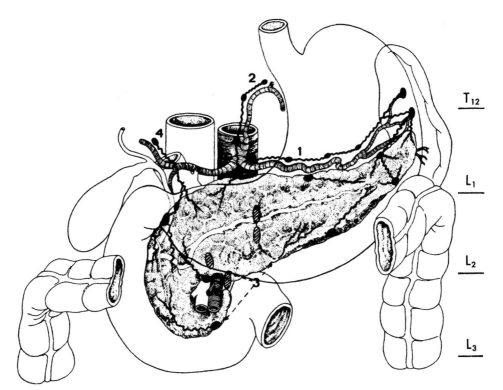

Figure 32-23. Anatomy and lymphatic drainage of the pancreas. Note the intimate relationship of the pancreas with the duodenum, stomach, transverse colon, spleen, and common bile duct. The four main trunks of lymphatic drainage. *1,* The left side drains along the tail into splenic hilar nodes; *2,* superior pancreatic lymph nodes and the celiac axis; *3,* inferior pancreatic, mesenteric, and left paraaortic nodes; *4,* right-side drainage to anterior and posterior pancreaticoduodenal nodes and right paraaortic nodes. *(From del Regato JA, Spjut HJ, Cox JD: Ackerman and del Regato's cancer: diagnosis, treatment, and prognosis, ed 6, St. Louis, 1985, Mosby.)*

Detection and Diagnosis

A thorough history and physical examination are extremely important. The abdomen should be assessed for palpable masses. The tumor's obstruction of the biliary system can result in an enlarged pancreas, gallbladder, or liver. Palpable supraclavicular nodes or rectal masses discovered during a digital rectal examination indicate peritoneal spread. All these signs suggest an advanced-stage disease. The presence or absence of jaundice is assessed by paying particular attention to the sclera, skin, and oral-cavity mucosa.[6,33]

The most valuable and important diagnostic test is a spiral CT scan of the abdomen. This scan provides a complete view of the abdominal structures most likely involved with the tumor. This image localizes the mass in the pancreas and depicts whether it is a head, body, or tail primary. The scan also demonstrates whether the tumor has invaded surrounding structures such as the duodenum, superior mesenteric vessels, or celiac-axis vessels. Spread to the regional lymph nodes, peritoneal implants, and distant metastasis to the liver can also be assessed.[4,43,54]

The resectability of the tumor can be determined by the information found on the CT scan. Liver metastasis and the involvement of the superior mesenteric artery or other major vessels are two contraindications to surgery. A CT-guided fine-needle biopsy of the primary tumor or metastatic lesions may be performed to establish the diagnosis.[6,33,43]

Endoscopic retrograde cholangiopancreatography (ERCP) is used in evaluating the obstruction and potential involvement of the biliary system. A biopsy of the ampulla or duodenum may be obtained at the time of the ERCP. This procedure is more beneficial for the diagnosis of a primary tumor of the biliary system. Ultrasonography has also been used to assess ductal obstruction, blood-vessel invasion, and liver metastasis.

EUS is a relatively new procedure used to image the pancreas. A transducer is passed down the esophagus to the duodenum adjacent to the pancreas. This examination is useful for visualizing small lesions in the head of the pancreas and to evaluate the potential involvement of lymph nodes and vasculature. EUS along with fine-needle aspiration is being evaluated as a tool to obtain tissue for diagnosis with less chance of tumor seeding as compared with a percutaneous approach. This procedure is not widely used because of the lack of experience of individuals with this technique.[43]

A laparoscopy performed before any surgical intervention may rule out small liver metastases (1 to 2 mm) that were undetectable on a CT scan.[33] According to a study done by Warshaw et al.,[65] laparotomies indicated that 40% of patients had small metastases in the liver or on parietal peritoneal surfaces. These patients were spared the morbidity of unnecessary abdominal surgery. If the patient's tumor appears to be resectable, based on the diagnostic workup, exploratory surgery and a biopsy are performed to determine the histology of the pancreatic mass.

Pathology and Staging

Adenocarcinomas comprise 80% of pancreatic cancers. Other histologic types include islet cell tumors, acinar cell carcinomas, and cystadenocarcinomas.[6,33,43]

A formal TNM staging system for pancreatic cancer is available. Most institutions, however, simply classify tumors as resectable or unresectable.

Routes of Spread

Cancers of the pancreas are locally invasive. Lymph node involvement or direct extension into the duodenum, stomach, and colon is not uncommon at the time of diagnosis. The tumor often encases or invades the superior mesenteric artery, portal vein, and celiac axis artery, rendering the tumor unresectable. Hematogenous spread to the liver via the portal vein is another common pathway of spread. Because of the propensity of these tumors to invade other abdominal structures, peritoneal seeding of tumor cells can also occur.[6,23,33,43]

Treatment Techniques

Surgery is the treatment of choice. Most tumors, however, are unresectable. Contraindications for undergoing a curative surgical procedure are liver metastasis, extra pancreatic serosal implantation, and invasion or adherence to major vessels.[6,43]

The most common potentially curative surgical procedure is a pancreaticoduodenectomy (Whipple procedure), which involves a resection of the head of the pancreas, entire duodenum, distal stomach, gallbladder, and common bile duct (Fig. 32-24). Reconstruction is done to maintain the continuity of the biliary-gastrointestinal system. The remaining pancreas, bile ducts, and stomach are anastomosed onto various sites of the jejunum (Fig. 32-25). The operative mortality rate from this procedure has greatly improved in recent years; it has been as high as 30%, but it is now less than 5%. The surgeon should place clips outlining the extent of the tumor to assist the radiation oncologist in planning adjuvant radiation therapy fields.[6,33,43,54,56]

Palliative biliary bypass procedures are often performed for unresectable tumors to redirect the flow of bile from obstructed ducts back into the gastrointestinal system. Typically, this is done by anastomosing the uninvolved bile ducts into the jejunum. Resolving the obstruction provides patients with relief of jaundice.

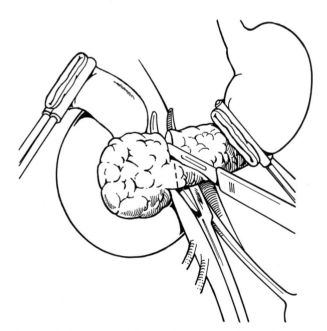

Figure 32-24. Pancreaticoduodenectomy (Whipple procedure); resection of the head of the pancreas, duodenum, distal stomach, gallbladder, and common bile duct. *(From Beazley RM, Cohn I Jr: Tumors of the pancreas, gallbladder, and extrahepatic ducts. In Murphy G, Lawrence W, Lenhard R: ACLS textbook of clinical oncology, 1995, American Cancer Society.)*

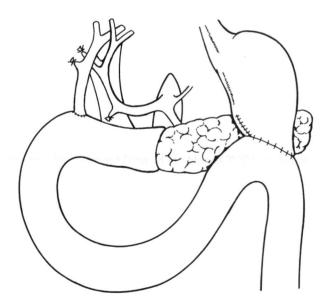

Figure 32-25. Reconstruction of the biliary and gastrointestinal system. The remaining pancreas, stomach, and bile ducts are anastomosed to the jejunum. *(From Beazley RM, Cohn I Jr: Tumors of the pancreas, gallbladder, and extrahepatic ducts. In Murphy G, Lawrence W, Lenhard R: ACLS textbook of clinical oncology, 1995, American Cancer Society.)*

Even with a potentially curative resection, the 5-year survival rate is usually less than 10%, with a median survival time of approximately 11 to 14 months.[23,39,41,56] This is due to a high local-regional recurrence rate and a high risk of distant metastases.[23,36,41]

Radiation therapy. Because of the high rate of distant metastasis and local-regional failure rate after surgery alone, combined-modality therapy versus observation was investigated in a randomized trial of patients with resected tumors. Adjuvant combined-modality treatment after surgery resulted in a significant improvement in the overall survival rate of 18 to 29 months compared with no further treatment. Chemoradiation, the delivery of radiation and chemotherapy simultaneously, has become the main method for the adjuvant treatment of pancreatic cancer.*

Radiation therapy and chemotherapy are considered the preferred treatments for locally advanced, unresectable pancreatic cancers. Studies comparing radiation alone with radiation and chemotherapy alone have demonstrated that the combined-modality treatment provides modestly improved survival rates.[4,43,50,54,56]

Specialized radiation therapy techniques have been investigated to determine whether higher doses to the tumor bed would translate into an increase in local control and better survival rates. One method of delivering a higher dose to the primary tumor is Intraoperative radiation therapy (IORT). A single dose of 20- to 25-Gy intraoperative electrons is delivered as a boost dose, following 50.4 Gy delivered by external beam radiation therapy. The main theoretical advantage of IORT is that it allows a higher dose to be delivered to the primary site than conventional external beam therapy because of the many dose-limiting structures located in the upper abdomen. Critical structures such as the kidney, liver, stomach, and small bowel can be moved out of the way or shielded during IORT. Studies evaluating the efficacy of this specialized boost technique have demonstrated an increase in local control when this method is added to the standard external beam therapy and chemotherapy treatment regimen. However, overall survival rates were not improved because of systemic failures in the liver or peritoneal seeding. Accordingly, IORT should not be used for pancreatic cancer in routine clinical practice. Different chemotherapy regimens are being investigated that may improve the systemic failures and increase survival rates.[4,22,23,43,54]

Chemotherapy. As mentioned, chemotherapy is used with radiation therapy as an adjuvant treatment in resected pancreatic tumors and as the primary treatment with radiation for unresectable disease. 5-FU is the drug of choice and is delivered concomitantly with the radiation. Even with combined-modality treatment, the overall survival rate of patients with pancreatic cancer is extremely poor. Different drug combinations and sequences are being investigated for improving survival rates. A new drug, gemcitabine, is being

evaluated for the treatment of unresectable pancreatic cancer. Preliminary results of the use gemcitabine have shown a slight improvement over 5-FU alone regimens, although more research is necessary to be conclusive.[4,23,39,43]

Field design and critical structures. A four-field technique is used for encompassing the primary tumor bed and draining lymphatics as defined by surgical clips or CT. A dose of 45 to 50 Gy is delivered in 1.8-Gy fractions with high-energy photons and a reduction in the field volume after 45 Gy. The upper abdomen contains many dose-limiting structures that must be considered for the designing and planning of radiation treatments. These structures include the kidneys, liver, stomach, small bowel, and spinal cord. The dose through the lateral fields is limited to 18 to 20 Gy because of the large volume of liver and kidneys in these fields.

Conformal 3D treatment planning and intensity modulated radiation therapy (IMRT) systems may allow higher doses of radiation to be delivered while keeping the dose-limiting structures within tolerance. 3D treatment planning permits the design of coplanar and non-coplanar beams that use a couch rotation to enter at unique angles to avoid critical structures allowing a higher dose to be achieved. Intensity-modulated systems use unique beam directions; however, they also vary the beam intensity and shape of the field with the use of multileaf collimators.[4,38]

Typical AP/PA field volumes for the head of a pancreatic lesion extend approximately from T10-T11 for inclusion of the tumor bed, draining lymphatics, and celiac axis (T12-L1). The width of the field should encompass the entire duodenal loop and the margin extending across the midline on the left. The lateral fields are designed to provide a 1.5- to 2-cm margin anteriorly beyond the known disease. Posteriorly, the field extends 1.5 cm behind the anterior vertebral body for adequate coverage of the paraaortic nodes (Fig. 32-26). For body or tail lesions the volume treated does not need to include the duodenal loop but must extend farther to the left to provide an adequate margin on the primary tumor and to include the splenic hilar nodes.[23,33]

For simulation the patient is placed in the supine position with the arms above the head for easier placement of the lateral isocenter marks. A vacuum device or foaming cradle immobilization device is made before the simulation. The device is measured to ensure it will fit in a CT scanner following the simulation procedure. A photograph of the patient in the device is taken to ensure reproducibility of the setup later. Preliminary borders and an isocenter are established and marked on the patient's skin. At many centers, renal contrast is injected, and a reference anteroposterior and/or lateral film is taken to determine the kidney location relative to other structures. This film assists in the design of custom shielding used to avoid unnecessary irradiation to the kidneys. The location of the kidneys may also be transferred from measurements of a CT scan onto the simulation film. For treating a head of pancreas lesion, approximately 50% of the right kidney is in the treated volume; therefore at least

---
*References 4, 22, 38, 41, 43, 54, 56.

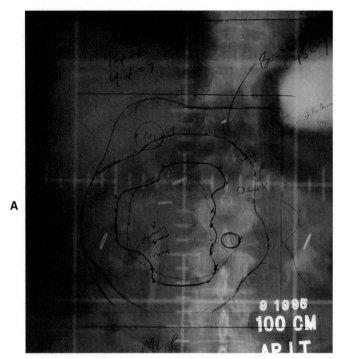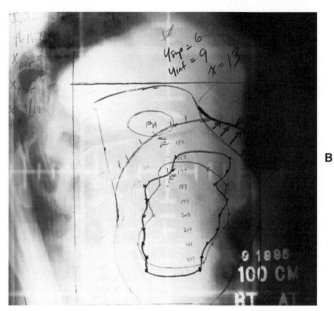

Figure 32-26. Radiation therapy treatment fields for pancreatic cancer. **A,** Anteroposterior/posteroanterior (AP/PA). **B,** Opposed laterals.

two thirds of the left kidney should be shielded to preserve normal kidney function.

After the films for kidney localization are completed, the patient is instructed to drink barium for localization of the duodenum and stomach. This is done to ensure adequate margins on the duodenum, especially for unresectable head of pancreas lesions. Another set of anteroposterior and lateral radiographs are then taken. This final set of films is representative of the actual volume to be treated. Shielding blocks or MLC are designed to block as much as possible of the kidneys, liver, and stomach on the AP/PA fields, and the lateral film is used to shield the spinal cord and small bowel.[33]

If a CT simulation is done, the patient is positioned with arms above the head in an immobilization device. The device is measured to ensure that it fits inside the scanner and a photograph of patient setup is taken. The CT simulation also requires that contrast be administered. With this simulation, the patient is instructed to drink contrast 30 minutes to 1 hour before the scan. Some centers may inject contrast for kidney localization although the kidneys can be visualized on the scan without contrast.

The radiation therapist will place reference marks on the patient's abdomen before scanning. A scan from above the diaphragm to below the iliac crest will be obtained. The physician can digitize in the location of the target volume, lymph nodes, porta hepatis, and the superior mesenteric artery to ensure coverage of these structures in the treatment field. The dose-limiting structures, kidneys, liver, stomach, small bowel, and spinal cord, may be outlined on the DRRs as well

(Fig. 32-27). Once the treatment isocenter has been identified, the radiation therapist will make the appropriate shifts from the reference isocenter and mark the final three points to be used for treatment. The CT images are then sent to the dosimetrist for 3D conformal planning (Fig. 32-28).

Side effects. The most common complaints of patients receiving radiation for pancreatic cancer are nausea and vomiting. Antiemetics may be given to mitigate these adverse effects. Other potential acute side effects include leukopenia, thrombocytopenia, diarrhea, and stomatitis. Long-term side effects, such as renal failure, are rare and suggest the possibility of improper shielding of the kidney.[3,50]

Case Study

A 55-year-old man presented with episodes of fever and dark urine. He was found on endoscopy to have a polypoid lesion in the periampullary region of the pancreas that was biopsied and found to be a grade 3 adenocarcinoma. His CT scan demonstrated no evidence of metastatic disease in the liver or upper abdomen. The patient underwent a pylorus-sparing pancreatic duodenectomy. At the time of surgery the tumor had invaded minimally into the pancreas and 1 of 16 nodes were found to be positive for tumor. Because of the high risk of local and distant failure with surgery alone, he was referred to radiation oncology for adjuvant chemoradiation. The patient underwent a CT simulation and a 3D treatment plan was performed to provide adequate dose to the tumor bed and regional nodes while minimizing dose to sensitive organs such as the kidneys, liver, and spinal cord. The patient was treated with a four field with a shrinking field coned-down boost to 5040 cGy.

Gynecologic Tumors

George M. Uschold

Outline

Key Terms

Interstitial implant
Intrauterine tandem
Midline block
Parametrium
Pelvic inlet
Perineum

Sensitive test
Specific test
Vaginal colpostats
Vaginal cuff
Vaginal cylinder implant

This chapter provides radiation therapists with basic knowledge of gynecologic malignancies. An initial section on epidemiology and etiology discusses the relative number of cancers and deaths resulting from the various sites. This section is followed by a site-specific discussion regarding the populations at risk and various risk factors. The anatomy of the pelvic gynecologic structures is then reviewed. Knowledge of radiation tolerances and lymphatic drainage is of critical importance in radiation therapy treatment planning. These issues are discussed in depth.

Following this general review, the organ areas (vulva, vagina, cervix, endometrium, and ovaries) are discussed in individual sections. Each section begins with a clinical presentation that includes symptoms, data regarding lymphatic spread, and prognostic features. This is followed by a brief description of the clinical workup, expected pathology, and staging. To minimize confusion, the staging is limited to the system provided by the International Federation of Gynecology and Obstetrics (FIGO).[21] Treatment considerations specific to each organ are then presented. This is done to orient the radiation therapist to required modifications in the treatment design beyond the basic pelvic treatment plan and to provide the rationale for these modifications. Each section closes with a case study that synthesizes the principles presented.

After the sections concerning specific organs, general principles of external beam radiation therapy and brachytherapy are discussed in detail. The goal is to promote a clear knowledge of the basic design of treatment fields and enable the radiation therapist to understand the rationale underlying the various simulations. Dose schedules are presented generally and with the specific sites. In general, the radiation therapist should be able to use data in this section to understand and critique most gynecologic treatment plans.

The chapter closes with a discussion of expected side effects from radiation therapy and the radiation therapist's role in evaluating and managing these sequelae. The radiation therapist has three main functions during the course of therapy: treatment delivery, ongoing patient assessment, and patient reassurance.

EPIDEMIOLOGY AND ETIOLOGY

An estimated 94,000 patients develop gynecologic cancer in the United States. This type of malignancy is divided into endometrial (48%), ovarian (29%), cervical (16%), and other gynecologic cancers (7%). An estimated 27,000 deaths occurred, with ovarian being the most prevalent (53%), followed by endometrial (25%), cervical (17%), and other gynecologic cancers (5%).[9]

Alternatively, considering the ratio of deaths to new cases, ovarian cancer has the highest death rate at 59%, followed by cervical cancer (excluding carcinoma in situ) at 34%, and endometrial cancer at 17%. Although there are 24% more endometrial than ovarian cancers, ovarian cancer deaths are 250% the incidence of endometrial-related deaths. The high death rate for ovarian cancer is primarily due to the relatively nonspecific early symptoms with a consequent diagnosis of later-stage disease. A secondary reason is less effective treatment. Endometrial cancer has a relatively higher cure rate because the early symptom of postmenopausal bleeding usually results in a physical evaluation at an earlier stage, during which effective local therapy can be initiated.

Overall, cervical carcinoma is more prevalent than other gynecologic cancers among younger women; however, although cervical intraepithelial neoplasia affects mainly younger women, invasive cervical cancer rates reach their peak in women aged 50 to 60.[25] In addition, women of lower socioeconomic status have a greater than average risk of developing cervical cancer and a less than average participation rate in cancer screening programs.[43] Early sexual activity, multiple partners, and multiple pelvic infections (especially with genital warts and human papillomaviruses [HPVs] and herpes simplex type 2 [HSII]) have been associated with an increase in the risk of this disease and an earlier onset. Incidence is also higher among wives of men with penile cancer.[22] As with vaginal cancers, there is an increased risk of clear cell adenocarcinoma and abnormalities of the stratified epithelium in women whose mothers used diethylstilbestrol (DES) during the early months of pregnancy.[45] However, all women are at some risk and need effective and safe screenings. The widespread use of Papanicolaou smears has resulted in early detection; two thirds of cervical cancers are now detected in the noninvasive stage and are therefore highly curable with local therapy.

The prevalence of endometrial cancer has increased as a result of the aging population, high-calorie and high-fat diets, and the use of unopposed estrogen in the 1960s and 1970s. The incidence peaks at about 58 years, and more than 75% of patients are women older than 50. Diabetes and hypertension are both linked with an increase in prevalence of endometrial cancer.[46] Women who are 50 pounds overweight have a ninefold increase in risk.[39] A higher risk also results from an increase in estrogen or the estrogen-to-progesterone ratio, as occurs with nulliparity, infertility secondary to anovulation (with a deficit in progesterone), dysfunctional bleeding during menopause (secondary to estrogen overstimulation), or prolonged hormone replacement therapy (HRT). In the case of HRT, the increased risk seems to be treatment duration dependent.[4]

Vaginal and vulvar cancers are rare and usually occur in older women. Vulvar carcinoma, which is three times as common as vaginal cancer, has been associated with diabetes and sexually transmitted diseases.[1] Atrophic-dysplastic changes in the normal vaginal lining, a loss of hormone stimulation, and poor hygiene may also be associated with vulvar cancers. An unusual clear-cell variant of vaginal cancer seen in young women (median age of 19) has been associated with DES use by their pregnant mothers while they were *in utero*.[45] If the cervix is involved with a vaginally located cancer, the tumor is instead classified as a cervical cancer with vulvovaginal spread and is treated in the same way as other advanced cervical cancers.

Ovarian carcinoma occurs primarily in women between the ages of 50 and 70. At approximately 14,000 estimated deaths annually, it is the fourth leading cause of cancer deaths in women, following lung (69,000), breast (40,000), and colon (29,000) cancer.[9] Risk factors include an older age; late or few pregnancies; late menopause; a lack of oral contraceptive use; a family history of ovarian cancer; and a personal history of breast, colon, or endometrial cancer.[38] Diets high in meat and/or animal fat and living in industrialized nations (except Japan) are risk factors. Screening is poor because the disease is only intermittently detectable during physical examinations, radiographic studies, and serologic tests and usually at an advanced stage. With the low prevalence of this disease, even a 100% **sensitive test** (0% false negative) for detecting tumors and a 99% **specific test** (1% false positive) for patients with disease result in over 100 laparotomies for every early ovarian cancer detected with an iatrogenic death rate equal or higher than the disease. For patients with hereditary ovarian cancer syndrome the lifetime risk increases from 1% to 40%, and a screening with an annual rectovaginal pelvic examination, CA 125 serum determinations, and transvaginal ultrasound* is recommended to reduce this significant risk.

ANATOMY AND LYMPHATICS

The vulva is the outermost portion of the gynecologic tract. The major parts include the labia majora and labia minora; the clitoris; and the area bound by these three, called the

---

*A test used to detect abnormalities in the reproductive system and possible complications with pregnancy by way of a vaginally inserted ultrasound transducer that emits high-frequency sound waves that are electronically converted to diagnostic images.

vestibule. The vestibule is triangular, is located anterior to the vaginal opening, and usually contains the urethral meatus, unless the meatus exits the outer third of the vaginal canal. The **perineum** refers to the area between the vulvovaginal complex and anal verge. The vagina is a muscular tube that extends 6 to 8 in. superiorly from the vulva and is located anterior to the rectum and posterior to the bladder. The cervix (the part of the uterus that extends into the apex of the vagina) is a firm, rounded structure from 1.5 to 3 cm in diameter. The cervix often protrudes into the vagina, producing lateral spaces in the vaginal apex called the fornices. A canal called the cervical os extends from the vagina, through the central cervix, and into the uterine cavity, or pelvic portion of the uterus. The uterus is a hollow, muscular structure that extends at a right angle from the vagina to overlie the bladder. Extending laterally from the superior uterus are the twin fallopian tubes. These are hollow structures designed to transmit the ova from the ovaries located adjacent to them. The **parametrium** refers to the area immediately lateral to the uterine body (Fig. 33-1).

Radiation therapy treatment requires an understanding of the radiosensitivity of the various gynecologic structures and their lymphatic drainage. The vulva and perineum usually show the most acute short-term side effects, partly because of their radiation sensitivity and the often parallel and tangential nature of the treatment beams applied to them. Doses above 40 Gy at standard fractions (1.8 to 2 Gy) often cause significant acute erythema and desquamation, and doses above 50 Gy cause late telangiectasis. Significant fibrosis can result from doses approaching 70 Gy. The vagina is more tolerant, with the upper vaginal mucosa tolerating up to 140 Gy and the lower up to 100 Gy before extensive fibrosis.[20] Early mucositis and later telangiectasis occur with much lower treatment-range doses (60 to 85 Gy). The uterus and cervix tolerate extremely high doses of radiation and allow the effectiveness of brachytherapy to the uterus. Low-dose-rate brachytherapy, in combination with fractionated external radiation therapy, can be delivered locally to the canal without necrosis when the total dose does not exceed 200 Gy.[18] The ovary is the most radiosensitive gynecologic structure. The dose response is age dependent. For example, a dose of 4 to 5 Gy produces the permanent cessation of menses in about 65% of women younger than 40, 90% of those aged 40 to 44, and 100% of those 50 years or older.[34]

Many other organs surrounding the gynecologic structures have dose tolerances that must be respected. The bladder, which is located anterior to the vagina and cervix and somewhat under the uterus, expands forward and away from

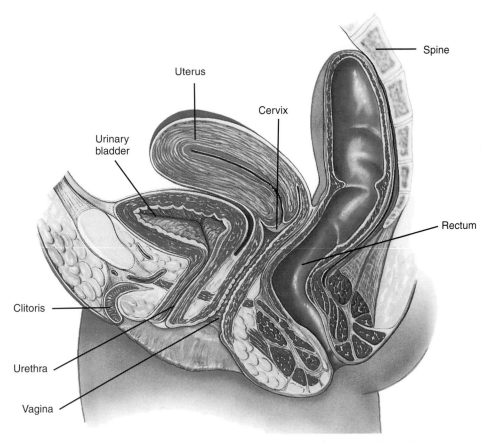

Figure 33-1. A sagittal view of the female pelvis. *(From Seely R: Essentials of anatomy and physiology, St. Louis, 1991, Mosby.)*

these structures when it is filled. The point tolerance is about 70 Gy, but whole-bladder treatment results in acute cystitis at doses as low as 30 Gy. This results in acute bladder irritation with dysuria, frequency, and urgency but usually resolves in a couple of weeks. Chronic cystitis occasionally occurs 6 months after radiation with doses above 50 to 60 Gy, and contracture and/or hemorrhagic cystitis occurs with doses above 65 Gy. The rectum, which is immediately posterior to the vagina and cervix, also has a point tolerance of about 70 Gy. The rectum continues superiorly with the sigmoid colon, with a whole-organ tolerance of about 50 Gy. Diarrhea, bleeding, urgency, and pain can occur acutely at 30 to 40 Gy. Stricture, bleeding, and perforation are late complications that occur with doses above the tolerance level. The small bowel is variably looped down in the pelvis and may overlie the uterus and bladder. This bowel has a lower tolerance at 45 Gy, can yield the same acute toxicity as the large bowel (but at lower doses), and is more likely to obstruct as a chronic complication.

The treatment design must consider the extent of the primary lesion and the probability of metastases to the draining lymph nodes. Lymphatic drainage includes the inguinal lymph nodes (external and internal), pelvic nodes (the internal iliac chain, which originates approximately with the obturator node, and external iliac chain), and periaortic nodes (Fig. 33-2). The deep inguinals drain into the external iliac chain, and the internal and external iliac chains join and then drain into the periaortics. Drainage is approximately contiguous. Therefore if involvement of the nodes occurs at one level, including the next higher nodal group in the treatment field may be appropriate.

Ovarian and upper endometrial lymphatics follow the ovarian blood supply to terminate in periaortic lymph nodes at the level of the kidneys and follow the round ligament to involve the inguinal lymphatics. The primary drainage pattern of the cervix and additional drainage patterns of the ovary and uterus are to the external iliac, obturator, and hypogastric chains. Upper vaginal drainage follows the cervical pathways. Lower vaginal drainage may follow the vulvar drainage into the inguinal nodes.

VULVA

Clinical Presentation

Vulvar cancer patients usually have a subcutaneous lump or mass. Patients with more advanced disease have an ulcerative exophytic mass. The disease is usually unifocal, with the labia majora as the most common location. Often, the patient has a long history of irritation. Lymphatic spread is predictable, involving the superficial inguinal nodes first, then the deep femoral nodes, and eventually the pelvic nodes. However, lymph nodes are falsely enlarged in about 40% of patients. The incidence of lymph node involvement is related to the depth of invasion (less than 10% at 1 to 3 mm and about 25% at 3 to 4 mm) and tumor size (38% for tumors greater than 5 mm and 46% for those greater than 20 mm).[36] Occult disease is common, as is inflammation, so a high level of false negatives and false positives are based on the examination and

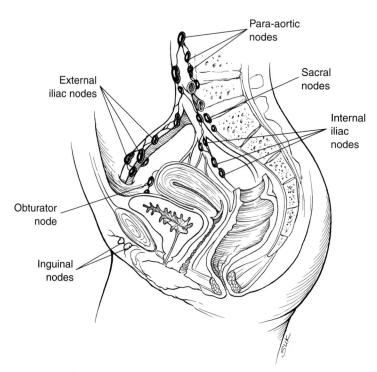

Figure 33-2. Lymph node drainage of the pelvis.

clinical suspicion alone. Prognostic factors include the size of the lesion, depth of invasion, and histologic subtype. The presence and extent of lymph node involvement is the strongest predictor of overall survival rates.

Detection and Diagnosis

A workup should include a biopsy, a cytologic examination, a history, a physical examination, blood counts and chemistries, a urinalysis, chest radiographs, an intravenous pyelogram (IVP) and/or a computed tomography (CT) scan, and a cystoscopy. Liver scans, a bone scan, a sigmoidoscopy, and a pelvic CT scan are usually performed if the tumor is advanced clinically or found on the other staging studies.

Pathology and Staging

Squamous cell carcinomas account for more than 90% of vulvar cancers, and adenocarcinomas represent the remaining cases.[38] Staging is as follows:

Stage I: Tumor confined to the vulva or vulva and perineum with a maximum diameter of 2 cm or less in greatest dimension

Stage II: Tumor confined to the vulva or vulva and perineum with a maximum diameter greater than 2 cm in greatest dimension

Stage III: Tumor of any size with contiguous spread to the lower urethra and/or vagina or anus

Stage IVA: Tumor invades any of the following: upper urethra, bladder mucosa, rectal mucosa, or is fixed to the pelvic bone

Treatment Considerations

Historically, treatment has involved a radical vulvectomy with a groin node dissection. For stage III disease with inguinal nodes positive for tumor, deep pelvic nodes must be addressed, either with a pelvic node dissection or pelvic irradiation. Recent studies have indicated that a more conservative approach using wide local excision with external irradiation of the primary and inguinal nodes produces similar tumor control, 5-year disease-free survival and overall survival rates, while causing less morbidity.[2,7,19]

Radiation therapy may be administered preoperatively, but it is seldom used as the sole treatment. (Simulation techniques are discussed at the end of the chapter.) For stages I and II disease, radiation therapy is usually given after a simple vulvectomy (50 Gy) and a wide local excision (60 Gy plus a 5- to 10-Gy boost if margins are positive for tumor). With radiation therapy alone, doses of 65 to 70 Gy are delivered.[37] For stage III disease, radiation therapy is given postoperatively if the primary is larger than 4 cm, margins are positive for tumor, or three or more lymph nodes are positive for tumor. A dose of 50 Gy is delivered to control microscopic disease, with a 15-Gy boost if margins are microscopically positive for tumor and 20 Gy for grossly involved margins. Boosts may be delivered using photons, en face perineal electrons, and via brachytherapy. The inguinal region (nodes) is treated to 45 to 50 Gy for control of microscopic disease and to 65 to 70 Gy for palpable disease. If the pelvic nodes are included, 45 to 50 Gy is delivered for microscopic disease and 60 Gy for macroscopic disease. Treatment interruptions are usually needed at 40 Gy or less if chemotherapy is given concomitantly. The vulva and perineum usually develop significant moist desquamation as a result of the decreased thickness of the region, the parallel delivery of the external beam, and the need for bolus.

The overall 5-year survival rate is about 70%,[23,26] and the disease-free survival rates in surgically treated patients with stages I through IV disease are 100%, 86%, 59%, and 25%, respectively.[31] Hacker et al.[19] have shown the influence of regional lymph node involvement, with actuarial 5-year survival rates of 96% for node negative for tumor, 94% with one node positive for tumor, 80% with two nodes positive for tumor, and 12% with three or more nodes positive for tumor.

Case Study

M.M. is an 83-year-old white woman with underlying vascular disease from her hypertension, diabetes, and hypercholesterolemia. She consulted her gynecologist and exhibited a 5-cm right labial mass. A wide local excision and bilateral lymph node dissections revealed no nodes positive for tumor. The mass recurred 6 months later on the right side, and the patient underwent a simple vulvectomy and rhomboid skin flap grafts. Because of the recurrence, deep invasion, and close margins, she was referred for postoperative radiation therapy. Her disease was considered stage II initially, before the recurrence.

The treatment design included anteroposterior/posteroanterior (AP/PA) lower pelvic fields and anteriorly treated inguinal fields. Initially, 6-MV photons were used with anterior bolus. The initial dose was 50.4 Gy at 1.8 Gy per fraction. The perineum and operative sites received a boost of 10 Gy with en face 9-MeV electrons at 2 Gy per fraction. The patient required several treatment breaks for moist desquamation and urethral irritation. Diarrhea was not a major problem.

M.M. remained free of disease for 18 months, until a recurrence in the periurethral area. An iridium **interstitial implant** was performed to a small volume surrounding the area of recurrence at a dose of 40 Gy over 4 days. This treatment controlled the local disease, but she experienced recurrence again in the peroneal body and anal canal. M.M. is considering some type of exenterative procedure.

VAGINA

Clinical Presentation

Vaginal cancer is a malignancy that arises in the vagina and does not extend to the vulva or cervix. This definition helps make vaginal cancer a rare disease that accounts for approximately 2% of all gynecologic cancers. No etiologic associations are definite, except for the rarer clear cell variant seen in 1 per 1000 women exposed to DES while they were in utero. The usual squamous cell carcinomas occur in older women (median age of 65), whereas clear cell carcinomas occur in young women between the ages of 15 and 27 (median age of 19 at diagnosis).[27] Abnormal vaginal bleeding and/or painful intercourse are the usual presenting symptoms. The most common location is the posterior upper third of the vagina. The risk of lymphatic involvement increases with the depth of invasion. Pelvic lymphatic involvement is similar to cervical cancer, with lesions of the lower third of the vagina also involving the inguinal nodes.

Detection and Diagnosis

The workup should include a biopsy, a cytologic examination, a careful history, a physical examination, blood counts and chemistries, a urinalysis, chest radiographs, an IVP or abdominopelvic CT scan, and a cystoscopy. If the disease is advanced, liver and bone scans, a sigmoidoscopy, and a pelvic CT scan are recommended.

Pathology and Staging

Squamous cell carcinomas total 80% to 90% of vaginal cancers. Malignant melanomas account for about 5% of vaginal cancers. Other vaginal cancers include sarcomas, malignant lymphomas, and clear cell adenocarcinomas. Staging is as follows:

Stage I: Tumor confined to the vagina

Stage II: Tumor invades the paravaginal tissue but not to the pelvic wall

Stage III: Tumor extends to the pelvic wall (muscle, fascia, neurovascular structures, or skeletal portions of the bony pelvis)

Stage IVA: Tumor invades the mucosa of the bladder or rectum and/or extends beyond the true pelvis

Treatment Considerations

Radiation therapy is the treatment of choice for most vaginal cancers. Surgery is used for recurrent or persistent squamous cell cancers and in young women who have early clear cell adenocarcinoma. For small, superficial lesions, only the vaginal tissues are treated (via local excision or brachytherapy), but for invasive lesions the entire pelvis must be treated. Doses of 45 to 50 Gy are given to the pelvis, and the entire vagina is included in the external beam field. If the tumor involves the middle or lower third of the vagina, the inguinal nodes are also treated as in vulvar cancer. Microscopic disease is treated to 50 Gy and macroscopic to 65 to 80 Gy. Brachytherapy implants are used to bring the primary and adjacent macroscopic disease to curative doses. Problems with early acute dermatitis are similar to those seen in vulvar cancer patients. *(Details concerning simulation, brachytherapy, and overall side effects are given in the final sections of this chapter.)*

Case Study

O.A. is a 61-year-old white woman with underlying chronic obstructive pulmonary disease (COPD) and hypertension. She complained to the gynecologist of 2 months of vaginal bleeding, especially after intercourse. A pelvic examination revealed a mass at the lateral aspect of the vagina and discontinuous from the cervix. A biopsy confirmed poorly differentiated, invasive squamous cell carcinoma. The results of other staging studies were negative for tumor. Her disease was classified as stage II (T2, N0).

Radiation therapy consisted of AP/PA pelvic and vaginal treatment, with 18-MV photons at 2 Gy per fraction to 20 Gy. A **midline block** (shielding block used to eliminate dose to centrally located anatomy) was then added, and she was treated to an additional 20 Gy. A reduced parametrial boost with midline blocking of the small bowel was given an additional 10 Gy.

Brachytherapy consisted of a **vaginal cylinder implant,** giving the mucosa 20 Gy over 2 days at the beginning of the midline-blocked pelvic treatment, and a second complex implant with a vaginal cylinder and right-sided interstitial needles given at the end of the initial pelvic treatment. The second implant yielded an additional 40 Gy to the vaginal mucosa and 25 Gy to the right-sided vaginal extension of the tumor.

The patient experienced some diarrhea, cystitis, and vaginal dryness but is still sexually active and free of disease 2 years later.

CERVIX

Clinical Presentation

Cervical cancer is a slowly progressive disease, with the earliest phase (noninvasive carcinoma in situ) occurring approximately 10 years earlier than invasive cancer. The earlier cervical cancer is detected, the better the local and overall control. Routine Papanicolaou smears have played a crucial role in the early detection of cervical cancer and in the improved overall survival rate. Screening should begin at age 18 or earlier in sexually active women.

Common presenting signs of invasive cancer are postcoital bleeding, increased menstrual bleeding, and discomfort with intercourse. A foul-smelling discharge, pelvic pain, and urinary or even rectal symptoms may accompany more advanced disease. Invasive cancer appears as a friable, ulcerative, or exophytic mass originating from or involving the cervix. The mass may extend into the vaginal canal and onto the vaginal sidewalls, or it may invade adjacent tissues such as the parametrium, bladder, or rectum. Lymphatic involvement is usually orderly, involving parametrial nodes, followed by pelvic, common iliac, periaortic, and even supraclavicular nodes. The incidence of pelvic and periaortic nodal involvement is local-stage dependent, with less than 5% and less than 1% for stage I, 15% and 5% for stage Ib, 30% and 15% for stage II, and 50% and 30% for stage III, respectively.[24] With periaortic nodal involvement, a 35% risk exists for supraclavicular spread.[6]

Survival rates and local control decrease as the stage and bulk of the disease increase. Ureter invasion has been associated with a reduction in 5-year survival rates from 92% to 54%.[29] Bulky or barrel-shaped cervical cancer is associated with a 15% to 20% increase in distant metastases and a decrease in local control.[41,42] For stages IB and IIA, the involvement of lymph nodes results in approximately a 50% reduction in survival rates.[12-14] Host factors associated with decreased local control or survival rates include anemia, which may affect aggressiveness of the tumor,[8,30] and a body temperature higher than 100° F.[15] In addition, a recent study by Milosevic et al.[28] found that patients with an interstitial fluid pressure (IFP) greater than 19 mm Hg had a significantly lower disease-free survival rate compared with those whose IFP was less than 19 mm Hg (34% vs. 68%, respectively).

Detection and Diagnosis

The workup should initially include a pelvic examination, Papanicolaou smear, and biopsy of any suspicious lesions. Further staging studies include a complete history, a physical examination under anesthesia, dilatation and curettage to assess uterine involvement, complete blood counts, chemistries, and a urinalysis. Chest radiographs, barium enema, and an IVP are used for FIGO staging. For more advanced disease, abdominopelvic CT or magnetic resonance imaging (MRI) scans, a cystoscopy, and a proctoscopy are recommended. A lymphangiogram and laparotomy may also be used to help with the treatment design but are not used for the initial staging. Surgical evaluation with lymph node dissection is associated with a significant increase in pelvic side effects, but a laparoscopic or CT-directed biopsy may be useful in designing treatment portals.

Pathology and Staging

Pathologically, most cervical, vaginal, and vulvar cancers are squamous cell types. Adenocarcinomas of the cervix arise from the mucous-secreting endocervical glands and account for about 8% of these tumors. Small cell and clear cell types account for about 2% of the remaining tumors and have a higher metastatic potential.[38] Staging is as follows:

Stage 0: Carcinoma in situ
Stage I: Cervical cancer confined to the uterus
Stage IA: Invasive carcinoma diagnosed only by microscopy. Stromal invasion with a maximum depth of 5.0 mm measured from the base of the epithelium and a horizontal spread of 7.0 mm or less. Vascular space involvement, venous or lymphatic, does not affect classification.
Stage IA1: Measured stromal invasion 3.0 mm or less in depth and 7.0 mm or less in horizontal spread
Stage IA2: Measured stromal invasion more than 3.0 mm and not more than 5.0 mm in depth and 7.0 mm or less in horizontal spread or horizontal spread greater than 7.0 mm
Stage IB: Clinically visible lesion confined to the cervix or microscopic lesion greater than IA2
Stage IB1: Clinically visible lesion 4.0 cm or less in greatest dimension
Stage IB2: Clinically visible lesion more than 4.0 cm in greatest dimension
Stage II: Cervical cancer invades beyond the uterus but not to the pelvic sidewalls or lower third of the vagina
Stage IIA: Tumor without parametrial invasion
Stage IIB: Tumor with parametrial invasion
Stage III: Tumor extends to the pelvic wall and/or to the lower third of the vagina, and/or causes hydronephrosis or nonfunctioning kidney

Stage IIIA: Tumor involves lower third of the vagina, no extension to pelvic wall
Stage IIIB: Tumor extends to the pelvic wall and/or causes hydronephrosis or nonfunctioning kidney
Stage IVA: Tumor invades mucosa of the bladder or rectum and/or extends beyond the true pelvis

Staging is based on a clinical examination before the initiation of therapy and may be supplemented by a blood analysis, chest radiographs, an IVP, a cystoscopy, a barium enema, and bone scans. A CT scan, laparotomy findings, an MRI scan, and lymphangiograms may modify treatment but do not change the FIGO staging. For statistical purposes the cancer is staged at the earlier level if disagreement or doubt exists.

Treatment Considerations

For early stage 0 (carcinoma in situ) and for stage Ia1 invasive cancer, the usual treatment is a total abdominal hysterectomy (TAH) with a small amount of vaginal tissue, known as the **vaginal cuff.** Alternately, a conization limited to the cervix may be performed in women who desire additional children. A tandem and ovoid implant, delivering 45 to 55 Gy to point A, is occasionally used for medically inoperable patients. For stage Ia2, TAH or a more aggressive modified radical hysterectomy is usually performed. In the medically inoperable patient, 60 to 70 Gy may be delivered with the use of a tandem and ovoid implant. Stages Ib and IIa are somewhat controversial because surgery and radiation therapy yield similar control and survival data. Because of the preservation of vaginal pliability and ovarian function, surgery is often used for younger women, whereas radiation is used for women who have a higher risk for surgical complications. Radiation is used with a combination of external beam therapy and implants. For bulky cervical disease, radiation therapy is the initial treatment of choice and may be delivered at doses slightly higher than usual or followed by a simple hysterectomy for barrel-type lesions. Postoperative irradiation is usually given for patients with pelvic nodes positive for tumor, disease more advanced than originally staged, margins positive for tumor, and if disease is an incidental finding in a less-than-definitive surgical procedure. Patients with stages IIb, III, and IVa are usually treated with irradiation, with or without chemotherapy. Total tumor doses are increased from 70 Gy for low-volume disease to 85 Gy for advanced or bulky disease. The external beam dose increases with more advanced disease, whereas the implant dose may stay the same or actually decrease, depending on critical organ doses. (External beam treatment, implant doses and techniques, and side effects are further discussed later in this chapter.)

Approximate 5-year survival rates are 95% for stage Ia cervical cancer, 85% for stage Ib, 70% for stage II, 50% for stage III, and less than 10% for stage IV. Local control rates are 92% for stage Ib, 85% for stage IIa, 75% for stage IIb, and 60% for stage IIIb.

Case Study

C.W. is a 42-year-old woman who had a 6-month history of slowly progressive bleeding after intercourse. Her periods were otherwise normal, and she did not have any pelvic or vaginal pain. She had Papanicolaou smears performed in her 20s and early 30s but none recently.

During an examination, the cervix was enlarged to about 5 cm, and an ulcerative lesion was seen extending from the inferior cervix into the posterior fornix. The Papanicolaou smear was positive for squamous cell carcinoma, and biopsies from the lesion, endocervix, and endometrium demonstrated invasive, poorly differentiated squamous cell carcinoma. A pelvic examination confirmed the bulky lesion, and the extension onto the vaginal wall was palpable; no appreciable parametrial extension was present (stage IIa). A chest radiograph and IVP were negative for metastatic disease. A pelvic CT scan confirmed the presence of an enlarged cervical mass, but no discernible pelvic adenopathy or masses were present.

Because of the lesion's bulk, the patient was not considered a surgical candidate and definitive radiation therapy was initiated. She received 4500 cGy via a four-field technique, with the treatment of customized 16 × 18.5 cm AP/PA and 14 × 18.5 cm right and left parallel-opposed fields. Photons of 15 MV were used to deliver 180-cGy daily fractions. She was evaluated during the fifth week, and marked shrinkage was noted in the tumor. The first tandem and ovoid implant procedure was performed 3 days after the completion of the 4500-cGy dose. The tandem was loaded with 15-, 10-, and 10-mg radium-equivalent cesium-137 (Cs-137) sources, and the small ovoids were each loaded with 15-mg sources. The point-A dose rate was 50 cGy per hour, and the implant was left in place for 48 hours. The dose rate at the pelvic sidewall was 12 cGy per hour, whereas the bladder and rectum maximum dose rates were 30 cGy per hour. The week after the first implant, 540 cGy was delivered in three fractions as a pelvic-sidewall boost via 16 × 16 cm AP/PA fields, with a midline (rectal and bladder sparing) block designed from the isodose distribution of the implant. A second, nearly identical implant was performed the week after the boost field, with a total implant time of 30 hours. The cumulative dose to point A was 8400 cGy, whereas the pelvic sidewall received 5980 cGy. The doses for the bladder and rectal points were each 6000 cGy.

Beginning the fourth week of treatment, the patient experienced diarrhea that was initially managed with a low-fiber diet and eventually required antidiarrheal agents. The diarrhea gradually improved through the implants, and the patient was without a complaint for 4 days after the second implant. She otherwise tolerated the treatment well.

At a follow-up 1 week after the second implant, the cervix's size was normal. Considerable necrotic debris was present at the vaginal apex, but bleeding did not occur during the examination. The following month she described a brown vaginal discharge with sparse matter that resembled coffee grounds. At her next examination, there were patchy, hypopigmented areas alternating with telangiectasis (fine, superficial blood vessels) of the vagina, and the cervix was nearly healed.

She continued to have control of the local disease and no pelvic side effects. About 1 to 1½ years after therapy, she exhibited multiple lung nodules. A chemotherapeutic regimen was begun, but the patient expired 5 months later.

ENDOMETRIUM

Clinical Presentation

Recent studies have highlighted the increased risk of endometrial cancer in women who take the drug tamoxifen, which has led some to suggest that surveillance of this subset of patients is warranted.[5,40] About 75% of women with endometrial cancer experience vaginal bleeding, and about 30% have a foul-smelling vaginal discharge. Approximately one third of postmenopausal bleeding is cancer related, usually cervical or endometrial. Most endometrial cancers are early stage, with about 70% in stage I and 10% each in stages II, III, and IV. Poor prognostic factors include higher grade, increased depth of invasion into the myometrial muscle, lymph node involvement, and cancer cells in the peritoneal fluid (peritoneal cytology positive for tumor) or on serosal surfaces.

Lymphatic spread occurs initially to the internal and external iliac pelvic nodes. For stage I disease, about 10% of patients have nodes positive for tumor. This increases to between 25% and 35% for stage II disease, a poorly differentiated histology, or a deep myometrial invasion. If pelvic nodes are involved, about a 60% chance exists for periaortic node involvement.

Detection and Diagnosis

Aspiration curettage has long been the gold standard of endometrial cancer screening, mostly because it improved on the accuracy of the Papanicolaou smear, a detection modality with only a 50% or less diagnostic accuracy in endometrial cancer.[11] However, it is increasingly the case that women with abnormal uterine bleeding are evaluated in the office setting using endometrial sampling or aspiration,[11] the latter of which has a reported sensitivity rate of 94% in some studies.[33] A thorough history is taken, and a physical examination is performed. Additional studies include chest radiographs, blood counts and chemistries, and a urinalysis. Surgery is most often the initial definitive management. Before proceeding, an ultrasound, a pelvic CT, or an MRI scan is often attempted to assess uterine invasion and lymph node involvement. Standard surgery includes an exploratory laparotomy with staging biopsies, washings, and a radical hysterectomy.

Pathology and Staging

Adenocarcinoma of the endometrial lining is the most common type of endometrial cancer. Adenosquamous cancer is a variant seen about 20% of the time and is usually more advanced in stage. Papillary serous adenocarcinoma is an extremely malignant form of endometrial carcinoma that tends to spread rapidly and widely throughout the abdominal cavity and usually has a poor outcome. Sarcomas rarely have a good outcome and deserve aggressive combined-modality therapy (usually surgery and radiation therapy). Staging is as follows:

Stage IA: Tumor limited to the endometrium

Stage IB: Tumor invading less than one half of the myometrium

Stage IC: Tumor invading one half or more of the myometrium

Stage IIA: Tumor limited to the glandular epithelium of the endocervix. No evidence of connective tissue stromal invasion

Stage IIB: Invasion of the stromal connective tissues of the cervix

Stage IIIA: Tumor involves serosa and/or adnexa and/or cancer cells in ascites or peritoneal washings

Stage IIIB: Vaginal involvement

Stage IVA: Tumor invades bladder mucosa and/or bowel mucosa

Treatment Considerations

Treatment can involve surgery and/or radiation therapy, depending on the stage, grade, medical condition of the patient, and experience of the institution administering the therapy. Preoperative therapy is given in some institutions for high grade and high clinical stages to downstage the patient before surgery. Usually, patients who have already undergone operations are referred for postoperative therapy, and nonoperative candidates are referred for definitive therapy. After a TAH, patients with stage Ia, grade 1 disease are not treated further. At many institutions, patients with stage Ib, grades 1 and 2 and sometimes stage Ia, grade 2 disease are treated postoperatively with brachytherapy alone. Low surface doses of 60 to 70 Gy are typically used in one application, or high doses of 5 to 7 Gy to a 0.5-cm depth are used for three applications. Patients with stage Ic (or higher) or grade 3 disease have an increased risk of pelvic node involvement, so external beam radiation therapy is a component of postoperative treatment. Minimal nodal doses of 45 to 50 Gy are supplemented with implants to bring the vaginal mucosa dose up to 80 Gy or more. Residual pelvic nodes or masses can be boosted up to 60 to 65 Gy with shaped, small-volume external fields.

Irradiation alone may be used for medically inoperable patients and for stages III and IV. Usually, at least a 50-Gy external beam pelvic dose is recommended with an implant sufficient to bring the tumor dose above 75 Gy. Bulky disease can be brought to 100 Gy with careful implant techniques and midline shielding. (See the section on simulation techniques at the end of the chapter.)

For stage I disease, the local recurrence rate can be reduced from 12% with surgery alone to 3% with preoperative radiation therapy, and to 0% with postoperative radiation therapy.[17] The 5-year survival rates are 64%, 76%, and 81%, respectively. Overall, there is a 90% 5-year survival rate for all stage I patients, including the most common and nonirradiated stage I, grade 1 patients. For stage II, 5-year disease-free survival rates are about 80% with surgery and radiation therapy versus 50% for radiation therapy alone. The 5-year survival rate for stage III disease treated with radiation therapy alone is only 25%. Overall, patients treated with surgery and radiation therapy have an overall survival rate of 81.6%, a 5-year disease-free survival rate of 80.7%, and a 5-year recurrence-free survival rate of 94.6%.[47]

Case Study

C.G. is a 62-year-old postmenopausal woman who had been having routine (biannual) Papanicolaou smears, which were normal. She developed intermittent vaginal bleeding and consulted her gynecologist the same week. Another Papanicolaou smear was normal, but an endometrial biopsy showed a moderately differentiated endometrial carcinoma. A chest radiograph, blood work, and a pelvic CT scan were normal. She underwent an abdominal hysterectomy and the removal of both ovaries. No lymph nodes were palpable during the surgery. A pathology report confirmed a moderately differentiated adenocarcinoma that invaded nearly the entire myometrium. The cervix and parametrial tissues were not involved, and her disease was classified as stage IC.

Her postoperative course was unremarkable, and she was referred for adjuvant radiation therapy. She was treated with 18-MV photons to 4500 cGy in 180-cGy daily fractions via a four-field technique with customized 16 × 16 cm AP/PA and 16 × 14 cm right and left parallel-opposed fields. After the external beam radiation therapy, she underwent a 60-hour vaginal cylinder implant. A 3-cm domed cylinder was placed and loaded with two 15-mg radium-equivalent Cs-137 sources, which delivered 60 cGy per hour at the vaginal surface. The patient tolerated the treatment well, experiencing mild diarrhea and fatigue at the completion of the external irradiation. The implant was well tolerated. About 6 years after treatment, she was without evidence of disease. She complained of having to urinate more frequently, but this was not problematic, and she was without dysuria. She had periodic rectal irritation, which responded after several days to steroid suppositories.

OVARIES

Clinical Presentation

Ovarian cancer is the most deadly of the gynecologic cancers because it has few symptoms until it is widely disseminated. The most common presenting symptoms are abdominal and/or pelvic pain, abdominal distention, or nonspecific gastrointestinal symptoms (e.g., nausea, constipation, and heartburn). These are due to the presence of the tumor or fluid in the abdominal cavity. Occasionally, ovarian cancer may be diagnosed in early stages as a palpable mass adjacent to the uterus.

The disease is most common in women 50 to 70 years old. It is considered early if confined to the ovaries. Progression occurs to the pelvis, abdominal cavity, and nodes. CA 125 is often elevated in the serum of epithelial ovarian cancer and has also been found to be a useful prognostic indicator of successful chemotherapy treatment.[3] In apparently early ovarian cancer, subclinical metastases are noted during surgery to the peritoneal fluid, periaortic nodes, and diaphragm in 33%, 10%, and 10% of the tumors, respectively.[41,42] About 80% of ovarian cancer patients have abdominal cavity involvement at the time of presentation. Spread occurs through the lymphatics and peritoneal fluid distributions. Survival rates are 90% at 5 years for stage I, 20% for stage III, and 5% for stage IV disease. About 22 months of increased survival time occurs with optimal versus suboptimal surgical reduction of intraabdominal disease.[32]

Detection and Diagnosis

Diagnosis and staging are surgical. The preoperative workup usually includes a history, a physical examination, liver and renal function blood work, chest radiographs, pelvic ultrasound (including transvaginal views), abdominopelvic CT or MRI scans, and serum CA 125. Some workups include a barium enema (BE), an endoscopy, and upper gastrointestinal (UGI) series. The surgical evaluation includes a cytologic evaluation of the peritoneal fluid, an intraoperative evaluation of adnexal masses, and an examination and biopsy of the peritoneal fluid drainage pathways. Removal of as much of the tumor as possible produces the best outcomes.

Pathology and Staging

About 90% of ovarian cancers are epithelial (from ovary surfaces), 7% are stromal, and 3% are from the ovarian germ cell. These include dysgerminomas, which are treated like seminomas. Staging is as follows:

Stage I: Tumor limited to the ovaries (one or both).
Stage IA: Tumor limited to one ovary, capsule intact, no tumor on ovarian surface. No malignant cells in ascites or peritoneal washings.
Stage IB: Tumor limited to both ovaries, capsules intact, no tumor on ovarian surface. No malignant cells in ascites or peritoneal washings.
Stage IC: Tumor limited to one or both ovaries with any of the following: capsule ruptured, tumor on ovarian surface. Malignant cells in ascites or peritoneal washings.
Stage II: Tumor involves one or both ovaries with pelvic extension and/or implants.
Stage IIA: Extension and/or implants on the fallopian tubes and/or uterus. No malignant cells in ascites or peritoneal washings.
Stage IIB: Extension to and/or implants on other pelvic tissues. No malignant cells in ascites or peritoneal washings.
Stage IIC: Pelvic extension and/or implants, with malignant cells in ascites or peritoneal washings.
Stage III: Tumor involves one or both ovaries with microscopically confirmed peritoneal metastases outside the pelvis.
Stage IIIA: Microscopic peritoneal metastases beyond the pelvis (no macroscopic tumor).
Stage IIIB: Macroscopic peritoneal metastases beyond the pelvis 2 cm or less in greatest dimension.
Stage IIIC: Peritoneal metastasis beyond the pelvis more than 2 cm in greatest dimension and/or regional lymph node metastasis.

Treatment Considerations

For epithelial tumors, the initial treatment involves surgical evaluation and debulking. Postoperative therapy may include single-agent or combination chemotherapy and/or whole abdominal and pelvic radiation therapy. Radiation therapy is controversial[10] and may include radioisotopes placed into the peritoneal cavity or all external beam treatment. For most epithelial tumors, postoperative therapy includes platinum-based chemotherapy, although abdominopelvic radiation therapy yields similar results.[12-14,16,32,38]

The two approaches are not additive, but toxicities are. Peritoneal radioisotope treatment is best not used in addition to external beam therapy for similar reasons.

For well-differentiated stages IA and IB, the 5-year survival rates are between 90% and 100%.[44] The 5-year survival rate for radiation-therapy–treated stage II is 74% for microscopic residual disease, 58% for residual disease less than 2 cm, and 39% for residual disease greater than 2 cm. Comparable results for stage III are 48%, 43%, and 18%.[12-14]

SIMULATION AND TREATMENT

Vulvar. Vulvar fields include the primary site and inguinal region. A pelvic field is added to the top or bottom of L5 if the primary is greater than 2 cm or if deep femoral nodes are positive for tumor. Pelvic fields should include the **pelvic inlet,** which is the opening in the pelvis into which a baby's head enters. The pelvic inlet includes the sacral promontory, the pelvic inner sidewalls, and the pubic bones, with a 2-cm lateral margin to cover pelvic lymph nodes. The patient is usually simulated in the "frog-leg" position, with wires over surgical scars and palpable nodes. Bolus is placed over the vulva and perineum. The fraction size is limited to 1.8 Gy, and frequent treatment breaks are often necessary by 40 Gy because of severe perineal reactions (Fig. 33-3). Inguinal nodes are best treated from the anterior to minimize doses to the femoral head and neck. Techniques to accomplish this include partial transmission blocks, weighting of the anterior field more heavily, anterior bolus, use of lower

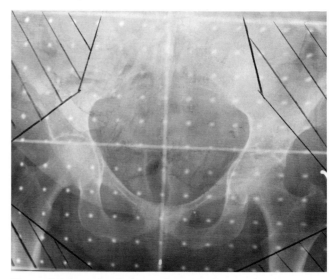

Figure 33-3. A simulation radiograph demonstrating a treatment field used to treat the vulva, pelvic, and inguinofemoral lymph nodes.

energies anteriorly and higher energies posteriorly, and anterior electron fields for boosts.

Vagina. Vaginal cancers are usually treated with radiation therapy. Surgery is most often reserved for recurrences, clear cell adenocarcinoma at an early stage, and persistent masses. Brachytherapy alone or as a boost depends on the size of the primary and nodal status. For carcinoma in situ and stage I well-differentiated cancer, the entire vagina can be treated via brachytherapy alone with a dose to 60 Gy through a device called a vaginal cylinder, which is a canal-filling cylinder into which an isotope can be placed to ensure an even dose to the vaginal mucosa. Further brachytherapy can be done as a boost of 20 Gy to minimal disease, with the cylinder and/or another brachytherapy device consisting of needles placed directly into the at-risk tissues (an interstitial implant) for more deeply invasive tumors. For more aggressive lesions other than early stage I, doses of 45 to 50 Gy are given to a pelvic field and the entire vagina. AP/PA fields with anterior weighting are customarily used to cover the at-risk tissues, to make blocking easier, and to deliver a lower dose to the femoral head and neck. The inguinal nodes are included for tumors involving the lower two thirds of the vagina. Brachytherapy implants are used to bring the primary and adjacent macroscopic disease to doses up to 65 to 85 Gy (Fig. 33-4, *A* and *B*). Perez recommends a midline block after 20 Gy for earlier invasive disease and after 40 Gy for stages IIb or greater so that a greater tumor-to-critical structure (bladder-rectum) dose can be given.[35,36] A midline block consists of a block placed in an AP/PA field to shield tissues that will be or already are treated by a brachytherapy device. Often the edges of the block have different value layers of blocking material to feather the junction of tissues treated with teletherapy and brachytherapy. Deeply invasive disease requires boosting with combination implants that include an interstitial component (Fig. 33-5, *A-C*).

Cervix. Radiation therapy is the best treatment for cervical cancer. Surgery is reserved for medically operable patients in earlier stages (I to IIa) for whom cure rates are similar and morbidity may be less. For bulky cervical disease, radiation may be followed by an extrafascial hysterectomy. Conversely, surgery may be followed by radiation therapy for pelvic nodes positive for tumor, margins positive for tumor, and disease more advanced than originally suspected. Patients with stages IIb, III, and IVa are usually treated with irradiation alone or in combination with chemotherapy.

Cervical fields can be administered via a four-field or high-energy AP/PA technique. The lower border is at the bottom of the obturator foramen, unless the vagina is involved, in which case the lower extent of the border is at least 4 cm below the lowest extent of the disease (some include the entire vaginal length). The upper border is usually at the top or bottom of L5 or may be extended upward to L4 for a portion of the treatment if nodal involvement is suspected. The lateral borders are 1.5 to 2.0 cm lateral to the pelvic sidewall

in the AP/PA plane. Laterally, the anterior border is at or anterior to the pubic symphysis, with a block designed to include the external iliac nodes; the posterior border includes S3. In patients with anterior or posterior extension, AP/PA fields alone or widening of the laterals to extend anterior to the pubis or posterior to include S4 and S5 is necessary. AP/PA fields allow midline blocking early so that a greater percentage of the dose is given with brachytherapy and less of the dose is given to the rectum and bladder. The four-field technique allows exclusion of the anterior bladder and posterior rectum in patients for whom brachytherapy plays a lesser role (e.g., bulkier disease) (Fig. 33-6, *A-E*). In patients with a high risk for periaortic involvement, matching AP/PA fields

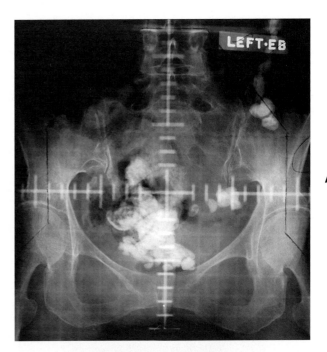

A

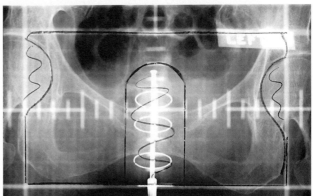

B

Figure 33-4. Radiographs of vaginal simulation and brachytherapy implant procedures. **A,** A typical anteroposterior/posteroanterior (AP/PA) simulation portal for a vaginal cancer treatment. **B,** A brachytherapy implant using a domed-cylinder technique. Note that the midline is blocked. The parametrial boost field with midline block is also shown.

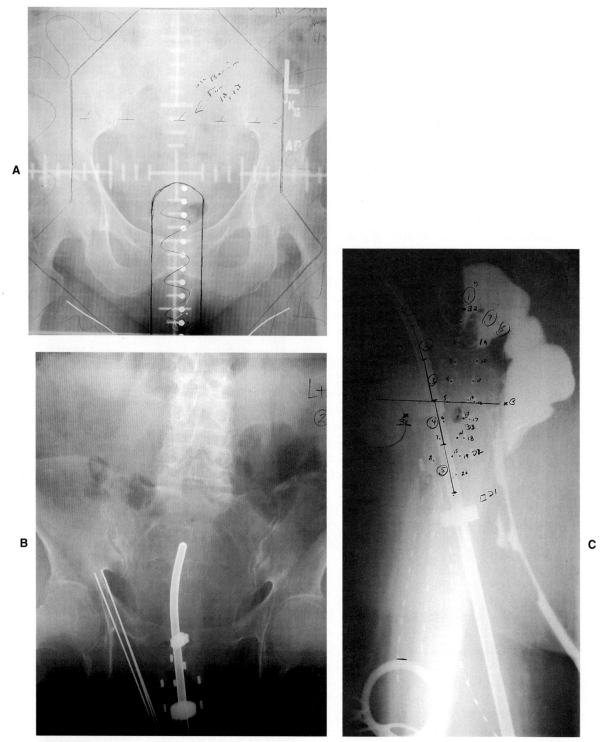

Figure 33-5. Treatment of vaginal cancer. **A,** Pelvic anteroposterior/posteroanterior (AP/PA) ports with a midline block. This particular arrangement used a 6-MV anterior field and an 18-MV posterior field. **B,** An AP view of an intrauterine tandem, vaginal cylinder, and interstitial needles used during a brachytherapy boost. **C,** A lateral view of an intrauterine tandem, vaginal cylinder, and interstitial needles used during a brachytherapy boost.

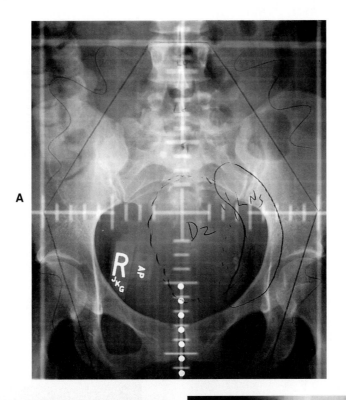

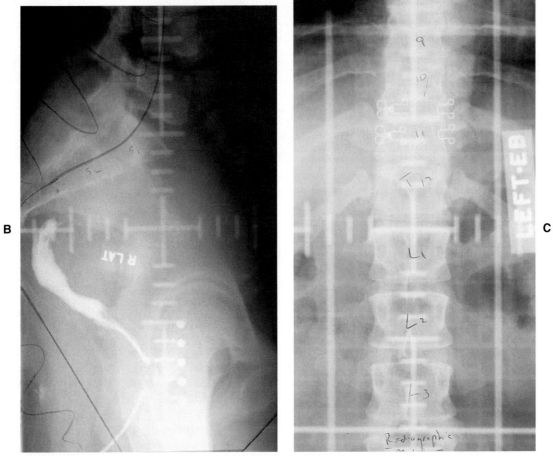

Figure 33-6. Radiographs of cervical simulation and implant procedures. **A,** Anteroposterior/posteroanterior (AP/PA) radiographs of a four-field technique for a bulky cervical cancer. Note the vaginal marker in place. **B,** A lateral view of a four-field technique for a bulky cervical cancer with rectal contrast and a vaginal marker. **C,** Matched AP/PA paraaortic fields used in the treatment of lymphatic drainage involved in regionally advanced cervical cancer.

continued

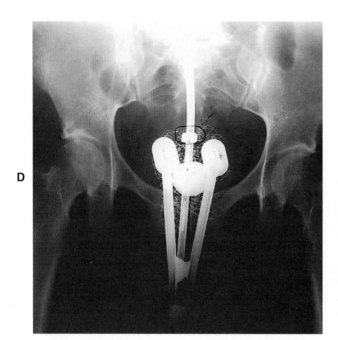

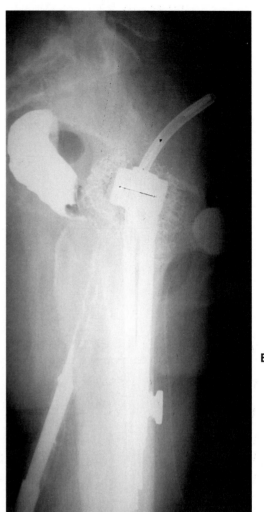

Figure 33-6, cont'd. D, An AP view of an intrauterine tandem and a vaginal colpostat cervical implant.
E, A lateral view of an intrauterine tandem and a vaginal colpostat cervical implant.

can be constructed and even lateral boosts can be given for a small portion of the treatment (Fig. 33-7).

Anal markers, rectal barium, vaginal markers, and bladder contrast can be used to help delineate critical structures during the simulation process. Often, placing the patient prone with a belly board or full bladder allows the exclusion of the small bowel without jeopardizing the tumor coverage. Small bowel contrast can allow minor field reductions that prevent complications, while allowing higher tumor or nodal doses.

Doses are escalated, depending on the stage and volume of the disease. The higher the volume of the tumor, the later implants are done in the course of treatment. Also, the greater the bulk and stage, the smaller the percentage of the dose contribution from implants. These two factors allow better coverage of the tumor by the implant and partially compensate for the poor geometry associated with increased volume disease. A standard **intrauterine tandem** (a small, hollow, curved cylinder that fits through the cervical os into the uterus) and **vaginal colpostats** (two golf-club–shaped, hol-

low tubes placed laterally to the tandem into the vaginal fornices) implants can also be supplemented with interstitial or cylinder components. Numerous dose, field, and timing arrangements are possible for external beam radiation therapy and brachytherapy. The actual protocol used is based on the radiation oncologist's clinical experience. Examples of doses and configurations include the following: a 70-Gy tumor dose via an implant alone for stage Ia disease, 75 Gy via 40-Gy pelvic radiation therapy plus 10 Gy with midline blocking plus a 35-Gy tumor dose from brachytherapy for stages Ib and IIa disease, 80 Gy via 40-Gy pelvic radiation therapy plus 20 Gy with midline blocking plus 40 Gy from brachytherapy for stages IIb and IIIa disease, and 85 Gy via 40-Gy pelvic radiation therapy plus 20 Gy with midline blocking plus 45 Gy from brachytherapy for stages IIIb and IVa disease. Some centers give a greater percentage of the dose with midline blocking to allow higher implant doses, and some give higher pelvic radiation therapy doses without midline blocking to cover the volume more evenly and sacri-

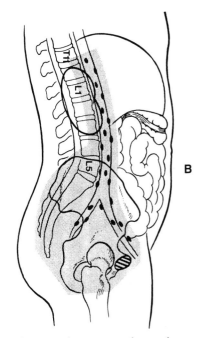

Figure 33-7. Extended field irradiation. **A,** Anterior and posterior portals. **B,** Lateral portals. *(From Russel A, et al: High dose para-aortic lymph node irradiation for gynecological cancer: technique, toxicity and results, Int J Radiat Oncol Biol Phys 13:267-271, 1987.)*

fice the amount of the brachytherapy dose. Low-dose-rate implants are usually paired (i.e., two are given approximately 2 weeks apart to achieve higher tolerated doses and allow further tumor regression). This also allows some correction in imperfections in the first implant dose distribution and in the patient's geometry. High-dose-rate implants are further fractionated for biologic reasons. The goal is to deliver 50 to 60 Gy to microscopic disease, 60 to 70 Gy to small macroscopic disease, and 70 to 90 Gy to large macroscopic disease while limiting the volume and dose to the bladder, colorectal tissues, and small intestine. Central doses are prescribed to the point A prescription point, usually defined as 2 cm superior to the cervical os and 2 cm lateral to the endocervical canal. Point B is 3 cm lateral to point A.

Uterine. Most endometrial cancers are seen postoperatively. For stage Ib, grades 1 and 2 and sometimes stage Ia, grade 2, a vaginal cylinder or colpostats alone are used to treat the vaginal cuff. Typical low-dose-rate doses, a 60- to 70-Gy surface dose, or high-dose-rate doses of 5 to 7 Gy to a 0.5-cm depth are prescribed. For stage Ic or higher or for grade 3 disease, an increased risk of pelvic nodal involvement exists and pelvic radiation therapy is given. Fields are similar to cervical fields, and midline blocking may be used if brachytherapy is included as part of the preoperative, postoperative, or definitive treatment. Heyman capsule techniques or an intrauterine tandem is used if a uterus is still available for implantation. Domed cylinders or vaginal colpostats are used if brachytherapy is necessary and a uterus is

no longer available. Pelvic nodal doses of 50 to 60 Gy are recommended, with boosting up to 65 Gy for gross involvement. The endometrial cavity can be taken to 75 to 90 Gy with brachytherapy, but the bladder and rectum must be kept to about 60 to 65 Gy or less maximally, and the small bowel must be kept at or below 50 Gy maximally (Fig. 33-8).

Ovary. Ovarian fields are also treated postoperatively after maximal debulking and staging by the gynecologic oncologist. The entire peritoneal cavity must be covered, and an open-field technique is preferred. When no liver shielding is used, the upper abdominal dose is limited to 25 to 28 Gy in 1.0- to 1.2-Gy fractions. Partial renal blocking is used to limit the dose to a total of 18 to 20 Gy. The pelvis is then boosted up to a total dose of 50 Gy at 1.8 Gy per fraction. Higher energy photons are recommended with AP/PA fields to limit the dosage variation to less than or equal to 5% (Fig. 33-9, *A* and *B*).

SIDE EFFECTS OF TREATMENT

Acute side effects of pelvic radiation therapy include fatigue, diarrhea, dermatitis, and dysuria. Fatigue can occur the first week of treatment and can be exacerbated or complicated by anemia and depression as the patient comes to grips with the disease. Rest, reassurance, adequate nutrition, and antidepressants can make the course of treatment easier. Anemia, secondary to the disease or its treatment or as a separate problem, should be corrected to at least maintain a hemoglobin level above 10 g/dl and ideally above 11 g/dl. Diarrhea

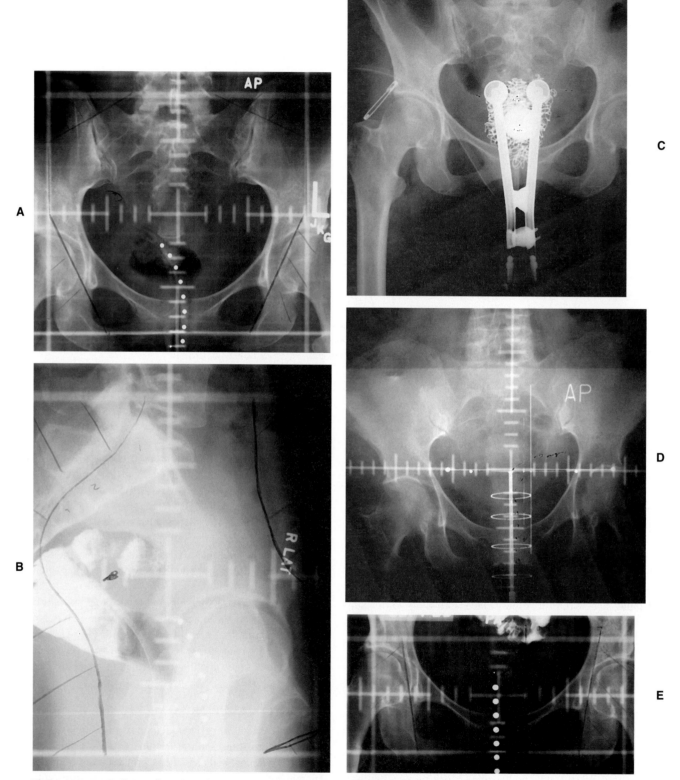

Figure 33-8. Radiographs of endometrial simulation and implant procedures. **A,** Anteroposterior/posteroanterior (AP/PA) simulation radiographs of a four-field treatment for postoperative endometrial cancer. Note the placement of the vaginal marker. **B,** A right and left lateral radiograph of a four-field treatment for postoperative endometrial cancer. Note the placement of the vaginal marker along with rectal contrast. **C,** A brachytherapy implant for postoperative endometrial cancer using colpostats. **D,** A brachytherapy implant using a high-dose-rate domed cylinder. **E,** A midline-blocked parametrial boost (small bowel excluded).

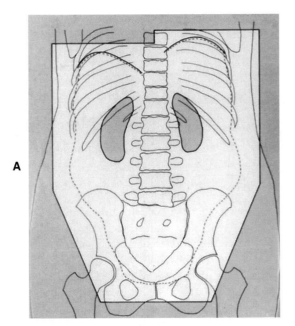
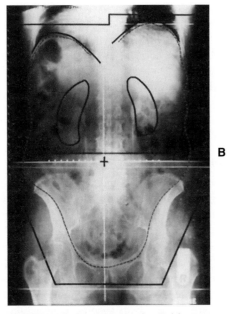

Figure 33-9. A line drawing **(A)** and prone simulator radiograph **(B)** showing the field margin for abdominopelvic irradiation *(nonshaded area)*, peritoneal outline *(dotted line)*, and renal shields. The pelvic boost field is not shown. *(From Cox JD: Moss' radiation oncology: rationale, techniques, results, ed 7, St. Louis, 1994, Mosby.)*

usually occurs the second or third week of treatment and is related to large and small bowel treatment. Chemotherapy can significantly worsen this problem. Low-fiber diets, sucralfate (Carafate) as a small bowel coating agent, diphenoxylate (Lomotil), and loperamide are useful in alleviating this problem. Excluding as much bowel as possible from the radiation therapy fields also helps. This is done with the use of belly boards, the prone position with a full bladder on smaller fields, custom shielding, and serial field-size reduction. Dermatitis is more common with low-energy treatment, AP/PA fields, perineal flash or bolus when indicated, and concomitant chemotherapy. Domboro soaks, Aquaphore ointment, and natural care gels can lessen the severity and speed healing. The prevention of local infection and correction of anemia and nutritional problems can also speed healing. Dysuria usually occurs during the third or fourth week of treatment and can be lessened by treatment with a full bladder, partial bladder exclusion on lateral fields, and maintenance of a partially full bladder during brachytherapy. Medications such as phenazopyridine (Pyridium) and Urised can be used to anesthetize the bladder, or oxybutynin (Ditropan), hyoscyamine (Levsin), and terazosin (Hytrin) can be used to relax the bladder. Infections should be treated aggressively. Bleeding can also complicate the treatment from anal irritation, bladder irritation, and a hemorrhagic tumor. Superficial en face radiation therapy can be applied directly to vaginal and cervical tumors with a large fraction size and not count against the total prescribed dose. (This can rapidly correct tumor bleeding.) Rectal irritation can be treated with hemorrhoidal preparations, steroids, topical anesthetic agents, and sitz baths.

Subacute side effects can include menopause, vaginal dryness and shrinkage, chronic cystitis, proctosigmoiditis, enteritis, and obstruction. Menopausal symptoms can be treated with cyclic hormonal therapy, vaginal dryness can be treated with moisturizing agents such as Replens or hormonal creams, and shrinkage can be prevented with vaginal dilators or regular sexual activity. The inflammatory problems listed can be treated with local medications, pentoxifylline (Trental), nutritional support, antiinflammatory agents, and pain medications. Obstruction is a surgical problem.

Abdominal fields can also cause diarrhea, nausea, and upper gastrointestinal bleeding. Nausea can be treated prophylactically with agents such as prochlorperazine (Compazine) or granisetron (Kytril), and gastritis can be treated with H_2 blockers (e.g., Tagamet, Zantac, Pepcid, and Axid), sucralfate, or other acid inhibitors.

ROLE OF RADIATION THERAPIST

Treatment Delivery

The primary role of the radiation therapist in the control of disease is simulation and treatment delivery. Patient positioning is an important component. Radiation therapists must often rely on their own experience regarding the way to position a particular patient for optimal comfort and stability. The pelvis can present considerable difficulty for simulation and reproducibility, especially when body habitus requires marking placement on loose skin overlying fat folds. The meticulous assessment of the patient's rotation is critical to prevent the shifting of the marks. Reminding the patient to maintain a full bladder when it is used to exclude the small bowel, encouraging the patient to remain on a low-residue diet when diarrhea is a problem, and remaining open and responsive to patient concerns helps to get the patient through treatment in the shortest possible time (optimal cure) and with minimal discomfort.

Patient Assessment

The radiation therapist is a critical link in patient assessment. The radiation therapist is in daily contact with the patient, allowing monitoring of early changes in the patient's physical status. In addition, there is often better, closer communication between the patient and radiation therapist compared with the physician. Concerns and observations should be communicated to the medical staff members initially for more in-depth assessment. In some institutions, standing orders are written with specific expectations for suggestions to the patient and communications with medical staff members. Knowledge of institutional policy is important.

The skin should be carefully assessed beginning the third week of radiation therapy. The gluteal and inguinal folds are the earliest to show a skin reaction. Pelvic irradiation can cause diarrhea, with consequent weight loss and electrolyte imbalance. A loose or soft stool is common, but the primary concern is watery diarrhea, which should be communicated immediately to medical staff members.

Reassurance

The radiation therapist has a responsibility to maintain a caring, professional atmosphere. Questions should be answered as much as knowledge permits, and medical staff members should be kept aware of patient concerns and questions. Chart rounds are an excellent format for this communication, but when in doubt, the radiation therapist should communicate with the nurse or physician.

SUMMARY

Gynecologic malignancies are common and can account for a significant proportion of the routine workload at a radiation oncology facility. For no other group of malignancies are the treatment options so diverse. The basic knowledge presented should enhance the radiation therapist's role in managing these patients while enabling a deeper understanding of the treatment rationale and potential outcome.

Review Questions

1. Which is the most radiotolerant gynecologic structure?
   a. Vulva
   b. Uteral canal

c. Endocervix
d. Ovary
2. Which is the most radiosensitive gynecologic structure?
   a. Vulva
   b. Uteral canal
   c. Endocervix
   d. Ovary
3. The dose response for radiation side effects in gynecologic structures is dependent on which factor?
   a. Age
   b. Race
   c. Both a and b
   d. Neither a nor b
4. Gynecologic radiation therapy planning requires consideration of which drainage pattern(s) to ensure appropriate field coverage?
   a. Arterial and venous
   b. Lymphatic
   c. Both a and b
   d. Neither a nor b
5. Bladder and rectal doses are more important to gynecologic radiation therapy planning than kidney or ovarian doses.
   a. True
   b. False

Matching (Match the Average Age of Onset)

6. Ovarian cancer
7. Cervical cancer
8. Uterine cancer
9. Clear cell vaginal cancer
10. Vulvar cancer
    a. 48 years
    b. 60 years
    c. 19 years
    d. 58 years
    e. 65+ years

Questions to Ponder

1. Why is the point A dose more important in the treatment design for cervical cancer than in that for uterine cancer?
2. What important structures in and around the pelvis may custom blocking help to reduce the dose while allowing full doses to at-risk tissues?
3. What are the tolerated (expected to have minimal long-term toxic effects) radiation therapy doses to the various pelvic structures?
4. Why is surgery less important for moderately advanced cervical cancer than for endometrial cancer?
5. In the United States, is preoperative or postoperative radiation therapy more commonly used for endometrial cancer? Explain the potential rationale for the most common approach.

REFERENCES

1. Ansink AC, et al: Human papillomavirus, lichen sclerosis, and squamous cell carcinoma of the vulva: detection and prognostic significance, *Gynecol Oncol* 52:180-184, 1994.

2. Balat O, Edwards C, Delclos L: Complications following combined surgery (radical vulvectomy versus wide local excision) and radiotherapy for the treatment of carcinoma of the vulva: report of 73 patients, *Eur J Gynecol Oncol* 21:501-503, 2000.

3. Bast RC Jr, et al: CA 125: the past and the future, *Int J Biol Mark* 13:179-187, 1998.

4. Beral V, et al: Use of HRT and the subsequent risk of cancer, *J Epidemiol Biostat* 4:191-210, 1999.

5. Bergman L, et al: Risk and prognosis of endometrial cancer after tamoxifen for breast cancer. Comprehensive Cancer Centres' ALERT group. Assessment of liver and endometrial cancer risk following Tamoxifen, *Lancet* 356:881-887, 2000.

6. Buchsbaum HJ: Extrapelvic lymph node metastases in cervical carcinoma, *Am J Obstet Gynecol* 133:814-824, 1979.

7. Burke TW, et al: Vulva. In Hoskine WJ, Perez CA, Young RC, editors: *Principles and practices of gynecologic oncology,* ed 3, Philadelphia, 1997, JB Lippincott.

8. Bush RD: The significance of anemia in clinical radiation therapy, *Int J Radiat Oncol Biol Phys* 12:2047-2050, 1986.

9. *Cancer facts and figures—2003,* Atlanta, 2003, American Cancer Society.

10. Cardenes H, Randall ME: Radiotherapy in epithelial ovarian cancer: state of the art, *Forum* 10:335-352, 2000.

11. Chambers JT, Chambers SK: Endometrial sampling: when? where? why? with what? *Clin Obstet Gynecol* 35:28-39, 1992.

12. Dembo AJ: Abdominopelvic radiotherapy in ovarian cancer: a 10 year experience, *Cancer* 55:2285-2290, 1985.

13. Dembo AJ, Bush RD: Choice of postoperative therapy based on prognostic factors, *Int J Radiat Oncol Biol Phys* 8:893-897, 1982.

14. Dembo AJ, Thomas GM, Freidlander ML: Prognostic indices in gynecologic cancer, *Dev Oncol* 48:239-250, 1987.

15. Fukuhisa K: Study of prognostic factors in patients with cervix carcinoma treated by radiotherapy, *Jpn J Cancer Clin* 35:1603-1609, 1989.

16. Fyles AW, et al: A randomized study of two doses of abdominopelvic radiation therapy for patients with optimally debulked Stage I, II, and III ovarian cancer, *Int J Radiat Oncol Biol Phys* 41:543-549, 1998.

17. Graham J: The value of preoperative or postoperative treatment by radium for carcinoma of the uterine body, *Surg Gynecol Obstet* 132:855, 1971.

18. Grigsby PW: Late injury of cancer therapy on the female reproductive tract, *Int J Radiat Oncol Biol Phys* 31:1281-1299, 1995.

19. Hacker NF, et al: Management of regional lymph nodes and their prognostic influence in vulvar cancer, *Obstet Gynecol* 61:408-412, 1983.

20. Hintz BL, et al: Radiation tolerance of the vaginal mucosa, *Int J Radiat Oncol Biol Phys* 6:711-716, 1980.

21. International Federation of Gynecology and Obstetrics (FIGO) classification, *FIGO* 18:190, 1989.

22. Iverson T, et al: Squamous cell carcinoma of the penis and of the cervix, vulva and vagina in spouses: is there any relationship? An epidemiological study from Norway, 1960-1992, *Br J Cancer* 76:658-660, 1997.

23. Kohler U, Schone M, Pawlowitsch T: Results of an individualized surgical therapy of vulvar carcinoma from 1973-1993. *Zentralblatt fur Gynakologie* 119(S1):8-16, 1997.

24. Lanciano RM, Corn BW: Gynecologic cancer. In Coia LR, Moylan DJ, editors: *Introduction to clinical radiation oncology,* ed 2, Madison, Wisc, 1994, Medical Physics Publishing.

25. Lawson HW, et al: Cervical cancer screening among low-income women: results of a national screening program, *Obstet Gynecol* 92:745-752, 1998.

26. Magrina JF, et al: Primary squamous cell cancer of the vulva: radical versus modified radical vulvar surgery, *Gynecol Oncol* 71:116-121, 1998.

27. Melnick S, et al: Rates and risks of diethylstilbestrol-related clear-cell adenocarcinoma of the vagina and cervix. An update, *N Engl J Med* 316:514-516, 1987.

28. Milosevic M, et al: Interstitial fluid pressure predicts survival inpatients with cervix cancer independent of clinical prognostic factors and tumor oxygen measurements, *Cancer Res* 61:6400-6405, 2001.

29. Noguchi H, et al: Uterine body invasion of carcinoma of the uterine cervix as seen from surgical specimens, *Gynecol Oncol* 30:173-182, 1988.

30. Orbalic N, Bilenjki D, Bilbija Z: Prognostic importance od anemia related parameters in patients with carcinoma of the cervix uteri, *Acta Oncol* 29:199-201, 1990.

31. Origoni M, et al: Surgical staging of invasive squamous cell carcinoma of the vulva. Analysis of treatment and survival, *Int Surg* 81:67-70, 1996.

32. Ozols RF, et al: Epithelial ovarian cancer. In Hoskins WJ, Perez CA, Young RC, editors: *Principles and practice of gynecologic oncology,* ed 3, Philadelphia, 1997, JB Lippincott.

33. Paley P: Screening for the major malignancies affecting women: current guidelines, *Am J Obstet Gynecol* 184:1021-1030, 2001.

34. Peck WS, et al: Castration of the female by irradiation, *Radiology* 34:176-186, 1940.

35. Perez CA, Garipagaoglu M: Vagina. In Perez CA, Brady LW, editors: *Principles and practices of radiation oncology,* ed 3, Philadelphia, 1997, JB Lippincott.

36. Perez CA, Grigsby PW: Vulva. In Perez CA, Brady LW, editors: *Principles and practices of radiation oncology,* ed 3, Philadelphia, 1997, JB Lippincott.

37. Perez CA, et al: Definitive irradiation in carcinoma of the vagina: long term evaluation of results, *Int J Radiat Oncol Biol Phys* 15:1283-1290, 1988.

38. Perez CA, et al: Gynecologic tumors. In Rubin P, Williams JP, editors: *Clinical oncology: a multidisciplinary approach for physicians and students,* ed 8, Philadelphia, 2001, WB Saunders.

39. Pettigrew R, Hamilton-Fairley D: Obesity and female reproductive function, *Br Med Bull* 53:341-358, 1997.

40. *Physicians desk query 2002. Endometrial cancer: screening,* Bethesda, Md, 2002, National Cancer Institute.

41. Piver MS, Chung WS: Prognostic significance of cervical lesion size and pelvic node metastasis in cervical carcinoma, *Obstet Gynecol* 46:507-510, 1975.

42. Piver MS, Barlow JJ, Lele SB: Incidence of subclinical metastasis in stage I and II ovarian carcinoma, *Obstet Gynecol* 52:100, 1978.

43. Segnan N: Socioeconomic status and cancer screening, *IARC Sci Pub* 138:369-376, 1997.

44. Thigpen JT: Limited-stage ovarian carcinoma, *Semin Oncol* 26(6 S18):29-33, 1999.

45. Treffers PE, et al: Consequences of diethylstilbestrol during pregnancy: 50 years later still a significant problem, *Netherlands Tijdschrift voor Geneeskunde* 145:675-680, 2001.

46. Weiderpass E, et al: Body size in different periods of life, diabetes mellitus, hypertension, and risk of postmenopausal endometrial cancer, *Cancer Caus Contr* 11(2):185-192, 2000.

47. Yalman D, et al: Postoperative radiotherapy in endometrial carcinoma: analysis of prognostic factors in 440 cases, *Eur J Gynecol Oncol* 21:3311-3315, 2000.

BIBLIOGRAPHY

Greene FL et al., editors: *AJCC Cancer Staging Manual,* ed 6, New York, 2002, Springer-Verlag.

Male Reproductive and Genitourinary Tumors

Deborah A. Kuban

Outline

Key Terms

Bowen's disease
Bulbous urethra
Corpora cavernosa
Corpus spongiosum
Cryptorchidism
Fossa navicularis
Impotence

Morphology
Penile urethra
Prostate gland
Prostatic hypertrophy
Smegma
Superior surface
Trigone

PROSTATE

Epidemiology

Carcinoma of the prostate is one of the most common malignancies in males in the United States. Approximately 1 in 11 men develop prostate cancer. It is estimated that 221,000 new cases will be diagnosed in the United States, and approximately 29,000 men will die of the disease each year.[3] The incidence increases with each decade of life; 80% of prostate carcinomas occur in men older than 65 years. African-American men in the United States have the highest incidence of prostate cancer in the world, significantly higher than that of white men of comparable age.

Prognostic Indicators

Tumor stage and histologic differentiation. Strong prognostic indicators in prostate carcinoma are the clinical stage and pathologic grade of tumor differentiation. Larger and less-differentiated tumors are more aggressive and have a greater incidence of lymphatic and distant metastases.

Age. Conflicting reports on age as a prognostic factor have been published. A Radiation Therapy Oncology Group (RTOG) study found a higher locoregional failure rate in patients younger than 60 years; however, survival was not significantly correlated with age.[71] Men younger than 65 years had an equivalent outcome at 5 years, as measured by posttreatment prostate-specific antigen (PSA), as compared with men older than 65.[33,38] Both groups had similar stages and prognostic factors.

Race.   Although higher incidence and mortality rates have been reported for African-American males, they have also been shown to present with more advanced disease.[54] Zagars et al.[108] have compared outcome in white versus black patients after radiation and found no difference when stratified by pretreatment prognostic factors.

Prostate-specific antigen level.   Several reports strongly suggest a close correlation between pretreatment and also posttreatment PSA levels and the incidence of failure-free survival.[48,49] Although a rising PSA level after radiation is more predictive than a single value, the higher the posttreatment nadir, the greater the risk of failure. For example, patients with a nadir ≥0.5 ng/ml had a 17% risk of subsequent failure, and those with a nadir ≥1.0 ng/ml had a 32% risk as shown by a large, multiinstitutional study.[92]

Lymph node status.   The presence and location of lymph node metastases have great prognostic significance. Bagshaw et al.[6] reported 10-year disease-free survival rates of 75% in patients with localized disease and lymph nodes negative for tumor, versus 20% with pelvic nodes positive for tumor. The outcome with paraaortic nodal metastasis is worse still. Reporting on a group of more than 1000 patients treated by pelvic node dissection and iodine-125 (I-125) prostate implant, Leibel et al.[56] found lymph node involvement to be the most significant covariate affecting distant metastasis-free survival. At 10 years posttreatment, 90% of patients with nodes positive for tumor had developed distant disease.

Anatomy

The **prostate gland** surrounds the male urethra between the base of the bladder and the urogenital diaphragm. The prostate is a walnut-shaped, solid organ that consists of fibrous, glandular, and muscular elements. It is attached anteriorly to the pubic symphysis by the puboprostatic ligament and separated posteriorly from the rectum by Denonvilliers' fascia (retrovesical septum), which attaches above to the peritoneum and below to the urogenital diaphragm. The seminal vesicles and vas deferens pierce the posterosuperior aspect of the gland and enter the urethra at the verumontanum (Fig. 34-1).

Natural History of Disease

Local growth patterns.   Most prostate carcinomas are multifocal and develop in the peripheral glands of the prostate, whereas benign prostatic hyperplasia arises from the central (periurethral) portion. As the tumor grows, it may extend into and through the capsule of the gland, invade periprostatic tissues and seminal vesicles and, if untreated, involve the bladder neck or rectum. The incidence of microscopic tumor extension beyond the capsule of the gland, at the time of radical prostatectomy, in patients with clinical stages T1b/c or T2 disease ranges from 10% to 50% and is also very much dependent on tumor grade and PSA. Seminal vesicle involvement has been observed in 1% to 30% of patients with stage T1 tumors and in 1% to 38% of patients with stage T2 lesions depending on the grade and PSA

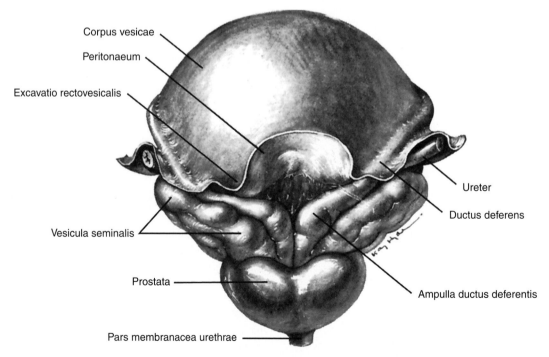

Figure 34-1. View of the posterior urinary bladder, illustrating the close relationship of the prostate and seminal vesicles. *(From Anson BJ, McVay CB: Surgical anatomy, vol 2, ed 5, Philadelphia, 1971, WB Saunders.)*

covariates.[68] The tumor may invade the perineural spaces, lymphatics, and blood vessels, producing lymphatic or distant metastases as well.

Regional lymph node involvement and distant metastases.   The tumor size and degree of differentiation affect the tendency of prostatic carcinoma to metastasize to regional lymphatics.

As smaller, nonpalpable tumors are diagnosed with the use of PSA screening, the incidence of metastatic pelvic lymph nodes decreases (Table 34-1). Periprostatic and obturator nodes are involved first, followed by external iliac, hypogastric, common iliac, and periaortic nodes (Fig. 34-2). Approximately 7% of patients have involvement of the presacral lymph nodes, including the promontorial and middle hemorrhoidal group, without evidence of metastases in the external iliac or hypogastric lymph nodes. Metastases to the paraaortic nodes occur in 5% to 25% of patients. Patients with pelvic lymph node metastases are more likely to develop distant metastases than those with nodes negative for tumor. The incidence of distant metastases ranges from 20% in stage T1b to 90% in stage N1-3.

Clinical Presentation

Patients with prostate carcinoma may complain of decreased urinary stream, frequency, difficulty in starting urination, dysuria, and infrequently even hematuria. These symptoms may also be caused by conditions other than cancer, such as benign **prostatic hypertrophy** (enlargement of the prostate gland, leading to narrowing of the urethra) and infection. Some tumors are diagnosed at the time of a transurethral resection (a surgical procedure of the prostate performed for lower urinary tract obstructive symptoms), although this procedure is being performed much less often. Bone pain or other symptoms associated with distant metastasis are seen less frequently at the time of the initial diagnosis.

Almost 40% of patients diagnosed with carcinoma of the

prostate 20 years ago had M1 disease (distant metastasis). Increasing awareness by the public and physicians and the growing use of PSA have reduced this percentage to less than 20%.

Detection and Diagnosis

Complete physical and rectal examination are mandatory. In most patients the seminal vesicles cannot be palpated, but a

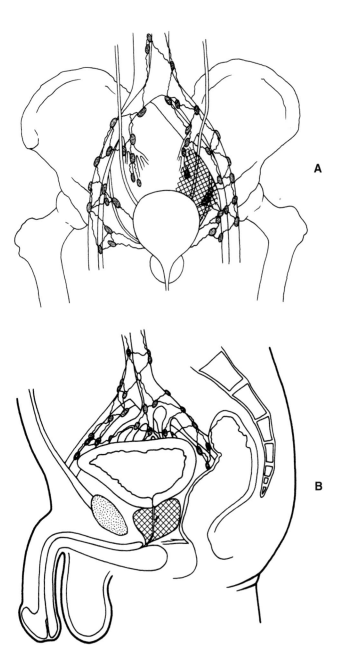

Figure 34-2. A, The location of lymph nodes most frequently involved in carcinoma of the prostate. The hatched area outlines the zone usually dissected in a limited staging lymphadenectomy. **B,** A sagittal view. (*A from Perez CA: Prostate. In Perez CA, Brady LW, editors: Principles and practice of radiation oncology, ed3, Philadelphia, 1998, Lippincott-Raven.*)

Table 34-1	Incidence of metastatic pelvic lymph nodes in carcinoma of the prostate	
Clinical Stage	**Nerve-sparing Radical Prostatectomy***	**Radiation Therapy Series: Lymph Node Dissection†**
A2 (T$_{1b}$)	2/61 (3.3%)	1/21 (5%)
B (T$_2$)	33/425 (7.8%)	38/135 (28%)
C (T$_3$, T$_4$)	—	48/95 (51%)

*Data from Petros J, Catalona WJ: Lower incidence of unsuspected lymph node metastases in 521 consecutive patients with clinically localized prostate cancer, *J Urol* 147:1574, 1992.

† Data from Hanks G, et al: Comparison of pathologic and clinical evaluation of lymph nodes in prostate cancer: implications of RTOG data for patient management and trial design and stratification, *Int J Radiat Oncol Biol Phys* 23:293, 1992.

T, Tumor.

firm area extending above the prostate suggests that the seminal vesicles are involved by malignancy. Approximately 50% of prostatic nodules found during rectal examination are confirmed to be malignant at the time of a biopsy.

The diagnosis of prostatic carcinoma can be obtained only through histologic confirmation. A transrectal ultrasound-guided needle biopsy is the standard method of diagnosis in the United States. In Europe, especially Scandinavia, an aspiration biopsy has been used for many years with impressive results.[7] False-negative diagnoses range from less than 5% to 30%.

The standard tests required in the evaluation of patients with prostatic carcinoma are listed in Box 34-1.

Some authors have concluded that in many cases there are no specific characteristics on transrectal sonograms that differentiate benign prostatic disease from malignancy. Therefore a biopsy is always required.[81] A sensitivity rate of 86% and a specificity rate of only 41% have been reported for ultrasound. Tumors less than 1 cm are the most difficult to detect.[13] Transrectal magnetic resonance imaging (MRI) is increasingly used in the evaluation of these patients.[88]

Screening.   Carcinoma of the prostate can be asymptomatic until reaching a significant size. An annual digital rectal examination of the prostate should be performed in all men older than 50 years. A digital rectal examination has a 70% sensitivity rate of 50% specificity rate in detecting prostate cancer. Radioimmunoassays for prostatic acid phosphatase, which have a sensitivity rate of only 10% and a specificity rate of 90% for malignant tumors, have been largely replaced by PSA testing.

PSA blood levels are routinely obtained in men older than 50 years. Prostatic antigen is detected in normal prostatic tissue, benign hyperplasia, malignant tumors, and seminal fluid and is measured by serum analysis. Although a normal PSA value, in general, is said to be ≤4 ng/ml, PSA level must be adjusted for age. For a 49-year-old man, a normal PSA would be ≤2.5 ng/ml, whereas a 70-year-old man would have a low risk of prostate cancer with a PSA of 6.5 ng/ml. As men age, prostate size increases, with higher PSA levels secondary to benign hypertrophy. An elevated PSA with no palpable disease of the prostate (Stage T1c) is now the most common presentation for this disease because of increased screening and awareness.

PSA in the selection of patients for therapy and post-treatment evaluation.   Several authors have shown a close correlation between PSA levels and clinical and pathologic tumor stage and lymph node status, especially in conjunction with Gleason score, the histologic tumor grade. A group of patients with a PSA level below 2.8 ng/ml and a Gleason score below 4 had an incidence of nodal disease or seminal vesicle involvement of approximately 1% at the time of prostatectomy, but 60% of patients with a PSA level above 40 ng/ml and a Gleason score above 8 had these findings[68] (Fig. 34-3). PSA is also of great value in the follow-up of patients treated with radical prostatectomy or radiation therapy.[19]

Pathology and Staging

Most malignant tumors of the prostate are adenocarcinomas. Gleason devised a quantitative histologic grading system based on the morphologic tumor characteristics.[34] The pathologist evaluates the predominant degree of differentiation of the tumor (primary pattern) and the less-frequent component (secondary pattern) based on the **morphology** of the lesion (e.g., glandular pattern, distribution of glands, stromal invasion) (Fig. 34-4, *A*). The primary and secondary tumor grades are each labeled from 1 to 5. The two grades are added for a Gleason score of 2 to 10. The Gleason score correlates closely with prognosis, lower scores representing more slowly growing, nonaggressive tumors and higher scores their more invasive, metastatic counterparts (Fig. 34-4, *B*). Perez et al.[70] found that the histologic differentiation of the tumor was strongly correlated with the incidence of distant metastases and survival but not as closely with locoregional failure.

Findings from the digital examination of the prostate and imaging studies determine the stage of the disease, which is classified according to the American Joint Committee on Cancer (AJCC)[29] (Box 34-2).

Stage T1 lesions are not detectable on digital rectal examination. T1a lesions are well-differentiated adenocarcinomas that are incidentally found during a transurethral resection of the prostate. They involve 5% or less of resected tissue. Stage T1b tumors are also subclinical, but they are more diffuse or have a larger volume, frequently with multifocal involvement of the prostate (>5% of tissue resected). T1c tumors are identified by a needle biopsy (e.g., because of elevated PSA levels).

Stage T2 tumors are palpable and confined within the capsule of the prostate gland. T2a tumors involve one lobe; T2b involve both lobes.

Stage T3 lesions are more locally extensive. T3a denotes

Box 34-1	Diagnostic Work-up for Carcinoma of the Prostate

Clinical
   History and clinical examination
   Rectal examination
Laboratory
   CBC and blood chemistry
   Serum PSA
Radiographic imaging
   Computed tomography or magnetic resonance imaging
     scan of the pelvis and abdomen
   Chest x-ray examination
   Radioisotope bone scan
   Transrectal ultrasonography
Biopsy
   Needle biopsy of prostate (transrectal, ultrasound guided)

CBC, Complete blood count; *PSA* prostate-specific antigen.

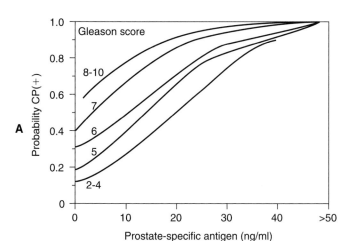

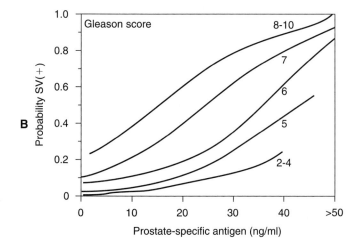

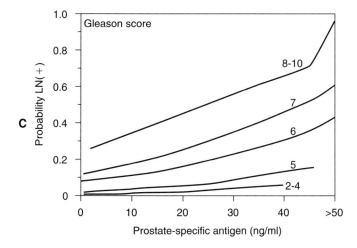

Figure 34-3. A, The probability of capsular penetration (*CP+*) as a function of the serum prostate-specific antigen (PSA) and preoperative Gleason score. **B,** The probability of seminal vesicle involvement (*SV+*) as a function of the serum PSA and preoperative Gleason score. **C,** The probability of lymph node involvement (*LN+*) as a function of the serum PSA and preoperative Gleason score. *(From Partin AW, et al: The use of prostate specific antigen, clinical stage and Gleason score to predict pathological stage in men with localized prostate cancer, J Urol 150:110-114, 1993.)*

extracapsular extension, either unilateral or bilateral. T3b indicates seminal vesicle invasion.

Stage T4 tumors are fixed to the pelvic sidewall or invade adjacent structures such as rectum or bladder. Regional nodal status is described as negative (N0) or positive (N1). Distant disease is designated M1a: nonregional nodes, M1b: bone, and M1c: other sites.

Treatment Techniques

Several areas of controversy surround the management of patients with prostatic carcinoma. The natural history of this tumor is variable and influenced by multiple prognostic factors. The different forms of therapy can affect the quality of life and sexual function to varying degrees.

In general, localized carcinoma of the prostate has a fairly slow clinical course. The National Cancer Institute Consensus Development Conference on Management of Localized Prostate Cancer concluded that radical prostatectomy and radiation therapy are clearly effective treatments in appropriately selected patients for tumors limited to the prostate.

Observation. Several authors have reported on patients who, after a histologic diagnosis of prostatic carcinoma, were managed conservatively and monitored without specific anticancer treatment until symptoms developed.[1,2,14,45] The literature indicates that the tumors that are not poorly differentiated can have a protracted course associated with significant competing mortality and marginal benefit from therapy at 10 years.[1,2,11] Observation is reasonable management for patients older than 75 years. It can also be offered to younger patients, 65 to 75 years old, with small, well-differentiated tumors. However, in today's health environment in the United States, most patients do not readily accept delaying definitive therapy unless they are very elderly with indolent-behaving disease or in very poor general health from other medical illness.

According to many urologists, stage T1a disease, which is found incidentally, requires no treatment; many years of natural evolution may pass before the disease becomes a clinical problem. According to one study, only 6.8% of 148 patients with this stage disease progressed.[8] A literature review showed a death rate of only 1.9% in 262 patients with stage T1a carcinoma. Some authors have noted decreased survival rates with poorly differentiated tumors, however.[14,45] In 313 patients treated with external irradiation, the 5-year survival rate was comparable to that of a matched-age normal male group but the 10-year survival rate was below the normal life expectancy, 51% versus 62%.[41] Both stage T1a and T1b (diagnosis by transurethral resection) prostate cancer have been more infrequently diagnosed since the introduction of PSA as a tool for screening in the mid-1980s. Patients with an elevated PSA, who are subsequently found to have prostate cancer on biopsy, are staged as T1c. Furthermore, benign prostate hypertrophy is now largely treated with medication, reserving transurethral resection for only the most severe cases.

Prostatectomy. Patients with resectable stage T1 or T2 prostate cancer who are in good general medical condition

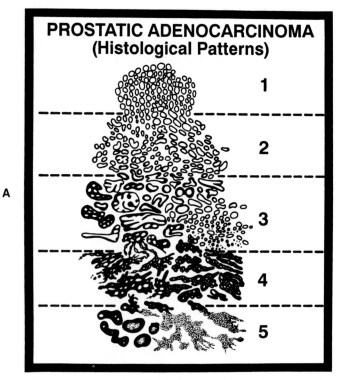

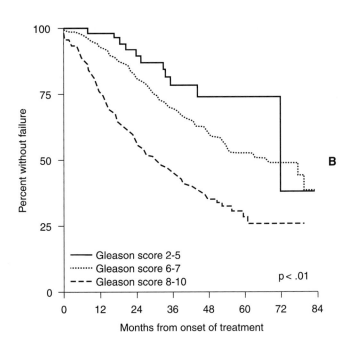

Figure 34-4. A, A simplified drawing of histologic patterns, emphasizing the degree of glandular differentiation and relation to stroma. The all-black area in the drawing represents the tumor tissue and glands with all cytologic detail obscured, except in the right side of pattern 4, where tiny open structures are intended to suggest the hypernephroid pattern. **B,** Survival correlated with the Gleason score ($N = 566$). (**A** *from Gleason DF, et al: Histologic grading and clinical staging of prostatic carcinoma. In Tannenbaum M, editor: Urologic pathology: the prostate, Philadelphia, 1977, Lea & Febiger;* **B** *from Pilepich MV, et al: Prognostic factors in carcinoma of the prostate: analysis of RTOG Study 75-06, Int J Radiat Oncol Biol Phys 13:339-349, 1987.*)

and have a life expectancy of at least 10 years are candidates for radical prostatectomy. Impetus has been given to the use of nerve-sparing surgery because an increasing number of tumors are being diagnosed at earlier stages, and a lower incidence of sexual **impotence** (the inability to obtain an erection) has been reported with this surgery (40% to 60%, depending on the patient's age and tumor extent) compared with classical radical prostatectomy (close to 100%).[12] Radiation therapy has been shown to provide very similar outcome for these patients. A recent report from the Cleveland Clinic compared stage T1 and T2 patients treated by surgery versus radiation.[51] For good prognosis patients (initial PSA ≤10 ng/ml, Gleason ≤6), 78% of irradiated patients and 80% of prostatectomy patients were disease-free 5 years after treatment by PSA criteria, which is the strictest and most objective measure. In those patients at higher risk for recurrence based on prognostic factors, 25% and 38% of those treated by radiation versus surgery, respectively, were PSA disease-free. This difference was not statistically significant. Of note is that these results were reported for patients treated by conventional radiation doses and techniques. Early reports of outcome for patients treated to higher doses using three-dimensional (3D) conformal or intensity modulated

radiation therapy (IMRT) techniques seem to indicate that even better results may be attainable.

For stage T3 disease most urologists and radiation oncologists agree that external beam radiation is the treatment of choice, usually with hormonal therapy. Because of the significant tumor bulk and high metastatic potential in this category, results with radiation alone have been less than satisfactory, 10% to 35% PSA disease-free survival at 10 years.[55] The addition of hormone therapy to radiation has markedly improved disease control. Zagars et al[109] report PSA disease-free survival of 78% versus 33% at 6 years dependent on hormonal therapy. Dose escalation studies have not shown nearly as marked a benefit to date for this group.

Radioisotopic implant is also an option for patients with early stage (T1c, T2a-b), low grade (Gleason ≤6), low PSA (≤10 ng/ml) prostate cancer. I-125 and palladium-103 (Pd-103) are the permanent sources used. The current technique is a transperineal template ultrasound guided approach. PSA disease-free survival appears to be equivalent to external beam therapy, 80% to 90% range, if candidates are carefully selected.[8,9]

Hormonal therapy. In 1941, Huggins et al[42] demonstrated prostate tumor regression and diminished serum acid phosphatase levels after orchiectomy or estrogen administra-

Box 34-2 — AJCC Staging System for Carcinoma of the Prostate

PRIMARY TUMOR (T)[1]

pT2	Organ confined
pT2a	Unilateral, one-half of one lobe or less
pT2b	Unilateral, involving more than one-half of lobe but not both lobes
pT2c	Bilateral disease
pT3	Extraprostatic extension
pT3a	Extraprostatic extension[2]
pT3b	Seminal vesicle invasion
pT4	Invasion of bladder, rectum

REGIONAL LYMPH NODES (N)

pNX	Regional nodes not sampled
pN0	No positive regional nodes
pN1	Metastases in regional nodes(s)

DISTANT METASTASIS (M)[5]

MX	Distant metastasis cannot be assessed (not evaluated by any modality)
M0	No distant metastasis
M1	Distant metastasis
M1a	Nonregional lymph node(s)
M1b	Bone(s)
M1c	Other site(s) with or without bone disease.

PRIMARY TUMOR (T)

TX	Primary tumor cannot be assessed
T0	No evidence of primary tumor
T1	Clinically inapparent tumor neither palpable nor visible by imaging
T1a	Tumor incidental histologic finding in 5% or less of tissue resected
T1b	Tumor incidental histologic finding in more than 5% of tissue resected
T1c	Tumor identified by needle biopsy (e.g., because of elevated PSA)

T2	Tumor confined within prostate[3]
T2a	Tumor involves one-half of one lobe or less
T2b	Tumor involves more than one-half of one lobe but not both lobes
T2c	Tumor involves both lobes
T3	Tumor extends through the prostate capsule[4]
T3a	Extracapsular extension (unilateral or bilateral)
T3b	Tumor invades seminal vesicle(s)
T4	Tumor is fixed or invades adjacent structures other than seminal vesicles: bladder neck, external sphincter, rectum, levator muscles, and/or pelvic wall

REGIONAL LYMPH NODES (N)

NX	Regional lymph nodes were not assessed
N0	No regional lymph node metastasis
N1	Metastases in regional nodes(s)

STAGE GROUPING

I	T1a	N0	M0	G1
II	T1a	N0	M0	G2, 3-4
	T1b	N0	M0	Any G
	T1c	N0	M0	Any G
	T1	N0	M0	Any G
	T2	N0	M0	Any G
III	T3	N0	M0	Any G
IV	T4	N0	M0	Any G
	Any T	N1	M0	Any G
	Any T	Any N	M1	Any G

HISTOLOGIC GRADE (G)

GX	Grade cannot be assessed
G1	Well differentiated (slight anaplasia) (Gleason 2-4)
G2	Moderately differentiated (moderate anaplasia) (Gleason 5-6)
G3-4	Poorly differentiated/undifferentiated (marked anaplasia) (Gleason 7-10)

With permission from American Joint Committee on Cancer (AJCC), Chicago, Illinois: *AJCC Cancer Staging Manual*, ed 6, New York, 2002, Springer-Verlag.

Notes
1. There is no pathologic T1 classification
2. Positive surgical margin should be indicated by an R1 descriptor (residual microscopic disease).
3. Tumor found in one or both lobes by needle biopsy, but not palpable or reliably visible by imaging, is calssified as T1c.
4. Invasion into the prostatic apex or into (but not beyond) the prostatic capsule is classified not as T3, but as T2.
5. When more than one site of metastasis is present, the most advanced category is used. pM1c is most advanced.

tion. Many types of hormonal therapy, all seeking to reduce the androgenic stimulation of prostatic carcinoma, have been used since then. Orchiectomy removes 95% of circulating testosterone and is followed by a prompt, long-lasting decline in serum testosterone levels. Estrogen appears to suppress pituitary gonadotropin, causing reduced stimulus for testicular testosterone synthesis, direct interference with hormonal synthesis, or a direct effect on the prostatic cell com-

peting with hormonal receptors. Gonadotropin-releasing hormone agonists such as goserelin (Zoladex) and leuprolide acetate (Lupron) cause an initial rise in gonadotropin levels, followed by a sharp decline within 2 to 3 weeks. Parallel changes occur in levels of circulating testosterone. Results with these compounds are similar to those obtained with bilateral orchiectomy.

Aminoglutethimide, which is administered with a glucocorticoid, inhibits the synthesis of all adrenal steroids and can further reduce serum testosterone levels in castrated patients.[104]

Flutamide (Eulexin) and bicalutamide (Casodex) are both nonsteroidal antiandrogens. Flutamide inhibits androgen uptake and nuclear binding in the prostate cancer cell, and bicalutamide competitively inhibits the action of androgens by binding to cytosol androgen receptors. Hormonal therapy has long been used to reduce metastatic tumor burden and palliate symptoms; however, more recently hormonal therapy has been added to radiation in locally advanced and high grade tumors. The RTOG 86-10 and 92-02 studies have shown an advantage in disease control and survival with short-term hormonal administration (2 months before and during radiation) in bulky Gleason score 2 to 6 tumors and with long-term hormonal therapy (2 years) in Gleason score 8 to 10 tumors. It appears that testosterone ablation helps by reducing tumor bulk locally and also by controlling microscopic, clinically undetected metastatic disease.[39,72]

Chemotherapy. Several drugs have been evaluated in patients for whom hormonal therapy has failed. Response rates with single-agent doxorubicin (Adriamycin) are 25% to 35%. With cyclophosphamide the rate of partial response plus stable disease ranges from 26% to 41%. In about 10% of patients 5-fluorouracil (5-FU) has induced partial responses. A partial response rate of only 8% was observed with hydroxyurea. Prospective randomized trials have not supported the superiority of combination chemotherapy over single drugs in metastatic prostate cancer. In five randomized studies of single-agent versus combination chemotherapy, there was no or minimal difference in the percentage of patients with partial response plus stable disease; the response duration and survival rates were essentially with the same. Less than 10% complete or partial response occurred in more than 3000 patients with advanced or recurrent metastatic carcinoma of the prostate treated with various chemotherapeutic agents.[25] The combination of paclitaxel (Taxol), etoposide, and estramustine is a newer regimen being investigated. Because patients with locally advanced, high-grade, high-PSA tumors typically have a poor outcome even with a combination of radiation and hormonal therapy, the RTOG recently initiated a protocol (RTOG 99-02) randomizing one arm to chemotherapy in addition to radiation and hormonal therapy. It is felt that effective cytotoxic systemic treatment will be necessary to truly eradicate the occult metastatic disease, which is so prevalent in this group.

External radiation. A decision must first be made regarding treatment volume and whether seminal vesicles and/or pelvic lymph nodes will be irradiated. Seminal vesicles are usually included in the treatment volume when the risk of involvement is at least in the 10% to 15% range. The risk of involvement can be calculated from an equation[82,83] or estimated from a table wherein surgically dissected patients are categorized by prognostic factors.[68] In general, these are usually patients with PSA greater than 10 ng/ml and tumors

with Gleason score greater than 6. Treating the seminal vesicles usually results in a larger volume of rectum irradiated. Although it would seem prudent to include the seminal vesicles under the conditions noted previously on the basis of general radiation therapy principles, there are no study results to date that document improved outcome.

Pelvic lymph node irradiation is controversial as well. Studies disagree as to the ultimate benefit in terms of disease progression and survival. An RTOG study addressing lymph node irradiation just reported preliminary results that were equivocal.[84] With longer follow-up, perhaps a more definite treatment recommendation will emerge. Currently, decisions on lymph node therapy are left to the discretion of the treating physician and institutional policy. In general, a risk of involvement in the 20% range would prompt therapy by those who believe it may be beneficial. When the pelvic lymph nodes are treated, the field size is usually 15 × 15 cm at the patient surface (16.5 cm at the isocenter) (Fig. 34-5, *A*). The reduced field for treatment of the prostate and seminal vesicles is determined by computed tomography (CT) scan, and therefore size will vary according to prostate and seminal vesicle size, usually in the range of 8 to 10 cm including margins. A final cone down may be done to encompass only the prostate. Location varies as well but is generally related to the pubic symphysis. The inferior margin may be determined by retrograde urethrogram, implanted marker, or CT scan. When CT scan is used, margins should be more generous because the inferiormost extent of the gland may be difficult to determine exactly. Blocking devices or multileaf collimation (MLC) are, of course, used to shape the fields.

A four-field box technique with lateral portals is usually used initially if lymph nodes are to be treated. Nodes can be mapped on CT scan and planning done individually, or a more standard field can be applied. With the latter technique, the upper border is at the midsacral level and the lower border determined by the inferior most aspect of the prostate. The lateral margins of the anterior field are 1.5 to 2 cm from the lateral pelvic brim (Fig. 34-5, *A*). For the lateral field, the anterior margin is 1 cm posterior to the projection of the anterior cortex of the pubic symphysis (Fig. 34-5, *B*). Small bowel is spared anteriorly at the upper aspect of the field being mindful of the location of the external iliac nodes. The posterior border is generally at the posterior ischium with shielding of the posterior rectal wall as appropriate. Barium or a plastic catheter with radiopaque markers can be used to define the rectum. The position of the seminal vesicles must be verified by CT scan, and the posterior field margin must allow for coverage of these structures with adequate margin. Typical simulation films for a pelvic nodal field are shown in Fig. 34-6, *A* and *B*.

Simulation. Patients are most often simulated in the supine position. Immobilization by a foaming cradle or vacuum bag is first carried out. If a conventional simulator is used, a standard isocenter can be marked (usually tattooed) on the patient. For a typical field to encompass the prostate or prostate and seminal vesicles, the isocenter is placed 1.5 to 2 cm below the top of the symphysis pubis, at midline on the anterior projection, and 5.5 to 6.5 cm posterior to the tip of the pubic symphysis on the lateral projection. If a CT simulator is available, a preliminary scan is done by obtaining slices every 5 mm from the inferior aspect of the sacroiliac joints through the inferior ischia. An isocenter is set within the prostate using the CT images. It is marked anteriorly and laterally, both right and left, with BBs. The patient is then scanned every 3 mm using the same superior and inferior margins with care to scan through the plane of the BBs. The

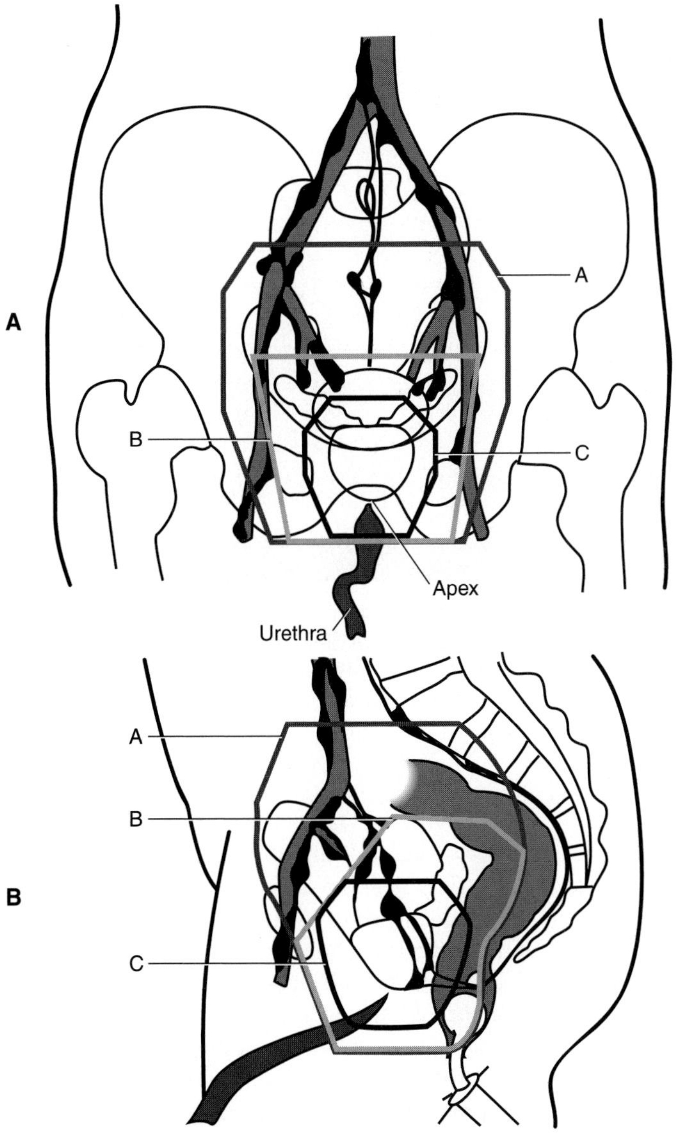

Figure 34-5. A, Anteroposterior (AP) fields for *(A)* prostate, seminal vesicles, and pelvic nodes, *(B)* prostate and seminal vesicles, *(C)* prostate only. **B,** Lateral fields for same regions. *(From Kuban DA, El-Mahdi AM: Cancers of the genitourinary tract. In Khan FM, Potish RA, editors: Treatment planning in radiation oncology, Baltimore, 1998, Williams & Wilkins.)*

isocenter is tattooed on the patient at the three points. Scans are transferred to the treatment-planning computer.

Because CT scan does not allow for very accurate visualization of the inferiormost extent of the prostatic apex because it appears to blend with the urogenital diaphragm, the field length is often overestimated to be sure that the entire prostate is well within the radiation portal. This can cause undue radiation of the penile bulb and perhaps a higher risk of impotence. In addition to CT scan, two other methods may be used to determine the inferior field margin. A retrograde urethrogram performed at the time of treatment simulation defines the apex of the urethra or the point where the urethra passes through the urogenital diaphragm, by a narrow point, or beak, in the column of contrast media (Fig. 34-6, *C*). The inferiormost aspect of the prostate is typically located approximately 1 cm above the urethral apex, and therefore by using the urethrogram an appropriate margin can be applied. The other method to localize the inferior extent of the prostate is to introduce two nonradioactive seeds through the perineum. These are positioned just posterior to the prostate apex and lateral to midline, to avoid the urethra, by prostatic palpation through the rectum. Comparison of this technique to prostatic apex localization by CT scan and retrograde urethrogram has shown that the latter two identify the apex of the gland as being 5 to 20 mm too far inferior in up to 30% of cases.[87]

Conformal three-dimensional treatment planning and delivery. The development of sophisticated radiation treatment-planning computers has allowed the planning CT to be reconstructed in three dimensions. The target (prostate or prostate and seminal vesicles) and the surrounding normal structures can be anatomically defined. These organs are outlined on each CT slice. Margins are generally dependent on intended dose, setup error, and internal organ motion. The latter two may vary depending on external immobilization and techniques for correcting internal movement such as fiducial markers, rectal balloon, or transabdominal ultrasound (B-mode acquisition technology [BAT]). In general, margins on the clinical target volume (CTV) to achieve the planning target volume (PTV), are usually in the range of 0.75 to 1.5 cm for standard conformal techniques and doses in the 70 to 72 Gy range and 0.5 to 1.0 cm for more specialized techniques and higher doses such as IMRT in conjunction with BAT.

Beam design may vary. A common technique is sixfields consisting of a right and left lateral pair and two parallel-opposed oblique pairs 45 degrees off lateral. If an anterior beam is used, mainly for the purpose of portal imaging, this may be referred to as a seven-field arrangement. A four-field, typical "box" approach, followed by sixfields as just described, is another technique frequently used, especially if lymph nodes are treated initially. To shape or conform each field cerrobend blocks or multileaf collimator settings on the treatment machine are applied as specified by the computer plan (Fig. 34-7). The dose to pelvic nodes is typically 50 Gy with 54 to 56 Gy to seminal vesicles at high risk but not

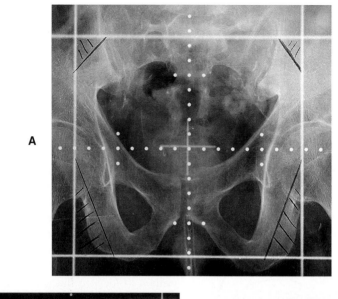

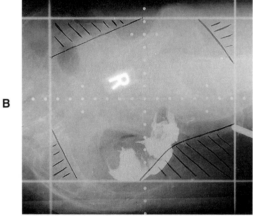

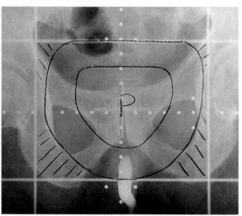

Figure 34-6. **A,** Anteroposterior (AP) simulation field to include pelvic nodes, seminal vesicles, and prostate. **B,** Lateral simulation field. **C,** AP urethrogram showing inferior field margin. *(From Kuban DA, El-Mahdi AM: Cancers of the genitourinary tract. In Khan FM, Potish RA, editors: Treatment planning in radiation oncology, Baltimore, 1998, Williams & Wilkins.)*

proven involved by tumor. Prostate doses may range from 70 to 80 Gy.

A word should be said about dose prescription. Care should be taken to define the prescription point. There can be up to a 5% difference depending on whether the total dose is prescribed to isocenter, the CTV, or PTV. Although doses prescribed to isocenter may appear higher on paper, the dose to the CTV and PTV is actually considerably lower. For definitions of tumor and planning volumes see Table 34-2.

IMRT is a more advanced technique, which specifies the chosen dose to the tumor volume as well as acceptable dose levels for surrounding normal structures such as bladder, rectum, and femoral heads. Although 6, 8, or 10 different beam angles are typically used, multileaf collimator settings change while each field is being treated, shielding the critical

structures a portion of the time and thus treating the tumor volume to a higher dose than the organs of lesser tolerance. Although this technique tends to produce extremely conformal fields with tight margins, inhomogeneity of dose tends to be greater with differentials in the 12% to 20% range. Care must be taken that the highest doses are within the tumor volume and not in normal structures where tolerance will be exceeded. It is with this technique that doses of 80 Gy or more can be delivered to the prostate. (Fig. 34-8) Dose-volume histograms (DVHs) must be constructed to determine the volume of the critical organs (rectum, bladder, and femur) receiving high doses. These parameters have been proven to be related to late radiation-induced complications.

Interstitial brachytherapy. Although prostate implant was done through an open retropubic technique similar to

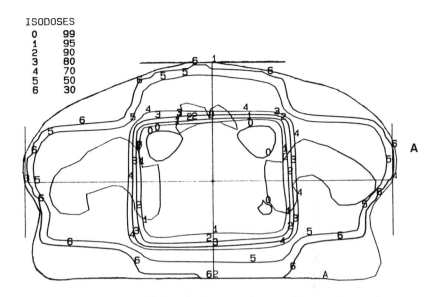

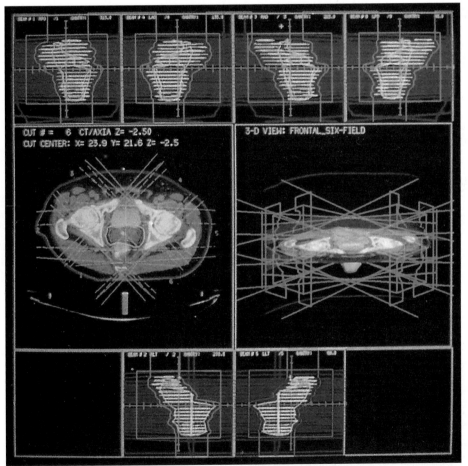

Figure 34-7. A, Isodose distribution for four-field box pelvic treatment technique. **B,** Three-dimensional beam's eye view treatment plan and fields. (**A,** From Kuban DA, El-Mahdi AM: Cancers of the genitourinary tract. In Khan FM, Potish RA, editors: Treatment planning in radiation oncology, Baltimore, 1998, Williams & Wilkins. **B,** Reprinted with permission from Ten Haken RK, et al: Boost treatment of the prostate using shaped, fixed fields, Int J Radiat Oncol Bio Phys 16:193-200, 1989.)

prostatectomy in the mid-1970s to mid-1980s, the advent of transrectal ultrasound permitted a less invasive transperineal template technique that was pioneered in the late 1980s. This procedure is done with either spinal or general anesthesia and uses a grid or template against the perineum with the patient

in the dorsal lithotomy position. Transrectal ultrasound is used to direct the needles, which are either preloaded or attached to the Mick applicator that deposits the radioactive seeds. Dosimetry planning may be done in advance by taking ultrasound images every 5 mm from the base of the prostate through the apex and then loading these into the treatment-planning computer. Seeds are then distributed throughout the prostate 1 cm apart. Isodoses are computed (Fig. 34-9, *A* and *B*). Alternatively, this planning can be done in the operating room just before the procedure. In general, for the average gland, approximately 25 needles and 100 or so seeds are used. The currently used permanent isotopes are I-125 (half-life 60 days) and Pd-103 (half-life 17 days). The usual dose for implant alone with iodine is 145 Gy and with palladium is 125 Gy. Postimplant dosimetry is done postoperatively by obtaining a CT scan, usually at approximately 30 days after the procedure to allow for edema to subside, and entering the seeds and prostate as seen on the scan into the treatment-planning computer. The prostate volume that receives 100% of the prescribed dose (V100) and the dose to 90% of the prostate volume (D90) are the parameters typically recorded. Outcome data suggests that recurrence rates increase with

Table 34-2	Volume definitions for treatment planning
Volume	**Definition**
GTV Gross tumor volume	Palpable or visible extent of tumor
CTV Clinical target volume	GTV plus margin for subclinical disease extension
PTV Planning target volume	CTV plus margin for treatment reproducibility (patient/organ movement, daily setup error)
Treatment volume	Volume enclosed by appropriate isodose in achieving the treatment purpose

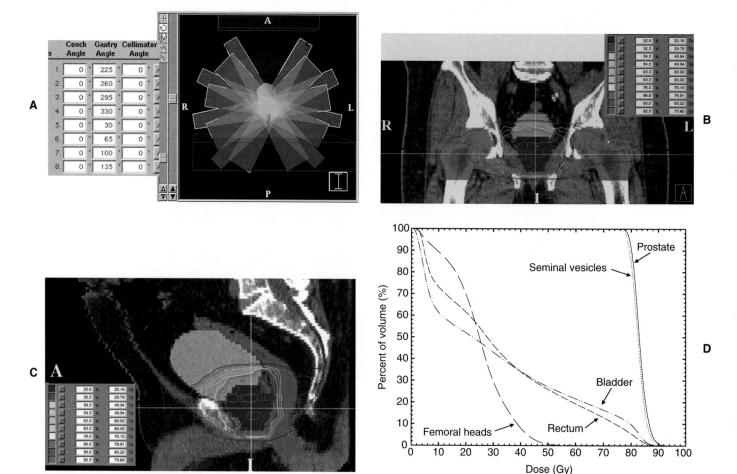

Figure 34-8. Intensity modulated radiation therapy (IMRT) prostate radiation. **A,** Beam angles (8). **B,** Coronal dose distribution. **C,** Sagittal dose distribution. **D,** Dose-volume histogram (DVH).

Continued

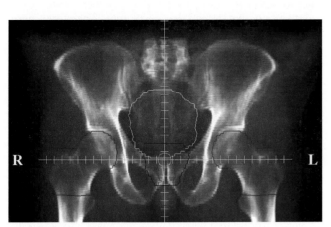

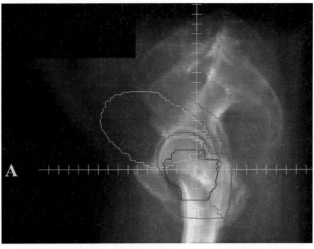

Figure 34-8, cont'd. E, Digitally reconstructed radiograph (DRR) for treatment setup, anterior view. **F,** DRR for treatment setup, left lateral view.

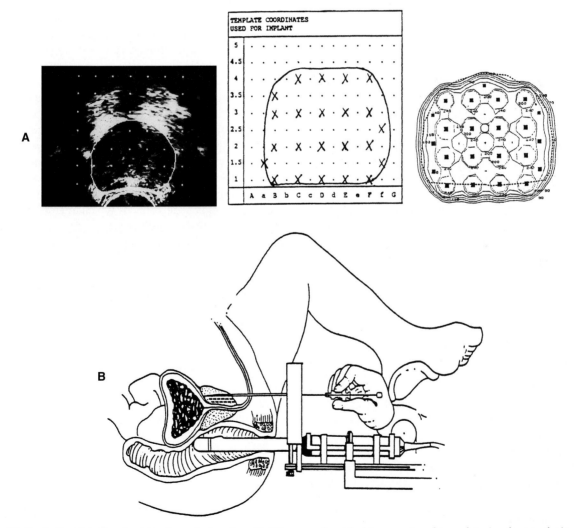

Figure 34-9. A, Prostate implant treatment planning. **B,** Ultrasound-guided transperineal template implant technique. *(From Kuban DA, El-Mahdi AM: Cancers of the genitourinary tract. In Khan FM, Potish RA: Treatment planning in radiation oncology, Baltimore, 1998, Williams & Wilkins.)*

D90s less than 145 Gy.[97] Implants with V100s of 80% or greater are considered good quality.

Interstitial implant can also be used as a boost after moderate dose external beam radiation. Patients chosen for this procedure are those with significant risk of tumor extension outside the prostate capsule. Typically, a dose of 45 Gy to the prostate, seminal vesicles, and possibly pelvic nodes is delivered with external beam. This is then followed 2 to 6 weeks later by an implant, as a boost, to the prostate. The implant dose is decreased to 110 Gy with I-125 and 100 Gy with Pd-103.

High-dose-rate (HDR) iridium is another way to deliver a boost following moderate dose external beam. As compared with I-125 and Pd-103, which are permanent implants, this is a temporary implant technique. Similar to permanent isotopes, a perineal template is used to introduce needles and catheters into the prostate. The catheters are left in place and the patient is hospitalized. Doses have ranged from 400 cGy in each of three fractions to 900 cGy for two fractions. This is generally delivered over 2 days. Total doses and fraction sizes have varied as radiobiologic dose equivalents of these large fraction sizes are being established.

Postprostatectomy radiation. Three situations arise in the postprostatectomy setting: (1) PSA does not decrease to the undetectable range immediately after prostatectomy, signaling that all tumor has not been removed; (2) PSA is undetectable postoperatively but tumor margins contain tumor or seminal vesicles are involved; and (3) PSA is undetectable immediately after surgery but after a period begins to rise. In the latter two circumstances, radiation to the prostate fossa is commonly applied. In the first situation, the PSA may still be detectable because of metastatic disease, and therefore local radiation would not be beneficial. Care must be taken to prove that the only disease remaining is in the surgical bed before local therapy is applied.

CT scan planning can be used similar to the procedure for an intact prostate. The surgical bed, or area where the prostate and seminal vesicles are normally found, is contoured as the target volume. Care is taken to include any site found worrisome by the surgeon or noted as being involved by the pathology report. Four-field or six-field conformal techniques are typically used. Field sizes tend to be in the 10 × 8 cm range. Doses for microscopic disease immediately postoperatively with undetectable PSA are generally at the 60 to 64 Gy level with higher doses, in the 70 Gy range, for rising PSA. Care must be taken to evaluate rectal and bladder DVHs. Following surgical removal of the prostate, the bladder and rectum tend to move into the prostatic space, necessitating inclusion of a significant portion of these organs if the area at risk is to be adequately treated. It is not unusual that desired dose levels are compromised by critical organ (rectum and bladder) tolerance.

Results of Treatment

Surgery. Overall survival is a poor measure of treatment outcome for prostate cancer therapy because this is a slowly progressive disease that many men die *with* but not because *of.* There are many other medical conditions in elderly men that affect the death rate. Therefore cause-specific survival based on death from cancer per se is a better measure. To evaluate a particular therapy and its efficacy in eradicating the disease, PSA disease-free survival is generally used in the case of prostate cancer. Because a rising PSA posttreatment signals disease recurrence, it is an objective and early measure of disease status. Outcome is also very much dependent on prognostic factors such as tumor stage, histologic grade (Gleason score), and pretreatment PSA. Patients who have had prostatectomy can be additionally classified according to pathologic features: extracapsular tumor extension, seminal vesicle involvement, and lymph node status.

For prostatectomy, overall PSA progression-free survival rates range from 70% to 85% at 5 years and 45% to 75% at 10 years. For those patients with the best prognosis, T1 to T2, PSA ≤10 ng/ml, Gleason ≤6, the PSA progression-free rate is 80% to 85% at 10 years.[23,67] On the contrary, however, the PSA progression-free rate at 10 years is only 50% for pretreatment PSA more than 10 ng/ml, 70% with extracapsular extension, 40% with seminal vesicle involvement, and 10% with lymph nodes positive for tumor.[23,67] Clinical disease usually becomes detectable long after the PSA rise. In the Hopkins surgical series, only 4% of men had local recurrence and 8% distant disease 10 years after prostatectomy.[67]

Radiation. Results with both external beam radiation and brachytherapy implant are much the same as for surgery if like groups are compared. When treating patients with radiation, we do not, of course, have the pathologic factors such as extracapsular extension, seminal vesicle involvement, and lymph node status by which to group patients into prognostic categories. Tumor stage, grade, and PSA, however, provide substantial information for comparison. With external beam therapy, the best prognostic group, T1 to T2, PSA ≤10 ng/ml, Gleason ≤6, has a PSA disease-free survival of 80% at 10 years just as for surgery[51]). Similar patients show PSA disease-free status 80% to 90% of the time with implant.[8,9] The implant patients tend to be a more highly select group with smaller amounts of disease, which may account for slightly better outcome statistics. Patients with more advanced disease, T3 or PSA greater than 10 ng/ml or Gleason 7 to 10, tend to have more guarded prognoses, once again, similar to those surgically treated.[55]

As radiation techniques become more highly conformal and doses are increased, early reports on outcome appear promising. The randomized study from UTMD Anderson Cancer Center comparing 70 with 78 Gy, reported a 27% absolute gain in PSA disease-free survival at 4 years for patients with pretreatment PSA greater than 10 ng/ml treated to 78 Gy (Fig. 34-10).[73] More recent update (unpublished as yet) shows this advantage has narrowed to 19% at 6 years but still remains significant. There was no advantage for higher dose in patients with pretreatment PSA ≤10 ng/ml. Other

Months	0	10	20	30	40	50	60
70 Gy	53	43	33	20	13	9	5
78 Gy	53	50	40	29	18	12	8

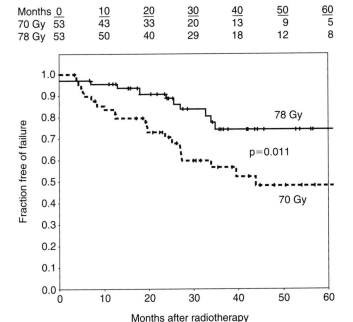

Figure 34-10. Kaplan-Meier Freedom from failure (FFF) curves for patients with PSA levels of more than 10 ng/mL by dose randomization (70 Gy vs. 78 Gy). The numbers of patients at risk at 10-month intervals are shown above the graphs. *(From Pollack A, et al: Preliminary results of a randomized radiotherapy dose-escalation study for prostate cancer, J Clin Oncol 18:3904-3911, 2000.)*

investigators have seen improved outcome results with higher doses as well (Table 34-3). Because serum PSA is a good marker for recurrent disease and has been shown to highly correlate with prostate biopsy results, routine postradiation biopsies are no longer done except on randomized trials. Biopsies become important, however, when local treatment for prostate recurrence is planned. Because these therapies, such as prostatectomy, cryotherapy, and repeat irradiation, usually carry significant complication rates, it is essential to ensure that there is, in fact, local disease present because a PSA rise could also be caused by nodal or distant disease.

Palliative radiation. Irradiation doses of 50 to 60 Gy may be effective in the treatment of massive locally extensive prostatic carcinoma or significant size pelvic lymph node disease, which may produce pain, hematuria, urethral obstruction, or leg edema.

Radiation is frequently used in the treatment of distant metastases secondary to carcinoma of the prostate. Marked symptomatic relief is noted in more than 80% of patients treated with doses of 30 Gy in 2 weeks. Most commonly, osseous sites are treated with localized fields. Although unusual, brain metastases may be successfully treated with doses of 30 Gy in 10 fractions to the entire cranial contents just as for other primary sites. Hemibody irradiation has been used for the palliation of widespread bony disease.

If multiple skeletal sites are involved by the tumor and produce symptoms, radioactive strontium-89 can be administered intravenously with some degree of pain relief occurring in 80% of patients.[74] Samarium-153 is a newer isotope that is also used for this purpose.[4]

Table 34-3	5-Year PSA disease-free survival with higher versus lower dose irradiation				

| | | | % 5-Yr PSA-DFS PSA (ng/ml) | | |
Study	Total No. of Patients	Dose (Gy)	≤10	10-20	< 20
Hanks	232	<71.5	ND	29	8
		71.5-75.7	ND	57	28
		≥75.7	ND	73	30
			≤10	>10	
Pollack	301	70	80	48	
		78	82	75	
			Favorable	Unfavorable	
Lyons	738	<72	81	41	
		≥72	98	75	
			Favorable	Intermediate	High
Zelefsky	1100	64.8-70.2	79	49	21
		75.6-86.4	90	67	50

Data from Hanks et al: *Int J Radiat Oncol Biol Phys* 41:501, 1998; Pollack, et al: *JCO* 18:3904, 2000; Lyons, et al: *Urology* 55:85, 2000; Zelefsky, et al: *J Urol* 166:876, 2001.
Favorable, PSA ≤10 ng/ml, Gleason ≤6, T1-T2; *intermediate,* one factor worse; *ND,* no difference based on dose; *PSA-DFS PSA,* prostate-specific antigen disease-free survival; *unfavorable or high,* ≥2 factors worse.

Side Effects and Complications

Surgery. With improved anesthesia and surgical techniques and the availability of antibiotics and other supportive care, operative mortality has been reduced to 1% or less. Wound infection, hematoma, or pelvic abscess occurs in less than 5% of patients. If a lymphadenectomy is done, patients may develop lymphocele (5%) or penile, scrotal, or lower extremity edema (less than 5%). Thrombophlebitis and pulmonary emboli rarely occur (less than 5%).[12] The most significant morbidity is incontinence and sexual impotence, which is related to the type of radical prostatectomy. Moderate stress incontinence requiring pads is reported to be 5% to 8% by major university centers.[23] Surveys of patients, however, show this rate to be considerably higher at 25% to 30%.[58] The preservation of potency is related to the tumor stage, unilateral or bilateral resection of the neurovascular bundle, and patient age. With a bilateral nerve sparing procedure, potency rates range from 76% in men younger than 60 years to 49% for those older 65. Potency rates are less, of course, if nerves can only be spared unilaterally because of close proximity to tumor or if the patient did not have full erectile function preoperatively.[23]

Radiation therapy. Acute gastrointestinal (GI) side effects of radiation include diarrhea, abdominal cramping, rectal discomfort, and occasionally rectal bleeding, which may be caused by transient proctitis. Patients with hemorrhoids may develop discomfort earlier than other patients, and aggressive symptomatic treatment should be instituted promptly. A higher incidence of both acute and late GI effects occurs when larger volumes of the pelvis are irradiated.

Severe late sequelae of treatment include persistent proctitis, rectal bleeding, and ulceration. Although the incidence of grade 2 (moderate) GI complications is low, 5%, with doses in the 64 to 70 Gy range, this rate more than doubles (14%) when higher doses of 75 to 81 Gy are used.[110] Storey et al.[98] have shown that the rectal complication rate is related to the amount of rectum treated to doses of 70 Gy or higher. Therefore attention to DVHs is imperative when dose escalating. Fortunately, severe grade 3 and 4 GI complications occur infrequently, in less than 2% of patients. Late urinary toxicity occurs at a similar rate, but to date no strong relationship to irradiated organ volume has been shown.

Sexual impotence (erectile dysfunction) has been observed in 30% to 60% of formerly potent patients treated with external irradiation and in 20% to 30% of those treated with interstitial implant.[5,58] These percentages are, of course, dependent on patient age, definition of potency, and degree of potency pretreatment. Data are also greatly influenced by physician versus patient reporting via survey. The latter tends to produce higher rates of dysfunction and complications.

PENIS AND MALE URETHRA

Epidemiology

Carcinoma of the penis is relatively rare in the United States; the estimated incidence is 1 per 100,000 each year, accounting for less than 1% of cancers in men. This tumor is extremely rare in circumcised Jewish men; circumcision performed early in life protects against carcinoma of the penis, but this is not true if the operation is done in adult life. The higher incidence in some areas of South America, Africa, and Asia and in African Americans seems to be related to the absence of the practice of neonatal circumcision. Phimosis (narrowing of the opening of the prepuce) is common in men suffering from penile carcinoma. **Smegma** (a white secretion that collects under the prepuce of the foreskin) is carcinogenic in animals, although the component of smegma responsible for its carcinogenic effect has not been identified.[16]

Carcinoma of the male urethra is also rare. There are no recognized racial nor geographic predisposing factors. Although the cause remains unknown, some correlation exists between the incidence of carcinoma of the urethra and chronic irritation and infections, venereal diseases, and strictures. The average age at the time of presentation is 58 to 60 years, although 10% of these tumors occur in men younger than 40 years.

Prognostic Indicators

The principal prognostic factors in carcinoma of the penis are the extent of the primary lesion and status of the lymph nodes. The incidence of nodal involvement is related to the extent and location of the primary lesion. Tumor-free regional nodes imply an excellent long-term disease-free survival rate, 85% to 90%.[17] Patients with involvement of the inguinal nodes do considerably worse, and only 40% to 50% experience long-term survival. Pelvic lymph node involvement implies an even worse prognosis; less than 20% of these patients survive. Tumor differentiation is another important prognostic factor.[32]

The overall prognosis for carcinoma of the urethra in males varies considerably with the location of the primary lesion. The prognosis for distal lesions is generally similar to that for carcinoma of the penis. Lesions of the bulbomembranous urethra are usually extensive and associated with a dismal prognosis. Tumors of the prostatic urethra have prognostic features similar to those of bladder carcinoma. Superficial lesions have a good prognosis and may be managed with a transurethral resection, whereas deeply invasive tumors have a greater tendency to develop inguinal or pelvic lymph node and distant metastases.

Anatomy and Lymphatics

The basic structural components of the penis include two **corpora cavernosa** and the **corpus spongiosum** (Fig. 34-11, *A*). These are encased in a dense fascia (Buck's fascia), which is separated from the skin by a layer of loose connective tissue. Distally, the corpus spongiosum expands into the glans penis, which is covered by a skin fold known as the *prepuce.*

Composed of a mucous membrane and the submucosa, the male urethra extends from the bladder neck to the external urethral meatus (Fig. 34-11, *B*). The posterior urethra is

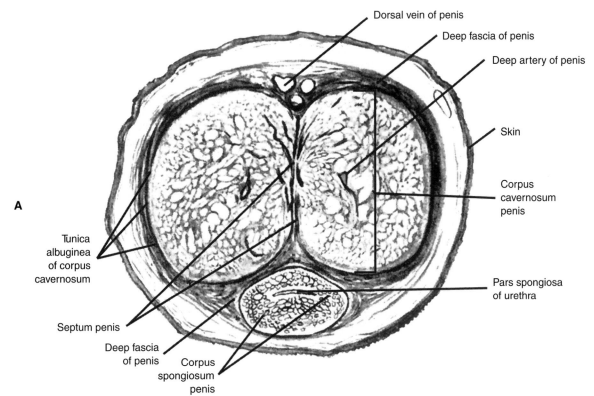

A

Dorsal vein of penis

Deep fascia of penis

Deep artery of penis

Skin

Corpus cavernosum penis

Pars spongiosa of urethra

Corpus spongiosum penis

Deep fascia of penis

Septum penis

Tunica albuginea of corpus cavernosum

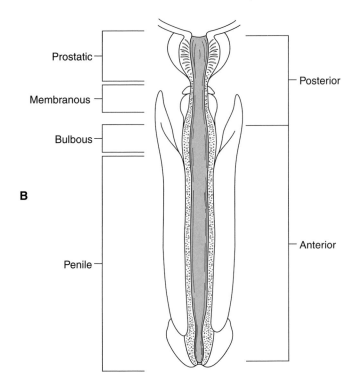

B

Prostatic

Membranous

Bulbous

Penile

Posterior

Anterior

Figure 34-11. A, A cross section of the penis shaft. **B,** Anatomic subdivisions of the male urethra. **(A** *from Sobotta/Becher, Atlas der Anatomie des Menschen, 17, Aufl., Urban & Schwarzenberg, 1972; **B** from Perez CA, Pilepich MV: Penis and male urethra. In Perez CA, Brady LW, editors: Principles and practice of radiation oncology, ed 2, Philadelphia, 1992, JB Lippincott.)*

urethra (which passes through the pendulous part of the penis), and the **bulbous urethra** (the dilated proximal portion of the anterior urethra).

The lymphatic channels of the prepuce and the skin of the shaft drain into the superficial inguinal nodes located above the fascia lata. For practical purposes lymphatic drainage may be considered bilateral. Some disagreement exists regarding whether the glands and deep penile structures drain into the superficial or deep inguinal lymph nodes. The lymphatics of the fossa navicularis and penile urethra follow the lymphatics of the penis to the superficial and deep inguinal lymph nodes. The lymphatics of the bulbomembranous and prostatic urethra may follow three routes: external iliac, obturator and internal iliac, and presacral lymph nodes. The pelvic (iliac) lymph nodes are rarely involved in the absence of inguinal lymph node involvement.

Clinical Presentation

The presence of phimosis may obscure the primary lesion. Secondary infection and an associated foul smell are common, whereas urethral obstruction is unusual. Inguinal lymph nodes are palpable at the time of presentation 30% to

subdivided into the membranous urethra, the portion passing through the urogenital diaphragm, and the prostatic urethra, which passes through the prostate. The anterior urethra passes through the corpus spongiosum and is subdivided into **fossa navicularis** (a widening within the glans), the **penile**

45% of patients.[17,26] However, the lymph nodes contain tumor in only half the patients; enlargement of the lymph nodes is often related to inflammatory (infectious) processes. Conversely, 20% of patients with clinically normal inguinal lymph nodes have occult metastases.

Patients with urethral carcinoma may exhibit obstructive symptoms, tenderness, dysuria, urethral discharge, and occasionally initial hematuria (blood in the urine). Lesions of the distal urethra are often associated with palpable inguinal lymph nodes at the time of presentation.

Detection and Diagnosis

Penile lesions can be seen on examination and documented by biopsy. Urethral lesions are evaluated by urethroscopy and cystoscopy. Inguinal lymph nodes should be thoroughly evaluated. Radiographic assessment of the regional lymphatics is of questionable value because of the extensive inflammatory changes often present in the lymph nodes. CT is useful in the identification of enlarged pelvic and paraaortic lymph nodes in patients with involved inguinal lymph nodes.

Pathology and Staging

Most malignant penile tumors are well-differentiated squamous cell carcinomas. No significant correlation between the histologic grade and survival time has been found.

Bowen's disease is squamous cell carcinoma in situ that may involve the shaft of the penis and hairy skin of the inguinal and suprapubic areas.

Erythroplasia of Queyrat is an epidermoid carcinoma in situ that involves the mucosal or mucocutaneous areas of the prepuce or glans. This carcinoma appears as a red, elevated, or ulcerated lesion. Some patients with erythroplasia of Queyrat have invasive squamous cell carcinoma at the time of the diagnosis.

Extramammary Paget's disease is a rare intraepithelial apocrine carcinoma. The most common sites are the scrotum, inguinal folds, and perineal region.

Primary lymphoma of the penis is extremely rare. Only five cases of secondary involvement of the penis by lymphoma have been reported in the literature.[105]

Cancers metastatic to the penis are also rare. The most common neoplasms metastasizing to the penis are carcinomas from the genitourinary organs, followed by carcinomas from the GI and respiratory systems. Priapism as an initial presenting feature or later development occurs in 40% of these patients.[75]

Approximately 80% of urethral carcinomas in males are well- or moderately differentiated squamous cell carcinomas.[69] Others include transitional cell carcinomas (15%), adenocarcinomas (5%), and undifferentiated or mixed carcinomas (1%). More than 90% of carcinomas of the prostatic urethra are of the transitional cell type. Adenocarcinomas occur only in the bulbomembranous urethra.

The AJCC staging systems for carcinoma of the penis and male urethra are shown in Boxes 34-3 and 34-4.[29]

Routes of Spread

Most carcinomas of the penis start in the preputial area, arising in the glands, the coronal sulcus, or the prepuce. Extensive primary lesions may involve the corpora cavernosa or even the abdominal wall. The inguinal lymph nodes are the most common site of metastatic spread. About 20% of patients with clinically nonpalpable inguinal nodes have micrometastases. Pathologic evidence of nodal metastases is reported in about 35% of all patients and in approximately 50% of those with palpable lymph nodes.[17,26] Distant metastases are uncommon, about 10%, even in patients with advanced locoregional disease. They usually occur in patients who have inguinal lymph node involvement.

The natural history of carcinoma of the male anterior urethra is similar to that of carcinoma of the penis. Most tumors are low grade and progress slowly at primary and regional sites rather than spread to distant areas. Tumors of the penile urethra spread to the inguinal lymph nodes, and tumors of the bulbomembranous and prostatic urethra metastasize first to the pelvic lymph nodes.[69]

Treatment Techniques

Carcinoma of the penis.   Therapy is usually performed in two phases: initial management of the primary tumor and later treatment of the regional lymphatics. Surgery for the primary tumor ranges from local excision or chemosurgery in a small group of highly selected patients, particularly those with small lesions of the prepuce, to a partial or total penectomy. Although surgical resection is usually a highly effective and expedient treatment modality, it may not be acceptable to sexually active patients.

Bowen's disease and erythroplasia of Queyrat can be treated with topical 5-FU (5% cream), a local excision, or superficial x-rays (4500 to 5000 cGy in 4 to 5 weeks). The principal advantage of radiotherapeutic management of the primary lesion in penile carcinoma is organ preservation. Many different techniques, doses, and fractionation schemes have been used.[26,69] Interstitial implants, molds, and contact orthovoltage and megavoltage irradiation have improved tumor control in some modern series and decreased the incidence of treatment-related sequelae. Most patients who experience local failure after radiation therapy can be salvaged surgically.

Nodal management by observation with delayed intervention when signs of nodal involvement appear has replaced elective nodal dissection for the following reasons: (1) the 1% to 3% surgical mortality rate, (2) the morbidity associated with lymphadenectomy, and (3) the relatively low incidence of metastatic disease (10% to 20%) in patients with clinically normal lymph nodes. Survival rates are high with this treatment.[86] Patients with lymph nodes clinically negative for tumor who are at risk for microscopic nodal metastases because of a primary tumor more advanced than stage I or a moderately to poorly differentiated histology can receive elective radiation to the inguinal lymph nodes (5000 cGy in 5 weeks) with a high

---

Box 34-3	AJCC Staging System for Carcinoma of the Penis

PRIMARY TUMOR (T)

TX	Primary tumor cannot be assessed
T0	No evidence of tumor
Tis	Carcinoma in situ
Ta	Non-invasive verrucous carcinoma
T1	Tumor invades subepithelial connective tissue
T2	Tumor invades corpus spongiosum or cavernosum
T3	Tumor invades urethra or prostate
T4	Tumor invades other adjacent structures

REGIONAL LYMPH NODES (N)

NX	Regional lymph nodes cannot be assessed
N0	No regional lymph node metastasis
N1	Metastasis in a single superficial inguinal lymph node
N2	Metastasis in a multiple or bilateral superficial inguinal lymph node
N3	Metastasis in deep inguinal or pelvic lymph node(s), unilateral or bilateral

DISTANT METASTASIS (M)

MX	Distant metastasis cannot be assessed
M0	No distant metastasis
M1	Distant metastasis

STAGE GROUPING

0	Tis	N0	M0
	Ta	N0	M0
I	T1	N0	M0
II	T1	N1	M0
	T2	N0	M0
	T2	N1	M0
III	T1	N2	M0
	T2	N2	M0
	T3	N0	M0
	T3	N1	M0
	T3	N2	M0
IV	T4	Any N	M0
	Any T	N3	M0
	Any T	Any N	M1

HISTOLOGIC GRADE (G)

GX	Grade cannot be assessed
G1	Well differentiated
G2	Moderately well differentiated
G3-4	Poorly differentiated or undifferentiated

With permission from American Joint Committee on Cancer (AJCC), Chicago, Illinois: *AJCC Cancer Staging Manual*, ed 6, New York, 2002, Springer-Verlag.

---

probability of tumor control and low morbidity. Generally, clinically involved and resectable regional lymph nodes are managed by radical lymphadenectomy. Some patients can be treated with combined radiation and lymphadenectomy and, if necessary, pelvic lymph node dissection.

Chemotherapy. The use of chemotherapy for carcinoma of the penis is limited. Some degree of tumor regression has been described with systemic agents, such as bleomycin, 5-FU, and methotrexate. A response to cisplatin has also been reported.[25] Systemic therapy is usually reserved for metastatic and recurrent disease or those lesions so advanced as to be incurable by surgery and radiation.

Carcinoma of the male urethra. Noninvasive carcinoma of the proximal urethra can be treated with a transurethral resection. For lesions of the distal urethra, results with penectomy or radiation therapy are similar to those for carcinoma of the penis, and the 5-year survival rates of 50% to 60% are comparable.[78] Involved regional lymph nodes are treated with lymphadenectomy. Most patients, however, exhibit advanced invasive lesions, which are difficult to manage with radical surgery or radiation therapy.

Radiation therapy techniques. If indicated, circumcision must be performed before the start of radiation therapy to minimize radiation therapy-associated morbidity.

External irradiation. External beam therapy requires specially designed accessories, including bolus, to achieve homogeneous dose distribution to the entire organ involved. One device consists of a plastic box with a central circular opening that can be fitted over the penis. The space between the skin and box must be filled with tissue-equivalent material (Fig. 34-12). This box can be treated with parallel-opposed megavoltage beams. An ingenious alternative to the box technique is the use of a water-filled container to envelop the penis while the patient is in a prone position.

A more complex device consists of a Perspex tube attached to a baseplate resting on the skin. This device is placed as close as possible to the base of the penis, and a flexible tube is connected to a vacuum pump. The suction effect keeps the penis in a fixed position during treatment. Appropriate bolus is placed outside the tube. The patient can also be treated in the prone position, with the penis hanging through a small hole placed in the Perspex's cylinder.

A well-established association exists between large fraction size and late tissue damage. The daily fraction in most reported series is 250 to 350 cGy for a total dose of 5000 to 5500 cGy, although a smaller daily fraction size, 180 to 200 cGy, and a higher total dose are preferable. A total dose of 6500 to 7000 cGy, with the last 500 to 1000 cGy delivered to a reduced portal, should result in reduced incidence of late fibrosis.

Regional lymphatics can be treated with external beam

Box 34-4	AJCC Staging System for Carcinoma of the Urethra

PRIMARY TUMOR (T) (MALE AND FEMALE)

TX   Primary tumor cannot be assessed
T0   No evidence of primary tumor
Ta   Non-invasive papillary, polypoid, or verrucous carcinoma
Tis   Carcinoma in situ
T1   Tumor invades subepithelial connective tissue
T2   Tumor invades any of the following: corpus spongiosum, prostate, periurethral muscle
T3   Tumor invades any of the following: corpus cavernosum, beyond prostatic capsule, anterior vagina, bladder neck
T4   Tumor invades other adjacent organs

UROTHELIAL (TRANSITIONAL CELL) CARCINOMA OF THE PROSTATE

Tis pu   Carcinoma in situ, involvement of the prostatic urethra
Tis pd   Carcinoma in situ, involvement of the prostatic ducts
T1   Tumor invades subepithelial connective tissue
T2   Tumor invades any of the following: prostatic stroma, corpus spongiosum, periurethral muscle
T3   Tumor invades any of the following: corpus cavernosum, beyond prostatic capsule, bladder neck (extraprostatic extension)
T4   Tumor invades other adjacent organs (invasion of the bladder)

REGIONAL LYMPH NODES (N)

NX   Regional lymph nodes cannot be assessed
N0   No regional lymph node metastasis
N1   Metastasis in a single lymph node 2 cm or less in greatest dimension
N2   Metastasis in a single node more than 2 cm in greatest dimension, or in multiple nodes
N3   Metastasis in deep inguinal or pelvic lymph node(s), unilateral or bilateral

DISTANT METASTASIS (M)

MX   Distant metastasis cannot be assessed
M0   No distant metastasis
M1   Distant metastasis

STAGE GROUPING

0a	Ta	N0	M0
0ais	Tis	N0	M0
	Tis pu	N0	M0
	Tis pd	N0	M0
I	T1	N0	M0
II	T2	N0	M0
III	T1	N1	M0
	T2	N1	M0
	T3	N0	M0
	T3	N1	M0
IV	T4	N0	M0
	T4	N1	M0
	Any T	N2	M0
	Any T	Any N	M1

HISTOLOGIC GRADE (G)

GX   Grade cannot be assessed
G1   Well differentiated
G2   Moderately well differentiated
G3-4   Poorly differentiated or undifferentiated

With permission from American Joint Committee on Cancer (AJCC), Chicago, Illinois: *AJCC Cancer Staging Manual*, ed 6, New York, 2002, Springer-Verlag.

megavoltage radiation. The fields should include bilateral inguinal and pelvic (external iliac and hypogastric) lymph nodes (Fig. 34-13). The posterior pelvis may be partially spared by anterior loading of the beams. Depending on the extent of nodal disease and proximity of the detectable tumor to the skin surface or presence of skin invasion, the application of a bolus to the inguinal area should be considered. If clinical and radiographic evaluations show no gross enlargement of the pelvic lymph nodes, the dose to these nodes may be limited to 5000 cGy. In patients with palpable lymph nodes, doses of 6500 to 7000 cGy in 7 to 8 weeks, 180 to 200 cGy per day, with reduced fields after 5000 cGy are advised.

Brachytherapy. A mold is usually built in the form of a box or cylinder with a central opening and channels for the placement of radioactive sources (needles or wires) in the periphery of the device. The cylinder and sources should be long enough to prevent under dosage at the tip of the penis. A dose of 6000 to 6500 cGy at the surface and approximately 5000 cGy at the center of the organ is delivered in 6 to 7 days. The mold can be applied continuously, in which case an indwelling catheter or intermittent catheterization is used. Single- or double-plane implants can also be used to deliver 6000 to 7000 cGy in 5 to 7 days. In extensive lesions involving the shaft of the penis (stage III), obtaining an adequate margin with brachytherapy procedures is difficult, similar to the situation seen in attempting a partial penectomy.

Results of Treatment

Carcinoma of the penis. Reports of treatment results are scarce because cancer of the penis is uncommon in the Western world. A significant proportion of patients have been

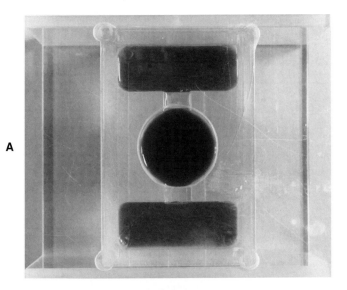

A

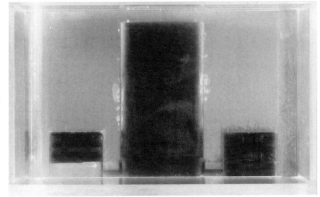

B

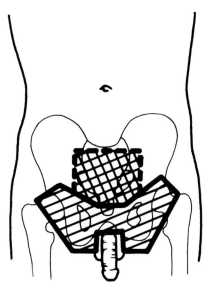

Figure 34-13. Portals encompassing the inguinal and pelvic lymph nodes. *(From Perez CA, Pilepich MV: Penis and male urethra. In Perez CA, Brady LW, editors: Principles and practice of radiation oncology, ed 2, Philadelphia, 1992, JB Lippincott.)*

Figure 34-12. A, A view from above of a plastic box with a central cylinder for external irradiation of the penis. The patient is treated in the prone position. The penis is placed in the central cylinder, and water is used to fill the surrounding volume in the box. The depth dose is calculated at the central point of the box. **B,** A lateral view. *(From Perez CA, Pilepich MV: Penis and male urethra. In Perez CA, Brady LW, editors: Principles and practice of radiation oncology, ed3, Philadelphia, 1998, Lippincott-Raven.)*

treated surgically, with 5-year survival rates ranging from 25% to 80%, depending on the stage of the primary tumor and inguinal lymph node involvement.[65,69]

A summary of tumor control rates achieved with irradiation is presented in Table 34-4. In patients 41 to 57 years old treated with various radiation techniques (mold, interstitial, and external beam), 5-year survival rates range from 45% to 68%. A 5-year survival rate of 66% and tumor control rate of 86% have been reported in patients with stage I carcinoma of the penis treated with radiation, compared with a 5-year survival rate of 70% and tumor control rate of 81% in surgically treated patients.[69] Survival and local control rates were only slightly affected by the treatment modality in stage II but were lower in stage III patients treated surgically. If radiation

did not control the primary lesion after 6 months, the penis was amputated and a significant number of patients were salvaged. Of patients initially treated surgically or with radiation, 8% and 20%, respectively, developed inguinal lymph node metastases. Overall, 8% of patients treated surgically and 10% of those irradiated died of inguinal lymph node metastases and tumor spread.

In one study, 80% of patients treated with radiation therapy had tumor control and conservation of the penis.[86] Although irradiation alone or combined with lymph node dissection controlled lymph node metastases smaller than 2 cm in four patients, radiation therapy was successful in controlling lymph node metastases in only one of seven patients who had N2 or N3 disease.

Duncan and Jackson[20] observed 3-year tumor-control rates of 90% with external beam irradiation and only 47% with mold therapy. Other authors have reported a 5-year survival rate of 92% in patients with stages I and II tumors treated with radium-226 or iridium-192 molds, compared with 77% in patients treated with partial penectomy.[86]

Table 34-5 shows a summary of treatment results correlated with the tumor stage, preservation of the organ, and morbidity.

Carcinoma of the male urethra. Most patients with male urethral carcinoma are treated surgically. In 11 patients with tumors at or anterior to the penoscrotal junction, 3 of 4 patients treated with total penectomy and perineal urethrostomy had tumor control.[10] Partial penectomy controlled the local tumor in two patients. Two patients were treated

Table 34-4

Overall control of primary carcinoma of the penis with radiation therapy

Author	Number of Patients	Treatment Method	Dose	Local Control (%)
Almgard and Edsmyr	16	Radium implant and external beam therapy		
Engelstad	72	Mold therapy and teleradium	3500-3700 R (500-700 R/day)	50
Jackson	39	Mold (most patients) and external beam therapy (some patients)	?	49
Marcial, et al.	25	External beam, interstitial, and mold therapy	4000 R in 2 weeks 5000 R in 4 weeks	
		Mold	5000-6000 R in 5-6 days	64
Murrell and Williams	108	External beam therapy	3000-6700 cGy (200 cGy/day)	52
Kelley, et al.	10	External beam therapy (electrons)	5100-5400 cGy (300 cGy/day)	100
Knudson and Brennhovd	145	Mold therapy	3500-3700 cGy in 3-5 days	32
Haile and Delclos	20	Mold therapy, implant, and External beam therapy	? 6000 cGy	90
Mazeron, et al.	23	Iridium-192 implant	6000-7000 cGy	78
Pointon	32	External beam therapy	5250-5500 cGy (16 Fx in 22 days)	84.4
Sagerman, et al.	15	External beam therapy	4500 cGy (15 Fx in 3 weeks) to 6400 cGy (32 Fx in 6.5 weeks)	60
Salaverria, et al.	41	Iridium mold therapy	6000 cGy over several days	84.3

Modified from Perez CA, Pilepich MV: Penis and male urethra. In Perez CA, Brady LW, editors: *Principles and practice of radiation oncology,* ed 2, Philadelphia, 1992, JB Lippincott.
R, Roentgen; *Fx,* fractions.

Table 34-5

Results of radiation therapy for carcinoma of the penis

Author	Modality	Tumor Control Stages I - II	Stages III - IV	Complications	Penis Preservation
Duncan and Jackson	Teletherapy	16/20 (80%)		2/20 (10%)	16/20 (80%)
Jackson	Mold therapy	20/45 (44%)		2/45 (4%)	20/45 (44%)
Haile and Delclos	External beam therapy Brachytherapy	6/6 (100%) 7/7 (100%)	2/2 (100%)	16/20 (80%)	
Kaushal and Harma	Cobalt-60	14/16 (88%)		2/16 (12%)	13/14 (93%)
Kelley et al.	Electron beam	10/10 (100%)			10/10 (100%)
Pierquin, et al.	Iridium implant	14/14 (100%)	12/31 (39%)	3/45 (6.7%)	
Sagerman, et al.	External beam therapy	9/12 (75%)	1/3 (33%)		2/15 (13%)
Salaverria, et al.	Mold brachytherapy	12/13 (92%)			10/13 (77%)

Perez CA, Pilepich MV: Penis and male urethra. In Perez CA, Brady LW, editors: *Principles and practice of radiation oncology,* ed 2, Philadelphia, 1992, JB Lippincott.

with radiation therapy and a third with a combination of preoperative irradiation (4500 cGy) and total penectomy. In four patients with inguinal lymph node metastases the regional disease was controlled with bilateral lymphadenectomy. All six patients in whom local and regional tumors were controlled were alive and disease free 1 to 20 years later. Urethral tumors arose posterior to the penoscrotal junction in 16 patients. A penectomy was performed in five of those patients, all of whom had tumor control and no evidence of recurrence 5 to 29 months after therapy. Two patients treated with a local excision died of disease within 18 months after surgery. Radiation was used in three patients unsuccessfully, and all died of cancer 13 to 31 months after therapy.

Side Effects and Complications

Irradiation of the penis produces brisk erythema, dry or moist desquamation, and swelling of the subcutaneous tissue of the shaft in almost all patients. Although they are uncomfortable, these reversible reactions subside within a few weeks with conservative treatment. Telangiectasia and fibrosis are usually asymptomatic, common, late consequences of radiation therapy.

Most strictures after radiation therapy are at the meatus. Meatal-urethral strictures occur with a frequency of up to 40%.[26,62] This incidence compares with that of urethral strictures after penectomy.

Ulceration, necrosis of the glans, and necrosis of the skin of the shaft are rare complications. Lymphedema of the legs has occurred after inguinal and pelvic radiation therapy, but the role of radiation in the development of this complication remains controversial. Many patients with this symptom have active disease in the lymphatics that may be responsible for lymphatic blockage.

URINARY BLADDER

Epidemiology

Approximately 57,000 new cases and 13,000 deaths from bladder cancer will be reported in the United States annually.[3] The incidence peaks in the seventh decade, and in men this cancer is the fourth most prevalent malignant disease. It occurs about three times more often in men than in women.

Prognostic Indicators

The tumor extent and depth of muscle invasion are important factors affecting the tumor's behavior and outcome of therapy. Tumor morphology is also important because papillary tumors are usually low grade and superficial with a favorable prognosis. Infiltrating lesions tend to be higher grade, sessile, and nodular; they invade muscle, vascular, and lymphatic spaces and generally have a worse prognosis. The degree of histologic differentiation must also be considered because well-differentiated tumors are less aggressive and have a better prognosis than poorly differentiated tumors, which are usually more invasive.[90]

Anatomy and Lymphatics

The urinary bladder, when empty, lies entirely within the true pelvis. The empty bladder is roughly tetrahedral; each of its four surfaces is shaped like an equilateral triangle. The base of the **superior surface** (the only surface covered with peritoneum) is behind, and the apex is in front. The apex of the bladder is directed toward the upper part of the pubic symphysis and is joined to the umbilicus by the middle umbilical ligament, the urachal remnant. The sigmoid colon and coils of the small intestine rest on the superior surface.

In the male, the rectovesical pouch separates the upper part of the bladder base from the rectum. The seminal vesicles and deferent duct separate the lower part of the base from the rectum.

The parietal peritoneum of the suprapubic region of the abdominal wall is displaced so that the bladder lies directly against the anterior abdominal wall without any intervening peritoneum.

The ureters pierce the wall of the bladder base obliquely. During the contraction of the muscular bladder wall the ureters are compressed, preventing reflux. The orifices of the ureters are posterolateral to the internal urethral orifice, and, with the urethral orifice, they define the **trigone** (the triangular portion of the bladder formed by the openings of the ureters and urethra orifice). The sides of the trigone are approximately 2.5 cm in length in the contracted state and up to 5 cm in the distended state (Fig. 34-14). In the male, the bladder neck rests on the prostate.

The epithelium, or urothelium, is transitional. The mucous membrane is only loosely attached to the subjacent muscle layer by a delicate vascular submucosa (lamina propria), except over the trigone, where the mucosa is firmly attached.

The lymphatics of the bladder form two plexuses, one in the submucosa and one in the muscular layer. They accompany the blood vessels into the perivesical space and ultimately terminate in the internal iliac lymph nodes. Some lymphatics may find their way into the external iliac nodes. From these nodes, the lymphatics progress to the common iliac and paraaortic lymph nodes.

Clinical Presentation

Most patients with bladder cancer, 75% to 80%, present with gross painless hematuria. Clotting and urinary retention may occur. Approximately 25% of patients have symptoms of vesical irritability, although almost all patients with carcinoma in situ experience frequency, urgency, dysuria, and hematuria.

Detection and Diagnosis

In addition to a complete history and physical examination, including rectal and pelvic examination, each patient should have a chest x-ray examination, urinalysis, complete blood cell count, liver function tests, cystoscopic evaluation, and bimanual examination performed under anesthesia. Biopsy is done for diagnosis. An intravenous pyelogram should be obtained before cystoscopy so that the upper tracts can be evaluated before retrograde pyelogram, ureteroscopy, brush biopsy, and cytology if indicated. CT or MRI is used to evaluate bladder-wall thickening and detect extravesical extension and lymph node metastases. Bone scans are obtained for patients with T3 and T4 disease and those with bone pain.

Pathology and Staging

Most bladder cancers (98%) are epithelial in origin. In the western hemisphere approximately 92% of epithelial tumors

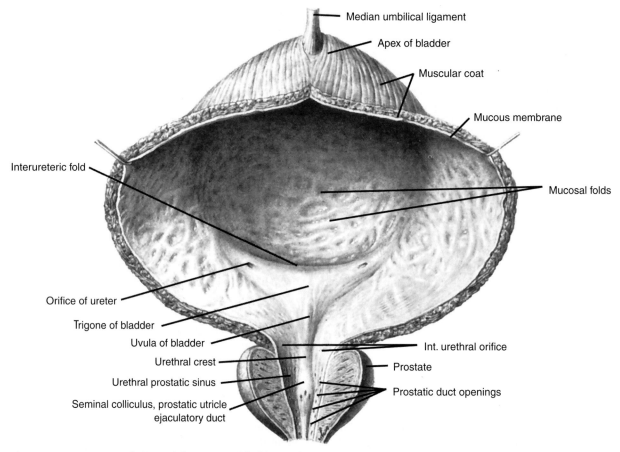

Figure 34-14. A ventral view of the urinary bladder and prostate, illustrating the location of the trigone of the bladder. *(From Sobotta/Becher, Atlas der Anatomie des Menschen, 17, Aufl., Urban & Schwarzenberg, 1972.)*

are transitional cell carcinomas, 6% to 7% are squamous cell carcinomas, and 1% to 2% are adenocarcinomas. Squamous or glandular differentiation can be seen in 20% to 30% of transitional cell carcinomas. Patients whose bladders are chronically irritated by long-term catheter drainage (e.g., paraplegics) or bladder calculi are at risk of developing squamous cell carcinoma.

Morphologically, bladder cancers can be separated into the following four categories: (1) papillary; (2) papillary infiltrating; (3) solid infiltrating; and (4) nonpapillary, noninfiltrating, or carcinoma in situ. At the time of diagnosis, 70% of these cancers are papillary, 25% show papillary or solid infiltration, and 3% to 5% indicate carcinoma in situ.

The TNM, AJCC V staging system is seen in Box 34-5.[29] This system combines histologic findings from transurethral resection specimens and clinical findings from bimanual examination under anesthesia. Pathologic staging is based on histologic examination of cystectomy specimens. In the AJCC system these stages are preceded by the prefix p (e.g., pT3).

The presence of muscle invasion categorizes the lesion as T2 to T4b. Although a bimanual examination with the patient under anesthesia and radiographic studies are helpful

in further separating the various stages, understaging is common.

Routes of Spread

Bladder cancer spreads by direct extension into or through the wall of the bladder. In a small proportion of cases the tumor spreads submucosally under intact, normal-appearing mucosa. Intraepithelial involvement of the distal ureters, prostatic urethra, and periurethral prostatic ducts is frequently found with multifocal or diffuse carcinoma in situ. Approximately 75% to 85% of new bladder cancers are superficial (Tis, Ta, or T1), and about 15% to 25% of patients have evidence of muscle invasion at the time of the diagnosis. Those with superficial disease can develop muscle invasion when tumors recur after conservative therapy. Of all patients with muscle-invasive bladder cancer, approximately 50% have evidence of muscle invasion at the time of the initial diagnosis, and the remaining 40% initially exhibit more superficial disease that later progresses. Perineural invasion and lymphatic or blood vessel invasion are common after the tumor has invaded muscle.

Lymphatic drainage occurs via the external iliac, internal iliac, and presacral lymph nodes. Published data correlate the

Box 34-5 — AJCC Staging System for Carcinoma of the Urinary Bladder

PRIMARY TUMOR (T)

TX	Primary tumor cannot be assessed
T0	No evidence of primary tumor
Ta	Non-invasive papillary carcinoma
Tis	Carcinoma *in situ*: "flat tumor"
T1	Tumor invades subepithelial connective tissue
T2	Tumor invades muscle
pT2a	Tumor invades superficial muscle (inner half)
pT2b	Tumor invades deep muscle (outer half)
T3	Tumor invades perivesical tissue
pT3a	microscopically
pT3b	macroscopically (extravesical mass)
T4	Tumor invades any of the following: prostate, uterus, vagina, pelvic wall, abdominal wall
T4a	Tumor invades prostate, uterus, vagina
T4b	Tumor invades pelvic wall, abdominal wall

REGIONAL LYMPH NODES (N)

NX	Regional lymph nodes cannot be assessed
N0	No regional lymph node metastasis
N1	Metastasis in a single lymph node 2 cm or less in greatest dimension
N2	Metastasis in a single lymph node, more than 2 cm but not more than 5 cm in greatest dimension; or multiple lymph nodes, none more than 5 cm in greatest dimension
N3	Metastasis in a lymph node, more than 5 cm in greatest dimension

DISTANT METASTASIS (M)

MX	Distant metastasis cannot be assessed
M0	No distant metastasis
M1	Distant metastasis

STAGE GROUPING

0a	Ta	N0	M0
0is	Tis	N0	M0
I	T1	N0	M0
II	T2a	N0	M0
	T2b	N0	M0
III	T3a	N0	M0
	T3b	N0	M0
	T4a	N0	M0
IV	T4b	N0	M0
	Any T	N1	M0
	Any T	N2	M0
	Any T	N3	M0
	Any T	Any N	M1

HISTOLOGIC GRADE (G)

GX	Grade cannot be assessed
G1	Well differentiated
G2	Moderately differentiated
G3-4	Poorly differentiated or undifferentiated

With permission from American Joint Committee on Cancer (AJCC), Chicago, Illinois: *AJCC Cancer Staging Manual*, ed 6, New York, 2002, Springer-Verlag.

Table 34-6 — Incidence of histologically positive lymph nodes correlated with pathological stage in bladder cancer

Pathological Stage	Number of Patients	Positive Lymph Nodes (%)
pT_1	41	5
pT_2	20	30
pT_{3a}	13	31
pT_{3b}	28	64
pT_4	8	50

Modified from Skinner DG, Tift JP, Kaufman JJ: High dose, short course preoperative radiation therapy and immediate single stage radical cystectomy with pelvic node dissection in the management of bladder cancer, *J Urol* 127:671-674, 1982.

incidence of pelvic lymph node metastases with the depth of tumor invasion in the bladder wall (Table 34-6).[94] The most common sites of distant metastasis are the lung, bone, and liver.

Treatment Techniques

For carcinoma in situ a radical cystectomy is usually curative. However, most patients and urologists prefer more con-servative initial management. For lesions that are smaller than 5 cm, reasonably well delineated, and without involve-ment of the bladder neck, prostatic urethra, or ureters, treat-ment consists of electrofulguration followed by intravesical chemotherapy or bacillus Calmette-Guérin (BCG).

Ta and T1 disease is usually treated with a transurethral resection and fulguration. Patients with diffuse grade 3, T1 disease or involvement of the prostatic urethra or ducts are difficult to treat locally and may be initially treated with a cystectomy.

Intravesical chemotherapy is often administered after a transurethral resection for T1, grade 2 or 3 lesions. Most physicians withhold intravesical treatment for patients with T1, grade 1 tumors. Some commonly used agents are thiotepa, mitomycin, doxorubicin, and BCG. Patients require close follow-up with cystoscopy, cytology, and resection as indicated.

Definitive treatment with transurethral resection is not applicable to most patients with muscle-invasive disease. Failure to completely eradicate high-grade disease, progression to muscle invasion, or involvement of the prostatic urethra or prostatic periurethral ducts usually signals the need for radical cystectomy.

Partial cystectomy. Carefully chosen patients with relatively small, solitary, well-defined lesions with muscle-invasion or superficial disease not suitable for transurethral resection may be treated by segmental resection. However, recurrence rates can be as high as 50% to 70%, and the primary lesion must be located at the bladder dome, right or left bladder wall, and well-removed from the ureteral orifices and trigone area such that partial cystectomy is technically feasible. Many patients who are disease-free 5 years after partial cystectomy owe their survival to salvage treatment with total cystectomy or radiation. In the Stanford series, radical cystectomy was the most successful salvage treatment.[28]

Radical cystectomy with or without preoperative radiation. Radical cystectomy is recommended for superficial disease (Tis, Ta, T1) in which all attempts at conservative management have proved unsuccessful. Patients are included whose recurrences after each successive transurethral resection and/or intravesical chemotherapy treatment increase in frequency or grade or progress to muscle invasion. Cystectomy is also indicated for patients with recurrent tumors in whom bladder capacity has been so reduced by repeated transurethral resections and intravesical chemotherapy treatments that the successful eradication of the tumor by conservative means, repeat fulguration or irradiation, would produce an unsatisfactory functional result.

For clinical stage T2, T3, and resectable T4a disease, radical cystectomy is commonly used. Preoperative radiation was recommended in years past for large tumors with deep muscle invasion because the risk of understaging was high and local recurrence rates were substantial. More recently, however, staging evaluation and surgical technique has improved such that local recurrence rates are in the 7% to 15% range.[63,93] Furthermore, neither the Southwest Oncology Group trial nor a meta-analysis of six randomized radiation trials showed a benefit associated with preoperative radiation.[43,95] Because most patients with bladder cancer fail therapy because of distant disease, attention was instead turned toward chemotherapy. For T3 and T4a disease, preoperative radiation may be used if resectability is questionable.[66] Although lower doses and shorter fractionation schedules have been used, 45 Gy in 25 fractions has the greatest potential for downstaging with the least complications.

Full-dose external beam radiation with surgery reserved for salvage. Patients treated with radical radiation ideally should have adequate bladder capacity without substantial voiding symptoms or incontinence. The completeness of transurethral resection before radiation may influence local control. Studies show that approximately 40% of patients will have a bladder free of tumor after radiation alone.[36,44] Doses are in the 65 to 70 Gy range.

After radiation, patients undergo cystoscopy every 3 months for 2 years and every 6 months thereafter. Some persistent or recurrent lesions, particularly low-grade tumors, that were downstaged with radiation therapy have been successfully managed with endoscopic resection. If a local tumor persists 3 months after resection, a cystectomy is indicated.[77]

Bladder sparing with chemotherapy plus irradiation. Because of the high rate of local recurrence after radiation alone and the high incidence of distant metastasis, several investigators began to administer chemotherapy concurrently with radiation in an attempt to sensitize the local tumor and address the metastatic component.[22,46,100] A trimodality approach was found to be effective: maximal transurethral resection, chemotherapy and radiation. Patients with T2 to T3 muscle-invasive tumors are candidates for this procedure. Those with poor renal function will not tolerate the necessary chemotherapy, and those with an irritable bladder may have severe symptoms secondary to radiation such that these factors must be considered before embarking on this treatment regimen.

A recent RTOG trial compared the classic regimen of methotrexate, cis-platinum, and vinblastine (MCV) given for two cycles before concurrent radiation and cis-platinum with radiation and cis-platinum alone.[91] There was no benefit in overall survival, survival with an intact bladder, or reduction of distant metastases secondary to the MCV. This regimen, as a neoadjuvant approach, has now been largely discontinued because it was also more difficult for patients to tolerate.

Doses with the previous regimen are typically 40 to 45 Gy to the larger pelvic field to include lymph nodes, followed by a boost to the involved area of the bladder for a total of 65 Gy. Cystoscopy with biopsy and cytology is done after the first 40 to 45 Gy, and, if residual tumor is documented and the patient is a surgical candidate, cystectomy is performed. Cystectomy can also be used for salvage should patients fail after completing the entire regimen.

Interstitial implants. Interstitial radiation therapy for bladder cancer is used more commonly in Europe than in the United States. This technique may be used alone, with external beam radiation, or following partial cystectomy. Suitable patients are those with solitary T1 high-grade to T3a lesions measuring less than 5 cm whose general medical condition permits a surgical procedure. In experienced hands, selected patients can achieve excellent local control and survival. Overall, however, results appear similar to external beam approaches and no comparative trials have been attempted.

Radiation Therapy

Initial target volume. Portals should include the total bladder and tumor volume, prostate and prostatic urethra, and pelvic lymph nodes. Typically, a four-field (anteroposterior/posteroanterior [AP/PA], laterals) pelvic technique is used. Fields extend 1 cm inferiorly to the caudal border of the obturator foramen and superiorly to just below the sacral promontory or just below the S1-L5 disk interspace on the AP projection. These fields include the perivesical, obturator, external iliac, and internal iliac lymph nodes but clearly not the common iliac nodes. The field widths should extend 1.5 cm laterally to the bony margin of the pelvis at its widest point. The irradiation portals are usually at least 12 × 12 cm to include the empty bladder.[27] The anterior boundary of the lateral fields should be at least 1 cm anterior to the most anterior portion of the bladder mucosa seen on an air contrast cystogram or CT scan or 1 cm anterior to the anterior tip of the symphysis, whichever is more anterior. Posteriorly, the fields should extend at least 2 cm posterior to the most posterior portion of the bladder or 2 cm posterior to the tumor mass if it present on a pelvic CT scan. The lateral fields should be shaped with corner blocks inferiorly to shield the tissues outside the symphysis anteriorly and to block the entire anal canal and as much of the posterior rectal wall as possible (Fig. 34-15). High-energy photons (10 to 20 MV) are most suitable.

Boost target volume. The contour of the primary

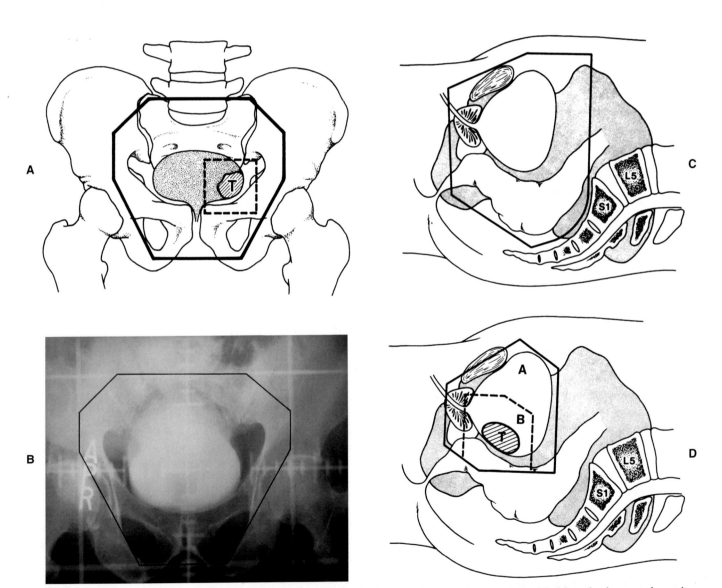

Figure 34-15. A, A diagram of the anteroposterior (AP) pelvic field used for carcinoma of the bladder. The boost volume is outlined with dashed lines. *T,* Residual primary tumor. **B,** Simulation film of the AP portal. **C,** A diagram of the lateral pelvic field encompassing the bladder and pelvic lymph nodes. **D,** Reduced portals after 4500 to 5000 cGy *(A)* and 6500 or 7000 cGy *(B).*

bladder tumor volume is obtained from findings gathered via a bimanual examination, cystoscopy, and CT scan. If the radiation oncologist is satisfied that all initial sites of the tumor are limited to one section of the bladder, the high-dose volume should exclude the uninvolved areas of the bladder (see Fig. 34-15). Treating the bladder while full can help in this regard. Lateral or oblique beams, arcs, or other field combinations can be used.

Simulation is performed with the patient in the supine position. A Foley catheter is inserted into the bladder through the use of sterile technique, and 150 to 250 ml of iodinated contrast material (20% concentration) is injected to outline the posterior portion of the bladder. For visualization of the anterior wall of the bladder on lateral (cross-table) radiographs, 100 to 150 ml of air is injected. Alternatively, CT scan planning can be used and is helpful for large tumor masses with extravesical extension.

Doses. The larger pelvic field to include the bladder and pelvic lymph nodes is generally treated to a dose of 45 to 50 Gy at 180 cGy per day, which requires 5 to 5½ weeks treatment. With chemotherapy, the nodal dose is usually kept at 45 Gy. A smaller boost volume, as previously described is taken to 65 Gy or possibly 70 Gy, if radiation alone is being used.

Results of Treatment

The rate of complete response for radical radiation alone for muscle-invasive bladder cancer is in the 45% range for all T stages.[21,61,77] Approximately 40% to 50% of patients who achieved complete response developed local recurrence later, yielding 5-year local control rates of approximately 25% to 30% for T2 and T3 lesions. The 5- and 10-year local control rates for T4 cancers are lower at 16%. A complete response is associated with significantly improved survival rates. Within each T stage, 5-year survival rates for patients with papillary, solid, or mixed tumors do not differ significantly after external beam irradiation alone.[77]

Using the trimodality bladder-sparing approach as described previously, maximal transurethral resection of the prostate (TURP), radiation, and concomitant chemotherapy, 5-year overall survival is 50% to 60% and with an intact bladder is approximately 40%.[22,46,91] Unfortunately, the distant metastatic rate remains high at 40%. Contrary to concern expressed by some urologists regarding a dysfunctional bladder and severe urinary symptoms following this regimen, quality of life remains good and bladder damage requiring cystectomy is very infrequent, 1.5% rate according to a large study.[46]

TESTIS

Epidemiology

The American Cancer Society estimates that 7600 new cases of testicular cancer and 400 deaths from the disease will occur each year in the United States.[3] The incidence of this tumor has been reported to be 3.8 per 100,000 in the United States. Although testicular tumors are relatively rare, they are the most common malignancy in men between 20 and 34 years of age.[102] The incidence is lowest in Asians, Africans, Puerto Ricans, and North American blacks. Higher rates are reported among whites in the United States, United Kingdom, and Denmark. The origin of testicular tumors may be related to gonadal dysgenesis, as strongly suggested by a higher incidence in men with undescended testes. **Cryptorchidism** (undescended testes) also increases the risk of intraabdominal testicular tumors. Patients with one testicular tumor are at increased risk for developing a contralateral malignancy; 5% may develop a contralateral lesion within 5 years.

Prognostic Indicators

In seminoma the tumor stage is a significant prognostic factor. The histologic subtype and elevation of serum beta human chorionic gonadotropin (HCG) have no prognostic implications. In stages II and III, the outcome is related to the bulk of the retroperitoneal disease, which is associated with an increased propensity for distant metastasis. Patients with stages III and IV disease have a worse prognosis because of the possibility of mediastinal and supraclavicular lymph node involvement or distant metastasis.

The prognosis of nonseminomatous tumors is related to the stage of the disease as well. Most patients with stage I or II disease survive with modern multiagent chemotherapy. In these patients, the levels of tumor markers and the volume of metastasis have some prognostic value. Patients with choriocarcinoma have a poor prognosis.

Anatomy and Lymphatics

The testes are contained in the scrotum and suspended by the spermatic cords. The left testis is usually longer than the right. The testis is invested by the tunica vaginalis, tunica albuginea, and tunica vasculosa. The functioning testis houses the spermatozoa in different stages of development and is responsible for testosterone production.

A close network of anastomosing tubes in a fibrous stroma at the upper end of the testis constitutes the rete testis and vasa efferentia. These small tubes converge in the vas deferens, a continuation of the epididymis, which is a hard, cordlike structure about 2 feet in length and 5 mm in diameter. The vas deferens enters the pelvis along the spermatic cord and empties into the seminal vesicles (two lobulated membranous pouches located on top of the prostate). The ejaculatory ducts, one on each side, begin at the base of the prostate, run forward and downward between its middle and lateral lobes, and end in the verumontanum after entering the prostate.[37]

The lymphatics from the hilum of the testes accompany the spermatic cord up to the internal inguinal ring along the cords of the testicular-spermatic veins. These lymphatics drain into the retroperitoneal lymph nodes between the level of T11 and L4 but are concentrated at the level of the L1 and

L3 vertebrae. They drain to the left renal hilum on the left side and to the pericaval lymph nodes on the right. Crossover from the right to the left side is common, but crossover in the opposite direction is rare. From the retroperitoneal lumbar nodes, drainage occurs through the thoracic duct to lymph nodes in the mediastinum and supraclavicular fossa and occasionally to the axillary nodes.

Clinical Presentation

Usually, a testicular tumor appears as a painless swelling or nodular mass in the scrotum and is sometimes noted incidentally by the patient or a sexual partner. Occasionally, patients complain of a dull ache, heaviness, or pulling sensation in the scrotum or an aching sensation in the lower abdomen. Approximately 10% of patients have acute and severe pain, which may be related to torsion of the spermatic cord. Frequently, patients relate the appearance of the mass to a previous trauma, although this is coincidental rather than etiologic. Rarely, patients exhibit symptoms of metastatic disease, such as a neck mass, respiratory symptoms, or low back pain. Gynecomastia occurs in approximately 5% of patients with testicular germ cell tumors.[24]

Detection and Diagnosis

A complete history and physical examination are mandatory. If a testicular tumor is suspected, a testicular ultrasound should be performed. The appropriate surgical procedure to make the diagnosis and remove the primary tumor is radical orchiectomy through an inguinal incision. Although beta HCG levels are slightly elevated in 17% of patients with pure seminoma, any elevation of alpha-fetoprotein (AFP) signals

nonseminomatous disease. Beta HCG and/or AFP levels are elevated in more than 80% of patients with disseminated nonseminomatous disease. Serum markers (beta HCG, AFP) are assayed before and after orchiectomy because they can be used to document persistent or recurrent cancer and may predict the responsiveness of nonseminomas to surgery or chemotherapy.

A chest radiograph and evaluation of the retroperitoneal lymphatics by CT or a pedal lymphangiogram are critical components of the staging process. A semen analysis and sperm banking should be considered for patients in whom treatment is likely to compromise fertility and who intend to have children in the future.

Pathology and Staging

A representation of the dual origin of testicular tumors is shown in Fig. 34-16. About 95% of testicular neoplasms originate in germinal elements. The most common type of testicular tumor is seminoma, which has three histologic subtypes: classical, anaplastic, and spermatocytic. The prognosis is not significantly different for the various subtypes. The nonseminomatous tumors include embryonal carcinoma, teratoma carcinoma, choriocarcinoma, and yolk sac tumor (embryonal adenocarcinoma in the prepubertal testis). The most common single-cell type is embryonal carcinoma. Yolk sac tumors are the most common in children. Sometimes nonseminomatous tumors contain more than one element; the most common combination is teratocarcinoma (teratoma and embryonal carcinoma). Choriocarcinoma accounts for about 1% of these tumors.

The European Organization for Research on Treatment of

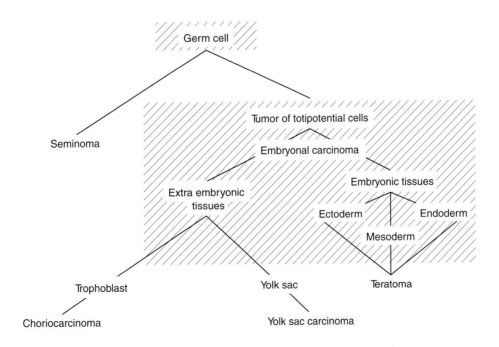

Figure 34-16. Dual origin for derivation of testes tumors.

Cancer/International Union Against Cancer (EORTC/UICC) and the AJCC staging systems are contained in Box 34-6. The EORTC/UICC or some modification is perhaps the most widely used.

Routes of Spread

Although the routes of dissemination are similar for seminoma and nonseminoma, the propensity for involvement of various sites differs. Pure seminoma has a much greater tendency to remain localized or involve only lymph nodes, whereas nonseminomatous germ cell tumors of the testes more frequently spread by the hematogenous route.

Seminoma spreads orderly, initially to the lymph nodes in the retroperitoneum. From the retroperitoneal nodes, the seminoma spreads to the next echelon of draining lymphatics in the mediastinum and supraclavicular fossa (stage III disease). Only rarely and late does pure seminoma spread hematogenously to involve the lung parenchyma, bone, liver, or brain (stage IV disease). Less than 5% of patients have stage III or IV disease at the time of presentation.[102] The orderly route of spread for pure seminoma has been confirmed by surveillance studies. A total of 255 patients participated in postorchiectomy surveillance studies. Of 33 patients with relapses, 29 had disease in the retroperitoneal lymph nodes. The site of the second relapse when infradiaphragmatic irradiation was used for the first relapse was the supra-diaphragmatic nodes.[18]

Nonseminomatous tumors that metastasize usually involve the lungs and liver.

Treatment Techniques

The initial management goal for a suspected malignant germ cell tumor of the testis is to obtain serum AFP and beta HCG measurements and, after staging procedures, to perform a radical inguinal orchiectomy with high ligation of the spermatic cord. Further management depends on the pathologic diagnosis of the stage and extent of the disease.

Seminoma. The most commonly applied treatment for patients with stage I seminoma is radical orchiectomy and postoperative irradiation of the paraortic and ipsilateral pelvic nodes. The standard dose is 2500 cGy in 160 to 180 cGy fractions (Fig. 34-17).[53] Because of the low incidence of pelvic nodal involvement, 0.5% to 3% as shown by the Leeds Conference and surveillance studies, it has been suggested that paraaortic radiation alone may be adequate.[59,99,101,103] Available reports to date, have shown equally as good results without pelvic radiation.[59,99] Surveillance studies performed in Canada and the United Kingdom with patients receiving no further treatment after orchiectomy have indicated recurrence rates of approximately 20%.[18,103] Of patients in whom the tumor recurred, 99.5% were salvaged by subsequent radiation or chemotherapy. If surveillance is chosen over radiation, consistent follow-up is mandatory.

For patients with stage IIA disease (<2 cm diameter mass), the radiation dose and portals for the paraaortic and ipsilateral

Box 34-6	Testis Staging Systems

EORTC	UICC/AJCC	
Primary tumor (T) (pathological classification)		
Stage I	pT_1	Tumor limited to testis (including rete)
	pT_2	Tumor invasion beyond tunica albuginea or into epididymis
	pT_3	Tumor invasion of spermatic cord
	pT_4	Tumor invasion of scrotum
Lymph nodes (N)		
Stage II		
IIA	N_1	Metastasis in single node (<2 cm maximum diameter)
IIB	N_2	Metastasis in a single node (2 to 5 cm in maximum diameter)
IIC, D	N_3	Metastasis in a lymph node (>5 cm in maximum diameter)
Stage III		Supradiaphragmatic and infra-diaphragmatic nodes: abdominal sites A, B, C, and D
Distant metastasis (M)		
	M_0	No distant metastasis
Stage IV	M_1	Distant metastases (specific site)
Stage groupings		
I	T_1, T_2, N_0, M_0	
II	T_3, T_4, N_0, M_0	
III	Any T, N_1, M_0	
IV	Any T, N_2 or N_3, M_0	
	Any T, any N, M_1	

EORTC, European Organization for Research on Treatment of Cancer; *UICC,* International Union Against Cancer; *AJCC,* American Joint Committee on Cancer.

pelvic lymph nodes are similar to those used for stage I disease including adequate margin to cover the enlarged nodes. For stage IIB disease (<5 cm diameter mass), the paraaortic and ipsilateral pelvic lymph nodes should be irradiated with appropriate modification of the treatment field to encompass the larger mass and higher doses. The dose to the entire nodal volume is 2500 cGy in 160- to 180-cGy fractions, with an additional boost of 500 to 1000 cGy in 180- to 200-cGy fractions with reduced portals to the gross tumor.[53]

The optimal therapy for patients with stage IIC retroperitoneal disease (5 to 10 cm in transverse diameter) must be individualized. If the mass is centrally located and does not overlap most of one kidney or significantly overlap the liver, primary radiation therapy can be applied, with chemotherapy reserved for relapse. However, if the location of the mass is such that the radiation volume covers most of one kidney or a significant volume of the liver, the potential morbidity

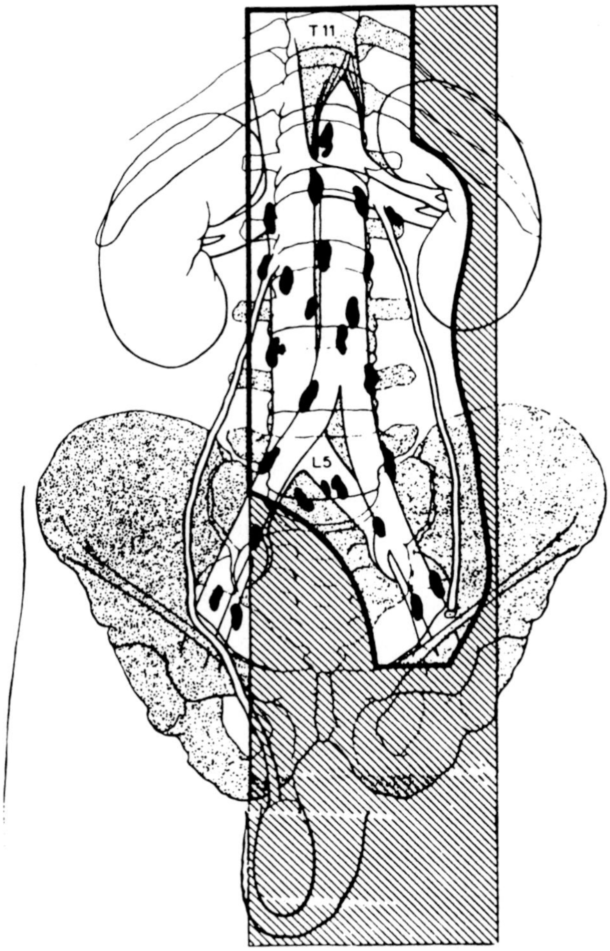

Figure 34-17. Contoured anterior and posterior radiation treatment fields for clinical stage I or IIA left testicular cancer. *(From Kubo H, Shipley WU: Reduction of the scatter dose to the testicle outside the radiation treatment fields, Int J Radiat Oncol Biol Phys 8:1741-1745, 1982.)*

of radiation therapy can be avoided by the use of primary cisplatin-containing combination chemotherapy.

Stage IID is rare. Patients in this stage should be treated with primary cisplatin-containing combination chemotherapy.

The current standard therapy for stages III and IV disease is four courses of cisplatin-containing combination chemotherapy. Often, residual masses may exist in the abdominal or mediastinal area after four cycles of chemotherapy. The 1989 Germ Cell Consensus Conference in Leeds, England, concluded from the available data that patients should be observed after appropriate chemotherapy and that further exploratory surgery or consolidative irradiation should be given only for overt disease progression.[101] This, however, is a controversial issue.

Nonseminoma. The initial treatment for nonseminoma is radical inguinal orchiectomy, followed by cisplatin-based chemotherapy. The most commonly accepted standard regimens include four courses of cisplatin, vinblastine, and

bleomycin (PVB) or bleomycin, VP-16, cisplatin (BEP). Several investigators are exploring the use of fewer courses of cisplatin-containing combination chemotherapy and the use of single-agent cisplatin, carboplatin, or ifosfamide. One third of chemotherapy-treated patients have a radiographically apparent residual mass or masses after chemotherapy. In general, these masses should be excised because approximately 40% are teratomas and another 10% to 15% are carcinomas. Presumptive evidence exists indicating that unresected teratomas may give rise to later relapse and that patients have a lower risk of recurrence after surgical excision. Patients with persistent carcinoma require additional chemotherapy but generally do well following treatment.

Irradiation has little role in the management of patients with disseminated nonseminoma, except in the palliation of brain and other metastatic sites. Chemotherapy is the mainstay of treatment in this advanced state.

Radiation therapy. Patients with stage I testicular seminoma should receive megavoltage irradiation to the paraaortic or paraaortic and ipsilateral pelvic lymph nodes. The top of the portal should be at the T9-T10 interface and the inferior border should be at the bottom of L5 or at the top of the obturator foramen, depending on whether pelvic nodes will be treated. The lateral border must include the paraaortic lymph nodes and ipsilateral renal hilum (usually 10 to 12 cm wide). A shaped field with 2-cm margins is designed to encompass the ipsilateral pelvic lymph nodes (see Fig. 34-17). Testicular shielding for decreasing primary and, to a lesser degree, scattered irradiation should be applied if the patient wants to preserve fertility.[31,50]

The recommended dose to retroperitoneal and pelvic lymphatics for stages I and IIA disease is 2500 cGy in fractions of 160 to 180 cGy with AP/PA fields given 5 days per week and both fields treated daily. For stages IIB and IIC tumors, the portals are the same as those in stages I and IIA, except that the fields should be modified to cover the palpable or radiographic mass with an adequate margin. The first 2500 to 3000 cGy to the entire nodal volume is delivered in fractions of 160 to 180 cGy. A boost of 500 to 1000 cGy in 180- to 200-cGy fractions is given to a reduced field to encompass the mass with an adequate margin of at least 2 cm.

If the primary radiation therapy field encompasses most of one kidney, care must be taken to protect at least two thirds of the kidney from receiving doses higher than 1800 cGy. The initial shrinkage of large masses is often rapid, and the abdominal CT scan should be repeated after the first 3 weeks of radiation therapy to determine possible field reduction. Care should also be taken to limit the radiation dose to a significant volume of the liver to less than 3000 cGy.

Controversial Issues

Scrotal or inguinal irradiation. A standard recommendation has been to modify the treatment volume to include both inguinal regions if there has been previous inguinal surgery and to include the scrotum if it has been violated. Reports from the Princess Margaret and Royal Marsden Hospitals demonstrated that previous inguinal or scrotal violation without irradiation of these sites results in little increased risk of relapse. The 1989 Consensus Conference in Leeds, England, recommended that inguinal or scrotal irradiation be omitted even if scrotal interference has occurred.[101]

Mediastinal irradiation. In the 1960s and early 1970s, using prophylactic mediastinal irradiation to treat patients who had stage I or II testicular seminoma was common. Compiled data from six series suggest that supradiaphragmatic relapse is extremely rare, even for relatively poorly staged patients with stage IIA or IIB disease, if prophylactic mediastinal irradiation is withheld. Mediastinal relapse occurred in only 8 of 250 patients, and 7 of 8 patients were salvaged with radiation. Because the possible survival benefit of elective mediastinal irradiation is only 0.4%, most radiation oncologists have abandoned its use for stages IIA and IIB disease.[85]

Paraaortic versus ipsilateral iliac and paraaortic irradiation. There is growing interest in Europe and the United Kingdom in reducing the radiation volumes for the treatment of stage I disease by omitting irradiation of the pelvic lymph nodes. Less than 3% of patients have involved pelvic nodes, and it is unlikely that the reduction of the irradiated volume will cause a significant increase in relapse rate. Furthermore, salvage chemotherapy is very effective. The most commonly used field in the United States, however, still encompasses both paraaortic and ipsilateral pelvic nodes (see Fig. 34-17).

Results of Treatment

Rates of disease-free survival for stage I testicular seminoma are in the 95% to 97% range at 5 years according to multiple studies.[30,99,103,106] Corresponding cause-specific survival is 100%.

For patients with stage IIA and IIB disease, rates of disease-free and cause-specific survival are 90% and 95%, respectively.[53,85,107]

Survival for patients with stage IIC, IID, and III disease depends on the initial bulk of the tumor and the therapeutic approach. With radiation alone, tumor-free survival rates range from 30% to 50%, and primary chemotherapy yields a progression-free survival rate of 91%. Chemotherapy is highly effective as salvage treatment for failure after radiation as well.

Side effects and complications. In general, paraaortic and pelvic radiation is well tolerated. Patients often develop nausea and occasionally diarrhea during the treatment course, which is usually controlled with appropriate medication. Severe dyspepsia or a peptic ulcer occurs in only 3% to 5% of irradiated patients.[30]

Patterns of case studies have shown that a significant increase in late complications occurred with wide-field irradiation for seminoma and Hodgkin's disease with doses greater than 2500 cGy. However, no late complications were reported with lower doses.[15] The complication rate increased to 2% with 3500 cGy and to 6% with 4000 to 4500 cGy.

Approximately 50% of patients with seminoma have decreased sperm count at the time of diagnosis. Further decreases are noted after pelvic and paraaortic irradiation, even if gonadal shielding is used. Typically, the uninvolved testicle receives 1% to 2% of the prescription dose because of scattered radiation through the body tissues.[31] Spermatogenesis may be affected by doses as low as 50 cGy, and cumulative doses above 200 cGy will likely induce permanent sterility.[89]

Second primary malignancy. A 5% to 10% incidence of second malignancy has been reported in patients treated with radiation therapy for testicular seminoma. These second malignancies arise from inside and outside the radiation treatment portal. Whether they result from radiation treatment, the predisposition of patients with testicular seminoma to develop a second primary, or a combination of both is not clear. The incidence of second malignancies among patients in surveillance studies is invaluable in clarifying this issue. However, because of the relatively short duration of follow-up for surveillance studies, the true relative risk of second malignancies in patients with testicular seminoma remains unclear.

KIDNEY

Epidemiology

Renal cell carcinoma. The estimated number of new cases of kidney and renal pelvis cancers in the United States is 32,000, which will result in approximately 12,000 deaths, representing 2% of all new cancers and cancer deaths annually.[3] The average age at the time of diagnosis is 55 to 60 years, with a male-to-female ratio of 2:1.

Several environmental, occupational, hormonal, cellular, and genetic factors are associated with the development of renal cell carcinoma.[57] Cigarette and tobacco use, obesity, and analgesic abuse (i.e., phenacetin-containing analgesics) have been correlated with an increased risk and incidence of kidney cancer. A higher incidence of renal cell carcinoma has also been reported among leather tanners, shoe workers, and asbestos workers. Exposure to cadmium, petroleum products, and thorium dioxide (a radioactive contrast agent used in the 1920s) causes renal cell carcinoma in humans.

The association of renal cell cancer and von Hippel-Lindau disease has long been established. Various tumor-produced growth factors have been described in the initiation or progression of renal cell carcinoma.[57]

Renal pelvic and ureteral carcinoma. About 7% of all renal neoplasms and less than 1% of all genitourinary tumors are transitional cell carcinomas of the upper urinary tract.[79] For renal pelvic tumors the incidence of men to women is 3:1, and the peak incidence is in the fifth and sixth decades of life. About one third of patients with upper urinary tract tumors develop bladder carcinoma. Etiologic factors for renal pelvic and ureteral cancer are similar to those for tumors of the urinary bladder. Urban residency, cigarette and tobacco use, aminophenol exposure (e.g., benzidine, β-naphthylamine), renal stones, and analgesics (e.g., chronic phenacetin abuse) have been associated with an increased risk of developing upper urinary tract tumors.

Prognostic Indicators

Renal cell carcinoma.   The major prognostic factors for the survival in patients with renal cell carcinoma are the stage and histologic grade of the tumor. Reported 5-year survival rates are 88% for stage I, 67% for stage II, 40% for stage III, and 2% for stage IV disease.[35] Renal vein or vena cava involvement, without corresponding regional lymph node metastasis, is not a poor prognostic sign if the entire tumor thrombus is removed. The mean survival time for patients with metastasis at the time of diagnosis is approximately 4 months, and only about 10% of patients survive 1 year.[76]

Renal pelvic and ureteral carcinoma.   Stage and grade are important prognostic factors in carcinoma of the renal pelvis and ureter. One report noted that 54 patients with transitional cell carcinoma of the renal pelvis and ureter had a median survival time of 91.1 months for early-stage tumors and 12.9 months for more advanced tumors.[41] When patients were stratified according to low or high tumor grade, the median survival time was 66.8 months versus 14.1 months, respectively.

Anatomy and Lymphatics

The kidneys and ureters and their vascular supply and lymphatics are located in the retroperitoneal space between the parietal peritoneum and the posterior abdominal wall. The kidneys are located at a level between the eleventh rib and the transverse process of the third lumbar vertebra. The renal axis is parallel to the lateral margin of the psoas muscle. Each kidney is about 11 to 12 cm in length, with the right kidney usually 1 to 2 cm lower than the left. Gerota's fascia envelops the kidney in its fibrous capsule and the perinephric fat.

The collecting system lies on the anteromedial surface of the kidney and forms a funnel-shaped apparatus that is continuous with the ureter. The ureters course posteriorly, parallel to the lateral border of the psoas muscle, until they curve anteriorly in the pelvis to join the base of the bladder.

The lymphatic drainage of the kidney and renal pelvis occurs along the vessels in the renal hilum to the paraaortic and paracaval nodes. The lymphatic drainage of the ureter is segmented and diffuse, involving any of the following: renal hilar, abdominal paraaortic, paracaval, common iliac, internal iliac, or external iliac nodes.

The topographical relationship of the kidneys, renal pelvis, and ureters to other abdominal organs is illustrated in Fig. 34-18.

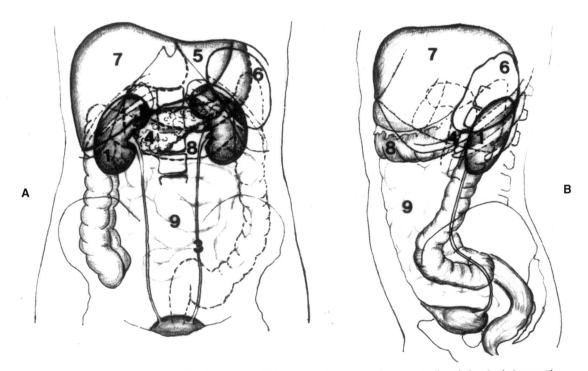

Figure 34-18. Anatomical relationships of the kidneys, renal pelvis, and ureters to the abdominal viscera. The surrounding structures as numbered (*1,* right kidney; *2,* left renal pelvis; *3,* left ureter; *4,* pancreas; *5,* stomach; *6,* spleen; *7,* liver; *8,* transverse colon; *9,* small bowel) become dose-limiting factors in the planning of abdominal or retroperitoneal irradiation. **A,** An anteroposterior view. **B,** A lateral view. *(Courtesy Peter P. Lai, MD)*

Clinical Presentation

Renal cell carcinoma. Renal cell carcinoma may appear as an occult primary tumor or with signs and symptoms. In one report the classic triad of gross hematuria, a palpable abdominal mass, and pain occurred in only 9% of patients. Two of three components of the triad occurred in 36% of patients, whereas hematuria, gross or microscopic, was noted in 59% of patients.[76] Several paraneoplastic syndromes or systemic symptoms of renal cell carcinoma have been described, and the tumor may masquerade behind a variety of symptom patterns.

Renal pelvic and ureteral carcinoma. Gross or microscopic hematuria is the most common sign in patients who have a renal pelvic or ureteral tumor, occurring in 70% to 95% of cases.[79] The other less common symptoms include pain (8% to 40%), bladder irritation (5% to 10%), and other constitutional symptoms (5%). Approximately 10% to 20% of patients have a flank mass secondary to the tumor or associated hydronephrosis. Otherwise, physical findings are unremarkable.

Detection and Diagnosis

Renal cell carcinoma. The diagnosis of renal cell carcinoma is established clinically and radiographically in most patients. After a radiographic diagnosis is made, a thorough staging workup is performed to determine resectability. A metastatic workup that includes a bone scan, chest radiograph, and CT or MRI scan of the abdomen and pelvis should be performed before surgery. If metastatic lesions are detected, a histologic confirmation of the most easily accessible lesion should be obtained.

An intravenous pyelogram (IVP) can identify the tumor, determine its location, and show the function of the contralateral kidney when surgery is contemplated. However, an IVP is not sensitive or specific for small to medium tumors. Ultrasonography provides accurate anatomical detail of extrarenal extension of the tumor. In addition, it differentiates solid from cystic renal lesions. If the lesion is cystic, a percutaneous cyst puncture can be done via ultrasound or CT guidance to rule out malignancy. Renal arteriography detects neovascularity, arteriovenous fistula, and pooling of contrast medium, and it accentuates capsular vessels. Contrast-enhanced or dynamic CT provides extremely accurate information about the location and size of the tumor and lymph node enlargement. CT plus digital subtraction angiography provides adequate diagnostic and anatomic details with much less morbidity than arteriography. Inferior venacavography is sometimes used to detect the extent of the tumor thrombus involvement within the vena cava. MRI provides a 3D picture of renal cell carcinoma.

Renal pelvic and ureteral carcinoma. Excretory urography is frequently used to evaluate patients with renal pelvic carcinoma. The most common finding is a filling defect in the renal pelvis or collecting system. Retrograde pyelography accurately delineates upper-tract filling defects and defines the lower margin of the ureteral lesion. CT or MRI of the abdomen and pelvis before and after contrast gives useful information regarding tumor extension. Angiography is not often used. Endoscopic ureteroscopy with percutaneous nephroscopy is a recently developed technique. A brush cytology or biopsy from such an endoscopic retrograde procedure has a diagnostic accuracy of 80% to 90%.[57]

Pathology and Staging

The proximal tubular epithelium is the tissue of origin for renal cell carcinoma. Clear cell carcinoma is the predominant subtype. Some reports indicate that spindle cell (sarcomatoid variant) carcinoma is associated with a poor prognosis. A tumor's high nuclear grade is associated with an increased incidence of lymph node involvement and a short survival time.[76]

Transitional cell carcinoma accounts for more than 90% of malignant tumors of the renal pelvis and ureter, and squamous cell carcinoma accounts for 7% to 8%.[57] Adenocarcinoma of the upper urothelial tract is rare. Squamous cell carcinoma of the renal pelvis is often deeply invasive and is associated with a worse prognosis than transitional cell carcinoma. High-grade renal pelvic or ureteral tumors are associated with poor survival rates.[41]

The AJCC system for the classification of renal cell carcinoma of the kidney is shown in Box 34-7. T1 and T2 refer to cancers that are intrarenal and have not invaded through the capsule. T3 and T4 cancers are based on the local extension of the primary tumor. The N classification depends on the size and number of involved lymph nodes and not on laterality.

The AJCC staging classification for renal pelvic and ureteral carcinoma is shown in Box 34-8. The grouping of the T categories depends on the tumor's extent with regard to depth of penetration of the lesion.

Routes of Spread

Renal cell carcinoma. A tumor may spread in the following ways: (1) by local infiltration through the renal capsule to involve the perinephric fat and Gerota's fascia; (2) by direct extension in the venous channels to the renal vein or inferior vena cava; (3) by retrograde venous drainage to the testis; (4) by lymphatic drainage to the renal hilar, paraaortic, and paracaval nodes; and 5) by hematogenous route to any part of the body, including the lung, liver, central nervous system, skeleton, and other organs. The incidence of lymph node metastasis is 12% to 23%.[57]

Approximately 45% of patients with renal cell carcinoma have localized disease, 25% have advanced disease, and 30% have radiographic evidence of metastasis at the time of the diagnosis.[57] Approximately 50% of patients with renal cell carcinoma eventually develop metastasis. Common metastatic sites include the lung (75%), soft tissue (36%), bone (20%), liver (18%), cutaneous areas (8%), and central nervous system (8%).[60]

Box 34-7	AJCC Staging Classification for Cancer of the Kidney

PRIMARY TUMOR (T)

TX	Primary tumor cannot be assessed
T_0	No evidence of tumor
Tis	Carcinoma in situ
T_a	Papillary noninvasive carcinoma
T_1	Tumor invasion of subepithelial connective tissue
T_2	Tumor invasion of muscularis
T_3	Tumor invasion beyond muscularis into periureteric-peripelvic fat or renal parenchyma
T_4	Tumor invasion of adjacent organs or through the kidney into perinephric fat

REGIONAL LYMPH NODES (N)

NX	Regional lymph nodes cannot be assessed
N_0	No regional lymph node metastasis
N_1	Metastasis in a single lymph node (2 cm or less in greatest dimension)
N_2	Metastasis in a single lymph node (more than 2 cm but not more than 5 cm in greatest dimension) or multiple lymph nodes (none more than 5 cm in greatest dimension)
N_3	Metastasis in a lymph node (more than 5 cm in greatest dimension)

DISTANT METASTASIS (M)

MX	Distant metastasis cannot be assessed
M_0	No distant metastasis
M_1	Distant metastasis

STAGE GROUPING

Stage 0	Tis	N_0	M_0
	T_a	N_0	M_0
Stage I	T_1	N_0	M_0
Stage II	T_2	N_0	M_0
Stage III	T_3	N_0	M_0
Stage IV	T_4	N_0	M_0
	Any T	N_1, N_2, N_3	M_0
	Any T	Any N	M_1

HISTOPATHOLOGICAL GRADE

GX	Grade cannot be assessed
G1	Well differentiated
G2	Moderately well differentiated
G3-4	Poorly differentiated or undifferentiated

With permission from American Joint Committee on Cancer (AJCC), Chicago, Illinois, *AJCC Cancer Staging Manual*, ed 6, New York, 2002, Springer-Verlag.

Box 34-8	AJCC Staging Classification for Renal Pelvic and Ureteral Cancer

PRIMARY TUMOR (T)

TX	Primary tumor cannot be assessed
T_0	No evidence of tumor
Tis	Carcinoma in situ
T_a	Papillary noninvasive carcinoma
T_1	Tumor invasion of subepithelial connective tissue
T_2	Tumor invasion of muscularis
T_3	Tumor invasion beyond muscularis into periureteric-peripelvic fat or renal parenchyma
T_4	Tumor invasion of adjacent organs or through the kidney into perinephric fat

REGIONAL LYMPH NODES (N)

NX	Regional lymph nodes cannot be assessed
N_0	No regional lymph node metastasis
N_1	Metastasis in a single lymph node (2 cm or less in greatest dimension)
N_2	Metastasis in a single lymph node (more than 2 cm but not more than 5 cm in greatest dimension) or multiple lymph nodes (none more than 5 cm in greatest dimension)
N_3	Metastasis in a lymph node (more than 5 cm in greatest dimension)

DISTANT METASTASIS (M)

MX	Distant metastasis cannot be assessed
M_0	No distant metastasis
M_1	Distant metastasis

STAGE GROUPING

Stage 0	Tis	N_0	M_0
	T_a	N_0	M_0
Stage I	T_1	N_0	M_0
Stage II	T_2	N_0	M_0
Stage III	T_3	N_0	M_0
Stage IV	T_4	N_0	M_0
	Any T	N_1, N_2, N_3	M_0
	Any T	Any N	M_1

HISTOPATHOLOGICAL GRADE

GX	Grade cannot be assessed
G1	Well differentiated
G2	Moderately well differentiated
G3-4	Poorly differentiated or undifferentiated

With permission from American Joint Committee on Cancer (AJCC), Chicago, Illinois, *AJCC Cancer Staging Manual*, ed 6, New York, 2002, Springer-Verlag.

Spontaneous regression of metastatic renal cell carcinoma after nephrectomy has been reported but is extremely rare.

Renal pelvic and ureteral carcinoma. Upper urinary tract carcinoma is a multifocal process; patients with cancer at one site in the upper urinary tract are at greater risk of developing tumors elsewhere.

Transitional cell carcinoma of the upper urothelial tract may spread by direct extension or blood lymphatics. The implantation of tumor cells in the bladder has been demonstrated, especially in previously traumatized areas.[80]

Treatment Techniques

Renal cell carcinoma. Standard treatment for patients with localized renal cell carcinoma T1 and T2 is radical nephrectomy, which consists of the complete removal of the intact Gerota's fascia and its contents, including the kidney, adrenal gland, and perinephric fat. Regional lymphadenectomy is often performed at the time of radical nephrectomy.

The role of preoperative radiation therapy before nephrectomy has not been defined. Tumor shrinkage and increased resectability have been reported in patients who received preoperative irradiation, but no survival benefit has been noted.[52]

Definitive radiation treatment may be indicated if the patient is not a candidate for surgical resection. It is limited, of course, by the inability to deliver high doses of radiation to the upper abdomen, where most surrounding structures have low tolerance.

Chemotherapy and immunotherapy, such as interferon and interleukin, are used although survival gains are marginal.

Patients with a solitary bony metastasis are at risk of developing multiple metastases, but these patients also have a 30% to 40% chance of surviving for 5 years.[47] Thus high-dose palliative radiation therapy to metastatic bony lesions should be performed to ensure a long symptom-free survival time for these patients.

Renal pelvic and ureteral carcinoma. Management of renal pelvic and ureteral carcinoma consists of nephroureterectomy with the excision of a cuff of bladder and bladder mucosa. Less aggressive surgery, such as nephrectomy and partial ureterectomy, is accompanied by a ureteral stump recurrence rate of 30%. More conservative surgical excision has been advocated for patients with low-stage, low-grade, and solitary lesions. The survival rate of patients with solitary, well-differentiated tumors after surgical resection is greater than 90%.[64]

Combination chemotherapy consisting of methotrexate, vinblastine, doxorubicin [Adriamycin], and cis-platinum (MVAC) produces an objective response of more than 70% in limited groups of patients who have metastatic transitional cell carcinoma of the bladder, ureter, or renal pelvis.[96] For patients who have high-stage and high-grade tumors with local extension or patients with regional lymph node metas-

tases, combination chemotherapy and radiation offer the best chance of disease control.

Radiation Therapy Techniques

Renal cell carcinoma. Radiation is most commonly delivered in the postoperative setting when tumor is left behind or for recurrence following surgery. The treatment volume includes the renal fossa and site of gross recurrence, if present, along with the paraaortic nodal drainage sites in the adjuvant setting.

Postoperative radiation doses range from 4500 to 5500 cGy; the usual recommended dose that can be safely given to the upper abdomen with an acceptable complication rate is 5040 cGy at 180 cGy per fraction over 5 to 6 weeks. A boost of 540 cGy in three fractions to a smaller volume may be added, with special care, to bring the total tumor dose to 5580 cGy. The remaining kidney should not receive doses above 1800 cGy. For a right-sided tumor a field reduction may be needed at 3600 to 4000 cGy to ensure that no more than 30% of the liver parenchyma is irradiated to a higher dose. The nominal dose for the spinal cord should be limited to 4500 cGy with 180-cGy fractions. No attempt is made to include the entire surgical incision in the treatment field for patients who receive postnephrectomy irradiation, unless specific knowledge exists of significant wound contamination by tumor spillage.[52] Fig. 34-19 shows an intact kidney and the potential lymph node drainage sites involved by renal carcinoma. This is the same general area that would be treated postoperatively with individualization dependent on the surgical findings.

The patient is usually treated via isocentric, parallel-opposed AP/PA-shaped fields. CT planning is often used to define the area at risk and normal structures. Treatment plans include (1) equal weighting of parallel-opposed AP/PA fields, (2) bias loading (i.e., 3:1 or 2:1 posterior loading), and (3) other wedge pair techniques. A shrinking-field technique should be used to reduce exposure to dose-limiting adjacent structures. High-energy photons, 10 MV or higher, should be used. An example of a typical postoperative treatment field and technique is shown in Fig. 34-20. Although the kidney is shown, this would, of course, constitute the renal bed after surgical removal.

Radiation can also be used to palliate a symptomatic renal mass that is unresectable or the patient who is inoperable. Depending on the patients symptoms and longevity, a shorter treatment scheme can be used. Similar treatment plans encompassing the kidney are applied.

Renal pelvic and ureteral carcinoma. Postoperative radiation has been applied to patients with renal pelvic and ureteral carcinoma. The treatment portal usually includes the entire renal fossa, ureteral bed, and ipsilateral bladder trigone. The extent is dictated by clinical information obtained at the time of surgery and a pathologic analysis of the resected specimen (Fig. 34-21). Because of the high inci-

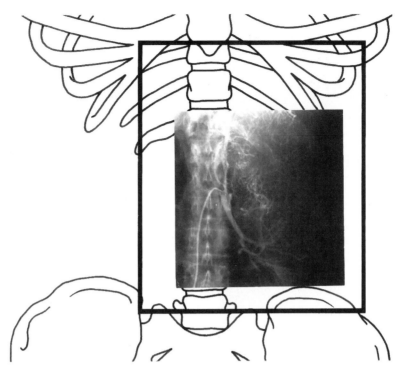

Figure 34-19. A radiation portal for large, left-sided renal cancer. The primary tumor and bilateral lymph nodes are included. *(From Lai PP: Kidney, renal pelvis, and ureter. In Perez CA, Brady LW, editors: Principles and practice of radiation oncology, ed 2, Philadelphia, 1992, JB Lippincott.)*

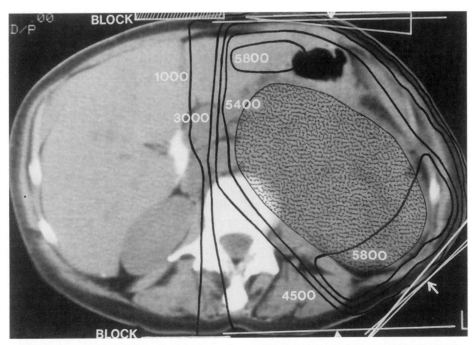

Figure 34-20. Radiation dose distribution corresponding to the treatment portal in Fig. 34-19. Notice that a combination of anteroposterior/posteroanterior (AP/PA) plus oblique portals with wedges is used to encompass the entire lesion with an isodose curve of 5400 cGy. The spinal cord dose is less than 4150 cGy. *(From Lai PP: Kidney, renal pelvis, and ureter. In Perez CA, Brady LW, editors: Principles and practice of radiation oncology, ed 2, Philadelphia, 1992, JB Lippincott.)*

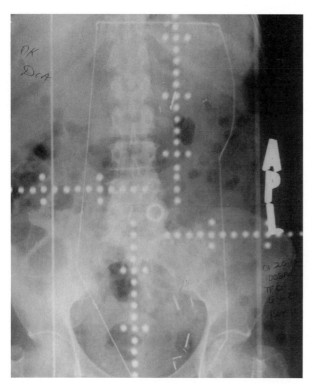

Figure 34-21. A postoperative radiation portal for cancer of the renal pelvis and ureter. Usually, the entire renal fossa, ureteral bed, and ipsilateral trigone are included; the exact extent is determined by pathologic information. *(From Lai PP: Kidney, renal pelvis, and ureter. In Perez CA, Brady LW, editors: Principles and practice of radiation oncology, ed 2, Philadelphia, 1992, JB Lippincott.)*

dence of lymph node involvement, the treatment portal should also include the paraaortic and paracaval areas. As in renal cell carcinoma of the kidney, the postoperative radiation dose is limited by the tolerance of normal tissues in the treatment field. The usual dose is 5040 cGy in 180-cGy fractions, with a possible boost of an additional 540 cGy in three fractions to a reduced volume. The technique is generally AP/PA parallel opposed for the large field with the same technique or oblique beams for the boost.

Results of Treatment

Results of studies of postoperative radiation therapy for renal cell carcinoma have varied, making it difficult to draw conclusions regarding efficacy (Table 34-7). Survival benefit remains questionable. Of note is that locoregional failure is rarely reported and compared. Older treatment techniques without CT planning were used, oftentimes, with severe or even fatal complications. Therefore postoperative radiation is not widely applied for renal, renal pelvis, and ureteral malignancies. Sufficient evidence of residual disease from evaluation of surgical findings and specimens must be present to warrant postoperative radiation. Similarly, preoperative radi-

ation has shown questionable benefit in past studies and is generally no longer applied.

Side effects. The side effects and complications from radiation treatment of cancer of the kidney, renal pelvis, and ureters are similar to those expected from irradiation of the abdomen and pelvis. Acute side effects include nausea, vomiting, diarrhea, and abdominal cramping, which usually respond to conservative medical management.[52] The complication rate is related to the total dose and fraction size. With careful attention given to the treatment technique and dose-volume distribution, many complications can be eliminated.

ROLE OF RADIATION THERAPIST

Treatment Plan Implementation

Accurate dose delivery, daily observation of the patient's tolerance to therapy, and the psychologic needs of the patient are important aspects of the radiation therapist's role. Reproducibility of the daily treatment is of prime importance because the patient's outcome depends on accurate dose delivery to the target volume and the sparing of critical structures. A positive outcome, however, can be overshadowed if the patient is unhappy because of a lack of appropriate psychologic support and understanding of potential side effects during the course of therapy.

Treatment Information and Psychologic Support

Accurate dose delivery is important for the control of disease. However, patients are just as concerned with potential side effects of radiation treatments and the way that the side effects affect their daily routine and interaction with family and friends. The potential side effects of treatment to the abdomen and pelvis are similar to those of other sites treated with radiation, including skin reaction, fatigue, weight loss, nausea and vomiting, diarrhea, and hair loss in the area being treated.

Skin changes caused by radiation exposure depend on the beam energy and dose. Because most tumors in the abdomen and pelvis (>85%) are treated with a beam energy greater than 6 MV, skin reactions are usually not more severe than dry desquamation or slight tanning. Single or parallel-opposed treatment fields given with lower beam energies may produce more severe skin reactions because of higher surface doses and the thick body parts involved. Patients should be instructed to avoid the use of harsh creams or soaps in the irradiated area. Topical preparations usually provide some comfort.

Many patients are more easily fatigued during radiation treatments because much of the body's energy is being used to fight the disease process or repair the effects of radiation on normal tissues. The therapist should counsel patients not to be alarmed if they are more easily tired during the course of treatment; patients should be told to maintain good nutrition and get plenty of rest to minimize weight loss and

Table 34-7	Renal cell carcinoma: 5-year survival rates after nephrectomy or postoperative irradiation and nephrectomy

Author	Stage	Number of Patients	Radiation Dose/Fraction Size (cGy)	Treatment	5-year Survival Rate	Local Recurrence (%)
Peeling, et al. (1969)*		96		N	52% (50/96)	
		68		N+RT	25% (17/68)	
Rafla (1970)†	All	96		N	37% (35/94)	
		94		N + RT	57% (46/81)	
	Renal vein	36		N	30% (11/36)	
	± others	40		N + RT	40% (14/35)	
	Renal pelvis	50		N	32% (16/49)	
	± others	60		N + RT	60% (30/50)	
	Renal capsule	52		N	28% (15.52)	
	± others	69		N + RT	57% (34/59)	
Rafla and Parikh (1984)‡		135		N	18% (24/135)	
		105	4500	N + RT	38% (40/105)	
Finney (1973)§		48		N	47% (17/35)	7
		52	5500/204	N + RT	36% (14/39)	7
Kjaer et al. (1987)¶		33		N	63%§	1
		32	5000/250	N + RT	38%‖	0

Modified from Lai PP: Kidney, renal pelvis, and ureter. In Perez CA, Brady LW, editors: *Principles and practice of radiation oncology,* 1992, JB Lippincott.
N, Nephrectomy; *RT,* postoperative radiation therapy.
*This is a retrospective study with incomplete staging information and no description of the radiation dose or technique. The endpoint was 5-year survival, with no mention of local recurrence.
†This is the only report that described the benefits of irradiation with survival *and* local recurrence as endpoints. Unfortunately, there was no description of the radiation dose or technique. The study was performed in the pre-CT era; therefore local recurrence is an underestimate. Subgroup analysis (involvement of renal vein, renal pelvis, renal capsule + others) indicated an effect of radiation therapy on survival.
‡The authors also showed some data attesting to the benefits of radiation therapy in patients with renal capsular, renal vein, and regional lymphatic involvement.
§This is a randomized study, but no staging information is available. The incidences of local recurrence and distant metastasis are similar. However, there are four fatal liver complications among the patients who received radiation therapy.
¶In this randomized study 27 or 32 patients assigned to the irradiation arm completed treatment; 12 of 27 (44%) reported significant complications, with five fatal complications related to irradiation.

fatigue. If the patient encounters problems with nausea, vomiting, or diarrhea, the physician can prescribe medications to alleviate these symptoms. Fatigue may also be caused by treatment induced anemia. Blood counts should be checked.

Hair loss can occur in the irradiated field because of the sensitivity of the follicles to radiation. This hair loss may be permanent, depending on the dose of radiation.

The therapist should encourage the patient and family to discuss with the physician any problems concerning treatment. Problems dealing with transportation, work, or financial concerns should be referred to social service personnel to minimize the patient's emotional stress. A pleasant, friendly, and helpful attitude can also provide good emotional support.

Treatment Planning and Delivery

The basic steps in the planning and delivery of the physician's treatment plan generally apply to all sites. However, some issues that improve the daily reproducibility of the treatment apply specifically to abdominal and pelvic sites.

For example, rectal and bladder filling can have a significant effect on prostate position. Procedures should be developed and followed to improve consistency in the setup between simulation and treatment units.

Simulation

Immobilization. The construction of immobilization devices, an important part of the treatment-planning process, should be accomplished during the initial simulation. The patient's treatment position must be established, and appropriate immobilization and repositioning devices should be constructed before any simulation images are taken or treatment-planning CT data are obtained. This helps ensure agreement in the transfer of information between the simulator and treatment unit.

Reproducibility of the patient setup can be improved with a treatment position that the patient can maintain through proper immobilization and repositioning devices. The methods most commonly used for immobilization during treatment of abdominal and pelvic sites are polyurethane foam molds or vacuum devices with the patient in the supine position. However, thermal plastic molds are also being used at some facilities with the patient in the prone position. These immobilization devices may extend from the chest through the thighs for abdominal fields or the hips to the feet for pelvic fields. The length tends to vary between institution. Of greatest importance is that the therapists are experienced and comfortable with a device which consistently provides a reproducible setup.

Simulation and treatment variations. Daily isocenter variation in the AP/PA direction can be reduced by setting the isocenter based on the digital couch height or lateral lasers rather than using the optical distance indicator projected on the patient's skin surface. The depth of the isocenter should be checked daily for consistency and verification that the depth of calculation is not changing as a result of weight loss or bloating. Daily fluctuations of 1 to 2 cm in the skin's isocenter depth for an anterior abdominal or pelvic field are not uncommon. If the depth of calculation is consistently off in one direction, the physicist and physician should be notified so that the resulting change in dose may be evaluated for a new monitor unit calculation. Differences in the skin's isocenter depth on lateral or posterior fields are generally less than 1 cm when patients are carefully aligned with the sagittal lasers and the vertical height is set with a digital readout or lateral lasers. Variations in laser marks placed on the lateral aspect of the pelvis can also be reduced by placing a rubber band around the feet to hold them together.

Systematic errors can also occur from differences in the alignment of lasers and optical distance indicators from the simulator and the treatment unit. A tolerance of 2 mm on the laser alignment or optical distance indicator can result in a 4-mm discrepancy in the setup from the simulator to the treatment unit. Similar discrepancies can occur from differences in the alignment of blocking trays from machine to machine caused by worn or damaged parts.

Studies of variation in the daily setup of portals relative to bony landmarks in treatment of the prostate show greater maximum and average variation without versus with foam-mold immobilization devices.

Treatment Verification

Portal images of the treatment fields should be taken before treatment on the first day and compared with the simulation images for correct field placement. The first-day images serve as a guide for subsequent images taken during the course of therapy. Both portals for parallel-opposed beams should be taken on the same day with a fiducial grid in place to distinguish block-mounting errors from patient-positioning or patient-movement errors. The fiducial grid provides a means for determining the magnification factor on the portal image so that required adjustments can be made easily. Interpreting anatomic changes resulting in a magnification change of corresponding anatomy on each of the images is also much easier with a fiducial grid in place.

Most conformal treatment techniques use multiple oblique beam arrangements, which are difficult to interpret for anatomical coverage and positional accuracy of the isocenter. For these reasons conformal beam arrangements are best evaluated from a set of orthogonal films that allow vertical and horizontal shifts in the isocenter position to be viewed separately. A set of portal images taken with the exact treatment angles may still be useful for documentation and comparison with the simulation images for anatomic coverage.

Dose-verification measurements can be taken on all photon portals through the use of a diode detector or thermoluminescent dosimeter. The dose measurements are meant to discover large-dose errors resulting from incorrect or missing wedges, compensating filters, or incorrect monitor unit calculations.

Record-and-verify systems are also highly recommended to ensure that daily setups are consistent and correct.

Site-Specific Instructions

Some type of immobilization or repositioning device is always used for patients with conformal techniques. Immobilization is not always used in treatments to the whole pelvis or abdomen with parallel-opposed techniques. However, lasers are always used to aid in repositioning of the patient. Typical simulation procedures are listed in the simulation section.

Prostate. Patients should be treated when they have a full bladder to minimize the amount of bladder in the treatment portals. The rectum is often simulated empty to ensure that a full rectum does not move the prostate anteriorly during simulation. An empty rectum during treatment would then allow the prostate to move posteriorly, outside the treatment field. Transabdominal ultrasound (BAT) is also used to align a daily image with the planning CT. Field changes can then be made to follow the internal movement of the gland.

Bladder. Patients should be treated with an empty bladder when the entire bladder is being treated to maintain an adequate margin. During a boost field, a full bladder will reduce the amount of bladder treated to the boost dose.

Kidney. Considerations relative to abdominal treatments should be applied to treatment of the kidney. Tolerance of abdominal organs is relatively low.

Penis. The treatment approach depends on the need to treat only the penis or the penis and regional lymphatics. External beam therapy requires specially designed accessories, including bolus, to achieve homogeneous dose distribution to the entire organ involved.

Review Questions

1. What is the most common pathology of malignant tumors of the prostate?
   a. Squamous cell carcinoma
   b. Adenocarcinoma

c. Transitional cell carcinoma

d. Burkitt's cell carcinoma

2. What is the most common type of kidney tumor?

a. Transitional cell lymphoma

b. Choriocarcinoma

c. Adenocarcinoma

d. Seminoma

3. Which of the following has the highest incidence rate for males?

a. Prostate cancer

b. Penile cancer

c. Kidney and ureteral cancer

d. Lung cancer

4. Which of the following are common immobilization-repositioning devices used in the treatment of prostate cancer?

I. Polyurethane molds

II. Plaster/Thermoplastic casts

III. Belly board

IV. Rubber bands around the feet

a. I and III only

b. I and IV only

c. II and III only

d. I, II, and IV only

5. For patients with bladder cancer the bladder should be _____ during whole-bladder radiation.

a. Empty

b. Partially full

c. Full

d. Localized with contrast material

6. _____is a side effect associated with the treatment of prostate cancer, in which the adult male is unable to obtain an erection.

a. Benign prostatic hypertrophy

b. Transurethral resection of the prostate

c. Impotence

d. None of the above

7. The prostate gland is located _____ to the rectum?

a. Posterior

b. Anterior

c. Superior

d. Both a and c

8. Of the following tumors of the male reproductive and genitourinary system, which would require the lowest dose to control the disease?

a. Prostate

b. Kidney

c. Testis

d. Bladder

9. Which of the following tumors of the male reproductive and genitourinary system would a brachytherapy implant be most likely used to control the disease?

a. Prostate

b. Kidney

c. Testis

d. Bladder

10. Which of the following testicular tumor pathologies is most common?

a. Seminoma

b. Choriocarcinoma

c. Teratoma

d. Embryonal carcinoma

Questions to Ponder

1. Discuss the role of a digital rectal examination and prostate-specific antigen (PSA) in the screening of the prostate cancer.

2. Compare and contrast the following prognostic indicators related to carcinoma of the prostate: tumor stage, grade, PSA level, and race.

3. Examine the following specific treatment options for carcinoma of the prostate: surgery, external beam radiation therapy, brachytherapy, hormonal therapy, and chemotherapy.

4. Discuss the general management of cancer of the urinary bladder, surgery versus radiation.

5. Compare the treatments for testicular seminoma and non-seminoma.

6. Discuss the role of the radiation therapist in the treatment of patients with genitourinary tumors.

REFERENCES

1. Adolfsson J, Steineck G, Whitmore WF Jr: Recent results of management of palpable clinical localized prostate cancer, *Cancer* 72:310-322, 1993.

2. Albertsen PC, et al: Competing risk analysis of men aged 55 to 74 years at diagnosis managed conservatively for clinically localized prostate cancer, *JAMA* 280:975-980, 1998.

3. American Cancer Society: *Cancer facts and figures: 2003,* Atlanta, 2003, American Cancer Society.

4. Anderson PM, et al: High-dose samarium-153 ethylene diamine tetramethylene phosphonate: low toxicity of skeletal irradiation in patients with osteosarcoma and bone metastases, *J Clin Oncol* 20:189-196, 2002.

5. Arterbery VE, et al: Quality of life after permanent prostate implant, *Semin Surg Oncol* 13:461-464, 1997.

6. Bagshaw MA, Ray GR, Cox RS: Radiotherapy of prostatic carcinoma: long- or short-term efficacy (Stanford University experience), *Urology* 25:17-23, 1985.

7. Benson MC: Fine-needle aspiration of the prostate, *NCI Monogr* 7:19-24, 1988.

8. Blasko JC, et al: Prostate specific antigen based disease control following ultrasound guided 125iodine implantation for stage T1/T2 prostatic carcinoma, *J Urol* 154:1096-1099, 1995.

9. Blasko JC, et al: Palladium-103 brachytherapy for prostate carcinoma, *Int J Radiat Oncol Biol Phys* 46:839-850, 2000.

10. Bracken RB, Henry R, Ordonez N: Primary carcinoma of the male urethra, *South Med J* 73:1003-1005, 1980.

11. Byar DP, Veterans Administration Cooperative Urological Research Group: Survival of patients with incidentally found microscopic cancer of the prostate: results of a clinical trial of conservative treatment, *J Urol* 108:908-913, 1972.

12. Catalona WJ, Bigg SW: Nerve-sparing radical prostatectomy: evaluation of results after 250 patients, *J Urol* 143:538-544, 1990.

13. Chodak GW, et al: Comparison of digital examination and transrectal ultrasonography for the diagnosis of prostate cancer, *J Urol* 135-951-954, 1986.

14. Chodak GW, et al: Results of conservative management of clinically localized cancer, *N Engl J Med* 330:242-248, 1994.

15. Coia LR, Hanks GE: Complications from large field intermediate dose infradiaphragmatic radiation: an analysis of the Patterns of Care Outcome Studies for Hodgkin's disease and seminoma, *Int J Radiat Oncol Biol Phys* 15:29-35, 1988.

16. Crawford ED, Dawkins CA: Cancer of the penis. In Skinner DG, Lieskovsky G, editors: *Diagnosis and management of genitourinary cancer,* Philadelphia, 1988, WB Saunders.

17. DeKernion JB, et al: Carcinoma of the penis, *Cancer* 32:1256-1262, 1973.

18. Duchesne GM, et al: Orchidectomy alone for stage I seminoma of the testis, *Cancer* 65:1115-1118, 1990.

19. Dugan TC, et al: Biopsy after external beam radiation therapy for adenocarcinoma of the prostate: correlation with original histological grade and current prostate specific antigen levels, *J Urol* 148:1565-1566, 1992.

20. Duncan W, Jackson SM: The treatment of early cancer of the penis with megavoltage X-rays, *Clin Radiol* 23:246-248, 1972.

21. Duncan W, Quilty PM: The results of a series of 963 patients with transitional cell carcinoma of the urinary bladder primarily treated by radical megavoltage x-ray therapy, *Radiother Oncol* 7:299-310, 1986.

22. Dunst J, et al: Organ-sparing treatment of advanced bladder cancer: a 10-year experience, *Int J Radiat Oncol Biol Phys* 30:261-266, 1994.

23. Eastham JA, Scardino PT: Radical prostatectomy for clinical stage and T2 prostate cancer. In Volgelzang NJ, et al, editors: *Comprehensive textbook of genitourinary oncology,* ed 2, Philadelphia, 2000, Lippincott Williams & Wilkins.

24. Einhorn LH, Richie JP, Shipley WU: Cancer of the testis. In DeVita VJ Jr, Hellman S, Rosenberg SA, editors: *Cancer: principles and practice of oncology,* ed 4, Philadelphia, 1993, JB Lippincott.

25. Eisenberger MA: Chemotherapy for prostate cancer, *NCI Monogr* 7:151-163, 1988.

26. Ekstrom T, Edsmyr F: Cancer of the penis: a clinical study of 229 cases, *Acta Chir Scand* 115:25-45, 1958.

27. Emami BE, Pilepich MV: Anatomic considerations in radiotherapeutic management of bladder cancer, *Am J Clin Oncol (CCT)* 6:593-597, 1983.

28. Faysal MH, Freiha FS: Evaluation of partial cystectomy for carcinoma of bladder, *Urology* 14:352-356, 1979.

29. Fleming ID, et al: *Manual for staging of cancer,* ed 5, Philadelphia, 1997, Lippincott-Raven.

30. Fossa SD, Aass N, Kaalhus O: Radiotherapy for testicular seminoma stage I: treatment results and long-term post-irradiation morbidity in 365 patients, *Int J Radiat Oncol Biol Phys* 16:383-388, 1989.

31. Fraas BA, et al: Peripheral dose to the testes: the design and clinical use of a practical and effective gonadal shield, *Int J Radiat Oncol Biol Phys* 11:609-615, 1985.

32. Fraley EE, et al: Cancer of the penis: prognosis and treatment plans, *Cancer* 55:1618-1624, 1985.

33. Freeman GM, et al: Young patients with prostate cancer have an outcome justifying their treatment with external beam radiation, *Int J Radiat Oncol Biol Phys* 35:243-250, 1996.

34. Gleason DF, Veterans Administration Cooperative Urological Research Group: Histologic grading and clinical staging of prostatic carcinoma. In Tannenbaum M, editor: *Urologic pathology: the prostate,* Philadelphia, 1977, Lea & Febiger.

35. Golimbu M, et al: Renal cell carcinoma: survival and prognostic factors, *Urology* 27:291-301, 1986.

36. Gospodarowicz MK, et al: Radical radiotherapy for muscle invasive transitional cell carcinoma of the bladder: failure analysis, *J Urol* 142:1448-1454, 1989.

37. Gray HG: *Anatomy, descriptive and surgical,* 1901 ed, Philadelphia, 1974, Running Press.

38. Hanks GE, et al: The outcome of treatment of 313 patients with T-1 (UICC) prostate cancer treated with external beam irradiation, *Int J Radiat Oncol Biol Phys* 14:243-248, 1988.

39. Hanks GE, et al: RTOG Protocol 92-02: A phase III trial of the use of long term total androgen suppression following neoadjuvant hormonal cytoreduction and radiotherapy in locally advanced carcinoma of the prostate, *Int J Radiat Oncol Biol Phys Suppl* 48(3):112, 2000.

40. Heaney JA, et al: Prognosis of clinically undiagnosed prostatic carcinoma and the influence of endocrine therapy, *J Urol* 118:283-287, 1977.

41. Huben RP, Mounzer AM, Murphy GP: Tumor grade and stage as prognostic variables in upper tract urothelial tumors, *Cancer* 62:2016-2020, 1988.

42. Huggins C, Stevens RE, Hodges CV: Studies on prostatic cancer II. The effects of castration on advanced carcinoma of the prostate gland, *Arch Surg* 43:209-223, 1941.

43. Huncharek M, Muscat J, Gesehwind JF: Planned preoperative radiation therapy in muscle invasive bladder cancer: results of a meta-analysis, *Anticancer Res* 18:1931-1934, 1998.

44. Jenkins BJ, et al: Reappraisal of the role of radical radiotherapy and salvage cystectomy in the treatment of invasive bladder cancer, *Br J Urol* 62:343-346, 1988.

45. Johansson JE, et al: High 10-year survival rate in patients with early, untreated prostatic cancer, *JAMA* 267:2191-2196, 1992.

46. Kachnic LA, et al: Bladder preservation by combined modality therapy for invasive bladder cancer, *J Clin Oncol* 15:1022-1029, 1997.

47. Kjaer M: The treatment and prognosis of patients with renal adenocarcinoma with solitary metastasis 10 year survival results, *Int J Radiat Oncol Phys* 13:619-621, 1987.

48. Kuban DA, El-Mahdi AM, Schellhammer PF: Prostate-specific antigen for pretreatment prediction and posttreatment evaluation of outcome after definitive irradiation for prostate cancer, *Int J Radiat Oncol Biol Phys* 32:307-316, 1995.

49. Kuban DA, El-Mahdi AM, Schellhammer PF: PSA for outcome prediction and post-treatment evaluation following radiation for prostate cancer: do we know how to use it? *Semin Radiat Oncol* 8:72-78, 1998.

50. Kubo H, Shipley WU: Reduction of the scatter dose to the testicle outside the radiation treatment fields, *Int J Radiat Oncol Biol Phys* 8:1741-1745, 1982.

51. Kupelian P, et al: External beam radiotherapy versus radical prostatectomy for clinical stage T1-2 prostate cancer: therapeutic implications of stratification by pretreatment PSA levels and biopsy Gleason scores, *Cancer J Sci Am* 3:78-87, 1997.

52. Lai PP: Kidney, renal pelvis, and ureter. In Perez CA, Brady LW, editors: *Principles and practice of radiation oncology,* ed 2, Philadelphia, 1992, JB Lippincott.

53. Lai PP, et al: Radiation therapy for stage I and IIA testicular seminoma, *Int J Radiat Oncol Biol Phys* 28:373-379, 1993.

54. Landis SH, et al: Cancer statistics, 1998, *CA Cancer J Clin* 48:6-29, 1998.

55. Lee RW, Hanks GE, Schultheiss TE: Role of radiation therapy in the management of stage T3 and T4 prostate cancer: rationale, technique, and results. In Volgelzang NJ, et al., editors: *Comprehensive textbook of genitourinary oncology,* ed 2, Philadelphia, 2000, Lippincott Williams & Wilkins.

56. Leibel SA, et al: The effects of local and regional treatment on the metastatic outcome in prostatic carcinoma with pelvic lymph node involvement, *Int J Radiat Oncol Biol Phys* 28:7-16, 1993.

57. Linehan WM, Shipley WU, Longo DL: Cancer of the kidney and ureter. In DeVita VT, Hellman S, Rosenberg SA, editors: *Cancer: principles and practice of oncology,* ed 3, Philadelphia, 1989, JB Lippincott.

58. Litwin MS, et al: Quality of life outcomes in men treated for localized prostate cancer, *JAMA* 273:129-135, 1995.

59. Logue JP, et al: Para-aortic radiation for stage I seminoma of the testis. *Int J Radiat Oncol Biol Phys* 48(suppl):208 (abstract no 192), 2000.

60. Maldazys JD, deKernion JB: Prognostic factors in metastatic renal carcinoma, *J Urol* 136:376-379, 1986.

61. Mameghan H, et al: Analysis of failure following definitive radiotherapy for invasive transitional cell carcinoma of the bladder, *Int J Radiat Oncol Biol Phys* 31:247-254, 1995.

62. Mandler JI, Pool T: Primary carcinoma of the male urethra, *J Urol* 96:67-72, 1966.

63. Montie JE, Straffon RA, Stewart RH: Radical cystectomy in men treated for localized prostate cancer, *JAMA* 273:129-135, 1995.

64. Mufti GR, et al: Transitional cell carcinoma of the renal pelvis and ureter, *Br J Urol* 63:135-140, 1989.

65. Narayana AS, et al: Carcinoma of the penis: analysis of 219 cases, *Cancer* 49:2185-2191, 1982.

66. Parsons JT, Million RR: Planned preoperative irradiation in the management of clinical stage B2-C (T3) bladder carcinoma, *Int J Radiat Oncol Biol Phys* 14:797-810, 1988.

67. Partin AW, Walsh PC: Management of stage B (T1c-T2) prostate cancer. Surgical management of localized prostate cancer. In Radhavan D, et al., editors: *Principles and practice of genitourinary oncology,* Philadelphia, 1997, Lippincott-Raven.

68. Partin AW, et al: Combination of prostate specific antigen, clinical stage and Gleason score to predict pathological stage in men with localized prostate cancer, *JAMA* 277:1445-1451, 1997.

69. Perez CA, Pilepich MV: Penis and male urethra. In Perez CA, Brady LW, editors: *Principles and practice of radiation oncology,* ed 2, Philadelphia, 1992, JB Lippincott.

70. Perez CA, et al: Factors influencing outcome of definitive radiotherapy for localized carcinoma of the prostate, *Radiother Oncol* 16:1-21, 1989.

71. Pilepich MV, et al: Prognostic factors in carcinoma of the prostate: analysis of RTOG Study 75-06, *Int J Radiat Oncol Biol Phys* 13:339-349, 1987.

72. Pilepich MV, et al: Androgen deprivation with radiation therapy compared with radiation therapy alone for locally advanced prostatic carcinoma: a randomized comparative trial of the Radiation Therapy Oncology Group, *Urology* 45:616-623, 1995.

73. Pollack A, et al: Preliminary results of a randomized radiotherapy dose-escalation study comparing 70 Gy with 78 Gy for prostate cancer, *J Clin Oncol* 18:3904-3911, 2000.

74. Porter AT, et al: Results of randomized phase III trial to evaluate the efficacy of strontium-89 adjuvant to local external beam irradiation in the management of endocrine metastatic prostate cancer, *Int J Radiat Oncol Biol Phys* 25:805-813, 1993.

75. Powell BL, Craig JB, Muss HB: Secondary malignancies of the penis and epididymis: a case report and review of the literature, *J Clin Oncol* 3:110-116, 1985.

76. Pritchett TR, Lieskovsky G, Skinner DG: Clinical manifestations and treatment of renal parenchymal tumors. In Skinner DG, Lieskovsky G, editors: *Diagnosis and management of genitourinary tumors,* Philadelphia, 1988, WB Saunders.

77. Quilty PM, et al: Results of surgery following radical radiotherapy for invasive bladder cancer, *Br J Urol* 58:396-405, 1986.

78. Radhavaiah NV: Radiotherapy in the treatment of carcinoma of the male urethra, *Cancer* 41:1313-1316, 1978.

79. Reitelman C, et al: Prognostic variables in patients with transitional cell carcinoma of the renal pelvis and proximal ureter, *J Urol* 138:1144-1145, 1987.

80. Richie JP: Carcinoma of the renal pelvis and ureter. In Skinner DG, Lieskovsky G, editors: *Diagnosis and management of genitourinary tumors,* Philadelphia, 1988, WB Saunders.

81. Rifkin MD, et al: Comparison of magnetic resonance imaging and ultrasonography in staging early prostate cancer: results of a multi-institutional cooperative trial, *N Engl J Med* 323:621-626, 1990.

82. Roach M: The use of prostate specific antigen, clinical stage and Gleason score to predict pathological stage in men with localized prostate cancer, *J Urol* 150:1923-1924, 1993.

83. Roach M, et al: Predicting the risk of lymph node involvement using the pre-treatment prostate specific antigen and Gleason score in men with clinically localized prostate cancer, *Int J Radiat Oncol Biol Phys* 28:33-37, 1994.

84. Roach M III, et al: A phase III trial comparing whole-pelvic (WP) to prostate only (PO) radiotherapy and neoadjuvant to adjuvant total androgen suppression (TAS): preliminary analysis of RTOG 9413, *Int J Radiat Oncol Biol Phys* 51(suppl 1, abstract plenary 5):3, 2001.

85. Sagerman RH, et al: Stage II seminoma: results of postorchiectomy irradiation, *Radiology* 172:565-568, 1989.

86. Salaverria JE, et al: Conservative treatment of carcinoma of the penis, *Br J Urol* 51:32-37, 1979.

87. Sandler HM, et al: Localization of the prostatic apex for radiation therapy using implanted markers, *Int J Radiat Oncol Biol Phys* 27:915-919, 1993.

88. Schnall MD, et al: Prostate cancer: local staging with endorectal surface coil MR imaging, *Radiology* 178:797-802, 1991.

89. Shapiro E, et al: Effects of fractionated irradiation on endocrine aspects to testicular function, *J Clin Oncol* 3:1232-1239, 1985.

90. Shipley WU, et al: Full-dose irradiation for patients with invasive bladder carcinoma: clinical and histological factors prognostic of improved survival, *J Urol* 134:679-683, 1985.

91. Shipley WU, et al: Phase III trial of neoadjuvant chemotherapy in patients with invasive bladder cancer treated with selective bladder preservation by combined radiation therapy and chemotherapy: Initial results of RTOG 89-03, *J Clin Oncol* 16:3576-3583, 1998.

92. Shipley WU, et al: Radiation therapy for clinically localized prostate cancer—a multi-institutional pooled analysis, JAMA 281:1598-1604, 1999.

93. Skinner DG, Liekovsky G: Management of invasive and high grade bladder cancer. In Skinner DG, Liekovsky G, editors: *Diagnosis and management of genitourinary cancer,* Philadelphia, 1988, WB Saunders.

94. Skinner DG, Tift JP, Kaufman JJ: High dose, short course preoperative radiation therapy and immediate single stage radical cystectomy with pelvic node dissection in the management of bladder cancer, *J Urol* 127:671-674, 1982.

95. Smith JA, et al: Treatment of advanced bladder cancer with combined preoperative irradiation and radical cystectomy versus radical cystectomy alone: a phase III intergroup study, *J Urol* 157:805-808, 1997.

96. Sternberg CN, et al: Preliminary results of M-VAC (methotrexate, vinblastine, doxorubicin and cisplatin) for transitional cell carcinoma of the urothelium, *J Urol* 133:403-407, 1985.

97. Stock RG, et al: A dose-response study for I-125 prostate implants, *Int J Radiat Oncol Biol Phys* 41:101-108, 1998.

98. Storey MR, et al: Complications from dose escalation in prostate cancer: preliminary results of a randomized trial, *Int J Radiat Oncol Biol Phys* 48:635-642, 2000.

99. Sultanem K, et al: Para-aortic irradiation only appears to be adequate treatment for patients with stage I seminoma of the testis, *Int J Radiat Oncol Biol Phys* 40:455-459, 1998.

100. Tester W, et al: Combined modality program with possible organ preservation for invasive bladder carcinoma: results of RTOG protocol 85-12, *Int J Radiat Oncol Biol Phys* 25:783-790, 1993.

101. Thomas G, et al: Consensus statement on the investigation and management of testicular seminoma 1989, *EORTC Genitourinary Group Monogr* 7:285-294, 1990.

102. Thomas GM, Williams SD: Testis. In Perez CA, Brady LW, editors: *Principles and practice of radiation oncology,* ed 2, Philadelphia, 1992, JB Lippincott.

103. Warde P, et al: Stage I testicular seminoma: results of adjuvant irradiation and surveillance, *J Clin Oncol* 13:2255-2262, 1995.

104. Worgul TJ, et al: Clinical and biochemical effect of aminoglutethimide

in the treatment of advanced prostatic carcinoma, *J Urol* 129:51-55, 1983.

105. Yu GSM, Nseyo UO, Carson JW: Primary penile lymphoma in a patient with Peyronie's disease, *J Urol* 142:1076-1077, 1989.

106. Zagars GK: Stage I testicular seminoma following orchidectomy: to treat or not to treat, *Eur J Cancer* 14:1923-1924, 1993.

107. Zagars GK, Babaian RJ: The role of radiation in stage II testicular seminoma, *Int J Radiat Oncol Biol Phys* 13:163-170, 1987.

108. Zagars GK, Pollack A, Pettaway CA: Prostate cancer in African-American men: outcome following radiation therapy or without adju-vant androgen ablation, *Int J Radiat Oncol Biol Phys* 42:517-523, 1998.

109. Zagars GK, Pollack A, Smith LG: Conventional external-beam radia-tion therapy alone or with androgen ablation for clinical stage III (T3, NX/N0, M0) adenocarcinoma of the prostate, *Int J Radiat Oncol Biol Phys* 44:809-819, 1999.

110. Zelefsky MJ, et al: High dose radiation delivered by intensity modu-lated conformal radiotherapy improves the outcome of localized prostate cancer, *J Urol* 166:876-881, 2001.

Breast Cancer

George M. Uschold

Outline

Key Terms

HISTORICAL PERSPECTIVE

The recorded history of the treatment of breast cancer dates back 5000 years to a document known as the "Edwin Smith Papyrus." Written between 3000 and 2500 BC, the papyrus discusses surgical and other treatments for illnesses afflicting the ancient Egyptians. A translation of the document, first published in 1930, reveals that at the time there was thought to be no treatment for what were most likely malignant tumors of the breast.

Several millennia later, Hippocrates (460 to 370 BC), the revered Greek physician who gave the name carcinoma to malignant disease, referred only twice to breast cancer. Both references describe advanced disease that resulted in the patient's death. He felt that it was better not to treat deep-seated cancer, because in his experience, treatment only hastened death. Hippocrates taught that cancer was caused by an excess or imbalance of "black bile" in the body.[34] Therefore medical belief of the day was that cancer is a systemic disease and essentially incurable.

During the Roman Empire, physicians performed surgery for breast cancer, sometimes using an extremely aggressive approach that included removal of the pectoralis muscles. This approach was later discouraged by Aulus Celsus, an important scholar of the early first century AD, argued that cancer of the breast was "irritated" by the surgeon's intervention, which hastened the patient's death; therefore he recommended treatment with "mild medicines."

Leonidus, a Greek physician from the first century AD, described the surgical procedure he used for breast cancer. He removed the breast with a margin of normal-appearing tissue and was careful to stop the bleeding during surgery through the use of cautery (heat).

Claudius Galen (138-201 AD), a physician who was educated in Greece and practiced in Rome, became the authority on medicine for the next 1000 years. Galen subscribed to Hippocrates' black bile theory of the systemic nature of cancer, and he recommended no intervention in the course of the disease.

During the 1000 years that comprised the Medieval period, or Dark Ages, which followed the fall of the Roman Empire, essentially no advances were made in the scientific understanding of cancer or any human illnesses. This was a period of political and religious activity, to the exclusion of scientific endeavor. Restrictions placed on the study and practice of medicine by religious authorities and adherence to the teachings of Galen as all encompassing left the world of medicine basically unchanged for a millennium. Despite the lack of advancement between 500 and 1500 AD, knowledge of medicine and an appreciation for learning were kept alive in monasteries. Eventually, the foundations for future progress were laid in the eleventh century, when several medical schools came into existence in cities such as Paris and Oxford.

In the middle of the sixteenth century, Andreas Versalius published *De Humani Corporis Fabrica,* the work that established the science of human anatomy. Humans were no longer bound by religious dictum and centuries of tradition. Increasingly, extensive surgical techniques were developed. The seventeenth century saw the treatment of breast cancer evolve to include the excision of enlarged axillary lymph nodes at the time of mastectomy. However, in the days before anesthesia and asepsis, surgery of any kind was fraught with danger for patients, many of whom died from overwhelming infection.

A revolution in thinking relative to the nature of breast cancer occurred in the mid-eighteenth century, when French surgeons Henri Le Dran and Jean Louis Petit theorized that the disease originated locally in the breast and was not initially systemic. They believed the malignancy spread from its primary site in the breast to involve regional lymph nodes and ultimately to disseminate widely via the circulatory system. As a result, physicians of the day realized an opportunity to cure patients if the cancer could be removed early in its course and if local control could be established. Therefore wide surgical excision with axillary dissection and removal of the pectoralis muscle was advised.

With the advent of anesthesia, antisepsis, and the ability to examine tissue microscopically in the mid-nineteenth century, radical breast surgery evolved rapidly. William Stewart Halsted perfected the technique of radical mastectomy at the end of the nineteenth century (Fig 35-1). For the first time, a dramatic improvement in local recurrence and overall survival rates could be demonstrated. The Halstedian approach remained preeminent until the mid-twentieth century.

Current concepts in the treatment of breast cancer include a much less radical role for surgery and the emergence of radiation therapy and systemic drug treatment, all of which have permitted a conservative, breast-preserving approach for women with relatively early disease. However, although great strides have been made in the detection and treatment of breast cancer, it remains a disease that defies complete control. Approximately 22% of women who have breast cancer die of the disease.[40] Therefore the need exists for continued research into improved treatment modalities, earlier diagnoses, and ultimately, the prevention of breast cancer.

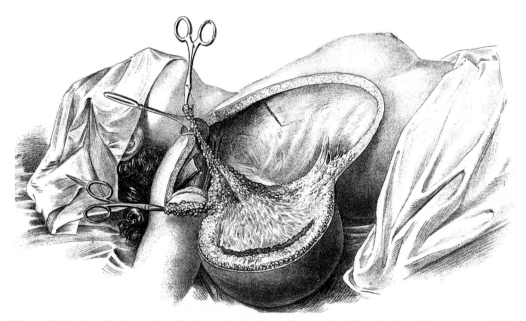

Figure 35-1. A technique of radical mastectomy at the end of the nineteenth century at John Hopkins. This is where Dr. William Halsted perfected the technique of radical mastectomy. *(Courtesy The Alan Mason Chesney Medical Archives of the John Hopkins Medical Institution, Baltimore, Maryland.)*

EPIDEMIOLOGY

Incidence

According to American Cancer Society (ACS) statistics, breast cancer is the most common malignant disease in American women, affecting an estimated 213,000 new patients each year in the United States.[1] In addition, breast cancer is diagnosed in about 1300 men each year. Current data indicate that every woman has approximately a one in eight chance of developing breast cancer over her lifetime.[1] The incidence rate has steadily risen since the 1980s, correlating with diagnostic advances and the increased use of mammography. In women, breast cancer is the second major cause of cancer death, preceded only by lung cancer. Despite a rise in incidence, early detection and treatment advances have maintained stable mortality rates over the past 50 years.

Risk factors

Gender. The most significant risk factor for breast cancer is gender. The female-to-male incidence ratio is approximately 100:1.[1] In men, breast cancer represents less than 1% of all malignancies.[20] Major risk factors for women are listed in Box 35-1.

Age. Older women have the highest probability of developing breast cancer. Women 60 to 79 years old have an incidence rate of 468 per 100,000. This is double the rate for women 40 to 59 years old, whose incidence rate is 258 per 100,000.[30] Although incidence rates are higher for older persons, these patients represent only a small number of the total cases.

Incidence rises steadily during the reproductive years after age 30. The median age of onset is approximately 55 years, with the predominant age-group between 40 and 70 years.[14] A slight decrease in incidence occurs in the perimenopausal years, followed by a gradual rise during postmenopausal years. The decrease in incidence is attributed to hormonal changes that occur during menopause.

Family history. Genetic associations and racial differences in breast cancer rates suggest inherited tendencies toward development of the disease. Although hereditary patterns may be partially attributed to shared risk factors such as dietary and environmental factors, a genetic association is strongly suggested. Family history appears to be significant because female relatives of women with breast cancer have a higher incidence than the general population. Indeed, a recent population-based, case-control study concluded that 33% of breast cancer cases in patients age 20 to 29 are genetically attributable. This rate, however, markedly decreases in older patients, down to nearly 2% in patients age 70 to 79.[8]

The probability of developing breast cancer is highest for women whose mothers and/or sisters (first-degree relatives) have the disease, especially if the family members were premenopausal. Overall, these women have two to three times the usual risk of developing breast cancer.[26] Women with a strong family history of breast cancer must follow a good breast health program.

The gene *BRCA1* and *BRCA2* is associated with a 100% likelihood of breast cancer development. This particular type of heritable breast cancer accounts for less than 4% of all cases. Currently, women of families with multiple cases of breast cancer may be tested for this gene so that the risk will be known.

Hormonal factors. Risk factors for breast cancer are influenced by hormonal variables, as listed in Box 35-2. These risk factors appear to reflect menstrual and childbearing history. Early **menarche** (the beginning of menstruation) and late **menopause** (the ending of menstruation) increase breast cancer risk. **Oophorectomy** (removal of one or both ovaries) before age 50 appears to reduce risk.[40] These facts lead to a general assumption that the overall length of ovarian function is related to breast cancer risk.

Women who have given birth to a child (parous women) have less risk than women who have never been pregnant (nulliparous women). Pregnancy later in life increases the risk more than nulliparity. Women who give birth to their first child after age 35 are twice as likely to develop breast cancer as women who give birth to their first child before age 20.[40]

Box 35-1	**Major Risk Factors for Breast Cancer**

- Gender
- Age
- Family history
- Hormonal factors
- History of other malignancies
  Previous breast cancer
  Colon, thyroid, uterus, ovary, and salivary gland
- History of benign breast disease
  Atypical hyperplasia
  Lobular carcinoma in situ

Box 35-2	**Hormonal Influences on Breast Cancer Risk**

- Ovarian function
  Age at menarche
  Age at menopause
  Oophorectomy
- Parity
- Hormonal manipulation

Hormonal manipulation, relative to progesterone and estrogen, has also been associated with an increased incidence of breast cancer. Women who are taking hormone replacement therapy (used to alleviate menopausal symptoms) are at an increased risk of being diagnosed with breast cancer, and this risk further increases with prolonged use.[10] However, any increased risk disappears approximately 5 years after cessation of therapy. Women taking oral contraceptives (used to prevent ovulation) are at a slightly increased risk of being diagnosed with breast cancer during use and within 10 years of cessation of oral contraceptive use, but there is no increased risk noted after 10 years.[9]

History of malignancy. A history of breast cancer, either invasive or ductal **carcinoma in situ** (DCIS) (cancer confined to the breast), in one breast increases the risk for development of cancer in the opposite breast. This risk increases for women treated curatively for breast cancer at a relatively young age. Breast cancer patients must be closely monitored for the development of a contralateral breast malignancy.

Women with a history of malignant tumors of the colon, thyroid, uterus, ovary, or major salivary glands have also demonstrated an increased risk for breast cancer. Patients with these malignant diagnoses may share some of the dietary and hormonal factors that appear to influence breast cancer risk.

History of benign breast disease. Benign breast disease encompasses a variety of histologic subcategories associated with varying degrees of cancer risk. Women with **atypical hyperplasia** or lobular carcinoma in situ have an increased risk of developing breast cancer. These abnormal findings, in association with a family history of breast cancer, may increase the risk between 20% and 25% at 15 years.[7,41]

Dietary and environmental factors. International differences in breast cancer rates have been well documented. Incidence rates are higher in Europe, Canada, and the United States and lower in Asia and developing countries such as Mexico. White women have a higher incidence of breast cancer than nonwhite women. Increased incidence has been observed for women who migrate from low-incidence areas to high-incidence areas, indicating that environmental and dietary factors influence the level of risk.[7] Dietary fat intake, long suspected as a risk factor for breast cancer, has been found to have no association.[24]

Moderate consumption of alcohol (more than two drinks per day) appears to increase the risk of breast cancer development. The exact level of consumption relative to risk remains controversial. Alcohol consumption appears to have the greatest effect on breast cancer risk in women younger than 30.[39]

Radiation exposure. Radiation exposure causes breast cancer. However, the issue is complicated by numerous variables, including the type and quality of radiation, frequency of exposure, and magnitude of dose. Retrospective studies of women exposed to low levels of radiation for the monitoring of tuberculosis or treatment of benign conditions such as postpartum mastitis or fibroadenomas of the breast indicate increased breast cancer incidence. Subsequently, the treatment of nonmalignant conditions with radiation has been almost completely abandoned.

Much information on cancer induction by radiation exposure has been gained from the study of Hiroshima and Nagasaki atomic bomb survivors. A series of reports have been prepared by the National Research Council's committees on the biological effects of ionizing radiations (BEIR). The BEIR V report indicates that radiation-induced cancer is dose and time dependent and that the latent period appears to be relatively long (between 20 and 30 years).[11] The risk of breast cancer resulting from radiation appears to be greatest for women exposed at a relatively young age.

A threshold dose for breast cancer induction by radiation has not been determined. It is possible that exposure at levels similar to that of natural background radiation carries no risk. Based on current knowledge, the risk of radiation-induced breast cancer rarely contraindicates medically necessary radiation exposure.

PROGNOSTIC INDICATORS

Box 35-3 lists prognostic indicators for breast cancer; however, the list continues to expand through clinical and laboratory research. The pathologic staging system incorporates the most important factors, including the lymph node status, extent of the tumor, and presence of distant metastasis.

Lymph Node Status

The number of axillary lymph nodes involved by a tumor is the most important prognostic indicator and is a significant aspect of staging. A higher number of involved nodes correlates with an increased recurrence rate and a decreased survival rate. At least 10 axillary nodes must be evaluated to separate low risk (fewer than three nodes positive for tumor) from high risk (four or more nodes positive for tumor). The prognosis for patients with more than 10 axillary lymph nodes positive for tumor is extremely poor.

The involvement of internal mammary (IM) lymph nodes by cancer, with or without axillary lymph node involvement, further reduces disease-free survival rates. Similarly, supraclavicular lymph node involvement implies a poor prognosis.

Box 35-3	Prognostic Indicators for Breast Cancer

- Lymph node status
- Tumor extent
- Histology
- Estrogen and progesterone receptor status
- Flow cytometry
- Other laboratory studies

Tumor Extent

The size of the primary tumor is another aspect of the staging system that serves as a prognostic indicator. Larger tumors increase the likelihood of involvement of the skin, muscle, chest wall, and regional lymph nodes, resulting in a worse overall prognosis. The 5-year survival rate for patients with lesions less than 0.5 cm is 99%, whereas the rate associated with lesions larger than 0.5 cm is 82%. With regional lymph node metastasis, 4.5-cm tumors have a 70% incidence rate of nodal involvement, whereas 1.5-cm tumors have a 38% incidence rate.[39]

Although tumor location by quadrant influences the pattern of lymph node metastasis, no evidence indicates that the location of the primary tumor directly affects the prognosis. The fixation of a mass to the chest wall involves significant negative staging and prognostic implications.

Histology

Infiltrating ductal carcinoma is the most common histologic type of breast malignancy, accounting for 70% of all breast cancers. Infiltrating lobular carcinoma is the next most common type, comprising about 5% to 10% of breast cancers.[17]

There are several other relatively rare types of infiltrating breast cancer, such as mucinous or colloid, tubular, and papillary carcinoma. These lesions have distinct histologic characteristics and tend to yield a more favorable prognosis.

Inflammatory Carcinoma

Tumors classified as inflammatory carcinoma yield an extremely poor prognosis. The diagnosis of inflammatory cancer is based on pathologic evidence of malignancy and clinical findings of breast tenderness and enlargement, *peau d'orange* appearance, erythema, warmth, and diffuse induration of the skin.

Estrogen and Progesterone Receptor Status

Samples of tumor tissue should be analyzed to determine the effect of estrogen and progesterone on the cells. This information and other factors indicate the potential response to hormonal therapy. Patients who are receptor positive are more likely to respond to hormonal therapy. However, a receptor-negative status does not automatically indicate a lack of response to hormonal therapy. In general, patients with receptor-positive tumors have a better outcome than those with receptor-negative tumors.[40]

Flow Cytometry

Deoxyribonucleic acid (DNA) from breast cancer cells is routinely evaluated for prognostic information. The content of the DNA is studied for **ploidy** (pertaining to a cell that has the complete set of chromosome sets) status because **aneuploid** (pertaining to a cell that does not have an exact multiple of the normal number of chromosomes [variation may occur through individual chromosomes]) tumors are associated with a poorer prognosis than diploid tumors. Cell-cycle indicators are an even more sensitive marker for prognosis than ploidy status. Tumors with a high proportion of cells in the S phase of the cell cycle tend to be much more aggressive.

Other Laboratory Studies

Thymidine labeling indices, growth regulators, oncogene amplification, protein levels, and the use of monoclonal antibodies are under investigation for their prognostic and predictive value. These laboratory tests indicate the tumor cell proliferation, DNA content (ploidy), and fraction of tumor cells in the S phase of the cell cycle. Knowledge of such predictive factors influences treatment-management decisions.

Survival

Advancements in methods of detection and treatment of breast cancer have resulted in improved survival rates at all stages. The overall 5-year survival rate, as indicated by women who survive 5 years after the initial diagnosis (regardless of disease status), is 85%. The 5-year survival rate decreases to 77% if evidence exists of regional spread and to 21% if distant metastasis is present at the time of the diagnosis.[1] Survival rates correlate with early detection, tumor characteristics, the treatment approach, and the patient's general condition.

However, 5-year survival is not the best indicator of survival for breast cancer patients. Because of breast cancer's systemic nature, patients may relapse up to 20 years or more after treatment, and few options are available for cure after relapse. According to surveillance, epidemiology, and end result (SEER) statistics, the 10-year breast cancer survival rate is 75.7%, and the 15-year survival rate is 57.7%.[30]

ANATOMY

Embryology

The breast evolves from sudoriferous (sweat) gland tissue. Early in human fetal development the galactic band or milk streak develops, extending bilaterally from the axilla to the inguinal region. The portion of the band located on the thoracic trunk continues to develop, with the appearance of cells that form the nipple, areola, and ultimately all tissues of the breast. The remainder of the band regresses and disappears.

Location and Extent

The protuberant portion of the adult breast is located between the second and sixth ribs in the sagittal plane and extends from the sternochondral junctions to the midaxillary line in the axial plane. Additional breast tissue is often present beyond these margins, particularly medially and superiorly. Breast tissue is also in the axilla, which is referred to as the axillary tail of Spence. The average diameter of the gland at its base is 10 to 12 cm, and the average central thickness is 5 to 6 cm.

Structure

The breast parenchyma consists of 15 to 20 sections or lobes that are embedded in adipose (fat) tissue. Each lobe is drained by a system of ducts that open at the nipple. In each lobe are numerous lobules that contain the milk-producing alveoli. The subcutaneous tissues of the breast also include fat, connective tissue, circulatory and lymphatic vessels, and nerve supply (Figs. 35-2 and 35-3).

The skin overlying the breast is thin and contains sweat glands, hair follicles, and sebaceous (oil) glands. The circular, pigmented area surrounding the nipple is the areola. The nipple and areola are largely composed of smooth muscle tissue and contain sweat and sebaceous glands.

Musculature

The breast is contiguous with or in close proximity to several functionally important muscles: the pectoralis major and minor, serratus anterior, and latissimus dorsi. The breast lies over the pectoralis major and serratus anterior muscles and is attached to them by a layer of connective tissue, the deep pectoral fascia. The superficial pectoral fascia encompasses the breast tissue and is attached to the deep fascia by bands of connective tissue called Cooper's suspensory ligaments, which support the breast. Surgical approaches to breast cancer have historically involved the removal of several of these muscles, at times producing significant disfigurement and functional deficit.

Blood Supply

Arteries. The major arterial supply to the breast is via the branches of the IM artery. Several branches of the axillary artery provide blood to the lateral aspect of the breast, most notably the lateral thoracic artery.

Veins. The deep venous drainage of the breast lies along three major routes that play significant roles in the development of bloodborne metastasis from breast cancer. The IM vein, axillary vein, and intercostal veins empty into the pulmonary capillaries via the superior vena cava, allowing metastatic spread into the lung.

In addition, the intercostal veins communicate with the vertebral plexus of Batson, a system of small veins running vertically through and around the vertebral column. This system drains the proximal humeri, shoulders, skull, vertebral bodies, bony pelvis, and proximal femurs. Venous blood can flow in both directions in this system because of the absence of valves and low pressure in the channels. Malignant cells in the blood draining through the intercostal veins from the breast can therefore enter the axial skeleton, resulting in metastatic disease.

Lymphatic Drainage

Lymph vessels. Two sets of lymphatic channels are associated with the breast. These were first delineated in the

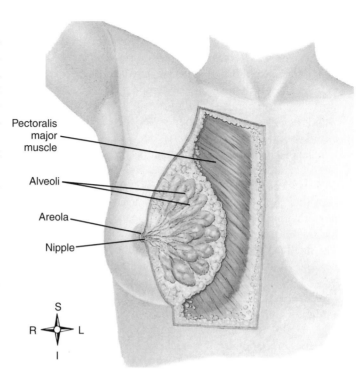

Figure 35-2. Dissected view of the breast. *(From Thibodeau GA, Patton KT: Anatomy and physiology, ed 3, St. Louis, 1996, Mosby.)*

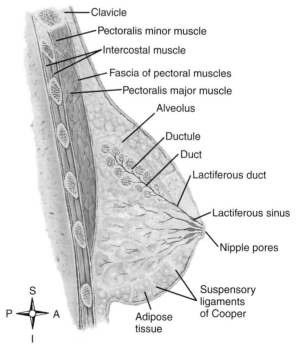

Figure 35-3. Sagittal section of the breast. *(From Thibodeau GA, Patton KT: Anatomy and physiology, ed 3, St. Louis, 1996, Mosby.)*

late eighteenth century by Cruikshank and Mascagni, who used injections of mercury on cadavers to visualize the lymphatics of this area.[12,28] The first group of lymphatics is superficial and drains the skin covering the breast. The second is a deep group that drains the internal breast tissues. The superficial and deep groups of lymphatics communicate with each other extensively, a fact that has implications for the management of breast cancer.[19] Fig. 35-4 illustrates lymphatic channels of the breast.

Axillary lymph nodes. Primary deep lymphatic drainage of the breast occurs to the ipsilateral axilla. Between 10 and 38 lymph nodes are in each axilla. These can be divided into three major sections (levels I, II, and III) based on location and sequential drainage patterns. Nodes in level I are located lowest, or most superficially, in the axilla and represent the first station of drainage from the breast. These are followed by nodes in levels II and III, which are positioned at increasing height in the axilla.[20] Studies in the 1800s first demonstrated that 70% of the lymphatic drainage of the breast occurs to the axilla, with 30% going to the IM nodes.

Internal mammary lymph nodes. The IM lymph nodes are located near the edge of the sternum, embedded in fat in the intercostal spaces. Most IM nodes are in the first, second, and third intercostal spaces, with the average person having approximately eight small nodes (four per side).[20]

Supraclavicular lymph nodes. In addition to direct drainage to the previously mentioned nodal groups, lymphatic drainage occurs from the breast to the supraclavicular nodes, liver, and contralateral IM nodes.

NATURAL HISTORY

Sites of Origin

The location of a primary breast tumor is best described by dividing the breast into quadrants. As shown in Fig. 35-5, approximately 48% of breast cancers arise in the upper-outer quadrant, 15% in the upper-inner quadrant, 11% in the lower-outer quadrant, 6% in the lower-inner quadrant, and 17% in the subareolar area (around the nipple, where the ducts converge); an additional 3% are multicentric.[40] The higher frequency of cancers in the upper-outer quadrant is explained by the fact that more breast tissue is contained in this area. Breast cancer rarely appears in both breasts (bilaterally).

The term *multicentric* describes tumors that appear in several areas of the breast. Multifocal breast cancer denotes a situation in which elements of a tumor are contained in tissue near the primary lesion in the same quadrant. Multifocal breast cancer is more common than multicentric cancer and is prognostically more favorable.[40]

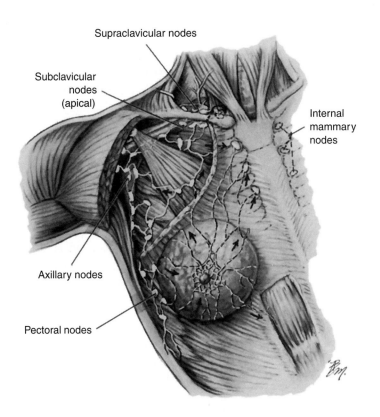

Figure 35-4. Lymph drainage and lymph node groups of the breast. *(From Cox JD, editor: Moss' radiation oncology: rationale, technique, results, ed 7, St. Louis, 1994, Mosby.)*

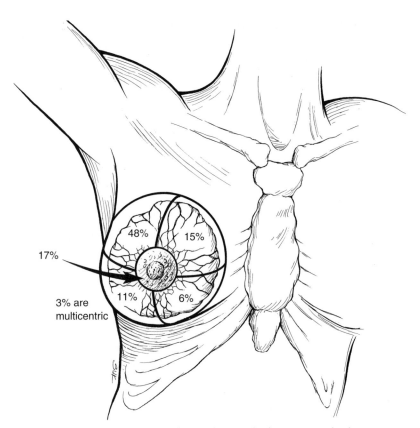

Figure 35-5. Frequency of breast lesions by location in the breast.

Tumor Progression

Breast cancer tends to grow locally, involving the ducts and adjacent tissues, and may spread to local and regional lymphatics. Left untreated, the cancer can become fixed in position, and the overlying skin may become infiltrated by the tumor, eventually causing ulceration. Disease involving the dermal lymphatics is a sign of inflammatory cancer.

The involvement of axillary lymph nodes occurs in an orderly and progressive manner. Large tumor size and multicentricity are highly associated with axillary lymph node involvement. Lesions of the upper-outer quadrant more frequently metastasize to the axillary lymph nodes, whereas lesions of the medial quadrants and central area have a tendency to metastasize to the IM lymph nodes. Progressive involvement of supraclavicular lymph nodes may also occur.

Recurrence

Breast cancer can recur in the breast (local recurrence), in the lymphatics (regional recurrence), or at distant metastatic sites. Patients with local recurrence after conservative treatment can be treated with additional surgery. Patients who experience regional recurrence are usually treated with systemic therapy and, if possible, surgical resection.

Distant Metastasis

Breast cancer can spread to distant sites via invasion of the blood vessels, followed by hematogenous spread to other sites. Distant metastatic sites include bone, brain, liver, lung, eyes, ovaries, and adrenal and pituitary glands.

CLINICAL PRESENTATION

With early detection, breast cancer is one of the most curable malignant diseases. A three-step breast health program is recommended for all women. This program includes a monthly self-examination, an annual clinical examination by a qualified medical professional, and a routine mammographic examination as defined by established guidelines. Women must pay careful attention to breast cancer warning signs. Presenting symptoms of breast cancer are listed in Box 35-4.

Although most changes of the breast are benign, 20% of all masses are malignant. The potential for a diagnosis of malignancy, combined with the shortness of breast tumor doubling time, warrants immediate attention and close follow-up of women with breast complaints. Women who follow a good breast health program and seek medical attention promptly after the detection of breast changes may benefit from an early diagnosis and treatment, ultimately leading to a better outcome.

Breast Mass

The most common presentation of breast cancer is a painless lump. Unfortunately, by the time a breast lesion is palpable it has already grown to about 0.5 cm. Small lesions can be difficult to detect, especially if they are deep within breast tissues. The assessment of a breast mass must address the size, shape, consistency, mobility, pain or tenderness, location in the breast, and relation to skin and surrounding tissues. The opposite breast should be compared for asymmetry. A clinical history relative to known risk factors, a physical assessment of the mass, and a biopsy of a suspicious lesion are critical to the proper management of a patient who has a breast mass.

In premenopausal women, glandular breast tissues tend to change throughout the menstrual cycle. For this reason the evaluation of a breast mass over one or two menstrual cycles may be necessary. An aspiration, biopsy, or both may be recommended for a persistent mass.

Because benign breast conditions (including cysts) are more rare postmenopausally, the finding of palpable breast masses in postmenopausal women tend to be highly suspicious. In these instances a biopsy is strongly recommended.

Nipple Discharge or Retraction

The sudden onset of nonlactational serous discharge from one breast is the second most common symptom of breast cancer. Nipple retraction and tenderness or pain in the nipple may also suggest cancer. Nipple changes must also be investigated for benign diagnoses, including cystic mastopathy, intraductal papilloma, and Paget's disease.

Skin Changes and Alterations in Breast Contour

Changes in skin texture, dimpling, irritation, increased warmth, scaling, pain, and ulceration of the skin are breast cancer symptoms requiring careful evaluation. Other types of symptomatic changes include distortion of the normal breast contour, swelling, and thickening of subcutaneous tissues. *Peau d'orange,* a condition in which the skin develops an orange peel appearance, is a clinical sign of inflammatory breast cancer.

Lymphadenopathy

Occasionally, the first sign of breast cancer is the enlargement of an axillary lymph node. Cervical, supraclavicular, and axillary lymph nodes drain breast tissues and require careful assessment. Arm edema may also be a sign of lymph node involvement.

Mammographic Abnormality

A mammogram and a clinical examination of the breast can detect small, discreet lesions and chest wall involvement. On a mammogram, breast cancer typically appears as an ill-defined, opacified lesion with or without spiculated margins, as demonstrated in Fig. 35-6.

Mammographic breast cancer screening is recommended for improving survival rates through early detection. Patients with an incidental finding of breast cancer through a mammography tend to have the best prognosis.

Distant Metastasis

Distant metastasis (most commonly in the form of bone, brain, lung, or liver involvement) may be present at the time of the diagnosis. Patients with distant metastasis (stage IV disease) have an extremely poor prognosis. Discomfort from

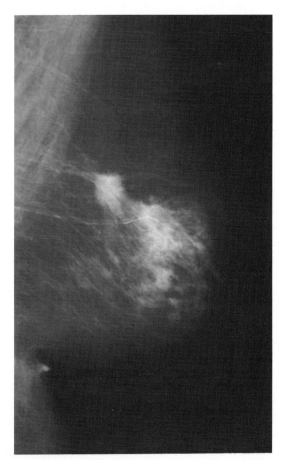

Figure 35-6. Mammogram demonstrating a malignant lesion.

the metastatic site is usually not the patient's only symptom; however, it provides the patient with the impetus for seeking medical attention. As a result of improvements in health education, awareness, detection, and diagnosis, fewer patients exhibit distant metastasis at the time of the diagnosis.

DETECTION AND DIAGNOSIS

As the most common malignancy in women, cancer of the breast affects one in every eight women in the United States.[1] Such a widespread disease merits the continued development of screening and detection methods that provide the earliest possible diagnosis because early lesions can be highly curable.[23,33] Important features of breast cancer screening and detection methods include cost effectiveness, accuracy, **specificity** (the probability that a test will be negative for an instance when no disease if present), safety, and availability.

The medical community has made great progress in this regard. As recently as several decades ago most breast cancer patients were first treated in an advanced stage of disease. Fear and ignorance played a large role in preventing earlier diagnoses. Women were not cognizant of the need to examine their own breasts and thus were often not aware of any change until it became obtrusive. In addition, women were not anxious to hear that they needed a radical mastectomy, and they often delayed seeking medical attention. Surgical treatment for breast cancer was perceived as disfiguring and defeminizing and was often psychologically traumatic for the patient.

Detection

As a result of public education campaigns by the ACS and other groups, many breast cancers are diagnosed early (i.e., at a smaller size and before involvement of the lymph nodes). Such tumors can often be successfully treated without removal of the breast.

The ACS periodically publishes updated recommendations for the detection of breast cancer. The current cornerstones of breast cancer detection are breast self-examination (BSE), clinical breast examination, and mammographic screening.

Breast self-examination. BSE is widely regarded as a simple and effective means of familiarizing women with the consistency and feel of their breasts, thereby allowing them to detect changes. The ACS recommends that women examine their breasts monthly, particularly at the same point each month relative to their menstrual cycle.

Varying reports describe the effectiveness of BSE in terms of its influence on the stage of disease at the time of the diagnosis and on survival rates. Some retrospective studies found a lower mortality rate among women who had breast cancer and practiced BSE. One reported that women who had been given a brochure on BSE had somewhat smaller tumors at the time of diagnosis.

BSE can be effective only if performed correctly. Educational materials are available that describe the technique, the frequency of examinations, the position of the body during an examination, and the way to palpate the breast and axillary tissue.

Clinical breast examination. A clinical breast examination is an important aspect of breast cancer detection. Physicians and other health professionals perform this procedure, which can detect tumors as small as 0.5 cm in diameter. The skin over the breast is evaluated for color and textural changes. With the patient in the sitting and supine positions, the breast is examined visually and by palpation for mobility and the presence of a mass. The presence of chest wall fixation is assessed through a series of muscle-tensing maneuvers by the patient. Dimpling of the skin, nipple discharge, and axillary lymph node enlargement are evaluated during the clinical examination.

Mammographic screening. Mammography is a powerful tool in the quest for early detection of breast cancer. However, aspects of mammographic screening remain controversial. One of the major sources of contention is disagreement concerning the ideal interval for mammographic screening. The ACS and American College of Radiology (ACR) recommend that a baseline mammogram be obtained between ages 35 and 39 in asymptomatic women who are at an average risk for developing breast cancer. Women between 40 and 49 years of age should have a mammogram every other year, and women older than 50 are advised to get annual mammograms.

Numerous prospective, randomized trials have demonstrated the efficacy of mammography in the screening of asymptomatic women for breast cancer. In addition, mammography remains the only modality that routinely detects breast cancer if the lesion is too small to feel during a clinical examination.

Mammography is not without limitations. Mammograms miss 10% to 15% of small and moderate-size breast cancers. This is often due to radiographic overlap between glandular and tumor tissue, rendering the tumor difficult to discern. Because of the relative radiographic similarity of glandular and tumor tissue, mammographic findings are often not specific for malignancy, resulting in numerous invasive diagnostic procedures (biopsies) that are negative for malignancy. Several studies have shown as few as one biopsy positive for tumor for every seven performed. Other series show that approximately one out of three and one half biopsies are positive for cancer. Most centers today have similar results.

Another problem affecting the efficacy of mammography as a screening tool is the lack of its access for many women. Not all insurance policies cover mammographic screening, and uninsured women in lower socioeconomic strata are often unable to pay the cost of screenings. Through the efforts of many individuals and organizations, low-cost screening programs have been made available, but a pressing need for services remains for millions of economically disadvantaged women.

Many factors are involved in the production of an optimal mammographic study. These include the age, upkeep, and type of equipment and the competency of the radiographer, mammographer, and radiologist. Proper positioning of the breast is essential to produce a useful mammogram. Even the film processor must be appropriately maintained to avoid the appearance of artifacts and to optimize the quality of the mammogram. For many years the ACR conducted a voluntary program that granted accreditation to mammographic facilities meeting their quality standards. Since October 1994, the U.S. Food and Drug Administration (FDA) has required the certification of all mammographic facilities. The major agency approved by the FDA to grant mammography accreditation is the ACR.

The two primary modalities of mammography are low-dose film and screen mammography and xerography. The standard low-dose film mammogram involves exposures in two views, a cranio-caudad and medial-lateral view. Although the current maximum acceptable radiation dose from a two-view mammogram is 0.01 Gy, the average optimally performed procedure delivers only 0.002 Gy. With radiation doses at this level, mammography presents a favorable risk-benefit ratio to patients.

Xerography is a technique of mammography that provides greater visualization of the area close to the chest wall but lacks the detail of good quality film mammography. As a result, xerography is reserved for obtaining additional detail in the patient whose lesion is adjacent to the chest wall.

Ultrasound. Ultrasound (US) has been used fairly extensively in breast cancer detection. US is currently used as an adjunct to mammography for its ability to distinguish between cystic and solid masses and to guide biopsy procedures. US is not a suitable screening modality for breast cancer for several reasons. It cannot detect microcalcifications, it is not sensitive enough to detect small breast cancers, and it can miss subtle structural irregularities indicative of breast malignancy.

Thermography. Thermography is a procedure that uses one of several methods to produce an image of the temperature of the skin overlying the breast. In theory, a malignant lesion radiates heat, which is then detected by one of these techniques. The image produced corresponds to the location of cancer cells in the breast. However, there is a high incidence of false-positive and false-negative results with this modality. Therefore it is not currently recommended as a breast cancer screening tool.

Transillumination. Transillumination, or diaphanography, is a procedure that involves the transmission of light of various wavelengths through breast tissue for detecting masses. Theoretically, a malignant tumor absorbs more of the light passing through the breast than the surrounding normal tissue, thereby casting a shadow on the opposite skin surface. The technique, first described about 60 years ago, has evolved to include computer enhancement but has not demonstrated accuracy or specificity in the detection and/or differentiation of breast malignancies. Transillumination is not currently accepted as a screening method for breast cancer.

Magnetic resonance imaging. Magnetic resonance imaging (MRI) of the breast has been used for approximately a decade. It has been of some value in women with silicone breast implants, extremely dense breast tissue, or changes in the breast secondary to radiation treatment. MRI of the breast has several significant limitations, including its inability to detect microcalcifications and its high cost. Recent advances in the development of surface coils have resulted in several studies on the efficacy of MRI for breast cancer, but additional clinical trials are necessary to further define its role.

Computed tomography. The expense of computed tomography (CT) is sufficiently high to rule out its use as a screening method. However, it is an important tool for the evaluation of local and regional disease in selected patients who have an established diagnosis of breast cancer.

Diagnosis

A definitive diagnosis of breast cancer can only be made through a microscopic examination of tissue removed from the breast. This tissue is obtained from a biopsy through one of several techniques.

Fine-needle biopsy. Fine-needle biopsy involves the careful placement of a relatively small-gauge needle into the suspicious tissue in the breast. The needle is attached to a syringe in which the evacuated blood and/or tissue is collected. This material is prepared on slides for cytologic evaluation.

Core-needle biopsy. Core-needle biopsy is similar to fine-needle biopsy in that a syringe and a larger-gauge needle are used to aspirate a core of tissue from the breast mass. The pathologist then examines this tissue histologically.

Incisional biopsy. An incisional biopsy involves the partial removal of a breast mass to make a histologic diagnosis. This procedure is usually performed if the mass is too large to be completely removed without compromising subsequent surgical treatment.

Excisional biopsy. Excisional biopsy, sometimes referred to as lumpectomy, removes the mass in its entirety with or without a portion of surrounding normal tissue. This has become the method of choice for removing small breast masses. The placement of the surgical incision is extremely important. Cosmetic effect and treatment considerations (radiation therapy and surgical) are directly related to the type and placement of the incision. Curvilinear rather than radial incisions must be used.[19] The incision should be placed directly over the mass to avoid tunneling through breast tissue (a situation with implications for the placement of the boost field during radiation treatment).

PATHOLOGY

Two basic methods are used for obtaining pathologic information. Gross examination is performed to record the dimensions of the specimen, the size of the tumor, and the tumor's relationship to the excisional margin. Microscopic examination is performed through an analysis of the specimen under a microscope whereby tumor margins are assessed to evaluate the adequacy of the excision. In addition, the pathologist determines the tumor histology and presence of associated DCIS and lymphatic invasion, if any.

Histopathologic types of breast cancer are listed in Box 35-5. Most breast cancers arise in the terminal ductal lobular units of the breast and are classified as ductal or lobular, depending on the specific site of origin. The specific type is defined based on cytologic features and growth patterns. Carcinoma in situ (CIS) is also classified as ductal or lobular and is characterized by a proliferation of malignant epithelial cells that do not invade the basement membrane.

More than 70% of invasive breast cancers are infiltrating ductal carcinoma. These tumors usually contain some component of DCIS and tend to spread to the axillary lymph nodes. Infiltrating lobular carcinoma comprises about 5% to 10% of breast cancers.[40] The prognosis and likelihood of lymph node involvement is similar to that of ductal carcinoma.

Inflammatory breast cancer can be composed of any histologic cell type. However, its clinical features are distinct. Accounting for less than 1% of all breast cancer, it is characterized by obvious skin changes such as *peau d'orange,* erythema, thickening, increased warmth, and diffuse induration caused by dermal lymphatic involvement. The entire breast may be tender and enlarged. Inflammatory cancer involves a grave prognosis, with a survival time of less than 2 years. It tends to be aggressive and fast growing. Therefore combined-modality treatment (including surgery, chemotherapy, and radiation therapy) is used for these patients.

In addition to defining the histologic type of breast cancer, the pathologist can assess the tumor grade. The degree of differentiation assesses the morphologic features of tubule formation, nuclear pleomorphism, and mitotic count of the tissue being reviewed. In the assessment of these components, a value of 1 (favorable) to 3 (unfavorable) is assigned for each feature and is then added together. A combined score of 3 to 5 points is a grade 1, a combined score of 6 to 7 is grade 2, and a combined score of 8 to 9 is grade 3. The higher the grade the more undifferentiated the disease, which equates to a more aggressive disease (Box 35-6).

STAGING

Patients with breast cancer are staged for a variety of reasons. Staging aids in the selection of the treatment technique, allows the evaluation of treatment methods, and indicates the prognosis. The two methods of staging breast cancer are clinical and pathologic. Clinical staging involves all physical, operative, and gross pathologic findings used to establish the diagnosis, including the primary tumor, breast, skin, chest wall, lymph nodes, and any sites of metastasis. Pathologic staging includes all these factors plus microscopic assessment of the tumor margin. If gross involvement of the tumor margin is present, then the true extent of the primary tumor cannot be assessed and is therefore coded as TX. Level I axil-

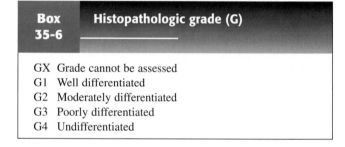

Box 35-5	Histopathologic types of breast cancer

Cancer, NOS
  Ductal
  Intraductal (in situ)
  Invasive with predominant intraductal component
  Invasive, NOS
  Comedo
  Inflammatory
  Medullary with lymphocytic infiltrate
  Mucinous (colloid)
  Papillary
  Scirrhous
  Tubular
  Other
Lobular
  In situ
  Invasive with predominant in situ component
  Invasive
Nipple
  Paget's disease, NOS
  Paget's disease with intraductal carcinoma
  Paget's disease with invasive ductal carcinoma
Other
  Undifferentiated carcinoma

NOS, Not otherwise specified.

Box 35-6	Histopathologic grade (G)

GX   Grade cannot be assessed
G1   Well differentiated
G2   Moderately differentiated
G3   Poorly differentiated
G4   Undifferentiated

lary lymph nodes should also be pathologically assessed for staging purposes.

The currently accepted staging system is that of the American Joint Committee on Cancer (AJCC), which is based on tumor, node, metastasis (TNM) definitions and stage groupings (Box 35-7). The primary tumor, regional lymph node status, pathologic classification status, and distant metastasis are parameters used to place patients into four main groups. With simultaneous bilateral breast cancers, the tumors are staged independently.

ROUTES OF SPREAD

Cancer of the breast is a relatively slow disease process, with distant metastases sometimes occurring decades after

Box 35-7	AJCC Staging System for Breast Cancer

PRIMARY TUMOR (T)

Tx   Primary tumor cannot be assessed

T0   No evidence of primary tumor

Tis   Carcinoma in situ

Tis   (DCIS) Ductal carcinoma in situ

Tis   (LCIS) Lobular carcinoma in situ

Tis   (Paget's) Paget's disease of the nipple with no tumor
Note: Paget's disease associated with a tumor is classified according to the size of the tumor

T1   Tumor 2 cm or less in greatest dimension

T1mic   Microinvasion 0.1 cm or less in greatest dimension

T1a   Tumor more than 0.1 cm but not more than 0.5 cm in greatest dimension

T1b   Tumor more than 0.5 cm but not more than 1 cm in greatest dimension

T1c   Tumor more than 1 cm but not more than 2 cm in greatest dimension

T2   Tumor more than 2 cm but not more than 5 cm in greatest dimension

T3   Tumor more than 5 cm in greatest dimension

T4   Tumor of any size with direct extension to
(a) chest wall or
(b) skin, only as described below

T4a   Extension to chest wall, not including pectoralis muscle

T4b   Edema (including peau d'orange) or ulceration of the skin of the breast, or satellite skin nodules confined to the same breast

T4c   Both T4a and T4b

T4d   Inflammatory carcinoma

REGIONAL LYMPH NODES (N)

NX   Regional lymph nodes cannot be assessed (e.g., previously removed)

N0   No regional lymph node metastasis

N1   Metastasis in a movable ipsilateral axillary lymph node(s)

N2   Metastasis in ipsilateral axillary lymph node(s) fixed or matted, or in clinically apparent[1] ipsilateral internal mammary nodes in the *absence* of clinically evident axillary lymph node metastasis

N2a   Metastases in ipsilateral axillary lymph node fixed to one another (matted) or to other structures

N2b   Metastasis only in clinically apparent[1] ipsilateral internal mammary nodes in the *absence* of clinically evident axillary lymph node metastasis

N3   Metastasis in ipsilateral infraclavicular lymph node(s) with or without axillary lymph node involvement, or in clinically apparent[1] ipsilateral internal mammary node(s) and in the *presence* of clinically evident axillary lymph node metastasis; or metastasis in ipsilateral supraclavicular lymph node(s) with or without axillary or internal mammary lymph node involvement

N3a   Metastasis in ipsilateral infraclavicular lymph node(s) and axillary lymph node(s)

N3b   Metastasis in ipsilateral internal mammary lymph node(s) and axillary lymph node(s)

N3c   Metastasis in ipsilateral supraclavicular lymph node(s)

REGIONAL LYMPH NODES (pN)[2]

pNX   Regional lymph nodes cannot be assessed (e.g., previously removed, or not removed for pathologic study)

pN0   No regional lymph node metastasis histologically, no additional examination for isolated tumor cells (ITC)[3]

pN0(i–)   No regional lymph node metastasis histologically, negative IHC

pN0(i+)   No regional lymph node metastasis histologically, positive IHC, no IHC cluster greater than 0.2 mm

pN0(mol–)   No regional lymph node metastasis histologically, negative molecular findings (RT-PCR)[4]

pN0(mol+)   No regional lymph node metastasis histologically, positive molecular findings (RT-PCR)[4]

pN1   Metastasis in 1 to 3 axillary lymph nodes, and/or in internal mammary nodes with microscopic disease detected by sentinel lymph node dissection but not clinically apparent[5]

pN1mi   Micrometastasis (greater than 0.2 mm, none greater than 2.0 mm)

pN1a   Metastasis in 1 to 3 axillary lymph nodes

pN1b   Metastasis in internal mammary nodes with microscopic disease detected by sentinel lymph node dissection but not clinically apparent[5]

pN1c   Metastasis in 1 to 3 axillary lymph nodes and in internal mammary lymph nodes with microscopic disease detected by sentinel lymph node dissection but not clinically apparent[5,6]

pN2   Metastasis in 4 to 9 axillary lymph nodes, or in clinically apparent[1] internal mammary lymph nodes in the *absence* of axillary lymph node metastasis

pN2a   Metastasis in 4 to 9 axillary lymph nodes (at least one tumor deposit greater than 2.0 mm)

pN2b   Metastasis in clinically apparent[1] internal mammary lymph nodes in the *absence* of axillary lymph node metastasis

pN3   Metastasis in 10 or more axillary lymph nodes, or in infraclavicular lymph nodes, or in clinically apparent[1] ipsilateral internal mammary lymph nodes in the *presence* of 1 or more positive axillary lymph nodes; or in more than 3 axillary lymph nodes with clinically negative microscopic metastasis in internal mammary lymph nodes; or in ipsilateral supraclavicular lymph nodes

pN3a   Metastasis in 10 or more axillary lymph nodes (at least one tumor deposit greater than 2.0 mm), or metastasis to the infraclavicular lymph nodes

pN3b   Metastasis in clinically apparent[1] ipsilateral internal mammary lymph nodes in the *presence* of 1 or more positive axillary lymph nodes; or in more than 3 axillary lymph nodes in internal mammary lymph nodes with microscopic disease detected by sentinel lymph node dissection but not clinically apparent[5]

pN3c   Metastasis in ipsilateral supraclavicular lymph node

continued

Box 35-7	AJCC Staging System for Breast Cancer—cont'd

DISTANT METASTASIS (M)

MX Distant metastasis cannot be assessed
M0 No distant metastasis
M1 Distant metastasis

STAGE GROUPING

0	Tis	N0	M0
I	T1[7]	N0	M0
IIA	T0	N1	M0
	T1[7]	N1	M0
	T2	N0	M0
IIB	T2	N1	M0
	T3	N0	M0
IIIA	T0	N2	M0
	T1[7]	N2	M0
	T2	N2	M0
	T3	N1	M0
	T3	N2	M0
IIIB	T4	N0	M0
	T4	N1	M0
	T4	N2	M0
IIIC	Any T	N3	M0
IV	Any T	Any N	M1

Note: Stage designation may be changed if post-surgical imaging studies reveal the presence of distant metastases, provided that the studies are carried out within 4 months of diagnosis in the absence of disease progression and provided that the patient has not received neoadjuvant therapy.

HISTOLOGIC GRADE (G)

All invasive breast carcinomas with the exception of medullary carcinoma should be graded. The Nottingham combined histologic grade (Elston-Ellis modification of Scarff-Bloom-Richardson grading system) is recommended. The grade for a tumor is determined by assessing morphologic features (tubule formation, nuclear pleomorphism, and mitotic count), assigning a value of 1 (favorable) to 3 (unfavorable) for each feature, and adding together the scores for all three categories. A combined score of 3-5 points is designated as grade 1; a combined score of 6-7 points is grade 2; a combined score of 8-9 points is grade 3.

HISTOLOGIC GRADE (NOTTINGHAM COMBINED HISTOLOGIC GRADE IS RECOMMENDED)

GX Grade cannot be assessed
G1 Low combined histologic grade (favorable)
G2 Intermediate combined histologic grade (moderately favorable)
G3 High combined histologic grade (unfavorable)

With permission from American Joint Committee on Cancer (AJCC), Chicago, Illinois: *AJCC Cancer Staging Manual*, ed 6, New York, 2002, Springer-Verlag.
Notes

1. Clinically apparent is defined as detected by imaging studies (excluding lymphoscintigraphy) or by clinical examination.
2. Classification is based on axillary lymph node dissection with or without sentinel lymph node dissection. Classification based solely on sentinel lymph node dissection without subsequent axillary lymph node dissection is designated (sn) for "sentinel node," e.g., pN0(i+)(sn).
3. Isolated tumor cells (ITC) are defined as single tumor cells or small cell clusters not greater than 0.2 mm, usually detected only by immunohistochemical (IHC) or molecular methods but which may be verified on H&E stains. ITCs do not usually show evidence of metastatic activity (e.g., proliferation or stromal reaction.)
4. *RT-PCR*, reverse transcriptase/polymerase chain reaction.
5. Not clinically apparent is defined as not detected by imaging studies (excluding lymphoscintigraphy) or by clinical examination.
6. If associated with greater than three positive axillary lymph nodes, the internal mammary nodes are classified as pN3b to reflect increased tumor burden.
7. T1 includes T1mic.

definitive treatment of the primary tumor.[20] Some researchers believe that cancer of the breast is a systemic disease, even in the earliest clinical stages, based on the following facts: (1) little change has occurred in long-term survival rates since the radical mastectomy was developed and (2) late distant metastases continue to appear, even with the use of advanced treatment techniques.[22]

Extension in the Breast

A basic therapeutic tenet of this disease is that all ipsilateral breast tissue is at risk and requires treatment. This is due to the fact that extension throughout the breast is possible as a result of the following mechanisms:
1. Direct invasion into surrounding breast tissue
2. Extension via the duct system
3. Spread along the lymphatic channels in the breast

Direct extension of a primary breast lesion can be demonstrated mammographically. The tumor has fingerlike projections that extend into the parenchyma of the breast (Fig. 35-7). Without treatment, such lesions ultimately involve the skin of the breast and/or the chest wall.

Cancer also spreads in the breast by progressive involvement

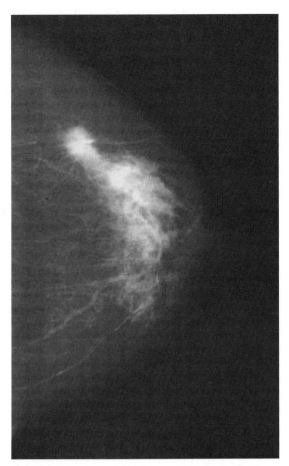

Figure 35-7. Mammographic demonstration of a primary breast lesion.

of the ducts. Whether this process represents actual direct extension along the ducts or a more generalized development of cancer in multiple ducts simultaneously is not fully understood.

The extensive lymphatic system of the breast provides an avenue for the primary spread of tumor cells in breast tissue. Cells can migrate via lymphatic channels deep into the chest wall or central portion of the breast beneath the nipple-areola complex.

Regional Lymph Node Involvement

Lymph nodes in the axillary and IM areas are the most likely sites of regional involvement of breast cancer. The supraclavicular nodes are only occasionally involved. The presence or absence of disease in these nodal groups is an important factor in treatment decisions and as an indicator of the prognosis.

Axillary lymph node involvement. Lymph nodes located in the axilla represent the primary lymphatic drainage of the breast. Half of all patients with breast cancer have microscopic involvement of the axillary nodes.[19] The inci-

dence of axillary lymph node involvement is a function of several factors, including the following:
1. Size of the primary tumor—as tumor size increases, so does the likelihood of axillary node involvement.[7]
2. Quadrant location of the primary tumor—lesions located in the upper-outer or lower-outer quadrants have a greater chance of axillary node involvement.[16]

Lymph nodes in the axilla can be divided into three subsections. Because of the sequential drainage pattern, the lowest (level I) nodes are the first and most likely to be involved, followed by levels II and III. Occasionally, lymph nodes in a higher level may be involved while the nodes in the lower level(s) are negative for tumor, a situation referred to as skip metastasis. The two largest series studying this process demonstrated a 3.5% rate of skip metastasis in patients with axillary lymph node involvement.[31,37]

Internal mammary lymph node involvement. IM lymph nodes are the second most common nodal site of involvement from breast cancer. Of all breast cancer patients, 20% have IM nodes positive for tumor.[19] The incidence of IM involvement is directly related to axillary node involvement and the size of the primary tumor. The age of the patient also influences IM node involvement, with younger patients demonstrating a higher incidence.[36] Most studies also show that the primary tumor location in the medial quadrants or center of the breast increases the incidence of IM involvement.

Assessing the status of IM nodes as a result of their intrathoracic location, which is relatively inaccessible for a biopsy, can be difficult. CT and lymphoscintigraphy are used to image the IM nodes.

Supraclavicular lymph node involvement. Supraclavicular lymph node involvement from breast cancer is correlated with extensive axillary metastasis and medial quadrant location.[20] The involvement of IM and supraclavicular nodes is considered a grave prognostic indicator in breast cancer.

Distant Metastasis

Breast cancer has a propensity to metastasize to distant sites, most commonly bone, lung, and liver.[4,32,38] The mechanism of this type of dissemination is embolization (i.e., spread via tumor cells entering the circulatory system and traveling to a distant organ). The length of time between the initial diagnosis and discovery of distant metastasis varies widely in this disease but can be extremely long, measured sometimes in decades. The development of distant metastasis is linked to the size and histology of the primary tumor and extent of lymph node involvement.

TREATMENT MANAGEMENT

A multidisciplinary approach that includes surgery, radiation therapy, and chemotherapy is required for breast cancer treatment. Historically, breast cancer was treated aggressively via radical mastectomy with or without radiation therapy. In addition to single-institution studies, large national cooperative groups, such as the National Surgical Adjuvant Breast and Bowel Project (NSABP) and the Radiation Therapy Oncology Group (RTOG), contribute to continuing breast cancer research and the development of treatments. The research of these and other groups (carried out over the last 30 years) indicates that breast cancer appears to be systemic in its progression. Historically, aggressive local treatment via radical mastectomy has not improved survival rates. Therefore current surgical and radiation treatment techniques are more conservative. Chemotherapy has been used increasingly to address microscopic, lymphatic, and systemic disease. When indicated, radiation therapy is usually delivered postoperatively.

Decisions regarding treatment are influenced by the extent of the primary tumor, the patient's general medical condition, and the patient's personal preference. Although limited surgery (breast conservation) with or without radiation treatment is popular, it is not appropriate for all patients. If the breast is small relative to the tumor or multicentric tumor involvement is present, then a mastectomy may be the best treatment choice. In addition, limited surgery is not an option for patients with advanced breast cancer.

Surgery

Radical mastectomy.   Introduced by William S. Halsted in the late 1800s, the Halsted radical mastectomy was the treatment of choice for breast cancer through the 1970s. Before this, patients were more likely to have large, bulky tumors, and early, limited surgical techniques were ineffective in reducing the incidence of chest wall recurrence. To address the high incidence of chest wall recurrence and lymph node involvement, Halsted devised the radical mastectomy, which involves the removal of the breast with its overlying skin, all the axillary lymph nodes, and the pectoral muscles (Fig. 35-8).

Although the Halsted radical mastectomy did not lead to improved long-term survival rates, chest wall recurrences were reduced, which accounts for the procedure's initial popularity. Unfortunately, the complication rate from radical mastectomy is high and complications can be severe, often leaving the patient with a concave chest wall, arm weakness, shoulder stiffness, and lymphedema (arm swelling). Eventually, the extent of surgery was reduced because radical mastectomy did not reduce the incidence of metastatic disease and because of the high risk of complications. Currently, radical mastectomy is rarely performed, comprising less than 2% of all breast surgeries in the United States.

Modified radical mastectomy.   Radical mastectomy was subsequently modified to preserve muscle, some skin, lymphatics, and blood vessels, thereby improving cosmetic results, reducing arm edema, and improving arm strength. Modified radical mastectomy involves removal of the breast and some or all of the axillary lymph nodes. It may also include removal of the pectoralis minor muscle, while preserving the pectoralis major (Fig. 35-9). Sometimes the

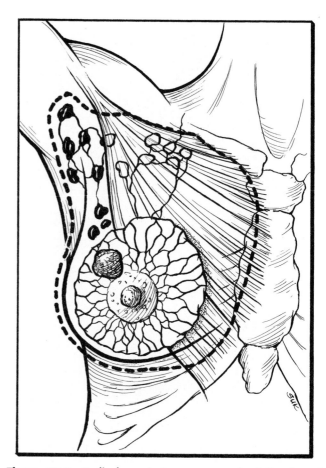

Figure 35-8. Radical mastectomy: removal of the breast with its overlying skin, the axillary lymph nodes, and the pectoralis major and minor muscles.

lymph nodes are sampled through a separate axillary incision. The use of modified radical mastectomy resulted in survival rates similar to those for radical mastectomy; therefore this modified procedure eventually replaced the more extensive operation.

Lumpectomy.   The excisional biopsy of a breast mass is sometimes referred to as lumpectomy, tylectomy, or tumorectomy. This procedure involves removal of the tumor with a margin of normal-appearing tissue (Fig. 35-10). Overlying skin and underlying tissue are left intact. Lymph nodes are sampled through a separate axillary incision.

Axillary dissection.   Removal of a sample of axillary lymph nodes in the axilla on the side of the involved breast (ipsilateral) is necessary for staging the patient's disease. The pathologic status of axillary lymph nodes influences the selection of the treatment technique and helps indicate the prognosis.

Breast reconstruction.   Breast reconstruction, which may be an option for women who have undergone a mastectomy, is achieved through the gradual expansion of existing skin and muscle and the subsequent placement of an artificial

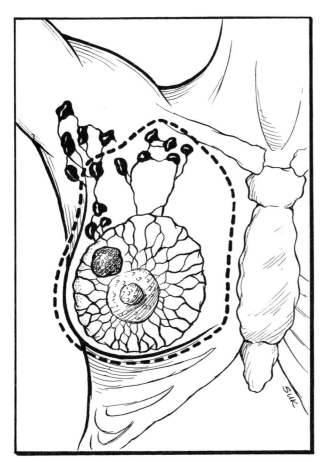

Figure 35-9. Modified radical mastectomy: removal of the breast with its overlying skin, some or all of the axillary lymph nodes. The pectoralis minor muscle may be removed, leaving the pectoralis major muscle intact.

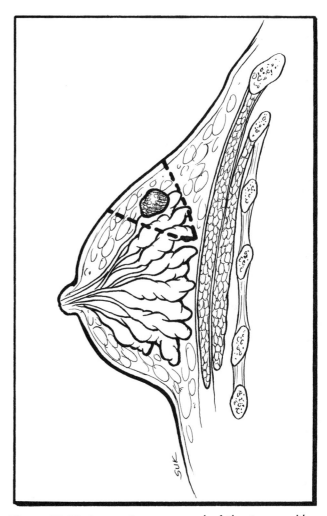

Figure 35-10. Lumpectomy: removal of the tumor with a margin of normal-appearing tissue.

breast implant. If remaining tissues are inadequate for expansion after a mastectomy, then skin and muscle may be transferred to the chest area from other parts of the body. A normal breast contour may be obtained by matching the size and shape of the implant with that of the opposite breast. It is possible to reconstruct just the contour of the breast or, in some patients, the entire breast, including the nipple and areola. A plastic surgeon performs the procedure, which may require several operations over 6 to 12 months.

Systemic Therapy

Systemic therapy may be combined with surgery and/or radiation therapy and consists of chemotherapy or endocrine therapy (hormonal manipulation). The goal of systemic treatment is the destruction, prevention, or delay of tumor spread to distant sites in the body. When systemic therapy is used with surgery or radiation, it is referred to as **adjuvant therapy.**

Chemotherapy. Chemotherapy consists of the following cancer-killing agents (used alone or in combination): cyclophosphamide (C), 5-fluorouracil (F), methotrexate (M),

doxorubicin (Adriamycin) (A), vinblastine, mitoxantrone, and mitomycin C. Combination chemotherapy is the use of several agents together. For example, combination chemotherapy consisting of CMF means that cyclophosphamide, methotrexate, and 5-fluorouracil are used together.

A treatment regimen is defined according to the order of administration, specific agent(s), dosages, routes of administration, and exact administration schedule. Drugs can be administered through the patient's mouth or via an injection into a vein or muscle. A schedule of administration indicates whether the drugs are given daily, weekly, or monthly. The duration of treatment is expressed in terms of months or years. Chemotherapy may be administered before or after surgery, before or after radiation therapy, or with radiation treatment. The sequence of chemotherapy, surgery, and radiation therapy continues to be studied for its effect on local control and survival. In addition, a variety of adjuvant treatment regimens are under investigation.

Endocrine therapy.   Current endocrine therapy consists of a variety of drugs used to deprive cancer cells of the hormones needed for growth. The most commonly used agents are tamoxifen and megestrol acetate (Megace). Tamoxifen is frequently a component of adjuvant therapy for postmenopausal women. It is used alone or with other chemotherapeutic agents. The estrogen receptor status also plays a role in the selection of hormonal therapy as an element of treatment.[25]

Treatment approach.   Each patient is considered unique, and management depends on the patient's stage of disease, lymph node status, estrogen receptor and progesterone receptor (ER/PR) status, and menopausal status. Although no single treatment exists that is best for any group of patients, some general comments can be made. In general, stage I breast cancer patients have a low incidence of relapse; therefore chemotherapy is reserved for high-risk patients in this group. For stages II and III breast cancer patients, systemic therapy is useful in reducing relapse rates and increasing overall survival rates. Multiagent chemotherapy is the present treatment of choice for premenopausal women with ipsilateral lymph node involvement, whereas tamoxifen alone or with chemotherapy is beneficial for postmenopausal women.[18,22,25] A combination of systemic and local treatment is usually required for patients with advanced disease (stage IV).[25] For patients with unresectable tumors, chemotherapy is frequently sequenced first to achieve a systemic effect and to potentially downstage the tumor. Although data suggest that delaying irradiation during chemotherapy increases the risk of local failure, this risk may be acceptable for patients with locally advanced disease because distant metastasis is a predictor of overall survival. Optimal sequencing of chemotherapy, surgery, and radiation therapy has not yet been determined.

Treatment of advanced breast cancer.   For metastatic breast cancer, current chemotherapy can often prolong the survival time or inhibit progression of the disease. For some patients chemotherapy is used as a palliative measure.

Treatment efforts involving high-dose chemotherapy and autologous bone marrow transplantation for patients with advanced breast cancer (more than 10 involved lymph nodes) are under investigation. Initial results from several institutions indicate that the 2-year relapse-free survival rate for patients with advanced disease treated with this approach appears to be superior to results for similar patients treated with adjuvant chemotherapy. Continued research efforts involving randomized clinical trials and longer follow-up evaluations contribute to determining the optimal treatment management of advanced breast cancer.

Side effects.   Endocrine and chemotherapeutic agents can also affect healthy tissues, causing side effects such as nausea and vomiting, loss of appetite, fatigue, change in menstruation, mouth ulcers, and hair loss. The type of side effects the patient experiences depends on the agent(s) used and the patient's response to the drugs. For example, some patients may experience hot flashes (a short-term side effect of tamoxifen) as a result of lowered levels of estrogen. Most side effects are acute, resolving after the completion of treatment. A few side effects are permanent. For example, doxorubicin may cause cardiac damage. In addition, a small chance exists that the chemotherapy will cause a second cancer.

Radiation Therapy

Conservative breast cancer management.   Current methods for conservative breast cancer management have been well established. The ACR adopted "Standards for Breast Conservation Treatment" in 1992. The American College of Surgeons, the College of American Pathologists, and the Society of Surgical Oncology have endorsed this document. A variety of research efforts have provided the evidence necessary to conclude that mastectomy and breast conservation treatment (lumpectomy, ipsilateral axillary lymph node dissection, and radiation therapy) are equally effective for selected patients with early-stage breast cancer (stages I and II). In addition, these studies revealed no difference in the rate of development of metastasis or contralateral breast cancer.[13]

As defined by ACR standards, the four critical elements used to select patients for breast conservation are as follows:
1. The patient's history and a physical examination are used to establish familial patterns and assess physical findings.
2. A mammographic evaluation is used to define the extent of the tumor, investigate the potential presence of multicentric or multifocal disease, and evaluate the contralateral breast.
3. A pathologic evaluation of the tumor including a gross and microscopic examination and additional data such as ER/PR analysis, extent of CIS, DNA ploidy, S phase fraction, and mitotic grade are obtained.
4. An assessment of the patient's needs and expectations is a difficult but essential consideration. Long-term survival, possibility and consequences of local recurrence, treatment options for potential local recurrence, follow-up procedures, physical and cosmetic outcomes, psychologic adjustment, and quality of life are factors requiring careful consideration.

Although properly staged and selected patients may be eligible for conservative treatment, some contraindications have been identified. First- and second-trimester pregnancy, multicentric disease, and a history of prior breast irradiation of significant dosage are absolute contraindications of breast conservation treatment. A history of vascular disease, a large tumor in a small breast, an extremely large or pendulous breast, and the specific location of the tumor in the breast are factors requiring special consideration and potentially contraindicating the use of a conservative approach to treatment.

Total gross removal of the tumor and a margin of surrounding tissue with maintenance of good cosmesis is the main goal of conservative breast surgery. A separate axillary dissection is performed, which minimally involves the removal of level I lymph nodes. Based on the size and histology of the tumor, removal of level II or III lymph nodes may be appropriate.

After a 2- to 4-week surgical recovery, radiation therapy may begin. Proper simulation and treatment planning are critical factors in establishing an appropriate treatment technique. Special attention to physical and technical considerations substantially reduces the risk of complications. Specific techniques are addressed in the following section. Generally, however, lower megavoltage beam energies (4 to 8 MV) and tissue compensators are used to improve dose homogeneity. Tangential fields are used to encompass the entire breast and chest wall. The amount of lung projected at the center of the tangential fields should be limited to between 1.0 and 3.4 cm, thereby reducing the risk of radiation pneumonitis. If peripheral lymphatic irradiation is required, then overlapping or excessive gapping between fields must be avoided. If the axillary dissection includes level III, then axillary irradiation should be avoided so that lymphedema does not result.

Fields are treated daily with standard fractionation (180 to 200 cGy per fraction) to a total dose of 4500 to 5000 cGy. A boost dose may be delivered with an electron beam or interstitial technique, increasing the total dose to the primary tumor site to 6000 to 6600 cGy. Although precise indications for performing the boost remain controversial, patients with margins positive for tumor or close margins of surgical resection usually receive boost irradiation.

Follow-up assessment of patients receiving conservative breast treatment is carefully scheduled to evaluate new or recurrent disease status, treatment sequelae, and cosmetic outcome. The patient's medical history, physical examination, and follow-up mammograms contribute to the evaluation process. The RTOG and European Organization for Research on Treatment of Cancer acute and late radiation morbidity scoring schemes are provided in Tables 35-1 and 35-2. An assessment of the cosmetic result is based on the physician's evaluation (using a four-point scoring index) and the patient's perception.

Postoperative management of breast cancer. Currently, the role of radiation therapy in postoperative breast cancer treatment is not well defined. Radiation therapy was initially used in breast cancer management as an adjuvant to radical mastectomy for the purpose of prophylaxis. The main goal was to reduce the local recurrence rate, thereby improving survival. The risk of radiation-induced cardiac damage and the evolution of the role of chemotherapy have reduced the use of radiation therapy in postoperative patients. The tumor size and location, number of axillary lymph nodes positive for tumor, tumor involvement of the skin or supraclavicular lymph nodes, and hormone receptor status may be indications for adjuvant radiation therapy.

If radiation therapy is indicated, then the chest wall is treated via tangential fields with lower megavoltage beam energies, using tissue compensators as necessary. Peripheral (supraclavicular and/or axillary) lymphatic irradiation may also be required. Fields are treated daily with standard fractionation (180 to 200 cGy per fraction) to a total dose of 4500 to 5000 cGy. Patients with IM lymph nodes positive for tumor are usually treated with chemotherapy. However, if radiation therapy is indicated, wider tangential ports that extend across the midline may be used. Another technique for treating the IM nodes combines photon and electron treatment, helping to limit the cardiac dose. Adjoining fields must be carefully planned to avoid overdosage or underdosage of tissues in these areas, leading to potential match-line **fibrosis** (abnormal formation of fiberlike scarring) or local recurrence, respectively.

Radiation Treatment Technique

Radiation treatment for primary breast malignancy is one of the more technically challenging and relatively high-volume procedures performed in a radiation oncology department. Therefore straightforward, reproducible techniques are advantageous, affording optimal target-volume-dose homogeneity and acceptable dose limits for normal structures.

There are almost as many techniques for breast irradiation as there are radiation oncology centers. Many techniques are only slight variations on a theme. Current standard of practice incorporates several essential elements in the treatment of breast cancer. This section presents these elements and details one specific technique.

Positioning and immobilization. Radiation treatment of breast cancer is demanding, requiring stringent positioning and immobilization techniques. One of the key elements involves the mobility of the patient's arm. Many postoperative patients (whether the surgery involved a mastectomy or an axillary dissection) experience initial difficulty in raising the arm to an acceptable position for radiation treatment. Most patients who encounter this problem can correct it with exercise in several days. Therefore the simulation and start of therapy should be delayed until the patient's arm moves appropriately. If the patient is simulated before mobility is restored, then the shoulder girdle will assume a different position for treatment than for simulation, leading to poor reproducibility of the treatment fields. At the time of consultation, before the simulation appointment, the radiation oncologist can give the patient a handout detailing exercises and explaining their necessity.

Many commercially available devices are available to assist in patient positioning for treatment of breast cancer. These range from custom-molded foam casts to boards with adjustable head and arm supports. One such device is illustrated in Fig. 35-11. An important element of reproducibility in immobilization is the ability to index the patient to the immobilization device exactly the same way daily.

For this type of treatment the patient should, at minimum, disrobe from the waist up. The patient lies supine in the selected positioning device on the simulator-treatment table. The patient's body must be straight (in the sagittal plane) and level from side to side. Laser triangulation points are marked on the patient's anterior and side surfaces in the area between the waist and inframammary fold to assist in the daily positioning process.

Table 35-1	**RTOG acute radiation morbidity scoring criteria**				

Organ Tissue	Grade 0	Grade 1	Grade 2	Grade 3	Grade 4
Skin	No change over baseline	Follicular, faint, or dull erythema; epilation; dry desquamation; decreased sweating	Tender or bright erythema and patchy, moist desquamation; moderate edema	Confluent, moist desquamation other than skin folds and pitting edema	Ulceration; hemorrhage; necrosis
Mucous membrane	No change over baseline	Injection; possible experience of mild pain not requiring analgesic	Patchy mucositis that may produce an inflammatory serosanguineous discharge; possible experience of moderate pain requiring analgesia	Confluent fibrinous mucositis; possibility of severe pain requiring narcotic	Ulceration; hemorrhage; necrosis
Eye	No change over baseline	Mild conjunctivitis with or without scleral injection; increased tearing	Moderate conjunctivitis with or without keratitis requiring steroids and/or antibiotics; dry eye requiring artificial tears; iritis with photophobia	Severe keratitis with corneal ulceration; objective decrease in visual acuity or in visual fields; acute glaucoma; panophthalmitis	Loss of vision (unilateral or bilateral)
Ear	No change over baseline	Mild external otitis with erythema and pruritis secondary to dry desquamation not requiring medication; audiogram unchanged from baseline	Moderate external otitis requiring topical medication; serous ototis medius; hypoacusis on testing only	Severe external otitis with discharge or moist desquamation; symptomatic hypoacusis; tinnitus, not drug related	Deafness
Salivary gland	No change over baseline	Mild mouth dryness; slightly thickened saliva; possibility of slightly altered taste, such as metallic taste (these changes not reflected in alteration in baseline feeding behavior, such as increased use of liquids with meals)	Moderate to complete dryness; thick, sticky saliva; markedly altered taste	—	Acute salivary gland necrosis
Pharynx and esophagus	No change over baseline	Mild dysphagia or odynophagia; possible requirement of topical anesthetic or nonnarcotic analgesics and soft diet	Moderate dysphagia or odynophagis; possible requirement of narcotic analgesics and puree or liquid diet	Severe dysphagia or odynophagia with dehydration or weight loss (>15% from pretreatment baseline) requiring NG feeding tube, intravenous fluids, or hyperalimentation	Complete obstruction; ulceration; perforation; fistula
Larynx	No change over baseline	Mild or intermittent hoarseness; cough not requiring antitussive; erythema of mucosa	Persistent hoarseness but ability to vocalize; referred ear pain, sore throat, patchy fibrinous exudate or mild arytenoid edema not requiring narcotic; cough requiring antitussive	Whispered speech and throat pain or referred ear pain requiring narcotic; confluent fibrinous exudate and marked arytenoid edema	Marked dyspnea; stridor or hemoptysis with tracheostomy or intubation necessary
Upper gastrointestinal system	No change	Anorexia with ≤5% weight loss from pretreatment baseline; nausea not requiring antiemetics; abdominal discomfort not requiring parasympatholytic drugs or analgesics	Anorexia with ≤15% weight loss from pretreatment baseline; nausea and/or vomiting requiring antiemetics; abdominal pain requiring analgesics	Anorexia with >15% weight loss from pretreatment baseline or requiring NG tube or parenteral support. Nausea and/or vomiting requiring tube or parenteral support; abdominal pain (severe despite medication; hematemesis or melana; abdominal distention (flat plate radiograph demonstrates distended bowel loops)	Ileus, subacute or acute obstruction, perforation, and bleeding requiring transfusion; abdominal pain requiring tube decompression or bowel diversion

NG, Nasogastric.

Table 35-2

RTOG and EORTC late radiation morbidity scoring scheme

Organ Tissue	Grade 0	Grade 1	Grade 2	Grade 3	Grade 4
Skin	None	Slight atrophy; pigmentation change, some hair loss	Patch atrophy; moderate telangiectasia; total hair loss	Market atrophy; gross telangiectasia	Ulceration
Subcutaneous tissue	None	Slight induration (fibrosis) and loss of subcutaneous fat	Moderate fibrosis but asymptomatic; slight field contracture; <10% linear reduction	Severe induration and loss of subcutaneous tissue; field contracture >10% linear measurement	Necrosis
Mucous membrane	None	Slight atrophy and dryness	Moderate atrophy and telangiectasia; little mucus	Marked atrophy with complete dryness; severe telangiectasia	Ulceration
Salivary glands	None	Slight dryness of mouth; good response on stimulation	Moderate dryness of mouth; poor response on stimulation	Complete dryness of mouth; no response on stimulation	Fibrosis
Spinal cord	None	Mild Lhermitte's sign	Severe Lhermitte's sign	Objective neurologic findings at or below cord level treated	Mono; paraquadraplegia
Brain	None	Mild headache; slight lethargy	Moderate headache; great lethargy	Severe headaches; severe central nervous system dysfunction (partial loss of power or dyskinesia)	Seizures or paralysis; coma
Eye	None	Asymptomatic cataract; minor corneal ulceration or keratitis	Symptomatic cataract; moderate corneal ulceration; minor retinopathy or glaucoma	Severe keratitis; severe retinopathy or detachment; severe glaucoma	Panopthalmitis; blindness
Larynx	None	Hoarseness; slight arytenoid edema	Moderate arytenoid edema; chondritis	Severe edema; severe chondritis	Necrosis
Lung	None	Asymptomatic or mild symptoms (dry cough); slight radiographic appearances	Moderate symptomatic fibrosis or pneumonitis (severe cough); low-grade fever; patchy radiographic appearances	Severe symptomatic fibrosis or pneumonitis; dense radiographic changes	Severe respiratory insufficiency; continuous O_2; assisted ventilation
Heart	None	Asymptomatic or mild symptoms; transient T wave inversion and ST changes; sinus tachychardia >110 (at rest)	Moderate angina on effort; mild pericarditis; normal heart size; persistent abnormal T wave and ST changes; low QRS	Severe angina; pericardial effusion; constrictive pericarditis; moderate heart failure; cardiac enlargement; electrocardiogram abnormalities	Tamponade; severe heart failure; severe constrictive pericarditis
Esophagus	None	Mild fibrosis; slight difficulty in swallowing solids; no pain on swallowing	Inability to take solid food normally; swallowing semisolid food; possible indication for dilatation	Severe fibrosis; ability to swallow only liquids; possibility of pain on swallowing; dilation required	Necrosis; perforation; fistula
Small and large intestine	None	Mild diarrhea; mild cramping; bowel movement five times daily; slight rectal discharge or bleeding	Moderate diarrhea and colic; bowel movement >5 times daily; excessive rectal mucus or intermittent bleeding	Obstruction of bleeding requiring surgery	Necrosis; perforation; fistula
Liver	None	Mild lassitude; nausea, dyspepsia; slightly abnormal liver function	Moderate symptoms; some abnormal liver function tests; serum albumin normal	Disabling hepatic insufficiency; liver function tests grossly abnormal; low albumin; edema or ascites	Necrosis; hepatic coma or encephalopathy
Kidney	None	Transient albuminuria; no hypertension; mild impairment of renal function; urea 25-35 mg%; creatinine 1.5-2.0 mg% creatinine clearance >75%	Persistent moderate albuminuria (2+); mild hypertension; no related anemia; moderate impairment of renal function; urea >36-60 mg%; creatinine clearance (50%-74%)	Severe albuminuria; severe hypertension; persistent anemia (<10%); severe renal failure; urea >60 mg%; creatinine >4.0 mg%; creatinine clearance<50%	Malignant hypertension; uremic coma; urea >100%
Bladder	None	Slight epithelial atrophy; minor telangiectasia (microscopic hematuria)	Moderate frequency; generalized telangiectasia; intermittent macroscopic hematuria	Severe frequency and dysuria; severe generalized telangiectasia (often with petechiae); frequent hematuria; reduction in bladder capacity (<150 ml)	Necrosis; contracted bladder (capacity >100 ml); severe hemorrhagic cystitis
Bone	None	Asymptomatic; no growth retardation; reduced bone density	Moderate pain or tenderness; growth retardation; irregular bone sclerosis	Severe pain or tenderness; complete arrest of bone growth; dense bone sclerosis	Necrosis; spontaneous fracture
Joint	None	Mild joint stiffness; slight limitation of movement	Moderate stiffness; intermittent or moderate joint pain; moderate limitation of movement	Severe joint stiffness; pain with severe limitation of movement	Necrosis; complete fixation

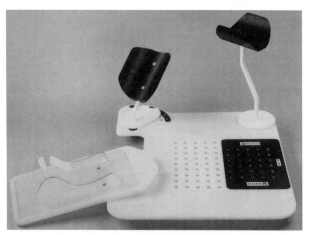

Figure 35-11. Diacor immobilization device used to assist in patient positioning for radiation treatment. *(Courtesy Diacor, Salt Lake City.)*

The arm on the uninvolved (contralateral) side should rest on the tabletop with the hand palm down. Patients must not place the contralateral hand on the abdomen or grasp the belt or waistband of their clothing. Such a position of the contralateral hand and arm (particularly in large-breasted women) can result in distortion of the thoracic anatomy, including rotation and/or displacement of the uninvolved breast into the treatment field.

The ipsilateral arm is raised and supported far enough in a cephalad direction to allow the tangential radiation beam to treat the breast or chest wall while avoiding the patient's upper arm. Adjustment of the patient's arm position can help reduce or eliminate skin folds in the axilla and supraclavicular areas.

The patient's head should be straight if treatment is limited to the breast or chest wall. If the peripheral lymphatics also require irradiation, then the head should be turned slightly to the contralateral side. Identical daily positioning of the patient's arm and head is extremely important for the accuracy of the treatment process.

The feet should be held together with a band or masking tape around the toes. This helps eliminate rotation of the patient's lower abdomen, thereby enhancing setup reproducibility. A triangular sponge or bolster may be placed under the patient's knees to relieve pressure on the lumbar region. The same immobilization devices must be used each time the patient is treated.

When lying supine, patients with large and/or pendulous breasts often have breast tissue displaced up into the infraclavicular area. These patients can be positioned on an incline board so that their head and thorax are elevated relative to their pelvis and lower extremities. This position can be useful in keeping the breast tissue in a more normal location, which is necessary to adequately irradiate the breast and avoid treating the upper arm. This position can also help alle-

viate the problem of deep skin folds in the supraclavicular area. Care must be taken, however, to avoid overtilting the patient and causing redundancy of the skin in the inframammary area.

The patient position should be well documented and explained in the setup instructions. For patients with unusual conditions or situations in which the setup needs further clarification, Polaroid photographs or digital images of the patient in the treatment position are essential.

Intact breast or chest wall treatment technique. Women who require only breast or chest wall irradiation are treated with tangential (glancing) fields. The purpose of this field arrangement is to maximize coverage of the tissues at risk and minimize the radiation dose to underlying structures, primarily the lung and heart. Radiation beams produced by lower energy linear accelerators (4 to 6 MV) and cobalt units are ideally suited to this type of treatment. Considerations for field margins for tangential fields are as follows:

Superior, at the most cephalad of the following points:
- First intercostal space
- As far cephalad as possible without including the arm
- Superior extent of the palpable breast tissue
- Cephalad (>2 cm) to original location of the mass

Inferior
- Caudad (1 to 2 cm) to the inframammary fold
- In a postmastectomy patient, this can be extrapolated from inframammary fold of contralateral breast

Medial
- At midline of patient, as determined by palpation of suprasternal notch and xiphoid process
- Exceptions include patient whose mass or incision extends to or beyond midline and patient who will receive IM lymphatic irradiation

Lateral
- Corresponding to midaxillary line (a line drawn from the center of the patient's axilla in a caudad direction)
- Including drain sites or incisions considered at risk, original tumor bed, and appropriate amount of lung margin

Most current techniques use an isocentric method of tangential field irradiation. In these techniques the isocenter is placed at some depth in the patient's breast or chest wall. At many institutions the isocenter is placed approximately halfway between the ribs and skin, at a point approximately midway between the medial and lateral entrance points of the beam. Other techniques place the isocenter at the deep edge of the tangential field and split the radiation beam in half, blocking the deep half of the beam.

An important feature of the tangential field arrangement is the **coplanar** nature of the deep (or posterior) margin of the ports (Fig. 35-12). In coplanar fields, the deep border of the medial tangent and the deep border of the lateral tangent form a single plane. This is important in ensuring a dose as homogeneous as possible throughout the treatment volume. Coplanar tangential fields may be achieved with a split-beam technique, as just mentioned, or an unblocked technique.

Asynchronous jaws or MLC provides the best result with a split-beam technique. Suspended blocks are least desirable

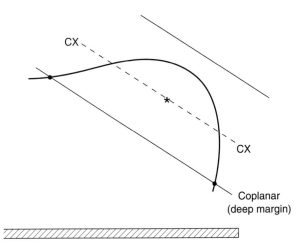

Figure 35-12. Tangential breast irradiation field arrangement features a coplanar deep margin.

between the superior and inferior borders, and mark this point on the patient. This is identified as point a on the contour and is the anterior setup point (Fig. 35-13). Measure the separation at this point by raising the table top to the isocenter, reading the SSD and subtracting this number from the source-axis distance (SAD) (e.g., an SSD of 78 subtracted from an SAD of 100 results in a separation of 22).
3. Measure the height of the lateral border relative to the tabletop. This is identified as point b on the contour.
4. Measure the separation between the medial and lateral margins with a caliper.
5. Obtain a contour through the plane of the field center, marking the medial (point a) and lateral (point b) borders on the contour material.
6. Indicate the patient's separation (step 2) and height of the lateral border from the table top (step 3) as horizontal planes on the graph paper. These will correlate with points a and b.
7. Draw line ab, which is equal in length to the separation measured in step 4 (Fig. 35-14).

because of transmission through the block and scatter that reaches the contralateral breast. Unintended irradiation of the contralateral breast is of concern, especially in younger patients. Several investigators have demonstrated a small but finite incidence of radiation-induced cancer in the contralateral breast of women who received radiation treatment for breast cancer.[5,12]

Perhaps the most desirable method of treating coplanar tangential fields (from the standpoint of limiting dose to the contralateral breast) is the unblocked isocentric technique. Coplanar tangential fields are not parallel opposed. The number of degrees from parallel opposition is a function of field size and may be calculated.

Planning tangential fields can be a relatively complex process. Several techniques described in the literature over the past 20 years have become well-established methods for planning comprehensive radiation treatment of the breast or chest wall and peripheral lymphatic areas.[28,32,35,36] Techniques used at many institutions today are exact replicas or variations of these themes. Several commercial vendors market systems that include immobilization devices and programmable calculators capable of performing the necessary mathematical calculations. Other techniques use factors that are derived empirically.

The following empirical isocentric method is reproducible, satisfies all essential criteria, and incorporates the advantage of a stable setup point. Tangential fields are set up with a mark on the anterior chest overlying the sternum. The table is then raised to a specified source-skin distance (SSD) and shifted laterally to place the isocenter at the appropriate location in the breast or chest wall. Steps in patient simulation with this technique are as follows:
1. Mark superior, inferior, medial, and lateral margins on the patient.
2. Set the field center at the midline of the chest, halfway

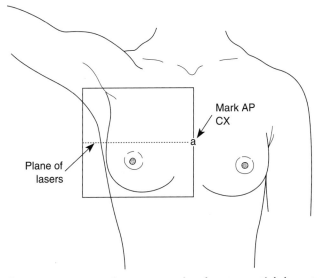

Figure 35-13. Anterior setup point for tangential breast fields.

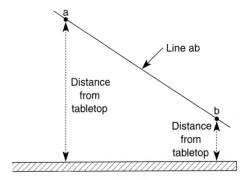

Figure 35-14. Line ab, which is equal in length to the oblique separation at the deep (coplanar) edge of the tangential fields.

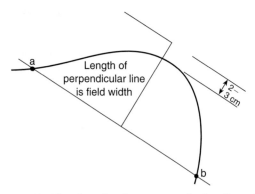

Figure 35-15. The length of a perpendicular line, drawn from the midpoint of line *ab*, and extending approximately 2 to 3 cm above the apex of the breast, is the field width.

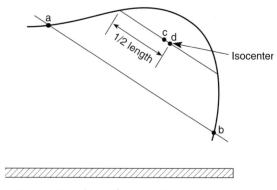

Figure 35-17. Based on the anterior setup point, vertical and horizontal table shifts are determined with reference to point *d*.

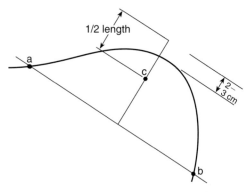

Figure 35-16. A line is drawn parallel to line *ab* through point *c*.

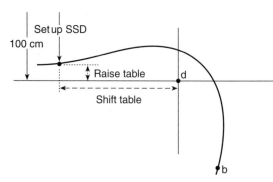

Figure 35-18. Based on the anterior setup point, vertical and horizontal table shifts are determined with reference to point *d*.

8. Trace the contour outline onto the paper, taking care to align points a and b of the contour material with points a and b on the graph paper.

9. Draw a perpendicular line from the midpoint of line ab, extending approximately 2 cm above the apex of the breast. This 2-cm extension allows for flash of the tangential field and accommodates tissue swelling during treatment. The length of the perpendicular line equals the field width (Fig. 35-15).

10. Measure the perpendicular line, and mark point c at the midpoint.

11. Draw a line parallel to ab, through point c (Fig. 35-16).

12. Mark point d on the parallel line at the midpoint between the contour of the medial and lateral skin surfaces. Point d is the isocenter of the tangential fields (Fig. 35-17).

13. The horizontal distance between point a (the anterior setup point) and point d (the isocenter) is the distance the table is shifted laterally (Fig. 35-18).

14. The vertical distance between point a and point d is subtracted from the SAD (100 or 80 cm) and is the setup SSD.

15. Align the patient to the anterior setup point. Apply the vertical and horizontal adjustments from steps 13 and 14 by shifting the table.

16. Place lead markers on the medial and lateral field borders, as marked on the patient.

17. To align the medial tangent field, rotate the gantry via fluoroscopy until the two lead markers are superimposed (coplanar). There should be 1 to 3 cm of lung in the field.

18. Rotate the collimator so that the medial field edge is parallel to the chest wall. Image this field (Fig. 35-19).

19. To align the lateral tangent field, rotate the gantry approximately 180 degrees, and confirm via fluoroscopy that the two lead markers are superimposed (coplanar). Adjustment of the gantry may be necessary to obtain superimposition. There should be 1 to 3 cm of lung in the field. Rotate the collimator the same number of degrees in the opposite direction of that used in step 18. Image this field (Fig. 35-20).

20. The amount of lung included in the tangential fields should be carefully considered. If insufficient lung is in the field, adjust the lateral border in a posterior direction (if clinically allowable). If there is too much lung, move the lateral border anteriorly (if clinically allowable). It may also be possible to adjust the medial border, depending on the location of the lesion. If adjustments are necessary, return to step 3 and continue.

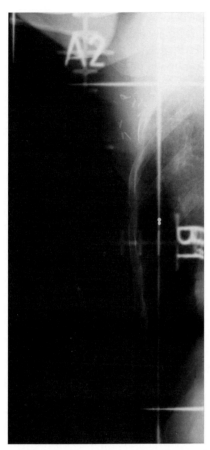

Figure 35-19. Simulation radiograph of the medial tangential field.

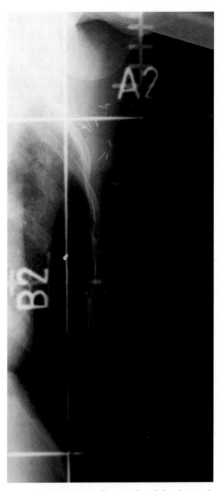

Figure 35-20. Simulation radiograph of the lateral tangential field.

21. Mark the setup points and field borders on the patient for accurate realignment of the fields for treatment.
22. Complete the setup documentation form.

Computerized treatment planning of the tangential field pair is necessary to visualize the dose distribution throughout the treatment volume. Based on the isodose plot, a decision is made regarding the use of wedges to improve dose homogeneity. In the conservatively managed patient, it may be advantageous to obtain computer-generated isodose plots in up to three planes (one at the central ray or widest part of the breast and one each closer to the superior and inferior field margins). This assists in evaluating dose variation in the breast as a result of the changing contour. Skin doses are adequate because of their inherent reduction from tangentially configured radiation beams; therefore bolus is not usually required.

Comprehensive breast or chest wall and peripheral lymphatics-treatment technique. One critical aspect of comprehensive irradiation for breast cancer is the avoidance of junctional inconsistency between the peripheral lymphatic fields (i.e., supraclavicular-axillary and tangential fields). If overlap occurs, hot or overdosed areas result from a combination of divergence and geometrical distortion of the radia-

tion beams. Such excess dose can lead to match-line fibrosis and a poor cosmetic result. Conversely, a cold or underdosed area provides the potential for tumor recurrence. Avoidance of junctional irregularities can be achieved through the establishment of a vertical straight edge in the axial plane, perpendicular to the floor where the fields meet.

Supraclavicular field. When used, the supraclavicular field is planned before the tangential fields. Considerations for field margins for the supraclavicular field are as follows:
Superior
- Approximately 5 cm above the suprasternal notch (SSN)
- Avoidance of flash over the skin of the supraclavicular area
Medial
- Midpoint of the SSN
Lateral
- Approximately 2 to 3 cm of the humeral head
Inferior, at one of the following:
- Approximately at the angle of Louis
- Just above the superior extent of the palpable breast tissue
- A point >2 cm cephalad to the original location of the mass
The central ray of the supraclavicular field is placed at the

inferior margin of the volume to be treated. The inferior half of the beam is blocked by multileaf collimation, an asymmetrical jaw, or a suspended block, creating a vertical straight edge at the inferior border of the supraclavicular field. The gantry is angled 10 to 15 degrees mediolaterally to avoid exiting through the spinal cord. A simulation film of the supraclavicular field is provided in Fig. 35-21.

Posterior axillary boost field. A posterior axillary boost (PAB) field is sometimes used to increase the midaxillary dose to the prescribed level in a subset of patients who have not had dissection of the level III lymph nodes. This is done because at midplane the radiation dose from an anterior supraclavicular field alone may be insufficient. A simulation film of the PAB field is provided in Fig. 35-22.

The PAB field should be parallel opposed to the supraclavicular field and uses the identical inferior margin, preserving the vertical straight edge. Considerations for field margins of the PAB field are as follows:

Superior
■ Mid- to upper-clavicle

Medial
■ A strip of lung approximately 1 cm wide

Lateral
■ Approximately 1 to 2 cm of the humeral head, which is subsequently blocked

Inferior
■ Corresponding to the inferior border of the supraclavicular field

Its relatively small total dose notwithstanding, the PAB should be treated with the same fractionation scheme as the supraclavicular field. Considering larger boost fractions (about 1.8 or 2.0 Gy delivered over a few days) may be tempting; however, this dose must be considered as additive to that being delivered via the supraclavicular field, and a large boost fraction would result in an extremely large daily dose to the PAB site.

Tangential breast or chest wall fields. The tangential photon fields in comprehensive irradiation for breast cancer are planned in the same way as those described in the section on tangential breast or chest wall irradiation, with several notable additions necessary for an appropriate junction with the supraclavicular-axillary fields. To establish a vertical straight edge at the superior border of the tangential fields, correction must be made for the divergence of the tangential fields into the supraclavicular-axillary field and for geometrical distortion of the radiation beam. The couch assembly is rotated in such a way that the patient's feet are directed away from the collimator and a block is placed at the superior edges of the tangential fields. This is done to force correspondence to the vertical straight edge created by the inferior border of the supraclavicular-axillary field pair. The exact location of the block can be determined by placing a rod with a dependent chain on the patient's skin at the level of the supraclavicular field's inferior border. Steps in comprehensive breast irradiation are as follows:

1. After imaging the supraclavicular-axillary fields, follow steps 1 through 17 of the previously described tangential technique with some modification. A device composed of a metal rod with an attached chain is used to help define the inferior border of the supraclavicular-axillary field. The metal rod is taped to the patient's skin at the level of the inferior border of the supraclavicular-axillary field, allowing the dependent chain to hang freely over the patient's side. In step 1, add approximately 3 cm to the superior edge of the tangential

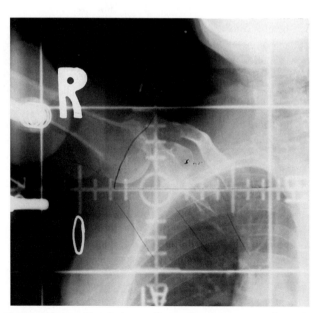

Figure 35-21. Simulation radiograph of the supraclavicular field.

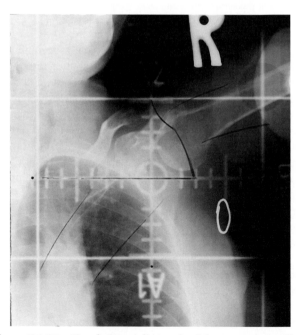

Figure 35-22. Simulation radiograph of the posterior axillary boost field.

field. This overlap into the supraclavicular field will be blocked for treatment.

2. Rotate the collimator so that the medial field edge is parallel to the chest wall.
3. Rotate the couch until fluoroscopic images of the rod and chain are superimposed. Film this field (Fig. 35-23).
4. To align the lateral tangent field, rotate the gantry approximately 180 degrees, and confirm via fluoroscopy that the two lead markers are superimposed (coplanar). Adjustment of the gantry angle may be necessary to obtain superimposition. There should be 1 to 3 cm of lung in the field (Fig. 35-24). Rotate the collimator the same number of degrees in the opposite direction of that used in step 2.
5. Mark the edge of the lateral tangential light field on the patient's skin.
6. Rotate the couch in the opposite direction from that in step 3 until fluoroscopic images of the rod and chain are superimposed.
7. Readjust the gantry and collimator angles to match the line marked on the patient in step 5.
8. Verify superimposition of the medial field edge markers and the rod and chain via fluoroscopy. Image this field.
9. Mark the setup points and field borders on the patient for accurate realignment of the fields for treatment.
10. Complete a setup documentation form.

Internal mammary lymph nodes. A relatively small proportion of patients with breast cancer may be at risk for involvement of the IM lymph nodes.[17,38] Whether to irradiate the IM nodes remains controversial, partly because current techniques are potentially damaging to normal tissues. One method of irradiating the IM nodes is the extended or deep tangential field configuration. Rather than placing the edge of the medial tangential field at the patient's midline, the field is extended beyond the midline to the contralateral side by approximately 3 cm. Although this arrangement is usually successful in encompassing the ipsilateral IM nodes, it results in a significant increase in the volume of lung irradiated. The extended tangential field also encroaches on the contralateral breast tissue, causing an increase in scattered dose to the breast. Furthermore, in the treatment of left-sided lesions, a fairly large portion of the heart is often included in the extended tangential field.

An alternative method of irradiating the IM nodes involves the use of an en face (perpendicular to the skin surface) IM field with a combination of electrons and photons. This field arrangement is subject to the difficulties of matching en face and tangential fields, as well as the problems of joining photon and electron ports, and may result in a hot or cold spot at the junctional area. In addition, an increased

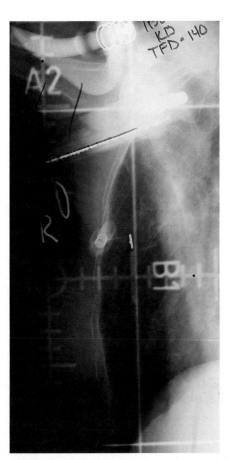

Figure 35-23. Simulation radiograph of the medial tangential field, illustrating the use of the rod and chain.

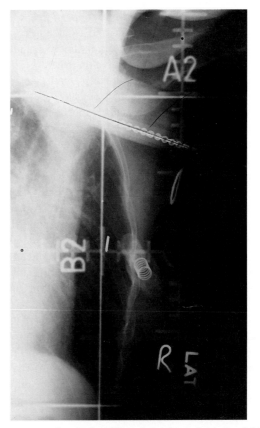

Figure 35-24. Simulation film of the lateral tangential field, illustrating the use of the rod and chain.

volume of cardiac tissue is included in the en face configuration. The photon portion of the IM node treatment contributes exit dose to the vertebral bodies and spinal cord. Conversely, if electrons are used for most or all of the IM treatment, the skin dose may be unacceptably high, contributing to acute and chronic sequelae and potentially a less acceptable cosmetic result.

Breast boost. Patients with conservatively managed breast cancer usually receive additional radiation treatment to the tumor bed immediately after the completion of tangential irradiation. This boost may be delivered with electron teletherapy or radioactive implantation. Electrons are the technique of choice at most institutions because of patient convenience, cost, and cosmetic considerations. In planning the electron boost, care must be taken to ensure that the treatment volume adequately encompasses the tumor bed. The assumption that the location and length of the scar accurately reflect the position and size of the tumor bed may be inaccurate.[2,29,35] If the surgeon places clips on the tumor bed at the time of resection, then the position and size of the electron field can be optimized via fluoroscopy and/or radiographs obtained in the simulator room.

Occasionally, the tumor-bed boost is delivered via radioactive implantation. Potential indications for this method include the presence of a gross residual tumor at the time of resection, a deep-seated lesion in an extremely large breast, and rarely, patient preference. Because implantation is invasive, relatively expensive, and labor intensive, and because it requires anesthesia and sometimes inpatient admission, current practice does not routinely include boosting the tumor bed with a radioactive implant.

Special problems. Occasionally, patients requiring radiation therapy for breast malignancy have special circumstances that render planning and treatment difficult. These include a lack of arm mobility, extreme breast size, and very pendulous breasts.

Lack of arm mobility. When planned appropriately in terms of energy selection, field placement, and junction considerations, electron beams offer a viable method of treating postmastectomy patients who have severely compromised arm mobility, as in instances of brachial plexopathy. Because electron fields are treated en face as opposed to tangentially, the problem of avoiding the patient's arm is circumvented. The ideal candidate for this technique has a relatively flat chest wall of uniform thickness. The patient's arm can rest on the treatment table, at her side, and in as abducted a position as the patient can manage. Typically, a minimum of two electron fields are used to encompass the chest wall margins listed previously. One field treats the anterior-medial chest wall, and the other covers the lateral chest wall. The precise matching of adjacent electron field edges can be difficult, so care must be taken to shift the match-line or use junctional wedges or some other means of enhancing dose uniformity where the fields meet.

Some postoperative patients are completely unable to

abduct the arm, usually as a result of advanced disease. These individuals can be treated with their arm in an abducted position through the use of an anterior photon field that encompasses the supraclavicular, axillary, and lateral chest wall regions in a single field. The anterior chest wall can be treated with an en face electron field.

Extreme breast size and pendulous breasts. Patients with extremely large and/or pendulous breasts are particularly challenging to treat. Numerous devices and techniques have been developed to stabilize the breast and position it on the chest, permitting a reasonably accurate setup and treatment. Elastic netting can be placed over the breasts; however, this works best on smaller breasts because the material is not strong enough to support an extremely large breast on the chest wall. Systems that use thermoplastic materials to mold the breast into an appropriate position are available commercially. Thermoplastic sheets may also be molded to the patient and fastened around the patient's back with bandage material. A simple ring can be placed around the breast to immobilize and retain the breast in position on the anterior chest.[3] A Styrofoam crutch can also be fashioned and positioned to support pendulous breast tissue located far to the patient's lateral chest.

Side effects. The aim of radiation therapy to the breast is the complete eradication of tumor cells with minimal structural and functional damage to normal tissue. A compromise of accepting a certain degree of acute and chronic tissue damage in return for a potential cure is necessary. In every situation, careful planning and treatment delivery are essential to minimize side effects.

Combining radiation treatment and chemotherapy may intensify toxicity. In breast cancer patients, the use of doxorubicin is of particular concern. When used concomitantly, radiation and doxorubicin may be hazardous. If doxorubicin is given after radiation therapy, then a recall phenomenon may occur in previously treated areas, displayed by exacerbation of reactions of the esophagus, skin, lungs, and heart.

Skin changes. Skin and subcutaneous tissue changes are expected in the irradiated treatment volume. The skin dose depends on the exact treatment technique used for each patient. Variables in the treatment plan that affect the skin dose include the type of radiation (photons or electrons), beam energy, boost technique (external beam or brachytherapy), wedge, bolus, fraction size, total dose, and physical conformation of the patient.

Special consideration must be given to the physical conformation of the patient. Skin folds tend to intensify skin reactions as a result of bolus effect and are therefore the most sensitive areas. Proper positioning is necessary to help minimize folds in potential problem areas. Axillary folds may be minimized by adjusting arm abduction. Skin folds in the inframammary, supraclavicular, and neck areas may be altered or eliminated by increasing or decreasing the cephalocaudad incline of the patient. Obese patients or those with large, pendulous breasts may require netting or thermoplastic material for the immobilization and reduction of skin folds.

During a standard radiation treatment schedule, skin reaction intensifies according to the escalating dose. The RTOG categorizes acute and chronic skin reactions, as shown in Tables 35-1 and 35-2. Dryness and redness (erythema) of the skin are common after a skin dose of about 3000 cGy (3 to 4 weeks into treatment). Dry desquamation, which involves flaking of superficial layers of the epidermis, may appear after the delivery of about 4000 cGy to the skin. Moist desquamation, involving the loss of superficial and deep epidermal layers, occurs when doses to the skin exceed 5000 cGy. Moist desquamation may arise earlier in treatment in areas where skin folds or bolus intensify the prescribed dose. Treatment of the large breast is more difficult secondary to such acute effects and can result in a less acceptable cosmetic outcome.

Care of irradiated skin varies according to the type and severity of the reaction. Patients should be advised regarding measures that protect the skin from further irritation and damage. The treatment area must be kept clean through normal, gentle cleansing, and sun exposure should be avoided. Cornstarch is often recommended as a soothing agent for early skin reactions and as a substitute for commercial deodorant. The use of lotions, creams, deodorants, or powders in the treatment area should be discouraged because they may contain irritating agents such as perfumes, alcohol, or metals. Shaving under the arm is not recommended, and clothing should be soft and loose fitting. Extreme temperatures from hot water bottles, heating pads, and ice packs should also be avoided over the skin of the treated area.

Patients experiencing moist desquamation may require daily skin care to help prevent infection and minimize fluid loss. Gentle cleansing may be performed with a solution of hydrogen peroxide diluted by sterile water and dabbed carefully onto the affected area. Proper wound dressing using nonstick bandaging techniques is essential to promote healing. Care must be taken to avoid placing bandage adhesives or tape in the treatment area. Cornstarch should never be used in areas of moist desquamation because it may promote fungal growth and increase the risk of wound infection.[21]

Severe acute reactions may result in a longer healing time and higher incidence of chronic skin changes. Such skin changes progress slowly and can persist for months or years after irradiation. Most chronic skin changes are cosmetic and rarely problematic, and they include hyperpigmentation (excessive coloration), hair loss, epidermal thinning, **telangiectasia** (permanent dilation of vessels, producing small, red lesions), and subcutaneous fibrosis. Rare cases of delayed wound healing, ulceration, and **necrosis** (death of skin cells) may occur after skin doses of over 70 Gy.[15]

Fatigue. Most patients receiving radiation therapy complain of generalized fatigue. The incidence appears to be related to the radiation dose, treatment volume, and site of involvement. Breast cancer patients may experience a comparatively minor degree of fatigue. Other factors (such as a history of recent surgery or chemotherapy, the patient's general medical and psychologic condition, current medications, pain, or anemia) may contribute to fatigue.

Cardiac effects. Portions of the heart are sometimes necessarily included in the radiation fields used in breast cancer treatment. Tangential fields used to treat the left chest wall may include a small to moderate volume of the heart, depending on the patient's anatomy and physical configuration. A larger volume of the heart may be included during irradiation of the IM lymph nodes. Although the myocardia (heart muscle) is relatively radioresistant, the risk of promoting arteriosclerosis, leading to pericarditis, is of concern. The incidence of pericarditis is less than 5% for small heart volumes treated to 60 Gy with standard fractionation or for large heart volumes treated to 40 Gy.[6,15] In addition, larger fraction sizes may intensify cardiac damage.

Pulmonary effects. Tangential fields used to irradiate the breast and/or chest wall always include a small volume of lung tissue. Peripheral lymphatic fields may also irradiate lung tissue. Some degree of **radiation pneumonitis** (inflammation of the lung tissue) and fibrosis can be expected after the administration of more than 2500 cGy to any portion of lung via standard fractionation.[27] These effects are directly related to the total dose, fraction size, and irradiated lung volume. The incidence of pulmonary damage grows as the volume, dose, and fraction size increase. The time of onset and degree of severity also vary depending on the volume, dose, and fraction size of lung irradiated.

Although initial morphologic changes are not clinically manifested, symptoms may appear after a latent period of 1 to 3 months.[27] These symptoms may include coughing, dyspnea, sputum production, fever, and night sweats and may subside after several months. Scarring or fibrosis may begin 3 to 7 months after irradiation, and depending on its severity, chronic respiratory distress may develop. The degree of severity can be monitored via a chest radiograph, CT scan, and pulmonary function tests. Fortunately, the incidence of chronic pulmonary effects is rare in breast cancer patients because of the small volume of lung irradiated.

Lymphedema. Lymphedema of the arm may occur as a result of axillary lymphatic obstruction. Some acute lymphedema usually occurs immediately after breast surgery and axillary dissection. The severity and risk of lymphedema are directly related to the extent of the axillary dissection and may be further complicated by radiation and chemotherapy. Approximately 25% to 30% of patients receiving radiation therapy after level III axillary lymph node dissection experience arm edema. Tumor infiltration, infection, inflammation, scarring of the lymph nodes, and radiation-induced fibrosis (alone or in combination) may cause lymphatic obstruction. If a collateral circulatory pathway develops in response to the obstruction, allowing for lymphatic drainage, then the edema will resolve. Where the obstruction is severe or the damage is irreparable, lymphatic circulation may be permanently compromised, resulting in chronic edema of the arm.

Radiation-induced lymphedema is relatively rare and similar to other chronic effects in that the incidence and severity are directly related to the radiation dose and treatment volume. Depending on the degree of edema, this condition may be disfiguring and uncomfortable and may impair mobility and function of the arm.

Brachial plexopathy. The brachial plexus (a network of nerves supplying the upper extremities) originates between C5 and T1 and extends downward over the first rib, behind the middle of the clavicle, and into the axilla. Damage to these nerves in the form of fibrosis is termed brachial plexopathy. High doses of radiation (5500 to 6000 cGy) may lead to this condition.[3,21] Fortunately, standard dose levels prescribed for breast cancer treatment do not exceed 4500 to 5400 cGy and rarely result in this complication. The incidence of brachial plexopathy may also be related to surgery and chemotherapy. Symptoms include a loss of motor function (paresthesia of the arm and hand), weakness, and pain, for which the only treatment is symptomatic pain relief.

Myelopathy. Although the spine is usually avoided entirely during breast irradiation, portions of the cervical and thoracic spine may need to be included in the IM and supraclavicular fields. Care must be taken not to exceed the spinal cord's tolerance dose to avoid delayed complications of chronic progressive myelopathy (ranging from severe to fatal). The TD 5/5 (minimal tolerance dose) is 4500 to 5000 cGy for instances in which portions of the spinal cord are irradiated with standard fractionation.[3,15]

The supraclavicular field may be angled 10 to 15 degrees mediolaterally to avoid the spinal cord completely. The IM chain field may be treated via expanded tangential fields that entirely avoid the spinal cord or with a combination of en face photons and electrons to reduce the spinal cord dosage. Any adjoining of fields over the spinal cord must be planned carefully to avoid overlap, which can result in an overdose of radiation to the spinal cord.

Osteoradionecrosis. Tangential treatment fields of the chest wall may incidentally deliver a relatively high dose of radiation to the ribs. The incidence of a resulting rib fracture is relatively low (less than 1%), and the ribs appear to heal on their own.

SUMMARY

Breast cancer represents an enigmatic yet fascinating challenge in cancer management. The incidence of breast cancer is widespread, and it is sometimes fatal, recurring sometimes two or three decades after the initial diagnosis and treatment. Breast cancer is especially important because it affects a part of the female anatomy that is functionally and culturally associated with beauty, femininity, sexuality, and nurturing. With recorded history dating back several millennia, the pendulum of breast cancer treatment has swung between extremes of belief that breast cancer is an incurable systemic disease and the notion that it is a local therefore curable prob-

lem. This debate continues today, with many researchers occupying a rational middle ground in which each patient is evaluated against the backdrop of multiple prospective and retrospective analyses to maximize survival potential.

Review Questions

1. The pathologic staging system for breast cancer incorporates which of the following?
   I.   Lymph node status
   II. Tumor extent
   III. Distant metastasis
   a. I and II
   b. II and III
   c. I and III
   d. I, II, and III
2. What is the most common presenting symptom of early-stage breast cancer?
   a. Nipple discharge
   b. Pain
   c. Palpable mass
   d. Ulceration
3. Which of the following is proper advice for a patient receiving radiation treatment to the breast?
   I.   Do not wear restrictive clothing
   II. Avoid using commercial deodorant
   III. Avoid sun exposure to the skin of the treated area
   a. I and II
   b. II and III
   c. I and III
   d. I, II, and III
4. To what does TD 5/5 refer?
   a. Minimal tolerance dose
   b. Maximum tolerance dose
   c. Tumor dose of 5 Gy in 5 days
   d. Tumor dose of 5 cGy in 5 days
5. What is the TD 5/5 for the spinal cord delivered through standard fractionation?
   a. 1500 cGy
   b. 3000 cGy
   c. 4500 cGy
   d. 6000 cGy
6. Which of the following is NOT currently a standard technique for breast surgery?
   a. Radical mastectomy
   b. Modified radical mastectomy
   c. Lumpectomy
   d. Tylectomy
7. Chemotherapy for breast cancer may consist of which of the following?
   I.   Drug therapy
   II. Endocrine therapy
   III. Immunotherapy

a. I and II
b. II and III
c. I and III
d. I, II, and III

8. In treating a breast cancer patient via tangential fields plus an electron field boost, what is the usual total dose to the tumor bed delivered through a standard fractionation schedule?
   a. 4000 to 4600 cGy
   b. 5000 to 5600 cGy
   c. 6000 to 6600 cGy
   d. 7000 to 7600 cGy

9. Which of the following techniques may be used to adequately irradiate the internal mammary lymph nodes on a patient with left breast cancer and simultaneously deliver the least cardiac dose?
   a. Anterior photon field, 50 Gy in 5 weeks
   b. Anterior photon-electron fields, equally weighted, 50 Gy in 5 weeks
   c. Wide tangential fields, extending 5 cm across the midline, 50 Gy in 5 weeks
   d. Anterior electron field, 50 Gy in 5 weeks

10. The skin usually reacts in a pattern that is dose dependent. Which of the following would you expect to see first for radiation administered using a standard fractionation schedule?
    a. Dry desquamation
    b. Erythema
    c. Moist desquamation
    d. Radiation pneumonitis

Questions to Ponder

1. Discuss the significant prognostic indicators for breast cancer.
2. Describe the signs of inflammatory breast cancer.
3. Describe the acute effects experienced by patients undergoing radiation treatment to the breast.
4. Define the three elements of treatment in conservative management of early-stage breast cancer.
5. Describe the field arrangements most commonly used for patients receiving conservative management of breast cancer.
6. Discuss important considerations for positioning the conservatively managed patient for breast irradiation.
7. Describe the methods for detection and diagnosis of breast cancer.
8. Identify the common presenting symptoms of breast cancer.
9. Discuss the importance of staging breast cancer.
10. Describe the primary lymphatic drainage of breast tissue.

REFERENCES

1. American Cancer Society: *Cancer facts and figures—2003,* Atlanta, 2003, American Cancer Society.
2. Bedwinek J: Breast conserving surgery and irradiation: the importance of demarcating the excision cavity with surgical clips, *Int J Radiat Oncol Biol Phys* 26:675-679, 1993.
3. Bentel GC, Nelson CE, Noell KT: *Treatment planning and dose calculation in radiation oncology,* ed 4, Elmsford, NY, 1989, Pergamon Press.
4. Boag JW, et al: The number of patients required in a clinical trial, *Br J Radiol* 44:122-125, 1971.
5. Boice JD, et al: Risk of breast cancer following low dose radiation exposure, *Radiology* 131:589-597, 1979.
6. Byhardt RW, Moss WT: The heart and blood vessels. In Cox JD, editor: *Moss' radiation oncology rationale, technique, results,* ed 7, St. Louis, 1994, Mosby.
7. Carter C, Allen C, Henson D: Relation of tumor size, lymph node status, and survival in 24,740 breast cancer cases, *Cancer* 63:181-187, 1989.
8. Claus EB, et al: The genetic attributable risk of breast and ovarian cancer, *Cancer* 77:2318-2324, 1996.
9. Collaborative Group on Hormonal Factors in Breast Cancer: Breast cancer and hormonal contraceptives: collaborative reanalysis of individual data on 53,297 women with breast cancer and 100,239 women without breast cancer from 54 epidemiological studies, *Lancet* 347:1713-1727, 1996.
10. Collaborative Group on Hormonal Factors in Breast Cancer: Breast cancer and hormonal replacement therapy: collaborative reanalysis of individual data on 53,297 women with breast cancer and 100,239 women without breast cancer from 54 epidemiological studies, *Lancet* 350:1047-59, 1997.
11. Committee on the Biological Effects of Ionizing Radiations, Board on Radiation Effects Research, Commission on Life Sciences, National Research Council: *Health effects of exposure to low levels of ionizing radiation BEIR V,* Washington, DC, 1990, National Academy Press.
12. Cruikshank WC: *The anatomy of the absorbing vessels of the human body,* London, 1786, G. Nicol.
13. Cumberlin RL, Dritchilo A, Mossman KL: Carcinogenic effects of scattered dose associated with radiation therapy, *Int J Radiat Oncol Biol Phys* 17:623-629, 1989.
14. Donegan WL, Spratt JS: *Cancer of the breast,* ed 4, Philadelphia, 1995, WB Saunders.
15. Emami B, et al: Tolerance of normal tissue to therapeutic radiation, *Int J Radiat Oncol Biol Phys* 22:109-122, 1991.
16. Fisher B, et al: Location of breast carcinoma and prognosis, *Surg Gynecol Obstet* 129:705-716, 1969.
17. Fox MS: On the diagnosis and treatment of breast cancer, *JAMA* 241:489-494, 1979.
18. Goldhirsch A, Gelber RD: Understanding adjuvant chemotherapy for breast cancer, *N Engl J Med* 330:1308-1309, 1994.
19. Haagensen CD: *Diseases of the breast,* ed 3, Philadelphia, 1986, WB Saunders.
20. Harris JR, et al: *Diseases of the breast,* ed 2, Philadelphia, 2000, Lippincott Williams & Wilkins.
21. Hassey Dow K, Hilderley L: *Nursing care in radiation oncology,* ed 2, Philadelphia, 1997, WB Saunders.
22. Henderson IC: Adjuvant systemic therapy for early breast cancer, *Cancer Suppl* 74(1):401-408, 1994.
23. Henderson IC, Canellos GP: Cancer of the breast: the past decade, *N Engl J Med* 302:17-30, 1980.
24. Hunter DJ, et al: Cohort studies in fat intake and the risk of breast cancer: a pooled analysis, *N Engl J Med* 334:356-361, 1996.
25. John MJ, et al: *Chemoradiation: an integrated approach to cancer treatment,* Malvern, Pa, 1993, Lea & Febiger.
26. Kelsey JL: A review of the epidemiology of human breast cancer, *Epidemiol Rev* 1:74-109, 1979.
27. Komaki R, Cox JD: The lung and thymus. In Cox JD, editor: *Moss'*

radiation oncology: rationale, technique, results, ed 7, St. Louis, 1994, Mosby.

28. Mascagni P: *Vasorum lymphaticorum corporis humani historia et ichnographia,* Siena, Italy, 1787, P. Carli.
29. Regine WF, et al: Computer-CT planning of the electron boost in definitive breast irradiation, *Int J Radiat Oncol Biol Phys* 20:121-125, 1991.
30. Ries LAB, et al., editors: *SEER cancer statistics review, 1973-1998,* Bethesda, Md, 2001, National Cancer Institute.
31. Rosen PP, et al: Discontinuous or "skip" metastases in breast carcinoma: analysis of 1228 axillary dissections, *Ann Surg* 276-283, 1983.
32. Saphillo O, Parker MI: Metastases of primary carcinoma of the breast with special reference to spleen, adrenal glands and ovaries, *Arch Surg* 42:1003, 1941.
33. Schottenfeld D, et al: Ten-year results of the treatment of primary operable breast carcinoma, *Cancer* 38:1005, 1976.
34. Shinkin MB: *Contrary to nature,* Washington, DC, 1977, United States Printing Office.
35. Solin LJ, et al: A practical technique for the localization of the tumor volume in definitive irradiation of the breast, *Int J Radiat Oncol Biol Phys* 11:1215-1220, 1985.
36. Veronesi U, et al: Prognosis of breast cancer patients after mastectomy and dissection of internal mammary nodes, *Ann Surg* 202:702-707, 1985.
37. Veronesi U, et al: Distribution of axillary node metastases by level of invasion: an analysis of 539 cases, *Cancer* 59:682-687, 1987.
38. Warren S, Wittman EM: Studies on tumor metastases: the distribution of metastases in cancer of the breast, *Surg Gynecol Obstet* 57:81, 1937.
39. Wilson JF: The breast. In Cox JD, editor: *Moss' radiation oncology: rationale, technique, results,* ed 7, St. Louis, 1994, Mosby.
40. Winer EP, et al: Cancer of the breast. In DeVita VT, Hellman S, Rosenberg SA, editors: *Cancer principles and practice of oncology,* ed 6, Philadelphia, 2001, Lippincott Williams & Wilkins.
41. Wise L, Johnson H: *Breast cancer: controversies in management,* Armonk, NY, 1994, Futura Publishing.

BIBLIOGRAPHY

Bentel GC, Marks LB: A simple device to position large/flaccid breasts during tangential breast irradiation, *Int J Radiat Oncol Biol Phys* 29:879-882, 1994.

Breasted JH: *The Edwin Smith surgical papyrus,* Chicago, 1930, University of Chicago Press.

Cox JD, Winchester DP, editors: Standards for breast conservation treatment. Adopted by the Board of Chancellors, American College of Radiology, and endorsed by the Board of Regents, American College of Surgeons, *CA Cancer J Clin* 42(3):134-162, 1992.

Fowble B, et al: Frequency, sites of relapse, and outcome of regional node failures following conservative surgery and radiation for early breast cancer, *Int J Radiat Oncol Biol Phys* 17:703-710, 1989.

Halsted WS: The results of operations for the cure of cancer of the breast performed at Johns Hopkins Hospital from June 1889 to January 1894, *Johns Hopkins Hosp Bull* 4:297, 1894-1895.

Hanke BF, Steinhorn SC: Long term patient survival for some of the more frequently occurring cancers, *Cancer* 50:1904-1912, 1982.

Harness JK, et al: *Breast cancer, collaborative management,* Chelsea, Mich, 1988, Lewis Publishers.

Harris JR, Hellman S: Observations on survival curve analysis with particular reference to breast cancer treatment, *Cancer* 57:925-928, 1986.

Lichter AS, et al: A technique for field matching in primary breast irradiation, *Int J Radiat Oncol Biol Phys* 9:263-270, 1982.

Rosenow UF, Valentine ES, Davis LW: A technique for treating local breast cancer using a single set-up point and asymmetric collimation, *Int J Radiat Oncol Biol Phys* 19:183-188, 1990.

Siddon RL, et al: Three field technique for breast irradiation using tangential field corner blocks, *Int J Radiat Oncol Biol Phys* 9:583-588, 1983.

Svensson GK, et al: A modified three-field technique for breast treatment, *Int J Radiat Oncol Biol Phys* 6:689-694, 1980.

Veronesi U, Vallagussa P: Inefficacy of internal mammary node dissection in breast cancer surgery, *Cancer* 47:170-175, 1981.

Pediatric Solid Tumors

Jeffrey Young

Outline

Key Terms

Alopecia
Astrocytomas
Craniospinal irradiation (CSI)
Ependymomas
Germ cell tumors
Histiocytosis X
Medulloblastoma
Neuroblastoma

Oncogene
Palliation
Residua
Retinoblastoma
Rhabdomyosarcomas
Second malignant neoplasm
  (SMN)
Wilms' tumor

Although older groups dominate the patient population of radiation oncology centers, childhood cancer (age 14 or younger) is a significant problem. An estimated 9000 new cases are expected to occur each year among children aged 0 to 14. An estimated 1500 deaths are expected annually, about one third of them from leukemia.[3] The treatments, cure rates, and types of cancers that develop in children are distinctively different than those of the adult population (Table 36-1). Predisposing genetic conditions include xeroderma pigmentosa, ataxia telangiectasia, Bloom and Fanconi's syndromes, neurofibromatosis, and gene abnormalities such as *p53*.[33] Cytogenetic and molecular markers that correlate to prognosis are being increasingly identified, which allow treatment intensity stratification. Acute leukemias and lymphomas account for about 40% of pediatric cancers. Central nervous system (CNS) tumors are the most frequent solid tumors, and radiation has a critical role in their treatment. Although a shift toward other effective therapies has taken place, radiation is still involved with patients who have soft tissue sarcoma, Wilms' tumor, neuroblastoma, and other benign and malignant conditions.

The treatment of childhood malignancies is always multidisciplinary and requires close attention to the physical and emotional needs of the child and family. Care is coordinated with medical, surgical, and nursing oncologic colleagues and supported from social services, physical therapists, nutritionists, educators, and others. This team approach usually requires referral to a specialized children's cancer program. (This is especially true outside the United States.) More than 50% of patients are involved in clinical trial investigations led by the Pediatric Oncology Group

Table 36-1	Cancer in Children	
Cancer Type	Percentage Occurring in Children	Predominant Age at Occurrence
Acute leukemia	31.0	2-8 years
Acute lymphoblastic leukemia	21.0	2 years, then stable
Other	10.0	2-18 years
Central nervous system	19.0	Varies with histology
Malignant lymphoma	8.0	Varies with type
Hodgkin's disease	6.0	Increases with age
Neuroblastoma	8.0	0-3 years
Wilms' tumor	6.0	< 5 years
Soft tissue sarcomas	5.0	< 5 years > 10-12 years
Bone sarcomas	5.0	Increases with age > 10 years
Retinoblastoma	2.5	0-2 years
Germ cell tumors	2.5	< 1 year; > 8-10 years
Liver tumors	2.5	4 years

From Cox JD, Ang KK: *Radiation oncology, rationale, technique, result,* St. Louis, 2003, Mosby.

Table 36-2	Relative incidence of brain tumors	
Type of Tumor		Percentage of Total
SUPRATENTORIAL (45%-50%)		
Low-grade astrocytoma		25
Anaplastic astrocytoma, glioblastoma, and PNET		10
Ependymoma		3
Pineal and germ cell tumors		4
Pituitary and craniopharyngioma		5
INFRATENTORIAL (50%-55%)		
Medulloblastoma		25
Low-grade astrocytoma		15
Ependymoma		5
Brainstem glioma		10

Data from Duffner PK, et al: Survival of children with brain tumors: SEER program, 1973-1980, *Neurology* 36:597-601, 1986.
PNET, Primitive neuroectodermal tumor.

(POG) and Children's Cancer Group (CCG) in the United States and Societe Internationale d'Oncologie Pediatrique (SIOP) in Europe. Therapists have special demands for such protocol patients, for example, data guidelines, ongoing chemotherapy, and anesthesia. Because many radiation therapists do not see pediatric patients, the remainder of this chapter highlights selected childhood cancers and their unique treatments.

BRAIN TUMORS

Epidemiology

CNS cancer cases annually involve a wide spectrum of lesions histologically and anatomically. In children (compared with adults) low-grade and infratentorial (posterior fossa) tumors are more frequent, metastatic lesions from non-CNS primaries are rare, and late effects of treatment are a major concern. Table 36-2 illustrates relative incidences from a combination of patient series. Neurofibromatosis is linked to risk of low-grade glioma, and retinoblastoma suppressor gene defects on chromosome 13 can be inherited, leading to a high risk of bilateral disease. However, most benign and high-grade tumors occur sporadically. Because the disease and its treatment can have major long-term side effects for children, individualized multidisciplinary care involving neurosurgery, endocrinology, pediatric and radiation oncology, rehabilitation, social work and other services is a must.

Low-grade Astrocytoma

Astrocytomas are tumors originating from the nonneuronal-supporting cells of the brain. These tumors can be histologically similar to normal glial cells but continue slow, relentless growth. They occur about equally in the cerebrum and posterior fossa. A long history of mild symptoms dependent on the area of brain involved is the usual course. Headaches, degenerating coordination, visual impairment, or poor school performance can worsen subtly for months or years, and seizures can eventually develop. Radiologically, a cystic component may be present, and there is less surrounding edema than with high-grade lesions (Fig. 36-1, *A*).

If discovered in an extremely young child without major neurologic deficits, a low-grade brain tumor can be followed with serial physical and radiologic examinations. After the child reaches an age at which the brain is more mature (usually 3 to 5 years old), neurosurgery is the primary treatment. If the lesion can be completely removed, the long-term prognosis is excellent. A recurrence-free survival rate of 90% to 100% has been achieved.[44] Although historically felt to be resistant, modern chemotherapy has induced responses in low-grade gliomas allowing delay and, rarely, avoidance of radiation.

Radiation therapy has been reserved for surgically inaccessible or recurrent lesions and those with postsurgical **residua** (pertaining to the portion that remains after the surgical procedure that removed the bulk of the tumor). A dose of 5000 to 5500 cGy at 180 cGy per day is routinely used. Because infiltration of surrounding brain is limited, only a 2-cm margin around the lesion is necessary. Radiation has enhanced the long-term control of residual tumors in most series,[4] but progression may occur years later. Stereotactic

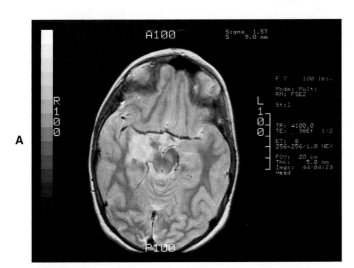
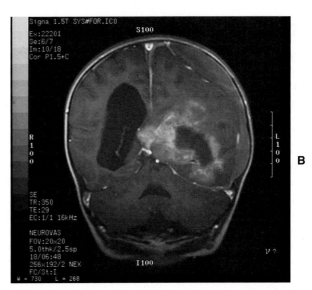

Figure 36-1. A, Low-grade astrocytoma. Note the regular border and minimal edema. **B,** Glioblastoma multiforme. Invasive borders, edema, and shift of normal structures.

radiosurgery and three-dimensional (3D) conformal and intensity modulated radiation therapy (IMRT) treatment have been used for focal lesions.

High-grade Astrocytoma

In contrast to their low-grade counterparts, high-grade astrocytomas definitely behave malignantly. They grow rapidly, invade and destroy adjacent brain tissues, and can spread through the CNS or distantly. Neuropathologists commonly classify high-grade gliomas in order of escalating malignancy as anaplastic astrocytoma, glioblastoma multiforme, and malignant primitive neuroectodermal tumor (PNET). High-grade gliomas are usually supratentorial, with neurologic symptoms progressing quickly. Headaches and lethargy are followed by motor or sensory loss, seizures, and intracranial hemorrhage. Radiologically, these lesions have indistinct borders, areas of necrosis, and much surrounding edema (Fig. 36-1, *B*). Steroids are used to reduce edema before surgery. Staging has been proposed according to tumor size, ventricle or brainstem invasion, and metastases; however, staging is not routinely used.

Neurosurgery is the important first step of multidisciplinary treatment for high-grade brain tumors. Surgery yields the histologic diagnosis, removes the gross tumor, and decompresses adjacent structures, but residual tumor invariably remains. Chemotherapy and radiation are standardly used postoperatively. The optimal sequencing is still uncertain, but cooperative research groups have demonstrated improvements in survival rates with various combinations.[18] Chemotherapy is especially vital in infants to delay the need for radiation while the brain matures, which reduces late sequelae.

The radiation technique requires large fields. Anaplastic astrocytomas may be treated with a margin of 3 cm or more.

Glioblastoma and PNET usually receive whole-brain radiation therapy to a dose of 3000 cGy or more, followed by a tumor boost of 6000 cGy and higher. Because of the occasional occurrence of cerebrospinal fluid (CSF) seeding, some pediatric radiation oncologists recommend **craniospinal irradiation (CSI)** initially. CSI involves irradiation of all CNS and CSF regions from behind the eye down to the midsacrum. The overall prognosis is poor, even with aggressive treatment. Neither hyperfractionated radiation to over 7000 cGy nor high-dose chemotherapy with stem cell transplant have made a major impact on cure. The survival rate at 5 years is 20% to 35% in many series.[21] Local control is still a major problem.

Optic Glioma

Optic tract and hypothalamic gliomas are usually extremely low-grade astrocytomas and some authors argue they are benign. Children with neurofibromatosis are at a much higher risk. Because visual and hormonal functions can be impaired, they frequently require treatment. The POG had a study with observation for asymptomatic patients. Those who progressed radiologically or developed symptoms received carboplatin chemotherapy or radiation. Potential bilateral, chiasmatic, and distal optic tract involvement must be considered during radiation therapy. In such instances larger tailored fields with about 2-cm margins are required, and the prognosis is worse. Long-term follow-up is required before any conclusions can be made about the treatment of this indolent disease.

Benign Tumors of the Central Nervous System

Pituitary adenomas usually occur in adolescents and adults but can also be seen in young children. These patients can have excessive hormone production, visual disturbance from pressure on the optic chiasm, or diabetes insipidus (DI). Transphenoidal hypophysectomy or medical management with bromocriptine used to counteract hormone production usually supplants radiation in the treatment of children. Localized radiation therapy with multiple fields or stereotactic radiation therapy with a dose of 4500 cGy can be given if other methods fail and can control more than 70% of tumors.[9]

Craniopharyngiomas arise from embryologic remnants of pharyngeal pouch tissues. These tumors eventually enlarge (usually with a prominent cystic component) and disrupt the hypothalamic pituitary axis (DI or precocious puberty), impair vision, or induce seizures. Surgery and focal radiation can be effective with the goal of reducing visual or late side effects. External radiation portals and doses are similar to those for pituitary adenomas. Because subsequent panhypopituitarism almost always develops, a pediatric endocrinologist must be included on the management team for these patients. Some physicians have injected radionuclides into the cysts, with good results in selected patients.[56] Meningiomas and acoustic neuromas are histologically benign lesions that occur far more often in patients who have neurofibromatosis. These lessons are treated by observation or surgery if they progress and cause neurologic symptoms. Arteriovenous malformations in surgically difficult regions were treated with proton beam therapy many years ago. Now they are the predominant lesions treated in some stereotactic radiosurgery programs. Usually 1500 to 2000 cGy is delivered in a single fraction, with control of potentially deadly rebleeding in 80% of patients.[22]

Medulloblastoma

Epidemiology.   **Medulloblastoma** is the prototype posterior fossa malignancy and constitutes about 25% of all childhood brain tumors. It usually occurs in children 2 to 12 years old, with a peak at 5 years.[10] It rarely occurs in adults. Medulloblastoma is believed to arise from primitive neuroepithelial cells and histologically appears as small, round, blue cells forming pseudorosettes.[48] The tumor usually arises in the midline of the cerebellum, can invade the fourth ventricle and brainstem, and has a high propensity to spread throughout the CSF.

Diagnosis and staging.   The presenting symptoms of medulloblastoma usually occur over a period of weeks to a few months. Several symptoms develop as a result of the invasion and compression of the fourth ventricle, thus stopping the inferior flow of CSF with resultant hydrocephalus. Headaches and early-morning vomiting occur intermittently at first and then become more steady. Later findings are ataxia and cranial nerve abnormalities from invasion of the brainstem. Computed tomography (CT) and magnetic resonance imaging (MRI) scans show a round, central cerebellar-enhancing mass (Fig. 36-2), and hydrocephalus is often noted. Steroids and a ventriculostomy can be used to reduce

pressure in the acute situation. Because of the propensity for CSF seeding, imaging the entire CNS via myelography or MRI is important. Supratentorial and spinal cord drop metastases can be present in up to 25% of patients.[14] CSF cytology for tumor cells can be performed from a ventriculostomy or lumbar puncture preoperatively.

Chang et al[8] initially developed a staging system at Columbia University that related to tumor size, invasion of the fourth ventricle and brainstem, and amount of CSF spread. With the known importance of surgical debulking, therapy is now based on residual tumor of greater than 1.5 cc and the extent of CSF or gross neuroaxis metastases. Medulloblastoma is one CNS tumor that can develop distant metastases, usually in bone. The intense, technical multidisciplinary therapy necessary for medulloblastomas must be performed in a center with pediatric cancer expertise.

Treatment techniques.   After the patient is stabilized neurologically, every attempt should be made for neurosurgical removal of the gross tumor. A posterior occipital craniotomy is used. The purple, friable, bulging tumor is usually quickly evident. Although the central mass is removed easily, it is the anterior extent into the brainstem or into the cervical spinal cord inferiorly that often leads to residua. Most studies have demonstrated a survival benefit with gross total removal, but surgery is not curative. The routine use of ventriculoperitoneal (VP) shunts is discouraged because of the risk of tumor seeding into the peritoneal cavity.

The benefit of postoperative radiation therapy was documented by Patterson and Farr[45] as early as 1953. CSI is a technical challenge, and several methods have been used. The most common technique uses lateral-opposed fields for the brain and CSF spaces from the retroorbital space down through the midcervical cord. Careful shielding must be done

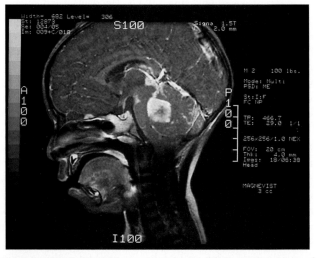

Figure 36-2. Magnetic resonance imaging (MRI) scan of medulloblastoma. Pressure on the brainstem and cerebrospinal fluid (CSF) obstruction are evident. Diffuse CFS seeding is present.

for the anterior globe, oropharynx, and neck. The treatment couch is angulated a few degrees to compensate for divergence over the spinal cord. The divergence of the spinal radiation field determines the collimator angle for the brain field. Depending on the height of the child, one or two posterior fields are used to encompass the spine down to the level of the second or third sacral segment. This technique is illustrated in Fig. 36-3.[52] Some centers have used electrons to treat the spinal cord, avoiding radiation exposure to anterior tissues; however, this requires precise physics and extensive tissue compensators. Usually, 4- to 6-MV x-rays are used for each field. Present physics recommendations are for a 0- to 0.5-cm gap between the spinal field and lateral brain fields. Usually, this junction and the one between the two spine fields in taller children are moved superiorly and inferiorly

1 cm daily or weekly. This prevents excessive dose gradients at the junctions with the potential for a spinal cord overdose or a cold spot that can allow tumor cells to survive. These children should be immobilized in a prone position unless doing so is deemed unsafe. Custom head holders or body cradles are helpful. Reproducible positioning of the head and careful marking of treatment portal edges are paramount. If sedation is needed, the anesthesia staff members may require some modifications of the previous technique for airway safety and monitoring equipment.

CSI can usually proceed at 150-180 cGy per day. Premedication for nausea is often needed because of the exit beam of the spinal field interacting with the gastrointestinal tract. Because of late sequelae, an attempt has been made to reduce the CSI dose or use chemotherapy as a substitute.

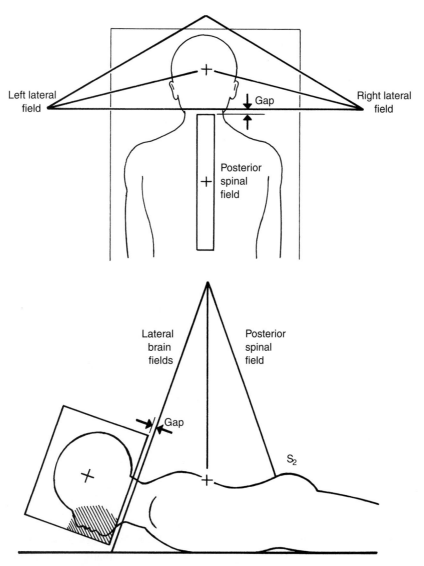

Figure 36-3. Radiation portal alignment for medulloblastoma. The brain portal collimator angle is adjusted for spinal field divergence. The junction gap is moved 1 cm daily or weekly.

However, in the United States a recent study by POG and CCG found increasing relapses outside the posterior fossa with a dose of 2340 cGy versus 3600 cGy.[54] Because the primary site of recurrence is still the posterior fossa, that region is boosted with lateral-opposed fields after CSI. This boost field should extend from the posterior clinoids to the back of the skull and from beyond the superior aspect of the tentorium (usually over halfway from the skull's base to its top) down to the level of C2. 3D treatment planning can avoid excessive doses to the cochlea and ear canals improving hearing. The daily fraction is usually 180 cGy per day up to a total of 5580 cGy. Dose response in earlier studies noted lower control rates with doses under 5000 cGy.[50] There are some proponents for radiosurgery to an even higher dose if gross residua is present. The entire radiation treatment course for medulloblastoma is 6 to 7 weeks, even without any treatment breaks that are possible due to surgical complications, low blood counts and infection, or gastrointestinal toxicity. In addition to weekly blood counts, nutrition must be carefully monitored in these children. The psychologic trauma of **alopecia** (hair loss) and a daily hospital trip are not insignificant. Despite the rigors of the treatment, the addition of radiation brought survival rates to more than 60%.[32]

Chemotherapy was initially used in relapsed patients, and some lasting responses were seen. Over the last few years cooperative research groups in Europe and the United States have added chemotherapy in a randomized fashion to standard surgery and radiation. In most studies a 10% to 20% benefit has been noted with chemotherapy, with most of the improvement in T3, T4, or M1 situations.[25] The sequencing of chemotherapy before or after radiation is still under evaluation. High-dose chemotherapy and stem cell transplant has salvaged some relapsed patients.

Ependymoma and Other Cerebrospinal Fluid Seeding Tumors

Ependymomas arise from the ventricular linings and can be cerebral or posterior fossa in location. CSF metastatic seeding is far more likely in infratentorial and anaplastic ependymomas. Although neuropathologists debate the grading of ependymomas, a definite relationship exists with higher rates of CSF seeding and primary tumor relapse in highly malignant histology lesions.[35] Staging of the entire brain and spinal cord is necessary. If CSF seeding is noted or high-risk histology exists, CSI with techniques similar to medulloblastoma are needed. Supratentorial and low-grade tumors can be treated with a 2- to 3-cm margin. Doses of about 5500 cGy to the primary mass are recommended. Chemotherapy is being used in some investigational trials, but the value has yet to be established.

Germ cell tumors (which develop from embryologic rests of tissue in the midline from the brain down to the ovaries and testes) and pineal-region tumors may also seed the CSF. Germinomas and pineoblastomas may require CSI. Before neurosurgical biopsy became safe, empirical treatment of the tumor mass with radiation was common. If the tumor regressed after 1500 to 2000 cGy, the assumption was made that the tumor was a germinoma or high-grade pineal lesion, and craniospinal therapy was initiated. In most instances a biopsy can now be performed to guide the radiation oncologist. Although lower CSI doses are reasonable, the primary lesion is best controlled with 5000 cGy. Because these histologic types are sensitive to chemotherapeutic agents, the need for CSI may be supplanted except with gross CSF involvement.[2]

Brainstem Glioma

Brainstem gliomas typically involve cranial nerve deficits that can affect vision, facial nerves, and swallowing. Most of these lesions are diffuse in the pons and thus are entirely unresectable. Biopsy has been possible lately, and most of these pontine tumors are high-grade astrocytomas. Posterior expansion of the pons can create hydrocephalus.

The mainstay of treatment is radiation therapy. The fields should cover the entire brainstem and midbrain region, reaching from about 4 cm superior to the clinoids down to at least the level of C1. Doses of 180 cGy per day have historically been delivered with lateral-opposed fields, although this truly central lesion can be treated with rotational fields or 3D conformal therapy. Doses of 5500 cGy in the past resulted in poor cure rates. The use of hyperfractionation with doses escalated to 7800 cGy delivered at 100 to 117 cGy twice daily and concomitant chemotherapy yielded no improvement. Unfortunately the survival rate in diffuse lesions is only 10%.[24]

Rarely the brainstem glioma is an exophytic lesion extending from the posterior aspect of the brainstem. These lesions tend to have a low-grade histology and are amenable to surgical resection by select pediatric neurosurgeons. The survival rate for patients with these lesions is more than 50%.[31]

Late Effects of Treatment

The treatment of large areas of the brain and spinal cord can have a variety of devastating late sequelae. These effects are definitely worse the younger the child's age at the time of treatment. Because survival rates were so poor for many decades, only now are these factors being assessed. Postsurgical deficits of motor-sensory loss, poor coordination, or cranial nerve dysfunction can last a lifetime. Parents are always extremely concerned about the child's subsequent intellectual abilities. Changes of cortical atrophy and basal ganglia calcifications can occur, even with lower doses used in leukemic CNS prophylaxis, but do not correlate with neurologic impairment. Whole-brain radiation with high doses for high-grade gliomas and CSF seeding tumors has decreased the median intelligence quotient of survivors 10% to 20%.[30] Cisplatin and radiation can decrease hearing. Doses over 2000 cGy to the pituitary and hypothalamus can cause delayed decreases in pituitary hormones. Thyroid and growth hormone deficits are most likely and with early detection can be reversed via supplemental hormones.[43] CSI can decrease the height of vertebral bodies, leading to a short-waisted adult. The acute hair loss can be psychologically traumatic, and high doses of radiation can lead to permanent hair loss for some children. Second malignancies may develop many years later in the CNS, bones and soft tissues, or bone marrow from the damage that earlier radiation and chemotherapy induces. Careful follow-up and early intervention, medically and educationally, can lessen many of the late effects just mentioned. Although doing so may frighten parents, mentioning the risks for late effects when obtaining informed consent for a child's radiation treatment is necessary. Despite these risks, parents are almost always ecstatic that even an impaired child has survived a life-threatening brain tumor.

RETINOBLASTOMA

Epidemiology

Although **retinoblastoma** (the primitive neuroectodermal tumor of the retina) is the most common intraocular tumor in young children, it only occurs about 250 times annually in the United States. Most retinoblastomas occur in children 6 months to 4 years of age.[1] A well-documented hereditary pattern is present in 25% to 35% of patients. The retinoblastoma gene is located on chromosome 13 (13q-14 deletion) and is a tumor-suppressor gene. Therefore both halves of the chromosome must suffer a deletion of the gene for retinoblastoma to occur. These patients account for most cases of bilateral retinoblastoma and have a significant risk of development of later nonocular cancers. At least 65% of retinoblastomas are unilateral and without evidence of inheritance.[6]

Diagnosis and Staging

Retinoblastoma is usually discovered as a result of an abnormal retinal light reflex (white rather than red). This tumor may be noted from a flash photograph or during the pediatrician's routine examination. An ophthalmologist should examine both eyes with the child under anesthesia to document multifocality or bilaterality. A biopsy is not done because of the risk of vitreous seeding. CT of the brain and orbit can detect unusual cases with extraocular extension or simultaneous supratentorial-pineal lesions (trilateral retinoblastoma). The CSF is assessed by lumbar puncture cytology, and a bone marrow biopsy may be indicated. Clinical staging systems have developed to suggest preferred treatments and predict success rates. The foremost system is that of Reese-Ellsworth,[47] which highlights multifocality, tumor size and location, vitreous involvement, and bilaterality (Box 36-1).

Treatment Techniques

As mentioned, the pediatric ophthalmologist must detail the extent of local disease. With small focal tumors away from the optic disc and macula, photocoagulation or cryosurgery may yield control. With more extensive but unilateral retinoblastoma not involving the optic nerve, enucleation leads to almost certain cure while sacrificing the globe.

Radiation has classically been used in cases of bilateral or inoperable unilateral disease. If both eyes are involved, they must be treated with organ-sparing intent because visual preservation may occur on the side with more advanced initial disease. It is a technical challenge with external beam therapy to treat the entire retina, which extends anterior to the lateral bony canthus, and still spare the cornea and lens.

Box 36-1	Reese-Ellsworth Staging System for Retinoblastoma

Group I (quite favorable)
  a. Solitary tumor (less than 4 dd at or behind the equator)
  b. Multiple tumors (none over 4 dd at or behind the equator)
Group II (favorable)
  a. Solitary lesion (4-10 dd at or behind the equator)
  b. Multiple tumors (4-10 dd behind the equator)
Group III (doubtful)
  a. Any lesion anterior to the equator
  b. Solitary lesions (larger than 10 dd behind the equator)
Group IV (unfavorable)
  a. Multiple tumors (some larger than 10 dd)
  b. Any lesion extending anteriorly to the ora serrata
Group V (quite unfavorable)
  a. Massive tumors involving over half the retina
  b. Vitreous seeding

Modified from Reese A: *Tumors of the eye,* Hagerstown, PA, 1976, Harper & Row.
dd, Disc diameter (equal to 1.6 mm).

Methods include (1) combined lateral and anterior fields with a divergent hanging lens block, (2) a suction cup to displace the anterior globe (popular in Europe), or (3) 3D conformal volumes especially when tumor is beyond the globe. Daily general anesthesia is required, with specialized dosimetry verifying doses in such small-shaped radiation portals. The usual dose is 180 to 300 cGy, delivered three to five times weekly. Several series report local control and visual preservation ranging from 30% to 100%, depending on the stage (Table 36-3). If the tumor masses are less extensive, radiation implant plaques can be used. Cobalt-60 and iodine-125 are the most widely used radionuclides. Doses of 4000 to 6000 cGy over 1 week are delivered, with a cure rate of more than 80% and visual preservation in most patients.[28] Implants reduce radiation exposure to the bones, contralateral globe, and anterior structures, with a resultant decrease in long-term effects.

Because retinoblastoma is a small blue cell tumor of neuroectodermal origin, a good response to chemotherapeutic agents is expected. Vincristine, cyclophosphamide, and the platinols have shown good response rates when extraocular or disseminated disease is present. Newer trials involve neoadjuvant chemotherapy in hope of avoiding external radiation therapy sequelae.

Late Effects of Treatment

Long-term sequelae of retinoblastoma therapies include the cosmetics of the face, effects on vision, and a high risk of a **second malignant neoplasm** (SMN), a new cancer developing years after treatment of the initial tumor. After enucleation is chosen the child will require several prosthetic eyes as growth occurs and limited orbital growth maybe noted. Because external radiation uses doses of 4000 cGy or more and occurs in children who are young, facial growth will definitely be impaired. As adults, these patients have small orbits, which are narrow between the temples. Cured tumors can leave blind spots. Radiation retinitis, dry eyes from decreased tear gland function, and cataracts can limit useful vision. However, overall survival rates and visual acuity are often excellent (Table 36-3).

As noted earlier, the retinoblastoma gene is a tumor-suppressor gene. If this gene is absent, other cancers (especially osteosarcomas) develop later in life with alarming frequency. Sarcomas can be induced in the radiation therapy portal but occur outside the radiation therapy field more often. Eng et al[19] reported a 25% incidence at 30 years.

NEUROBLASTOMA

Epidemiology

Neuroblastoma is a small, round, blue cell tumor derived from cells of neural crest origin. These cells migrate embryologically to form paravertebral sympathetic ganglia and the adrenal medulla. Neuroblastoma-like cells occur in fetal adrenals and in 1% of infant autopsies. Because only about

Table 36-3	Visual preservation per Reese group after radiation therapy for retinoblastoma		
Institution	Preservation for Group I	Preservation for Groups II and III	Preservation for Group IV and V
Columbia University	84%	68%	20%
Stanford University	88%	63%	30%
Utrecht University	100%	89%	58%

Data from Cassady JR, et al: Radiation therapy in retinoblastoma, *Radiology* 93:405-409, 1969; Egbert PR, et al: Visual results and ocular complication following radiotherapy for retinoblastoma, *Radiology* 96:1826-1830, 1978; and Schipper J, Tan KE, Von Peperzeel HA: Treatment of retinoblastoma by precision megavoltage radiation therapy, *Radiother Oncol* 3:117-132, 1985.

500 such tumors develop in the United States annually, most of these precursor lesions must spontaneously regress. However, neuroblastoma is the second most common solid tumor (after brain tumors). Patients range from newborns to children several years old, with a median age of younger than 24 months.[34]

Like the normal adrenal tissues, neuroblastoma cells can manufacture epinephrine-like compounds such as vanilmandelic acid (VMA) and homovanillic acid (HVA), which can be detected in the urine. Molecular genetic studies have demonstrated a deletion on the short arm of chromosome 1 in up to 80% of patients.[6] Surprisingly, neuroblastomas with an excessive or aneuploid number of chromosomes yield a better prognosis. The **oncogene** (a gene regulating the development and growth of cancerous tissues) primarily associated with neuroblastoma is n-*myc*. This gene occurs on the short arm of chromosome 2 and is a promoter of growth. Thus when excessive copies of this gene are present (called n-*myc* amplified tumors), aggressive growth and poor survival are typical.[7]

Diagnosis and Staging

Most neuroblastomas occur in the abdomen, with the origin in the adrenal gland or paraspinal ganglia. A lethargic, ill-appearing child younger than 2 years with an abdominal mass is common. The invasion of the spinal canal in a dumbbell fashion from a paravertebral neuroblastoma can cause symptoms of neurologic compromise such as Horner's syndrome (ptosis, meiosis, and anhydrosis) and spinal cord compression Flushing and diarrhea occur in response to the vasoactive peptides. In the newborn a large abdominal mass or liver metastases usually cause respiratory compromise, necessitating emergency intervention.

Unfortunately, many children present with symptoms of metastatic disease. Patients older than 18 months have a 70% chance of developing metastatic disease.[34] Weakness and anemia from bone marrow invasion, painful bony metastases, blue skin lesions, or massive liver involvement may occur, even with a small primary tumor. In general, these patients are younger and sicker than those with a corresponding-sized **Wilms' tumor** (the childhood embryonal kidney cancer). The radiologic evaluation depends on the presentation in the abdomen or chest. Abdominal ultrasound or CT and chest CT are appropriate. Sometimes calcifications are visible in the mass on a CT scan. The lungs and liver must be assessed for metastases. MRI of the spine is used for paravertebral masses to delineate spinal canal invasion. A bone marrow biopsy is required and a bone scan is done to look for bone cortex lesions. More recently, radioiodinated catecholamine precursors have been used to detect occult metastatic involvement. Staging systems have historically evolved based on radiographic and surgical findings. Initially, Evans and D'Angio developed such a prognostic staging system. The POG and an international staging committee have included surgical guidelines. These systems are summarized in Table 36-4.

As mentioned, the age at the time of presentation is extremely important regarding the prognosis. The special category IV-S predominantly occurs in infants younger than 1 year. Many of these patients spontaneously regress, and the cancerous elements turn benign if acute situations can be managed.[13] Increasingly, molecular genetic markers (especially n-*myc* amplification) are being used to predict clinical behavior. Although this technique has not yet been included in universal staging systems, it is certainly directing the aggressiveness of therapy in most clinical research groups. Variations in molecular genetics may explain the differential age prognosis observed clinically. A novel approach to early detection has shown benefits in Japan. Urine samples from diaper pads of infants were analyzed for catecholamine excretions and led to earlier stage presentations and higher cure rates in initial evaluations.[42]

Treatment Techniques

The therapy for neuroblastoma remains an enigma to most pediatric oncologists. Although it may spontaneously regress

---

Table 36-4	**Neuroblastoma staging systems**

EVANS AND D'ANGIO

Stage I—Tumor confined to the organ or structure of origin

Stage II—Tumor extending in continuity beyond the organ or structure of origin but not crossing the midline; regional lymph nodes on the ipsilateral side

Stage III—Tumor extending in continuity beyond the midline; possible involvement of regional lymph nodes bilaterally

Stage IV—Remote disease involving the skeleton, bone marrow, soft tissue, and distant lymph node groups, etc. (see stage IV-S)

Stage IV-S—Patients who would otherwise be in stage I or II but have remote disease confined to the liver, skin, or bone marrow (without radiographic evidence of bone metastases on a complete skeletal survey)

PEDIATRIC ONCOLOGY GROUP

Stage A—Complete gross resection of primary tumor, with or without microscopic residual; intracavitary lymph nodes, not adhered to and removed with primary (nodes adhered to or within tumor resection may be positive for tumor without upstaging patient to stage C), histologically free of tumor; if primary in abdomen or pelvis, liver histologically free of tumor

Stage B—Grossly unresected primary tumor; nodes and liver same as in stage A

Stage C—Complete or incomplete resection of primary; intracavitary nodes not adhered to primary histologically positive for tumor; liver as in stage A

Stage D—Any dissemination of disease beyond intracavitary nodes (i.e., extracavitary nodes, liver, skin, bone marrow, bone)

INTERNATIONAL

Stage 1—Localized tumor confined to area of origin; complete gross excision, with or without microscopic residual disease; identifiable ipsilateral and contralateral lymph nodes negative microscopically

Stage 2A—Unilateral tumor with incomplete gross excision; identifiable ipsilateral and contralateral lymph nodes negative microscopically

Stage 2B—Unilateral tumor with complete or incomplete gross excision; with positive ipsilateral regional lymph nodes; identifiable contralateral lymph nodes negative microscopically

Stage 3—Tumor infiltrating across the midline with or without regional lymph node involvement; unilateral tumor with contralateral regional lymph node involvement; or midline tumor with bilateral regional lymph node involvement

Stage 4—Dissemination of tumor to distant lymph nodes, bone, bone marrow, liver, and/or other organs (except as defined in stage 4S)

Stage 4S—Localized primary tumor as defined for stage 1 or 2, with dissemination limited to liver and skin

---

Data from Brodeur GM, et al: International criteria for diagnosis, staging and response to treatment with neuroblastoma, *J Clin Oncol* 6:1874-1881, 1988; Evans AE: Staging and treatment of neuroblastoma, *Cancer* 45:1799-1802, 1980; and Hayes FA, study coordinator: *Comprehensive care of the child with neuroblastoma: a stage and age oriented study,* Chicago, 1982, Pediatric Oncology Group.

in the newborn, neuroblastoma often has a progressive metastatic course in older children. Individual masses may regress well with low doses of chemotherapy or radiation, but cure of the usual advanced disease presentation is infrequent. Completely resected localized disease without nodal metastases is often cured with surgery alone. In 1967 Lingley et al.[38] showed 100% local control and long-term survival in 8 of 13 patients after they underwent incomplete surgery followed by radiation. The use of multiagent chemotherapy has supplanted radiation in most resected patients, even with nodal metastases or microscopic residua. More extensive stage III tumors definitely benefit from tumor bed irradiation, usually to doses of 2000 to 3000 cGy.[39] Radiation is directed to residua after surgery and chemotherapy, rather than to all areas of initial disease.

The likelihood of children older than 2 years developing metastatic disease demands the use of multiagent chemotherapy. In Europe and the United States, aggressive regimens involving platinum compounds, vincristine, doxorubicin (Adriamycin), etoposide, and cyclophosphamide have been used. Although such treatment has improved the previously almost uniformly fatal stage IV results, overall survival rates have been disheartening (Table 36-5). Newer efforts involve therapeutic radionuclides and the use of high-dose chemotherapy stem cell transplant up to three consecutive times show promise in pilot studies

Radiation therapists can also be called on to palliatively treat patients who have progressive metastatic disease. Low doses of 1000 cGy may achieve pain relief or regression of soft tissue masses, which are important for short-term quality of life to terminally ill patients and their families.

Late Effects of Treatment

Because neuroblastoma patients are often infants, the late effects of radiation can be significant. In the acute situation with a newborn, doses of only 500 cGy may be effective with almost no long-term side effect. In older patients receiving 2000 to 3000 cGy the bones and soft tissues of the treated region will have decreased growth. This may cause asymmetry as the child grows. Kidney and liver tissues must be

Table 36-5	5-year survival rates in 550 neuroblastoma patients on POG protocols, 1981-1989	
Stage	Children Less than 1 Year Old	Children More than 1 Year Old
A and B	95%	85%
C	80%	60%
D	50%	15%

Modified from Ries LAG et al, editors: *SEER Cancer Statistics Review, 1973-1991: tables and graphs,* NIH Pub. No. 94-2789, Bethesda, Md, 1994, National Cancer Institute.
POG, Pediatric Oncology Group.

shielded from the highest doses of radiation to prevent impaired function. Lung fibrosis can occur with thoracic radiation. The intense doses of multiagent chemotherapy and stem cell transplants used for neuroblastoma can adversely affect many organ systems. Although late second malignancies are always a risk after radiation and chemotherapy, the oncogenes associated with neuroblastoma do not exacerbate the risk to an alarming level.

WILMS' TUMOR

Epidemiology

Wilms' tumor is a malignant embryonal cancer of the kidney. It was first described in the German medical literature in 1899. Nearly 500 cases occur annually in the United States and about 5% are bilateral. The average age at the time of presentation is 3 or 4 years, and almost all such tumors occur before the age of 8. A higher risk of Wilms' tumor occurs in patients with multiple genitourinary (GU) abnormalities, hemihypertrophy and aniridia, and the facial abnormality syndrome Beckwith-Wiedemann. A Wilms' tumor gene has recently been discovered and represents a deletion on chromosome 11p13.[16] Benign embryonal rests called nephroblastomatoses can be associated with malignant Wilms' tumor, especially in bilateral cases. Wilms' tumors can contain renal tubular, glomerular, and connective tissue elements. Unfavorable histologic appearances occur in up to 15% of patients and include highly anaplastic, clear cell sarcomas, and rhabdoid tumors. These unfavorable tumors have a cure rate only half that of their usual histologic Wilms' tumor counterpart and metastasize to bone or brain.[5]

Diagnosis and Staging

Wilms' tumor most often appears as a painless abdominal mass noted at the pediatrician's examination or when parents bathe the child. As the cancers enlarge, they can cause pain and pressure on the gastrointestinal tract. They may even hemorrhage and rupture. Despite large tumors, children do not often appear severely ill. A differential diagnosis includes neuroblastomas, lymphomas, sarcomas, and liver tumors.

After the physical examination an abdominal ultrasonogram is usually the first step in making a diagnosis. In the United States this is followed by a CT scan of the chest and abdomen because of the tendency for lymph node and pulmonary metastases. Because Wilms' tumor can be bilateral, the contralateral kidney must be carefully examined (Fig. 36-4, *A*). With right-sided tumors, direct liver invasion can mimic liver metastases. The unfavorable histologies of clear cell sarcomas and rhabdoid tumors can metastasize to bone and brain. The initial staging system recommended by Cassady focused on tumor size, tumor spill or postoperative residua, and metastases. The National Wilms' Tumor Study Group (NWTS) was formed in the United States to investigate treatment options; members have conducted protocol study no. 5. The staging system of the NWTS is based on

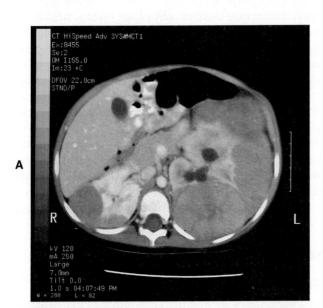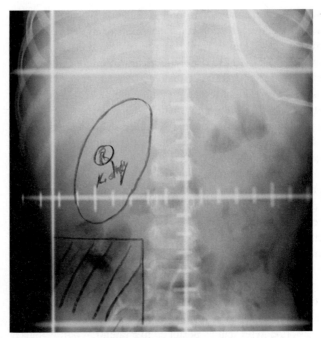

Figure 36-4. Wilms' tumor. **A,** Preoperative computed tomography (CT) scan of a bilateral Wilms' tumor in a 3-year-old girl. **B,** Postoperative radiation portal received 1200 cGy to the left tumor bed and remaining involved right kidney. Note the shielding for the bowel and pelvic structures inferiorly on the right side.

Box 36-2	The National Wilms' Tumor Study Staging System

Stage
I   Tumor limited to kidney and completely excised
II   Tumor beyond kidney but completely excised
     Local tumor spillage or vessel invasion permitted but resected
III Residual nonhematogenous tumor confined to abdomen
     Involved lymph nodes, diffuse tumor spillage, or grossly unresected tumor
IV   Hematogenous metastases
     Usually lung, liver, bone, or brain
V   Bilateral kidney involvement at time of diagnosis

operative findings and is listed in Box 36-2. These stages relate to prognosis and direct the aggressiveness of treatment options.

Treatment Techniques

In the United States the removal of the malignant kidney via nephrectomy is nearly always the first step. Careful examination of the other kidney for bilateral tumors is done intraoperatively. A biopsy is performed on the lymph nodes, and tumor thrombi in the renal vein or inferior vena cava can be removed during surgery. Because large Wilms' tumors are often soft and necrotic, rupture of the mass and tumor spill into the abdominal cavity are risks. Because widespread tumor spill

adversely affects the prognosis and demands more subsequent treatment, SIOP studies usually use chemotherapy or radiation preoperatively. In the first SIOP cooperative study this method reduced intraoperative tumor spill from 32% to 4%.[37] In patients with bilateral disease a partial resection can be done on the minimally affected side. Because surgery alone led to cure rates of less than 30% many years ago, radiation therapy by the 1940s and chemotherapy by the 1960s have greatly increased survival rates.

Radiation was initially used to cover the entire tumor bed and abdomen. If tumor spill occurred, the whole abdomen was treated. Doses higher than 3000 cGy were successful but led to significant late effects. The first four NWTS studies have resulted in conclusions for less radiation. With the addition of effective chemotherapy routine radiation for completely removed stages I and II tumors is not necessary. Data from NWTS 3 indicated no significant difference in local control between 1080 and 2000 cGy.[55] This lower dose is still indicated for residual disease, lymph node metastases, bilateral disease, and pulmonary metastases. All cases of unfavorable histology are treated as high-stage lesions and uniformly irradiated. Known areas of residual disease are usually boosted to at least 2000 cGy.

In designing the radiation portals, it is important to use the preoperative imaging and surgeon's intraoperative findings to delineate the radiation portal. If treating only unilateral disease, it is still important to cover the entire width of the vertebral body plus 1 to 2 cm contralaterally. This allows periaortic nodal coverage and homogeneous irradiation of the vertebral bodies to reduce the risk of scoliosis. At the low dose of 1080 cGy, which is often used now, the risk of bony or visceral toxicity (including the remaining kidney) is minimal. Still, it is wise to shield the growth plates of long bones. Fig. 36-4, *B,* represents a postoperative radiation portal for a bilateral Wilms' tumor patient whose large left-sided cancer was removed. Because abdominal recurrence is still a major problem in an unfavorable histologic Wilms' tumor, the fields are similar but doses are usually 2000 cGy or more.

Farber[20] first reported the encouraging survival improvement associated with Wilms' tumor by using actinomycin-D in 1966. The addition of vincristine and doxorubicin for advanced stages led to cure rates of 80% to 100% in later NWTS studies. Even patients with metastatic disease can be cured more than 70% of the time (Table 36-6). Patients with late pulmonary metastases can often be salvaged with chemotherapy, lung irradiation, and lung resections. With the high overall cure rates, the present aim of studies is to reduce late effects and find more successful multidisciplinary combinations for patients who have advanced disease and unfavorable histology.

Late Effects of Treatment

Historically, when doses of 3000 to 4000 cGy of orthovoltage radiation were used, atrophy of soft tissues on the treated side and scoliosis were common. With modification of the technique to include the entire vertebral body plus the margin and the use of doses less than 2000 cGy, such late effects should rarely occur now. For the treatment of pulmonary metastases, doses must be kept below 1500 cGy to prevent diffuse lung fibrosis. If thoracic radiation is needed for a prepubertal female, breast development can be impaired. High doses of actinomycin-D have resulted in liver damage. SMNs have occurred in a small percentage of long-term survivors. Because these children go through life with only one kidney, any urinary tract symptoms must be addressed quickly to prevent infections, stones, or other diseases from damaging the remaining kidney.

SOFT TISSUE SARCOMAS

Epidemiology

Soft tissue sarcomas arise from mesenchymal tissues and can occur anywhere in the body. At Children's Hospital in Philadelphia a decade of oncology cases were reviewed and 8% were soft tissue sarcomas. A wide variety of histologic appearances can be seen, but **rhabdomyosarcomas** and undifferentiated sarcomas constitute more than 60% of cases. No dominant chromosomal abnormality has been noted, but familial cases may be related to the *p53* oncogene mutation, as noted by Li and Fraumeni. About 75% of soft tissue sarcomas occur before the age of 10. The rhabdomyosarcoma sites are nearly evenly divided between the head and neck area (including the orbit), GU region, and extremities and trunk.[46]

Rhabdomyosarcoma has distinct histologic variants. A more favorable embryonal type tends to occur in the orbit and GU regions. The alveolar subtype has a worse prognosis and a predilection for extremities and the trunk.[41] Other undifferentiated sarcomas are often treated along guidelines established by the Intergroup Rhabdomyosarcoma Study Group (IRS).

Diagnosis and Staging

The presenting symptoms of soft tissue sarcomas depend on the area of involvement. A painless mass can enlarge relatively asymptomatically in an extremity, whereas a small mass in the orbit can cause pain, tearing, and outward displacement of the globe, known as proptosis. The GU occurrences in the prostate and bladder in males cause urinary difficulties. A fleshy, exophytic mass extruding from the vagina in young girls has been called sarcoma botryoides because of its resemblance to clusters of grapes.

The staging of rhabdomyosarcomas and other soft tissue sarcomas has historically included size and resectability, nodal involvement, and metastases. The latter are most likely to occur in the lung and bone marrow. The IRS first developed a

Table 36-6	4-year survival rates of NWTS-3 patients	
Stage	**Relapse-Free Rate (%)**	**Overall Rate (%)**
I FH	90	96
II FH	88	92
III FH	79	86
IV FH	75	82
I-III UH	65	68
IV UH	55	55

Modified from Green DM, et al: Wilms' tumor. In Pizzo PG, Poplack DG, editors: *Principles and practice of pediatric oncology,* ed 2, Philadelphia, 1993, JB Lippincott.
FH, Favorable histology; *NWTS-3,* National Wilms' Tumor Study Group protocol study no. 3; *UH,* unfavorable histology.

clinical grouping system based on surgical findings, but some experts now favor the TGNM system (Table 36-7), which also includes the histology (a known prognostic factor). After the histologic diagnosis is obtained from an incisional biopsy, staging includes a physical examination and ultrasound, CT, or MRI scans to determine the tumor's size and involvement of adjacent structures. A bone marrow biopsy and chest CT scan are done to detect metastases. The stage and histology dictate the treatment regimen in IRS and other international studies. Metastatic disease is extremely rare with orbital presentations but may be present in about 25% of patients who have tumors in the extremities and trunk.[40]

Treatment Techniques

After the biopsy and staging the surgical possibilities must be assessed. The first choice, if possible, is the complete removal of the mass with appropriate margins without the destruction of precious anatomy. The initial IRS study proved that small, fully resected lesions have good curability without additional treatment. In more advanced cases the local relapse rate was extremely high with surgery alone. The original approach of removing the entire organ or extremity is no longer necessary because of multidisciplinary treatment including chemotherapy and radiation. The removal of a child's eye or GU structures is generally not preferred and has led to organ-sparing combined treatments.

Radiation improves local control and organ preservation in all rhabdomyosarcoma groups, except small and fully excised lesions. Some authors have reported increased local control with doses of 5000 cGy versus less than 4000 cGy. Fortunately, the frequently unresectable areas of the orbit and pelvis are usually the more favorable embryonal histology, and local control rates of 90% or more have been obtained with combinations of chemotherapy and radiation.[53]

Originally the margins of radiation fields included the entire muscular compartment. More recently, the IRS has decreased margins to 5 cm or sometimes 2 cm if critical normal tissues can be spared. Around the orbit a wedge pair alignment or mixed beam with electrons can spare the contralateral eye, facial bones, optic chiasm, and most brain tissues. In the pelvis or along extremities the growth plates of the long bones must be shielded. With the routine use of chemotherapy the bone marrow in the pelvic wings should be spared if possible. For locally positive intraoperative margins and some surface gynecologic presentations, brachytherapy implants have been used with success.[26] In general, the external beam radiation portals include the prechemotherapy tumor volume with at least a 2-cm margin. Standard doses have been 180 cGy per day to a total of 5040 cGy. IRS-IV included hyperfractionated radiation twice daily at 110 cGy per treatment to a total of 5940 cGy to decrease long-term effects but maintain a high local control rate. No advantage was noted in group III (gross disease) for hyperfractionated therapy with both regimens yielding 70% relapse free survival at 5 years.[15]

Table 36-7	Intergroup Rhabdomyosarcoma Study staging systems
Clinical system	**TGNM system**

I. Localized, completely resected
II. Grossly resected with microscopic residue or involved lymph nodes
III. Gross residual tumor
IV. Distant metastases
	Tumor
	T_1—Confined to site origin
	T_2—Extension to surrounding tissues
	  a. <5 cm
	  b. ≥5 cm
	
	Histology
	G_1—Favorable: embryonal, undifferentiated, mixed
	G_2—Unfavorable: alveolar
	
	Nodes
	N_0—Not clinically involved
	N_1—Clinically involved by tumor
	
	Metastases
	M_0—No distant metastases
	M_1—Metastatic disease at time of diagnosis

Modified from Raney RB et al: Rhabdomyosarcoma and other undifferentiated sarcomas. In Pizzo PA, Poplack DG, editors: *Principles and practice of pediatric oncology,* Philadelphia, 1989, JB Lippincott.
TGNM, Tumor, Grade, Node, Metastases.

Chemotherapy was initially used only for metastatic disease, but its subsequent use postoperatively led to higher survival rates because of the elimination of occult metastatic disease.[29] In serial IRS studies, vincristine and actinomycin-D have been effective. New regimens have combined these agents with etoposide and ifosfamide. With good tumor reduction some inoperable cancers can be resected or radiation fields greatly reduced. Surgery or radiation therapy must be performed for local control early in the overall treatment because resistant clones of cells can lead to tumor growth and lost opportunities. Local control procedures are usually at 2 to 3 months into the overall treatment program of about 1 year. The tumor's histology, stage, and location affect survival rates (Table 36-8). Although the survival rate for patients with orbital lesions is more than 90%, patients with large unresectable pelvic masses or metastatic disease still fare poorly.

Late Effects of Treatment

The long-term sequelae of rhabdomyosarcoma and other soft tissue sarcoma treatment depends on the tumor's location and treatment modality. Amputations and pelvic exenterations are generally reserved for the salvaging of organ-sparing treatment failures. However, some patient's family prefer

Table 36-8	Actuarial survival rates at 3 years: Results of the Intergroup Rhabdomyosarcoma Studies I and II	
Prognostic Factors	**IRS Study I (%)**	**IRS Study II (%)**
CLINICAL GROUP		
I	79	88
II	68	77
III	42	68
IV	18	32
HISTOLOGIC TYPE		
Embryonal	—	69
Alveolar	—	56
Other	—	66
PRIMARY SITE		
Orbit	91	93
GU	74	—
GU (mainly group III)	—	64
Cranial parameningeal	53	71
Other head or neck areas	59	69
Trunk	53	57
Extremity	53	56
Retroperitoneum and pelvis	39	46

Modified from Pizzo PA, et al: Solid tumors of children. In DeVita T, Hellman S, Rosenberg SA, editors: *Cancer: principles and practice of oncology,* ed 4, Philadelphia, 1993, JB Lippincott.
GU, Genitourinary; *IRS,* Intergroup Rhabdomyosarcoma Study Group.

bladder removal rather than the long-term effects of radiation on their young daughter's reproductive structures. With the high radiation doses, bone and soft tissue growth is affected unless the growth points of bones can be excluded. In the head and neck region, invasion of the cranial contents can occur, necessitating CNS radiation to 3000 cGy or more. (Its well-known side effects are listed in the brain tumor section.) Treatment of the orbit and facial structures causes bony growth decreases. Dryness of the treated eye or retinal damage from chemotherapy and radiation sometimes necessitates enucleation, even if the rhabdomyosarcoma is cured. The appropriate use of brachytherapy implants can spare many of the surrounding normal tissues from damage. Chemotherapeutic agents can cause acute and chronic neurologic, kidney, heart, and liver damage. The risk of SMNs after cytotoxic therapy is present. As survivors grow to adulthood, fertility is questionable after chemotherapy and highly unlikely for those receiving pelvic radiation.

UNUSUAL CHILDHOOD TUMORS

Germ Cell Tumors

According to embryologic development, benign and malignant germ cell tumors can occur anywhere in the midline, from the CNS through the mediastinum and retroperitoneum,

down to the ovaries and testicles. Sacrococcygeal teratomas often occur in newborns. The majority of these tumors are histologically benign and are almost always cured by surgery. Tumors affecting older children in this region have a higher risk of malignancy but can usually be controlled with chemotherapy. Radiation is rarely used in this young age-group. Ovarian and testicular tumors that occur in adolescents differentiate along seminoma-dysgerminoma or nonseminomatous lines. The latter group includes embryonal carcinoma, choriocarcinoma, and yolk sac tumors. The nonseminomatous tumors often produce alpha-fetoprotein (AFP) or human chorionic gonadotropin (HCG), which can be used as chemical markers for response to therapy. Surgical removal of the testicles or ovaries is done first and is often curative in stage I disease. Chemotherapy with regimens containing cisplatin, bleomycin, etoposide, and vinblastine have led to a high rate of success. Moderate doses of radiation in the 2000- to 2500-cGy range prevents pelvic and periaortic nodal relapse in seminoma-germinoma patients[36] and is used most often in older adolescent males. CNS germ cell tumors are discussed in the brain tumor section.

Liver Tumors

Liver tumors appear as right upper quadrant abdominal masses, much like Wilms' tumor or neuroblastoma. Ultrasound or CT scanning can usually determine the organ of origin. Benign vascular or fetal remnant tumors can be observed if they are small, or if necessary because of their large size, they can be resected with excellent results. Hepatoblastoma is a malignancy usually occurring in patients younger than 2 years. Hepatocellular carcinoma occurs in the second decade of life and can be multifocal. AFP can be elevated in both hepatic malignancies.[23]

Primary surgical resection is the goal. If this is not possible or postoperative residua is present, chemotherapy with doxorubicin and cisplatin is often used. Radiation has demonstrated some good response but is rarely used, especially in infants. However, overall survival rates (usually less than 50%) are poor.[27]

Histiocytosis X Syndromes

Histiocytosis X is a spectrum of diseases that involves abnormal proliferation of the histiocytic immune system's Langerhans' cells. Sometimes a single bone is involved with a lytic lesion in a situation called eosinophilic granuloma. Infants can have multifocal visceral disease involving the lung, skin, liver, and bone marrow. This is a life-threatening condition known as Letterer-Siwe. Individual histiocytosis lesions may vary over time and occasionally spontaneously regress. Focal bony lesions can be treated via surgical curettage with success. If an impending fracture is a concern or the lesion is in a surgically unresectable region such as the base of skull or spinal column, low doses of radiation are usually effective. Although no direct dose-response curve has been substantiated, doses from 400 to 1200 cGy can be effective.[32] Steroids, vinblastine, or cyclophosphamide can be effective as well.

Miscellaneous Tumors

Male adolescents may develop nasopharyngeal angiofibromas. Usually, vascular embolization and surgical resection are used. Moderate doses of radiation (such as 3000 cGy) can control relapses.[12] Undifferentiated nasopharyngeal carcinomas can occur and require high-dose radiation, as they do in adults. Recently, chemotherapy has been used to reduce radiation fields and resultant long-term side effects.

Benign and malignant thyroid tumors can arise in adolescents (more often in girls). These tumors are surgically approached, and even lymph node metastases do not imply a bad prognosis. External radiation is rarely used, but iodine-131 can be helpful for thyroid ablation or treatment of metastatic lesions.

Keloids and fibromas can be bothersome and cosmetically disfiguring for young people. If repeated resections and steroid injections are not successful, the best control is obtained via resection, followed immediately by low-dose radiation (900 to 1200 cGy in 3 fractions).[51] Unfortunately, the human immunodeficiency virus (HIV) infection epidemic has led to the occurrence of Kaposi's sarcoma in children. Focal painful or disfiguring lesions can be palliated with single doses of 700 cGy, although more lasting results are obtained by a short course to a total dose of more than 2000 cGy.[11]

PALLIATIVE RADIATION

Despite the obvious goal of cure for pediatric malignancies, **palliation** or symptom-relieving treatments are sometimes necessary. The Children's Hospital of Philadelphia reported 13% of their patients from 1988 to 1994 were referred for emergency radiation.[49] Mediastinal malignancies may cause airway or vascular compromise. Spinal cord compression at the time of presentation or late in the course of the illness demands immediate treatment to reduce pain and avoid paralysis.

The palliative needs of children in the final stages of cancer must be addressed carefully and compassionately. The goal of such treatments is much different than the usual curative protocols. The attempt must be made to relieve symptoms quickly with a minimum number of treatments to limit the hospital personnel's invasion of the family's remaining time together. The successful treatment of painful or disfiguring masses can reduce the need for narcotics or hospitalization and improve cosmetics and quality of life during precious final days or weeks. In these instances immobilization and simulation techniques are altered in deference to the comfort of the child. Frequently, high daily doses are used for rapid palliation when long-term effects are not of concern.[57] Although this is a difficult time for radiation staff members, such palliative efforts in times of great need are of immeasurable importance to the children and their families.

ROLE OF RADIATION THERAPIST

Almost all patients in radiation oncology centers are adults. In addition to the diseases and their treatment, the personal needs of pediatric patients pose a challenge. Immobilization, small treatment fields, and techniques such as CSI are technically demanding. For general anesthesia, treatment techniques may need to be altered for anesthetic safety. Close cooperation among radiation therapists, nurses, and anesthesia staff members is necessary for patient positioning and visibility of monitors. This takes much longer than a normal treatment time, so blocking out the schedule sufficiently is important. Usually, this is done early in the morning to reduce disruption of the child's feeding patterns and avoid conflicts. Therapists often must juggle an already crowded schedule of adults, but most patients are willing to change in deference to children and their families.

Most pediatric patients are on an investigational protocol, requiring careful documentation of treatment setups, daily doses, and quality assurance. Clear instructions between the radiation therapist on the simulator and treatment machine are essential. Polaroid pictures or digital images of patient positioning, verification of initial portal films, and dose calculations are usually sent for immediate review by national clinical research groups. Careful adherence to protocol

Table 36-9	5-year survival trends for cancers in children ages 0 to 14 years		
Diagnosis	**Survival Rate (%) for 1960-1963**	**Survival Rate (%) for 1974-1976**	**Survival Rate (%) for 1986-1991**
Acute lymphocytic leukemia	4.0	52.4	78.0
Brain tumor	35.0	53.7	60.0
Neuroblastoma	25.0	51.9	61.0
Wilms' tumor	33.0	74.3	92.0
Hodgkin's disease	52.0	78.7	92.0
All sites	28.0	55.2	70.0

Modified from Parker SL, et al: Cancer statistics, 1996, *CA Cancer J Clin* 46:5-27, 1996.
*Since 1975 the mortality rate for childhood cancer has declined by approximately 47%.[3]

guidelines reflects positively on the quality of a radiation oncology department.

The psychosocial elements of pediatric oncology can be immense. Families who are constantly at the hospital have an extremely difficult time maintaining jobs and homes. In addition, children evoke sympathy and compassion from everyone involved. However, behavorial limits may need to be placed on patients or families to ensure quality treatments. Rewards such as stickers or toys should not be used daily, but therapists are the best judges of when a difficult or sick child needs an uplifting gift. When terminal cancer children come for palliation, it is an especially difficult time. However, the value of the radiation therapist's technical expertise and heartfelt compassion cannot be overstated.

SUMMARY

The multidisciplinary protocol approach to pediatric oncology is always a learning experience. This strategy has led to dramatic increases in cure rates for childhood cancers over the past 40 years (Table 36-9) to reach an overall survival rate of nearly 70%. However, numerous late sequelae must be considered. In addition to organ toxicities and risk of second malignancies, childhood cancer survivors have psychologic scars. Social, employment, and insurance discrimination may exist throughout adulthood. The Children's Oncology Group (formed from the combination of IRSG, NWTSG, CCG, and POPG) not only directs clinical trials and research but also advocates for survivors of childhood cancer. For the radiation therapist, the treatment of children can truly be the most joyous or sorrowful portion of the job.

Review Questions

1. Which of the following tumors does not spread through the entire central nervous system?
   a. Medulloblastoma
   b. Craniopharyngioma
   c. Ependymoma
   d. Dysgerminoma

2. What is the approximate survival rate for patients with stage IV Wilms' tumor?
   a. 10%
   b. 30%
   c. 50%
   d. 70%

3. Which factor is related to survival in neuroblastoma cases?
   a. Age
   b. Stage
   c. n-*myc* amplification
   d. All of the above

4. The retinoblastoma gene is a _____.
   a. Tumor promoter
   b. Tumor suppressor
   c. Active haploid
   d. Inactive haploid

5. Successful treatment of histiocytosis X lesions requires _____ cGy.
   a. 200-400
   b. 400-1200
   c. 1500-2500
   d. More than 4000

6. The usual dose for occult Wilms' tumor is approximately _____ cGy.
   a. 1000
   b. 2000
   c. 4000
   d. 6000

7. The tolerance of the kidney is about _____ cGy.
   a. 100
   b. 1000
   c. 1500
   d. 3000

8. The most likely second malignant neoplasm after radiation for retinoblastoma is _____.
   a. Leukemia
   b. Lung cancer
   c. Lymphoma
   d. Osteosarcoma

9. Which of the following has the highest incidence in children?
   a. Retinoblastoma
   b. Neuroblastoma
   c. Leukemia
   d. Wilms' tumor

10. Craniospinal irradiation (CSI) is usually administered to which of the following?
    a. Retinoblastoma
    b. Neuroblastoma
    c. Leukemia
    d. Medulloblastoma

Questions to Ponder

1. Why is shifting the junction between the brain and spinal fields important during craniospinal irradiation?
2. Discuss the characteristics of stage IV-S neuroblastoma.
3. Detail some technical considerations for the simulation of craniospinal irradiation.
4. List examples of chromosome and gene abnormalities associated with pediatric cancer.
5. What types of counseling and advice are needed for long-term survivors of childhood cancer?
6. Note possible long-term effects of high-dose brain radiation, and discuss remedies.
7. What organ-sparing techniques are possible by combining chemotherapy, radiation, and surgery?

REFERENCES

1. Abramson DH: Retinoblastoma: diagnosis and management, *CA Cancer J Clin* 32:130-140. 1982.
2. Allen JC, Kim JH, Packer RJ: Neoadjuvant chemotherapy for newly diagnosed germ cell tumors of the central nervous system, *J Neurosurg* 67:65-70, 1987.
3. American Cancer Society: *Cancer facts and figures 2003,* Atlanta, 2003, American Cancer Society.
4. Bouchard J: *Radiation therapy of tumors and diseases of the nervous system,* Philadelphia, 1988, Lea & Febiger.
5. Breslow N, et al: Prognosis for Wilms' tumor patients with nonmetastatic disease at diagnosis: results of the Second National Wilms' Tumor Study, *J Clin Oncol* 3:521-531, 1985.
6. Brodeur GM, Sekhon GS, Goldstein MN: Chromosomal aberrations in human neuroblastomas, *Cancer* 40:2256-2263,1977.
7. Brodeur GM, et al: Gene amplification in human neuroblastomas: basic mechanisms and clinical implications, *Cancer Genet Cytogenet* 19:101-111, 1986.
8. Chang CH, Housepian EM, Herbert C: An operative staging system and a megavoltage radiotherapeutic technique for cerebellar medulloblastoma, *Radiology* 93:1351-1359, 1969.
9. Chun MS, Masko GD, Hetelekidis S: Radiation therapy in the treatment of pituitary adenomas, *Int J Radiat Oncol Biol Phys* 15:305-309, 1988.
10. Cohen ME, Duffner PK: *Brain tumors in children: principles of diagnosis and treatment,* New York, 1984, Raven Press.
11. Cooper JS, Fried PR: Defining the role of radiotherapy for epidemic Kaposi's sarcoma, *Int J Radiat Oncol Biol Phys* 13:35-39, 1987.
12. Cummings BJ, Blend R: Primary radiation therapy for juvenile nasopharyngeal angiofibroma, *Laryngoscope* 94:1599-1605, 1984.
13. D'Angio GJ, Evans A, Koop CE: Special pattern of widespread neuroblastoma with a favorable prognosis, *Lancet* 1:1046, 1971.
14. Deutsch M: The impact of myelography on the treatment results of medulloblastoma, *Int J Radiat Oncol Biol Phys* 10:999-1003, 1989.
15. Donaldson SS, et al: Results from the IRS-IV trial of hyperfractionated radiotherapy in children with rhabdomyosarcoma: a report from the IRSG, *Int J Radiat Oncol Biol Phys* 51:718-28, 2001.
16. Douglas EC, et al: Abnormalities of chromosome 1 and 11 in Wilms' tumor, *Cancer Genet Cytogenet* 14:331-338, 1985.
17. Druja TP, et al: Homozygosity of chromosome 13 in retinoblastoma, *N Engl J Med* 310:550-553, 1984.
18. Duffner PK, Cohen ME: Treatment of brain tumors in babies and very young infants, *Pediatr Neurosci* 12:304-310, 1986.
19. Eng C, et al: Mortality from second tumors among long term survivors of retinoblastoma, *J Natl Cancer Inst* 85:1121-28, 1993.
20. Farber S: Chemotherapy in the treatment of leukemia and Wilms' tumor, *JAMA* 138:826,1966.
21. Finley JL, Uteg R, Giese WL: Brain tumors in children. II. Advances in neurosurgery and radiation oncology, *Am J Pediatr Hematol Oncol* 9:256-263, 1987.
22. Flickinger JC, Kondziolka D, Lunsford LD: Radiosurgery of benign lesions, *Semin Radiat Oncol* 5:220-224, 1995.
23. Fraumeni JF, Miller RW, Hill JA: Primary carcinoma of the liver in childhood: an epidemiologic study, *J Natl Cancer Inst* 40:1087-1099, 1968.
24. Freeman CR, et al: Hyperfractionated radiation therapy of brainstem tumors, *Cancer* 68:474-481,1991.
25. Friedman HS, Schold SC: Rational approaches to the chemotherapy of medulloblastoma, *Neurol Clin* 3:843-854, 1985.
26. Gerbaulet A, et al: Iridium afterloading curietherapy in the treatment of pediatric malignancies, *Cancer* 56:1274-1279, 1985.
27. Giacomantonio M et al: 30 years of experience with pediatric primary malignant liver tumors, *J Pediatr Surg* 19:523-526, 1984.
28. Hernandez JC, et al: Conservative treatment of retinoblastoma: the use of plaque brachytherapy, *Am J Clin Oncol* 16:397-401, 1993.
29. Heyn RM, et al: The role of combined chemotherapy in the treatment of rhabdomyosarcoma, *Cancer* 34:2128-2142,1974.
30. Hirsch JE, et al: Medulloblastoma in childhood: survival and functional results, *Acta Neurochir* 48:1-15, 1979.
31. Hoffman HJ, Becker I, Craven MA: A clinically and pathologically distinct group of benign brainstem gliomas, *Neurosurgery* 7:243-248, 1980.
32. Hughes EN, et al: Medulloblastoma at the Joint Center for Radiation Therapy between 1968 and 1984, *Cancer* 61:1992-1998, 1988.
33. Israel MA: Molecular and cellular biology of pediatric malignancies. In Pizzo PA, Poplack DG, editors: *Principles and practice of pediatric oncology,* Philadelphia, 1989, JB Lippincott.
34. Kissane JM, Smith MG: *Pathology of infancy and childhood,* St. Louis, 1967, Mosby.
35. Kun LE: Patterns of failure in tumors of the central nervous system, *Cancer Treat Symp* 2:285-294, 1983.
36. Lawson AP, Adler GF: Radiotherapy in the treatment of ovarian dysgerminoma, *Int J Radiat Oncol Biol Phys* 14:431-434. 1988.
37. Lemere J, et al: Effectiveness of preoperative chemotherapy in Wilms' tumor: results of SIOP clinical trials, *J Clin Oncol* 1:604-610,1983.
38. Lingley JF, et al: Neuroblastoma: management and survival, *N Engl J Med* 277:1227-1230, 1967.
39. Mathey KK, et al: Patterns of relapse after ABMT for neuroblastoma, *Proc ASCO* 10:312, 1991.
40. Maurer HM, et al: The Intergroup Rhabdomyosarcoma Study-I: a final report, *Cancer* 61:209-220, 1988.
41. Newton WA Jr, et al: Histopathology of childhood sarcomas, IRS I and II: clinicopathologic correlation, *J Clin Oncol* 6:67-75,1988.
42. Nishi M, et al: Effects of the mass screening of neuroblastoma in Sapporo city, *Cancer* 60:433-436, 1987.
43. Oberfield SE, et al: Thyroid and gonadal function and growth of long

term survivors of medulloblastoma/PNET. In Green DM, D'Angio GJ, editors: *Late effects of treatment for childhood cancer,* New York, 1992, Wiley-Liss.

44. Palma L, Guidetti B: Cystic pilocytic astrocytomas of the cerebral hemispheres: surgical experience with 51 cases and long term results, *J Neurosurg* 62:811-815, 1985.

45. Patterson E, Farr RF: Cerebellar medulloblastoma: treatment by irradiation of the whole central nervous system, *Acta Radiol* 39:323-336, 1953.

46. Raney B: Soft tissue sarcoma in adolescents. In Tebbi CK, editor: *Adolescent oncology,* Mt. Kisco, NY, 1987, Futura Publishing.

47. Reese A: *Tumors of the eye,* Hagerstown, Md, 1976, Harper & Row.

48. Rorke L: The cerebellar medulloblastoma and its relationship to primitive neuroectodermal tumors, *J Neuropathol Exp Neurol* 42:2-15, 1983.

49. Rudoler S, et al: Patterns of presentation, treatment, and outcome of children referred for emergent/urgent therapeutic irradiation. Presented at the Evolving Role of Radiation in Pediatric Oncology Conference, Philadelphia, 1995.

50. Silverman CL, Simpson JR: Cerebellar medulloblastoma: the importance of posterior fossa dose to survival and patterns of failure, *Int J Radiat Oncol Biol Phys* 8:1869-1876, 1982.

51. Stevens KR Jr: The soft tissue. In Moss WT, Cox JD: *Radiation oncology: rationale, techniques, results,* ed 6, St. Louis, 1989, Mosby.

52. Tarbell NJ, Buck BA: *Postgraduate advances in radiation oncology: the treatment of medulloblastoma,* Berryville, Va, 1990, Forum Medicum.

53. Tefft M, Wharam M, Gehan E: Local and regional control of rhabdomyosarcoma by radiation in IRS II, *Int J Radiat Oncol Biol Phys* 15(suppl 1):159, 1988.

54. Thomas PRM: Personal communication, 1994.

55. Thomas PRM, et al: Validation of radiation dose reductions used in the Third National Wilms' Tumor Study, *Proc ASCO* 29:227, 1988.

56. Van den Berge JH, et al: Intracavitary brachytherapy of cystic craniopharyngiomas, *J Neurosurg* 77:545-550, 1992.

57. Young JA, Eslinger P, Galloway M: Radiation treatment for the child with cancer, *Issues Comp Pediatr Nurs* 12:159-169, 1989.

BIBLIOGRAPHY

D'Angio GJ, et al: *Practical pediatric oncology,* New York, 1989, Raven.

Green DM, D'Angio GJ, editors: *Late effects of treatment for childhood cancer,* New York, 1992, Wiley-Liss.

Halperin EC, et al: *Pediatric radiation oncology,* New York, 1989, Raven.

Kun LE: Childhood cancer. In Cox JD, and Ang KK editors: *Radiation oncology: rationale, techniques, results,* St. Louis, 2003, Mosby.

Perez CA, Brady LK: *Principles and practice of radiation oncology,* Philadelphia, 1998, Lippincott-Raven.

Pizzo PA, et al: *Principles and practice of pediatric oncology,* Philadelphia, 1993, JB Lippincott.

Rubin P: Clinical Oncology: *A multidisciplinary approach for physicians and students,* Philadelphia, 2001, Saunders.

Skin and Melanoma

Charles M. Washington, Todd A. Blobe

Outline

Key Terms

Actinic (solar) keratoses
Basal cell carcinoma
Dermis
Desquamation
Epidermis
Erythema
Keratin
Keratinocytes
Keratoacanthoma

Melanin
Melanocytes
Mohs' surgery
Mycosis fungoides
Nevus
Squamous cell carcinoma
Subcutaneous layer
Telangiectases
Xeroderma pigmentosum

D uring a lifetime, the skin, one of the most visible and vulnerable organs of the body, is subjected to many external influences, including cold, heat, friction, ultraviolet (UV) light, pressure, and chemicals. As a result, the skin is especially susceptible to trauma, infection, and disease.

This chapter focuses on the three main types of skin cancer: basal cell carcinoma (BCC), squamous cell carcinoma, and malignant melanoma. Basal cell and squamous cell carcinomas are commonly referred to as *nonmelanoma cancers of the skin.*

SKIN AND MELANOMA

Epidemiology

Cancer of the skin is the most common type of malignancy. Approximately 50% of all people who live to age 65 will develop at least one skin cancer during their lifetime.[7] In 2003 the incidence of basal cell and squamous cell skin cancer is estimated to be more than 1,000,000 new cases (basal cell cancers outnumber squamous cell cancers of the skin approximately five to one), whereas malignant melanoma of the skin was expected to account for 54,200 new cases, an increase seen over the last few years.[5] Fig. 37-1 shows the estimated new melanoma cases per year for the last 6 years. The reason that such a large range for nonmelanoma skin cancer estimates exists is that many early skin cancer lesions are easily treated by primary physicians and dermatologists and are not reported to the various cancer-tracking agencies.

Unfortunately, the incidence of skin cancers and melanomas is rising. "During the past decade, the annual increase in malignant melanoma was approximately 7 percent *per year,* the most rapidly increasing rate for any cancer in the United States."[55] For adults between the ages of 25 and

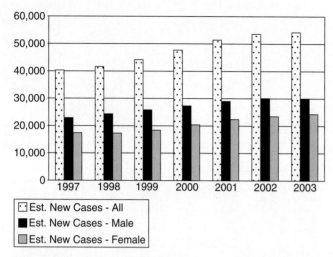

Figure 37-1. Estimated new melanoma cases per year in the United States. *(Compiled from 1997-2003 Cancer facts and figures on the American Cancer Society's web site http://www.cancer.org/docroot/STT/STT_0.asp)*

29 and men aged 30 to 40, melanoma now displaces other cancers in occurrence. In women between the ages of 30 and 40, only breast cancer outnumbers the cases of melanoma. The number of basal cell and squamous cell skin cancers have also increased by as much as 65% since 1983,[48] and more young people are being affected. A few theories that might account for this trend are as follows:

1. The "healthy tan" has become fashionable in recent years. Crowded beaches and the proliferation of tanning salons seem to indicate people are interested in that look.
2. Clothing trends have changed in recent years. Every day fashions and swimwear have become more liberal, allowing for more skin to be exposed to the sun's rays.
3. The depletion of the ozone layer has diminished the atmosphere's ability to protect the earth and its inhabitants from the sun's harmful UV rays. Rays that were formerly filtered by the ozone layer now reach the earth's surface and its inhabitants. "According to the latest projections, a one percent decrease in ozone heralds a 2.6 percent increase in basal and squamous cell cancers."[53]

In contrast to increasing rates of incidence, death rates as a result of skin cancer have stayed virtually the same over the last 6 years (Fig. 37-2). Melanoma mortality for the most recent period is increasing slightly in white men, and it has stabilized in white women.[5] Nonmelanomas, however, have experienced a decreasing death rate. The fact that death rates are so low and declining for nonmelanoma skin cancer is good news, but the comparatively higher death rates for melanomas are concerning.

Melanomas are much more lethal than their nonmelanoma counterparts. About 7400 people (4700 males and 2700 females) will die from melanoma each year. Although nonmelanomas outnumber melanomas approximately 30:1, more people die each year from melanoma than from nonmelanoma skin cancers.

Some individuals are more prone to skin cancer than others. Tendencies for people to develop skin cancers and melanomas can be grouped into four main categories: geographic location, skin type, multiplicity, and gender.

Geographic location. People who live near the equator have a high chance of developing skin cancer because the sun's rays are intense and direct. At latitudes away from the equator, the sun's rays are angled and are not as intense. This angulation causes the rays to travel through more of the atmosphere, allowing it to absorb more harmful rays in areas away from the equator than those at the equator itself (Fig. 37-3). Table 37-1 shows annual UV levels in selected cities, with Anchorage's level as an arbitrary baseline. On average, the closer a city is to the equator, the higher the UV exposure. The higher the UV exposure, the higher the rates for skin cancer. For example, melanoma rates in Honolulu are twice those in Detroit. This difference corresponds roughly with that in the UV index. Similarly, people living at high altitudes are more prone to develop skin cancer because high levels have fewer atmospheres to filter the sun's rays. Each 1000-foot climb in elevation is accompanied by a 4% to 5% increase in UV radiation exposure.[53]

Skin type. Individuals with fair complexions are 10 times more likely to develop skin cancer than those with dark skin. Especially susceptible are albinos, people with freckles or light-colored eyes, and people who suffer from **xeroderma pigmentosum** (a genetic condition caused by a defect in mechanisms that repair deoxyribonucleic acid [DNA] damage caused by UV light, characterized by the development of pigment abnormalities and multiple skin cancers in body areas exposed to the sun). These people tend to tan poorly and burn easily.

People with dark skin have greater quantities of **melanin**

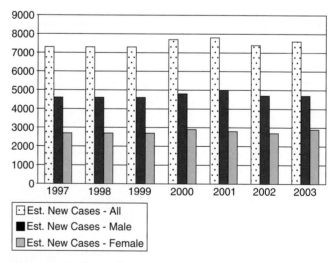

Figure 37-2. Estimated new melanoma deaths per year in the United States. *(Compiled from 1997-2003 Cancer facts and figures on the American Cancer Society's web site, http://www.cancer.org/docroot/STT/STT_0.asp)*

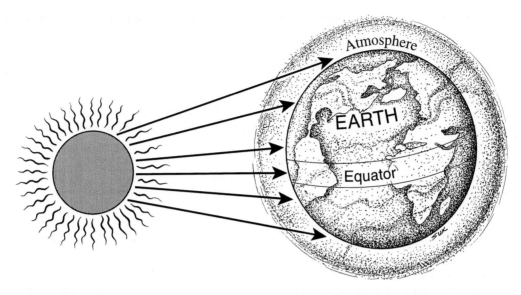

Figure 37-3. Areas near the equator receive more direct sunlight than areas closer to the poles. Notice the way the angled rays near the poles are filtered through larger amounts of the atmosphere before they reach the earth.

Table 37-1	Comparison of latitude on ultraviolet exposure		
City	Degrees of latitude	Elevation (ft)	Ultraviolet index
Anchorage	61	118	100
Seattle	47	10	477
Detroit	42	585	630
Philadelphia	40	100	656
Boise*	43	2704	715
Phoenix	33	1090	889
Denver*	39	5280	951
Houston	29	40	999
Miami	25	10	1028
Honolulu	21	21	1147

Modified from Roach M, Hastings J, Finch S: Sun struck: here's the hole story about the ozone and your chances of getting skin cancer, *Health* 11:40, May-June, 1992.
*UV readings for Boise and Denver seem to be out of place, but in comparing the elevations of those two cities, a significant difference is evident. High elevations also contribute to higher UV exposures.

(a natural protective substance that gives color to the skin, hair, and iris of the eye) in their skin, giving them more protection from the UV rays of the sun. This does not mean that dark-skinned individuals are free of skin cancers, but they get them less often and in more unusual places, such as on the palm of the hand, on the sole of the foot, or in the mucous membranes. Among African Americans, squamous cell carcinoma is more common than BCC. Squamous cell carcinoma tends to occur in sites not exposed to the sun and is often aggressive.[48]

Multiplicity. Prior skin cancer occurrence increases the odds that a second primary skin cancer will develop. Reasons for this may include the following: (1) other areas of the skin may have been exposed to the same carcinogens that caused the initial skin cancer and (2) the individual may have a weakness in the immune system that hinders the ability to fight off skin cancers naturally.

A previous melanoma of the skin increases the risk of another primary melanoma by five to nine times. The rate of second primary melanomas is higher in persons younger than 40 years at the original time of diagnosis compared with persons diagnosed at age 40 or older. The risk is highest in the first year after the original diagnosis but remains highly elevated long afterward.[52]

For individuals with at least one nonmelanoma cancer occurrence, the chances of developing a second malignancy are 17% within 1 year and 50% within 5 years.[30] Because of these elevated risks, any patient diagnosed with skin cancer should be closely monitored for signs of recurrence or new primaries.

Gender. Rates for melanoma skin cancers are slightly more for men than women, but men are three times more likely than women to develop nonmelanomas, except on the legs, where women have higher rates of nonmelanoma skin cancers.[40] This trend seems to be related to skin care habit differences between the genders rather than genetics. Men tend to work outside more often and do not wear sunscreens as often (50% less) as women. Also, men have a more nonchalant attitude about sun exposure and its effects. In general, women seem to pay more attention to their skin than men.[32]

Etiology

Many factors are directly and indirectly responsible for the development of the various forms of skin cancer, but the major cause is exposure to UV light.

UV light. The American Cancer Society estimates that approximately 90% of all skin cancers would be prevented if people protected their skin from the sun's rays.[7] The risk of developing melanoma increases four to five times after three or more blistering sunburns during adolescence.[4] The time between the initial stimulus (sunburn) and the appearance of a melanoma is believed to be between 10 and 20 years.[56] At greatest risk for developing a malignant melanoma is the person who primarily stays indoors and receives occasional sun exposure. In contrast, people who spend a majority of the time in the sun (e.g., farmers, construction workers) are most apt to develop basal cell or squamous cell carcinomas.

Sunlight contains two types of UV rays that are harmful to the skin: ultraviolet A (UVA) and ultraviolet B (UVB). Their wavelengths are between 290 and 320 nanometers (UVA) and between 320 and 400 nanometers (UVB).[55]

UVB is thought to cause cancer by damaging DNA and its repair systems, resulting in mutations that may lead to cancer. It is also thought to play a role in cellular immunity by impairing T-cell function and increasing suppressor T-cell numbers.[48]

UVA rays have long been considered relatively harmless compared with UVB rays. In fact, "most tanning equipment emits ultraviolet A light."[48] Recent studies have shown that the stratum corneum absorbs UVB (see anatomy and physiology section in this chapter), whereas 50% of UVA radiation is able to penetrate to the highly mitotic basal layer of the skin, where the potential for malignant changes and premature aging of the skin exists. Evidence also suggests that UVA acts to promote tumors initiated by UVB.[56]

Like many other cancers, skin cancer is a disease of aging. Most skin cancers appear after age 50, but the damaging effects of the sun's rays are accumulated over a lifetime. However, skin cancers can develop in infants, children, and young adults, especially those with high-risk factors (e.g., xeroderma pigmentosum, giant hairy nevi).

Other factors associated with nonmelanoma skin cancers. Other factors that contribute to nonmelanoma skin cancers include exposure to arsenic (an element used in medicines and poisons) and therapeutic or occupational exposure to radiation. After irradiation the risk to the exposed individual is up to 20%, and latent periods may extend up to 50 years beyond the initial exposure. Squamous cell carcinomas account for two thirds of these radiation-induced lesions, which tend to be aggressive and result in a 10% mortality rate.[17]

Besides xeroderma pigmentosum, another genetic condition associated with the formation of BCCs is called basal cell nevus syndrome (a genetically linked condition that appears during the late teen years). Symptoms include multiple BCCs of the skin, cysts of the jaw bones, pitting of the palms and soles, and skeletal anomalies (particularly of the ribs).[7]

Squamous cell carcinomas of the skin have also been associated with the following[61]:
- Human papillomavirus infection
- Immunosuppression as a result of organ transplant, lymphoma, or leukemia

- Thermal or electrical burns and chronic heat exposure
- Scars or chronic inflammatory conditions
- Hydrocarbons derived from coal and petroleum
- Areas of chronic drainage (e.g., fistulas, sinuses)

Smoking is a proven cause of squamous cell carcinoma of the lip. It has also been linked to the development of squamous cell skin cancer in other anatomic areas. However, it is not known whether cigarette smoke acts directly as a skin carcinogen or has an adverse effect on the immune system, inhibiting the body's ability to defend itself from cancer.[30]

Other factors associated with melanoma skin cancers. Melanomas tend to develop from **melanocytes** (the skin cells that produce melanin), which grow in clusters to form a mole, or **nevus**. Moles can be broadly classified according to when they are acquired: congenital melanocytic nevi (those present at birth) and common acquired nevi (those that develop later in life).

Congenital melanocytic nevi can be classified into three sizes: small (less than 1.5 cm in diameter), medium (1.5 cm to 19.9 cm in diameter), and large (20 cm or more in diameter). Large nevi (Fig. 37-4) are accompanied by an approximate 6%

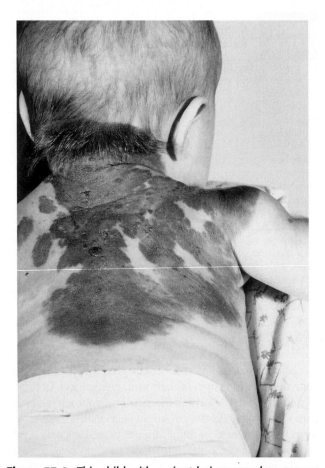

Figure 37-4. This child with a giant hairy nevus has approximately an 8% chance of developing a melanoma within the first 15 years of life. Because of the high risk, this lesion will be removed in a series of prophylactic surgical procedures. *(Photo and information courtesy R. Dean Glassman, MD.)*

to 8% risk of developing melanoma compared with a 1% risk in the general population. Accordingly, some surgeons believe that these moles should be removed prophylactically before malignant changes can occur. Prophylactic removal of small and medium lesions should be made individually because the chance of malignant change in them is small.[24]

Melanocytic nevi can be grouped into three main categories: junctional, compound, and intradermal. Junctional nevi tend to be small (usually less than 6 mm), well-circumscribed, flat lesions with smooth surfaces that are uniformly brown or black and circular. The melanocyte clusters in junctional nevi are found above the basement layer. Compound nevi contain melanocyte clusters in the dermis and epidermis. They appear as small, well-circumscribed, slightly raised papules that often contain excess hair. The surface is rough and color ranges from tan to brown throughout. Over time, these lesions may take on a nodular appearance. Intradermal nevi are small, well-circumscribed, dome-shaped lesions that range from flesh to brown. They too may contain excess hair. Melanocytic clusters are found only in the dermal layer in these moles.[24]

The propensity of a mole to develop into a melanoma is related to the location of the melanocytic clusters found in the moles. Intradermal nevi rarely transform into melanomas; the likelihood of junctional and compound nevi transforming into melanomas is far greater. One theory for this pattern is that melanocytes located in the dermis do not receive as much UV exposure because they are located deep in the skin. Melanocytes in junctional and compound nevi are closer to the skin's surface and receive higher amounts of melanoma-inducing UV radiation.

Dysplastic nevi, also known as B-K or atypical moles, are acquired pigmented lesions of the skin that have one or more of the clinical features of melanoma—asymmetry, border irregularity, color variation, or a diameter greater than 6 mm.[24] "The presence of dysplastic moles marks an individual as having a seven-fold to seventy-fold increased risk of melanoma. Even a single dysplastic mole appears to be a significant risk factor for melanoma."[52]

The number of moles a person has also influences the chances of acquiring melanoma. One study showed that "persons who have twelve moles at least 5 mm in diameter have an estimated 41-fold increased risk of melanoma while those who have fifty or more moles at least 2 mm in diameter have a 64-fold increased risk of melanoma."[52]

People with a family history of melanoma have an eight-fold increase in their chances of acquiring the disease.[52] Several studies have pinpointed a region on the short arm of chromosome 9 (9p) as one involved in the early-stage development of melanoma tumors.[16] Genetic material from this area is thought to play a vital role in the suppression of tumor formation. Without this material a person may be more susceptible to tumor formation because one of the normal defense mechanisms may be missing. Other chromosomal abnormalities associated with melanomas can be found on chromosomes 1, 6, 7, 11, and 19.[28]

"Some families are affected with an inherited familial atypical mole and melanoma (FAM-M) syndrome, also known as B-K mole syndrome or dysplastic nevus syndrome (DNS). The syndrome is defined by (1) occurrence of melanoma in one or more first- or second-degree relatives; (2) large number of moles (often 50+), some of which are atypical and often variable in size; and (3) moles that demonstrate certain distinct histologic features. Persons with this syndrome have a markedly increased risk of developing melanoma. Their lifetime risk may be as much as 100%."[43] These patients require close monitoring because of the high risks involved. This syndrome has also been described in the nonfamilial setting.[24]

"Hormones, pregnancy, birth control pills, and certain environmental exposures have also been linked to the development of malignant melanoma, but these factors need further study."[6]

Anatomy and Physiology

The skin is the largest organ of the body, covering about 22 sq ft and weighing 10 to 12 lb on the average person. The skin provides many functions, including the following:

- Regulates body temperature through perspiration (as perspiration evaporates, it carries heat away from the body) and blood flow through vessels located in the skin (the skin allows heat carried by the blood to radiate off its surface)
- Acts as a barrier between the external environment and the body, offering protection against factors such as trauma, UV light, and bacterial invasion
- Participates in the production of vitamin D, which is vital to the process enabling the body to absorb and use calcium in the gastrointestinal tract
- Provides receptors for external stimuli such as heat, cold, pressure, and touch, allowing the body to be aware of its environment

The skin is an example of an epithelial membrane, a connective tissue covered by a layer of epithelial tissue. The connective tissue layer in the skin is called the **dermis;** the epithelial layer is called the **epidermis** (Fig. 37-5). These layers are held together by an intermediate layer called the basement membrane.[59]

The dermis is the deeper layer of the skin composed of connective tissue that contains blood and lymphatic vessels, nerves and nerve endings, sweat glands, and hair follicles. It contains mainly elastic and collagen fibers that allow for the flexibility and strength of the skin. The upper 20% of the dermis is referred to as the papillary region and contains dermal papillae, ridges that are responsible for the formation of fingerprints. The lower 80% of the dermis is the reticular region and contains many accessory structures of the skin, such as the following: hair follicles, sebaceous (oil) and sudoriferous (sweat) glands and their ducts, nerve endings, and blood vessels.[59]

A **subcutaneous layer** containing nerves, blood vessels, adipose (fat) tissue, and areolar connective tissue lies beneath the dermis. Because the epidermis is avascular, the blood vessels of the dermis and subcutaneous layer are responsible for the nutritional status of the epidermis.

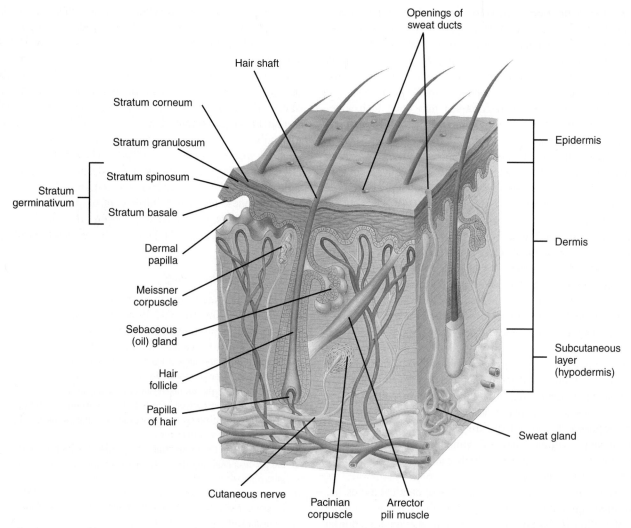

Figure 37-5. This cross section of the skin shows the relationship between the epidermis, dermis, and subcutaneous layers. Notice how thick the dermis is compared with the epidermis. Also shown are the various accessory structures of the skin and their location. *(From Thibodeau GA, Patton KT: Anatomy and physiology, ed 3, St. Louis, 1996, Mosby.)*

The epidermis is the extremely thin outer layer of the skin, composed of four to five layers (depending on its location). These layers are as follows, from deepest to most superficial[59]:

1. **Stratum basale (stratum germinativum)**—this is the basal layer containing stem cells capable of producing **keratinocytes** (stratified epithelial cells, which comprise 90% of the epidermal cells of the skin and provide a barrier between the host and the environment, prevent the entry of toxic substances from the environment and the loss of important constituents from the host) and cells that give rise to glands and hair follicles. This layer also contains melanocytes (which comprise 8% of the epidermal cells of the skin), cells with branching processes that produce the pigment melanin. In hairless skin a third type of cell, Merkel's cells, can also be found. Together with a flattened portion of a neuron called a tactile (Merkel's disc), Merkel's cells function in the sensation of touch.

2. **Stratum spinosum**—this layer contains 8 to 10 rows of keratinocytes, which have a spiny appearance microscopically.

Branches from the melanocytes reach into this layer, allowing the keratinocytes to absorb the protective pigment melanin via exocytosis.

3. **Stratum granulosum**—this layer contains three to five rows of somewhat flattened cells. The keratinocytes begin to produce a substance called keratohyalin, which is a precursor to a waterproof protein called **keratin.**

4. **Stratum lucidum**—this layer is normally found only in areas in which thick skin is present (soles and palms) and contains three to five rows of clear, flat cells that contain eleidin, another keratin precursor.

5. **Stratum corneum**—this layer forms the skin surface and contains 25 to 30 rows of flat, dead, scaly (squamous) cells that are completely filled with keratin and have lost all their internal organelles, including nuclei. The lower layers of cells are closely packed and adhere to each other, whereas the upper layers of cells are loosely packed and continually flake away from the surface.

Basically, the outer, protective layer of the skin is composed of dead cells filled with keratin. Each day, millions of these cells are sloughed off and continually replaced by cells from the lower layers of the epidermis. Germ cells in the stratum basale give rise to keratinocytes, which go through a process called keratinization as they are pushed toward the surface by new cells. As the cells are relocated, they accumulate keratin to the point that the cells can no longer function and dies. The mature keratinocytes serve their protective function and are eventually shed from the surface of the skin. The time necessary for the cell to travel from the germ layer to the surface is approximately 2 to 4 weeks. This cycle continually repeats itself.

Melanin is a pigment that serves a protective function of the skin. It is produced by the melanocytes and absorbed by the keratinocytes in the stratum spinosum layer of the epidermis. UV light damages the keratinocytes by inhibiting synthesis of DNA and ribonucleic acid (RNA) (genetic material in the cell), leading to cell dysfunction or death. The melanin absorbed by the keratinocytes is placed in the cell so that it lies between the skin surface and nucleus of the cell, thus protecting it from the sun's rays like an umbrella (Fig. 37-6).

Melanin is one of the pigments responsible for differences in skin color among individuals. The more melanin a person's skin contains, the darker the skin. The number of melanocytes is about the same in all races. Differences in skin darkness are attributed to the amount of melanin that the melanocytes produce. The systemic release of melanocyte-stimulating hormone (MSH) from the anterior pituitary gland controls overall skin darkness. The more MSH released by the pituitary, the more melanin the melanocytes produce and the darker the person's skin. Variations in skin darkness can occur in localized areas of the body as a result of exposure to UV light. Brief exposure to UV light causes melanin already present in the epidermis to darken considerably, whereas long-term exposure causes melanocytes to increase melanin production. Both processes result in darker or tanned skin. A tan is actually a response by the body to damage caused by UV light.[53] In the absence of UV stimulation, melanocytes decrease melanin production to normal levels and the skin returns to normal color.[63]

Skin cancers can be classified according to the cell of the skin from which they originate. Malignant melanoma, the most lethal form of skin cancer, arises from the melanocytes located in the stratum basale. The most common sites for melanoma are the legs of women and the trunk and face of men. Melanomas can also arise in other areas of the body, such as the choroid or ciliary body of the eye, the eyelids, the mucosa of the oral cavity, the genitalia, and the anus.

Basal cell carcinoma (BCC), a slow-growing form of skin cancer that does not tend to metastasize, arises from the stem cells of the stratum basale. It is the most prevalent cancer in humans and, if left untreated, can cause extensive damage.

Squamous cell carcinoma, a faster-growing cancer than the basal cell type with a higher propensity for metastasis,

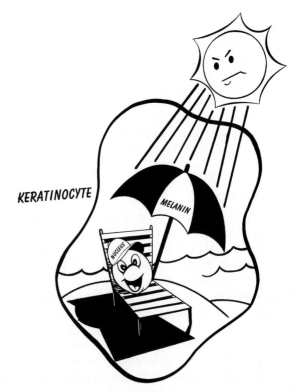

Figure 37-6. This cartoon depicts the way melanin is strategically placed inside the keratinocyte between the nucleus and sun's rays, protecting it from ultraviolet radiation.

arises from the more mature keratinocytes of the upper layers of the epidermis. This type of nonmelanoma skin cancer can arise anywhere on the body but is especially common on sun-exposed areas such as the head, neck, face, arms, and hands.

Other types of cancers can arise in the skin but are not covered in detail in this chapter. These include, but are not limited to, the following[45]:

1. **Adenocarcinoma of the sebaceous and sudoriferous glands—** this type of cancer arises in the dermal layer of the skin and is a slow-growing lesion capable of metastasis. It tends to be radioresistant; therefore surgery is the treatment of choice.

2. **Cutaneous T-cell lymphoma,** including **mycosis fungoides—** this is a disease of the T lymphocytes. It resembles eczema or other inflammatory conditions and tends to remain localized to the skin for long periods. Total-body irradiation with electrons and topical nitrogen mustard has been used to control early stages of the disease.

3. **Kaposi's sarcoma—**this is a slow-growing, temperate tumor thought to arise from vascular tissue. The associated nodular purple lesions are often multifocal and common in individuals affected with acquired immunodeficiency syndrome (AIDS) and those living in the Mediterranean region. Surgical excision is indicated for individual lesions and radiation therapy for multiple lesions.

The AIDS epidemic has introduced an aggressive variant of this disease. Although associated lesions are radiosensitive, AIDS patients who acquire this disease have a poor prognosis and are best treated systemically with chemotherapy. Radiation therapy is used to palliate local areas.

4. **Merkel's cell carcinoma**—this is a rare tumor thought to arise from Merkel's (tactile) cells. It is known for high rates of recurrence after surgical excision, frequent involvement of regional lymph nodes, and distant metastatic failure. These tumors are structurally similar to small cell carcinomas and appear as firm, nontender, pink-red nodular lesions with an intact epidermis.[46] These types of cancers are often treated with a combination of chemotherapy and radiation therapy or surgery.

Clinical Presentation

Although skin cancers and melanomas occur in a wide variety of shapes, sizes, and appearances, similarities exist that facilitate lesion classification. Following is a discussion concerning the tumors seen most often and premalignant growths that may precede them.

Nonmelanoma precursors and characteristics. Premalignant lesions are those that, if left untreated or not closely monitored, can develop into cancer. Squamous cell carcinomas tend to arise more often from precursor lesions compared with BCCs.[62] The American Cancer Society classifies some of the precancerous lesions for nonmelanomas as follows[7]:

1. **Actinic (solar) keratoses**—These are warty lesions or areas of red, scaly patches occurring on the sun-exposed skin of the face or hands of older, light-skinned individuals (Fig. 37-7). Because actinic keratoses have a 5% to 10% chance[31] of degrading into squamous cell carcinoma, some physicians remove them surgically or treat them with 5-fluorouracil (5-FU), liquid nitrogen, or electrodesiccation to destroy them and eliminate the possibility of cancerous change.[17]
2. **Arsenical keratoses**—These are multiple, hard, cornlike masses on the palms of hands or soles of feet resulting from long-term arsenic ingestion.
3. **Bowen's disease**—This is a precancerous dermatosis or carcinoma in situ characterized by the development of pink or brown papules covered with a thickened, horny layer (Fig. 37-8).
4. **Keratoacanthoma**—This is a rapid-growing lesion that can

appear suddenly as a dome-shaped mass on a sun-exposed area (Fig. 37-9). Microscopically, the nodules are composed of well-differentiated squamous epithelia with a necrotic center or central keratin mass. They can be difficult to distinguish from squamous cell cancer and usually resolve themselves if left untreated.

Nonmelanoma skin cancers have a multitude of appearances (Figs. 37-10 and 37-11). BCCs tend to arise as smooth, red, or milky lumps and have a pearly border and multiple **telangiectases** (tiny blood vessels visible on the skin's surface). BCCs can be shiny or pale. About 80% of BCCs occur on the head and neck. Squamous cell carcinomas tend to have a scaly, crusty, slightly elevated lesion that may have a cutaneous horn. Approximately 80% of UV-induced squamous cell carcinomas develop on the arms, head, and neck.[48] Other symptoms possibly indicating a basal cell or squamous cell carcinoma include a sore that takes longer than 3 weeks to heal, a recurrent red patch that may itch or be tender, and a wart that bleeds or scabs. Some BCCs may contain melanin, causing the lesion to appear black and resemble a melanoma. In general, any new growths that persist or change in appearance should be reported to a physician.

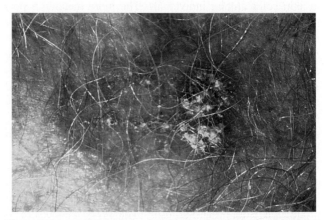

Figure 37-8. Bowen's disease. *(Courtesy Mark McLaughlin, MD.)*

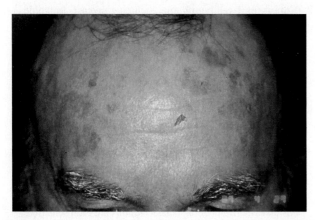

Figure 37-7. Actinic keratosis. *(Courtesy Mark McLaughlin, MD.)*

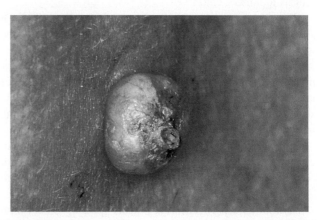

Figure 37-9. Keratoacanthoma. *(Courtesy Mark McLaughlin, MD.)*

Melanoma precursors and characteristics. Approximately 70% of melanomas occur as the result of a change in a preexisting nevus. The other 30% arise from de novo melanomas, growths not associated with previously observed nevi.[17] The American Cancer Society[7] has released the ABCD rules for early detection of melanoma (Fig. 37-12). These are as follows:

A, *Asymmetry*—melanomas tend to be asymmetrical; most benign moles tend to be symmetrical.

B, *Border*—melanomas tend to have notched, uneven borders; most benign moles tend to possess clearly defined, smooth borders.

C, *Color*—melanomas can contain different shades of black, brown, or tan; benign moles tend to be uniformly tan or brown.

D, *Diameter*—most melanomas have a diameter greater than 6 mm; most benign moles tend to be less than 6 mm in diameter.

In addition to the ABCD rules, the following changes in the appearance of a mole should be monitored as possible signs of melanoma[41]:

1. Change in color—red, white, and/or blue areas in addition to black and tan

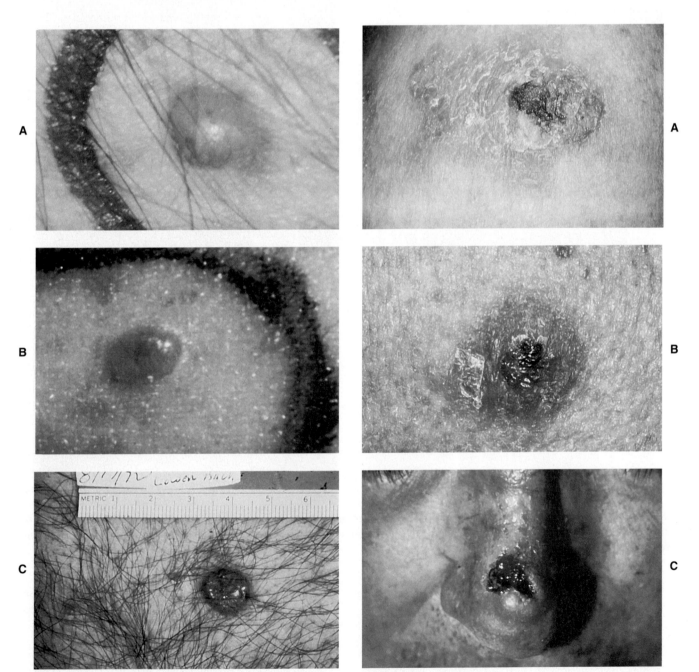

Figure 37-10. A, B, and **C,** Examples of basal cell carcinomas. *(**A, B,** and **C** courtesy the National Cancer Institute.)*

Figure 37-11. A, B, and **C,** Examples of squamous cell carcinomas. *(**A, B,** and **C** courtesy the National Cancer Institute.)*

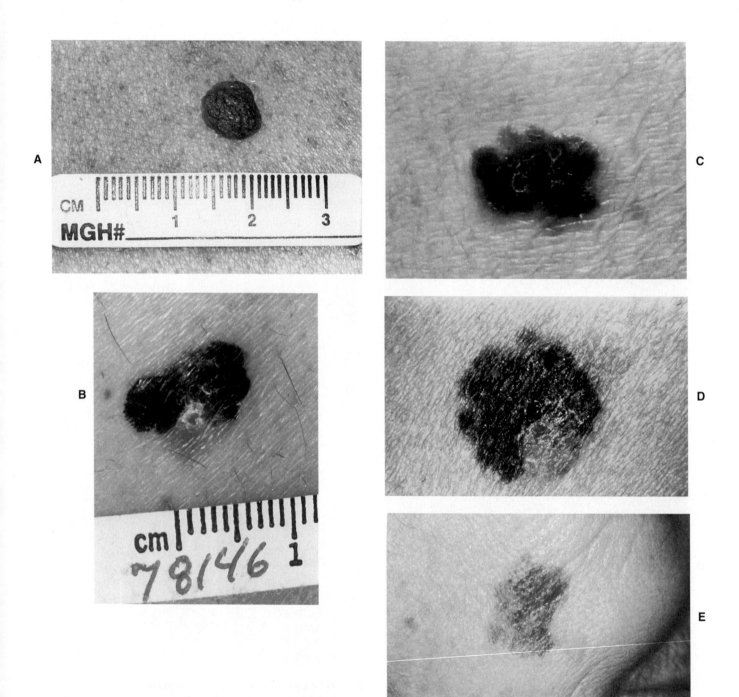

Figure 37-12. A, Normal mole. **B,** Melanoma showing asymmetry. **C,** Melanoma showing irregular borders. **D,** Melanoma showing uneven color. **E,** Melanoma showing a large diameter. *(A to D courtesy the American Cancer Society; E courtesy the National Cancer Institute.)*

2. Change in surface—scaly, flaky, bleeding, or oozing moles or a sore that does not heal
3. Change in texture—hard, lumpy, or elevated moles
4. Change in surrounding skin—spread of pigmentation, swelling, or redness to surrounding skin
5. Change in sensation—unusual pain or tenderness in a mole
6. Change in previously normal skin—pigmented areas that arise in previously normal skin

A few pigmented lesions of the skin are benign, but these can be difficult to distinguish from melanoma.[24] They are as follows:

1. Simple lentigo—This is a small (1 to 5 mm), brown to black macule. It is round with sharply defined edges, and the surface is flat, similar to a freckle. Thought to be the precursor to the common mole, some simple lentigines are clinically indistinguishable from junctional nevi.

2. Solar lentigo—This is a small to medium, flat, lightly pigmented macule better known as a liver spot. It is especially common in older white people on areas of the skin chronically exposed to the sun.

3. Seborrheic keratoses—These are round or ovoid, wartlike papules ranging from a few to several millimeters. These growths tend to be raised (often with a warty, "stuck-on" appearance) and composed of proliferating epidermal cells, especially of the basal type.

4. Others—Some common moles may be difficult to distinguish from melanoma. For a description of common moles, see the section on etiology.

Although all these lesions tend to be benign, they should be watched for signs of malignant change. Questionable lesions should be biopsied and analyzed to rule out malignancy.

Detection and Diagnosis

Theoretically, no one should die from skin cancer because the skin lends itself easily to self-inspection and cancer detection. If people were educated on the way to detect skin cancer and actually took the time to inspect themselves, cancer should be found at an early stage and therefore be easily treatable. Following are some of the methods used to detect and diagnose skin cancer.

Everyone should inspect the total surface area of the skin monthly for signs of cancer (Box 37-1). High-risk individuals should have photographs of the skin taken to document existing moles to which they can refer when questions arise concerning factors such as the size, color, and shape of moles. Body charts indicating the location and size of moles may also be useful.

Inspections should take place in well-lighted areas. Familiarity with existing moles, freckles, and blemishes is important so that newly pigmented areas or blemishes can be distinguished from older ones. When surveying the skin, individuals should remember the ABCD rules. In addition, people should watch for sores that do not heal or other areas of unexplained changes in the skin.

Any unusual changes should be brought to the attention of a physician. The earlier skin cancer is detected, the better the chance it will be cured. People who find unusual lesions must not let their fears of pain, cost, and disfigurement get in the way of seeking a proper diagnosis and treatment. Skin cancer is obviously not something that will go away by itself.

A routine physical examination should include a thorough inspection of the skin's surface by the physician. Physicians must be knowledgeable in distinguishing between benign and malignant conditions. Also, regional lymph nodes should be inspected for signs or symptoms of metastasis.

A family history should be taken to determine whether a person is at a higher risk for developing melanoma because a family member previously had the disease. Patients with a family history of melanoma should be monitored closely.

Individuals should have a biopsy performed for unusual or suspicious lesions. Depending on the size and location of the lesion, the biopsy may be incisional (only a portion of the lesion is removed for tissue diagnosis—usually reserved for large lesions) or excisional (entire lesion is removed). Excisional biopsies (including punch, saucerization, or elliptical incision) may be indicated for suspected squamous cell carcinomas or melanomas to ascertain the depth of the tumor's penetration and should include a portion of the underlying subcutaneous fat for accurate microstaging. A shave or curettage may be adequate to diagnose BCC but is not recommended for lesions suspected to be melanoma.[43]

To the naked eye, some lesions are difficult to define as malignant or nonmalignant without a biopsy. A relatively new technique in diagnosing melanomas is in vivo (in tissue) epi-luminescence microscopy (ELM), or dermatoscopy. ELM is a noninvasive procedure that allows physicians to differentiate between benign and malignant lesions while they are in the early phases of development and have not yet begun to exhibit the features displayed by later melanomatous lesions. The procedure uses a dermatoscope (R), which looks similar to an ophthalmoscope. Mineral oil is placed on the surface of the lesion, causing the stratum corneum to become almost invisible and facilitating the examination of the epidermis, particularly the dermal-epidermal junction. ELM images can be digitized by primary care physicians and sent to ELM experts by telephone for quick analysis.[34] Digitized ELM images can also be fed into computers run by specially designed software. These programs evaluate lesions based on factors such as

---

Box 37-1	Performing a Skin Self-Examination

A simple skin self-examination performed regularly can aid in the early detection of cancer. The best time to do this self-examination is after a shower or bath. Check the skin in a well-lighted room using a full-length mirror and a handheld mirror. It is best to begin by noting the location of birthmarks, moles, and blemishes and what they usually look like. Check for anything new—a change in the size, texture, or color of a mole, or a sore that does not heal.

Check **all** areas, including the back, the scalp, between the buttocks, and the genital area.

Look at the front and back of your body in the mirror, then raise your arms and look at the left and right sides.

Bend your elbows and look carefully at your palms; forearms, including the undersides; and the upper arms.

Examine the back and front of your legs. Also look between your buttocks and around your genital area.

Sit and closely examine your feet, including the soles and the spaces between the toes.

Look at the face, neck, and scalp. Use a comb or a blow dryer to move hair to see better.

Modified from the National Cancer Institute: *What you need to know about skin cancer,* accessed from http://www.cancer.gov/cancerinfo/wyntk/skin#25 on April 15, 2003.

shape, size, color, and border and attempt to make an objective analysis on a previously subjective science.[24]

A dermatologist should be able to identify a type of lesion just by its appearance. Based on this information, the dermatologist should also have a good idea concerning the metastatic potential of the lesion. Again, BCCs have an extremely small chance of metastases, squamous cell carcinomas have a slightly higher chance, and malignant melanomas have the highest chance of all the major skin cancers.

If the physician suspects that a patient may have an advanced squamous cell carcinoma or melanoma, an evaluation for metastasis should be conducted. This evaluation should include the following:

- Physical examination of the patient to find evidence of lymphadenopathy, secondary lesions of the skin, or second primaries
- Evaluation of motor skills to detect possible brain involvement
- Chest x-ray examination to rule out lung metastasis
- Liver function tests to rule out liver involvement
- Evaluation of alkaline phosphatase levels and bone scan if patient complains of bone pain
- Complete blood counts (CBCs) to detect anemias that may be the result of gastrointestinal bleeding caused by metastasis
- Biopsy of regional lymph nodes to compare the number of lymph nodes positive for tumor with the total number of nodes in the biopsy

Computed tomography (CT) and magnetic resonance imaging (MRI) examinations, because of their cost, are often done only when signs and symptoms point to metastatic disease. Because melanoma can spread to virtually any part of the body, CT scans of the head, chest, abdomen, and pelvis may be ordered to rule out involvement of the brain, lung, liver, bowel, adrenals, and subcutaneous skin. MRI is often used as an adjuvant to CT.

Pathology and Staging

Melanoma. After it has been removed, the biopsy specimen is sent to a pathologist who examines it microscopically and provides much useful information that is used to diagnose, stage, and develop a prognosis for the patient. Essential to a pathology report for melanoma are the diagnosis (whether the biopsy specimen indicates cancer), thickness of the tumor, and status of the margins (whether tumor cells are present on the edges of the biopsy specimen). If cancer is diagnosed, additional information may include the following:

- Specific cancer subtype
- Depth of tumor penetration
- Degree of mitotic activity (reproductive rate of cells)
- Growth pattern (radial versus lateral)
- Level of host response (number of lymphocytes present in and/or around the tumor)
- Presence, if any, of tumor ulceration, tumor regression, or satellitosis (lymphatic extensions of the tumor that result in small lesions adjacent to the primary)[43]

Melanomas can be classified according to their growth patterns, and histologic appearances can be grouped into the following four major categories[17,19,45]:

1. Superficial spreading melanomas (SSMs), also called *radial spreading melanomas,* are the most common melanoma subtype, accounting for approximately 70% of all lesions. They generally arise on any anatomic site as preexisting lesions that evolve over several years and have a radial (horizontal) growth pattern. The periphery of these deeply pigmented lesions is often notched or irregular and colors in the tumors can vary from brown, black, red, pink, or white. Partial regression of the tumor is common. As time passes, the tumor tends to grow more vertically, resulting in a more elevated, irregular surface.

2. Nodular melanomas (NMs) account for approximately 15% of all lesions and can also occur on any anatomic site. They are twice as common in men than women. Lesions tend to be raised throughout and vary in color from dark brown, blue, or blue-black. Some lesions may not contain any pigment at all (amelanotic). These tumors are particularly lethal because they lack a radial growth phase, making an early diagnosis difficult. They tend to invade early and frequently show ulceration when advanced.

3. Lentigo maligna melanomas (LMMs), also called *Hutchinson's freckles,* account for approximately 5% of all lesions and tend to occur in chronically sun-exposed skin of older white people, especially females. LMM begins with a relatively benign radial growth phase that may last for decades before it enters its vertical growth phase. The appearance of an LMM is similar to that of an SMM but lacks the red hues and has minimal elevation during its vertical growth phase.

4. Acral lentiginous melanomas (ALMs) account for approximately 10% of all lesions and are found mainly on the palms, soles, nail beds, or mucous membranes. The ALM is the most common form of melanoma in black and oriental people and has a tan or brown flat stain on the palms or soles. An ALM can also appear as a brown to black discoloration under the nail bed and is often mistaken for a fungal infection.

Because melanocytes are found in the basal layer of the epidermis, melanoma formation takes place in this area. Most melanomas begin their development with a radial (horizontal) growth phase (Fig. 37-13), during which abnormal melanocytes form nests along the basal layer. Later, some of the melanocytes begin to migrate into and form nests in the upper layers of the epidermis. The horizontal phase can last as long as 15 years in instances of SSM, 5 years in instances of LMM, or an extremely short (or nonexistent) period in instances of NM.

The second phase of development is the vertical growth phase. During this phase melanocytes descend across the basal lamina and into the dermis. Also during this phase nodules can become raised on the skin's surface. After invasion into the dermis has taken place, inflammatory cells arrive to defend the body from foreign invaders. If these cells are successful, a spontaneous regression takes place. If they are not successful, the melanoma grows deeper into the dermis and may involve the blood and lymphatic vessels, thus possibly helping the melanoma spread to regional lymph nodes and/or virtually any organ of the body.[1]

Dr. Wallace Clark and Dr. Alexander Breslow developed

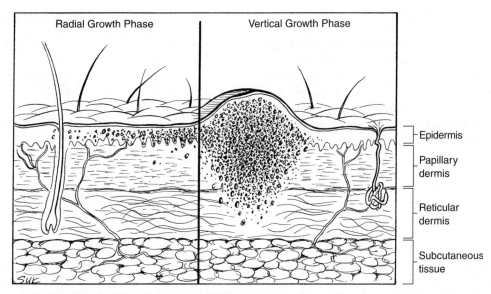

Figure 37-13. A cross section of a superficial spreading melanoma showing the radial growth phases indicative of most early melanomas *(left)*, and the vertical phase indicative of most late melanomas *(right)*.

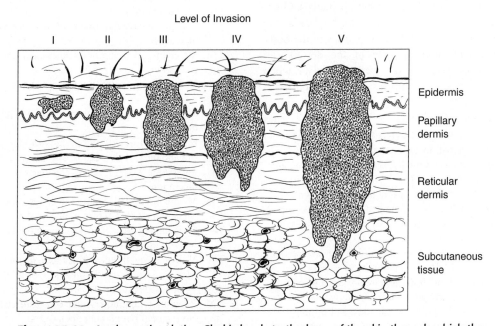

Figure 37-14. A schematic relating Clark's levels to the layer of the skin through which the tumor has penetrated.

the main microstaging systems for melanomas. Both systems are basically indirect measures of tumor volume. Clark's system categorizes melanomas based on their level of invasion through the epidermis and layers of the dermis. Clark's levels (Fig. 37-14) may indicate the potential for metastasis because the access of tumor cells to lymphatic and vascular structures are assessable. Also, the extent of invasion may indicate the tumor's progression from relatively harmless

radial growth to more aggressive vertical growth.[38] Clark's levels are as follows:

- Level 1—confinement to the epidermis above the basement membrane
- Level 2—invasion through the basement membrane to the papillary dermis
- Level 3—presence of tumor cells at the papillary-reticular junction of the dermis

- Level 4—invasion into the reticular dermis
- Level 5—invasion into subcutaneous fat

Breslow's system categorizes melanomas based on tumor thickness from the top of the granular layer of the epidermis or, if the primary tumor is ulcerated, from the ulcer surface to the deepest identifiable melanoma cell as measured by an ocular micrometer.[15] Fig. 37-15 demonstrates how melanoma thickness should be measured using Breslow microstaging. Breslow's microstaging levels are as follows:

- Level 1—melanoma in situ, limited to the epidermis
- Level 2—less than 0.75 mm
- Level 3—0.76 mm to 1.5 mm
- Level 4—1.51 mm to 4 mm
- Level 5—greater than 4 mm

Because Breslow's system has more to do with tumor bulk than penetration, the current thought is that this system is more reproducible and correlates more accurately with the risk of metastatic disease and prognosis than Clark's system. One problem that Clark's system does not address is the variation in skin thickness throughout the body. In contrasting the extremely thin skin of the eyelids with the extremely thick skin of the soles of the feet, a 0.75-mm lesion would be far more penetrating in the eyelid than on the sole of the foot, yet the size of the tumor is the same in both instances. Other problems that pathologists may encounter with Clark's system occur when specimens are taken from areas of the body where the papillary-reticular junction of the dermis (an important demarcation point) is not well defined or when the integrity of the tissue layers in the surgical specimen is compromised.[25]

The American Joint Committee on Cancer (AJCC) has recently revised its assessment system for malignant melanoma of the skin to reflect the following changes:

Melanoma thickness and ulceration, but not level of invasion, are used in all T categories except T1.

The number of metastatic lymph nodes, rather than their gross dimensions and the delineation of clinical occult (microscopic) versus clinically apparent (macroscopic) nodal metastases, are used in the N category.

The site of distant metastases and the presence of elevated serum lactic dehydrogenase (LDH) are used in the M category.

All patients with stage I, II, or III disease are upstaged when a primary melanoma is ulcerated.

Satellite metastases around a primary melanoma and in-transit metastases have been merged into a single staging entity that is grouped into stage IIIc disease.

A new convention for defining clinical and pathologic staging has been developed that takes into account the new staging information gained from intraoperative lymphatic mapping and sentinel node excision.[8]

With these changes, the TNM system has been modified to take into account these changes. Familiar to most radiation oncology professionals, this system for melanoma assesses primary tumor thickness, regional node status, and distant metastatic sites as follows:

Primary tumor (T)

TX   Primary tumor cannot be assessed

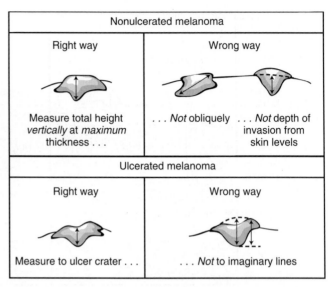

Nonulcerated melanoma	
Right way	Wrong way
Measure total height *vertically* at *maximum* thickness . . .	. . . *Not* obliquely . . . *Not* depth of invasion from skin levels

Ulcerated melanoma	
Right way	Wrong way
Measure to ulcer crater . . .	. . . *Not* to imaginary lines

Figure 37-15. Measuring melanoma thickness correctly and incorrectly for Breslow microstaging.

T0   No evidence of primary tumor

Tis   Melanoma in situ

T1   Melanoma ≤1.0 mm in thickness with or without ulceration

T1a   Melanoma ≤1.0 mm in thickness and level II or III, no ulceration

T1b   Melanoma ≤1.0 mm in thickness and level IV or V or with ulceration

T2   Melanoma 1.01-2.0 mm in thickness with or without ulceration

T2a   Melanoma 1.01-2.0 mm in thickness, no ulceration

T2b   Melanoma 1.01-2.0 mm in thickness, with ulceration

T3   Melanoma 2.01-4.0 mm in thickness with or without ulceration

T3a   Melanoma 2.01-4.0 mm in thickness, no ulceration

T3b   Melanoma 2.01-4.0 mm in thickness, with ulceration

T4   Melanoma greater than 4.0 mm in thickness with or without ulceration

T4a   Melanoma >4.0 mm in thickness, no ulceration

T4b   Melanoma >4.0 mm in thickness, with ulceration

Regional lymph nodes (N)

NX   Regional lymph nodes cannot be assessed

N0   No regional lymph node metastasis

N1   Metastasis in one lymph node

N1a   Clinically occult (microscopic) metastasis

N1b   Clinically apparent (macroscopic) metastasis

N2   Metastasis in two or three regional nodes or intralymphatic regional metastasis without nodal metastasis

N2a   Clinically occult (microscopic) metastasis

N2b   Clinically apparent (macroscopic) metastasis

N2c   Satellite or in-transit metastasis *without* nodal metastasis

N3   Metastasis in four or more regional nodes, or matted metastatic nodes, or in-transit metastasis, or satellite(s) with metastasis in regional node(s)

Distant metastasis (M)

MX Distant metastasis cannot be assessed

M0 No distant metastasis

M1 Distant metastasis

M1a Metastasis to skin, subcutaneous tissues or distant lymph nodes

M1b Metastasis to lung

M1c Metastasis to all other visceral sites or distant metastasis at any site associated with an elevated serum lactic dehydrogenase (LDH)

After it has been classified according to the TNM system, tumors are typically organized into specific stages. Stage groupings allow health care workers to assemble patients with similar disease patterns to aid physicians in treatment planning, facilitate information exchange, indicate disease spread risk and prognosis, and help evaluate treatment results. In assessing metastatic spread potential, stage I tumors demonstrate a low risk, stages II through IIIA have an intermediate risk, stage IIIB has a high risk, and stages IIIC and IV are at a very high risk.[8] The presence of melanoma ulceration upstages the prognosis of stages I to III patients compared with patients with melanoma of the same thickness without ulceration or those with nodal metastases arising from a nonulcerating melanoma. The clinical groupings that relate TNM and stage are as follows:

Stage 0	Tis	N0	M0
Stage IA	T1a	N0	M0
Stage IB	T1b	N0	M0
	T2a	N0	M0
Stage IIA	T2a	N0	M0
	T3a	N0	M0
Stage IIB	T3b	N0	M0
	T4a	N0	M0
Stage IIC	T4b	N0	M0
Stage III	Any T	N1	M0
	Any T	N2	M0
Any T	N3	M0	
Stage IV	Any T	Any N	M1

Survival rates for patients with an ulcerated melanoma are proportionally lower than those with a nonulcerated melanoma of the same T category, but similar to those for patients with a nonulcerated melanoma of the next higher T category.[8]

The two most significant characteristics of the primary melanoma are tumor thickness and ulceration. Other significant prognostic factors were age, site of the primary melanoma, level of invasion and gender, as noted in the following list:

1. Tumor thickness—thicker tumors yield a poorer prognosis.
2. Ulceration—ulcerated tumors have a worse prognosis than nonulcerated.
3. Age—the prognosis for older patients is worse than that for younger patients.[54]
4. Location of primary tumor—tumors located on the extremities, excluding the feet, have a better prognosis than tumors on the

head and neck, which have a better prognosis than a tumor found on the trunk.[19]

5. Depth of invasion—the deeper the level of penetration, the poorer the prognosis.
6. Gender—all things being equal, women have a 22% survival advantage over men when the disease is found before it has metastasized.[58]

Because the epidermis does not contain any blood vessels or lymphatics, skin cancers confined to that area have virtually no chance of spreading other than via direct extension. After a tumor invades the superficial lymphatic plexus of the dermis (which is devoid of valves characteristic of deeper lymphatic vessels),[36] it can spread in any direction from the tumor. Because melanomas can occur on a multitude of different locations throughout the body, physicians must be aware of the lymphatic drainage patterns of the specific area where the melanoma is found. Obviously, a melanoma found on the shoulder will affect different regional nodes than a melanoma found on the leg. Following are areas of the body and the regional nodes that may be affected if a melanoma developed there[8]:

- Ipsilateral preauricular, submandibular, cervical, and head and neck—supraclavicular nodes
- Thorax—ipsilateral axillary lymph nodes
- Arm—ipsilateral epitrochlear and axillary lymph nodes
- Abdomen, loins, and buttocks—ipsilateral inguinal lymph nodes
- Leg—ipsilateral popliteal and inguinal lymph nodes
- Anal margin and perianal skin—ipsilateral inguinal lymph nodes

Some melanomas do not fit into specific drainage categories but rather between drainage areas. In those cases, regions on both sides of the area containing the tumor must be considered potential drainage sites. Procedures have been developed to aid physicians in determining the actual lymphatic flow patterns from the primary melanoma site. A study called *lymphoscintigraphy* uses a radioactive isotope that is injected into the primary melanoma site. The isotope then filters through the lymphatic channels that drain the tumor, and the patient is scanned to determine which lymph node stations could potentially harbor malignant cells. Another procedure, called *intraoperative lymphatic mapping,* uses special dyes that are injected into the primary tumor. As these dyes are transported through the lymphatic channels, they stain the tissues that they contact. During surgery the physician can identify the draining lymphatics and follow them to the lymph node closest to the tumor, or the sentinel node. The most likely site of early metastases, the sentinel node is removed and analyzed to determine whether it contains malignant cells.[38]

Melanomas can spread to virtually any organ of the body and tend to spread in the following order: (1) direct extension of the primary, including invasion into the subcutaneous tissues; (2) regional lymphatics; (3) distant skin and subcutaneous tissues; (4) lung; and (5) liver, bone, and brain.

Nonmelanoma. After a biopsy is taken (incisional

or excisional) the cell type of the carcinoma must be determined.

The four main subtypes of BCC are as follows[19]:

1. Nodular-ulcerated BCC is the most common type and is found mainly on the head and neck. Lesions are generally smooth, shiny, and translucent and accompanied by telangiectasis, an abnormal dilation of capillaries and arterioles that may be visible on the skin's surface. Ulceration is common and lesions may be pigmented. Pigmented lesions may sometimes be mistaken for melanoma.
2. Superficial BCC is found mainly on the trunk and appears as a red plaque, which may develop areas of translucent papules as it spreads over the skin's surface. These lesions may also develop areas of pigmentation.
3. Morphea-form, or sclerosing, BCC often appears as a scar-like lesion, often with indistinct margins. This type of lesion is uncommon, is found mainly on the head and neck, and has a rather high propensity for invasion and recurrence after treatment.
4. Cystic BCC is an uncommon cancer that "undergoes central degeneration to form a cystic lesion."[17]

Although BCCs do not tend to metastasize, they are capable of extensive local invasion and destruction. They commonly follow the path of least resistance, although they have been known to destroy bone and cartilage if left untreated.

However, rare cases of metastatic BCC have been reported. The rate of metastasis is less than 1 per 4000 cases, and the condition is often detected 10 or more years after treatment of the primary. Tumors most likely to metastasize are large, ulcerated, resistant tumors found on the head or neck of middle-aged men.[48] Regional lymph nodes are usually involved, but the involvement of liver, lung, and bone has been reported.

Squamous cell carcinomas can take on a variety of appearances. As mentioned earlier, they can be scaly, slightly ulcerated, or nodular. Occasionally, tumors contain characteristics of BCC and squamous cell cancer.

A verrucous variety of squamous cell carcinoma has been described as a low grade, warty neoplasm with a greasy, foul discharge. These lesions are most commonly found on the sole of the foot.[22]

Squamous cell carcinomas have a higher propensity to metastasize than BCCs. This tendency is based on a variety of factors, including the following[48]:

1. Differentiation—poorly differentiated lesions have a higher propensity to metastasize than well-differentiated lesions.
2. Etiology—tumors developing in immunosuppressed patients or in areas of chronic inflammation, scar tissue, and radiation dermatitis have higher rates of metastasis compared with tumors that develop in sun-exposed areas.
3. Size and invasion—tumors greater than 1 cm in size and more than 4 mm deep have a higher propensity for metastasis, even in sun-exposed areas.

Most studies report a 3% to 10% rate of metastasis from squamous cell skin cancer, but patients with high-risk factors can have up to a 30% chance of developing metastasis. Regional lymph nodes are affected 85% of the time in metastatic patients, with possible involvement of liver, bone, brain, and especially lung.[48]

Because nonmelanoma skin cancers can occur anywhere on the skin's surface, multiple lymphatic regions may be affected. Lymphatic drainage patterns for nonmelanomas are the same as those for melanomas. The following describes the TNM categories for nonmelanomas:

Primary tumor (T)
  TX Primary tumor cannot be assessed
  T0 No evidence of primary tumor
  Tis Melanoma in situ
  T1 Tumor ≤ 2 cm in greatest dimension
  T2 Tumor >2 cm but ≤ 5 cm, in greatest dimension
  T3 Tumor >5 cm in greatest dimension
  T4 Tumor invades deep extradermal structures (bone, cartilage, etc.)
Regional lymph nodes (N)
  NX Regional lymph nodes cannot be assessed
  N0 No regional lymph node metastasis
  N1 Regional lymph node metastasis
Distant metastasis (M)
  MX Distant metastasis cannot be assessed
  M0 No distant metastasis
  M1 Distant metastasis

BCC and squamous cell cancer of the skin are not reportable diseases. In other words, physicians are not responsible for keeping accurate records concerning factors such as incidence and survival. Therefore a strong database does not exist for calculating survival rates stage by stage. Although the overall survival rate is not known, early nonmelanoma lesions are almost 100% curable.[42]

Treatment Techniques

Melanoma. Surgical excision has been the mainstay in the treatment of primary melanoma and typically consists of en bloc removal of the intact tumor or biopsy site with a margin of normal-appearing skin and underlying subcutaneous tissue.[11] Chemotherapy, immunotherapy, and biochemotherapy are often used as a treatment for melanomas that have metastasized. The role of radiation therapy is limited primarily to the palliative treatment of metastatic disease sites. Melanoma has a reputation for being a radioresistant tumor, but radiation therapy has been a successful adjuvant to surgery and as the primary treatment modality in selected tumors and tumor sites.

Although surgery is currently the only form of curative therapy for malignant melanoma, controversy exists concerning surgical margins and the use of prophylactic lymph node removal to help prevent the occurrence of metastasis. Although early retrospective data suggested less sensitivity to radiation delivered at a conventional dose rate per fraction, it is now well documented that regardless of fractionation schedule, melanoma cells are radioresponsive if adequate total doses are delivered.[12]

Until the late 1970s, wide local excisions with 5-cm margins of normal skin surrounding the tumor were routine, sometimes creating large defects requiring skin grafts to close the wound. There are two reasons for use of these wide margins: a field effect surrounding tumors with a radial growth phase and the possibility for small groups of melanoma cells arising near the main tumor mass. Recent studies, however, indicate that wide margins are not always required. The thickness of the tumor, site of the tumor, and potential morbidity of the operation should determine the margin size around the primary. The decision to use wider margins should be based on the chance of local recurrence because no clear evidence exists to prove that creating larger margins increases the likelihood of survival.[58] In all excisions, surgical margins should include subcutaneous tissue down to the fascia and should show no involvement of the tumor.

Biopsies of questionable lesions often encompass a 0.5-cm margin around the tumor. If at the time of the pathologic examination the lesion is found to be a malignant melanoma beyond the in-situ stage, the surgeon must go back and create the proper margins. In the case of subungual lesions (found beneath the nail beds), all but the earliest lesions are treated by the amputation of the complete digit.

The key to melanoma treatment is the eradication of the tumor before it has a chance to metastasize. Although a tumor may be removed with clear margins, a few stray cells that can lead to recurrence or metastasis may be left behind. This is the area in which chemotherapy and immunotherapy play a role. These agents will hopefully cause the destruction of stray cells before they can reseed. (Specifics concerning chemotherapy and immunotherapy are discussed in the section concerning metastatic disease.)

Patients with proven lymph node metastasis should undergo a complete excision of regional lymph nodes, removing as much of the soft tissue and its associated lymphatics as possible between the tumor site and the regional lymph nodes. Even with such treatment the risk of distant metastasis is typically high.[22]

Patients who have melanomas on an extremity have been treated with isolated limb perfusion, which combines chemotherapy with hyperthermia. With this technique the extremity is isolated with a tourniquet while the blood in the limb circulates through a machine that pumps, oxygenates, and heats it. Because this blood is cut off from the rest of the body, large doses of chemotherapy can be introduced and circulated through the limb. Melphalan (L-PAM) is the agent of choice in most instances, although cisplatin (DDP) has been used successfully.[30] Because melanoma cells cannot survive above 105.8° F, the heating action provides an extra mode of cell killing to the process. After about 1 hour of treatment the treated blood is completely drained and the tourniquet is removed, allowing the normal blood supply to return to the limb.[53]

For patients who have developed distant metastasis, no successful curative treatment options are available. The options available are for symptomatic relief and the prolongation of life.

Surgery can be used to remove local recurrences and localized metastatic areas such as nonregional lymph nodes, distant skin lesions, and subcutaneous metastases. Because surgery of this type is palliative, it is normally performed on patients whose quality of life would be enhanced with few side effects. Radiation therapy can also be used for palliation. It can be used to relieve symptoms caused by skin, soft tissue, bone, brain, and spinal cord metastases.

Chemotherapy has been successful in producing remissions in some patients, but its use in the treatment of malignant melanoma is largely palliative. Dacarbazine (DTIC) as a single agent is the drug of choice, although nitrosoureas and vinca alkaloids have also been used. "Tumors of the skin, lymph nodes, and soft tissues respond better to drugs than do visceral metastasis."[33] Unfortunately, the response rate is low and lasts an average of 4 to 6 months.[18,22] The problem with cytotoxic regimens is their lack of tumor specificity. They affect the surrounding tissue as much as they do the tumor, causing serious complications in when administered in large doses. Through the study of the biochemical properties and behavior of melanomas, the addition of cytokines (immune system mediators) to a chemotherapeutic regimen improves the outcome of metastatic melanoma by increasing the time to progression of the disease.[14]

Studies have shown that some melanomas contain estrogen (hormones affecting the secondary sex characteristics as well as systematic effects such as the growth and maturity of long bones) receptors, allowing for responses to antiestrogen therapy. Antiestrogens block receptor sites for estrogen, denying the cell the effect that estrogen would have had on the cell. Research has shown that dacarbazine plus tamoxifen (TAM), an antiestrogen, is more effective than dacarbazine alone in terms of response rate and median survival. The effects of tamoxifen-aided treatment are more pronounced in women and in men and postmenopausal women with higher than normal body mass indexes (weight divided by height).[18] Tamoxifen also has a synergistic effect on cisplatin.[33]

A bone marrow transplant using high-dose chemotherapy and autologous, or self-donated, marrow can also improve the response to chemotherapy treatment. Although improvements in short-term survival have been seen, long-term survival has not been affected.[33]

Immunotherapy also plays a role in metastatic melanoma treatments. Melanomas have a history of spontaneous regression in which the body is somehow able to fend off the disease using its own natural defenses. Basically, immunotherapy attempts to take advantage of this phenomenon and bolster the body's immune system so that it is able to fight off the melanoma on its own.

Immunotherapy can be divided into the following five major types[37]:

1. Active—stimulation of the body's natural defenses
   ■ Nonspecific—use of microbial or chemical adjuvants to activate macrophages, natural killer cells, and other nonspecific defenses; stimulation of the immune system in general

- Specific—use of tumor cells or tumor-associated antigens sometimes mixed with haptens, viruses, or enzymes to activate T cells, macrophages, or other cells the body uses to fight specific tumor cells; stimulation of particular areas of the immune system
2. Adoptive—transfer of cells with antitumor properties into the tumor-bearing host to directly or indirectly cause tumor regression
3. Restorative—replacement of depleted immunologic subpopulations, such as T cells, or inhibition of the body's natural suppressor mechanisms (suppressor T cells or suppressor macrophages) to allow the body to replace the depleted subpopulations on its own
4. Passive—transfer of antibodies or other short-lived antitumor factors into the tumor-bearing host to control tumor growth
5. Cytomodularitive—enhancement of tumor-associated antigens and histocompatibility (HLA) antigens on the surface of tumor cells to make them more recognizable as foreign invaders by the body's immune system

Other agents used to promote a general immune response are interferons and interleukins. Interferons are special proteins that activate and enhance the tumor-killing ability of monocytes and produce chemicals toxic to cells. Interferons tend to be toxic to the patient and are not often used in single-agent therapy.[28] Interleukins are substances that act as costimulators and intensifiers of immune responses.

Although the results of immunotherapy are not curative, the fact that the body is able to cause tumor regression at all gives researchers hope that someday immunology will play a bigger role in the fight against melanoma and other cancers.

Nonmelanoma. Patients with basal cell or squamous cell carcinomas of the skin have several treatment options. The technique selected depends on factors such as previous methods of treatment (if any), the location on the body, the risk of recurrence and metastasis, and the volume of tissue invasion. The number one goal of treatment is eradication of the tumor, followed by good cosmetic results. In instances in which cure rates are similar but the cosmetic results will differ, the modality offering better cosmetic results should be used. If control rates are similar and cosmetic results are similar or unimportant, the most cost-effective and/or quickest treatment method is preferred.[39]

Surgery can be performed to remove nonmelanoma skin cancers from areas where scarring is acceptable and patients want expedient results. Often, the original excisional biopsy contains all the tumor with acceptable margins, and no further treatment is needed. Otherwise, the surgeon may have to operate on the site a second time to ensure that safe margins around the tumor have been created. Although a uniform recommendation does not exist concerning the size of margins, many surgeons use 3- to 5-mm margins for small, well-defined lesions and at least 1-cm margins for larger or more aggressive tumors.[48]

For large, salvageable, eroding tumors, extensive surgery may be needed to remove not only the tumor but also additional tissue that may have been invaded, such as bone or muscle tissue. Such intervention may include the use of skin grafts and/or prosthetic devices.[17]

A more precise type of surgery, referred to as **Mohs' surgery** (developed by Dr. Fredric Mohs at the University of Wisconsin), is used in areas where normal tissue sparing is important; in areas of known or high risk of cancer recurrence; in areas where the extent of the cancer is unknown; or in instances of aggressive, rapidly growing tumors.[27]

Mohs', or microscopic, surgery is different from conventional surgery in that the tumor is completely mapped out through the examination of each piece of removed tissue to determine the presence and extent of any tumor. Through the removal of only tissue containing a tumor a major amount of tissue is preserved versus conventional surgery. Mohs' surgery is indicated for recurrent basal and squamous cell carcinomas, those in known high-risk sites for recurrence, and those with aggressive histologic subtypes.[50]

This surgery is performed on an outpatient basis with a local anesthetic. The tumor is removed one layer at a time and examined under a microscope. From the microscopic sample the surgeon knows where to obtain the next sample. This process repeats itself until the tumor is excised completely. The wound is then stitched or allowed to heal on its own.[27] Of all therapeutic modalities, Mohs' surgery has the greatest success rate.[17]

One reason that Mohs' surgery has not replaced conventional surgery in the treatment of nonmelanoma skin cancers is that it is a time-consuming and expensive process. Cancers that are not viewed as problematic are treated almost as effectively and more inexpensively with conventional surgery.

Curettage and electrodesiccation are often used to treat BCC and early squamous cell carcinoma. With the patient under local anesthesia, the cancer is scooped out with a curette, an instrument in the form of a loop, ring, or scoop with sharpened edges. The destruction of any remaining tumor cells and stoppage of bleeding is carried out through a process called electrodesiccation, which uses a probe emitting a high-frequency electric current to destroy tissue and cauterize blood vessels. The advantage of this method, also known as electrosurgery, is that it often leaves a white scar, which is less noticeable on people with fair skin.[40]

Another method of treating early nonmelanoma skin lesions is cryosurgery, in which liquid nitrogen or carbon dioxide is applied to a lesion, lowering its temperature to around −50° Celsius and thereby freezing and killing the abnormal cells. This procedure may have to be repeated once or twice to completely eliminate the tumor. Again, a white scar is generally formed as a result. Cryosurgery is not recommended for lesions of the scalp or lower legs because of poor healing in those areas.[22]

Lasers (light amplification by stimulated emission of radiation) can also be used to treat early BCCs and in-situ squamous cell carcinomas. Lasers use highly focused beams of light that are able to destroy areas of a tumor with pinpoint accuracy while preserving the surrounding normal tissue.

Advantages of laser surgery include little blood loss or pain because the blood vessels and nerves are instantly sealed. In addition, laser surgery provides faster healing than conventional surgery.

Radiation therapy is used on BCC and squamous cell carcinoma located in places of cosmetic significance, such as the eyelids, lips, nose, face, and ears. It is also used on tumors in which surgical removal is difficult or in areas of recurrence. The major advantage of radiation therapy is normal tissue sparing. Disadvantages include its considerable cost, multiple treatments, and late skin changes in the treatment area. Doses and fractionation schedules should be carefully planned to avoid these late changes, which could include scarring, necrosis, and chronic radiation dermatitis.[22]

Finally, early nonmelanoma skin cancers can be treated with 5-FU in the form of a solution or cream. Applying 5-FU to the affected area daily for several weeks causes the area to become inflamed and irritated during treatment, but scarring does not usually result.[40]

A few investigational therapies are being researched that may someday be used to treat nonmelanoma skin cancers. In photodynamic therapy (PDT), a photosensitizing agent is injected into the body and absorbed by all cells. The agent is quickly discharged from normal cells but is retained longer by cancer cells. Light from a laser is directed on the tumor area, causing a reaction within the cells containing the photosensitizing agent that destroys the cell.[40]

As with melanomas, immunotherapy is also being researched for use against nonmelanoma cancers. Intralesional interferon alpha has been used, but because of side effects such as local pain, skin necrosis, and an influenza-type syndrome, it is not expected to be a major player in the treatment of skin cancer.[48]

Radiation Therapy

Nonmelanoma. Radiation therapy is effective in the treatment of nonmelanoma skin cancers, especially in the treatment of small tumors in which cosmetic results are important or in areas of extensive disease where the primary tumor and affected lymph nodes can be included in the radiation field. Because most skin lesions tend to be superficially located, electrons and kilovoltage x-rays are often used in their treatment. Megavoltage x-rays are rarely used in the treatment of skin cancers but may be used with or without electrons for special circumstances such as scalp lesions or tumors that are deeply infiltrating.[35]

Brachytherapy, including temporary implants or superficial molds using iridium-192 or cesium-137 sources and permanent implants using gold seeds, has produced good curative and cosmetic results. However, brachytherapy does not possess any significant advantages over external beam radiation therapy. There are disadvantages in the use of brachytherapy for skin cancer: cost, trauma, and length of stay required for the procedure; radiation exposure to personnel; uncertain dose distribution; and risk associated with anesthesia.[39]

Radiation therapy is often used to treat lesions on the lips, nose, eyelids, face, and ears because they are highly visible and cosmetic results are important. The choice between treatment with kilovoltage x-rays and electrons comes down to the size of the treatment volume, depth of the lesion, underlying anatomic structures, physician preference, and equipment availability. Modern radiation therapy departments have linear accelerators capable of producing a wide range of electrons with energies from 3–4 MeV to more than 20 MeV; kilovoltage machines dedicated to therapy are becoming scarce.

Each modality has advantages and disadvantages that can be compared by using the following four main categories[3]:

1. **Field size**—For the treatment of next-to-critical structures such as the eye, kilovoltage x-rays allow the target volume to be covered with a smaller field size compared with that of a field producing similar effects near the skin surface through the use of electrons. Because of its physical properties, the electron field must be opened considerably to cover the same as the kilovoltage machines. One solution to help minimize this problem with electrons is to increase the field size and use tertiary collimation on the skin's surface.

2. **Depth of maximum dose (D_{max})**—A surface dose less than 90% to 95% is generally unacceptable in the treatment of skin cancer.[47] The characteristics of the beam to be used must be known for each specific setup to ensure that the skin surface is receiving the correct dose. This is relatively easy with low-energy x-rays because D_{max} is always at the surface regardless of field size or collimation technique. The D_{max} of electrons, in contrast, is a function of field size, location of secondary collimation, and surface contour. Because the D_{max} of electron beams is a function of energy and is usually found at a depth beneath the skin's surface, bolus material of appropriate thickness is often used to bring the dose toward the surface.

3. **Deep-tissue dose**—A characteristic of electrons is their rapid falloff; they penetrate the tissue to a certain point and dissipate, allowing for the sparing of some of the underlying tissues. Kilovoltage x-rays penetrate much deeper, however, and affect a greater volume of underlying tissue.

4. **Differential bone absorption**—Gram for gram, the absorbed dose is higher in bone and cartilage than in soft tissue with the use of kilovoltage x-rays. This can result in underlying bone and cartilage receiving higher doses than the dose at D_{max}. No significant difference exists between bone and soft tissue doses for electrons used in clinical practice.

5. **Cosmesis and control rates**—A study by Perez, Lovett, and Gerber[47] indicated excellent or good cosmesis in 95% of patients treated with kilovoltage x-rays, compared with 80% of patients treated with electrons. Also, cosmetic results were superior for patients in whom less than 50% of the dose was delivered with bolus.

Both electron and orthovoltage treatment use various cones to collimate the treatment field, although the shielding cutouts for each type of beam are manufactured by different processes. In electron therapy most departments manufacture custom cutouts by using low melting point alloys like Cerrobend. These cutouts outline the field and protect normal tissues as the radiation oncologist outlines. Custom cutouts may be substituted with a series of lead strips layered to produce the desired outline. These strips rest on the lower part of the cone and are commonly taped into position. Orthovoltage treatment requires a different type of blocking scheme. Instead of being attached to the machine, the blocking material typically rests on the patient's skin (Fig. 37-16). Because lead is a soft metal, it can be formed into thin sheets that are somewhat pliable. These sheets can be contoured to the patient's anatomy, and holes can be cut into the sheets, creating the field through which the radiation passes. This type of blocking scheme can also be used as tertiary shielding in electron beam therapy. Regardless of the type of radiation used, the transmission factor for the blocking material should not exceed 5%.[29]

Radiation fields as a general rule should include a 2-cm margin completely surrounding the tumor to cover possible microscopic extension.[2] A 1-cm margin may be adequate for small, superficial BCCs. Tumors and their full margins should receive a majority of the dose, with a boost field encompassing the clinical tumor to deliver the full dose to the tumor. In doing so the amount of normal tissue treated is reduced, and the cosmetic effect is improved.[23] Although surgery accounts for the major means of management for most nonmelanomas, radiation therapy still plays a role with doses vary according to the size and penetration of the tumor and will differ from institution to institution.

Rapid fractionation schemes may be used in areas where late cosmetic results are not important or in instances in which transportation to and from the treatment site is difficult for the patient. Fraction size is the dominant factor in producing adverse reactions in late-responding normal tissue (the higher the daily dose, the greater the likelihood of adverse late effects).[60]

Depending on the area to be treated and type of radiation used, special considerations exist, including the following:

- Carcinomas of the skin overlying the pinna of the ear or nasal cartilages require special care in dose fractionation. Poorly designed treatment regimens can result in painful chondritis, which may require excision.[39]
- Bolus may be used with electron therapy to fill in gaps on uneven surfaces, maximize the surface dose, or reduce the underlying tissue dose.
- Lip—cancers that cross the vermilion border of the lip have a higher risk of nodal metastasis, possibly indicating the need for prophylactic neck irradiation.[2] In the designing of a radiation field for the lip, a lead shield should be created to protect the teeth and gums. Paraffin wax on the outside of the shield helps prevent electron backscatter, reducing the dose to the buccal mucosa.
- Nose—radiation treatments for skin cancers involving the nose should also include a wax-coated lead strip in the nostril to help protect the nasal septum. For more invasive lesions, tissue-equivalent material should be inserted into the nostril to remove the air gap and create a more uniform dose to the deeper tissues.
- Eye—for the treatment of carcinomas of the eyelid with radiation, the lens of the eye should be protected with an

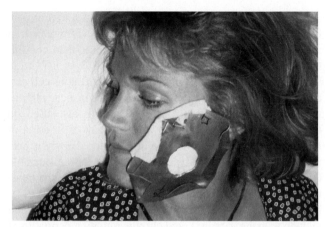

Figure 37-16. Blocking material for orthovoltage equipment often consists of a thin strip of lead shielding that rests directly on the patient's skin.

appropriately sized eye shield. Small-to-medium shields can be placed between the eyelid and eye, whereas larger shields can be used to cover the eyelid. A thin film of antibacterial ointment can be applied to the inside of the shield before insertion to aid in the prevention of infection and help protect against scratching of the lens. Concern about the increase in lid dose from backscatter is avoidable by coating the outer surface of the shield with a low-atomic-number material such as wax or dental acrylic.[29] The lens of the eye is one of the most radiosensitive structures. A single dose of 200 cGy may cause the development of cataracts (a loss of transparency in the lens of the eye).[13] Larger doses are required for cataractogenesis in fractionated regimens. The latent period between irradiation and the appearance of cataracts is also dose related. The latency is about 8 years after exposure to a dose in the range of 250 to 650 cGy.[26]

- Ear—in the treatment of skin cancers of the ear with radiation, treatment planning should be done so that doses to the inner ear do not exceed 1000 cGy.[23] Because of the unique and varied shape of the external ear and depending on the location and extent of the tumor, bolus material may be necessary to "flatten" the surface of the ear or get rid of the air gap behind the external ear in tumors involving the base of the auricle.

Malignant melanoma. Traditionally, malignant melanoma has been considered a radioresistant tumor when treated with conventional dose fraction sizes; radiation therapy was reserved mainly for the treatment of metastases. Recently, however, the role of radiation therapy has expanded to that of an adjuvant and, in some instances, the primary treatment modality.

Researchers have discovered that treatment results improve with the use of larger fractions. Because of the initial shoulder of the cell survival curve of melanoma cells exposed to radiation, standard fraction sizes of 180 to 200 cGy are not effective. Larger doses per fraction are needed to overcome the apparent repair processes that melanoma cells seem to possess.[9,49]

Radiation therapy as the primary treatment modality is limited to large facial lentigo maligna melanomas for which wide surgical resection requires extensive reconstruction.

Most of these lesions are controllable with proper fractionation, but up to 24 months may be necessary for the lesion to regress completely.[9]

One of the problems physicians face in the treatment of melanoma patients with bad prognostic features (i.e., ulcerative lesions or positive nodes) is local recurrence or regional relapse after wide local excision with or without limited neck dissection. Physicians at the M.D. Anderson Cancer Center in Houston, Texas, continue to use radiation therapy as an adjuvant to surgery. Their aim is to reduce the morbidity associated with local-regional recurrences such as ulceration, disfigurement, and pressure symptoms and possibly improve the survival rate of a small subgroup of patients by helping to contain the disease before it has a chance to spread to distant sites. Patients were treated with five fractions of 600 cGy delivered twice per week via electron beams of appropriate energies when possible.[10]

The role of radiation therapy is greatest in the treatment of metastatic or recurrent disease. The role of megavoltage x-rays is also increased as deeper levels of tissue become involved or major organs become affected. Fractions of at least 500 cGy should be used to treat cutaneous, subcutaneous, lymph node, or visceral metastases in small treatment volumes or in areas in which late effects are irrelevant. When affected lymphatics or organs require large treatment volumes or if late effects may be detrimental, lower daily doses of 200 to 400 cGy may be used up to normal tissue tolerance or hyperfractionation may be used (115 cGy × 2 per day to a total dose of 3500 to 4000 cGy). The therapeutic outcome is based on the tumor size and dose per fraction.[19,49]

Side effects. A major difference between megavoltage x-ray treatment of internal structures and kilovoltage x-ray or megavoltage-electron treatment of skin lesions is the location of the D_{max}. For the treatment of internal structures, having the D_{max} at least 0.5 cm beneath the skin surface is preferable for maintaining the skin-sparing effect (i.e., if the maximum dosage of radiation is absorbed beneath the skin, the epidermal layer receives a much smaller percentage of radiation and produces fewer side effects as a result). For the treatment of skin cancers, just the opposite should occur. Maximum doses should be applied at or near the skin surface where tumors are located, whereas underlying tissues are spared. As a result, skin reactions can be expected to be worse during the treatment of primary skin cancers than during the properly planned treatment of internal structures.

Radiation reactions can be divided into acute (early) or chronic (late) changes. The severity of the reaction depends on the volume, dose, and protraction of the treatment. High doses to large volumes in short amounts of time result in more severe reactions than low doses to small volumes over long periods.

Early reactions that can be expected during the course of radiation treatment for skin cancers include the following:

- **Erythema** (inflammatory redness of the skin) is usually the first sign of the effects of irradiation. This condition is caused by the swelling of the capillaries of the dermal layer, increasing the blood flow to the skin.[39]
- Pigmentation is caused by the increased production of melanin by the melanocytes, causing the skin to become darker. The melanocytes respond to x-rays and electrons the same way that they do to UV rays and try to protect the young epithelial cells in the same fashion.
- Dry **desquamation**, or shedding of the epidermis, appears at intermediate doses of radiation. The radiation affects the sensitive basal cells, and, although not all are killed, enough are compromised that the basal layer has a hard time replacing the cells naturally sloughed off. The result is an abnormal thinning of the epithelial layer.[39]
- Moist desquamation* appears at the high-dose levels necessary to control skin cancer. As a result of these high doses, nearly all the cells of the basal layer are destroyed. After the cells of the epidermis have gone through their normal cycle, no cells from the germinal layer exist to replace them. The dermis then becomes exposed and begins producing a serous oozing from its surface. The epidermis is thought to be ultimately repopulated from more radioresistant cells surrounding hair follicles or sweat glands.[46]
- Temporary hair loss (alopecia) appears after moderate doses of radiation. Higher doses may result in permanent hair loss.
- Sebaceous (oil) and sudoriferous (sweat) glands may show decreased or absent function when subjected to curative doses for skin cancer.[46]

Late reactions that can be expected after a curative course of radiation therapy include the following[51]:

- The skin seldom returns to its previous state. Damage to the dermal layer results in fibrosis, giving the skin a firmer, rougher appearance. Capillaries are dilated and fewer, resulting in telangiectasia. Also, the epithelial layer is thin and more susceptible to injury. Damage to melanocytes results in hypopigmentation and increased sensitivity to the sun.
- Necrosis is a common effect in patients who receive large doses in short amounts of time. The incidence of necrosis in carefully planned treatment regimens should not exceed 3%.

Prevention

Skin cancer is one of the few malignancies in which the causes are readily identifiable and preventable. About 90% of skin cancers can be avoided if people take proper precautions against the sun's rays.[7] If people take the time to educate themselves concerning skin cancer prevention and detection and follow through on that knowledge, the trend of rising skin cancer incidence could be reversed.

Exposure to UV light is the main triggering mechanism for skin cancer, so any type of preventive measures will stress ways to avoid UV exposure. Sun exposure also causes photoaging of the skin, including processes such as premature freckling, fine wrinkling, and dilation of the capillaries. Irregular pigmentation, commonly referred to as liver spots, often develops during later years in photodamaged skin.

---

*Moist desquamation is a skin reaction that can occur with exposure to radiation that is characterized by breakdown of the epidermis and presence of a white or yellow color. Raw skin may be apparent, and bleeding may occur.

The ozone layer is the portion of the atmosphere that protects the earth from harmful UV rays. In recent years this natural defense mechanism has been under attack by manmade substances such as chlorofluorocarbons, automobile exhaust, and other agents. The National Aeronautics and Space Administration (NASA) estimates a 2% increase in UV radiation for every 1% loss of the ozone layer.[51] Efforts are under way by many governments throughout the world to limit the release of these destructive agents into the atmosphere. Through the preservation of the ozone layer the amount of UV light that reaches the earth's surface can be limited.

With or without a healthy ozone layer, plenty of UV light reaches the planet's surface and is a potential cause of skin cancer. Not all sun exposure is bad, however. The human body needs sunlight to aid in the production of vitamin D, which is essential for calcium absorption in the intestines and may help protect against certain types of cancer. Not much sun exposure is needed; only about 5 minutes a day is required to produce sufficient amounts of vitamin D. Also, a little time in the sun after an extended period of cloudy days can often give a person a psychologic boost.[51]

Following are some potential UV light sources about which people should be aware[53]:

- Strong sun—avoid exposure to the sun between 10 AM and 2 PM because the rays are directly overhead and considered strongest during this time. In the continental United States, the UV intensity is reduced by half at 3 hours before and 3 hours after peak exposure time. The peak exposure time is 12:00 noon during standard time and 1:00 PM during daylight saving time.[20] One way to judge the amount of UV exposure is by looking at a person's shadow. The longer the shadow, the lower the intensity of the UV rays. The shorter the shadow, the higher the intensity.[21]
- Reflected light—snow, sand, water, and cement are capable of reflecting UV light. Added to the direct rays of the sun, the reflective rays can increase overall exposure rates. Even people who wear hats or sit under umbrellas must be aware of the exposure risks of reflected light.
- Cloudy skies—UV rays can penetrate through clouds. Depending on cloud conditions, between 20% and 80% of UV rays still reach the ground. Proper precautions are needed even on cloudy days.
- Fluorescent lights—fluorescent lights emit small amounts of UVA radiation, potentially boosting a desk worker's annual exposure by approximately 6%.
- Tanning lamps—although most tanning salons and tanning equipment manufacturers would like the public to believe that tanning beds are safe, most emit UVA rays capable of skin injury, including skin cancer, premature skin aging, blood vessel damage, and immune system effects. A tan is the body's natural response to damage caused by UV light, whether that light is made by humans or nature.

If avoiding sources of UV light is impossible, certain protective measures must be undertaken. Slacks, long-sleeved shirts, hats, and visors offer excellent protection from UV light. Care must be taken to protect areas of the skin not directly covered by the various articles. These areas include the ears, tops of the feet, and backs of the knees.

Sunscreens are effective in protecting against UV exposure. The blocking ability of sunscreens is indicated by its sun-protection factor (SPF), which tells how long a person can stay in the sun with protection versus without protection before a sunburn develops. For example, a sunscreen with an SPF of 15 enables a person wearing it to stay in the sun 15 times longer than if the person was wearing no sunscreen.

Sunscreens contain different ingredients to protect against UVA and UVB rays. Agents that can block both types of rays are referred to as broad-spectrum sunscreens. The use of sunscreens and their role in the prevention of skin cancers is controversial. Some think that although the protective capacity of sunscreens against UVB is good, the protective capacity against UVA is lacking.

Some people think that the use of sunscreens may be counterproductive. They theorize that people using sunscreens are able to stay out in the sun for longer periods than without sunscreen because the UVB rays are being effectively blocked. With a minimum number of UVB rays available to cause the skin to feel burned, people are able to stay in the sun for longer periods. Because sunscreens are not as effective in blocking UVA, people are being exposed to higher levels of UVA than before sunscreens were developed. Increased UVA exposure can promote previous UVB damage or cause other types of damage on its own.

The American Academy of Dermatology, the Australian College of Dermatology, and the Canadian Dermatology Association strongly disagree with these views, stating, "One of the most powerful weapons in our fight against (skin cancers) is sun avoidance through the combination of protective clothing and sunscreens."[56] In fact, the Australians have initiated the "Slip, Slap, Slop" program, encouraging individuals to slip on protective clothing, slap on a hat, and slop on some sunscreen. Babies are very susceptible to sunburn and should be kept out of the direct sun. Therefore they require extra sun protection.[44]

A sunscreen with an SPF of at least 15 is the best choice. Sunscreen should be applied at least 15 minutes before going outside to allow the skin to absorb it. Also, sunscreen should be reapplied every 2 hours and after swimming or heavy physical activity. Because the lips do not contain melanin and are a prime site for skin cancer, they should be protected with a lip balm or block having an SPF of 15.

Certain types of medications, such as antibiotics and diuretics, can increase a person's sensitivity to the sun. Before taking any medications, people should always consult drug labels, the physician, or the pharmacist regarding possible side effects, including those caused by UV exposure.

In 1994 the National Weather Service (NWS), the United States Environmental Protection Agency (EPA), and the Centers for Disease Control and Prevention (CDC) introduced the ultraviolet (UV) index to inform the public about the type of UV conditions to expect so that proper precautions can be taken. The index is a next-day forecast of the likely exposure to UV radiation for a specific location during the peak hour of sunlight around noon. The UV index ranges from 0 to 15; the higher the number, the more intense the sun intensity. Although there is no direct link between SPF and UV index, the UV index can inform us what level of protection we should consider.[57] The index uses a set of four skin-type categories into which the public is divided based on the normal color of the persons skin and its propensity for sunburn. These are shown in Table 37-2.

In addition to analyzing primary protection against UV rays, the National Cancer Institute is researching chemoprevention of nonmelanoma skin cancer. Chemoprevention is the use of natural and manmade substances to prevent cancer. High doses of vitamin A, beta carotene, and isotretinoin, (a synthetic form of vitamin A) may help individuals who lack natural defenses (persons with albinism and xeroderma pigmentosum) to fight skin cancer.

Helping people to realize the dangers of overexposure to the sun and the importance of early detection remains a major hurdle in skin cancer prevention. Young people especially feel invulnerable to the damaging and aging effects of the sun. To many, the short-term gratification a tan provides outweighs the seemingly small risks of the sun exposure that provides it. They think that skin cancer is for old people. In a way they are correct, because skin cancer usually shows up as people grow older. However, they do not realize that the cause of skin cancer is overexposure to the sun during a person's younger years.

Currently, mass media campaigns, educational posters, and brochures are aimed at educating the public concerning the dangers of sun exposure and the importance of early screening and detection. Health care institutions are trying to help by providing skin cancer screenings as a part of public health care fairs. Again, rising skin cancer rates can be reversed if people become educated on the prevention and detection of skin cancers and follow through on the recommendations.

Role of Radiation Therapist

The radiation therapist plays a prominent role in the management of skin cancer patients being treated with ionizing radiation. Patient education, technical expertise, assessment, and therapeutic communication are as important for the therapist to pay attention to as in treating any other cancer patient. The therapist typically blends their technical and psychosocial skills to achieve the best possible patient outcome.

The radiation therapist reiterates the physician instructions for the patient undergoing treatment, particularly the management of sensitive and injured skin during treatment. As they note changes in the integrity of skin being treated, that information can be relayed to the appropriate member of the patient care team so that any issues or problems are addressed.

It is not uncommon for patients to need to be reminded about cleaning treatment areas and keeping any treatment lines placed on their skin. This being the case, the daily interactions that the therapist has with the patient serves as a unique opportunity to remind them about such things as line management and skin care and to assess how the patient is coping with treatment, mentally and physically.

Technical skills and treatment delivery competencies in skin cancer treatment are paramount in the radiation therapist's role. Seeing the patient each day and delivering potentially dangerous doses of radiation require great attention to detail and careful consideration of each step of treatment. This end provider of care is the link to successful delivery of a planned course of therapy; the best plan delivered incorrectly does not serve the patient well.

Case Study

A 29-year-old white man had a 3-year history of a nonhealing ulceration just above the vermilion border of the right lip. He saw a physician, who gave the patient a prescription for acyclovir (Zovirax) in case the ulceration was a fever blister, but the condition never resolved. He was referred to a dermatologist but never kept his appointment. Finally, his primary physician performed a biopsy, which revealed a BCC.

The biopsy report described the lesion as an incompletely excised BCC, so further treatment was necessary. Because of the location of the lesion, the physician referred the patient to a radiation oncologist for definitive treatment. Radiation therapy offered a high probability for cure and a good chance of excellent cosmetic results.

A physical examination revealed a healthy, white man without supraclavicular, cervical, or preauricular adenopathy. A 12-mm lesion without

Table 37-2	The four skin phototypes		
Skin phototypes	**Skin color in unexposed area**		**Tanning history**
Never tans, always burns	Pale or milky white; alabaster		Develops red sunburn; painful swelling occurs; skin peels
Sometimes tans, usually burns	Very light brown; sometimes freckles		Usually burns; pink or red coloring appears; can gradually develop light brown tan
Usually tans, sometimes burns	Light tan, brown, or olive; distinctly pigmented		Infrequently burns; shows moderately rapid tanning response
Always tans, rarely burns	Brown, dark brown, or black		Rarely burns; shows very rapid tanning response

discrete edges but with some central ulceration was found on the upper lip. No other lesions were seen on the face or neck.

The patient's history was unremarkable for specific sun exposure or other skin problems. He did not smoke and was an occasional drinker. His medical history included eye surgery as a child and trauma to the lip as a youth. His family history was significant because a grandmother had breast cancer.

The patient was simulated in the supine position with a B headrest and an Aquaplast mask. A 3 × 3.5 cm electron field with a 4 × 4 cm cone was mapped out and encompassed the right half of the right upper lip and the surrounding tissue. He was to receive a 240-cGy D_{max} dose each day, 5 days per week for a total dose of 6000 cGy, with a 0.5-cm bolus every other day. A mouth shield was constructed to protect the teeth and gums.

The course of therapy was unremarkable until the patient was at the 3840-cGy level. The outside of the lip became red and dry; the patient was given 4 days of rest for a skiing vacation and was instructed to use Vaseline on the area to keep it moist.

After the vacation, the treatment was resumed and carried to the 6000-cGy level. At the completion of treatment a scab was present externally and moist desquamation internally in the treatment area. The patient reported little pain and good function in spite of the treatment.

The patient was seen for a follow-up visit 1 month after the completion of the radiation regimen. The skin over the lip was completely reepithelialized and flat, and no ulceration was visible around the upper lip internally or externally. He had no submental, preauricular, or cervical adenopathy and was declared clinically disease free.

About 3 months after the completion of the radiation therapy, the patient visited the radiation oncologist unexpectedly, complaining of a 2-week history of thickening in the treatment area. An examination showed a 2-mm area of swelling just above the vermilion border. The patient admitted he had been picking at the area and was encouraged to stop. He was also instructed to use Vaseline on the treated area three times a day for 3 weeks. If this condition were to persist or enlarge, a biopsy might determine the presence or absence of a recurrent tumor.

The patient was seen 4 weeks later, and no irritation, thickening, or irregularity was found to suggest recurrence. The patient was told to continue to use lotion in the treatment area and return for a follow-up visit in 6 months. He is expected to be fully cured.

Because of the young age at which this patient developed his skin cancer, he will be at high risk for developing future lesions. He was encouraged to contact a dermatologist to begin baseline skin screenings. The use of sunscreens and protective lip balms was also stressed.

Despite a 3-year history of skin cancer, this patient was lucky and has an excellent chance of cure. If the skin cancer had been a squamous cell carcinoma or melanoma, the patient may not have been so fortunate. Again, any suspicious lesions that do not resolve over a few weeks should be checked by a physician.

Review Questions

1. Which layer of the epidermis contains cells most sensitive to radiation?
   a. Stratum basale
   b. Stratum granulosum
   c. Stratum lucidum
   d. Stratum corneum

2. Which of following diseases is occasionally treated by total skin irradiation with electrons?
   a. Kaposi's sarcoma
   b. Malignant melanoma
   c. Mycosis fungoides
   d. Glandular adenocarcinoma

3. What are the layers of the skin, starting with the most superficial to the deepest?
   I.   Subcutaneous layer
   II. Epidermis
   III. Dermis
   IV. Basement layer
   a. I, III, IV, II
   b. II, IV, III, I
   c. II, III, I, IV
   d. IV, I, III, II

4. Melanocytes are found in which layer of the skin stratum?
   a. Basale
   b. Granulosum
   c. Spinosum
   d. Corneum

5. What is the treatment of choice for most melanoma skin cancers?
   a. Surgery
   b. Isolated limb perfusion
   c. Chemotherapy
   d. Radiation therapy

6. What is the technique in which the tumor is removed and examined one layer at a time?
   a. Curettage and electrodesiccation
   b. Mohs' surgery
   c. Cryosurgery
   d. Laser surgery

7. Tanning of the skin in the treated area after a course of radiation therapy is caused by which of the following?
   a. Damage to the basal layer
   b. Increased vascularity of the epidermis
   c. Stimulation of the melanocytes
   d. Inflammation of the dermis

8. With the use of shielding to protect the eye during irradiation, backscatter can be minimized by which of the following?
   a. Using a shield composed of Cerrobend
   b. Using a shield at least 1.7 mm in thickness
   c. Using a larger diameter shield
   d. Coating the outer surface of the shield with a low-atomic-number material such as wax

9. The use of kilovoltage x-rays allows the target volume to be covered with a smaller field size compared with a field that would produce similar effects near the skin through the use of electrons.
   a. True
   b. False

Questions to Ponder

1. Describe the latest trends in the rates of incidence and rates of death in nonmelanoma and melanoma skin cancers.
2. Analyze circumstances that would render individuals more susceptible to developing skin cancer.
3. Contrast the microstaging systems for melanoma developed by Drs. Wallace Clark and Alexander Breslow.
4. Describe and outline the prognostic factors for malignant melanomas.
5. Compare the advantages and disadvantages of electron beam therapy versus kilovoltage x-rays in the treatment of nonmelanoma skin cancer.

REFERENCES

1. Ackerman AB: Malignant melanoma: a unifying concept, *Hum Pathol* 11:591-595, 1980.
2. Ackerman S: Personal interview, August, 1994.
3. Amdur RJ, et al: Radiation therapy for skin cancer near the eye: kilovoltage x-rays versus electrons, *Int J Radiat Oncol Biol Phys* 23:769-779, 1992.
4. American Cancer Society: *Cancer facts and figures 2003,* Atlanta, 2003, American Cancer Society.
5. American Cancer Society: *Cancer response system: malignant melanoma,* no. 448257, Atlanta, American Cancer Society.
6. American Cancer Society: *Cancer response system: skin cancer,* no. 473157, Atlanta, American Cancer Society.
7. American Cancer Society: *Prevention and early detection of malignant melanoma,* no. 3029-PE, Atlanta, 1990, American Cancer Society.
8. American Joint Committee on Cancer: *Manual for staging of cancer,* ed 6, Philadelphia, 2002, JB Lippincott.
9. Ang KK, et al: Postoperative radiotherapy for cutaneous melanoma of the head and neck region, *Int J Radiat Oncol Biol Phys* 30:795-798, 1994.
10. Ang KK, et al: Regional radiotherapy as adjuvant treatment for head and neck malignant melanoma, *Arch Otolaryngol Head Neck Surg* 116(4):169, 1990.
11. Balch CM, Sober AJ, Houghton H, editors: *Cutaneous melanoma,* ed 3, St. Louis, 1998, Quality Medical Publishers.
12. Ballo MT, et al: Adjuvant irradiation for axillary metastatic metastases from malignant melanoma, *Int J Radiat Oncol Biol Phys* 52:964-972, 2002.
13. Bentel GC: *Treatment planning and dose calculation in radiation oncology,* ed 4, New York, 1991, Elsevier Science.
14. Boggs W: *Biochemotherapy extends survival in metastatic melanoma,* available at http://www.oncolink.com/custom_tags/print_article.cfm?Page=2&id=8354&Section=Reuters_Articles (accessed August 20, 2003).
15. Breslow A: Cross-sectional areas and depth of invasion in the prognosis of cutaneous melanoma, *Ann Surg* 172:902, 1970.
16. Cannon-Albright LA: Assignment of a locus for familial melanoma, mlm, to chromosome 9p13-p22, *Science* 258:1148, 1992.
17. Casciato DA, Lowitz BB: *Manual of clinical oncology,* ed 4, Philadelphia, 2000, Lippincott Williams & Wilkins.
18. Cocconi G, et al: Treatment of metastatic malignant melanoma with dacarbazine plus tamoxifen, *N Engl J Med* 327:516, 1992.
19. De Vita VT, et al., editors: *Cancer: principles and practice of oncology,* ed 6, Philadelphia, 2001, Lippincott Williams & Wilkins.
20. Environmental Protection Agency: *Experimental UV index,* EPA 430-F-94-017, Washington, DC, June, 1994, Environmental Protection Agency.
21. Environmental Protection Agency: *The federal experimental ultraviolet index: what you need to know,* EPA 430-F-94-016, Washington, DC, June, 1994, Environmental Protection Agency.
22. Fink DJ, Holleb AI, Murphy GP: *American Cancer Society textbook of clinical oncology,* Atlanta, 1991, American Cancer Society.
23. Fletcher GH: *Textbook of radiotherapy,* ed 3, Philadelphia, 1980, Lea & Febiger.
24. Friedman RJ, et al: Malignant melanoma in the 1990's: the continued importance of early detection and the role of physician examination and self-examination of the skin, *CA Cancer J Clin* 41:201, 1991.
25. Glassman RD: Personal interview, June, 1994.
26. Hall EJ: *Radiobiology for the radiologist,* ed 4, Philadelphia, 1994, JB Lippincott.
27. *Healthcare update,* Roswell, Ga, May, 1994, Publications.
28. Hunger K, McClay EF: Melanoma: new biology, new therapy, *Crit Rev Oncol Hematol* 2:299, 1991.
29. Kahn F: *The physics of radiation therapy,* Philadelphia, 1994, Lippincott Williams & Wilkins.
30. Karagas MR, et al: Risk of subsequent basal cell carcinoma of the skin among patients with prior skin cancer, *JAMA* 267:3305, 1992.
31. Kartsonis J: Lecture, August, 1994.
32. Katarzyna W: Safe sun, *Forbes,* p. 212, July 19, 1993.
33. Malignant melanoma. Report of a meeting of physicians and scientists, University College London Medical School, *Lancet* 340(8825):948-951, 1992.
34. Melanoma detection: a new, improved method, *Patient Care* 13:xx, 1992.
35. Mendenhall WM, et al: T2-T4 carcinoma of the skin of the head and neck treated with radical irradiation, *Int J Radiat Oncol Biol Phys* 13:975, 1987.
36. Million RR, Cassisi NJ, editors: *Management of head and neck cancer,* ed 2, Philadelphia, 1994, JB Lippincott.
37. Mitchell MS: Chemotherapy in combination with biomodulation: a 5-year experience with cyclophosphamide and interleukin-2, *Semin Oncol* 19(2 suppl 4):80-87, 1992.
38. Morton DL, et al: Multivariate analysis of the relationship between survival and the microstage of primary melanoma by Clark level and Breslow thickness, *Cancer* 71:3737, 1993.
39. Moss WT, Cox JD: *Radiation oncology rationale, technique, results,* ed 6, St. Louis, 1989, Mosby.
40. National Cancer Institute: *Research report: skin cancers: basal cell and squamous cell carcinomas,* National Institutes of Health publication number 91-2977, Bethesda, Md, 1990, National Cancer Institute.
41. National Cancer Institute: *Research report: melanoma,* National Institutes of Health publication number 92-3020, Bethesda, Md, 1992, National Cancer Institute.
42. National Cancer Institute: *Physician's data query state of the art cancer treatment information,* Bethesda, Md, 1993, National Cancer Institute.
43. NIH consensus development panel on early melanoma, *JAMA* 268:1314, 1992.
44. Ontario Division—Canadian Cancer Society (29 October 2001) [Online]. *SunSense guidelines,* available at http://www.nb.cancer.ca/ccs/internet/standard/0%2C939%2C3172_273070_275853_langId-en%2C00.html (accessed April 25, 2003).
45. Osteen RT, editor: *Cancer manual,* ed 8, Boston, 1990, American Cancer Society, Massachusetts Division.
46. Perez CA, Brady LW: *Principles and practice of radiation oncology,* ed 2, Philadelphia, 1992, JB Lippincott.
47. Perez CA, Lovett RD, Gerber R: Electron beam and x-rays in the treatment of epithelial skin cancer: dosimetric considerations and clinical results, *Front Radiat Ther Oncol* 25:90, 1992.
48. Preston DS, Stern RS: Nonmelanoma cancers of the skin, *N Engl J Med* 327:1649, 1992.
49. Pyrhonen SO, Kajanti MJ: The use of large fractions in radiotherapy for malignant melanoma, *Radiother Oncol* 24:195, 1992.
50. Randle HW: *Management of basal and squamous cell carcinomas,* Mayo Clinic lecture material, Jacksonville, Fla, Mayo Clinic, 1995.

51. Reid K, Vikhanski L: The sun's ominous side: skin cancer, *Med World News* 33:18, February, 1992.

52. Rhodes AR, et al: Risk factors for cutaneous melanoma: a practical method of recognizing predisposed individuals, *JAMA* 258:3146, 1987.

53. Roach M, Hastings J, Finch S: Sun struck: here's the hole story about the ozone and your chances of getting skin cancer, *Health,* p. 40, May-June, 1992.

54. Shaw KE: Management of malignant melanoma, *Jacksonville Medicine* p. 200, May, 1991.

55. Skolnick AA: Melanoma epidemic yields grim statistics, *JAMA* 265:3217, 1991.

56. Skolnick AA: Sunscreen protection controversy heats up, *JAMA* 265:3218, 1991.

57. The ultraviolet index [Online], available at http://www.cpc.ncep.noaa.gov/products/stratosphere/uv_index/uv_what.html (accessed April 25, 2003).

58. Timmons MJ: Malignant melanoma excisions: making a choice, *Lancet* 340:1393, 1992.

59. Tortora GJ, Grabowski SR: *Principles of anatomy and physiology,* ed 7, New York, 1993, Harper Collins.

60. Travis EL: *Primer of medical radiobiology,* ed 2, St. Louis, 1989, Year Book Medical Publishers.

61. Weinstock MA: The epidemic of squamous cell carcinoma, *JAMA* 262:2138, 1989.

62. White JW: *Epidemiology of skin cancer,* Mayo Clinic lecture, Jacksonville, Fla, Mayo Clinic.

63. Williams PL, Warwick R, editors: *Gray's anatomy,* ed 36, Philadelphia, 1980, WB Saunders.

BIBLIOGRAPHY

Marx JL: Cancer vaccines show promise at last, *Science* 245:813, 1989.

Mitchell MS, et al: Effectiveness and tolerability of low-dose cyclophosphamide and low-dose intravenous interleukin-2 disseminated melanoma, *J Clin Oncol* 6:409, 1988.

Showers V: *World facts and figures,* ed 3, New York, 1989, John Wiley & Sons.

Sober AJ, Haluska FG: *American Cancer Society atlas of clinical oncology: skin cancer,* Hamilton, Ontario, 2001, BC Decker.

Wandycz W: Safe sun, *Forbes* 152:212, July 19, 1993.

abdominoperineal resection An anterior incision into the abdominal wall, with the construction of a colostomy followed by a perineal incision to remove the rectum and anus and draining lymphatics.

ablation The surgical excision or amputation of any part of the body.

absorbed dose Energy absorbed per unit mass of any material; units are the centigray or rad (older term) (100 ergs per gram) or **gray** (1 Gy = 1 joule per kilogram). 1 Gy = 100 cGy or 100 rad.

abstracting Gathering data for measuring and evaluating patterns of care and outcomes among the general population. In oncology centers this is done on an ongoing basis with a Tumor Registry system.

accelerated fractionation The technique in which the overall treatment time is shortened through the use of doses per fraction less than conventional doses two to three times per day.

accelerated hyperfractionation The technique in which there are more treatment days than accelerated fractionation. The total dose (cGy) of primary radiation is more than conventional fractionation, hyperfractionation, or accelerated fractionation.

accelerator structure The structure resembles a length of pipe and is the basic element of the linear accelerator. The accelerator structure allows electrons produced from a hot cathode to gain energy until they exit the far end of the pipe.

accreditation A process of voluntary external peer review in which a nongovernmental agency grants public recognition to an institution or specialized program of study that meets current qualifications and educational standards.

This recognition is determined through initial and subsequent periodic evaluation.

achalasia The loss of the normal peristaltic activity of the lower two thirds of the esophagus, resulting in dilation of the esophagus. This is a risk factor for the development of esophageal cancer.

actinic keratosis A warty lesion with areas of red, scaly patches occurring on the sun-exposed skin of the face or hands of older, light-skinned individuals.

active length In brachytherapy, the length of the area in which the radioactivity lies in the source.

activity rate At which a radioactive isotope undergoes nuclear decay; units are the Curie (Ci) or becquerel (Bq = 1 disintegration per second). 1 Ci = 3.7×10^{10} Bq.

ADCZ A combination of the following drugs: doxorubicin, dacarbazine, cisplatin, and vincristine commonly used in chemotherapy.

adenocarcinoma Epithelial cells that are glandular. An example is the tissue lining the stomach. A tumor originating in the cells of this lining is called adenocarcinoma of the stomach.

adenohypophysis The anterior lobe of the pituitary.

adjacent Refers to the length of the side of the right triangle that is close, or adjacent, to the specified angle.

adjuvant therapy The use of one form of treatment in addition to another.

advisory agency An organization that collects and analyzes data and information and makes recommendations.

advocate A supporter who can act as a professor and friend. The advocate assists patients by ensuring that their needs are fulfilled and their rights enforced.

affective Content that may be verbal or

nonverbal and comprises feelings, attitudes, and behaviors.

afferent lymphatic vessel Lymphatic vessels that flow into a lymph node. There are more afferent vessels than efferent vessels associated with each lymph node.

afterloading A system that was developed to allow devices known as applicators to be inserted into the treatment area first, then loaded with radioactivity quickly and safely. In this way, dose to personnel is kept to a minimum.

agreement state A state that enters into an agreement with the Nuclear Regulatory Commission to assume the responsibility of enforcing regulations for ionizing radiation.

akimbo The position in which the arms are bent by the side.

ALARA As Low As Reasonably Achievable.

algebraic equation A mathematical formula that describes a physical phenomenon based on the interaction of several factors or variables. Algebraic equations are typically used to find an unknown value when related factor values are known.

allergic reaction A reaction resulting from an immunologic reaction to a drug to which the patient has already been sensitized.

alopecia Hair loss. A partial or complete lack of hair.

Alpha Cradle Trade name for an immobilization device created from a Styrofoam shell and foaming agents.

alpha particle Particulate radiation, positively charged, which consists of two protons and two neutrons; emitted during nuclear decay.

American Joint Committee on Cancer (AJCC) A classification and anatomic staging system.

anaphylactic shock A severe reaction (marked by respiratory arrest and vascular shock) to a sensitizing substance such as insect stings, contrast media, and penicillin.

anaplastic A pathologic description of cells, describing a loss of differentiation and more primitive appearance.

analytical model Also referred to as an *engineering model*. Identifies the caregiver as a scientist dealing only in facts and does not consider the human aspect of the patient. The analytical or engineering model is a dehumanizing approach and is usually ineffective.

anatomic position Position in which the subject stands upright, with feet together flat on the floor, toes pointed forward, eyes looking forward, arms straight down by the sides of the body with palms facing forward, fingers extended, and thumbs pointing away from the body.

anemia A decrease in the peripheral red cell count.

anesthetic An agent that produces complete or partial loss of sensation with or without loss of consciousness.

aneuploid A condition in which the cells have an abnormal number of chromosomes.

Ann Arbor staging system A classification system used for non-Hodgkin's lymphomas and Hodgkin's disease.

anode The mechanism of the modern x-ray tube that becomes a target for the source of electrons (the cathode) that in turn allows an extremely high voltage necessary to move the electron cloud to flow at the velocity required to produce x-rays.

anorexia Loss of appetite resulting in weight loss.

ANSI (American National Standards Institute) The institute seeks to provide standardization of interfaces and data sources by outlining industry-specific requirements.

anterior Relates to anatomy nearer to the front of the body.

anterior resection An abdominal incision to remove an affected portion of the bowel with the margin plus the adjacent lymphatics. An end-to-end anastomosis is constructed, maintaining the continuity of the gastrointestinal tract (no colostomy).

antibody A protein substance manufactured by the immune system's plasma cells in a defensive response to the presence of a specific antigen.

antigen A substance or pathogen that is viewed as foreign by a person's immune system and induces the formation of antibodies.

anxiety The response to a perceived threat at an emotional level with an increased level of arousal associated with vague, unpleasant, and uneasy feelings. Anxiety is one of the critical psychologic factors that affect a patient's response to pain and ability to tolerate and cope with pain because anxiety often increases pain.

applied dose The applied dose is the dose delivered at the depth of D_{max} for a single treatment field. Sometimes referred to as *given dose*.

Aquaplast Trade name for a thermoplastic that is frequently used as an immobilization device.

articular cartilage A thin layer of hyaline cartilage covering the joint surface of the epiphyses.

asepsis A condition free from germs.

ASP (Application Service Providers) Providers who maintain computer servers.

aspect of care Those activities considered to be of the most importance in providing health care services.

assault The threat of touching in an injurious way. If patients feel threatened and believe they will be touched in a harmful manner, justification may exist for a charge of assault. To avoid this, professionals must always explain what is going to happen and reassure the patient in any situation involving the threat of harm.

astrocytoma A central nervous system tumor originating from the nonneuronal supporting cells. It can be low grade or anaplastic.

asymmetric collimation A process using collimators in which the blade pairs are capable of independent movement.

asymptomatic The absence of symptoms. A patient who does not have or experience symptoms is asymptomatic.

atlas First cervical vertebral body with the specialized function of supporting the skull and allowing it to turn.

atom The smallest unit of an element that retains the properties of that element.

atomic mass unit (AMU) A quantity that describes the very small masses of subatomic particles. The mass of an atom of carbon 12 is exactly 12.000 AMU.

attenuation The removal of photons and electrons from a radiation beam by scatter or absorption as it travels through a medium, typically tissue or tissue equivalent materials.

attributable risk Risk that can be linked to a specific disease.

atypical hyperplasia The proliferation of unusual-appearing cells in a normal tissue arrangement.

auer rods Structures in the cytoplasm of myeloblasts, myelocytes, and monoblasts.

autoclave A device used for sterilization by steam under pressure.

autologous bone marrow transplant (ABMT) A technique of using a patient's own previously removed bone marrow to rescue the patient from the potentially fatal hematologic toxicity of extremely high-dose chemotherapy and radiation.

autonomy The quality or state of being self-governing; self-directing freedom, especially moral independence.

autoradiograph A signature exposure of a radioactive source obtained by placing the source on an unexposed x-ray film for a period of time long enough to darken the film. The film may be scanned to check for dose uniformity.

axillary lymphatic pathway (principal pathway) Comes from trunks of the upper and lower half of the breast and moves toward the underarm.

B symptoms A group of symptoms (fevers, night sweats, weight loss) associated with lymphomas.

backscatter factor The ratio of the dose rate with a scattering medium (water or phantom) to the dose rate at the same point without a scattering medium (air).

backup timer setting The backup timer device refers to a safety device that will stop the treatment if the primary timer device fails.

Barrett's esophagus A condition in which the distal esophagus is lined with a columnar epithelium rather than a stratified squamous epithelium. It usually occurs with gastroesophageal reflux. This condition is associated with an increased risk in the development of adenocarcinomas of the distal esophagus.

barium sulfate Heavy metal salt; the most commonly used contrast agent for examinations of the gastrointestinal tract.

basal cell carcinoma A slow-growing, locally invasive, but rarely metastasizing neoplasm derived from basal cells of the epidermis or hair follicles.

base A special number discovered by Euler, a mathematician. This special number is represented by the letter *e* and is called Euler's constant or the "base of the natural logarithms." Numerically, *e* is equal to 2.718272..... Logarithms based on e are called "natural logarithms." Exponential function is the terminology used to describe *e* raised to a power.

baseline study An initial study performed so that future studies can be compared with the original values.

battery The touching of a person without permission.

beamlet A small photon intensity element, also referred to as a bixel, used to subdivide an IMRT beam for calculation purposes.

beam modifiers Devices that change the shape of the treatment field or distribution of the radiation at depth.

beam-restricting diaphragms Devices made of 2 mm to 3 mm of lead, the diaphragms (also called x-ray shutters, blades, or collimators) define both the size and the axis of the x-ray beam.

beam's eye views (BEVs) A visualization perspective that is "end-on" or positioned as if looking at a volume from the source or radiation. Made possible from collected CT data, this perspective is essential in 3-dimensional planning.

becquerel (Bq) A Standard International (SI) unit of radioactivity that equals 1 disintegration per second.

bending magnet Used in high-energy linear accelerators to bend the electron stream within the head of the gantry, sometimes at right angles.

beneficence The doing or producing of good; acts of kindness and charity.

benign Tumors that are generally well differentiated and do not metastasize or invade surrounding normal tissue. Benign tumors are often encapsulated and slow growing. Although most benign tumors do little harm to the host, benign tumors of the brain (because of their location) are considered behaviorally malignant because of the adverse effect on the host.

benign prostatic hypertrophy (BPH) An enlargement of the prostate gland common in men older than 50 years. It generally causes a narrowing of the urethra.

beta particle Electrons (B⁻, negatively charged) or positrons (B⁺, positively charged) emitted during nuclear decay.

betatron A megavoltage unit that can provide x-ray and electron therapy beams from less than 6 to more than 40 MeV.

bimodal Occurring with two peaks of incidence. With Hodgkin's disease the disease occurs with greater frequency during the young adult years and then again in the fifth or sixth decade of life.

biopsy The surgical removal of a small tissue sample from a solid tumor to determine the pathology for the diagnosis of disease.

bite block An object placed between the patient's teeth to assist in immobilization and to position the tongue.

bitemporal hemianopsia The loss of peripheral vision.

blocked field size The equivalent rectangular field dimensions of the open treated area within the collimator field dimensions. The blocked field size is the actual area treated. Therefore the blocked field size is normally smaller than the collimator field size.

blood-brain barrier (BBB) The barrier system that hinders the penetration of some substances into the brain and cerebrospinal fluid. The BBB exists between the vascular system and brain. Its purpose is to protect the brain from potentially toxic compounds. Substances that can pass through the BBB must be lipid soluble.

body cavities The spaces within the body that contain internal organs.

body habitus The physique of the human body. The internal anatomy of a person varies with the physique. The four standard body habiti are hypersthenic, sthenic, hyposthenic, and asthenic.

Bohr atom The Bohr atom model states that the electrons surrounding the nucleus exists only in certain energy states or orbits, and when an electron moves from one orbit to another it must gain or lose energy. This model has been replaced with complex quantum mechanical models of the atom, but it is still an excellent way to derive a mental picture of the atom's structure.

bolus Tissue equivalent material that is usually placed on the patient to increase the skin dose and/or even out irregular contours in the patient. When bolus is placed on the skin surface for megavoltage irradiation, skin sparing is lost.

boost fields Fields that are used to deliver a high dose to a small volume. With boost fields the radiation dose is generally delivered to the gross tumor volume only, excluding regional lymph nodes.

Bowen's disease A precancerous dermatosis or form of intraepidermal carcinoma characterized by the development of pink or brown papules covered with a thickened, horny layer.

brachytherapy Radiation treatment of disease accomplished by inserting radioactive sources directly into the tumor site.

Bragg peak A sharp increase in the dose distribution curve of a charged particle at a particular depth.

bremsstrahlung German term for "braking" radiation. The principal interaction in x-ray production results in the output of bremsstrahlung radiation. Bremsstrahlung accounts for approximately 75% to 80% of the tube's output and is produced by the sudden deceleration of the high-speed electron as it is deflected around the nucleus of the tungsten atom.

bronchogenic carcinoma Cancer of the lung that arises in the anatomy of the bronchial tree.

build-up region The region between the skin surface and the depth of D_{max}. A build-up region is a characteristic of megavoltage irradiation. In this region the dose increases with depth until it reaches a maximum at the depth of D_{max}.

bulbous urethra The dilated proximal portion of the anterior urethra.

cachexia A state of general ill health and malnutrition with early satiety; electrolyte and water imbalances; and progressive loss of body weight, fat, and muscle.

caliper A graduated ruled instrument with one sliding leg and one that is stationary is used to figure out the thickness of the patient's tissue.

calvaria The part of the skull that protects the brain.

carcinoma in situ Malignant changes at the cellular level in epithelial tissues without extension beyond the basement membrane.

carfusion A dyelike liquid usually containing silver nitrate and phenol in a fuchsin base; magenta liquid that can be painted onto patients by using thin sticks or swabs.

carina The area in which the trachea divides into two branches.

carrier A person who carries a specific pathogen but is free of signs or symptoms of the disease and yet is capable of spreading the disease.

case manager A member of the health care team who is assigned to manage the continuum of care for the patient.

cassette The cassette provides the light-tight conditions necessary for x-ray film and intensifying screens to work properly. The cassette, which opens like a book, is made of material with a low atomic number such as cardboard, plastic, and carbon fiber.

cathode One of the electrodes found in the x-ray tube that represents the negative side of the tube. The cathode consists of two parts: the filament and focusing cup. As a first step in x-ray production, the primary function of the cathode is to produce electrons and focus the electron stream toward the metal anode.

cell cycle The sequence of recurring biochemical and morphologic events observed in a population of reproducing cells.

cellular differentiation The degree to which a cell resembles its cell of origin in morphology and function.

centigray Unit of energy absorbed per unit mass of any material. 1 cGy = 1 rad.

central axis It is the central portion of the beam emanating from the target; the only part of the beam that is not divergent.

cerebellum The part of the brain that plays a role in the coordination of voluntary muscular movements located in the occipital region.

cerebrospinal fluid (CSF) The fluid that flows through and protects the brain and spinal canal.

cerebrum The largest part of the brain, consisting of two hemispheres. The functions of the cerebrum include interpretation of sensory impulses and voluntary muscular activities; it is the center for memory, learning, reasoning, judgment, intelligence, and emotions.

certification A process by which a governmental or nongovernmental agency or association grants authority to an individual who has met predetermined qualifications to use a specific title.

cervical cancer A slowly progressive disease, with the earliest phase (noninvasive carcinoma in situ) occurring approximately 10 years earlier than invasive cancer.

cervix The part of the uterus that protrudes into the cavity of the vagina.

cesium A radioactive isotope with a half-life of 30 years that is commonly used as a low-dose brachytherapy source.

characteristic radiation Radiation that is created by the direct interaction of cathode electrons with inner-shell electrons of the target material.

chemotherapeutic agents Chemotherapeutic agents that are classified by their action on the cell or their source and include alkylating agents, antimetabolites, antibiotics, hormonal agents, nitrosoureas, vinca alkaloids, and miscellaneous agents.

chemotherapy The use of chemical agents to induce specific effects on disease.

chief complaint The patient's reason for visiting with the clinician. The chief complaint is recorded by the clinician.

childhood cancer The incidence of malignancies in people less than 18 years old.

chin to SSN measurement A measurement taken between the anatomic landmarks of the tip of chin and the suprasternal notch (SSN).

chromophobe adenomas Nonfunctioning pituitary tumors.

chromosomes The gene-bearing protein structures in the nucleus of animal cells.

chronic ulcerative colitis Extensive inflammation and ulceration of the bowel wall resulting in bloody mucoid diarrhea several times a day. It is associated with an increased risk of the development of colorectal cancer.

circulator One of four major components housed in the drive stand (a stand containing the apparatus that drives the linear accelerator). The circulator acts much like the valves found in human veins and the lymphatic system, which are designed to prevent the backflow of blood and lymphatic fluid. The circulator prevents backflow of microwave power.

civil law The law that governs relationships between individuals.

Clarkson integration or Clarkson technique A method used to calculate the dose in an irregularly shaped field.

clinical target volume (CTV) The visible (imaged) or palpable tumor plus any margin of subclinical disease that needs to be eliminated through the treatment planning and delivery process.

cobalt-60 A radioactive isotope with a half-life of 5.26 years that is used as a

source for external-beam radiation therapy.

cognitive Pertaining to an individual's basic reasoning processes.

cold thyroid nodule A nodule having no uptake.

collegial model A cooperative method of pursuing health care for the provider and patient. It involves sharing, trust, and consideration of common goals.

collimation The definition of radiation beam size and dimensions.

collimator An arrangement of shielding material designed to define the dimensions of the beam of radiation. The collimators are located in the treatment head. The secondary collimators are used to set the field size.

collimator assembly The collimator assembly provides support for the x-ray tube aperture, field-defining wires, light field indicator, beam-limiting diaphragms, an accessory holder, and other essential equipment within the head of the gantry.

collimator field size The unblocked or open field size as defined by the collimator setting and projected at the reference distance, usually the isocenter of the machine.

colonization The presence of an agent that is infectious but does not initiate an immune response.

colostomy The surgical construction of an artificial excretory opening from the colon on the surface of the abdominal wall.

combination chemotherapy The selection of drugs that act on the cell during different phases of the cell cycle, increasing the cell killing potential. In addition, drugs with known toxicities are used for maximum effectiveness, resulting in fewer side effects.

common iliac nodes Nodes that lie at the bifurcation of the abdominal aorta at the level of L4. These nodes directly drain the urinary bladder, prostate, cervix, and vagina.

communication The ability to transfer concrete and abstract information from one person to another person or a group of people while keeping the same meaning. Communication can be verbal, nonverbal, or a combination of the two techniques.

compensator A beam modifier that changes radiation output relative to loss of attenuation over a changing patient contour.

compensatory vertebral curves Specific sections of the curvature of the vertebral column that form after birth because of the development of muscles as an infant grows. The cervical and lumbar curves are compensatory curves.

complex immobilization devices Individualized devices that restrict patient

movement and ensure reproducibility in positioning.

computer-based patient record (CPR) An electronic patient record stored digitally. CPR systems provide patient data when and where it is needed, regardless of the source. They provide access to clinical and administrative data; support physician ordering and data entry; support and coordinate clinical communication between multiple organizations; and are capable of providing clinical decision support including clinical guidelines, drug interactions, and alerts for abnormal test results.

concomitant The situation in which two types of treatment take place at the same time.

conformal radiation therapy Therapy that, with the use of three-dimensional treatment planning, allows the delivery of higher tumor doses to selected target volumes without increasing treatment morbidity.

consequentialism (the theory of utility) Evaluates an activity by weighing the good against the bad or the way a person can provide the greatest good for the greatest number.

contact therapy unit A machine that operates at potentials of 40 to 50 kV and uses an extremely short source-skin distance.

contiguous Systematic and predictable, as in the spread of Hodgkin's disease.

continuous quality improvement (CQI) Same as for quality improvement; it is an ongoing improvement of health care services through the systematic evaluation of processes.

contour contralateral The opposite side of the body.

contour corrections (obliquity corrections) Corrections for beam incidence onto surfaces other than flat surfaces and for angles of incidence other than 90 degrees ("normal" incidence).

contractual model A model that maintains a business relationship between the provider and patient; a sharing of information and responsibility.

contrast media High-density substances used radiographically to visualize internal anatomy for diagnostic imaging.

convalescence The period of recovery after an illness.

conventional fractionation Fractionation in which the total dose of radiation is typically divided into 180 or 200 cGy increments and delivered once a day, 5 days a week.

coplanar A geometrical principle describing two radiation fields configured in such a way that the beam edges lie in the same plane. (The central ray is not parallel opposed.)

coronal plane Perpendicular (at right angles) to the sagittal plane and vertically divides the body into anterior and posterior sections.

corpora cavernosa One of the basic structural components of the penis that is encased in a dense fascia (Buck's fascia), which is separated from the skin by a layer of loose connective tissue.

corpus spongiosum One of two basic structural components of the penis. The other basic structural component is the **corpora cavernosa** of which there are two. These components are encased in a dense fascia (Buck's fascia), which is separated from the skin by a layer of loose connective tissue. Distally, the corpus spongiosum expands into the glans penis, which is covered by a skin fold known as the prepuce.

cortex The outer portion of a structure as in the adrenal gland. The inner portion of the adrenal gland is the medulla. The cortex and the medulla have distinct histologic features and physiologic functions.

cosine One of three of the most common functions associated with the right triangle. The other two functions are the sine and tangent.

covenant model A model that deals with an understanding between the patient and health care provider and is based on traditional values and goals.

craniospinal irradiation (CSI) Complex irradiation of all central nervous system and cerebrospinal fluid regions from behind the eye down to the midsacrum for treatment of medulloblastoma and other cerebrospinal fluid seeding tumors.

critical structures Normal tissue whose radiation tolerance limits the deliverable dose.

critical thinking The cognitive process that allows mastery of theory and uses practical experiences. Critical thinking incorporates the use of cognitive, affective, and psychomotor domains. The art of critical thinking helps the therapist question and critique each step of a patient's treatment, thereby ensuring an understanding and accurate administration of the treatment.

cryotherapy The use of cold temperatures to treat a disease.

cryptorchidism Undescended testes.

CT simulator/virtual simulation A type of simulation that operates along with a three-dimensional (3D) geometric planning computer. The extension of a CT system (usually a high-performance spiral CT acquisition system) allows the single acquisition of many thin slices over a required treatment area. Virtual simulation is a geometrical planning function. It is not a 3D radiation treatment planning function, because it does not include or require dose computation. To complete the process of simulation, true virtual simulation systems allow the generation of digitally reconstructed radiograph (DRR) on an interactive basis.

CT simulator A computed tomography scanner equipped with software that can provide information needed to design the patient's treatment parameters. CT based planning allows more spatial orientation information required for 3-dimensional treatment planning.

cumulative effect An effect that develops if the body is unable to detoxify and excrete a drug quickly enough or if too large a dose is taken.

curie (Ci) A historical unit of radioactivity that equals 3.7×10^{10} Bq.

curriculum The body of courses and formally established learning experiences presenting the knowledge, principles, values, and skills that are the intended consequences of a program's formal education.

customer (external, internal) An *external* customer is a person who is not employed by the particular institution or hospital that employees come in contact with. A patient is an example of an external customer. An *internal* customer is a person who is also employed by the particular institution and might be another employee from a different department or area in the company.

cyclotron A charged particle accelerator used mainly for nuclear research and more recently for generating proton and neutron beams.

cystectomy Surgical removal of the bladder.

cytoplasm All the cellular protoplasm except the nucleus and its contents. It consists of a watery fluid (cytosol) in which numerous organelles are suspended.

cytotoxic The ability to kill cancer cells. Cytotoxic drugs are used to destroy cells of the primary tumor and those that may be circulating through the body.

CYVADIC A chemotherapy program that consists of the combination of the following drugs: cyclophosphamide (Cytoxan), vincristine, doxorubicin (Adriamycin), and dacarbazine. CYVADIC is one of the most used drug programs in chemotherapy.

daily treatment record A document recording the actual treatment delivery.

debulking surgery Surgical procedure used to reduce tumor size, reduce tumor burden, and increase the opportunity to obtain a pathologic diagnosis.

decay constant The total number of atoms that decay per unit time.

definitive A course of radiation therapy in which the objective is to cure by eradication of the disease.

de novo A Latin term that means "anew."

densitometer A special device that measures the degree of blackening on the film. The readings from the densitometer, plotted on logarithmic graph paper, correlate to the characteristics of the film.

deontology One of three ethical theories. The other two are consequentialism and virtue ethics. Deontology uses formal rules of right and wrong for reasoning and problem solving. A few gray areas exist in this theory, which make it difficult to use in our society because varieties of life experiences make formal rules of right and wrong impossible to define.

deoxyribonucleic acid (DNA) A large, double-stranded nucleic acid molecule that carries the genetic material of the cell on the chromosomes. This genetic information is composed of a sequence of nitrogen bases and molecular subunits.

depression The perceived loss of self-esteem resulting in a cluster of affective behavioral (e.g., change in appetite, sleep disturbances, lack of energy, withdrawal, and dependency) and cognitive (e.g., decreased ability to concentrate, indecisiveness, and suicidal ideas) responses.

depth The distance beneath the patient's skin to the point of calculation.

dermis The deeper layer of the skin composed of connective tissue that contains blood and lymphatic vessels, nerves and nerve endings, sweat glands, and hair follicles.

desquamation An acute effect of irradiation characterized by shedding of the epidermis.

diaphysis The shaft or long axis of the bone.

DICOM (Digital Imaging and Communications in Medicine) Standards produced by a joint committee of the National Electrical Manufacturers Association (NEMA) and the American College of Radiology (ACR) and affiliated with several international agencies. This committee was formed to provide communication standards for sharing image information regardless of manufacturer and has included radiation therapy treatment information. This facilitates the use of picture archival and communications systems (PACS) and allows diagnostic images to be widely distributed.

digitally reconstructed radiograph (DRR) Based on acquired CT information, these are images that render a beam's eye view display of the treatment field anatomy and areas of treatment interest. These images resemble conventional radiographs.

dimensional analysis A process that involves assessment of units of measure used in calculating some scientific quantity. This practice involves canceling of common units in an effort to leave the specified unit.

direct proportionality Relationship between measurable quantities and factors; as one increases, the other increases and vice versa.

divergence Divergence is the spreading out of the beam of radiation. The farther from the source, the more the beam has spread. We need to be aware of beam divergence when setting up adjacent fields or where field edges are near critical structures. The divergence of the beam is taken into account when performing field size calculations and many dose calculations.

D_{max} The depth at which electronic equilibrium occurs for photon beams. This is also the depth of maximum absorbed dose and ionization, for photons, from a single treatment field. The depth of maximum ionization and maximum absorbed dose are usually not the same depth for electrons.

Do A graphic representation of the cell's radiosensitivity.

doctrine of foreseeability A principle of law that holds a person liable for all consequences of any negligent acts to another individual to whom a duty is owed and should have been reasonably foreseen under the circumstances.

doctrine of personal liability The doctrine stating that all persons are liable for their own negligent conduct.

doctrine of *res ipsa loquitur* ("the thing speaks for itself") A doctrine, which is an accepted substitute for the medical expert, requiring the defendant to explain an incident and convince the court that no negligence was involved.

doctrine of respondent superior A legal doctrine that holds an employer liable for negligent acts of employees occurring while they are carrying out their orders or otherwise serving their interests.

domain A group of job activities related on the basis of required skills and knowledge.

dose calculation matrix A grid of points at which dose is computed and subsequently displayed.

dose distributions Spatial representations of the magnitude of the dose produced by a source of radiation. They describe the variation of dose with position within an irradiated volume.

dose equivalent Product of the absorbed dose and a quality factor (QF), which takes into account the biologic effects of different types of radiation on humans; units are the rem (1 rem = 1 rad × QF) or sievert (1 Sv = 1 Gy × QF). 1 Sv = 100 rem.

dose rate Also known as output, the dose rate of a treatment machine is the amount of radiation exposure produced by a

treatment machine or source as specified at a reference field size and at a specified reference distance.

dose-volume histogram (DVH) A plot of target or normal structure volume as a function of dose. It is, in essence, a frequency distribution of the number of target or normal-structure voxels (volume elements) receiving a certain dose. In its most common form (the "cumulative" DVH), it is a plot of volume versus the minimum dose absorbed within that volume.

dosimetrist Radiation therapy practitioner responsible for production of the patient's treatment plan and any associated quality assurance components.

drop metastases Secondary tumors that occur via the cerebrospinal fluid.

droplet nuclei The residual remains of airborne pathogens after the evaporation of moisture.

drug Any substance that alters physiologic function, with the potential for affecting health.

drug interactions The mutual or reciprocal action or influence between drugs and/or food that can create positive or negative effects in the body.

dynamic wedge The use of a moving collimator jaw to produce a wedged field.

dysphagia Difficulty in swallowing. The sensation of food sticking in the throat.

dysplopia Double vision.

dyspnea Difficult, labored, or uncomfortable breathing.

EAM External auditory meatus.

ecchymoses The escape of blood into the tissues, causing large, blotchy areas of discoloration.

edema Excessive accumulation of fluid in a tissue, producing swelling.

effective dose equivalent The dose equivalent weighted by the proportionate risk for various tissues. That is, it is the sum over specified tissues of the products of the dose equivalent in a tissue and the weighting factor for that tissue.

effective field size (EFS) Another term for blocked field size (BFS). The effective field size is the equivalent rectangular field dimensions of the open or treated area within the collimator field dimensions. The effective field size is the actual area treated.

efferent lymphatic vessels Lymphatic vessels that flow out of the hilum of a lymph node.

elapsed days The total time over which treatment is delivered (protracted).

electrical charge A measure of how strongly the particle is attracted to an electrical field and can be either positive or negative.

electrocautery An instrument for directing a high-frequency current through a local tissue area.

electron binding energy The amount of energy required to remove an electron from its orbit in an atom.

electron density Number of electrons per unit mass.

electron gun The electron gun is responsible for producing electrons and injecting them into the accelerator structure.

electronic medical record (EMR) A patient's medical record stored on and accessed from a computer.

electronic portal imaging devices (EPID) A system producing near real-time portal images on a computer screen for evaluation.

electrons Negatively charged subatomic particles that can be accelerated by a variety of machines or are emitted from decaying isotopes and used for external beam treatment and brachytherapy.

electron shields "Cutouts" that collimate and shape the electron treatment field.

empathy Identifying with the feelings, thoughts, or experiences of another person.

en bloc A French term meaning "in one block." In surgical cancer care, it means "in one specimen."

endocavitary radiation therapy A sphincter-sparing procedure in which the radiation treatment is delivered by a 50-kVp contact unit inserted into the rectum. Only a select group of people with low-middle-third rectal lesions that have small exophytic tumors confined to the bowel wall are eligible candidates for this treatment.

endometrial cancer Cancer of the endometrium or uterus.

endophytic pattern A growth pattern that invades within the lamina propria and submucosa.

endoplasmic reticulum A continuous membrane in the cellular cytoplasm containing the ribosomes.

engineering model A model that identifies the caregiver as a scientist dealing only in facts and does not consider the human aspect of the patient.

ependymoma Tumors arising from the ependymal cells lining the brain ventricles and central spinal canal. They may be low or high grade.

epidemiology The study of defining the distribution and determinants causing disease and injury in human populations.

epidermis The extremely thin outer layer of the skin composed of four to five distinct layers of cells.

epiphyseal line Cartilage at the junction of the diaphysis and epiphysis in young bones that serves as a growth area for long-bone lengthening.

epiphyses The knoblike portions of a long bone made up of spongy bone. It is located at either end of a long bone.

epistaxis A nosebleed.

equivalent square The square field that has the same percentage depth dose and output of a rectangular field.

erythema This acute radiation effect, manifested by redness and inflammation of the skin or mucous membranes, is caused by capillary congestion, caused by dilation of the superficial capillaries.

erythroplasia Reddened, velvetlike patches on the mucous membranes.

esophagitis Inflammation of the esophagus. Patients complain of substernal pain and food sticking. Esophagitis may begin after 2 weeks of radiation therapy and continues for 2 to 4 weeks after treatment.

ethics The discipline dealing with what is good and bad, with a concern for moral duty and obligations; a set of moral principles or values; a theory or system of moral values; the principles of conduct governing an individual or professional group.

etiology The study of the causes of disease.

excisional biopsy The removal of the entire tumor by cutting it out so that a diagnosis can be made.

exenteration (pelvic) The radical removal of most or all pelvic organs.

exit dose The term exit dose is used for the dose at the exit surface of the patient or to a depth that is the equivalent of the depth of D_{max}.

exophytic A noninvasive neoplasm that projects out from an epithelial surface.

exponent An exponent, or "power," is a shorthand notation that represents the multiplication of a number by itself a given number of times.

exposure Amount of ionization produced by photons in air per unit mass of air; units are the roentgen (R) or Coulomb per kilogram (C/kg). $1 R = 2.58 \times 10^{-4}$ C/kg.

extended distance setup An extended distance setup occurs when the setup source-skin distance (SSD) is greater than the reference SSD. The reference SSD is normally 80 cm for cobalt-60 treatment machines and 100 cm for linear accelerators.

extrapolation number (n) Part of a graphic representation of a cell-survival curve, determined by extrapolating the linear portion of the curve back until it intersects the y-axis.

extravasation Accidental leakage into the surrounding tissues; a discharge or escape (e.g., of blood) from a vessel into the tissues.

false imprisonment The intentional confinement without authorization by a person who physically constricts another with force, threat of force, or confining clothing or structures.

false positive/false negative Screening tests may yield false-positive or false-negative readings. A false-positive reading indicates disease when in reality none is present. A false-negative reading is the reverse; the test indicates no disease when in fact the disease is present.

familial adenomatous polyps (FAP) A hereditary disease in which the entire large bowel is studded with polyps. If left untreated, the patient develops a cancer of the large bowel.

feathering The migration of a gap between treatment fields through the treatment course.

fibrosis The abnormal formation of fibrous tissue caused by alterations in the structure and function of blood vessels.

fiducial marker Fiducial markers may include natural anatomy or be artificial markers placed internally or at the skin surface or fixed external to the patient to document location.

fiducial plate Plastic trays imbedded with lead markers at regular intervals. These trays, sometimes referred to as a reticule or beaded trays, are positioned in the head of the gantry between the field-defining wires and accessory holder.

field-defining wires They are small tungsten wires (also called delineators) located in the collimator assembly that represent the edge of the treatment field.

field size The dimensions of a treatment field at the isocenter (usually represented by width × length).

filament A small coil of wire made of thoriated tungsten, which has an extremely high melting point (3380 °C).

file server A central computer where the database and program executables reside.

film badge A device for measuring dose. It makes use of the following phenomenon: when film is exposed to radiation and subsequently developed, the amount of blackening is proportional to the dose delivered to the film. Therefore metal and plastic filters in the film badge holder are used to allow discrimination of the energy levels of the radiation.

film speed The reciprocal of the exposure in roentgens needed to produce a density of 1.0.

flatness The difference between the maximum and minimum intensity of the central 80% of the profile and specifying this difference as a percentage of the central axis intensity. The degree of evenness of dose across a beam profile.

flow chart A diagram illustrating a sequence of steps to be used in the completion of a process.

focal spot The section of the target at which radiation is produced.

focusing cup A small oval depression in the cathode assembly.

fomite Any inanimate object (vehicle) involved in the transmission of disease.

forward planning The process of entering dose-altering parameters and beam modifiers into the treatment plan by the planner.

fractionation Radiation therapy treatments given in daily fractions (segments) over an extended period of time, sometimes up to 6 to 8 weeks.

free radical An atom or atom group in a highly reactive transient state that is carrying an unpaired electron with no charge.

free space Term used for dosimetry measurements using a build-up cap or miniphantom.

friable tumors Tumors that are easily broken or pulverized.

gadolinium A noniodine-based intravenous contrast agent used for computed tomography and magnetic resonance imaging scans. Gadolinium helps differentiate between edema and a tumor.

gamma rays Electromagnetic radiation emitted from decaying isotopes and used for external-beam treatment and brachytherapy.

gamma rays High-energy electromagnetic radiation of no mass and no charge emitted during nuclear decay.

gantry On a simulator, it is a mechanical C-shaped device that supports the x-ray tube and collimator device at one end and an image system at the other and allows the duplication of treatment unit motions.

gap The distance between the borders of two adjacent fields. The gap is usually measured on the patient's skin. The skin gap is usually calculated to verify the depth at which the two adjacent fields abut.

Gardner's syndrome An inherited disorder (similar to familial adenomatous polyps) consisting of adenomatous polyposis of the large bowel, upper gastrointestinal polyps, periampullary tumors, lipomas, fibromas, and other tumors. This condition is associated with an increased risk in the development of colorectal cancer.

generic name The drug name coined by the original manufacturer.

genetically significant dose The dose equivalent to the gonads weighted for the age and sex distribution in those members of the irradiated population expected to have offspring; units are the rem or sievert.

genome The complete complement of hereditary factors as found on a haploid distribution of chromosomes.

germ cell tumors Tumors developing from embryologic nests of tissue located throughout the body, from the brain down to the ovaries and testes.

germ theory The hypothesis that microorganisms cause disease.

given dose The given dose (GD) is the dose delivered at the depth of D_{max} through a single treatment field. Also known as applied dose or D_{max} dose.

golgi apparatus A cytoplasmic organelle consisting of flattened membranes that modify, store, and route products of the endoplasmic reticulum.

grade The **grade** of a tumor provides information about its biological aggressiveness and is based on the degree of cell differentiation. For some tumors, such as a high-grade astrocytoma, grade is the most important prognostic indicator.

gradient The change in position with the rate of change of a value (dose).

grenz ray Low-energy x-ray in the range of 10 to 15 kV.

grid A device constructed with thin lead foil strips and plastic spacers. It should be employed during simulation both to absorb the scattered radiation emitted from the thicker body parts and to allow the use of beam energies needed to maximize differential absorption between similar tissues.

gross tumor volume (GTV) The gross palpable or visible tumor.

ground state The minimum amount of energy needed to keep the atom together.

half-life The time period in which the activity decays to one half of the original value. It is the essential value to employ the decay formula for a particular isotope.

half-value layer The thickness of absorbing material necessary to reduce the x-ray intensity to half its original value.

health care organization A generic term used to describe all types of groups that provide health care services.

hematuria A common symptom of bladder and kidney tumors with an abnormal presence of blood in the urine.

hemiglossectomy The surgical removal of half the tongue.

hereditary nonpolyposis colorectal syndrome The frequent occurrence of colorectal cancer in families without adenomatous polyposis. This syndrome is associated with an increased risk of developing a second malignancy of the colon and adenocarcinomas of the breast, ovary, endometrium, and pancreas.

high-dose-rate (HDR) brachytherapy The delivery of brachytherapy on an outpatient basis using HDR brachytherapy equipment. The actual treatment delivery lasts about 5 to 10 minutes in contrast to a hospital stay that might take several days for low-dose-rate brachytherapy.

high osmolality A high number of particles in solution.

hilum The area of an organ where blood, lymphatic vessels, and nerves enter and exit.

hinge angle The measure of the angle between central rays of two intersecting treatment beams.

HIPPA (Health Insurance Portability and Accountability Act) Congress passed HIPPA in 1996. HIPAA guidelines and regulations require security precautions not only to restrict access but also to keep records of who is accessing information.

histiocyte A phagocytic cell found in loose connective tissue.

histiocytosis X A spectrum of diseases caused by abnormal proliferation of a variety of immune cells affecting single or multiple organs.

history and physical Initial presentation and plan for assessment and treatment that becomes part of the patient's medical record.

history of present illness A clinician records, through conversation with the patient, a history of the present illness, and this becomes part of the patient's medical record.

HL7(Health Level 7, Inc.) An ANSI-accredited organization that develops standards for exchanging clinical and administrative data. Specifically, HL7 defines standards for "the exchange, management and integration of data that supports clinical patient care and the management, delivery and evaluation of healthcare services." HL7 interfaces allow sharing of information available used across the entire health care facility.

Horner's syndrome A condition caused by paralysis of the cervical sympathetic nerves. It may cause sinking in of the eyeball, ptosis of the upper eyelid, slight elevation of the lower lid, constriction of the pupil, and flushing of the affected side of the face.

hospice A program that provides care for patients who have limited life expectancy. The care is provided in the patient's home or a hospital setting.

hot thyroid nodule A nodule having a radionuclide uptake much higher than the rest of the thyroid gland.

hyperfractionation Fractional doses smaller than conventional, delivered two or three times daily to achieve an increase in the total dose in the same overall time.

hyperparathyroidism A condition, caused by a tumor in the parathyroid, in which calcium is leaked from the bones, resulting in softening and deformity as the mineral salts are replaced by fibrous connective tissue.

hyperpigmentation Excessive coloration to the skin.

hyperthyroidism Hyperactivity of the thyroid gland.

hypertrophic pulmonary osteoarthropathy A frequently seen phenomenon associated with lung cancer, which is manifested by clubbing of the distal phalanges of the fingers.

hypophysis The pituitary gland.

hypotenuse The length of the longest side of the triangle.

hypothesis A prediction of the relationship between certain variables.

hypothyroidism Underactivity of the thyroid gland.

iatrogenic Disease or illness created as a result of the treatment or diagnosis of another condition.

idiosyncratic response (effects) The inexplicable and unpredictable symptoms caused by a genetic defect in the patient.

image fusion The process of combining images from different modalities with a CT image. Properly fused images combine the enhanced imaging capabilities of MRI and/or PET with the spatial accuracy of CT. Anatomy can be defined on any of the image data sets and can then be displayed on the CT image.

image intensifier It is a useful tool during fluoroscopy, because it converts an x-ray image into a light image.

immobilization The process of ensuring that a patient does not move out of treatment position, thus allowing for reproducibility and accuracy in treatment.

immobilization device A device that reproduces the treatment position while restricting movement (i.e., casts, masks, or bite blocks).

immune serum globulin A serum-containing antibody; a form of artificial immunity.

immunity The ability of the body to defend itself against infectious organisms, foreign bodies, and cancer cells.

immunoglobulin The system of closely related, although not identical, proteins capable of acting as antibodies. Humans have five main types.

immunotherapy Therapy producing or increasing immunity.

impotence A significant side effect associated with the treatment of prostate cancer in which the adult male is unable to obtain an erection or ejaculate after achieving an erection.

IMRT (Intensity Modulated Radiation Therapy) Therapy that delivers nonuniform exposure across the beam's eye view (BEV) using a variety of techniques and equipment.

incidence The occurrence of a particular disease over a period of time in relationship to the entire population.

incident Any happening not consistent with the routine operation of the hospital or routine care of a particular patient.

incisional biopsy The act of cutting into tissue to remove part of the tumor so that a diagnosis can be made.

incubation The time interval between exposure to infection and the appearance of the first sign or symptom characteristic of the disease.

induration The process of becoming hard and firm in soft tissues.

inferior Toward the feet.

infiltration A swelling around the injection site accompanied by cool, pale skin and possibly hard patches or localized pain.

information system department A department that may employ several computer specialists in areas ranging from hardware to network to application support for managing the array of requirements, from running the computer system to ensuring that it is employed efficiently by clinicians and staff.

informed consent An assurance that the purpose, benefit, risk, and any alternative options have been explained and understood and a disclaimer (which will not always hold up in court) releasing the caregiver and facility from liability if complications develop or the treatment fail.

infundibulum Stalklike structure that attaches the pituitary to the hypothalamus.

intensifying screens Used to convert the invisible energy of an x-ray beam into visible light energy.

interdisciplinary All the disciplines cooperating in the management of the disease process, as in the cancer-management team.

interlocks Safety switches blocking or terminating radiation production.

internal mammary lymphatic pathway Lymphatic chain that runs toward the midline and passes through the pectoralis major and intercostal muscles close to the body of the sternum (T4 to T9).

interpolation To estimate values between two measured, known values. A mathematical process used in radiation therapy in which unlisted values in tables can be derived.

interstitial brachytherapy Treatment technique that is characterized by the placement of radioactive sources directly into a tumor or tumor bed. Interstitial implants can be either permanent or temporary.

interstitial implant The application of a brachytherapy implant directly into the tissues via devices such as needles, ribbons, or seeds placed in the at-risk tissues.

interstitial radiation therapy The insertion of radioactive sources into the tissue to treat the disease.

intracavitary brachytherapy In this aspect of brachytherapy, radioactive sources are placed within a body cavity for treatment. This type of brachytherapy has been the mainstay in treatment of cervical cancer for more than 50 years.

intradermal A shallow injection between the layers of the skin.

intrahypophyseal tumors A pituitary tumor that stays in the pituitary gland.

intraluminal brachytherapy Closely associated with interstitial brachystherapy, intraluminal brachytherapy places sources of radiation within body tubes such as the esophagus, uterus, trachea, bronchus, and rectum. Many high dose rate applications are performed for intraluminal applications.

intra-muscular (IM) An administrative route for chemotherapy agents. It is used for large amounts or quick effects.

intraoperative radiation therapy (IORT) A boost technique in which a single dose of 10 to 20 Gy is delivered directly to the tumor bed with electrons or photons. The tumor bed has been surgically exposed, allowing critical normal structures to be shielded or displaced out of the radiation beam.

intrasellar lesions Pituitary tumors that grow within the confines of the sella.

intrathecal An injection that requires drugs to be instilled into the space containing cerebrospinal fluid. Although most chemotherapy drugs can be administered by the patient or a nurse, intrathecal administration is only done by a physician.

intrauterine tandem A brachytherapy device placed through the cervical os into the uterus and subsequently afterloaded to give the dose application directly to the cervix, uterus, and upper vagina.

intravascular brachytherapy A rapidly emerging treatment modality that introduces radioactive source(s) through vascular routes.

intravenous An injection directly into the bloodstream providing an immediate effect.

intravenous pyelogram (IVP) A radiographic procedure using contrast media to outline the kidneys, ureters, and bladder.

invasion of privacy Revealing confidential information or improperly and unnecessarily exposing a patient's body.

inverse planning Treatment planning in which the clinical objectives are specified mathematically and computer software is used to determine the best beam parameters (mainly beamlet weighting) that will lead to the desired dose distribution.

inverse proportionality Relationship between measurable quantities and factors, in that as one increases, the other decreases, and vice versa.

inverse square law A mathematical relationship that describes the change in beam intensity as the distance from the source changes. The change in intensity is primarily caused by the divergence of the beam.

involved field radiation Radiation that includes only the affected lymph node region such as the supraclavicular, ipsilateral cervical, or the inguinal nodes.

ionic contrast media Media having high osmolality or a high number of particles in isolation. The large amount of iodine provides greater contrast but also increases toxicity and viscosity. Meglumine iodine salts and various sodium iodine salts are the most common ionic iodides used.

ionizing radiation Radiation with sufficient energy to separate an electron from its atom.

ipsilateral Refers to a body component on the same side of the body.

iridium A radioactive isotope with a half-life of 74 days. It is used in wire form for interstitial brachytherapy.

irradiated volume The volume of tissue receiving a significant dose (e.g., >50%) of the specified target dose.

ISO Acronym for International Standards Organization. An organization that accredits various specialty organizations that produce standards for industry specific requirements.

isocenter The point of intersection of the three axes of rotation (gantry, collimator, and base of couch) of the treatment unit.

isocentric technique Also called the source-axis distance (SAD) approach, which is a strategy in which the isocenter is placed within the target volume with the aid of fluoroscopy and other imaging modalities.

isodose curve The plotted percentage depth dose at various points in the beam along the central axis and elsewhere.

isodose distributions Two-dimensional spatial representations of dose.

isodose lines Lines connecting points of equivalent relative radiation dose.

isthmus Connects the lobes of the thyroid gland.

Joint Commission on the Accreditation of Healthcare Organizations An independent, not-for-profit organization dedicated to improving quality of care in organized health care settings. It is the accrediting body for health care organizations.

jugulodigastric The group of high neck nodes below the mastoid tip.

justice The quality of being just, impartial, or fair; treatment that is fair or adequate.

Karnofsky performance scale (KPS) A scale that measures the neurologic and functional status. KPS allows measuring of the quantity and quality of neurologic defects. The scale ranges from 1 to 100.

keratin An extremely tough, waterproof, protein substance in hair, nails, and horny tissue.

keratinocyte Any one of the cells in the skin that synthesizes keratin.

keratoacanthoma A papular lesion filled with a keratin plug that can resemble squamous cell carcinoma. It is benign and usually subsides spontaneously within 6 months.

keratosis A lesion on the epidermis marked by the presence of a circumcised overgrowth of the horny layer.

kilovoltage units Equipment carrying out external-beam treatment by using x-rays generated at voltages up to 500 kVp.

kilovolts peak (kVp) Unit of measurement for x-ray voltages. (1 kV equals 1000 V of electrical potential.)

klystron Equipment that converts kinetic energy to microwave energy in the linear accelerator. Klystrons are high-vacuum devices that use a well-focused pencil electron beam that directs the stream through a number of microwave cavities, which are tuned at or near the operating frequency of the tube. Conversion takes place as a result of the amplified RF input signal, causing the beam to form "bunches." These "bunches" give up their energy to the high-level induced RF fields at the output cavity. The simplified signal is extracted from the output cavity through a vacuum window.

kwashiorkor Protein malnutrition that includes an adequate intake of carbohydrates and fats but an inadequate intake of protein.

kyphosis An excessive curvature of the vertebral column that is convex posteriorly.

LAN A local area network is geographically confined to an area in which a common communication service may be used. For larger geographic areas or when multiple LANs are to be connected, a wide area network is used.

lasers Each positional laser projects a small red or green beam of light toward the patient during the simulation or treatment process. This provides the therapist several external reference points in relationship to the position of the isocenter.

latent period The time between the exposure and incidence of an abnormality.

lateral Toward one side or the other.

law of Bergonié and Tribondeau The law stating that ionizing radiation is more effective against cells that are (1) actively mitotic, (2) undifferentiated, and (3) have a long mitotic future.

LD 50/30 The lethal effect of acute whole-body exposure in which 50% of the total population exposed is affected in 30 days.

legal concepts The sum of artificial rules and regulations by which society is governed in any formal and legally binding manner.

legal ethics The study of the law mandating certain acts and forbidding others under penalty of criminal sanction.

LET (linear energy transfer) The average energy deposited per unit path length to a

medium by ionizing radiation as it passes through that medium.

leukoencephalopathy Widespread demyelinating lesions of the brain, brainstem, and cerebellum.

leukopenia An abnormal decrease in the white blood cell count, usually below 5000 cells per mm^3.

leukoplakia Small, white, raised patches on the mucous membrane.

Lhermitte's syndrome Pain resembling sudden electric shock throughout the body. It is produced by flexing of the neck or some cervical trauma.

libel Written defamation of character.

licensure A process by which an agency or government grants permission to an individual to work in a specific occupation after finding that the individual has attained the minimal degree of competency to ensure the health and safety of the public.

life experiences Life experiences can be described as information gathered through a normal day's activity that is useful to enhance an existing cognitive knowledge base. Life experiences can be used to promote knowledge and elevate functionality.

light cast A fiberglass tape that contains resin, which can be molded around a patient. When exposed to ultraviolet light, it hardens, creating a rigid immobilization device.

limb salvage surgery or limb sparing surgery (LSS) Radical or wide en bloc resection for soft tissue masses that requires a 1- to 3-cm normal tissue margin that allows the limb and extremity to remain intact (avoids amputation).

linear accelerator A radiation therapy treatment unit that accelerates electrons and produces x-rays or electrons for treatment.

linear interpolation The process of calculating unknown values from known values.

localization The geometrical definition of the tumor and anatomic structures using surface marks for reference.

logarithm The inverse or exponential notation. The exponent that indicated the power to which a number is raised to produce a given number.

low-dose rate (LDR) brachytherapy Brachytherapy that is delivered in a conventional low dose rate regimen that lasts several days and requires a hospital stay.

low osmolality This refers to contrast agents in which the iodides remain intact instead of splitting, and therefore they agitate the cells less.

lymph Excessive tissue fluid consisting mostly of water and plasma proteins from capillaries.

lymphangiography A radiographic study that uses special injected dyes that aid in

visualizing the lymphatic system on x-ray.

lymphatic system Consists of lymphatic vessels, lymphatic organs, and the fluid that circulates through it, called lymph. The system is closely associated with the cardiovascular system and is composed of specialized connective tissue that contains a large quantity of lymphocytes.

lysosome A membranous sac containing hydrolytic enzymes and found in the cellular cytoplasm. It functions in intracellular digestion.

lytic Pertaining to the destruction of cells.

magnetic resonance imaging (MRI) A diagnostic, nonionizing means of visualizing internal anatomy through noninvasive means. Imaging is based on the magnetic properties of the hydrogen nuclei.

MAID One of the most often used chemotherapy drug programs consisting of the following drugs: methotrexate, doxorubicin, ifosfamide, and dacarbazine.

malignant Tumors that are malignant often invade and destroy normal surrounding tissue and, if left untreated, can cause the death of the host.

malignant melanoma The most lethal form of skin cancer, which arises from the melanocytes found in the stratum basale of the epidermis.

mantle field The radiation field that treats the lymph nodes superior to the diaphragm.

mantoux tuberculin skin test A purified protein derivative (PPD) of tuberculin used in skin tests to show if a person has ever been "infected" by tuberculosis (TB) germs.

marasmus Calorie malnutrition that is observed in patients who are slender or slightly underweight and characterized by weight loss of 7% to 10% and fat and muscle depletion.

mass equivalence A measure of the mass of photons used to help explain related physical characteristics.

mass stopping power The sum of all energy losses. This includes both losses caused by collisions of electrons with atomic electrons (S/p)col and radiation losses or bremsstrahlung production (S/p)rad. The expression for the total mass stopping power (S/p)tot is as follows: (S/p)tot = (S/p)col + (S/p)rad

mastoid process An extension of the mastoid temporal bone at the level of the ear lobe.

Mayneord's factor Used to convert the percentage depth dose at the reference distance to the percentage depth dose at a nonreference distance. This would occur, for example, at extended distance setups.

mean life The average lifetime for the decay of radioactive atoms. It is the time period for a hypothetical source that decays at a constant rate equal to its initial activity to produce the same number of disintegrations as the exponentially decaying source that decays for an infinite period of time. It is primarily applicable to dose calculations in permanent implants, typically gold-198 (^{198}Au) and iodine-125 (^{125}I).

medial Toward the midline of the body.

median sagittal plane Also called the midsagittal plane, divides the body into two symmetric right and left sides. There is only one median sagittal plane.

mediastinum Tissue and organs separating the lungs. The mediastinum contains the heart and its large vessels, trachea, esophagus, thymus, lymph nodes, and other structures.

medical record All components used to document chronologically the care and treatment rendered to a patient.

medication A drug administered for its therapeutic effects.

medulla The inner portion of the adrenal gland.

medullary The cavity within the bone that contains fats or yellow bone marrow.

medulloblastoma A highly malignant cerebellar tumor usually arising in the midline with the propensity to spread via the cerebrospinal fluid.

megavoltage equipment Units using x-ray beams of energy 1 MeV or greater.

melanin The pigment that gives color to the skin and hair and serves as protection from ultraviolet light.

melanocyte The melanin-forming cell found in the stratum basale of the epidermis.

melanoma A dark pigmented malignant tumor arising from the skin.

menarche The beginning of a woman's first menstrual period.

menopause The end of a woman's menstrual activity.

menorrhagia Pain during menstruation.

mesothelioma Malignant tumors that develop in the mesothelial lining, the pleura, and possibly the pericardium.

metastases The spread of cancer beyond the primary site.

metastasize The process of tumors spreading to a site in the body distant from the primary site.

meter setting Used for the monitor unit setting for linear accelerators and the minute setting for cobalt-60 treatment machines.

microadenomas Neoplasms that are less than 1.0 cm.

midline block Shielding device used to spare the midline structures like the spinal cord from the effects of radiation.

milliamperes (mA) Units of measurement for x-ray currents in which the ampere (Å) is a measure of electrical current.

misadministration Incorrect application or delivery of a prescribed dose of radiation therapy, which can be minor or major and may cause death or serious injury to the patient depending on the extent of the dose.

mitochondria A cytoplasmic organelle serving as the site of cellular respirations and energy production.

mitosis Cell division involving the nucleus and cell body.

Mohs' surgery A surgical method in which the tumor is removed one layer at a time and examined microscopically. It is used for tumors in high-risk sites for recurrence and those with aggressive histologic subtypes. Mohs' surgery is known for its high success rate.

monitor unit (MU) A unit of output measure used for linear accelerators. The accelerators are calibrated so that one MU delivers 1 cGy for a standard, reference field size at a standard reference depth at a standard source-to-calibration point.

monoclonal antibody An antibody derived from hybridoma cells that can be used to identify tumor antigens.

moral ethics The study of right and wrong as it relates to conscience, God, a higher being, or a person's logical rationalization.

morphology The glandular pattern, distribution of glands, and stromal invasion of the tumor.

multicentric Arising from many foci and having multiple origination.

multidisciplinary The use of several disciplines at the same time.

multidisciplinary Having two or more modalities in a combined effort to treat a disease process.

multileaf collimator (MLC) A distinct part of the linear accelerator that allows treatment field shaping and blocking through the use of motorized leaves in the head of the machine. The use of MLCs can reduce or eliminate the use of Cerrobend shielding devices.

Musculoskeletal Tumor Society (MTS) A surgical staging system—classification and anatomic staging system used for soft tissue sarcomas.

mutation Change; transformation.

mycosis fungoides A chronic, progressive lymphoma arising in the skin. Initially, the disease stimulates eczema or other inflammatory dermatoses. In advanced cases, ulcerated tumors and infiltrations of lymph nodes may occur.

myelosuppression A reduction in bone marrow function.

nadir The lowest point and the time of greatest depression of blood values.

nasion The center depression at the base of the nose.

natural background radiation Ionizing radiation from natural sources including cosmic rays from outer space and the sun, terrestrial radiation from radioactive materials in the earth, and internal radiation from radioactive materials normally present in the body.

natural history The normal progression of a tumor without treatment.

necrosis Death or disintegration of a cell or tissue caused by disease or injury.

NED (no evidence of disease) At the time of patient follow up examination, there is no residual cancer noted.

negligence The neglect or omission of reasonable care or caution.

neuroblastoma Cancer of neural crest tissues, usually adrenal medulla or spinal ganglia, with frequent metastases.

neurohypophysis The posterior lobe of the pituitary.

neutrons Neutral subatomic particles found in the nucleus of an atom.

nevus A benign, localized cluster of melanocytes arising in the skin, usually early in life.

nonionic contrast media Media having low osmolality. The iodides remain intact instead of splitting; therefore they agitate the cells less. These agents are equally effective but cost much more than ionic agents.

nonmaleficence Not doing wrong or harm to an individual.

nosocomial Infection acquired in a hospital.

nuclear binding energy The total amount of energy that it takes to hold a nucleus together and is measured in MeV (10^6 electron volts).

nuclear energy level High energy states of the atom.

nuclear force The major force that holds the nucleus of an atom together.

nuclear medicine The branch of medicine that uses radioisotopes in the diagnosis and treatment of disease.

nuclear membrane The membranous envelope enclosing the nucleus and separating it from the cytoplasm.

nucleoli A rounded internuclear organelle serving as the site of construction of the ribosomes.

nucleoside A compound composed of a nitrogenous base and a five-carbon sugar. With the addition of a phosphate group, a nucleoside becomes a nucleotide.

nucleotide A compound composed of a nitrogenous base, five-carbon sugar, and phosphate group. Nucleotides are the basic building blocks of the nucleic acids RNA and DNA.

nucleus A conspicuous cytoplasmic organelle containing most of the genetic material (a small amount is located in the mitochondria) and nucleolus.

obliquity corrections Corrections for

beam incidence onto surfaces other than flat surfaces and for angles of incidence other than 90 degrees ("normal" incidence).

occupancy factor (T) The fraction of time that an area adjacent to a source of radiation is occupied.

Occupational Safety and Health Administration (OSHA) An administrative regulatory agency requiring employers to ensure the safety of workers.

odontalgia A toothache.

odynophagia Painful swelling.

Ohngren's line The line that connects the medial canthus of the eye with the angle of the mandible. It divides the maxillary antrum into anterior-inferior and superior-posterior halves.

oncogene A gene that regulates the development and growth of cancerous tissues.

oophorectomy The surgical removal of the ovaries.

oophoropexy Fixation of the ovaries behind the uterus.

opposite The length of the side of the right triangle that is opposite the specified angle in equations.

optical distance indicator (ODI) Sometimes called a rangefinder, it projects a scale onto the patients' skin, which corresponds to the source-skin distance (SSD) used during the simulation or treatment process.

optimal contrast When technical factors (primarily kVp) are selected that maximize the rate of differential absorption between body parts of varying tissue density and effective atomic number.

organelle One of many membrane-bound particles suspended in the cytoplasm of cells and having specialized functional characteristics.

organ segmentation The process of identifying structures, target volumes or normal tissues, by creating contours around them.

orthogonal films/radiographs Two films taken 90 degrees apart. They are required for treatment-planning purposes to define the location and relationship of various anatomic structures relative to the field's isocenter.

orthopnea Difficulty breathing, except in an upright position.

orthovoltage therapy (deep therapy) Treatments using x-rays produced at potentials ranging from 150 to 500 kV.

osmolality A property of a solution that depends on the concentration of the solute per unit of solvent.

osseous Composed of bone or resembling bone; bony.

osteoblastic Bone-forming cells.

osteomyelitis Infection of bone and marrow caused by the growth of germs in the bone. Infection may reach the bone

through the bloodstream or by direct injury.

otalgia An earache.

outcomes The result of the performance, or lack of performance, of a process.

output Referred to as the dose rate of the machine. Dose rate should be specified for field size, distance, and medium.

output factor The ratio of the dose rate of a given field size to the dose rate of the reference field size.

ovarian cancer Cancer of the ovaries.

ovoid Also called colpostats, these applicators are oval-shaped and insert into the lateral fornices of the vagina. They can hold radioactive sources and shielding material and are used in the treatment of gynecologic tumors.

oxygen-enhancement ratio (OER) The comparison of the response of cells to radiation in the presence and absence of oxygen:

$$OER = \frac{\text{Radiation dose under hypoxic/anoxic conditions.}}{\text{Radiation dose under oxic conditions to produce the same biologic effect.}}$$

Paget's disease A disease characterized by excessive and abnormal bone reabsorption and formation. It may affect any part of the skeletal system but primarily strikes the spine, pelvis, femur, and skull.

palliation Noncurative treatment to relieve pain and suffering when the disease has reached the stage at which a cure is no longer possible.

palpation The use of touch to acquire information about the patient. The physician palpates the patient by using the tips of the fingers. Light palpation is used for a superficial examination. Heavy pressure may be necessary for deep-seated structures. Through palpation the physician tries to distinguish between hard and soft, rough and smooth, and warm and dry.

pancoast tumor A malignant superior sulcus tumor in the apex of the lung with clinical symptoms that includes (1) pain around the shoulder and down the arm, (2) atrophy of the muscles of the hand, (3) Homer's syndrome caused by involvement of the brachial plexus, and (4) bone erosion of the ribs and sometimes vertebrae.

pantograph The most widely used and most accurate mechanical contouring device.

papilledema Swelling of the optic disc, usually associated with increased intracranial pressure.

para-aortic field The radiation field that treats the subdiaphragmatic nodes.

para-aortic nodes Efferent to the cisterna chyli, which is the beginning of the thoracic duct. These nodes run adjacent to the abdominal aorta from T12 to L4. This major section of the lymphatic

system eventually receives lymph from most of the lower regions of the body.

parallel-opposed field set The most common combined-field geometry in which two treatment fields share common central axes, 180 degrees apart.

parametrium Tissues lateral to and around the uterus.

paranasal sinuses Air spaces in the skull, lined by mucous membranes, that reduce the weight of the skull and give the voice resonance. The four paranasal sinuses are the ethmoid, maxillary, sphenoid, and frontal.

paraneoplastic syndrome A collective term for disorders arising from metabolic effects of cancer on tissues remote from the tumor. Such disorders may appear as endocrine, hematologic, or neuromuscular disorders.

parenteral Medication bypassing the gastrointestinal tract. Taken literally, this would include the topical and some mucous membrane routes, but the word has come colloquially to mean "by injection."

parity Viable pregnancy (500-g birth weight or 20-week gestation), regardless of the outcome.

pathogenicity The ability of an infectious agent to cause disease.

patient couch One of the mechanical components of the conventional simulator. The treatment couch, sometimes mounted on a turntable, allows rotation about a fixed axis that passes through the isocenter.

patient positioning aids Devices that place the patient in a particular position for treatment but do not ensure that the patient does not move.

patient support assembly (PSA) Also called a "couch" or "table," it allows the tabletop its mobility, permitting the precise and exact positioning of the isocenter during simulation or treatment. A standard feature allows the tabletop to mechanically move vertically, radially, horizontally, and in a lengthwise direction.

peak scatter factor The peak scatter factor is a backscatter factor sometimes normalized to a reference field size, usually 10×10 cm, for energies of 4 MV and above.

peer review An evaluation by health care professionals with the same credentials in which standards of practice are applied to evaluate professional performance and processes. This evaluation may be conducted by health care professionals within the same organization or from another health care organization.

pelvic inlet The upper entrance into the pelvis, bordered by the sacral promontory, medial pelvic sidewalls, and pubic bones.

pendant A set of handheld local controls

suspended from the ceiling or attached to the treatment couch that mimic those of the treatment unit.

penile urethra The urethra that passes through the pendulous part of the penis.

penumbra An area or region at the beam's edge where the radiation intensity falls to 0.

percentage depth dose (PDD) The ratio, expressed as a percentage, of the absorbed dose at a given depth to the absorbed dose at a fixed reference depth, usually D_{max}.

perineum The part of the body dorsal to the pubic arch; ventral to the tip of the coccyx; and lateral to the inferior rami of the pubis, ischium, and sacrotuberous ligaments. These are the tissues surrounding the genitals and anal opening.

periosteum The glistening-white, double-layered membrane covering the outer surface of the diaphysis.

peritoneal cytology Pathologic examination of cells obtained from the fluid surrounding the abdominal wall and its contained viscera.

peritoneal seeding The shedding or sloughing of tumor cells into the abdominal (peritoneal) cavity.

peroxisome An intracellular enzyme-containing body that participates in the metabolic oxidation of various substrates.

petechiae Minute red spots caused by the escape of small amounts of blood.

Peyer's patches Extra lymphatic tissue located within the submucosal layer in the distal ileum.

pharmacodynamics The way drugs affect the body.

pharmacokinetics The way drugs travel through the body to their receptor sites.

pharmocology The science of drugs and their sources, chemistry, and actions.

pharynx A membranous tube that extends from the base of skull to the esophagus and connects the oral and nasal cavities with the larynx and esophagus.

phase I, II, III studies A series of studies performed to assess the risk, benefits, and effects of proposed treatment options. A phase I study is the first step in testing a new treatment in humans, assessing the best way to give a new treatment and the best dose. The dose is usually increased a little at a time to find the highest dose that does not cause harmful side effects. A phase II study tests whether a new treatment has an appropriate tumoricidal effect against certain cancers. A phase III study compares the results of people taking a new treatment with the results of people taking the standard treatment to prove the safety and efficacy of a new treatment.

phlebitis Inflammation of a vein.

photoelectric effect This interaction, sometimes described as true absorption, occurs when the incident photon penetrates deep into the atom and ejects an inner-shell electron from orbit.

photon Small packet of electromagnetic energy (e.g., radiowaves, visible light, and x-rays and gamma rays).

phototiming A form of automatic exposure control (AEC) in which one or more ionization cells automatically stop the exposure during the creation of a simulation image.

pigmentation Coloration of the skin caused by the presence or absence of melanin.

pixels Small, discrete elements that make up an image.

planning target volume (PTV) The volume that indicates the clinical target volume (CTV) plus margins for geometric uncertainties, such as patient motion, beam penumbra, and treatment setup differences.

ploidy The number of chromosome sets in a cell. (Haploid cells have one set, and diploid cells have two sets.)

Plummer-Vinson syndrome Iron-deficiency anemia characterized by esophageal webs and atrophic glossitis. It predisposes an individual to the development of esophageal cancer.

pluripotent Pertaining to an embryonic cell that can form different kinds of cells.

pocket ionization chamber (pocket dosimeter) A device for measuring exposure. It uses the phenomenon that, when air is irradiated, the ions formed partially discharge the static electricity on a fine filament, allowing it to move across a scale. The filament and scale can be visualized by holding the cylindrical device up to a light and looking through one end.

polypeptide A chain of many amino acids linked by peptide bonds. Polypeptides are the subunits of proteins.

polyurethane mold An immobilization-repositioning device in which polyurethane (a synthetic rubber polymer) foam hardens and shapes to the patient's body build.

portal verification The documentation of treatment portals through radiographic images or electronic portal imaging devices.

positioning devices Common or customized devices that assist in ensuring patient treatment location during treatment.

positioning lasers Lasers that project a small red or green beam of light toward the patient during the simulation process. These lasers provide the therapist several external reference points in relationship to the position of the isocenter.

positron emission tomography (PET) Positron emission tomography is a beneficial diagnostic tool that may be useful in determining differences between necrosis and malignancy, which are associated with areas of high metabolism. PET is useful in determining the physiology of the organ in question.

positrons Positively charged electrons.

premalignant Physiologic characteristics of predisposing factors that may lead to malignancy.

prevention An effective strategy for saving lives lost from cancer and diminishing suffering. Prevention includes measures that stop cancer from developing.

priestly model A model that provides the caregiver with a godlike, paternalist attitude by making decisions for the patient and not with the patient.

primary site compartment Natural anatomic boundaries surrounding the soft tissue sarcoma primary. It is composed of common fascia plane(s) of muscles, bone, joint, skin, subcutaneous tissues, and major neurovascular structures.

primary tumor The main, or initial, source of malignant or benign tumor location, without reference to secondary sites of spread.

primary vertebral curves Vertebral curves that are developed *in utero* as the fetus develops in the C-shaped fetal position, and they are present at birth.

profile A description of radiation intensity as a function of position across the beam at a given depth.

progenitor Originator or precursor.

prognosis The estimation of life expectancy.

proliferation The rapid and repeated reproduction of a new part (e.g., through cell division).

proportion Two ratios that are equal. A proportion can also be an equation relating two ratios.

prospective study A study in which the theory of the cause of a condition or disease is tested by examining those who have a particular characteristic or trait. The population to be examined is selected in the beginning of the study.

prostate A walnut-shaped organ that surrounds the male urethra, located between the base of the bladder and urogenital diaphragm.

prostate gland The gland that surrounds the male urethra between the base of the bladder and the urogenital diaphragm.

prostate hypertrophy Enlargement of the prostate gland, leading to narrowing of the urethra.

prostate-specific antigen (PSA) PSA is a glycoprotein that is produced by epithelial cells in the prostate. Serum PSA level has been roughly correlated with prostate tumor volume. Testing that involves an evaluation of plasma levels. Prostatic antigen is found not only in prostate tissue and seminal fluid, but also in the sera of patients with benign prostatic hypertrophy or cancer.

protein A complex biologic compound composed of amino acids. Linked together in a determined, three-dimensional sequence, 20 different amino acids are commonly found in proteins.

protocols A specified treatment regimen. It describes the specifics of the type of treatment, the time schedule of the treatment, the total dose of the treatment, and specific areas to be included in the treatment.

protraction The time over which total dose is to be delivered.

protractor A gantry angle scale that is located at the central point of rotation of the gantry arm. It is an instrument in the shape of a graduated circular device. It is used to measure the gantry angle, which may range from 0 to 360 degrees.

pruritus Itching.

pseudocapsule Soft tissue sarcomas that are surrounded by compressed normal tissue, reactive inflammation, and fibrosis to give the gross anatomic appearance of a capsule.

psychosocial Psychologic support of the patient during the course of disease, with the recognition that social aspects of the treatment and disease prognosis may require special care.

purpura Blotchyness and red spots caused by petechiae and ecchymoses.

quality assessment The systematic quality analysis and review of patient care data.

quality assurance (QA) A systematic monitoring of the quality and appropriateness of patient care with an emphasis on performance levels.

quality-assurance (QA) program A series of activities and documentation performed with the goal of optimizing patient care.

quality audit A review of the radiation therapy process that is routinely and continuously measured, the results analyzed, and corrective action taken as required to ensure quality patient care.

quality control (QC) A component of quality assurance used in reference to the mechanical and geometrical tests of the radiation therapy equipment.

quality improvement (QI) The continuous improvement of health care services through the systematic evaluation of processes.

quality indicator A measurement tool used to evaluate an organization's performance.

quality of life A person's subjective sense of well-being derived from current experience of life as a whole.

radiation necrosis Tissue death resulting from the effects of radiation.

radiation oncologist The physician that reviews the medical findings with the patient and discusses treatment options and the benefits of radiation therapy as well as the possible side effects. The

physician makes a treatment plan and sends the patient on for treatment planning and/or simulation. During treatment, the radiation oncologist generally sees the patient once a week to ensure that the treatment is progressing as expected.

radiation oncology team A group consisting of all staff employees in radiation oncology who come in contact with the patient and/or family members throughout the course of radiation treatments.

radiation therapist The medical practitioner on the radiation oncology team who sees the patient daily and is responsible for treatment delivery and daily assessment of patient tolerance to treatment.

radiation therapy domain The confines of the radiation therapy department and the socialization that takes place inside. It is a limited physical environment in which a wide sampling of ethnicity gathers daily and creates a miniature society in which many social interactions occur among clusters of patients and between patients and staff members.

radiation therapy prescription A legal document written by a radiation oncologist that provides the therapist with the information required to deliver the appropriate radiation treatment. It defines the treatment volume, intended tumor dose, number of treatments, dose per treatment, and frequency of treatment.

radical resection Surgical removal of structures.

radioactive decay The process of an unstable nuclei emitting radiation.

radioactivity The emission of energy in the form of electromagnetic radiation or energetic particles.

radiographic cassette A holder for radiographic film used in portal imaging or simulation.

radiographic contrast The element of imaging that provides visual evidence of the all-important differential absorption rates of various body tissues. Radiographic contrast has been described as the tonal range of densities from black to white or the number of shades of gray in the radiograph.

radiographic density The degree of darkening on the film. A radiograph of high density is dark, and a radiograph of low density is light.

radiolysis The initial event in the radiolysis (splitting) of water involves the ionization of a water molecule, thus producing a water ion.

radiopaque marker A material with a high atomic number used to document structures radiographically.

radioprotectors Certain chemicals and drugs that diminish the response of cells to radiation.

radiosensitizers Chemicals and drugs

that help enhance the lethal effects of radiation.

radium substitute Any isotope used for brachytherapy whose dosimetry is based on the original radium work.

random error Variation in individual treatment setup.

randomization A method by which patients are blindly assigned to participate in specific portions of a protocol called an arm. The use of randomization ensures an equitable distribution of patients in each arm without prejudices that can later be blamed for unfair patient selection and can be detrimental to the outcome of the trial.

randomize To make random for scientific experimentation.

ratio A mathematical comparison of two numbers, values, or terms that denotes a relationship between the two.

recombinant deoxyribonucleic acid (DNA) A DNA molecule in which rearrangement of the genes has been artificially induced.

recombinant DNA technology (genetic engineering) Techniques that facilitate the manipulation and duplication of pieces of DNA.

Reed-Sternberg cell A giant multinucleated connective tissue cell that is characteristic of Hodgkin's disease.

regeneration The repair, regrowth, or restoration of a part (as tissue).

regulatory Requirements for limits of exposure to radiation for various groups.

regulatory agency An organization that may promulgate rules and regulations that have the force of law, license users, and provide inspection and enforcement actions.

rehabilitation The dynamic process with the goal of enabling persons to function at their maximal level within the limitations of their disease or disability in terms of physical, mental, emotional, social, and economic potential.

relative biologic effectiveness (RBE) RBE equals dose from 250 keV x-ray divided by dose from test radiation to produce the same biologic effect.

reproductive failure A decrease in the reproductive integrity or the ability of a cell to undergo an infinite number of divisions after radiation.

rest mass The mass (weight) of the particle when it is not moving.

restricted mass collisional stopping power A refinement of the total mass stopping power. The restricted mass collisional stopping power better describes the absorbed dose by accounting for energy transferred by delta rays.

retinoblastoma A primitive neuroectodermal tumor of the retina that may be inherited. It usually occurs in children younger than 4 years.

retrospective studies A study of a group of individuals all having the same disease and common characteristics that might have caused the disease.

review of systems Includes the patient's description of the signs and symptoms that lead the patient to present to the doctor, including subjective report of overall feelings of wellness.

rhabdomyosarcoma (RMS) A malignancy of skeletal muscle origin that can occur in many areas of the body and disseminates early.

ribosome An organelle constructed in the nucleolus and concerned with protein synthesis in the cytoplasm.

right angle A three-sided polygon on which one corner measures 90 degrees.

right lymphatic duct Serves only the right arm and right side of the head and neck and drains into the right subclavian vein. This duct is about 1 to 2 cm in length.

risk management The process of avoiding or controlling the risk of financial loss to the staff members and hospital or medical center.

room's eye view An image rendering technique that demonstrates the geometric relationship of the treatment machine to the patient. The room's eye view allows clear visualization of the entrance and exit of the beam through the patient. This view may also help prevent possible orientations of the beam that could result in collisions with the patient.

Rouvier's node A node located just inferior to the base of the skull and medial to the internal carotid artery.

sarcoma A malignancy arising from other than epithelial tissues of the body.

scanning beams The narrow "pencil beam" of electrons is scanned by magnetic fields across the treatment area. This constantly moving pencil beam distributes the dose evenly throughout the field.

scatter Radiation that changes direction.

scatter air ratio (SAR) The ratio of the scattered dose at a given point to the dose in free space at the same point. The scatter air ratio is the difference between the tissue air ratio for a given field size and the tissue air ratio for a zero field size. An equation can be written for the SAR: SAR = TAR(d,r1) − TAR(d,0); where d is the depth of calculation and $r1$ is the field size at the depth. TAR(d,0) represents the primary component of the beam. There is no dose from the scatter components in TAR(d,0).

scattering foil The most common method of producing an electron beam wide enough for clinical use is to use a scattering foil. A scattering foil is a thin sheet of a material that has a high Z number placed in the path of the "pencil beam" of electrons. A second scattering foil may be added to create a "dual scattering foil" arrangement. The first scattering foil is used to widen the beam; the second is used to improve the flatness of the beam.

scattering This is produced when an x-ray photon interacts with an outer-shell orbital electron with sufficient energy to eject it from orbit and alter its own path. The classic analogy is seen in the game of billiards, in which the cue ball collides with another ball and both fly off in different directions. In Compton scattering, the freed electron likely travels only an extremely short distance before attaching itself to another atom.

scientific notation A special use of exponents that uses base 10 notation. It is used to represent either very large or very small numbers.

scientific revival The intellectual resurgence of the sixteenth century.

scope of practice The body of courses and formally established learning experiences presenting the knowledge, principles, values, and skills that are the intended consequences of formal education; the defining document to guide radiation therapists through the day-to-day responsibilities of the profession.

screening Selecting appropriate tests and studies to check for disease.

secondary vertebral curves (compensatory vertebral curves) Vertebral curves that develop after birth as the child learns to sit up and walk. Muscular development and coordination influence the rate of secondary curvature development.

second malignant neoplasm (SMN) Cancer developing years after the treatment of an initial tumor related to genetics and previous carcinogenic chemotherapy and radiation.

seminoma The most common malignant testicular tumor.

sensitivity The ability of a test to give a true, positive result.

sensitometry The measurement of the film's response to exposure and processing.

sentinal node The primary drainage lymph node of a specific anatomic area. For example, the sentinel node for the breast is most commonly located near the axilla.

separation The measurement of the thickness of a patient along the central axis or at any other specified point within the irradiated volume.

serial response tissues Tissues in organs that can be affected by the incapacitation of only one element. The spinal cord is such an organ. The high-dose region of a serial-tissue dose-volume histogram (DVH) is of particular importance.

shelling A surgical procedure that removes the primary tumor and its pseudocapsule, giving it the gross appearance of having removed all viable tumor.

shielding block Field-shaping material that reduces beam transmission to less than 5% of the original intensity.

shine over The falloff of the radiation beam over a surface that misses tissue and projects in the air; also known as fall off.

shrinking fields A technique that reduces the treated field area one or more times during the course of treatment in response to a tumor that reduces in size and/or the need to limit doses to normal structures.

significant figures The number of figures in a measurement or calculation that are known with some degree of reliability. For example, the number 10.2 is said to have 3 significant figures. The number 10.20 is said to have 4 significant figures.

simple immobilization devices Devices that restrict movement but require a patient's voluntary cooperation.

simulated CT The extension and adaption of a conventional simulator to allow the acquisition of axial "slices." They simulate CT slices. Usually these are limited to a small number of thick slices and are adequate for localization and two-dimensional (2D) treatment planning but generate poor quality digitally reconstructed radiograph (DRR) images.

simulation A process carried out by the radiation therapist under the supervision of the radiation oncologist. It is the mockup procedure of a patient treatment with radiographic documentation of the treatment portals.

simulators Radiographic x-ray units that mimic all the movements and parameters of the treatment units. They are used for imaging the target volume during treatment planning.

simulators with a CT mode Simulators that incorporate the conventional benefits with the added benefits of cross-sectional information obtained during the simulation process.

sine One of three most common functions associated with the right triangle. The other two are the **cosine** and **tangent.** The sine of the angle is the ratio opposite of hypotenuse.

skin sparing A property of megavoltage irradiation where the maximum dose occurs at some depth beneath the skin surface.

skin squames Superficial skin cells that serve as vehicles for airborne pathogens.

slander Oral defamation of character.

smegma A white secretion located under the prepuce of the foreskin in the adult male. It is carcinogenic in animals.

SOAP note The initial presentation and plan for assessment and treatment described in the history and physical (H&P) may be referred to as a "SOAP note." The acronym SOAP is described as follows: <u>S</u>ubjective findings as reported by the patient; <u>O</u>bjective or observations of the clinician, including vital signs and physical examination; <u>A</u>ssessment of the disease or condition; and <u>P</u>lan for further examination and/or treatment. This information becomes part of the patient's medical record.

soft tissue sarcoma (STS) A malignant tumor arising primarily, but not exclusively, from mesenchymal connective tissues. The following are types of sarcomas:

liposarcoma—STS arising from fat
leiomyosarcoma—STS arising from smooth muscle
rhabdomyosarcoma—STS arising from striated muscle
fibrosarcoma—STS derived from collagen-producing fibroblasts
malignant fibrous histiocytoma (MFH)—Deep STS tumor showing partial fibroblastic and histiocytic differentiation with a variable pattern and giant cells
neurofibromatosis (von Recklinghausen's disease)—Small, discrete, pigmented skin lesions (cafe au lait spots and/or pigmented nevi) that develop into multiple neurofibromas along the course of peripheral nerves; may undergo malignant transformation.
schwannoma—Nonencapsulated tumor resulting from disorderly proliferation of Schwann cells that includes portions of nerve fibers; typically undergoes formation to malignant schwannomas

source-axis distance (SAD) The distance from the source of radiation to the axis of rotation of the treatment unit.

source head The housing for shielding that contains the device for positioning the cobalt-60 source.

source-skin distance (SSD) The distance from the source of radiation to the patient's skin.

specific activity The activity per unit mass of a radioactive material (Ci/g). The specific activity dictates the total activity that a small source can have.

specificity The ability of the test to obtain a true-negative result.

squamous cell carcinoma As it relates to skin cancer, it is a faster growing cancer than the basal cell type with a higher propensity for metastasis, arises from the more mature keratinocytes of the upper layers of the epidermis. This type of nonmelanoma skin cancer can arise anywhere on the body but is especially common on sun-exposed areas such as the head, neck, face, arms, and hands.

staging Cancer is "staged" after a histologic diagnosis is made. Staging helps determine the anatomic extent of the disease. Treatment decisions are based on the histologic diagnosis and extent of the disease.

staging laparotomy A surgical procedure that includes a splenectomy, lymph node biopsy, and bone marrow biopsy; used in staging lymphomas

standard precautions Precautions that should be followed because of potential contact with body fluids. These precautions include wearing gloves, a mask, and protective eyewear; properly handling needles; and disposing of used equipment into containers for biohazardous material.

stereotactic radiosurgery The use of a high-energy photon beam with multiple ports of entry convergent on the target volume.

stomatitis Inflammation of the mouth.

stratified Segregate populations according to certain specific characteristics.

striae Lines or bands elevated above or depressed below surrounding tissue.

stridor Harsh, rasping breath.

subcutaneous Tissue just below the skin.

subcutaneous injection A 45- or 90-degree injection into the subcutaneous tissue just below the skin.

subcutaneous layer A layer of areolar connective tissue and adipose tissue that lies beneath the dermis and contains nerves and blood vessels.

superficial therapy Treatment with x-rays produced at potentials ranging from 50 to 150 kV.

superior vena cava syndrome Edema of the face, neck, or upper arms resulting from increased venous pressures caused by compression of the superior vena cava. It is most commonly caused by a metastatic, mediastinal lymph node tumor in lung cancer.

suprasternal notch (SSN) A depression in the manubrium, which occurs at the level of T2 and articulates with the medial ends of the clavicles. This point is commonly used in measuring the angle of chin tilt in head and neck patients when thermoplastic immobilization masks are not used. It also serves as a palpable landmark when setting up a supraclavicular fossa field.

Surveillance, Epidemiology, and End Results (SEER) program A program initiated in 1973 to collect data in an effort to determine the epidemiology and etiology of cancer.

symmetry The maximum point-to-point difference in the central 80% of the profile.

synergistic A body organ, medicine, or substance that cooperates with another or others to produce a total effect greater than the sum of the individual elements.

systemic error Variation in the translation of the treatment setup from the simulator to the treatment unit.

systemic treatment Cancer management treatment that encompasses the patient's entire system, generally through venous means. Chemotherapy affects not only cancerous cells but others also because of the systemic nature of its delivery. Radiation therapy has a local and regional focus, meaning it only affects the locals that it is aimed at.

tabletop That part of the patient support assembly (PSA) on which a patient is positioned during treatment or simulation; may be called a treatment couch or patient tabletop.

tandem A long narrow tube that inserts into the opening of the cervix (cervical os) into the uterus. They can hold radioactive sources and are used in the treatment of gynecologic tumors.

tangent The tangent of the angle is equal to the length of the opposite side divided by the length of the adjacent side. The three most common functions associated with the right triangle are the sine, cosine, and tangent. Also refers to the treatment field commonly used to treat primary breast cancer with radiation therapy with medial and lateral tangents.

target volume An area of a known and presumed tumor.

TD$_{5/5}$ The dose of radiation that is expected to produce a 5% complication rate within 5 years.

TD$_{50/5}$ The dose of radiation that is expected to produce a 50% complication rate within 5 years.

telangiectasia Dilation of the surface blood vessels caused by the loss of capillary tone, resulting in a fine spider-vein appearance on the skin surface.

tenesmus Ineffective and painful straining during a bowel movement.

tennis racket This may be a square or rectangular section of the tabletop, similar to a tennis or racquetball racquet woven tightly together. After extended use, the "tennis racquet" section should be restrung to provide more patient support and reduce the amount of "sag" during simulation.

tensile strength Resistance in lengthwise stress, measured in weight per unit area.

thermionic emission In an oversimplification, x-rays are produced when a stream of electrons liberated from the cathode is directed across the tube vacuum at extremely high speeds to interact with the anode. These cathode electrons are freed from the tungsten filament atoms in a process called thermionic emission. This elaborate-sounding term makes perfect sense if broken down into its root forms: thermal refers to heat, ions are charged particles, and emission is release.

thermoluminescent dosimeter (TLD) A device for measuring dose. It uses the phenomenon that some solid materials, when irradiated, will subsequently give off light when heated. The amount of light emitted is proportional to the dose delivered to the crystal.

thoracic duct Located on the left side of the body, the thoracic duct is typically larger than the right lymphatic duct. It serves the lower extremities, abdomen, left arm, and left side of the head and neck and drains into the left subclavian vein. This duct is about 35 to 45 cm in length and begins in front of the second lumbar vertebra (L2) called the cisterna chyli.

three-dimensional (3D) conformal radiation therapy (3DCRT) 3D image visualization and treatment-planning tools are used to conform isodose distributions to only target volumes while excluding normal tissues as much as possible.

three-point setup Three marks placed on a patient to define the isocenter. It is used to position and level the patient daily to ensure reproducibility and consistency of the setup and treatment.

thrombocytopenia An abnormal decrease in the number of platelets.

tissue absorption factor The beam of radiation gives up energy as it travels through the body. The more tissue the beam traverses, the more it is attenuated. There are a number of different methods for measuring the attenuation of the beam as it travels through tissue. These are percentage depth dose, tissue-air ratio, tissue-phantom ratio, and tissue-maximum ratio. The first method used was percentage depth dose.

tissue-air ratio The ratio of the absorbed dose at a given depth in phantom to the absorbed dose at the same point in free space.

tissue-maximum ratio The ratio of the absorbed dose at a given depth in phantom to the absorbed dose at the same point at the level of D_{max} in phantom.

tissue-phantom ratio The ratio of the absorbed dose at a given depth in phantom to the absorbed dose at the same point at a reference depth in phantom. If the reference depth is chosen to be the depth of D_{max}, then the tissue-phantom ratio is called the tissue-maximum ratio.

titers A measurement of the number of specific antibodies in a person's body or blood specimen.

tolerance The body's adaptation to a particular drug and requirement of ever greater doses to achieve the desired effect.

topical brachytherapy Radioactive sources are placed on top of the area to be treated. Molds of the body part to be treated may be taken and prepared to place

the sources in definite arrangements to deliver the prescribed dose.

tort law The type of law that governs rights between individuals in noncriminal actions. This law deals with violations of civil as opposed to criminal law.

total nodal irradiation A system of radiating all the major lymph nodes.

total quality management (TQM) Professional performance standards that define activities in the areas of education, interpersonal relationships, personal and professional self-assessment, and ethical behavior.

transcription The process resulting in the transfer of genetic information from a molecule of DNA to a molecule of RNA.

transfer An understanding of a subject matter to a depth that allows transfer of knowledge from one event to deal with another event. The ability to use knowledge in more than one setting. The use of preexisting knowledge to problem solve.

translation The process resulting in the construction of a polypeptide in accordance with genetic information contained in a molecule of RNA.

transmission factor Any device placed in the path of the radiation beam will attenuate the beam. The transmission factor is the ratio of the radiation dose with the device to the radiation dose without the device. Examples of commonly used devices in radiation therapy are blocking trays, wedges, and compensators.

transmission filters Filters that allow the transmission of a predetermined percentage of the treatment beam.

transpectoral lymphatic pathway Lymphatic pathway that passes through the pectoralis major muscle and provides efferent drainage to the supraclavicular and infraclavicular fossa nodes.

transurethral resection (TURP) A surgical procedure of the prostate performed through the urethra.

travel time The length of time for a cobalt-60 source to advance and retract.

treatment console The operating center where timers and system-monitoring indicators are displayed.

treatment couch Part of the linear accelerator, the treatment couch is the area on which patients are positioned to receive their radiation treatment. Several unique features of the treatment couch provide the tabletop with mobility. A standard feature allows the tabletop to move mechanically in a horizontal and lengthwise direction. This movement must be smooth and accurate with the patient in the treatment position, thus allowing for precise and exact positioning of the isocenter during treatment positioning.

treatment field (portal) The volume

exposed to radiation from a single radiation beam.

treatment number Number of treatments delivered.

treatment planning The process by which dose delivery is optimized for a given patient and clinical situation.

treatment technique A defined method by which a treatment is delivered to the patient.

treatment time The amount of time required to deliver a prescribed dose of radiation, taking all pertinent treatment factors such as field size, energy, depth, and so forth into account. Treatment time is used in treatment with cobalt-60.

treatment verification A process using diagnostic quality radiographs of each treatment field from the initial simulation procedure to determine the accuracy of the treatment plan.

treatment volume Generally larger than the target volume, the treatment volume encompasses the additional margins around the target volume to allow for limitations of the treatment technique.

trigone The portion of the bladder (shaped like a triangle) formed by the openings of the two ureters and orifice of the urethra.

tuberculin skin test (Mantoux test) An intradermal injection of purified protein derivative (PPD) or tuberculin used to test for exposure to tuberculosis.

tumor localization This may involve the use of a simulator in determining the extent of the tumor and location of critical structures.

tumor registry A tracking mechanism for cancer incidence, characteristics, management, and results in cancer-treatment facilities for patients diagnosed with cancer.

tumorcidal dose A dose high enough to eradicate the tumor.

tumor staging A means of defining the tumor size and extension at the time of diagnosis. Tumor staging provides a means of communication about tumors, helps in determining the best treatment, aids in predicting prognosis, and provides a means for continuing research.

tumor-suppressor gene A gene whose presence and proper function produces normal cellular growth and division. The absence or inactivation of such a gene leads to uncontrolled growth or neoplasia.

ulceration A rare, late radiation reaction exhibited by an open sore on the skin or mucous membrane. It is caused by the shedding of dead tissue.

universal precautions The method of infection control in which any human blood or body fluid is treated as if it were known to be infectious.

urticaria Hives.

use factor (U) The fraction of time that the radiation beam is directed at a barrier; the use factor for scatter and leakage radiation is always 1.

Vac-lok Trade name for an immobilization device that consists of a cushion and a vacuum compression pump.

vacuole A membrane-bound cavity in the cytoplasm of a cell having a variety of storage, secretory, and metabolic functions.

vacuum-formed shell An immobilization device that is formed when a piece of plastic is molded over a plaster cast of a patient's anatomy.

vaginal cancer A malignancy that arises in the vagina and does not extend to the vulva or cervix. Vaginal cancer is a rare disease that accounts for approximately 2% of all gynecologic cancers.

vaginal colpostats Paired brachytherapy devices that allow insertion into the lateral vaginal fornices or apex of the vagina for intracavitary treatment. These are usually shielded anteriorly and posteriorly for greater lateral throw of the dose and often look like small golf clubs.

vaginal cuff The small rim of vaginal tissue at the apex of the vagina around the cervix. Some of this is removed during a hysterectomy, and some remains as the new apex of the vagina with surgical scarring.

vaginal cylinder implant A domed-ended tubular brachytherapy device used to give even dose distribution to the apex or entire vaginal surface. This resembles a candle with a central hollow canal for later afterloading.

Van de Graaff generator An electrostatic accelerator designed to accelerate charged particles. In radiation therapy procedures the unit produces high-energy x-rays typically at 2 MeV.

vector An animal, usually an arthropod, that carries and transmits a pathogen capable of causing disease.

venipuncture Puncture of a vein.

ventricles Cavities that form a communication network with each other, the center canal of the spinal cord, and the subarachnoid space. They are filled with cerebrospinal fluid (CSF).

verification A final check that each of the planned treatment beams does cover the tumor or target volume and does not irradiate normal tissue structures.

verification simulation A final check that each of the planned treatment beams covers the tumor or target volume and does not irradiate normal tissue structures.

virtual simulation The target is defined first, and then the fields are shaped to conform to the target during 3DCRT treatment planning.

virtue ethics The use of practical wisdom for emotional and intellectual problem solving.

virulence The relative power of a pathogen to cause disease. Severity expressed in terms of morbidity and mortality.

vital signs Information, such as blood pressure, pulse, and respiration, that may be gathered along with a chief complaint at the patient's initial encounter with a nurse or other clinical specialist.

voxel Volume elements.

vulva Female external genitalia composed of the mons veneris, labia majora, labia minora, vestibule of the vagina, and vestibular glands.

vulvar cancer Cancer of the outermost portion of the gynecologic tract. Vulvar cancer patients usually have a subcutaneous lump or mass. Patients with more advanced disease have an ulcerative exophytic mass.

Waldeyer's ring The ring of tonsillar tissue that encircles the nasopharynx and oropharynx: two palatine tonsils, lingual, and pharyngeal tonsils.

WAN An acronym for wide area network. For large geographic areas or when multiple LANs (local area networks) are to be connected, a WAN may be employed. WANs use a variety of communication services currently including telephone dial-up, T-1 or T-3 lines, or even the Internet to communicate over long or short distances.

warm thyroid nodule A nodule having a slightly higher concentration than the rest of the thyroid gland.

wave guide A hollow, tube-like structure within the linear accelerator that is used to accelerate injected electrons to near the speed of light prior to striking a target to produce photons.

wavelength of the wave The physical distance between peaks of the wave.

wave particle duality Photons exhibit the characteristics of a particle at times and the characteristics of a wave at other times.

wedge A beam modifier that changes. The angle is defined relative to the horizontal plane at depth.

wedge angle The angle between the slanted isodose line and a line perpendicular to the central axis of the beam.

wedge filter A tool that modifies the isodose distribution of a beam to correct for oblique incidence or tissue inhomogeneities by progressively decreasing beam intensity across the field irradiated.

wide resection A surgical procedure for soft tissue carcinoma. The procedure involves a wide en bloc excision for limb salvage and/or wide through-bone amputation.

Wilms' tumor Childhood embryonal kidney cancer.

wipe test A test done to evaluate the contamination or leakage of a sealed radioactive source.

workload (W) For superficial and orthovoltage units, the milliamperage (mA) used and beam on time per week; for high energy units, the Gy (rad) per week at isocenter.

xeroderma pigmentosum A rare disease of the skin starting in childhood and marked by disseminated pigment discolorations, ulcers, cutaneous and muscular atrophy, and death.

x-ray Electromagnetic radiation that is produced when a fast electron stream hits a target. The energy of the resultant x-ray beam increases with the voltage that accelerates the electrons.

x-ray generator A generator that provides radiographic and fluoroscopic control of the simulator through the selection of various exposure factors, which include focal spot, mAs, kVp, and time.

Answers to Review Questions

Chapter 1

1. Cellular differentiation
2. Antioncogenes
3. Sarcomas
4. Carcinomas
5. Tumor staging
6. a. Anatomic site
   b. Cell of origin
   c. Biologic behavior
7. a. Age
   b. Culture
   c. Support system
   d. Education
   e. Family background
8. a. Surgery
   b. Radiation therapy
   c. Chemotherapy
   d. Immunotherapy

Chapter 2

1. b
2. d
3. a
4. d
5. a
6. c
7. c
8. b
9. b
10. a

Chapter 3

1. d
2. a

3. c
4. b
5. d
6. c
7. a
8. c
9. b
10. d
11. a
12. d
13. d
14. d
15. a
16. b
17. c
18. d
19. c
20. a

Chapter 4

1. b
2. c
3. d
4. a
5. c
6. d
7. b
8. b
9. b
10. c

Chapter 5

1. b
2. b

3. a
4. c
5. a
6. b
7. c
8. a
9. d
10. d

Chapter 6

1. d
2. b
3. b
4. b
5. b
6. b
7. d
8. b
9. c
10. c

Chapter 7

1. a
2. b
3. b
4. b
5. b
6. a
7. c
8. b
9. a
10. b

Chapter 8

1. d
2. b
3. b
4. a
5. c
6. a
7. b
8. b
9. d
10. a

Chapter 9

1. a
2. a
3. c
4. d
5. b
6. b
7. c
8. d
9. b
10. d

Chapter 10

Multiple Choice
1. d
2. b
3. d
4. d
5. c
6. c

Fill in the Blank
7. Epidemiology
8. Carrier
9. OSHA
10. TB and hepatitis C
11. Incubation, clinical illness, convalescence
12. Ethylene oxide

Chapter 11

1. Assessment is a dynamic and continuous process that involves listening and hearing the concerns of patients at the physical, psychologic, emotional, and spiritual levels. It should include the determination of the problem, the selection of an intervention, and the evaluation of effectiveness.
2. Cognitive content includes the actual facts and words of the message. Example: "I only slept 2 hours last night."
3. Empathy is defined as identifying with the feelings, thoughts, or experiences of another person.
4. The ten most common verbal responses in reflective listening are minimal verbal response, reflecting, paraphrasing, probing, clarifying, interpreting, checking out, informing, confronting, and summarizing.
5. The daily assessment responsibilities of radiation therapists are as follows (complete answers on a chart titled "Components of Daily Physical Assessment"):
   Skin reactions—Monitor and give lotion instructions.
   Fatigue—Assess, probe reasons, and counsel.
   Sleep—Assess and evaluate patterns.
   Mouth changes—Inspect and instruct regarding diet.
   Pharyngitis and esophagitis— Evaluate pain, diet, and medication.
   Diarrhea—Assess bowel function, instruct regarding a low-residue diet, and check medications.
   Cystitis—Assess bladder function, infections, and medication.
   Nausea and vomiting—Assess antiemetic use and diet, and use visual imagery if needed.
   Alopecia—Instruct regarding the care of the scalp, and address body-image issues if needed.
   Pain—Assess the location and intensity of the pain, and evaluate the administration of medications.
   Skin pallor—Monitor CBC counts.
   Weight loss—Weigh weekly, monitor daily eating, and offer helpful suggestions.
6. Weight loss is often the first change indicating the possibility of cancer.
7. The duration and pattern of pain are the two most important characteristics of the cause of pain.
8. Leukopenia is a decrease in the white blood cell count, which increases the risk of infection.
9. The major symptoms of depression are changes in appetite, sleep disturbances, lack of energy, withdrawal, reduced ability to concentrate, indecisiveness, and suicidal ideas.
10. Recognize that cultural diversity exists.
    - Respect persons as unique individuals.
    - Evaluate your own cultural beliefs.
    - Be willing to modify health care delivery to honor the client's beliefs.
    - Do not expect every person in a culture to behave in exactly the same way.

Answers to Exercises for Recognizing and Identifying the Types of Major Verbal Responses (in Box 11-5)
1. reflecting
2. paraphrasing
3. probing
4. informing
5. summarizing
6. checking out
7. interpreting
8. clarifying
9. confronting
10. minimal verbal response

Answers to Exercise for Listening for Feelings (in Box 11-6)
1. Fear of illness or pleasure of attention from physician
2. Anxiety about the new social worker or excitement about meeting her
3. Discouragement or fear of not responding to treatment
4. Fear of rejection or loneliness
5. Anticipation of being finished or fear of losing the support that "doing something" gives

Chapter 12

1. Right patient, right drug, right dose, right time, and right route
2. c
3. c
4. b
5. d

6. d
7. b
8. a. V
   b. IV
   c. XI
   d. I
   e. X
   f. IX
   g. II
9. The discharge or escape of blood or fluid into tissues
10. Side effects are physiologic responses to a medication other than the desired response. Most drugs produce some side effects in some patients. Complications are unexpected reactions to medications and can range from mild to severe.

Chapter 13

1. c
2. a
3. c
4. a
5. b
6. d
7. b
8. c
9. a
10. b

Chapter 14

1. c
2. d
3. c
4. e
5. c
6. b
7. a
8. d
9. e
10. e

Chapter 15

1. d
2. c
3. b
4. a
5. c
6. d
7. b
8. c
9. a
10. c

Chapter 16

1. c
2. c
3. b
4. b
5. c
6. c
7. c
8. d
9. d
10. c

Chapter 17

1. a
2. c
3. a
4. b
5. b

Chapter 18

1. a
2. a
3. b
4. b
5. c
6. d
7. b
8. b
9. c
10. c

Chapter 19

1. c
2. d
3. a
4. a
5. d
6. b
7. c
8. c
9. a
10. b

Chapter 20

1. d
2. c
3. a
4. b
5. b
6. b
7. a
8. d
9. b
10. d

Chapter 21

1. b
2. a
3. b
4. c
5. c
6. c
7. b
8. a
9. a
10. b

Chapter 22

1. b
2. b
3. c
4. b
5. b
6. b
7. c
8. b
9. b
10. a

Chapter 23

1. The predominant mechanism of the interaction of electron beams in the 1 to 20 MeV energy range used in radiation therapy is collisional interactions. This is due to the low Z number of tissue that interacts with the electron beam.
2. Scattering foils are a relatively simple and reliable method of producing a clinically useful electron beam (when compared with the scanning beam method).
3. The depth of the 80% isodose line = MeV/3 by substitution, 16 MeV/3 = 5.3 cm
   The depth of the 90% isodose line = MeV/4 by substitution, 16 MeV/4 = 4.0 cm
4. The depth of the 80% isodose line = MeV/3 solving for the energy, MeV/3 = 4.0 cm, 3 × 4.0 = 12 MeV
5. E_r = MeV/2, range of an electron beam in tissue, by substitution 12 MeV/2 = 6
6. (1) A partial bolus should never be used with electron beams.
   (2) The "edge effect" (areas of increased and decreased dose) produced by a large bolus

with an edge perpendicular to the surface.

(3) Electron beams less than 12 MeV may require a bolus to increase surface dose.

(4) Bolus may also be used to shape isodose distributions to conform to the treatment volume or as a tissue compensator.

7. $E_o = C_4R_{50}$, by substitution, $E_o = 2.4 \times 5.0$ cm $= 12$ MeV

8. Shield thickness in millimeters of lead = MeV/2
By substitution $7/2 = 3.5$ mm
Note: Kahn suggests that an additional millimeter of lead should be added to the amount indicated by the rule of thumb as follows:
$7/2 = 3.5 + 1.0 = 4.5$ mm

9. This would result in an area of increased dose below the location where the two treatment fields adjoin or abut.

10. The output of this treatment field may require a calibration measurement because of the diameter of the treatment field being less than the practical range (E_r = MeV/2) of the treatment beam.

11. Because of the lateral constriction of the higher isodose lines at 15 MeV, a larger area on the surface must be irradiated to cover a given area at depth. A margin of 1 cm is recommended between the lateral edge of the target volume and the edge of the collimator.

Chapter 24

1. c
2. d
3. d
4. a
5. b
6. b
7. c
8. c
9. a
10. a

Chapter 25

1. c

2. d
3. c
4. b
5. a
6. d
7. c
8. a
9. c
10. c
11. b
12. e
13. d
14. d
15. c
16. d
17. a
18. d
19. d
20. a

Chapter 26

1. a
2. c
3. a
4. c
5. c
6. a
7. c
8. a
9. d
10. a

Chapter 27

1. a
2. b
3. c
4. b
5. b
6. c
7. d
8. c
9. d
10. b

Chapter 28

1. a
2. a
3. c
4. a, c
5. d
6. c
7. a
8. a
9. d
10. c

Chapter 29

1. Increased duration of smoking, increased use of unfiltered cigarettes, increased number of cigarettes consumed
2. Stage, performance (Karnofsky) status, weight loss
3. Mediastinal and intrapulmonic
4. 6000 to 7500 cGy
5. Dermatitis, erythema, esophagitis
6. d
7. c
8. d
9. b
10. c

Chapter 30

1. b
2. a
3. b
4. a
5. c
6. c
7. c
8. b
9. d
10. d

Chapter 31

1. b
2. c
3. d
4. a
5. d
6. c
7. a
8. a
9. d
10. d

Chapter 32

1. d
2. b
3. d
4. c
5. d
6. a
7. c
8. d
9. c
10. a

Chapter 33

1. c

2. d
3. a
4. c
5. a
6. b
7. a
8. d
9. c
10. e

Chapter 34

1. b
2. c
3. a
4. d
5. a
6. c
7. b
8. c

9. a
10. a

Chapter 35

1. d
2. c
3. d
4. a
5. c
6. a
7. a
8. c
9. b
10. b

Chapter 36

1. b
2. d
3. d

4. b
5. b
6. a
7. c
8. d
9. c
10. d

Chapter 37

1. a
2. c
3. b
4. b
5. a
6. b
7. c
8. d
9. a

Index

Page numbers followed by "t" indicate tables, "f" indicate figures, "b" indicate boxes.